Mosby's
Comprehensive review of
CRITICAL CARE

# Mosby's Comprehensive review of CRITICAL CARE

*Edited by*

Donna A. Zschoche, R.N., M.A.

Associate Director of Nursing and Director of Education,
Critical Care Units, Paramedic Training Program, and
Cardiopulmonary Center, University of California Irvine Medical Center;
Education Director, National Critical Care Institute
(NCCI) of Education, Orange, California

*with 185 illustrations*

Special art: Ian Wells
Special photography: Richard C. Farrell

Saint Louis

The C. V. Mosby Company

1976

Printed in the United States of America

Distributed in Great Britain by Henry Kimpton, London

**Library of Congress Cataloging in Publication Data**

Main entry under title:

Mosby's comprehensive review of critical care.

(Mosby's comprehensive review series)
Includes bibliographies and index.
1. Critical care medicine. I. Zschoche, Donna A. II. Title: Comprehensive review of critical care. [DNLM: 1. Critical care. 2. Intensive care units—Examination questions. 3. Emergency health services—Examination questions. WX218 M894]
RC87.M884 616'.025 75-37718
ISBN 0-8016-5695-8

CB/CB/B 9 8 7 6 5 4 3 2 1

# Contributors

**HOWARD N. ALLEN, M.D.**

Assistant Professor of Medicine,
University of California, Los Angeles;
Director, Cardiac Noninvasive Laboratory,
Cedars-Sinai Medical Center,
Los Angeles, Calif.

**PATRICIA ALLYN, R.N.**

Head Nurse, Burn Center,
University of California Irvine Medical Center,
Orange, Calif.

**BERNHARD G. ANDERSON, M.D.**

Assistant Professor of Medicine,
Boston University Medical Center,
Boston, Mass.

**ROBERT BARTLETT, M.D.**

Associate Professor, Surgery,
University of California, Irvine,
California College of Medicine, Irvine, Calif.;
Director, Burn Center,
University of California Irvine Medical Center,
Orange, Calif.

**THEODORE B. BERNDT, M.D.**

Department of Cardiology,
Stanford University School of Medicine,
Stanford University Medical Center,
Stanford, Calif.

**DAVID R. BOYD, M.D.**

Director, Emergency Medical Services,
Department of Health, Education, and Welfare,
Washington, D.C.

**JOYCE CARNES, M.D.**

Emergency Physician, Albany General Hospital,
Albany, Ore.

**EARLE DAVIS, Ph.D.**

Professor, Basic Science Department,
Southern California College of Optometry,
Fullerton, Calif.;
Lecturer, Department of Anatomy,
University of California, Irvine,
California College of Medicine,
Irvine, Calif.

**BERTRAM F. FELSHER, M.D.**

Chief of Hepatology,
Long Beach Veteran's Administration Hospital,
Long Beach, Calif.

**HARRY FRIEDMAN, M.D.**

Neurosurgeon,
Memphis Neurosurgical Clinic, P.C.,
Baptist Medical Plaza,
Memphis, Tenn.

**D. E. GENTILE, M.D.**

Associate Clinical Professor of Medicine (Renal),
University of California, Irvine,
California College of Medicine, Irvine, Calif.;
Co-Director, Hemodialysis Center,
St. Joseph's Hospital,
Orange, Calif.

**EMILY S. HACKLER, R.N., B.S.N.**

Head Nurse, Physical Medicine and
Rehabilitation,
University of California Irvine Medical Center,
Orange, Calif.

**DONALD C. HARRISON, M.D.**

Professor of Medicine,
Stanford University School of Medicine;
Chief of Cardiology,
Stanford University Medical Center,
Stanford, Calif.

**ROBERT F. HUXTABLE, M.D.**

Associate Professor and Director,
Neonatology Division,
Department of Pediatrics,
University of California, Irvine,
California College of Medicine,
Irvine, Calif.

**ROBERT E. INGHAM, M.D.**

Department of Cardiology,
Stanford University School of Medicine,
Stanford University Medical Center,
Stanford, Calif.

**STANLEY M. KEGEL, M.D.**

Assistant Clinical Professor of Pediatrics
(Cardiology),
University of California, Los Angeles,
Los Angeles, Calif.; Cardiologist,
Children's Hospital of Orange County,
Orange, Calif.

**WILLIAM F. KIELY, M.D.**

Associate Professor and Director,
Consultation-Liaison Service,
Department of Psychiatry,
University of Southern California,
Los Angeles County/University of Southern
California Medical Center,
Los Angeles, Calif.

**MILDRED LAWSON, R.N., B.S.N.**

Head Nurse, Progressive Cardiac Care Unit,
University of California Irvine Medical Center,
Orange, Calif.

**RICHARD C. LILLEHEI, M.D., Ph.D.**

Professor, Department of Surgery,
University of Minnesota Hospitals,
Minneapolis, Minn.

**CHESTER B. MARTIN, M.D.**

Professor of Obstetrics and Gynecology,
University of Southern California,
Los Angeles County/University of Southern
California Medical Center,
Los Angeles, Calif.

**IRENE MATOUSEK, R.N., M.S.**

Assistant Professor of Obstetrics and Gynecology,
University of Southern California,
Los Angeles County/University of Southern
California Medical Center,
Los Angeles, Calif.

**MARY ROBERTA McMAHON, R.N.**

Head Nurse, Hemodialysis Unit,
University of California Irvine Medical Center,
Orange, Calif.

**DENNIS L. MING, Pharm. D.**

University of California Irvine Medical Center,
Orange, Calif.

**EUGENE NAGEL, M.D.**

Professor and Vice Chairman,
Department of Anaesthesiology,
University of California, Los Angeles,
Los Angeles, Calif.;
Chairman, Department of Anaesthesiology,
Harbor General Hospital,
Torrance, Calif.

**THOMAS A. PRESTON, M.D.**

Associate Professor of Medicine,
University of Washington School of Medicine;
Co-Director, Cardiology Service,
U.S. Public Health Service Hospital,
Seattle, Wash.

**ALLAN PRIBBLE, M.D.**

Assistant Professor of Medicine,
University of Washington School of Medicine,
Seattle, Wash.;
Chief, Medical Service,
American Lake Veteran's Hospital,
Tacoma, Wash.

**TERESA L. ROMANO, R.N.**

Emergency Medical Systems Specialist,
Center for the Study of Emergency Health Care,
University of Pennsylvania,
Philadelphia, Pa.

**STANLEY M. ROSEN, M.D.**

Associate Professor of Medicine (Renal),
Department of Medicine,
University of California, Irvine,
California College of Medicine,
Irvine, Calif.

**EARLENE SCHARPING, R.N.**

Lecturer, Neonatology Division,
Department of Pediatrics,
University of California, Irvine,
California College of Medicine,
Irvine, Calif.

**STEPHEN R. SEVERANCE, M.D.**

Gastroenterologist,
Long Beach Veteran's Administration Hospital,
Long Beach, Calif.

**CLAYTON H. SHATNEY, M.D.**

Medical Fellow, Department of Surgery,
University of Minnesota Hospitals,
Minneapolis, Minn.

**MELVILLE I. SINGER, M.D.**

Associate Clinical Professor of Pediatrics (Cardiology),
University of California, Los Angeles,
Los Angeles, Calif.;
Chief of Cardiology,
Children's Hospital of Orange County,
Orange, Calif.

**PAUL E. STANLEY, Ph.D.**

Associate Director, Biomedical Engineering Center,
Purdue University Institute for Interdisciplinary Engineering Studies,
West Lafayette, Ind.

**ROBERT A. STEEDMAN, M.D.**

Assistant Clinical Professor of Surgery,
University of California, Irvine,
California College of Medicine,
Irvine, Calif.;
Chairman, Thoracic and Cardiovascular Surgery,
Santa Ana–Tustin Community Hospital,
Santa Ana, Calif.

**N. DABIR VAZIRI, M.D.**

Assistant Professor of Medicine,
University of California, Irvine,
California College of Medicine,
Irvine, Calif.

**BERNHARD A. VOTTERI, M.D.**

Assistant Clinical Professor of Medicine,
University of California, San Francisco,
San Francisco, Calif.;
Director, Critical Care and Pulmonary Department,
Sequoia District Hospital,
Redwood City, Calif.

**KARIN ZENK, Pharm. D.**

University of California Irvine Medical Center,
Orange, Calif.

**DONNA A. ZSCHOCHE, R.N., M.A.**

Associate Director of Nursing and Director of Education,
Critical Care Units, Paramedic Training Program, and Cardiopulmonary Center,
University of California Irvine Medical Center;
Education Director,
National Critical Care Institute (NCCI) of Education,
Orange, Calif.

## Editorial consultants

**DELORES CORNEJO, M.S.W.A.C.S.W.**

Clinical Social Worker, Social Service,
University of California Irvine Medical Center,
Orange, Calif.

**ALLAN GAZZANIGA, M.D.**

Associate Professor of Surgery,
University of California, Irvine,
California College of Medicine,
Irvine, Calif.

**ALAN GIBERSON, M.D.**

Fellow, Renal Division,
University of California Irvine Medical Center,
University of California, Irvine,
California College of Medicine,
Irvine, Calif.

**JOSEPHINE LUSSIER, R.N.**

Head Nurse, Neurosurgical Unit,
University of California Irvine Medical Center,
Orange, Calif.

**DONALD E. PINDER, M.D.**

Clinical Professor of Anatomy,
University of California, Irvine,
California College of Medicine,
Irvine, Calif.

**ELAINE SINER, R.N.**

Supervising Nurse, Paramedic Training Division,
University of California Irvine Medical Center,
Orange, Calif.

**GERALD WHIPPLE, M.D.**

Professor of Medicine and Chief of Cardiology,
University of California, Irvine,
California College of Medicine,
Irvine, Calif.

To

**BILL**

# Foreword

The need for care of the critically ill will always exist even though the ability to prevent disease improves as the years pass.

The prevention of disease should be the goal of every citizen, nurse, physician, and health worker. Unfortunately, the prevention of all disease is not yet possible for the following reasons: (1) Even though a certain illness may be preventable, the individual citizen may not cooperate in the effort of prevention. For example, everyone does not take the injections for tetanus immunization. (2) The knowledge that might enable prevention of a certain disease may be incomplete. For example, the prevention of coronary atherosclerosis cannot be promised to every person who eliminates all of the "risk factors." Since the preventive measures are difficult to implement and since they are not universally successful, it is difficult to "sell" the preventive concept to everyone (although I personally subscribe to it). (3) There is no satisfactory prevention for many conditions, such as a gunshot wound in the abdomen of a suburban housewife who is carrying her groceries to her car and is attacked by an unknown assailant.

The point is that acute, serious illnesses will always exist. We must not succumb to the trend of being in favor of preventive medicine *or* emergency medicine. The problem we face cannot be reduced to a simple either-or formula. The fact is that we must all support the work in preventive medicine *and* the efforts to improve emergency care for patients who are seriously and critically ill.

The medical advances of the last few years have produced intensive/critical care units of many types, a new profession of emergency and critical care for physicians, nurses, and other allied health professionals, and new educational programs for the care of the critically ill. Every physician knows that it is not possible to care for seriously ill patients without the help of informed and skilled nurses and technicians who have responded to the modern needs in many exciting ways—not the least of which is their intense interest in continuing education.

*Mosby's Comprehensive Review of Critical Care* was written by experts in many fields and will be read and reread by nurses, physicians, and technicians alike, but we must thank a nurse for conceiving and stimulating its creation.

**J. Willis Hurst, M.D.**
Professor and Chairman,
Department of Medicine,
Emory University School of Medicine,
Atlanta, Georgia

# Preface

While traveling and contacting critical care professionals throughout the country in search of the highest standards and methods of delivering critical care, I have been fortunate to discover some outstanding professionals who have been isolated within their own sections of the country, and I have been able to distinguish numerous predominating and ascending figures in critical care whose efforts in aggregate constitute this text.

This book is not intended to be a primer for the beginning critical care practitioner, but rather is designed to assist the practicing critical care clinician in maintaining currency of knowledge with subsequent currency in practice. That is not to say, however, that the novice entering the critical care arena for the first time would not reap great benefits from perusing its contents.

*Mosby's Comprehensive Review of Critical Care* is designed to serve as a resource and reference for anyone—physicians, nurses, and other allied critical care professionals—seeking expert opinion or instruction on a particular question or an entire subject. The format is a simple one, structured to pinpoint questions and answers, with emphasis on the flow of information and continuity.

The critical care practitioner who utilizes the whole-body system and multiple-organ approach in practice will benefit from the chapter devoted to anatomy, physiology, and pathophysiology as they relate to the altered regulatory mechanisms present in the seriously ill patient. Other chapters focus on the specific diagnosis and clinical care related to disease and trauma entities.

Professionals prepared to function at the entry level both in mobile intensive care and hospital critical care units, including the emergency department and operating and recovery rooms, continue to be a scarce commodity. So often it becomes the hospital's responsibility to provide basic critical care education for new employees. Thus one chapter is devoted to a recommended critical care course content that individual educators in community and state college and university systems, as well as hospital in-service programs, may utilize in developing a personalized curriculum.

We hope that this contribution will be of value to the reader and of long-term benefit to patients.

**Donna A. Zschoche**

# Acknowledgments

It is with the deepest respect and gratitude that I acknowledge and thank the contributing authors who have made the preparation of this text possible. Their generous contributions of time, expertise, and knowledge have appreciated the value of this book far above that which words may describe.

I am grateful for the thoughtful foreword prepared by Dr. J. Willis Hurst, and I am indebted to my secretary, Peggy Freuh, whose long hours of deciphering and transcribing were marked with good nature and devotion, and for the assistance of Mrs. Rose Lacher, executive secretary extraordinaire, who helped organize this work.

I also gratefully acknowledge the assistance of Pearl Crouch, Marcia Swanson, Jacqueline Paul, and Lillian Sunquist, paramedic nurse instructors of Mobile Intensive Care, County of Orange, California.

Gratitude and affection are expressed to one of my former preceptors and special critical care team member, Frederick P. Sattler, D.V.M., without whose contribution to both medical and nursing education it is doubtful that the biomedical instrumentation (physiological measurements) referred to throughout this text would have come into common clinical bedside use within this past decade.

I would be remiss if I did not acknowledge the support and continued encouragement provided by Lillian E. Brown, R.N., M.P.A., Director of Nursing Service at University of California Medical Center (formerly Orange County Medical Center), who has created an environment in which the concept of critical care has been conceived and nurtured and in which my own "becoming" has been realized.

# Contents

Mosby's
Comprehensive review of
CRITICAL CARE

*chapter 1*

# Critical care education

**DONNA A. ZSCHOCHE**

Critical care practice encompasses definitive care for the seriously ill and injured at the scene of an emergency, during transport, or at any place in the hospital where the application of critical care knowledge and techniques are required. The critical care practitioner should have expertise in resuscitation and treatment of the seriously ill or injured as well as a theoretical and practical understanding of the common disease states and injuries that result in life-threatening conditions. Care may be extended independently or as a part of a team effort; the team may be composed of any combination of the following persons: physician, registered professional nurse, vocational/practical nurse, pharmacist, respiratory therapist, critical care technician, or paramedic/emergency medical technician.

Any one individual member of the critical care team may be required to render or supervise technologic treatment involving physiologic measurements as well as to administer to the patient's psychologic, social, and environmental needs . . . total care! *Such areas are not the exclusive concern of one profession or discipline!*

Because critical care may be needed anywhere and should be available anywhere, each member of the critical care team should be able to demonstrate skills in emergency life support until more comprehensive restorative care is available. Therefore any critical care team member may at any time be required to resuscitate and/or maintain life-support systems until professional help arrives, and it is recommended that the preparation reflect a minimum level of performance.

This preparation commences with the study of the major organ systems, that is, the respiratory, cardiovascular, renal, central nervous, and endocrine systems, with a foundation of anatomy and physiology *as they relate to the altered regulatory mechanisms affecting the critically ill.* These sciences provide the theoretical base required to knowledgeably incorporate technology into practice.

Critical care specialists now accept the concept and need for a basic "core" of instruction—a preparatory base for entry into the critical care arena. The concept of the core or basic critical care preparation views the patient en toto; it focuses on the patient as a whole and is as basic as the concept of the critical care center and system itself. All subspecialties, which can include respiratory, coronary, burn, neonatal, pediatric, hemodialysis, and emergency/trauma medicine, revolve around this whole-body concept. A well-prepared clinician will think physiologically, correlating all body systems in both healthy and disease states and comprehending the many parameters that are or that should be monitored through gross observation or utilization of advanced biomedical instrumentation. The goal is expertise and management of the definitive therapy required in life support.

The basic critical care preparation may be derived from the core curriculum, which may be modified for various levels of practice. Optimum preparation for the critical care clinician should be supplemented by internship (or bedside clinical experience) in the care of both adult and pediatric patients undergoing shock, respiratory distress, pre- and postoperative heart catheterization, surgery, pacemaker implantation, myocardial infarction, major burns, and renal failure, as well as the care of certain other specifically selected critically ill patients. Inasmuch as the emergency department and mobile intensive care unit are staffed by front-line critical care professionals, internship in those areas should be scheduled if possible.

Through isolating the commonalties and precepts in all critical care subspecialties, the basic course content, or core curriculum, becomes a dynamic tool to serve the entry-level practitioner. The progress and development of critical care preparation is reinforced when the practitioner has a central base of knowledge. For example, we now recognize and acknowledge that arrhythmia identification and interpretative skills are equally as important in caring for the open-heart surgery patient (or the respiratory care, burn, or hemodialysis patient) as they were in the first coronary care unit. We know, too, that alveolar ventilation shares priority with data relative to cardiac output, central venous pressure, and arterial and pulmonary wedge pressures. Temperature control is seen to be as vitally important in the care of the neonate, the critically burned patient, or the neurosurgical patient as is renal function and fluid and electrolyte management.

Consideration should also be given to the critical care environment—the esoteric devices that sustain and measure; the plan of care that will serve to avoid sensory overload; dream deprivation; and time and space disorientation.

In our perception of the patient in the whole-body system the core curriculum encompasses consideration for eventual recovery and rehabilitation. Thus such entities as these constitute the core or basic preparation for practice.

With didactics drawn from a basic core of knowledge, clinical internship, and return demonstration, the prepared clinician has the ability to apply the skills learned in any of the subspecialties with a minimum of additional knowledge. This core of knowledge is a tremendous asset to hospitals where economics implicitly requires full utilization of staff. The well-prepared individual is consequently in a position to provide backup support for colleagues in other critical care units. Efficiency, effectiveness, and economy are also served when this practitioner/clinician serves in the preceptor role without requiring additional extensive specialized education or training.

The core curriculum has already been recognized in the in-service departments of acute care hospitals' continuing education programs and adopted by many community colleges and state universities. It is a product of a new era in medicine. As we see medicine moving toward new standards and with medical science still developing and hospital design changing, the commonalties between disciplines become clear. The multidisciplinary critical care team approach to patient care is evolving and stabilizing. As role changes emerge, it is important to establish guidelines and standards that will provide a measure of security for both the provider and the consumer.

Signaling the congruent roles of the physicians, nurses, and allied health professionals, studies are presently being conducted in some areas of the country that may provide for the more efficient and economic utilization of each team member. The recognized collaborative role of the team was born out of knowledge, skills, and acceptance. There has been a gradual transfer of specific functions, including accountability and responsibility for decision making, from physicians to other critical care professionals and technicians. Such role changes could not occur without reliance on the knowledges and skills found in the core curriculum. The core approach to education provides the foundation on which critical care can be practiced efficiently, effectively, and dynamically.

Explosive changes are occurring in medical practice and health care itself, and we can be certain of an increased acceleration of change in this decade. Toffler[1] describes the "transient age" in *Future Shock,* which is of marked relevance to health care practitioners. Preparation for these expectations will lessen the trauma, and a "standard" base of knowledge lends a certain degree of security to both the practitioner and the consumer of critical care.

The core course content outlined on the following pages is recommended for entry-level critical care team members as well as those currently in practice. *The educator is cautioned that this course content will not include the minute aspects of care, since it is assumed that the practitioners have a body of basic knowledge in their initial preparation, certification, or professional licensure.* For example, if individuals require a review in basic anatomy and physiology, this should be pursued through *independent study* and not be a part of the critical care curriculum; however, anatomy and physiology *as they relate to the altered regulatory mechanisms seen in the critically ill* should be included. The same is true of basic bedside techniques and approaches for care. Superfluous courses increase program costs and ultimately are reflected in increased hospitalization per diem charges.

The educator or in-service department instructor is encouraged to use the core curriculum as a base, altering or adding specific content and laboratory experience or internship for specializations, without sacrificing the whole-body system approach.

## RECOMMENDED COURSE CONTENT FOR USE IN CRITICAL CARE CURRICULA DEVELOPMENT*

I. Review of anatomy and physiology *as they relate to the altered regulatory mechanisms in the critically ill*
   See Chapter 2 for a review of the integrative levels at which the body functions in states of health, disease, and/or injury.

II. Cardiovascular system
   A. The heart
      1. Conduction system
         a. Sinoatrial (SA) node
         b. Atrial preferential pathways
         c. Anterior internodal tract
         d. Middle internodal tract
         e. Posterior internodal tract
         f. Atrioventricular (AV) node
         g. Bundle of His
         h. Left bundle branch
            (1) Anterior superior fascicle
            (2) Posterior inferior fascicle
         i. Right bundle branch
         j. Purkinje fibers
      2. Electrophysiology
         a. Resting membrane potential
         b. Depolarization
         c. Repolarization
         d. Action potential
         e. Integrity and maintenance of the membrane potential
         f. Refractory periods
            (1) Absolute
            (2) Relative (effective)
            (3) Supernormal (vulnerable)
         g. Membrane responsiveness
         h. Vectors
         i. Electrical axis
   B. Muscle mechanics (Chapter 2)
      1. Electrical activation and electromechanics
         a. Ionic exchange or sodium pump
         b. Electrical potential
         c. Electromechanical coupling
         d. Contractile process
         e. Muscle function principles
            (1) All-or-none principle
            (2) Frank-Starling law
   C. Variables related to cardiac contractility
      1. Pharmaceuticals
         a. Inotropic drugs
            (1) Calcium
            (2) Isoproterenol (Isuprel)

*The reader is also referred to the bibliography, which includes a number of excellent references related to the recommended critical care course content.

(3) Digitalis
(4) Catecholamines
b. Negative inotropic drugs
(1) Lidocaine
(2) Propranolol
(3) Alcohol
(4) Barbiturates
(5) Quinidine
(6) Procainamide (Pronestyl)
c. Other properties related to contractility
(1) Available oxygen
(2) Condition of cardiac muscle
(3) Afterload status
(4) Nervous control
(5) Electrical activation
(6) Irritability
(7) Automaticity
(8) Conductivity

D. Cardiac evaluation
1. Physical examinatioin and assessment
2. Cardiac auscultation
3. Cardiac catheterization
4. Coronary angiography
5. Cine- and coronary arteriography
6. Echocardiography
7. Phonocardiography
8. Tracings of bundle of His
9. Vectorcardiography

E. Physiologic measurements
1. Arterial pressure
2. Pulmonary artery and capillary (wedge) pressure
3. Central venous pressure
4. Cardiac output and cardiac index

F. Arrhythmia identification (Chapter 7)
1. Cardiac monitoring
2. Arrhythmia recognition and interpretation
3. Pacemaker
a. Long-term pacing
b. Emergency pacing
4. Drugs
5. Cardioversion (synchronized)

G. Bioelectronic instrumentation (Chapter 30)
1. Instrument safety
a. Basic principles
b. Safety in practice
c. Electrical hazards

H. Cardiac and/or respiratory arrest
1. Cardiovascular collapse and electromechanical dissociation
2. Ventricular fibrillation
3. Ventricular asystole
a. Cardiopulmonary resuscitation (adult, pediatric, and neonatal patient)
(1) Ventilation
(2) External cardiac compression
(3) Internal cardiac massage
b. Definitive therapy
(1) Drugs
(2) Airway adjuncts
(3) Counter shock
(4) Intravenous fluids
(5) Monitoring and control of dysrhythmia
(6) Care after resuscitation

I. Heart sounds
1. Sound characteristics
a. Duration
b. Pitch
c. Frequency
d. Timbre
e. Intensity
2. Heart sound origin
a. Blood flow
b. Muscle vibration
c. Muscle contraction
d. Valves
3. Cardiac auscultation and normal heart sounds
a. Phonocardiography
b. Stethoscopy
c. First ($S_1$)
d. Second ($S_2$)
e. Third ($S_3$)
f. Fourth ($S_4$)
g. Heart sound variants (splitting)
4. Abnormal heart sounds

a. Gallop rhythms
   (1) Ventricular diastole ($S_3$)
   (2) Atrial contraction ($S_4$)
   (3) Summation gallop (both atrial and ventricular)
b. Murmur classification
   (1) Systolic
      (a) Tricuspid insufficiency
      (b) Aortic stenosis
      (c) Mitral valve insufficiency
      (d) Pulmonic stenosis
      (e) Coarctation of aorta
      (f) Intraventricular septal defect (maladie de Roger)
      (g) Foramen ovale
   (2) Diastolic
      (a) Aortic insufficiency
      (b) Pulmonic insufficiency
      (c) Mitral stenosis
      (d) Tricuspid stenosis
   (3) Continuous
      (a) "Machinery" murmur (begins in systole and continues through diastole)
      (b) Types
         i) Aortopulmonary connections
         ii) Arteriovenous connections
         iii) Disturbance in flow patterns in arteries
         iv) Disturbance in flow patterns in veins
c. Murmur characteristics
   (1) Loudness
   (2) Quality
   (3) Intensity
   (4) Time
   (5) Pitch
   (6) Transmission
   (7) Location

5. Heart sound variations caused by dysrhythmias
   a. Atrial fibrillation
   b. Premature extrasystole
   c. Bundle branch block
   d. Complete heart block
6. Extracardiac sounds
   a. Mediastinal "crunch"
   b. Pericardial "friction rub"
   c. Ejection sounds
      (1) Pulmonary
      (2) Aortic
   d. Systolic click
   e. Systolic whoop or honk
   f. Opening snaps
      (1) Mitral valve
      (2) Tricuspid valve
   g. Pericordial knock
   h. Artificial valves

J. Electrochemical physiology
K. Electrocardiography
   1. Rhythm strip
   2. 12- and 13-lead ECG
   3. Esophageal leads
   4. Lewis leads
   5. Intra-atrial lead
   6. ECG leads
      a. Bipolar (extremities)
      b. Unipolar (augmented)
      c. Unipolar (precordial)
   7. Electrical axis
      a. Einthoven's triangle
      b. Axis calculation
   8. Vectorcardiography (future ECG's)
L. Arrhythmia identification and interpretation

   NOTE: The learner and/or instructor is referred to a number of excellent textbooks listed at the end of this chapter for basic information related to the electrocardiograph and arrhythmia identification.
M. Cardiac catheterization
   1. Patient preparation
   2. Care before and after catheterization

3. Diagnostic purpose
4. Technique
5. Complications
6. Diagnostic data obtained

N. Clinical management of medical emergencies (Chapters 7-9 and 14)
1. Review of pathophysiology, etiology, precipitaing factors, clinical manifestations, and physical signs
a. Myocardial infarction
b. Congestive heart failure
c. Hypertensive crisis
d. Thyroid storm
e. Cardiac tamponade
f. Pulmonary edema
g. Cardiogenic shock
h. Ventricular rupture
i. Cor pulmonale

O. Shock (Chapters 9 and 26)
1. Definition and diagnosis
2. Pathophysiology
3. Types
4. Clinical management

P. Pericarditis
1. Diagnosis
2. Clinical management

Q. Subacute bacterioendocarditis
1. Diagnosis
2. Clinical management

R. Cardiovascular surgery (Chapters 10-13)
1. Pre- and postoperative clinical management
2. Surgical procedures
a. Aneurysm
(1) Surgical resection
(2) Grafting
b. Occlusive lesions
(1) Surgical resection and grafting
(2) Revascularization (bypass grafting)
(3) Thromboendarterectomy
(4) Embolectomy
(5) Angioplasty (patch graft)
c. Pericardiectomy
d. Valve replacements
e. Ventriculectomy
f. Commissurotomy
g. Valve replacements
3. Cardiopulmonary bypass
a. Procedure complications (arrhythmias, conduction defects, shock, tamponade, etc.)
4. Extracorporeal oxygenation
5. Venous surgical intervention
a. Embolism (embolectomy) or vena cava ligation, etc.
b. Thrombosis (thrombectomy)
6. Ischemic heart disease
a. Myocardial revascularization
(1) Vein and artery grafts
(2) Internal mammary artery to coronary artery bypass
(3) Gas endarterectomy
(4) Congenital cardiac lesion repairs
(5) Aneurysmectomy

III. Pulmonary system

NOTE: Topics for classroom discussion should include the following conditions:

Acute respiratory distress syndrome (RDS)
Lung contusion
Coccidioidomycosis
Fat emboli
Oxygen toxicity
Chronic obstructive pulmonary disease
Status asthmaticus
Pulmonary edema
Neoplasms
Cor pulmonale
Tracheal or bronchial lacerations
Esophageal rupture
Pulmonary emboli
Embolectomy
Vena caval ligation
Vena cava umbrella
Carbon monoxide poisoning
Acute idiopathic polyneuritis (Guillain-Barré syndrome)
Tetanus (lockjaw)
Myasthenia gravis

Poliomyelitis
Tracheal esophageal fistula
Pneumonoconiosis

A. Respiration
   1. External respiration
   2. Internal respiration
   3. Gas diffusion
      a. Partial pressures
      b. Pressure gradients
      c. Inspired and expired gases
      d. Blood gases
         (1) Sampling
            (a) Arterial catheter
            (b) Arterial puncture
            (c) Analysis and assessment ($P_{O_2}$, $P_{CO_2}$, pH, $O_2$ saturation, base excess, bicarbonate, constant exhaled $CO_2$ monitoring)
   4. Oxygen and carbon dioxide transport
      a. Oxygen measurements
      b. Oxyhemoglobin and myoglobin dissociation curves
      c. Dissolved carbon dioxide measurements
      d. Carbon dioxide transport and elimination
         (1) Hydrogen ions, acids, and bases
         (2) Buffers
         (3) Acidosis and alkalosis
            (a) Respiratory
            (b) Metabolic
            (c) Compensated
            (d) Partially compensated

B. Ventilation
   1. Ventilation and perfusion ratios
      a. Shunting
      b. Diffusion barriers

C. Definition of terms used in pulmonary care

D. Nomograms used in pulmonary care
   1. Hastings-Singer
   2. Henderson-Hasselbalch equation
   3. Radford
   4. Sigaard-Andersen

E. Disease states leading to respiratory failure
   1. Obstructive and restrictive conditions
      a. Impaired ventilation
      b. Restricted defects
      c. Limited thorax expansion
      d. Decreased diaphragmatic movement

F. General respiratory insufficiency
   1. Bronchopulmonary disease
   2. Common parenchymal disease
   3. Neoplastic disease
   4. Cardiopulmonary disease
   5. Neuromuscular disease

G. Traumatic respiratory insufficiency
   1. Cerebral dysfunction
   2. Cardiovascular dysfunction
   3. Respirator dysfunction
   4. Biochemical dysfunction
   5. Thoracic trauma

H. Postoperative respiratory insufficiency
   1. Atelectasis
   2. Pneumonia
   3. Aspiration pneumonitis
   4. Pneumothorax
   5. Hemothorax

I. Pediatric insufficiency
   1. Congenital anomalies
   2. Infant (acute) respiratory distress syndrome
      a. Incidence
      b. Pathology
      c. Management
   3. Cystic fibrosis
   4. Croup syndrome (laryngotracheobronchitis)

J. Acute respiratory failure
   1. Definition
   2. Diagnosis
   3. Symptoms
      a. Hypoxia
      b. Hypoxemia
      c. Hypercapnia
   4. Clinical management
      a. Ensurance of patent airway
      b. Ventilatory support

c. Chest physiotherapy
d. Control of secretions and bronchospasms; initiation or discontinuance of drug therapy
e. Infection control
f. Maintenance of physiologic blood gases
g. Patient support
(1) Reassurance
(2) Alleviation of fears and apprehension
(3) Relief of anxiety
(a) Comfort measures
(b) Drug therapy

K. Physical examination of the chest
1. Inspection
2. Palpation
3. Percussion
4. Auscultation

L. Vital signs and level of consciousness

M. Airway management
1. Equipment
2. Procedure
3. Endotracheal pathway
4. Nasopharyngeal pathway
5. Esophageal pathway (Chapter 5)
6. Tracheostomy
a. Indications
b. Procedure
c. Complications
d. Clinical bedside care
7. Suctioning
a. Equipment
b. Procedure
(1) For intubated patients
(2) For nonintubated patients
c. Tracheostomy and tracheostomy tube management
d. Potential complications of suctioning
(1) Arrhythmias, cardiovascular collapse, and cardiac arrest
(2) Hypoxemia and atelectasis
(3) Airway trauma
8. Ultrasonic nebulization, therapeutic humidity, and aerosol treatment

N. Mechanical ventilators
1. Indications for use
2. Types
a. Pressure ventilators
(1) Bird Mark VII and VIII
(2) Puritan-Bennett PR II
b. Volume ventilators
(1) Emerson
(2) Bennett MA-1
(3) Ohio 560
c. Bourn
d. Drinker respirator (iron lung)
e. Rocking bed (gravity)
3. Assisted or controlled ventilation
4. Negative external pressure (iron lung)
5. Cuirass ventilation
6. Positive pressure
7. Side effects and complications of use
8. Lecture and demonstration and return demonstration on use

O. Special techniques
1. Indications for weaning and complications
2. Procedures and methods used
3. Positive end-expiratory pressure (PEEP)
4. Continuous positive air pressure (CPAP)
5. Intermittent mandatory ventilation (IMV)
6. Expiratory resistance

P. Postural drainage
1. Indications
2. Methods
3. Clinical support

Q. Chest physiotherapy
1. Percussion
a. Mechanical
b. Manual
2. Vibration
3. Breathing exercises

R. Clinical bedside management of

intravenous, arterial, and pulmonary artery lines

- S. Pharmaceuticals used in respiratory management
  1. Indication
  2. Action
  3. Contraindication
  4. Untoward reaction
  5. Dosage and administration

IV. Renal system

- A. Pathophysiology of renal failure (Chapter 15)
  1. Definition
     - a. Acute
     - b. Chronic
  2. Laboratory studies
     - a. Urinalysis
     - b. Specific gravity
     - c. Osmolality
     - d. Urinary pH
     - e. Glucose determination
     - f. Protein evaluation
     - g. Microscopic examination
     - h. Serum creatinine level
     - i. Creatinine clearance
     - j. Blood urea nitrogen concentration
     - k. Renal biopsy
       - (1) Precautions
       - (2) Complications
- B. Causes of renal failure
  1. Prerenal failure
     - a. Precipitating factors
       - (1) Fluid and electrolyte imbalance
       - (2) Shock
       - (3) Plasma or blood loss
       - (4) Decreased renal blood flow
       - (5) Decreased glomerular filtration rate
       - (6) Decreased blood pressure
       - (7) Tubular ischemia
       - (8) Accumulated metabolic waste products in blood (decreased secretion of solutes)
  2. Intrarenal failure
     - a. Acute tubular necrosis
     - b. Acute cortical necrosis
     - c. Chronic glomerulonephritis
     - d. Nephrosis
     - e. Kidney trauma
  3. Postrenal failure
     - a. Obstruction
     - b. Structural abnormalities
     - c. Vascular occlusion
     - d. Calculi
     - e. Blood clots
     - f. Uric acid crystals
  4. Uremia
     - a. Anemia (normocytic/normochromic)
     - b. Hypertension
     - c. Pericarditis
     - d. Gastrointestinal manifestations
     - e. Neurologic manifestations
     - f. Uremic pneumonitis
     - g. Dermatologic manifestations
     - h. Role of diet
- C. Management and treatment of renal failure
  1. Medical and bedside management of renal failure
  2. Diagnosis and treatment of underlying cause
  3. Special nutrition and total parenteral nutrition
  4. Protein catabolism (to be minimized)
  5. Hyperkalemia management
  6. Calcium and phosphorus control
  7. Fluid and electrolyte balance
  8. Blood transfusion reactions
  9. Hemodialysis (Chapters 16 and 17)
     - a. Acute
     - b. Chronic
  10. Peritoneal dialysis (Chapters 18 and 19)
     - a. Acute
     - b. Chronic
  11. Kidney transplant
- D. Kidney transplant
  1. Indication
  2. Patient preparation

a. Tissue typing
(1) Antigens
(2) Antibodies
b. Donor organ harvesting
3. Recovery period
4. Potential complications and their management
5. Organ rejection
E. Prevention of renal failure
F. Pharmaceuticals as they relate to the patient suffering renal failure
1. Narcotics and barbiturates
2. Salicylates
3. Diuretics (xanthine, osmotic, or mercurial types)
4. Sulfonamides
5. Spironolactone
6. Triamterene
7. Carbonic anhydrase inhibitors
8. Immunosuppressive agents
a. Azathioprine (Imuran)
b. Steroids
9. Antibiotics
10. Antacids
11. Vitamin and mineral supplements
G. Drug metabolism and renal failure
H. Fluids, electrolytes, and acid-base balance
I. Bedside physical assessment
1. Central nervous system status
2. Respiratory status
3. Cardiovascular system status
4. Renal system status
5. Psychosocial status
V. The nervous system (Chapter 21)
A. Neurologic evaluation
1. Physical examination
2. Assessment and diagnosis
a. Neurologic check
(1) Level of consciousness
(2) Corneal reflexes
(3) Pupil reaction
(4) Ciliospinal response (pinch neck, observe ipsilateral eye dilation)
(5) Gag reflex
(6) Motor and sensory responses
(7) Colorics
(8) Doll's eyes
3. Continuous intracranial monitoring
4. Psychologic and sociologic factors
5. Human evoked responses
B. Neurologic emergencies
1. Trauma
a. Spinal cord injuries
(1) Paralysis
(2) Loss of sensation
(3) Loss of reflexes
(4) Hyperflexia
b. Head and neck injuries
2. Vascular disorder
a. Epidural hematoma
b. Ruptured aneurysm
c. Subarachnoid hemorrhage
d. Subdural hematoma
e. Arterial-venous malformation
3. Supratentorial herniation
4. Tumors and brain abscesses
a. Pituitary
b. Hypothalamus
5. Microbial invasion
a. Guillain-Barré syndrome
b. Myelitis
c. Meningitis
6. Electrochemical disorders
a. Seizure disorders, status epilepticus
b. Myasthenia gravis
c. Parkinson's disease
C. Treatments
1. Neurosurgery
a. Craniotomy
b. Burr holes
c. Transphenoidal hypophysectomy
d. Ventriculostomy
2. Pre- and postoperative care
3. Complications
a. Intracranial pressure (Scott cannula)
b. Spinal shock hypotension
c. Pneumonia (respiratory insufficiency)
d. Urinary tract infection
e. Malnutrition

f. Decubiti
g. Spasms
h. Chronic pain
i. Chronic depression
j. Temporary and permanent motor and sensory losses (aphasia, paraplegia, hemiplegia, quadriplegia)
k. Thermal imbalance
l. Hemorrhage
m. Fluid and electrolyte imbalance
4. Radiation therapy
5. Hormone replacement
6. Drug therapy

D. Cerebrovascular disturbances
1. Contusion
2. Concussion
3. Subdural hematoma
4. Subarachnoid hemorrhage

E. Infection
1. Etiology
2. Pathology
3. Clinical evaluation and assessment
4. Diagnosis
5. Management modalities

VI. Endocrine and metabolic disorders (Chapter 14)

A. Diagnosis and management modalities
1. Adrenocortical insufficiency
2. Addison's disease
3. Acute adrenal crisis
4. Pheochromocytoma
5. Thyroid disorders
a. Thyrotoxic storm (hyperthyroidism)
b. Myxedematous coma (hypothyroidism)
6. Diabetic syndrome and ketoacidosis
7. Hyperglycemia, nonketotic coma, and insulin shock
8. Diabetes insipidus
9. Lactic acidosis
10. Inappropriate antidiuretic hormone syndrome

VII. Psychosocial aspects of critical care (Chapter 4)

NOTE: The critical care practitioner, whether physician, nurse, respiratory therapist, or other allied critical care team member, is prompted to recognize his or her personal impact on each situation or individual encountered in practice. Self-awareness along with in-depth perceptual skills relative to the dynamics of human behavior, communication, and environmental effects are vital therapeutic components of care. Consideration of the psychosocial aspects of care is an integral part of any critical care education program. It is therefore recommended that the aspects of care listed here be included in the case presentation portion of any critical care curriculum or course of instruction.

A. Interpersonal relationships (psychosocial dynamics)
1. Patient
2. Behavioral adaptation to pathophysiologic changes
3. Family
4. Health team

B. Effects of critical care environment
1. Patient
2. Sensory and/or dream deprivation
3. Sensory overload
4. Dependencies and/or independencies
5. Space and/or time orientation
6. Staff (personnel)
7. Families

C. The dying patient
1. Patient
2. Family
3. Health team

D. Progressive care and rehabilitation (Chapter 31)

VIII. Electrical hazards in critical care (Chapter 30)

A. Delineation
B. Prevention
C. Equipment
D. Precautions

IX. Legal aspects of critical care

A. Malpractice insurance
B. Laws and precedence

- C. Joint Commission on Accreditation of Hospitals (standards)
- D. Nurse, medical, and paramedical practice acts
- E. Registration, licensure, and certification

X. Emergency care (Chapters 5 and 6)
- A. Emergency medical care system (prehospital and in-hospital)
  1. Rural environment
  2. Urban environment
- B. Field personnel
  1. Mobile intensive care paramedics
  2. Emergency medical technicians
  3. Other paramedical assistants
  4. Physician and nurse
- C. Field evaluation
  1. Patient history (data base)
  2. Physical examination
  3. Observations in the field
  4. Diagnosis
  5. Intervention
- D. Emergency airway establishment and ventilation procedures
  1. Intubation
     - a. Endotracheal procedure
     - b. Esophageal airway
  2. Cricothyreotomy
     - a. Needle thyrotomy
     - b. Other procedures
  3. Heimlich maneuver (Chapter 5)
- E. Circulatory inadequacy
  1. Cardiopulmonary resuscitation in the field and hospital
     - a. Infant
     - b. Child
     - c. Adult
- F. Common emergencies (prehospital and in-hospital)
  1. Diagnosis and early management
     - a. Myocardial infarction
     - b. Diabetes and other endocrine or metabolic emergencies
     - c. Congestive heart failure
     - d. Asthma (status asthmaticus)
     - e. Coma (unconscious patient)
     - f. Anaphylaxis
     - g. Seizures
     - h. Drug overdose
     - i. Near drowning
     - j. Ingestion of chemicals
       - (1) Insecticides
       - (2) Weed killers
       - (3) Bleach and other household substances
       - (4) Other poisons
     - k. Reptile and animal bites
     - l. Facial injuries
     - m. Ocular emergencies
     - n. Ear, nose, and throat emergencies
     - o. Head and neck injuries
     - p. Spinal cord injuries
     - q. Orthopedic injuries
     - r. Chest trauma
     - s. Abdominal injuries
     - t. Impaled objects
     - u. Vascular injuries (hemorrhage control)
     - v. Shock
     - w. Burn
       - (1) Emergency care/initial resuscitation
       - (2) Inhalation of hot gases
       - (3) Treatment of chemical burns
       - (4) Treatment of flame burns
     - x. Obstetric and gynecologic emergencies (Chapter 23)
- G. Radiologic accidents (nuclear)
  1. Emergency handling of radiation accident victims and rescue personnel (involving hospital emergency department, emergency medical technicians or paramedics, and ambulance personnel)
  2. Precautionary measures to be employed when providing direct patient care in the hospital setting

XI. Pharmacology (Chapter 3)
- A. Analgesics
- B. Anesthetics
- C. Antiarrhythmics
- D. Antibiotics

E. Anticoagulants
F. Anticonvulsants
G. Antispasmodics
H. Cardiotonics
I. Diuretics
J. Drugs used in cardiac arrest
K. Drugs used in controlled ventilation procedures
L. Drugs used in electrolyte replacement
M. Drugs used in respiratory therapy
N. Nitrates
O. Vasodilators
P. Vasopressors
Q. Steroids

XII. Recommended clinical practice (return demonstration)
- A. Skills and techniques
  1. Laboratory data interpretation
  2. Venous and arterial catheters
  3. Central venous pressure and arterial pressure monitoring
  4. Pulmnary wedge pressure monitoring (PAP monitoring)
  5. Cardiopulmonary resuscitation (adult and infant)
  6. Defibrillation
  7. Arrhythmia identification and interpretation
  8. Electrocardiogram (ECG) monitoring (12-lead)
  9. Esophageal lead
  10. EEG monitoring
  11. Pacemakers and pacing
      a. Internal and external
      b. Intrathoracic pacing
  12. Synchronized cardioversion
  13. Care of chest tubes
  14. Hematocrit
  15. Determination of alveolar ventilation
      a. Tidal volume
      b. Minute volume
      c. Dead space
      d. Minute alveolar ventilation
  16. Spirometry
  17. Use of nomograms
  18. Blood gas sampling and measurement
  19. Arterial puncture
  20. Intubation
      a. Endotracheal procedure
      b. Esophageal airway
      c. Cricothyreotomy
         (1) Needle thyrotomy
         (2) Other procedures
  21. Heimlich maneuver
  22. Breath sounds (auscultation and percussion)
  23. Heart sounds
  24. Chest physiotherapy
      a. Vibration
      b. Percussion
      c. Tracheostomy care
      d. Suctioning and secretion management
      e. Sepsis control
      f. Postural drainage
  25. Use of mechanical ventilators
      a. Assisted and controlled ventilation
         (1) Volume control
         (2) Pressure limitation
         (3) Accessories and modifications
         (4) Intermittent positive pressure breathing (IPPB)
         (5) Continuous positive air pressure (CPAP)
         (6) Positive end-expiratory pressure (PEEP)
         (7) Intermittent mandatory ventilation (IMV)
  26. Use of manual ventilatory devices
  27. Peritoneal dialysis
  28. Hemodialysis
      a. Atrioventricular shunt care
      b. Fistula (bovine)
  29. Patient/family teaching

XIII. Recommended clinical experience
- A. In-hospital patient care experience
  1. Shock
  2. Heart catheterization (pre- and postcatheterization)
  3. Open heart surgery (pre- and postoperative)
  4. Pacemaker
  5. Myocardial infarction

6. Respiratory distress (adult and child)
7. Acute renal failure
8. Neuromedical and neurosurgical care
9. Severe burns
10. Acute pulmonary edema
11. Major trauma
12. Patient and family teaching

B. Bedside assessments
1. Patient data base (history)
2. Physical examination
3. Diagnosis
4. Plan of care
5. Observation
6. Interpersonal relationships (development of trust between nurse and patient)

C. Prehospital patient care experience
Mobile intensive care (field experience) is highly recommended. This to include experience in the following:
Patient data base (history)
Physical examination
Observations in the field
Diagnosis
Intervention
Transportation

## REFERENCE

1. Toffler, A.: Future shock, New York, 1970, Random House, Inc.

## BIBLIOGRAPHY

Abram, H. S.: Adaptation to open heart surgery: a psychiatric study of response to the threat of death, Am. J. Psychiatry **122:**659-668, 1965.

Abram, H. S.: Psychological aspects of the intensive care unit, Hosp. Med. **2:**22, 1969.

Adams, C. W.: Recognition and evaluation of cardiogenic shock, Heart & Lung **2:**893-895, 1972.

Altshuler, A.: Complete transposition of the great arteries, Am. J. Nurs. **71:**96-98, 1971.

Amacher, N. J.: Touch is a way of caring, Am. J. Nurs. **73:**852-854, 1973.

American College of Cardiology: Advanced cardiac nursing, Philadelphia, 1970, The Charles Press, Publishers.

Andreoli, K., Hunn, V. K., Zipes, D. P., and Wallace, A. G.: Comprehensive cardiac care, a text for nurses and other health professionals, ed. 3, St. Louis, 1975, The C. V. Mosby Co.

Artiss, K. L., and Levine, A. S.: Doctor-patient relation in severe illness, N. Engl. J. Med. **288:**1210-1214, 1973.

Aspinall, M. J.: Nursing the open heart surgery patient, New York, 1973, McGraw-Hill Book Co.

Ayres, S. M., and Laguson, J.: Pulmonary physiology at the bedside; $O_2$ and $CO_2$ abnormalities, Cardiovasc. Nurs. **9:**1-6, 1973.

Ayres, S. M., and Mueller, H.: The overall approach to the patient with hypotension, Heart & Lung **3:**463-476, 1974.

Beall, C., Braun, H., and Cheney, F., Jr.: Physiologic bases for respiratory care, Missoula, Mont., 1974, Mountain Press Publishing Co.

Beigelman, P. M., et al.: Severe diabetic ketoacidosis, J.A.M.A. **210:**1082-1087, 1969.

Beland, I.: Clinical nursing: pathophysiological and psychosocial aspects, New York, 1971, Macmillan Publishing Co., Inc.

Bendixen, H. H., et al.: Respiratory care, St. Louis, 1965, The C. V. Mosby Co.

Bergersen, B. S.: Pharmacology in nursing, ed. 12, St. Louis, 1973, The C. V. Mosby Co.

Bernard, H., and Huickers, W.: Dynamics of personal adjustment, Boston, 1971, Holbrook Press, Inc.

Bilodeau, C. B.: The nurse and her reactions to critical care nursing, Heart & Lung **2:**358-363, 1973.

Brown, E. L.: Newer dimensions of patient care, New York, 1964, Russell Sage Foundation.

Browne, I. W., and Hackett, T. P.: Emotional reactions to threat of impending death. A study of patients on the monitor cardiac pacemaker, Ir. J. Med. Sci. **6:**177-187, 1967.

Broughton, J. O.: Chest physical diagnosis for nurses and respiratory therapists, Heart & Lung **1:**200-206, 1972.

Bruno, F.: Psychology: a life-centered approach, Santa Barbara, Calif., 1974, Hamilton Publishing Co.

Burke, S.: Composition and function of body fluids, St. Louis, 1972, The C. V. Mosby Co.

Burrell, L. O., and Burrell, Z. L., Jr.: Intensive nursing care, ed. 2, St. Louis, 1973, The C. V. Mosby Co.

Bushnell, S. S.: Respiratory intensive care nursing, Boston, 1973, Little, Brown & Co.

Carini, E., and Owens, G.: Neurological and neurosurgical nursing, ed. 6, St. Louis, 1974, The C. V. Mosby Co.

Carlson, C. E.: Behavioral concepts and nursing intervention, Philadelphia, 1970, J. B. Lippincott, Co.

Cassem, N. H., and Hackett, T. P.: Psychiatric

consultation in a coronary care unit, Ann. Intern. Med. **75**:9-14, 1971.
Cassem, N. H., and Hackett, T. P.: Psychological rehabilitation of myocardial infarction patients in the acute phase, Heart & Lung **2**:382-388, 1973.
Cassem, N. H., Hackett, T. P., Bascom, C., and Wishnie, H. A.: Reactions of coronary patients to the CCU nurse, Am. J. Nurs. **70**:319-325, 1970.
Chernick, R. M.: Oxygen therapy (pharmacology for physicians), Philadelphia, 1967, W. B. Saunders Co.
Chernick, R. M., et al.: Respiration in health and disease, ed. 2, Philadelphia, 1972, W. B. Saunders Co.
Children's Hospital Medical Center, Boston: Manual of pediatric therapeutics, Boston, 1974, Little Brown & Co.
Chusid, J. G.: Correlative neuroanatomy and functional neurology, Los Altos, Calif., 1970, Lange Medical Publications.
Clark, N. F.: Pump failure, Nurs. Clin. North Am. **7**:529-539, 1972.
Cogen, R.: Cardiac catheterization: preparing the adult, Am. J. Nurs. **73**:77-79, 1973.
Cohen, R. G.: Providing emotional support, R.N. Magazine **37**:62-70, 1974.
Cole, J. S., and McIntosh, H. D.: Electroshock hazards in the coronary care unit, Heart & Lung **1**:481-486, 1972.
Colley, R., and Phillip, K.: Helping with hyperalimentation, Nursing '73 **3**:6-17, 1973.
Comroe, J. H.: The lung, Chicago, 1962, Year Book Medical Publishers, Inc.
Comroe, J. H.: Physiology of respiration, Chicago, 1973, Year Book Medical Publishers, Inc.
Conn, H. L., and Horwitz, O., et al.: Cardiac and vascular diseases, vol. I-II, Lea & Febiger, 1971.
Conover, M. H.: Cardiac arrhythmias: exercises in pattern interpretation, St. Louis, 1974, The C. V. Mosby Co.
Craven, R. F.: Anaphylactic shock, Am. J. Nurs. **72**:718-721, 1972.
Daly, C. R., and Kelly, E. A.: Prevention of pulmonary embolism: intracaval devices, Am. J. Nurs. **72**:2004-2006, 1972.
Devek, J. H.: Chronic cor pulmonale, Cardiovasc. Nurs. **3**:25-30, 1967.
DeVillier, B.: Preoperative teaching of the cardiovascular patient, Heart & Lung **2**:522-525, 1973.
Druss, R. G., and Kornfeld, D. S.: Survivors of cardiac arrest: psychiatric study, J.A.M.A. **201**:291-296, 1967.
Dubin, D.: Rapid interpretation of EKG's, ed. 2, Tampa, Fla., 1973, Cover Publishing Co.
Egan, D. F.: Fundamentals of respiratory therapy, ed. 2, St. Louis, 1973, The C. V. Mosby Co.
Escher, D. J.: Medical aspects of artificial pacing of the heart, Cardiovasc. Nurs. **8**:1-5, 1972.
Flint, T., and Cain, H. D.: Emergency treatment and management, Philadelphia, 1970, W. B. Saunders Co.
Foster, S. B.: Pump failure, Am. J. Nurs. **74**:1830-1834, 1974.
Friedberg, C. K.: Diseases of the heart, Philadelphia, 1966, W. B. Saunders Co.
Germain, C. P.: Helping your patient with an implanted pacemaker, R.N. Magazine **37**:3-35, 1974.
Gernert, C. F., and Schwartz, S.: Pulmonary artery catheterization, Am. J. Nurs. **73**:1182-1185, 1973.
Glaser, B. G., and Strauss, A. L.: Awareness of dying, Chicago, 1965, Aldine Publishing Co.
Goldman, M. J.: Principles of clinical electrocardiography, ed. 8, Los Altos, Calif., 1973, Lange Medical Publications.
Gould, E. P.: The emotional effects of surgical illness, Heart & Lung **2**:368-369, 1973.
Greyton, A.: Textbook in medical physiology, ed. 4, Philadelphia, 1971, W. B. Saunders Co.
Grinker, R., and Sahs, A.: Neurology, ed. 6, Springfield, Ill., 1966, Charles C Thomas, Publisher.
Gutch, C. F., and Stoner, M. H.: Review of hemodialysis for nurses and dialysis personnel, ed. 2, St. Louis, 1975, The C. V. Mosby Co.
Guyton, A.: Textbook of medical physiology, ed. 3, Philadelphia, 1968, W. B. Saunders Co.
Guyton, A.: Basic human physiology: normal function and mechanisms of disease, Philadelphia, 1971, W. B. Saunders Co.
Hackett, T. P., and Cassem, N. H.: Psychological reactions to life-threatening illness. In Abram, H. S., editor: Psychological aspects of stress, Springfield, Ill., 1970, Charles C Thomas, Publisher.
Hackett, T. P., Cassem, N. H., and Wishnie, H. A.: The coronary care unit . . . an appraisal of its psychologic hazards, N. Engl. J. Med. **279**:1365-1370, 1968.
Hamilton, W. P., and Lavin, M. A.: Decision making in the coronary care unit—a manual and workbook for nurses, St. Louis, 1972, The C. V. Mosby Co.
Harrington, J. D., and Brener, E. R.: Patient care in renal failure, Philadelphia, 1973, W. B. Saunders Co.
Hay, D., and Oken, D.: The psychological stress of ICU nursing, Psychom. Med. **34**:109-118, 1972.
Himathongkam, T., et al.: Acute adrenal insufficiency, J.A.M.A. **230**:1317-1319, 1974.
Horney, K.: The neurotic personality of our

time, New York, 1964, W. W. Norton & Co., Inc.
Hudak, C., Gallo, B. M., and Lohr, T.: Critical care nursing, Philadelphia, 1973, J. B. Lippincott Co.
Hurst, J. W., and Logue, R. B.: The heart, New York, 1970, McGraw-Hill Book Co.
Hurwitz, L. J.: Helping the aphasic to communicate again, Geriatrics **28**:102-106, 1973.
Isler, C.: Blood, the age of components, R.N. Magazine **36**:31-41, 1973.
Isler, C.: I. V. therapy, R.N. Magazine **36**: 23-31, 1973.
Jackson, B. S.: Chronic peripheral arterial disease, Am. J. Nurs. **72**:928-934, 1972.
Jones, B.: Inside the coronary care unit: the patient and his responses, Am. J. Nurs. **67**:2313-2320, 1967.
Kee, J. L., and Gregory, A. P.: The ABC's and mEq's of fluid imbalance in children, Nursing '74 **4**:28-36, 1974.
Kernicki, J., Bullock, B., and Matthews, J.: Cardiovascular nursing, New York, 1970, G. P. Putnam's Sons.
Kersten, L.: Chest tube drainage system—indications and principles of operation, Heart & Lung **3**:97-101, 1974.
King, J.: Denial, Am. J. Nurs. **66**:1010-1013, 1966.
Kintzel, K. C., et al.: Advanced concepts in clinical nursing, Philadelphia, 1972, J. B. Lippincott Co.
Korones, S. B.: High-risk newborn infants—the basis for intensive nursing care, St. Louis, 1972, The C. V. Mosby Co.
Kory, R. C.: Cardiac catheterization and related procedures, Cardiovasc. Nurs. **4**:17-22, 1969.
Kubler-Ross, E.: On death and dying, New York, 1969, Macmillan Publishing Co., Inc.
Kurihara, M.: Postural drainage, clapping and vibrating, Am. J. Nurs. **65**:76-79, 1965.
Larson, E. L.: The patient with acute pulmonary edema, Am. J. Nurs. **68**:1019-1021, 1968.
Lehman, J.: Auscultation of heart sounds, Am. J. Nurs. **72**:1242-1246, 1972.
Levine, R. R.: Pharmacology: drug actions and reactions, Boston, 1973, Little, Brown & Co.
Lillehei, R. C., et al.: The pharmacologic approach to shock. I. Defining traumatic, septic and cardiogenic shock, Geriatrics **27**:73-83, 1972.
Lillehei, R. C., et al.: The pharmacologic approach to shock. II. Diagnosis of shock and the plan of treatment, Geriatrics **27**:81-94, 1972.
Lindsay, A., and Budkin, A.: The cardiac arrhythmias, Chicago, 1969, Year Book Medical Publishers, Inc.
Littman, D.: Stethoscopes and auscultation, Am. J. Nurs. **72**:1238-1241, 1972.
Long, M. L., Scheuling, M. A., and Christian, J. L.: Cardiopulmonary bypass, Am. J. Nurs. **74**:860-862, 1974.
Marchiondo, K.: CVP: the whys and hows of central venous pressure monitoring, Nursing '74 **4**:21-24, 1974.
Maron, L., Bryan-Brown, C. W., and Shoemaker, W. C.: Toward a unified approach to psychological factors in the ICU, Crit. Care Med. **1**:81-84, 1973.
Marriott, H. L.: Practical electrocardiography, Baltimore, ed. 5, 1972, The Williams & Wilkins Co.
Maslow, A. H.: Personality development and the self. In Hamachek, E. E., editor: The self in growth, teaching and learning, Englewood Cliffs, N. J., 1965, Prentice-Hall, Inc.
Maslow, A. H.: Toward a psychology of being, New York, 1968, Van Nostrand Reinhold Co.
Meltzer, L. E., et al.: Textbook of coronary care, Philadelphia, 1973, The Charles Press, Publishers.
Metheny, N. M., and Snively, W. D., Jr.: Nurses handbook of fluid balance, ed. 2, Philadelphia, 1974, J. B. Lippincott Co.
Moore, V. B.: I.V. fluids, Nursing '73 **3**:32-40, 1973.
Mountcastle, V. B., editor: Medical physiology, vol. I-II, ed. 13, St. Louis, 1974, The C. V. Mosby Co.
National Critical Care Institute of Education: Radiological accidents; critical care update! Orange, Calif., 1975, The Institute.
National Tuberculosis and Respiratory Disease Association: Chronic obstructive pulmonary disease: a manual for physicians, 1965, The Association.
Nett, L., and Petty, T. L.: Acute respiratory failure: principles of care, Am. J. Nurs. **67**: 1847-1852, 1967.
Phibbs, B.: The cardiac arrhythmias, ed. 2, St. Louis, 1973, The C. V. Mosby Co.
Piaget, J., and Inhelder, B.: The psychology of the child, New York, 1969, Basic Books, Inc., Publishers.
Picklesiner, L.: The nurse-challenging syndrome DIC, R.N. Magazine **37**:46-47, 1974.
Pinneo, R.: Symposium concepts in cardiac nursing, Nurs. Clin. North Am. **7**:411-412, 1972.
Plum, F., and Posner, J. B.: Diagnosis of stupor or coma, Philadelphia, 1972, F. A. Davis Co.
Roberts, F. B.: The child with heart disease, Am. J. Nurs. **72**:20-27, 1972.
Robinson, J. R.: Fundamentals of acid-base

regulation, ed. 3, Philadelphia, 1967, F. A. Davis Co.

Rodman, T., Myerson, R. M., Lawrence, L. T., Gallagher, A. P., and Kaspar, A. J.: The physiologic and pharmacologic basis of coronary care nursing, St. Louis, 1971, The C. V. Mosby Co.

Rogers, C. R.: On becoming a person, Boston, 1961, Houghton Mifflin Co.

Sarason, I. G.: Abnormal psychology: the problem of maladjustive behavior, New York, 1972, Appleton-Century-Crofts.

Scalzi, C. C.: Nursing management of behavior responses following an acute myocardial infarction, Heart & Lung **2**:62-69, 1973.

Selkurt, E. E.: Basic physiology for the health sciences, Boston, 1975, Little, Brown & Co.

Shafer, K. N., Sawyer, J. R., McCluskey, A. M., Beck, E. L., and Phipps, W. J.: Medical-surgical nursing, ed. 6, St. Louis, 1975, The C. V. Mosby Co.

Sharp, M. A., et al.: Nursing in the coronary care unit, Philadelphia, 1970, J. B. Lippincott Co.

Silver, H. K., Kempe, C. H., and Bruyn, H. B.: Handbook of pediatrics, ed. 10, Los Altos, Calif., 1973, Lange Medical Publications.

Smith, C., editor: The critically ill child, Philadelphia, 1972, W. B. Saunders Co.

Smith, S. W., and Gips, C. D.: Care of the adult patient, ed. 3, Philadelphia, 1971, J. B. Lippincott Co.

Spencer, R. T.: Patient care in endocrine problems, Philadelphia, 1973, W. B. Saunders Co.

Sproul, C. W., and Mullanney, P. J., editors: Emergency care: assessment and intervention, St. Louis, 1974, The C. V. Mosby Co.

Stephenson, H. E., Jr., editor: Immediate care of the acutely ill and injured, St. Louis, 1974, The C. V. Mosby Co.

Stude, C.: Cardiogenic shock, Am. J. Nurs. **74**: 1636-1640, 1974.

Swan, H. J.: Complications of cardiac catheterization, Cardiovasc. Nurs. **4**:27-30, 1968.

Sweetwood, H.: Nursing in the intensive respiratory care unit, New York, 1971, Springer Publishing Co., Inc.

Tesler, M., and Hardgrove, C.: Cardiac catheterization: preparing the child, Am. J. Nurs. **73**:80-82, 1973.

Vinsant, M. O., Spence, M. I., and Chapell, D. E.: A commonsense approach to coronary care—a program, St. Louis, 1972, The C. V. Mosby Co.

Wade, J. F.: Respiratory nursing care—physiology and technique, St. Louis, 1973, The C. V. Mosby Co.

Weldy, N. J.: Body fluids and electrolytes—a programmed presentation, St. Louis, 1972, The C. V. Mosby Co.

Whipple, G., et al.: Acute coronary care, Boston, 1972, Little, Brown & Co.

Zalis, E. G., and Conover, M. H.: Understanding electrocardiography—physiological and interpretive concepts, St. Louis, 1972, The C. V. Mosby Co.

# chapter 2

# Anatomy, physiology, and altered regulatory mechanisms

EARLE DAVIS

Characteristic interrelationships coexist at different stages in the normal maturation of the body and during the existence of pathologic conditions in any individual's life cycle. Since the integration of these interrelationships involves physiologic anatomy at the cellular through body system levels, potentially involving the entire field of medicine, the degree of comprehension sought in understanding these processes will determine the extent to which the individual reader will search the references beyond the minimum coverage summarized at the end of this chapter. The relative weighting of the material in this chapter is based on the premise that, although all of the body systems are important to proper integration, treatment of the critically ill patient will commonly be more involved with a limited number of these systems.

## ■ What are the integrative levels at which the body functions?

The cell theory states that the body is made up of *cells* (Fig. 2-1) and cell products. Although the definition of the cell as "the unit of structure, function and heredity of which the body is composed" has the problems inherent in defining basic words, it nonetheless provides on a gross level a substantial basis for initiating discussion.

The living substance of the cell is known as *protoplasm.* It consists of a nucleus and cytoplasm and is surrounded by a plasma membrane. The nucleus exerts control over the cellular metabolic processes and transmits the genetic information. Cytoplasm constitutes that portion of the protoplasm other than the nucleus.

*Tissues* are collections of similar cells and cell products that are organized for the performance of a given function. The classic categories are epithelial, connective (general and special, for example, blood), muscle, and nerve.

*Organs* are collections of tissues organized for the performance of a given function. Examples are the stomach, for storing food, and the brain, for integrating the actions of the nervous system.

*Systems* are collections of organs organized for the performance of a given function. The classic categories are integumentary, musculoskeletal, circulatory, respiratory, digestive, urogenital, endocrine, and nervous.

The total energy expenditures within the body are referred to as *metabolism.* In this constant interchange of energy, there is a building up of some substances (anabolic processes) and a tearing down of others (catabolic processes).

## ■ What is the histologic nature of the cytoplasm and what are its functions?

Although a considerable portion of the volume of most cells consists of substances (the solutes) dissolved in water (the solvent), many undissolved substances are held in suspension. The passage of these substances through selectively permeable membranes by diffusion is known as *osmosis.*

Some of the cytoplasmic substances are

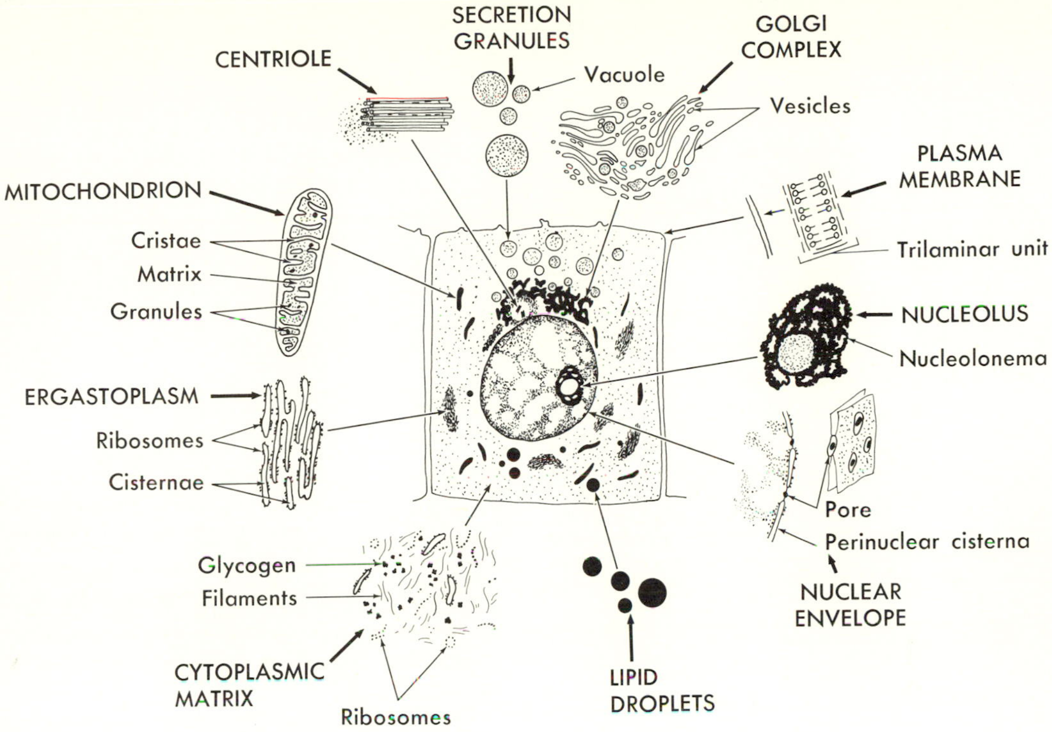


**Fig. 2-1.** Cell.

submicroscopic, that is, at the molecular level; others, known as *organelles* and *inclusions,* produce the characteristic features of specific cells as seen under the light microscope. It is significant that the submicroscopic and microscopic features of a cell and its chemical composition and pH vary according to the function(s) of the cell, that is, in the serous vs the mucous cells of a single submaxillary acinus or, more grossly, in muscle vs adipose tissue.

## ■ What are some examples of cytoplasmic organelles and what are their functions?

An *endoplasmic reticulum,* consisting of an irregular network of branching and anastomosing tubules and often associated with saccular structures called *cisternae,* attracts ribonucleoproteins called *ribosomes.* The ribosomes, some of which are also free in the cytoplasmic matrix, are the sites of protein synthesis.

Organelles known as *mitrochondria* generate a supply of *adenosine triphosphate* (ATP), which in turn acts as an energy source for many cellular chemical transformations.

The role of the *Golgi apparatus* is to add carbohydrate to proteins brought to the organelle from the endoplasmic reticulum. The glycoprotein formed is released into the cytoplasm (as enzymes or enzymatic precursors) in membranous vesicles known as zymogen granules and lysosomes. Ultimately the *zymogen granules* are released through the cell surface to carry on their enzymatic processes extracellularly, while the *lysosomes* remain within the cell, digesting substances brought in by phagocytosis or pinocytosis.

## ■ What is the structural and functional nature of the nucleus?

The nucleus contains *deoxyribonucleic acid* (DNA), or genetic material that determines the specific morphologic and biochemical characteristics of each cell type and controls each cell type's metabolic activities, including the cell division phenomena of mitosis and meiosis. Although aberrations at the level of the gene and/or chromosome become manifest as both anatomic and physiologic pathologies, in general these are not of the type involved with producing the critical illnesses discussed in this book.

### ■ How does the structure of the cell membrane (or plasmalemma) adapt itself for its functions?

Cytoplasmic membranes consist, theoretically, of bimolecular layers of lipids that orient themselves with their polar groups projecting into the polar solvent (water) on either side of the membrane and their nonpolar portions buried in the membrane interior. The membrane formed by these glyco- and phospholipids contains numerous motile proteins and glycoproteins embedded in it that act as enzymes or function as pumps, moving material into and out of the cell. It is the diversity of the protein activity that gives each particular membrane its characteristic distinctions. Although the basic principles of Donnan equilibrium underlie the cell's ultimate ionic balance, the processes of dialysis, ultrafiltration, and secretion each play a part in metabolism. The ease with which solutes pass through the plasmalemma is determined by such factors as polarity (nonpolar molecules pass through readily), temperature, lipid solubility (lipid-soluble compounds pass through readily), and size. The speed with which molecules diffuse across cell membranes implies that pores with an average diameter of about 8 Å occupy less than 1% of the total plasmalemma surface area.

All nutrients must enter the cell by crossing the membrane, and all substances synthesized by the cell as useful or waste products must leave the cell through the membranes.

### ■ What are pinocytosis and phagocytosis?

The additional methods by which substances may be moved through the plasma membrane are comparable to those used by protozoa in feeding. In these phenomena a portion of the cell membrane invaginates and then detaches itself from the surface, forming an intracellular vesicle. To what extent pinocytosis may occur with smaller particles in the lining of the digestive and respiratory systems or the endothelium of capillaries is currently unknown.

The phagocytic activity of leukocytes and macrophages of the reticuloendothelial system on bacteria has long been recognized. The production of acid hydrolases by lysosomes is implicit to the normal functioning of phagocytic cells and may be considered the self-destructive "suicide sac" of many cell series.

## BASIC CATEGORIES OF TISSUES

Tissues have been defined as specialized groups of cells organized for the performance of a given function. The four basic types of tissues are epithelial, connective, muscle, and nervous. The latter two will be discussed in association with their respective body systems.

### Epithelial tissues

### ■ What is the histologic nature of the basic types of epithelium and what are the functions of these basic types?

Epithelial tissues (Fig. 2-2) are classified (1) according to the shape of the individual cells, that is, squamosal, cuboidal, columnar, and transitional, and (2) as to whether they constitute a single cell layer, that is, nonstratified, or multiple cell layers, that is, stratified. The term "pseudostratified" applies to modified types of nonstratified epithelium.

*Cytologic metamorphosis* is seen in the follicle cells of the thyroid gland. When the follicle is distended with thyroxine, the cells assume a squamosal shape. As the follicle shrinks because of metabolic changes, the cells successively pass through stages in which they are cuboidal, then columnar. The process of modification in the internal epithelial lining of the ureters and bladder to accommodate size changes differs somewhat from that of the thyroid gland, involving the presence of *transitional cells.*

Cilia sometimes extend from the epithelial surfaces into adjacent lumina, providing a basis for using the terms "ciliated" and "nonciliated" epithelial tissues.

Squamosal cells lining body cavities form

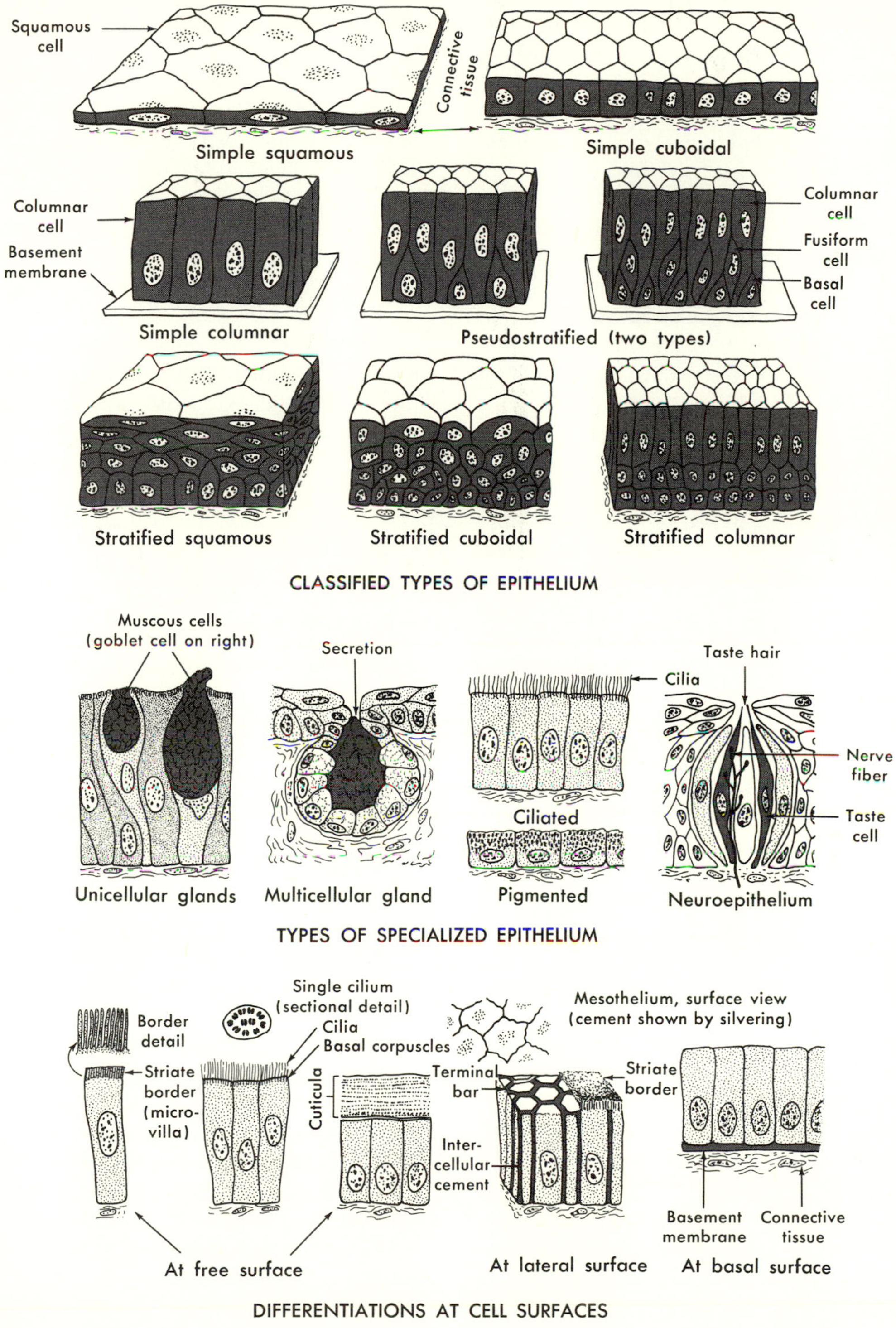


**Fig. 2-2.** Epithelial tissue. (From Arey, L. B.: Human histology, ed. 4, Philadelphia, 1974, W. B. Saunders Co.)

*mesothelia,* which are more commonly called *pleura* (in the chest) and *peritoneum* (in the abdominopelvic cavity). As the lining of a blood vessel, squamous cells form an *endothelium.*

Epithelium tissues exposed to the external environment, that is, those at the surface of the integument, lose their moisture content and replace it with the horny substance characteristic of *keratinized epithelium.* The presence of the cornified layer diminishes the dehydration of deeper cell strata. Where epithelial cells line the body's lumina, they remain moist (nonkeratinized) and can thus participate vigorously in the process of osmosis. By comparison, the inward penetration of substances from ointments is relatively slow at the surface.

## Connective tissues

The body is composed of three materials: cells, intercellular substances, and fluids. Intercellular substances are the prime constituents of connective tissue, being largely responsible for structural strength.

The relationship between various intercellular substances can be represented schematically.

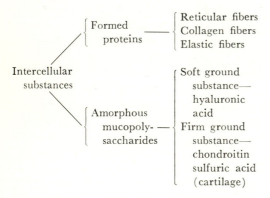

- Intercellular substances
  - Formed proteins —
    - Reticular fibers
    - Collagen fibers
    - Elastic fibers
  - Amorphous mucopolysaccharides —
    - Soft ground substance—hyaluronic acid
    - Firm ground substance—chondroitin sulfuric acid (cartilage)

### ■ What is the histologic nature of the formed intercellular substances and what are their functions?

Both reticular and collagen fibers are formed by the crystallization of tropocollagen. This takes place in the ground substance surrounding formative cells called *fibroblasts,* the number and arrangement of component fibrils and the relation of the fibrils to the intercellular cement being different in each particular type of connective tissue. The reticular fibers tend to form delicate networks, as in areolar tissue, and the collagen fibers form stronger structures, such as tendons and aponeuroses. Whereas collagen is relatively unyielding, elastin (of which elastic fibers are composed) can be stretched to 150% of its original length.

The design of the body is such that the relative amounts of collagen and elastin in a given structure relate directly to the function of that tissue. If tissues composing the origins and insertions of muscle contained much elastin, when the muscle belly contracted, stretching of the tendon would result rather than skeletal movement. Although a moderate amount of bone separation during flexion, extension, etc. is normal, an excessive stretching and separation of the joint would result under strain if the articular capsule of joints were composed primarily of elastin. This would result in ineffective muscle movement; therefore collagen predominates. On the contrary side, it is an advantage to have the skin loosely attached (by elastin) to the underlying epimysium in some places, for example, on the forearm, and firmly attached at others, as on the fingers.

*Cicatrix* is formed by a combination of the intercellular substances in which the white collagen fibers predominate. Keloid formation constitutes a familiar collagen disorder.

### ■ What is the histologic nature of the amorphous intercellular cement and what is its function?

The amorphous intercellular cement substances *chondroitin sulfuric acid* and *hyaluronic acid* act as adhesives to bind together cells and/or formed intercellular substances. Although chondroitin sulfuric acid is widely distributed throughout the body, it is proportionately in far greater abundance in cartilage. Since the amount of cartilaginous tissue in the body is relatively small, hyaluronic acid assumes the dominate role as the intercellular cement. Synovial fluid may be considered an example of hyaluronic acid admixed with an unusually high proportion of water. Since hyaluronidase (Wydase) decomposes the intercellular cement, it is used in injecting anesthetic drugs as an adjunct to speed up the drugs' diffusion to and through the epineurium. However, it also is equally able to break down the normal barrier of the blood vessel wall. Accordingly, rather than just producing local anesthesia, injections that include hyaluronidase may result in dramatic, sudden—and disconcertingly unexpected—total anesthesia if injected too near a vessel.

As in the case with other body tissues, intercellular substances are constantly being replaced and modified in type and composition as an adaptation to the environment. From the time of birth the process of aging consists of a gradual shift, with formed intercellular substances substituting more and more for amorphous substances, as is well evidenced in the wrinkling of the skin. This process is subject to considerable modification during pathologic processes, sometimes speeding up, sometimes slowing down, sometimes favoring the formation of one type of formed or amorphous intercellular substance, and sometimes sustaining another.

## ■ What is the histologic nature of loose connective tissue and what are the functions of its components?

The use of the terms "loose" and "dense" to describe connective tissue connotes the relative compactness of the formed intercellular substances collagen and elastin. The loose type is characterized by an admixture of fixed fibrous components (with their associated fibrocytes and adipose cells) and wandering cells, such as macrophages, plasma cells, mast cells, and white blood cells, that is, lymphocytes and eosinophils. Areolar tissue is the classic example. *Macrophages* (or *histiocytes*) are the equivalent of the phagocytic polymorphonuclear cells of the blood. Interstitial monocytes can develop into macrophages.

*Plasma cells* produce antibodies that in turn collect on mast cells. *Mast cells* produce histamine (and presumably inconsequential amounts of heparin). The combination of an antigen with an antibody causes histamine release, the subsequent contraction of smooth muscle, and the dilatation and increased permeability of capillaries that are associated with the anaphylactic phenomenon known as *allergy*. Considerable research is being done on the role of lymphocytes in rejecting tissue and organ transplants by activating destructive pyroninophilic cells.[1] Eosinophils phagocytize antigen-antibody complexes; basophils are also involved in allergic responses, containing about half of the histamine present in the blood.

It is generally believed that in adult tissues of mesodermal origin there typically remain a scattering of undifferentiated *mesenchymal* cells. Depending on the nature of the stimulus received, on occasion some of these cells may differentiate into tissue similar to that of the immediate area, for example, loose connective tissue. However, on receiving a different stimulus they may develop into another type of tissue of mesodermal origin, for example, bone. In addition to connective tissue and bone, mesoderm also gives rise to cartilage and muscle and, accordingly, they have the same propensities.

Normally one type of adult tissue, for example, loose connective tissue, does not form another type of adult tissue; for example, muscle does not become bone. However, under pathologic conditions such changes do occur and are referred to as *metaplasia*, a classic example being the replacement of pseudostratified ciliated columnar (respiratory) epithelium by stratified squamous epithelium.

## ■ What is the histologic nature of dense connective tissue and what are the functions of its components?

### *Tendons and aponeuroses*

In the form of tendons and aponeuroses dense connective tissue consists primarily of collagen with an admixture of collagen and elastin. Where more stretch is desired, proportionately more elastin is present. Where more nonyielding strength is desired, proportionately more collagen is present. The cornea is basically pure collagen; the nuchal ligament is basically pure elastin. In all of these tissues the intercellular cement is hyaluronic acid. Fibroblasts secrete both the hyaluronic acid and tropocollagen, the precursor of collagen. Although the origin of elastin is uncertain, it is believed to come from fibroblasts.

### *Cartilage*

Cartilage is simply dense connective tissue in which chondroitin sulfuric acid has substituted for hyaluronic acid, giving greater strength and rigidity to the tissue. Hyaline cartilage differs from fibrocartilage basically in that in hyaline cartilage the optic index of refraction of the intercellular cement is the same as that of the fibers, but the two optic indices are different in fibrocartilage. In elastic cartilage the elastic fibers and matrix also have different optical indices. Hyaline cartilage is located at the ends of long and short bones; elastic cartilage is found in the epiglottis and ear; fibrocartilage occurs in the symphysis pubis and intervertebral discs.

### *Bone*

Bone has achieved considerable strength, durability, and supporting power through the supplementation of the fibroelastin and cement complex with calcium phosphate salts. Since a review of the nature of both intramembranous and endochondral bone formation is essential to understanding the repair of fractures, bone transplants, malignancies, etc., the reader is encouraged to pursue appropriate details in a standard histology book.

## THE INTEGUMENTARY SYSTEM

The integumentary system consists of the skin (Fig. 2-3) and its modifications, which in man includes hair (variously modified to include the eyelashes and eyebrows) and the nails of the fingers and toes. Skin is stratified into a more superficial epidermis and a deeper dermis. The dermis is contiguous with the underlying hypodermis which, when rich with adipose tissue, is referred to as the superficial fascia. Depending on the area of the body considered, the hypodermis rests on the epimysium or aponeurosis of muscles, periosteum, or perichondrium.

■ **What is the histologic nature of the epidermis?**

The *epidermis* is unique in that its major purposes are achieved by producing dead cells. In the orderly accomplishment of this objective a stratification of cell layers results, in which new cells, constantly formed in the basal layer (in the stratum germinativum) are pushed to the surface, from which they are eventually sloughed off. Since the epidermis contains no blood vessels but is dependent on diffusion from the dermis for maintenance, the osmotic gradient established produces a gradual change in the shape and chemical composition of these cells. These cytologic stratifications are identifiable centripetocentrifugally as basal stratum germinativum (for cell replication), stratum granulosum, stratum lucidum, and stratum corneum, the latter being composed of anuclear keratinized cells.

■ **What is the histologic nature of the dermis?**

The *dermis* is composed of a more superficial papillary layer and a deeper reticular layer, the former possessing papillae that correspond to the epidermal ridges recognized, for example, as fingerprint lines. Sensory corpuscles for touch, pressure, and temperature plus capillaries are found in the papillae. Fibers for pain reception extend into the stratum granulosum. The basic tissue of the *papillary layer* is a closely interwoven mesh composed of thin collagen and elastic fibers, plus some reticular fibers.

The *reticular layer* is a densely interlacing fibroelastic layer varying from less than 0.5 mm (in the eyelid) to 4.0 mm or more (on the back). The roots of hair, sebaceous glands, and sweat glands originate in this layer.

■ **What is the histologic nature of the subcutaneous layer, the hypodermis?**

In adipose individuals considerable fat is stored in the *hypodermis,* or *superficial facia,* and the layer may attain considerable thick-

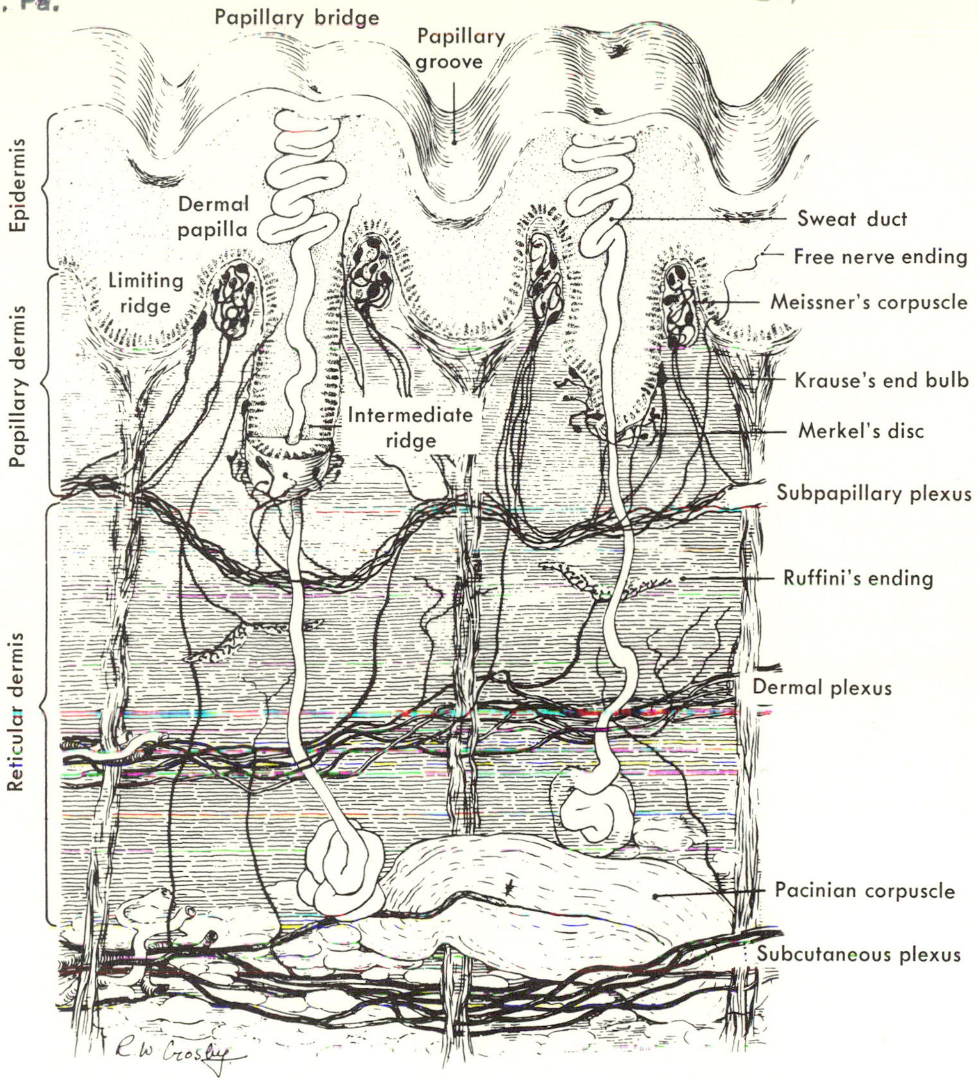


**Fig. 2-3.** Skin. (From Mountcastle, V. B.: Medical physiology, ed. 13, vol. 1, St. Louis, 1974, The C. V. Mosby Co.)

ness. With lesser amounts of fat the layer is thin and consists of a greater abundance of fibroelastic tissue.

## ■ What is the importance of the keratinized layer?

The horny nature of the stratum corneum acts as a physical barrier to the entrance of chemicals and foreign objects, such as splinters and disease-producing organisms (whole bodies or parts thereof). It also acts as a physical barrier to water, making it possible to bathe either in salt water, without losing water, or in fresh water, without the body becoming swollen. On the other hand, the use of dermal ointments indicates that the fact that a certain degree of absorption takes place through the skin is of therapeutic advantage.

## ■ Of what diagnostic value is the skin in medicine?

Many allergies and infectious diseases are identifiable by the skin rashes they produce. In certain vitamin deficiencies and hormonal imbalances the texture of the skin assumes characteristic features. The color of the skin may indicate jaundice, cyanosis, infection, hormonal imbalance, or malignancy. Skin temperature and/or the relative amounts of moisture are of diagnostic value also. In the event that the patient is unable to communicate or in the case of a cadaver, the character of the skin is often of value in determining the sites of mechanical trauma, burns, and frostbite.

### ■ How do skin wounds heal?[2]

In a V-shaped wound extending into the hypodermis some fibrin forms near the bottom, and the epidermis soon starts to grow down into the groove. About a week later the epidermis has extended well down the sides of the slit, attaching to the adjacent healthy tissue. Meanwhile, at the junction between the dermis and hypodermis a ridge of new tissue forms from fibroblasts and capillaries derived from the subcutaneous tissues. By the end of the second week the epidermal downgrowths on the two sides meet in the center, only to be pushed outward (toward the surface) during the next 2 weeks by the proliferating ridge until the area is flattened out.

### ■ What are the general categories of skin grafts?

Regardless of the type of tissue transplanted, transplants are classified as autologous grafts, homografts, or heterografts. In *autologous* grafts the tissue, usually skin, is moved from one part of the body to another site on the same individual. In *homografts* (or *allografts*) the tissue is transplanted from another individual of the same species. In *heterografts* the tissue is transplanted from another species. Homografts and heterografts do not "take," but are sometimes used as temporary filling until the patient can regenerate the tissue. This may involve skin or body organs.

### ■ What are the two general methods used in autologous grafting?

One method is to move skin from one part of the body to another without the transplant tissue ever being completely separated from its blood supply. There are two versions of this procedure. One is by "walking" the graft tissue from its original to its intended site by a series of retransplantations with a pedicle at one edge of the graft being left connected to its original blood supply until the other portion has established new vascular connections. Then the earlier pedicle is transected, a new one is created, and the patch is relocated again with the newly created pedicle. A modification of this method is to bring one part of the body close to another, freeing up the graft from the donor site, except for its pedicle, and suturing the graft to its recipient site. The transplant tissue is permitted to establish new anastomoses with the subjacent tissue of the recipient site before the pedicle is detached.

A second method is to use free skin grafts.

### ■ How are skin grafts performed and what is the rationale?

There are two general types of autologous skin grafts: split grafts and full-thickness grafts. In *split grafts* the skin to be transplanted may be cut at a level about halfway down the dermis and placed on the denuded area. Temporarily the transplanted tissue will derive its nourishment by diffusion from the raw surface to which it is transposed. In about a week capillaries in the graft bed will connect with capillaries of the transplant.

Concurrent with the take of the graft, the denuded area from which the graft was taken will be recovered with new epidermis that grows from the germinal cells of the external sheath of hair follicles and the ducts of sweat glands.[1]

In *full-thickness grafts* both dermis and epidermis are transplanted.

### ■ How is recovering of burned areas accomplished histologically?

In moderate burns the dermis may not be destroyed. Repair in these cases is comparable to that experienced in areas from which split grafts are removed, that is, as long as viable hair follicles and/or bases of the sweat glands remain, reepithelialization will take place. In more severe burns if grafting is not done, cicatrix will form, the fibroelastic plug being derived from fibroblasts located in the subcutaneous tissue and/or brought in on the surface of local capillaries.

## CARDIOVASCULAR SYSTEM

The cardiovascular system is committed to expediting the exchange of gases and of food and waste products involved in metabolism. This is achieved with the aid of a pump (the heart), a system of tubes (the blood vessels), and the blood itself. The food (energy) supply is made potentially available by being brought into the digestive tract and acted on by various enzymes. From there on, for further appropriate distribution, the body depends on the cardiovascular system. Less than 2% of the metabolic waste products are finally returned (by the bloodstream) to the digestive tract for elimination. Other by-products are eliminated via the lungs, the kidneys, and the skin, all of which are in turn dependent on the cardiovascular system for normal functioning (Fig. 2-4). Depending on the degree of finite knowledge of vessel distribution sought, the reader should select appropriate references.

### ■ What is the nature of plasma and what are its roles?

Blood consists of *cellular elements* and a liquid, *plasma,* in which the cellular elements are suspended. After an anticoagulant is added, if blood is permitted to stand or is centrifuged, the cells settle to the bottom 45% of the tube, constituting the hematocrit reading. The supernatant 55% is the plasma, which is 90% water by volume. When the fibrinogen is removed from plasma, the remaining fluid is known as *serum.*

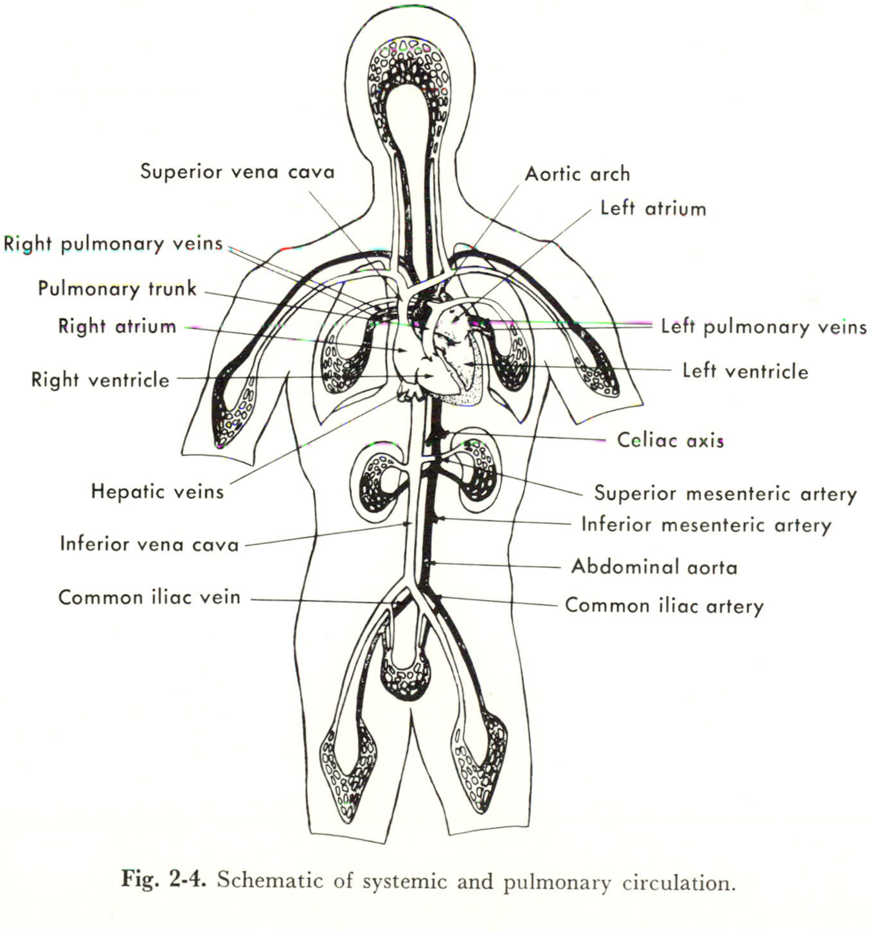


**Fig. 2-4.** Schematic of systemic and pulmonary circulation.

As the principal solvent in the blood, naturally most of plasma's functions relate to acting as a transport mechanism for respiratory gases, food, wastes, antibodies, hormones, electrolytes, and proteins. In addition, it acts as a suspensory agent for the blood's cellular elements and provides for fluid balance and temperature regulation, the latter being closely tied to the phenomenon of perspiring.

Plasma proteins are classified as albumins and globulins, and they are synthesized by the liver, except for the immunologically related gamma globulins, which are formed in the lymph nodes and spleen. Proteins used in cell synthesis are usually manufactured locally rather than drawn from the plasma proteins. Although proteins are the most abundant solute by weight, *osmolarity* depends on the number of particles. Accordingly sodium (144 mM/L) and secondly chloride (100 mM/L) are the most important determinants of plasma osmolarity, proteins falling in line with calcium (at 2.5 mM/L) after bicarbonate (4.4 mM/L) and potassium (4.4 mM/L).

## The heart

### ■ What is the basic course of the blood through the heart?

It is convenient clinically to speak of the heart as being composed of right and left halves, the blood vessels of the right half consisting of the venae cavae. After passing into the first chamber, the right atrium, blood passes through the right atrioventricular (tricuspid) valves to the right ventricle, and from there to the pulmonary trunk, backflow from which is prevented by semilunar valves. The trunk splits into right and left pulmonary arteries, which conduct the blood to the right and left lungs for an exchange of gases. Purified blood returns via the pulmonary veins to the left atrium. The right ventricle, pulmonary vessels, lungs, and left atrium constitute the *pulmonary system* of circulation. From the left atrium, blood passes through the left atrioventricular (bicuspid) valves into the left ventricle. In both the right and left halves of the heart the atrioventricular valves function to prevent regurgitation from the ventricles into the respective atria. From the left ventricle, blood flows out the aorta to be distributed to the nonpulmonary portions of the body, backflow being prevented by semilunar valves. The left ventricle, the aorta and its subdivisions, the associated venous network (including capillaries) returning blood to the heart, and the right atrium constitute the *systemic system*. Depending on the degree of finite knowledge of vessel distribution sought, the reader should select appropriate references on the systemic and/or pulmonary system(s).

### ■ On what does the heart depend for its mechanical effectiveness?

To derive its force as a pump the heart depends on the effective contraction of the cardiac muscle and the proper functioning of its valvular system. Effective contraction involves (1) proper stimulation of the cardiac myofibers, (2) the normal sequence of events associated with contraction of myofibers, and (3) an efficient transmission of the contractive force to propel the blood.

### ■ What is the nature of the contractile force of cardiac muscle?

The physiologic chemistry of cardiac myofiber contraction is basically similar to that of striated muscle, where the phenomenon has been worked out in greatest detail. Depolarization of the myofiber's T tubal system results in the critical release of calcium ions among the actinomycin filaments, activating adenosine triphosphatase (ATPase). The ultimate splitting of ATP and the associated release of energy cause the change in the shape of the myosin cross-bridges, which results in fiber contraction. Although the mechanism whereby the electric charge causes calcium ion to be released is unknown, clinically a proper balance of available ionic calcium is extremely important.

### ■ How is the rate of the heartbeat controlled?

In in vitro experiments dissociated heart cells each beat with their own independent rhythm. When two of them are joined, they assume the speed of the faster one. This intrinsic phenomenon is known as *autorhyth-*

*micity.* However, in the normal heart integration is achieved via the sinoatrial (SA) and atrioventricular (AV) nodes, the former located where the superior vena cava joins the right atrium and the latter situated on the posterior junction of the right atrium and ventricle near the interatrial septum.

The SA node is the normal pacemaker for the entire heart. Question exists as to whether there are special conduction fibers to the AV node. Atrial systole lasts approximately 0.1 seconds. There is a 0.1-second delay before the AV node is activated by atrial excitation, permitting the atria to contract before the ventricles do.

The AV node impulse travels down the interventricular bundle of His and spreads out in the Purkinje fibers. The impulse spreads over the right and left ventricles, resulting in ventricular systole, which lasts approximately four times as long as atrial systole—about 0.38 seconds.

## ■ What are the etiologies of some of the anomalous heartbeats?

*Atrial fibrillation* is associated with the development of ectopic atrial foci. *Ventricular fibrillation* is associated with unusual conduction routes, so that the main impulse constantly meets an area that is no longer refractory. For example, in electrocution the normal pathways conducting impulses of 60 beats/min are overwhelmed by 60 Hz.

In *partial cardiac blocks* only a fraction of the impulses reach the ventricles. As a consequence, there may be a rhythm of 85 beats/min in the atria, but only 65 beats/min in the ventricles, resulting in faulty filling. In *complete cardiac block* the atria may maintain a rhythm of 75 beats/min and the ventricles 25 to 40 beats/min, the two rhythms being completely independent.

*Cardiac blackouts* are associated with recurrent complete blocks, resulting in decreased flow to the brain and fainting.

## ■ What does the term "PQR-ST complex" mean?

The electromagnetic fields created by the beating of the heart are recorded as the electrocardiogram (ECG). In it P equals atrial depolarization; QRS, ventricular depolarization; and T, ventricular repolarization. Because it is masked by the QRS complex, atrial repolarization is not seen. Discussion of the PQR-ST waves receives appropriate detailed analysis in standard textbooks of physiology and/or cardiology.

## ■ What phenomena are associated with diastole and systole?

Typically when the terms "systole" and "diastole" are used without an adjective, for example, "during systole," reference is made to ventricular rather than atrial systole or diastole.

In *late diastole* the AV valves open, and 80% of ventricular filling takes place before atrial systole. The amount of blood in the ventricles just prior to systole is known as *end-diastolic volume.* During *systole* most of the blood is ejected rapidly, followed by a tapering off. The amount of blood remaining after contraction is the *end-systolic volume. Early systole* is the rapid ventricular filling taking place after the AV valves open. This is of considerable physiologic importance during periods of rapid heartbeat.

## ■ What are the common heart sounds and their causes?

In the normal heartbeat, *lub-dub,* the lub is caused by closure of the AV valves and coincides with the later part of the QRS wave. The dub is caused by closure of the semilunar valves and coincides with the T wave at the onset of diastole.

*Murmurs* are heard when the normal, smooth flow is caused to be turbulent. A *systolic murmur* results from a narrowed pulmonary or aortic valve or a hole in the interventricular septum. *Diastolic murmurs* are caused by faulty valve closure. *Atrial murmurs,* heard laterally, are produced by a patent foramen ovale.

## ■ How much is the normal cardiac output?

Cardiac output is determined by stroke volume and rate. The normal volume is about 60 ml/stroke, and the normal rate about 70 beats/min, thus totaling well over 4000 ml/min. (The concept of "a gallon a minute" is more meaningful to those on the English measuring system.)

■ **What mechanisms are involved in modifying the cardiac output?**

Among the factors modifying the cardiac activity are a series of sensors, the autonomic nervous system, response according to Starling's law of the heart, and restricting blood flow to certain organs according to the type of activity. *Baroreceptors* found in the carotid sinus and aortic arch respond reflexly to changes in arterial pressure, activating the sympathetic nerves to speed up the heart (if pressure is inadequate) or the parasympathetic nerves to reduce the speed (and the pressure). Reaching the heart by the vagus nerve, the parasympathetic nerves cause the SA and AV nodes to reach their thresholds more slowly. The sympathetic nerves, via the cardiac plexus, cause the pacemakers to reach their thresholds more rapidly. If both sympathetic and parasympathetic nerves are cut, the heartbeat goes to about 100 beats/min, illustrating the dominance of the parasympathetic system here.

According to *Starling's law of the heart,* there is a direct proportion between the diastolic volume and the contractile force of the following systole. With increased end volume there is increased stroke volume and vice versa. However, overstretching will produce a decreased contractile force and a reduction in stroke volume.

In exercise, because of increased heart rate and stroke volume, the flow of blood to skeletal muscle is increased. Additional compensation consists of decreasing the flow to the kidneys and decreasing the total peripheral resistance.

### Arteries

■ **How does the structure of arteries adapt them for their functions?**

Arteries and veins share the structural pattern of being composed of an outer tunica adventitia, an interposed tunica media, and an inner tunica intima.

The *tunica adventitia* is a relatively thin fibroelastic layer.

The *tunica media* varies with the size of the artery. In large arteries it is characterized by many layers of elastic membranes (to absorb the shock of the systolic pressure and begin the establishment of a smooth, steady blood flow to the capillaries). In smaller ("muscular") arteries, the tunica media consists of many layers of smooth muscle cells. There are gradual admixtures of elastic fibers and muscle cells in the tunica media of intermediate-sized vessels. The tunica media aids further in absorbing the pulsatile nature of the blood flow. Its musculature is under the control of the sympathetic nervous system.

The *tunica intima* is lined with a single layer of *squamosal endothelium* and may possess some subendothelial tissue.

■ **How is the structure of arterioles adapted to their functions?**

As compared with arteries, the major modifications of the three basic tunicae in arterioles is the prominence of the purely muscular tunica media. Relative to the lumen, the vessel wall is thicker than in any other blood vessel.

Although the elastic and muscular arteries do much toward removing the pulsatile nature of the blood flow, the sympathetic nerves, reacting to baro- and chemoreceptors, ultimately regulate peripheral resistance to meet local needs by setting the diameter of the arterioles (via the muscles of the tunica media). If less blood is needed, the medullary cardiovascular center increases sympathetic activity, and less blood passes through the narrowed arterioles; if more blood is needed, the sympathetic nerves are deactivated, and more blood passes through the dilated arterioles. There are probably also local effects produced by carbon dioxide ($CO_2$), lactic acid, epinephrine, angiotensin, and vasopressin.

In *surgical shock* there is a dilatation of the arteriolar bed, possibly from histamine released from injured tissues. The associated decrease in blood pressure causes a weak, rapid pulse and increased respiration.

Medically vasoconstriction may be brought about by the use of epinephrine and other sympathomimetic drugs. The vasodilatation sought for *pectoral angina* is induced with the aid of amyl nitrite.

### ■ What factors control the arterioles?

An obvious response to exercise is the increased blood supply to the muscles known as *hyperemia,* the increase in blood flow being directly proportional to increased activity. Unknown chemical factors probably underlie the cause of the phenomenon. Sympathetic fibers maintain a characteristic tone in the arterioles of all organs, usually releasing epinephrine as the neurohumor. (The amount of epinephrine released from the adrenal medulla is normally of no physiologic consequence.) Increased sympathetic activity causes increased vasoconstriction; decreased sympathetic activity results in dilatation. However, at the arterioles of skeletal muscles sympathetic fibers release acetylcholine (ACh), which causes vasodilatation and increased flow.

Histamine, released from mast cells at the time of injury, also causes vasodilatation.

### ■ How do the structure and distribution of capillaries adapt them to their functions?

The thin-walled structure, ubiquitous distribution, and total surface area provided by the capillaries are direct reflections of their functions in providing sites for the exchange of metabolites. Although the capillary lumen is only wide enough to pass the red blood cells (RBC's) in single file and although the tubule itself averages only 1 mm long, since no cell is more than 0.005 inch from a capillary, normally an adequate exchange of metabolites occurs. However, the ubiquitous network results in a total storage capacity of 7 L, considerably more than the 5 L constituting the total blood volume. An explanation as to why one "does not bleed to death into the capillaries" relates to the fact that most persons have a dual capillary system: arteriovenous shunts and true capillaries. The shunts connect arterioles and venules directly. The true capillaries are like branches of the shunts, each possessing a sphincter at its origin that opens and closes intermittently. At any one time most of the capillaries are closed, containing little, if any, blood. Although the total cross-sectional area of the capillary system is 800 times that of the aorta, the capillary flow rate is only 0.4 mm/sec, compared with 320 mm/sec in the aorta. The single layer of endothelial cells constituting the wall provides a minimum osmotic barrier consistent with retaining the circulating formed elements (RBC's, WBC's, and platelets) and preventing an infinite loss of fluids to the tissue spaces. It is not clear to what extent the diffusion of solutes is carried out from endothelial cell to subjacent cell as opposed to diffusion between the endothelial cells.

### ■ Why is there an exchange between the capillaries and the tissue fluid?

In arteries and arterioles and in veins and venules the thickness of the walls prevents significant osmotic exchange between the blood and adjacent extravascular cells. For capillaries the potentials for exchange that exist depend on the reciprocal interaction of blood pressure and osmotic strength. In the proximal end of the capillary there is typically found a relatively high blood pressure and a high concentration of crystalloids, plus the normal concentration of proteins. The capillary wall acts much like a highly porous filter, and a process of *ultrafiltration* takes place in which much of the plasma fluid and crystalloids leave the capillary, but the protein molecules remain because of their relatively large size. By the time the blood has reached the midpoint of the capillary the continued pressure of the capillary wall and the loss of fluid have further reduced the blood pressure and considerably elevated the concentration of the proteins, producing an equilibrium state. In the area of the distal capillary the difference in plasma protein and interstitial concentration produces an osmotic flow greater than the effect of the remaining capillary hydrostatic pressure, resulting in a return of crystalloids and water to the capillary and a reestablishment of a plasma concentration resembling the arteriolar state. Allowed for in the latter is the interposed exchange of metabolites of total equivalent isosmotic strength.

Any physiologic state, normal or pathologic, that increases the blood pressure causes the ultrafiltration to predominate, and edema results, as in exercise. Decreased blood pressure results in a movement of fluids from the tissues into the bloodstream. When protein synthesis decreases, as in liver disease, the resultant drop in plasma protein concentration causes an increased fluid accumulation in the tissues, edema. Edema may also result from changes in capillary permeability (as in trauma) or from obstruction of the lymphatics associated with node infection. Increased filtration from the capillaries as a result of elevated venous or capillary pressure may be the chief feature of ventricular failure.

Normally the interstitial fluid volume is three to four times the plasma volume.

## Veins

Systemic blood pressure drops steadily on its return to the heart; the values are arteries, 120/80 mm Hg; arterioles, 35 to 40 mm Hg; capillaries and venules, 15 mm Hg; veins, 10 mm Hg; and right atrium, 0 to 5 mm Hg.

### ■ What is the structural nature of veins?

Although veins are composed of the same basic layers that characterize arteries, the wall is proportionately thinner and the lumen correspondingly larger, the pressure being only one tenth that in the aorta. Compared with arteries, the tunica adventitia is proportionately much thicker; the tunica media is proportionately small and accordingly possesses less muscle. Unlike arteries, many veins possess valves to prevent the reflux of blood.

### ■ What part do veins play in regulating blood pressure?

The return of blood to the heart is constantly favored by the movements of the thorax and abdomen during respiration. During exercise veins are compressed by the adjacent musculature, propelling the venous blood toward the heart. Stimulation of the medullary cardiovascular center activates the venous as well as the arterial side of the circulatory system, raising the pressure within the veins. Consistent with the view that there is a direct relation between the diastolic volume of the heart and the force of contraction of the following systole—Starling's law of the heart—the rate of venous return directly relates to determining the stroke volume—and in turn to determining atrial pressure. However, concurrently the increased sympathetic activity also causes a more rapid and stronger ventricular contraction, resulting in a more complete ventricular ejection—lower end-diastolic volume. Accordingly, during exercise, although the blood pressure goes up, the normal heart usually does not distend.

## Lymphatic system

### ■ How are the structure and distribution of the lymphatic vessels related to their functions?

Histologically the lymphatic vessels begin as blind tubules, resembling capillaries in that they consist only of an endothelium. Their continuations toward the heart also resemble their venous counterparts in the relative increase in size of the tubules and associated tunicae (intima, media, and adventitia). As in the case of veins, these vessels are classified as superficial and deep and generally form chains that accompany the arteriovenous bundles. While they are also similar to veins in that they possess valves as an augmentation to lymph flow, they have in addition a series of nodes dispersed along their courses.

The lymphatic vessels from all of the lower half of the body and from the left upper half of the body drain into the junction of the left subclavian and left internal jugular veins. Lymphatic vessels from the right upper half of the body drain into the junction of the right subclavian and right internal jugular veins.

Over most of the body the lymphatic vessels act as adjuncts to the veins in returning tissue fluid to the heart. Once the tissue fluid enters the lymphatic vessels, it is called *lymph.* Compared with venous plasma, lymph is relatively rich in protein and lipids.

The nodes interspersed along the lymphatic chain act as filtering areas and add lymphocytes to the lymph. Lymphatic vessels that originate in the villi of the small intestine are called *lacteals*. Although they return a small amount of the local tissue fluid, their principal function is to transport lipids into the circulatory system in the form of *chyle*. They return collectively to nodes known as the *cisterna chyli,* which join the *thoracic duct* in returning their contents to the junction of the left subclavian and left internal jugular veins.

## RESPIRATORY SYSTEM

It is convenient to discuss the exchange of gases occurring in metabolism as *external respiration,* relating to the exchange of gases in the lungs and pulmonary circulation, and *internal respiration,* relating to events occurring in the systemic circulation between the blood and nonpulmonary tissues.

### ■ What is the course of air when traveling into the lungs?

From the nasal cavity, air travels through the nasopharynx to the oropharynx, where it is admixed with air drawn in through the mouth. It then passes through the larynx and into the trachea, which bifurcates within the chest into right and left bronchi, each of which enters its respective lung. The bronchi initiate a series of bifurcating branches that become progressively smaller and less complex in structure. The hierarchy of tubules thus established includes successively bronchi, bronchioles, respiratory bronchioles, alveolar ducts, atria, alveolar sacs, and alveoli.

### ■ What are the anatomic characteristics of the lungs?

The right lung is divided into three lobes, the left into two lobes. Lobes are composed of lobules, consisting of a bronchiole and its anatomic hierarchial subunits. The surface of the lung is covered by a mesothelium called the visceral pleura. (The inner lining of the chest wall is covered with a comparable parietal pleura.)

### ■ How does the microscopic structure of the alveoli adapt them for their physiologic functions?

The stroma of an alveolus consists of occasional septal cells, phagocytes, and elastic fibers. The parenchyma consists of capillaries covered with pulmonary epithelium, a basement membrane being interposed between the two. Accordingly, as interpreted with the aid of electron microscopy, air would have to pass through the epithelial cell, the basement membrane, and the capillary endothelium in admixing with the blood.

### ■ How is the flow of air created between the atmosphere and the alveoli?

The movement of air into the lungs is known as *inspiration;* the outward movement is *expiration.* The flow of air involved is created by the combined action of the diaphragm, the rib muscles, and surface tension.

The thoracic cavity is a closed compartment whose floor is formed by the diaphragm and sidewalls by the rib cage. At the end of expiration the lungs are deflated, the rib cage decreases in volume, and the diaphragm assumes a dome shape. In inhalation the size (volume) of the thoracic cavity increases because the diaphragm contracts (flattens out), and the intercostal muscles cause the ribs to move upward and rotate outward. A negative internal pressure results. Surface tension created between visceral and parietal pleurae causes the two layers to adhere, much as two sheets of glass would stick together if they were adjoined by a thin layer of water. Air rushes into the lungs until the internal and external pressures are equal.

When the diaphragmatic and intercostal muscles cease to contract, passive relaxation initiates exhalation, the elastic tissues surrounding the hierarchial subdivisions (from respiratory bronchiole to alveolus) supplementing the outflow by what is referred to as "elastic recoil."

Perforating the chest wall equalizes the intra- and extrathoracic pressures and causes lung collapse, a condition known as *pneumothorax.*

*Removal of a lung segment* results in classic symptoms: upward movement of the diaphragm, shifting of the mediastinum (heart) toward the side of the surgery, depression of the chest wall on the side of extirpation, and expansion of the adjacent lung segments.

■ **What are the respiratory volumes?**

*Tidal volume* is the amount of air moved into and out of the lungs with each breath and usually averages about 500 cc. Of the 500 cc, about 150 cc remains in the "anatomic dead space" of the trachea, bronchi, and bronchioles, resulting in only 350 cc of fresh air being exchanged within the alveoli. Increased depth of breathing is far more effective in elevating alveolar ventilation than an equivalent increase in breathing rate.

*Pulmonary ventilation* is computed by multiplying the tidal volume by the respiratory rate and averages about 5000 cc/min. Since the atmosphere is about 20% oxygen, about 1000 cc of oxygen is breathed per minute. However, only 200 cc is utilized, and the remaining 800 cc is returned to the atmosphere.

In respiratory therapy it frequently becomes necessary to know more of the patient's breathing capacity than just the normal rate of ventilation. Accordingly, a series of categories have been devised indicating the amount of air exchanged with varying depths of respiration.

The *inspiratory reserve volume* is the amount that can be forcibly inspired after the tidal volume has been taken in; this volume amounts to about 2500 cc. *Expiratory reserve volume* is the amount that can be forcibly expired after the tidal volume has been exhaled; it averages 1000 cc. *Vital capacity* is the cumulative volume of inspiratory and expiratory reserve plus tidal volume. *Residual volume* is the amount left in the lungs after the maximum forcible expiration and is estimated at 1000 cc. Thus the *total lung capacity* of the average individual is about 5000 cc.

■ **What clinical terms are applied to variations in the rate of ventilation?**

*Eupnea* is normal, quiet breathing and averages 15 to 18 times/min in the adult, varying with age and position. *Hyperpnea* is increased ventilation; *dyspnea* implies labored breathing; and *apnea* is the cessation of breathing.

■ **What is the significance of the respiratory quotient?**

The *respiratory quotient* (RQ) is the ratio of $CO_2$ produced compared with the amount of oxygen ($O_2$) used in a unit of time; or:

$$\frac{CO_2}{O_2} = RQ$$

where $CO_2$ and $O_2$ are measured in cubic centimeters. The RQ varies with the type of food utilized, being 1.0 for carbohydrates and 0.7 for fats and proteins. Whereas the brain has an RQ of 1.0, indicating that it uses only carbohydrates in respiration, the average for the body is 0.8.

■ **What is meant by the partial pressure of gases?**

The total of all gases in the dry atmosphere at 0° C creates a pressure of 760 mm Hg at sea level. Such a gas pressure measurement—dry atmosphere, 0° C, and at sea level—is said to be taken under "standard conditions," and appropriate corrections in calculations must be made for variations from the standard. Each gas exerts its own pressure independently of the others; the amount of pressure created by any one gas is referred to as its *partial pressure* (PP), for example, $P_{O_2}$ represents the PP of $O_2$. Since the air consists of about 79% nitrogen ($N_2$), the pressure exerted by $N_2$ is 79 × 760, or 600 mm (written $P_{N_2} = 600$). The $P_{N_2}$ remains relatively unchanged during respiration. Therefore it is common to speak of $O_2$ and $CO_2$ as though they were the only respiratory gases. At standard conditions the $P_{O_2}$ is about 159 mm Hg, and the $P_{CO_2}$ is about 0.3 mm Hg.

However, at sea level and 0° C the vapor pressure within the alveoli and/or blood

**Table 2-1.** Presence of oxygen and carbon dioxide in selected body components

| | $O_2$ | | $CO_2$ | |
|---|---|---|---|---|
| *Component* | *Vol%* | *Tension (mm Hg)* | *Vol%* | *Tension (mm Hg)* |
| Arterial blood | 20 | 100 | 50 | 40 |
| Venous blood | 15 | 40 | 58 | 46 |
| Tissues | | 30 | | 50 |

**Table 2-2.** Calculation of partial pressure for major respiratory gases

| *Alveolar air* | *% by volume* | *PP (mm Hg)* |
|---|---|---|
| $O_2$ | 14.0 | $14/100 \times 713 = 99.8$ |
| $CO_2$ | 5.5 | $5.5/100 \times 713 = 39.2$ |
| $N_2$ | 80.0 | $80/100 \times 713 = 570.4$ |

equals 47 mm, or approximately 6% of the total 760 mm. Therefore 47 is subtracted from 760, giving a figure of 713, in deriving the basis for calculating PP's within the body (Tables 2-1 and 2-2).

■ **What is meant by volumes percent of gases dissolved in water or blood?**

Within the alveoli 0.46 cc of $O_2$ and 3 cc of $CO_2$ can be dissolved in water. The physiologist would express this as 0.46 volume percent (vol%) of $O_2$ and 3 vol% of $CO_2$. A linear relationship exists between the amount of $O_2$ and $CO_2$ dissolved in pure water and the $O_2$ and $CO_2$ tensions.

■ **How do the principles of gas diffusion apply in respiration?**

Substances diffuse from areas of higher concentration to areas of lower concentration, and if a selectively permeable membrane is interposed between the two areas, the phenomenon is known as osmosis. Since $O_2$ is utilized and $CO_2$ produced in the process of metabolism, there is an ongoing inward movement of $O_2$ in accordance with the different $P_{O_2}$ gradients found in the atmosphere, the alveoli, the blood, and the tissues. The $P_{CO_2}$ gradient is established in the opposite direction, being greatest in the tissues, then successively less in the blood, the alveoli, and the atmosphere.

Atmospheric air contains 21% $O_2$ (at a PP of 159 mm Hg) and 0.04% $CO_2$ (at a PP of 0.3 mm Hg), whereas expired air contains 16% $O_2$ (at 120 mm Hg) and 4% $CO_2$ (at 32 mm Hg).

■ **What are some of the factors affecting the rate of gas diffusion?**

Any factors that affect the rate of diffusion (osmosis) of gases through the tissue would affect the rate of lung ventilation, lowering or raising it according to whether or not it hinders or abets the rate of diffusion. A decreased ambient $O_2$ (to 12% or less) or an increase in environmental $CO_2$ (to 2% or more) stimulates respiration (ventilation). There is an increased respiratory effort as a result of impaired diffusion. Emphysema, pulmonary edema, and beryllium poisoning (which causes a thickening of the alveolar walls) constitute clinical examples of this situation. Depending on the extent of stress, the total number of functional alveoli—total alveolar surface—and the total number of functional capillaries—total blood flow—will vary, increasing threefold if necessary. Finally, a number of chemical reactions involving the plasma and RBC's interrelate.

■ **How is $O_2$ transported in the blood?**

As stated previously, only 0.46 cc of $O_2$ can be dissolved physically in water or in the blood, which is 90% water. The rest of the $O_2$ in the blood is in chemical combination with hemoglobin, which can combine (at the 100 mm $P_{O_2}$ of arteriolar blood) at the ratio of 1.34 cc of $O_2$/g of hemoglobin. Since 100 cc of blood contains 13 to 15 g of hemoglobin, this provides a total of about 20 vol% of $O_2$ in arterial blood. In venous blood there are only 15 vol% of $O_2$, but the $P_{O_2}$ is only 40 mm Hg.

## ■ What is the significance of the $O_2$ dissociation curve?

Hemoglobin (Hb) is slightly acid. Combined with $O_2$, it forms oxyhemoglobin ($HbO_2$). The reaction is reversible and is regulated by the $P_{O_2}$, $P_{CO_2}$, temperature, and acidity, being more readily dissociated at higher temperatures and greater acidity.

If samples of blood are placed in a barometric (compression) chamber with air containing $O_2$ at various PP's, $O_2$ will continue to be absorbed until the $P_{O_2}$ reaches 150 mm Hg. At this point the blood hemoglobin is said to be 100% saturated. In contrast, at a $P_{O_2}$ of 0 mm Hg there would be no $O_2$ absorbed by the blood, and its percentage of saturation would be 0. However, a plot of the amount of $O_2$ in the blood against the PP's is not linear but is sigmoid, or S shaped (Fig. 2-5). At the alveolar $P_{O_2}$ the blood is 97% saturated. The reader should consider the physiologic advantages of having only 10% loss in available $O_2$ with a drop of environmental tension from 100 to 60 mm Hg, but a 50% dissociation between the blood and tissues as the $P_{O_2}$ drops from 60 to 20 mm Hg. (Tissue tension is 20 to 30 mm Hg.)

## ■ How is $CO_2$ transported in the blood?

About 5% to 8% of the $CO_2$ is dissolved in plasma and RBC's as $CO_2$. Usually more than 25% of the $CO_2$ combines with hemoglobin, forming carbaminohemoglobin ($HbCO_2$). The remaining 67% is carried in plasma as (sodium) bicarbonate.

## ■ In the lungs in external respiration, how do the physiochemical factors involved result in an exchange of gases?

For didactic purposes it is convenient to discuss respiration in two phases: external respiration (the exchange of gases taking place within the lungs) and internal respiration (the exchange of gases taking place within tissues other than the lungs).

As stated on p. 35, the relative pressure gradients in the alveoli and pulmonary capillaries result in an exchange of $O_2$ and $CO_2$. Additionally, the diffusion of $CO_2$ from the lung capillaries favors the combination of $O_2$ and hemoglobin, while concurrently oxygenation of the blood renders hemoglobin more acid and speeds up the release of $CO_2$. Within

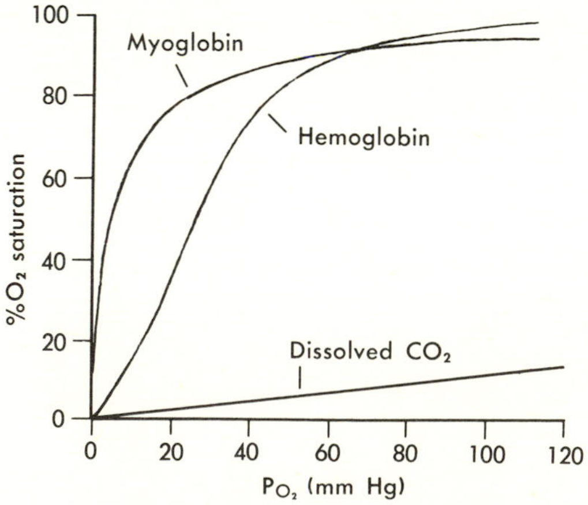


**Fig. 2-5.** Oxygen dissociation curve.

the RBC's the enzyme carbonic anhydrase expedites the intermediate, reciprocal exchange of $H_2CO_3$ with $CO_2$ and $H_2O$, speeding up the reaction approximately 5000 times. There is also a slow-acting local control in which an increase of $CO_2$ causes the bronchioles to expand, permitting more $O_2$ to enter; increased $O_2$, in turn, causes the arterioles to dilate. Decreases of $CO_2$ and $O_2$ have the opposite effect.

**■ In the tissues in internal respiration, how do the physiochemical factors involved result in an exchange of gases?**

As stated on p. 35, the relative pressure gradients in the tissue capillaries and systemic tissues results in an exchange of $CO_2$ and $O_2$. The loading of $CO_2$ in the capillaries and the unloading of $O_2$ are mutually helpful processes. An increase of capillary blood $P_{CO_2}$ with its attendant decrease of pH facilitates the unloading of $O_2$ *(Bohr effect)*. At the same time the unloading of $O_2$ facilitates the loading of $CO_2$ *(Haldane effect)*. As in external respiration, within the RBC the intermediate, reciprocal exchanges between $H_2O$, $O_2$, and $H_2CO_3$ are expedited 5000-fold by the enzyme carbonic anhydrase. For a detailed explanation of the chemical changes involved in internal and external respiration any standard physiology textbook may be consulted.

**■ What neurologic controls are involved in ventilation?**

During eupneic inhalation lung inflation receptors, acting through the *Hering-Breuer reflex,* carry afferent impulses from the stretching lungs through the vagus nerve to the respiratory center in the medulla, ultimately resulting in the cessation of inhalation. The neuronal relays that follow result in efferent impulses through the intercostal (T1-12) and phrenic (C3-5) nerves, producing contraction of the intercostal muscles and the diaphragm. In hyperpnea the pneumotaxic centers of the pons modify the rhythms of the medullary centers. For further details any standard physiology textbook may be consulted.

**■ What factors modify the action of the respiratory centers?**

One mechanism affecting the respiratory center is a system of $O_2$ sensors found in the carotid body and aortic bodies that monitor dissolved $O_2$. It is unfortunate that they do not monitor the $O_2$ associated with hemoglobin because in carbon monoxide (CO) poisoning the CO is combining with the hemoglobin, not with the dissolved $O_2$ being sensed. Another mechanism is sensitive to hydrogen ion, which increases as $CO_2$ increases. Actually the respiratory response in $CO_2$ accumulation is associated with an increase in pH and not with the $CO_2$ per se, as can be demonstrated experimentally.

Overventilating results in blowing off the $CO_2$ and a corresponding lack of respiratory stimulation.

**■ What are some additional clinical entities relating to the respiratory system?**

In *asthma* the allergic response produces both an edematous response and spasms of the bronchioles, doubly complicating the clinical picture. In *bronchitis* primarily the bronchi are inflamed.

*Emphysema* is characterized by a breakdown of alveolar walls and a corresponding reduction in the total surface area available for gaseous exchange. In contrast, tuberculosis, pneumonia, and lung cancer reduce the area for respiratory exchange by occlusion of the potential space with fibrosis, cellular hypertrophy, or fluid.

*Cheyne-Stokes breathing* is characterized by periods in which respirations increase in force and frequency alternating with gradual reversals to short periods of apnea. In addition to being associated with heart and kidney diseases, it may be caused by any damage to the brain stem from narcotics, anesthesia, or increase in intracranial pressure.

*Decompression sickness,* or *bends,* is experienced in deep underwater diving when the diver ascends too rapidly, forcing an abnormal amount of $N_2$ into the blood. Breathing pure $O_2$ during decompression assists in eliminating the $N_2$.

## URINARY SYSTEM

It is the function of the urinary system to regulate the levels of various substances within the body and to eliminate certain wastes. This is accomplished by the kidneys and their associated organs: the calyces, renal pelves, ureters, bladder, and urethra.

### ■ What is the general disposition and structure of the kidney and its proximal drainage system?

The kidneys are bilaterally disposed, bean-shaped organs about 4 to 5 inches long lying to the sides of the vertebral column in the lumbar region, with the right kidney disposed slightly lower than the left. The expanded, upper portion of the ureter, the *pelvis,* originates from the concave indentation on the medial border of the kidney known as the *hilus.* The hilus opens into a cavelike structure, the *renal sinus,* that houses the renal artery and vein and the calyces.

The interior of the kidney is almost wholly parenchyma and is divisible macroscopically into a peripheral *cortex* and a central *medulla.* The medulla consists of 10 to 15 pyramids whose apices point into the sinus. Some of the pyramids fuse, but whether or not this is the case, the single or fused apices are referred to as *papillae.*

In relation to each papilla is an infolded, double-walled cup, the *minor calyx,* whose inner wall fits over the papilla. Seven to 12 minor calyces are definable. Several adjacent minor calyces unite to form a total of two or three *major calyces.* Urine formed within the parenchyma drains by a system of tubules to the pyramidal papillae and into the lumina of the minor, and, in turn, the major calyces. The major calyces unite to form the ureteric pelvis. Each renal pelvis drains into a *ureter* that, in turn, drains into the bladder.

### ■ What is the anatomic functional unit of the kidney and what are its subdivisions?

The *nephron* constitutes both the anatomic and the functional unit of the kidney. There are approximately 1 million of these per kidney. Sequentially, the parts of a nephron include the renal (or malpighian) corpuscle, proximal convoluted tubule, descending tubule, Henle's loop, ascending tubule, and distal convoluted tubule. The distal convoluted tubules join collecting tubules that, much like branches of a tree, join the papillary ducts that open on the pyramidal apices. Each portion of the nephron has distinctive histologic features that are adaptive to its particular functions. The only one requiring further elucidation here is the corpuscle. For additional details concerning the other portions, any standard histology textbook may be consulted.

Bowman's capsule is like a partially inflated balloon into which a fist has been shoved. The indented surface of the balloon may be visualized as wrapping around the fingers, just as the inner visceral layer of Bowman's capsule wraps around the capillaries. The outer layer of the balloon would then be comparable to the peripheral parietal layer of Bowman's capsule, with the air space of the balloon being comparable to the lumen of Bowman's capsule, comparable to Bowman's space. The open end (or stump) of the balloon with its lumen would be continuous with the proximal convoluted tubule and its lumen.

### ■ What vascular patterns characterize the kidney?

After arising from the aorta the renal artery branches on entering the hilus. The branches pass between the pyramids and course to the plane separating the cortex and medulla, spreading out in this region as the arcuate artery and its branches. Since renal corpuscles (plus the proximal and distal convoluted tubules) are located in the cortex, about 95% of the arteries are directed peripherally into the glomeruli. Henle's loops and portions of the descending and ascending loops are found in the medulla, along with the collecting tubules and 5% of the total renal blood flow.

As the efferent arteriole leaves the capsule, it spreads out around the other components of the nephron, providing rich capillary networks to them. The venous return consists of arcuate veins and branches of the renal vein, which unite to form the main vein before returning to the inferior vena cava.

**■ What happens in the renal corpuscle?**

Of the three processes taking place in the kidney (glomerular ultrafiltration, tubular secretion, and tubular resorption), the first is characteristic of the malpighian corpuscle. The glomerulus acts as a type of filter, permitting approximately one fifth of the plasma to escape into Bowman's space, but retaining four fifths of the plasma, the cellular components, the proteins, and the large colloids. Although there is a glomerular capillary pressure of 90 mm Hg, there is a capsular hydrostatic pressure of 15 mm Hg resisting further filtration and an opposing osmotic gradient equivalent to 30 mm Hg caused by the high concentration of protein (28 mm Hg of the pressure is caused by the proteins, other colloids, and solutes in the capillaries). The net result is an outward force of about 45 mm Hg. Appropriate tests can be made for the *glomerular filtration rate* (GFR), which varies daily and with the state of health. Although the systemic blood pressure may vary, within limits the pressures in the glomerulus (and the GFR) are kept homeostatic by alterations in the size of the lumen of the efferent, as compared with the afferent, arteriole. Thus increased blood pressure results in narrowing of the afferent arteriole and expansion of the efferent arteriole, producing a reduced pressure to entering the glomerulus, less hydrostatic pressure, and less resistance to exiting via the efferent arteriole. A decreased blood pressure (BP) would be at least partially compensated for by opening the afferent arterioles and narrowing the efferent ones (but this would also result in an overall lower GFR if the pressure drop were significant).

**■ Of what significance is passive tubular reabsorption?**

On leaving Bowman's capsule the efferent arteriole distributes itself among the distal components of the nephron, forming extramural capillaries in relation to each of these structures. At the proximal convoluted tubule there is considerable (passive) osmosis of water and crystalloids, passing from the tubules into the capillaries in reestablishing the normal blood composition that has been temporarily imbalanced by the relatively high protein concentration left in the blood of the efferent arterioles. About 80% of the water that is reabsorbed is regulated in this way. In this process urea reabsorption is directly proportional to water reabsorption. Ultimately, of the 180 L of filtrate formed daily, about 178 L is reabsorbed.

**■ Of what significance is active reabsorption?**

In an effort to retain certain substances once they are secured, the body will expend energy to reabsorb them against a concentration gradient—the phenomenon of *active reabsorption.* A system of enzymes ("carriers") in the tubule wall with energy provided by ATP will actively transport these substances, such as sodium, bicarbonate, glucose, and amino acids, from the glomerular filtrate back into the capillary bloodstream. However, each material has a characteristic threshold or tubular maximum, and once this plasma saturation point has been reached, if additional amounts appear in the filtrate, they are permitted to pass on to become part of the urine—to "spill over." In *diabetes* the lack of insulin and consequent inability to utilize carbohydrates results in extremely high plasma glucose levels. The glucose in excess of the threshold spills over—glucosuria. There is *nothing wrong* with the tubular glucose transport mechanism. Since the threshold mechanism results in the release of the excess sugars, the diabetic occasionally experiences the compromising situation in which the injected insulin does not stop the reduction of blood sugar at its normal level. Weakness and prostration may result. In such cases it is necessary to administer glucose-containing substances and/or insulin. Under normal circumstances all of the glucose in the filtrate is reabsorbed, and no glucose is found in the urine.

## ■ What is the countercurrent mechanism?

Depending on the body's relative need to lose or conserve water, the loop of Henle is important in effecting the proper dilution or concentration. In the ascending limb of the loop sodium is actively reabsorbed by the metabolic pump, and chlorine follows to help maintain an electrolyte balance. The movement of electrolytes, however, results in a filtrate of lower and lower osmolarity, since the water is unable to enter the ascending limb unless the permeability of its cells is changed by a hormone known as antidiuretic hormone (ADH). The total result is that, as sodium chloride increases in the interstitial fluid, it diffuses back into the neighboring descending tubules, increasing the osmolarity of the filtrate moving toward the loop and creating a countercurrent.

## ■ What part do the kidneys play in acid-base balance?

Although some small amount of acid hydrogen ion ($H^+$) may be consumed as such in food, on a daily average the total net gain of $H^+$ comes primarily from protein degradation, for example, the formation of sulfuric acid on a high protein diet. (During the catabolism of carbohydrates and lipids $H^+$ may exist temporarily, but there is little, if any, net gain in $H^+$.) In normal respiration the $H^+$ temporarily released from carbonic acid is completely reincorporated into $H_2O$ molecules, and there is no real gain or loss of H. When $CO_2$ levels increase, there is an elevation in the ventilation rates, and more $CO_2$ is exhaled. However, in any lung disease causing inadequate elimination of $CO_2$ respiratory acidosis develops—free $H^+$ does accumulate.

Even in normal metabolism the body initially neutralizes the temporary excess of $H^+$ with its buffers (bicarbonate, proteins, phosphates, and hemoglobin) but must ultimately secrete the $H^+$ through the renal tubules to maintain homeostasis. Much of the significance of eliminating this excess $H^+$ relates to the fact that enzymes require optimal pH's in which to work, and without proper enzyme functioning the body would soon develop overwhelming complications. Since the actual elimination of $H^+$ from the body is normally performed only by the kidneys, it is imperative to understand the significant role played by the kidneys in this regard.

One process by which $H^+$ is secreted relates to the reciprocity between lungs and kidneys in eliminating $CO_2$, in which both organs utilize carbonic anhydrase to convert $CO_2$ and $H_2O$ to $H_2CO_3$. In the walls of the distal and collecting tubules the carbonic acid is dissociated into $H^+$ and bicarbonate ions ($HCO_3^-$). The $H^+$ is then secreted into the filtrate in exchange for sodium ions ($Na^+$). Once in the tubal cell the $Na^+$ and the $HCO_3^-$ diffuse into the capillary plasma.

Second, considering the process of ultrafiltration, in which $Na^+$ and $HCO_3^-$ enter the renal tubules, $Na^+$ is again exchanged for the secreted $H^+$. The $H^+$ combines with the filtrate's $HCO_3^-$, then dissociates into $CO_2$ and $H_2O$. Depending on the state of hydration, the water may diffuse back into the tubule. (About 10% to 15% of the filtrate $H_2O$ may be reabsorbed in the distal and collecting tubules.) If the $H_2O$ is voided, two $H^+$ have been eliminated. Since the $CO_2$ referred to in the preceding paragraph returned to the plasma with the $Na^+$ as $HCO_3^-$, the $CO_2$ alluded to in this paragraph may diffuse into the tubule as a substitute.

Third, when excess $HCO_3^-$ is formed, as in respiratory and/or metabolic alkalosis, the $HCO_3^-$ is flushed through the glomeruli, but, lacking sufficient $H^+$ to join it, the excess is voided and produces an alkaline urine. In the opposite case, excess $H^+$, phosphates (produced by the dissolution of bone salts and in the catabolism of phospholipids) can act as buffers. The dissociation of sodium phosphate releases two $Na^+$ and one phosphate ion. A secreted $H^+$ can exchange for one $Na^+$. The blood pH is raised because of the gain in sodium.

A fourth process for the elimination of $H^+$ relates to the fact that ammonia ($NH_3$) can diffuse through the tubule wall, but ammonia ion ($NH_4^+$) cannot. $NH_3$ is formed within the tubular cells primarily by the deamination of the amino acid glutamine. It then diffuses into the lumen, from which it may be excreted as $NH_3$. However, the $H^+$ secreted into the filtrate may convert $NH_3$ to $NH_4^+$, and the latter, in turn, may join with chloride ion ($Cl^-$). In states of metabolic acidosis, $NH_3$ may be eliminated as ammonium salts. However, it is usually excreted as urea, the principal end product of protein metabolism. (Urea normally comprises 80% to 90% of the total urinary nitrogen.) Its excretion is elevated whenever protein catabolism is increased, for example, with diabetes, fever, or excess adrenocortical activity.

### ■ How is hormonal control involved in renal function?

The hormonal influence is provided mainly by aldosterone and ADH. When the sodium concentration decreases, it stimulates certain renal cells to produce renin. Renin, in turn, is responsible for the formation of angiotensin. Angiotensin is a very potent vasoconstrictor, thereby causing increased BP, and also causes the adrenal cortex to release aldosterone. Aldosterone, in some unknown way, causes an increased absorption of sodium and a secretion of potassium.

ADH (or vasopressin) is produced by the hypothalamus and stored in the posterior lobe of the pituitary gland until released into the blood. It increases the size of the pores of the distal tubules and collecting ducts, permitting reabsorption of water from the filtrate and preventing diuresis. Absence of ADH results in diuresis and a lowering of the plasma level. Its release is determined conjointly by baro- and osmoreceptors located in the hypothalamus. The baroreceptors, being sensitive to changes in blood pressure, cause an increased release of ADH if the arterial and venous pressures are decreased, as would be the case in low plasma volume. If the plasma volume were low, the resultant stimulation of the hypothalamic osmoreceptors would also produce the release of ADH.

Alcohol inhibits the release of ADH, and as a result, diuresis occurs.

While assuring that the blood calcium level is high enough through regulating the movement of calcium into and out of bones and from the intestinal tract, parathormone (PTH) also increases the renal tubular reabsorption of calcium and reduces the tubular reabsorption of $PO_4^-$.

### ■ How does congestive heart failure relate to renal function?

In congestive heart failure the patient's low cardiac output results in a decreased GFR. There is also an unexplained increase of aldosterone, which results in increased sodium retention. The decreased GFR and increased sodium retention result in edema. The use of diuretics or drugs that inhibit tubular sodium reabsorption, for example, acetazolamide (Diamox), will result in greater water and sodium excretion.

### ■ What is the purpose of renal dialysis and how is it accomplished?

Typically substances found in the plasma exist in "normal" concentrations. However, in renal failure toxic substances and nitrogenous wastes that would ordinarily be excreted accumulate. To correct this, the patient's blood is passed through a hemodialysis machine, usually connected to the radial artery and the basilic or median vein. Blood from the artery flows into a device consisting of two plastic sheets surrounded by dialyzing fluid, whose consistency is determined in accordance with the findings of a prior blood analysis. The composition of the solution is adjusted so that hyperosmotic plasma substances will diffuse out of and substances in hyposmotic plasma concentration will diffuse into the blood through the cellophane. The pore size of the cellophane must permit diffusion without allowing plasma proteins and other desirable colloids to escape.

In the older peritoneal dialysis technique the abdominopelvic cavity substitutes for the machine, and a proper solution of osmotically balanced substances is introduced into the cavity for a period of 30 minutes, then withdrawn and discarded.

### ■ How does the anatomy of the ureters and bladder adapt them for the performance of their functions?

The bladder is shaped somewhat like a balloon shoved into the anteroinferior half of the pelvis, then partially deflated with the palm of the hand from above and behind, creating relatively triangular walls. The superior surface rises and falls according to the amount of urine contained and is slightly higher in the male than in the female because of the presence in the male of the prostate gland below the bladder. In the female it is circumscribed posteriorly by part of the vaginal wall and the uterus. The ureters and vesicular, or bladder, blood vessels travel from the pelvic wall to the lateral superior corners of the bladder in ligaments that help to hold the bladder (and prostate gland or uterus) in position. Urine drains from the bottom of the bladder into the proximal part of the urethra. On the internal aspect the triangular area on the posterior wall between the ureters and the origin of the urethra is recognized clinically as the *trigone*. While the histologic nature of the ureters and bladder is essentially similar to that of other abdominal and pelvic viscera, there are, of course, some modifications. Both ureters and bladder are lined internally with the type of transitional epithelium referred to on p. 20. This type of epithelium is an adaptation to the constantly changing size of the organs. The tunica muscularis of the bladder, called the *detrussor muscle,* is especially thick and is characterized by an intersecting of the smooth muscle cells of the basic laminae. It is modified at its junction with the urethra to form the internal urinary sphincter.

■ **How does the anatomy of the urethra adapt itself for its functions?**

The male urethra is divided into three parts. The prostatic portion is contained within the prostate gland. The membranous portion perforates the urogenital diaphragm, which, from its adjacent fibers, forms an external urinary sphincter around this portion of the urethra. Passing through the corpus spongiosum of the penis is the distal cavernous portion. For details of the structure and physiology of erection of the penis standard histology and general anatomy and physiology textbooks may be consulted.

The female urethra is comparatively short, since there is no prostate gland, and the portion distal to the urogenital diaphragm is only 3 to 5 cm long, lying immediately anterior to the vagina. It is because of this anatomic disposition that it is more susceptible to irritation and infection. However, the passage of catheters and cystoscopes is a much easier process.

As the bladder fills, it goes through a series of stages of stretching to accommodate the influx of urine. Both internal and external sphincters remain closed. When about 200 to 400 ml of urine have accumulated, the pressure receptors initiate a reflex in which the sphincters relax, and the detrussor muscle contracts (through innervation from the parasympathetics). The reflex is sustained until the voiding is complete. Abrupt, voluntary closure of the external sphincter helps to terminate the micturition.

## NERVOUS SYSTEM

The nervous and endocrine systems are specialized for integrating the body's activities. They accomplish this by providing secretions that stimulate the other organs and even other portions of their own systems. In the case of the endocrine system, the secretion (or stimulus), called a hormone, is released into the bloodstream, and the reaction produced is a relatively slow one. The secretion produced by nerves (neurosecretion) is released in the immediate proximity of the structure it will activate, producing almost instantaneous reaction in the structure "innervated," for example, the muscle innervated. The activation, or "excitation," of the nerve cell (called a *neuron*), to release its secretion is characterized by the propagation, or transmission, of an electrical impulse from one of its extremities to the other. Structures innervated by neurons include other neurons, myofibers, and gland cells. When one neuron innervates another, they are said to *synapse* with one another. Synaptic chains are formed when the first neuron in the chain, called a first-order neuron, stimulates a second, second-order neuron, which stimulates a third, third-order neuron, etc. Neurons interposed between the first and final order of neurons are referred to as internuncial, or intermediate, neurons. Of the 14 billion neurons in the body, 97% are internuncials.

## ■ What is a convenient system for classifying the component parts of the nervous system?

For didactic purposes it is convenient to divide the nervous system into the following categories:

| Central nervous system (CNS) | Peripheral nervous system (PNS) |
|---|---|
| Brain | Cranial nerves |
| Spinal cord | Spinal nerves |
| | Autonomic nervous system (ANS) |

## ■ What is the histologic nature of the neuron?

As shown in Fig. 2-6, in man the nucleus of a neuron is surrounded by a mass of cytoplasm, forming a *cell body* (synonyms are *soma* and *perikaryon*) from which project two or more processes, or *fibers,* called *axon(s)* and *dendrite(s)*. Embedded in the cytoplasm are neurofibrils, mitochondria, and Nissl bodies. The portion of the soma from which the axon originates is known as the *axon hillock,* or *initial segment*. Although some cells, called *bipolar cells,* possess only one dendrite and one axon, the majority of them, called *multipolar cells,* have many dendrites. The relative and absolute lengths of the axons and dendrites will vary, depending on the part of the body in which they are located. Unfortunately, many histologists have come to designate the nerve fiber, be it axon or dendrite, as the axon, which possesses a myelin sheath (p. 44). Consequently, their repeated reference to afferent "axons" of the arms and legs when they are talking technically of dendrites can be quite disconcerting to the uninitiated.

## ■ How do modifications of the peripheral ends of the dendrites adapt them to their functions?

The distal ends of dendrites and axons are called *end-organs* and are named, respectively, *receptors* and *telodendria*. While some receptors have free, naked endings, for example, pain receptors, in others there may be a fibrous capsule, variously shaped, surrounding the nerve tip. During the 1950's neurophysiologists espoused Müller's law of specific nerve energies, which maintained that any one neuron carried only one type of stimulus, for example, touch or temperature. This is no longer held to be true. For further details, standard texts of neurophysiology may be consulted.

## ■ How does the structure of axons adapt them for the performance of their functions?

The normal current flow of a neuronal impulse starts in a dendritic receptor, passes to and through the soma, and is distributed out the arborizations of the axon to the telodendria. While the branches of dendrites make angular junctions with one another, the branches of axons, called *collaterals,* leave the main trunk at right angles. Depending on their location, the total ("cable") length of the main axon and its collaterals may be less than, equal to, or greater than the total (cable) length of the dendrites. Each collateral branch is potentially capable of innervating some structure, that is, cell or cells. For example, the arborization of a neuron going to the biceps muscle of the thigh may have as many as 100 to 150 branches, each going to a separate myofiber, which it can activate. Furthermore, the myofibers innervated by any one neuron do not constitute a localized group but may have a considerable distribution throughout the muscle. Consequently, contraction is general throughout the muscle rather than local.

The exact structural nature of the telodendria and the structural relationship between a telodendron and the cell(s) it innervates take several forms. Some telodendria end by forming spirals around their effector cells. At myoneural junctions the telodendria form *motor end-plates*. Regarding synaptic chain connections, the telodendria of first-order neurons may form bulbous boutons that come into proximity either with the distal

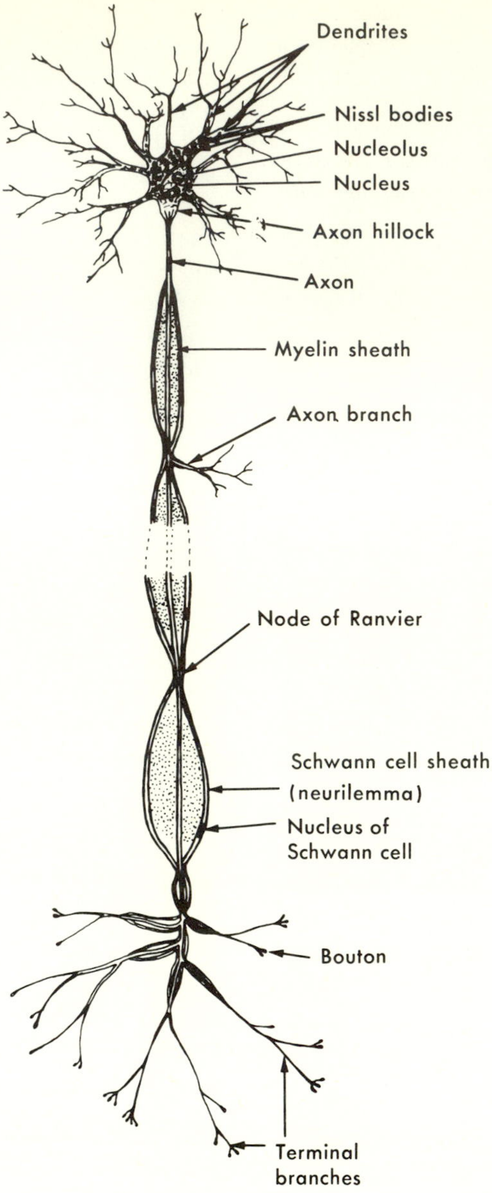


**Fig. 2-6.** Neuron.

ends or the sides of the second neuron's dendrites or with the soma of the second-order neurons.

■ **What are the sheath of Schwann (neurilemma or neurolemma) and myelin and what are their functions?**

Embryologically, as the axons and dendrites of the PNS grow toward the periphery, they are accompanied by *Schwann cells,* or *neurilemmae,* which invest themselves as a single-cell layer like a tunnel around the neuronal plasma membrane, somewhat like a capillary whose lumen is filled with a nerve fiber. The neurilemma is interrupted at regular intervals by *nodes of Ranvier,* the spaces between successive nodes being referred to as internodes. The nodes mark the areas of discontinuity between successive Schwann cells along the length of the fiber.

Although all nerves of both the CNS and PNS possess a neurilemma, some neurons, as they mature, remain gray whereas others become white. This depends on whether or not a myelin sheath develops. Electron microscopy (EM) has demonstrated that the *myelin* is actually part of the Schwann cell wrapped spirally around the neural plasma membrane so as to produce alternating layers of mixed lipids and proteins. The myelin sheath seems to act as an electrical insulator, enhancing the rate of impulse flow in neurons thus shielded.

Individual peripheral neurons, with or without myelin, are encompassed with reticular and fine collagen fibers; individual CNS fibers are similarly invested by *glial cells*. In each instance the surrounding structure is referred to as an *endoneurium* and may contain from a few to several thousand neurons. A number of nerves going to or coming from a specific area is usually grouped together as a bundle called a *fasciculus*. Each fasciculus also has a (collagen or glial) sheath around it, termed a *perineurium*. The classic "nerve" named in anatomy books, for example, the sciatic nerve, is composed of a number of fasciculi, the entire nerve being surrounded by an *epineurium*.

## ■ What processes are occurring in a patient who has traumatized a nerve?

If the peripheral portion of a nerve is devitalized by trauma, the portion of the nerve and neurilemma distal to the site of injury, referred to as the distal segment as compared with the proximal segment, will soon degenerate in a process known as *wallerian degeneration*. In this process the myelin and nerve fiber degenerate, then are consumed by macrophages, leaving a hollow tunnel within the endoneurium. Soon neurilemmal cells at the proximal and distal ends of the degenerate apex proliferate and grow toward one another, filling in the gap. Then the neuron sprouts into the slitlike spaces between the proliferating Schwann cells, toward the distal stump, and the Schwann cells spiral around the fiber, forming myelin. In the extremities proximal regeneration, for example, in the brachium, occurs at a rate of about 1 to 4 mm/week; more distal regrowth, for example, in the fingers, is slower. If a large nerve trunk is crushed, as the neurons regenerate they may grow back into the wrong endo- or even perineurium, for example, in the sciatic nerve, possibly to an entirely different group of muscles; accordingly, this requires that the patient be reeducated on the mental control over the muscle. Cicatrix may form at the site of injury, preventing reinnervation, and possibly even being associated with the growth of a neuroma. Even under the most favorable conditions, there will be anesthesia of the skin and some degree of paresis of the muscles normally innervated until the processes of wallerian degeneration and fiber regrowth have occurred.

In *nerve transplants* a sensory nerve, for example, the sural nerve, may be sacrificed and sewn into the position initially occupied by the motor nerve that has been destroyed. Surgically attention is directed to suturing the epineurium of the substitute to the epineurium of the remaining stumps in end-to-end anastomoses. Wallerian degeneration occurs in the neurons of the nerve transplant and the distal end of the injured nerve. Then the slow process of neural regeneration previously described takes place, with the same inherent problems that accompany normal regrowth.

## ■ How are nerve fibers classified?

As in the classification of many gross and microscopic anatomic structures and physiologic processes, there are numerous ways of categorizing the material, depending on the purpose(s). To indicate whether an impulse is going into or out of a structure, the neuron may be described as afferent (incoming) or efferent (outgoing). The terms *"presynaptic"* and *"postsynaptic"* are commonly used. Fibers carrying impulses toward a ganglion are *preganglionic;* those moving away from it are *postganglionic*. The impulse may be sensory or motor, depending on the nature of its stimulus. Impulses moving toward the brain are said to be *ascending;* those moving away from it are *descending.* Neurons surrounded by a myelin sheath are described as *myelinated;* those lacking the sheath are *nonmyelinated.* If the axon is long, as in peripheral neurons, the cell is referred to as a *Golgi type I neuron;* if it is short, as those within the gray matter of the cord, it is designated as a *Golgi type II neuron.*

The thicker the nerve, the faster impulses travel in it. Also, generally the thicker the nerve, the thicker is the myelin sheath. Combining these two characteristics, neurons may be classified as A, B, or C fibers, although they vary from one animal group to another with the criteria selected, among other factors, and, accordingly, provide a basis for the different statistics appearing in different books. Fibers of the A group[3] are heavily myelinated, 11 to 20 $\mu$ in diameter, and conduct at speeds of 5 to 120 m/sec. Included are somatic motor and proprioceptive fibers. Fibers of the B group are moderately myelinated, 5 to 10 $\mu$ in diameter, and conduct at speeds of 3 to 15 m/sec. In addition to fibers for touch and pressure, they include the preganglionic ANS fibers. C fibers are unmyelinated, 0.5 to 4 $\mu$ in diameter, and conduct at speeds of 0.5 to 4 m/sec. In addition to fibers for pain, temperature, taste, and touch, the C fiber group includes postganglionic ANS fibers.

**■ What are some of the terms the neurologist uses in discussing anatomic and physiologic nerve groups?**

In some regions of the body the nerves intertwine to form a complex network known as a plexus, for example, the brachial plexus.

The term *"ganglion"* is usually used in reference to a group of cell bodies lying outside the CNS, for example, dorsal root ganglion, autonomic ganglion, or ganglion of a cranial nerve. However, it has been used in reference to components of the CNS, for example, basal ganglion. Orthopedists also use the term in reference to fluid-filled cystic structures that are usually associated with fibrous tissue. The term *"nucleus"* is the typical counterpart of the term "ganglion" when the aggregate of cell bodies is found within the brain. Each cranial nerve possesses a nucleus—more specifically a right and a left nucleus for the right and for the left member of each pair of cranial nerves.

## Spinal cord and spinal nerves

**■ What are the gross characteristics of the spinal cord and the spinal nerves?**

The spinal cord, lying in the vertebral canal of the spinal column, is continuous through the foramen magnum with the medulla; it extends downward to the level of the second lumbar vertebra, where it ends as the medullary cone. At each vertebral level and attached to the sides of the cord are a pair (right and left) of spinal nerves that communicate with the periphery via openings between vertebra known as *intervertebral foramina.** The spinal nerves are named in relation to the associated vertebral level of their origins. The first pair of spinal nerves, indicated as C1, leave the canal between the base of the skull and the first cervical vertebra. The C2 pair emerges below the first cervical vertebra between the first and second; the C8 pair appears below the seventh cervical vertebra. T1 is found below the first thoracic vertebra, etc. In summary, there are eight pairs of cervical spinal nerves; 12 pairs of thoracic nerves, five pairs of lumbar nerves, five pairs of sacral nerves, and one pair of coccygeal nerves, totaling 31 pairs.

Each spinal nerve is divided into a dorsal (sensory or afferent) root and a ventral (motor or efferent) root near its attachment to the cord. In its dorsal root ganglion the sensory root possesses the cell bodies of the afferent neurons, the dendrites running distally and the axons proximally. The ventral root consists of the axons of motor neurons.

There is a cervical enlargement of the cord from the level of the fourth cervical vertebra to the second thoracic vertebra and a lumbar enlargement between the levels of the ninth and twelfth thoracic vertebrae be-

*Bony or ligamentous irregularities in the openings can apply pressure to the nerve, producing moderate to severe neurologic symptoms.

cause of the concentration of nerves passing to the arms and legs in these areas.

Since the cord ends at the level of the second lumbar vertebra, but its nerves are distributed as far as the coccyx, the nerves in the lower end of the cord become obliquely disposed as components of the cauda equina around a central nonsensory terminal filament lying in the midline.

Superficially the cord is divided longitudinally into right and left halves by a dorsal sulcus and a ventral fissure. In cross section a centrally disposed butterfly (or H-shaped) area of *gray matter* is seen to be surrounded by an area of *white matter*. The limbs of the H form the dorsal and ventral horns. In the regions of T1 to L2 and S2 to S4, intermediate gray columns house the cell bodies of autonomic neurons. A central canal that lies in the center of the gray matter runs continuously through the spinal cord, being continuous rostrally with the fourth ventricle of the medulla.

## ■ How does the anatomy of the spinal gray and white matter adapt them for their functions?

The gray matter consists primarily of cell bodies and, most commonly, the proximal portions of their associated axons and dendrites. Since cell bodies are unmyelinated, the area is gray. The myelin surrounding the axons and dendrites comprising the white matter is produced by oligodendrocytes, the counterparts of the Schwann cells of the PNS. Within the white matter the fibers are grouped into sensory or motor fasciculi that form ascending and descending *"tracts,"* going to or coming from certain parts of the brain and/or ascending or descending to various vertebral levels to make synapses within the cord. Fasciculi are grouped into dorsal, ventral, and lateral *funiculi.* For example, fibers of the dorsal funiculi are chiefly ascending (sensory), and their dysfunction, as in syphilis, results in tabes dorsalis, or locomotor ataxia, in which disturbances of joint and muscle sensation produce problems with walking. The virus producing infantile paralysis, or poliomyelitis, attacks the anterior horn cells, resulting in motor paralysis of the associated muscles.

As the (sensory) fibers from the periphery join the spinal cord, fibers from the lower part of the body lie most medially. Those entering at progressively higher levels are found progressively more laterally, the cord itself thickening in a caudocephalad direction as a result of this accretion. Conversely, part of the cephalocaudad reduction in diameter is because of the concurrent attrition in the cord's content of motor fibers.

## ■ What are the anatomic and functional characteristics of a reflex arc?

If the finger is burned, the arm is rapidly withdrawn. The impulse activated by the painful stimulus travels along the dendrites of the involved spinal nerve to the cell bodies located in the dorsal root ganglion and in turn via their axons into the spinal cord. For any one neuron, on reaching the cord, several collateral branches may be given off, including one going into the dorsal (gray) horn of the spinal level of entrance, as well as branches that may descend one or more vertebral levels or ascend one or more vertebral levels before entering the dorsal horn; some of the branches ascend to a portion of the brain known as the thalamus before synapsing. After entering the dorsal horn, the collateral synapses with a second-order neuron, called an internuncial or intermediate neuron, whose axon, in turn, may do any of the following:

1. Synapse with a third-order neuron whose cell body lies in the ipsilateral ventral (gray) horn
2. Cross over to the contralateral ventral horn to synapse with a third-order neuron
3. Split, one of its collaterals synapsing on the ipsilateral side and one on the contralateral side

The axon of the third-order neuron leaves the cord by the ventral root (also designated as the motor root because the nerve is carrying out a motor function), as contrasted with the dorsal sensory root, whose nerves perform sensory functions. The dorsal and ventral roots are also labeled as afferent and efferent because of the direction of impulse flow through them. Components of the ventral root join the main nerve to pass distally to an area containing muscles that would be involved in retracting the arm. Any one neuron would be distributed to 100 or so myofibers of some specific muscle, for example, the brachialis muscle, to participate in the reflex withdrawal.

## The brain

In studying any of the body systems some knowledge of anatomy is necessary to developing a meaningful concept of the physiology of that system. This principle is especially applicable to the nervous system in view of its relative complexity. Whether a fundamental or advanced knowledge of the nervous system is sought, some appreciation of neurologic embryogenesis is inherent to making any sense of the maze of pathways and interrelationships.

Early in its development the forerunner of the brain and spinal cord is a hollow neural tube that enlarges at one (the cephalic) end. This swelling develops two transverse strictures, producing three bulbous structures identified serially as the *prosencephalon, mesencephalon,* and *rhombencephalon.* The pros- and rhombencephalon in turn also develop transverse strictures, dividing the prosencephalon into a *telencephalon* and a *diencephalon* and the rhombencephalon into a *metencephalon* and a *myelencephalon.* The *neuroblasts* (formative cells) in the five initial blastema develop in different anatomic patterns and at different speeds, resulting in the formation of (1) swollen and constricted areas; (2) discrete aggregates of cell bodies, which will form the thalamus, cranial nuclei, etc., vs more homogeneous areas; and (3) rostral modifications of the original central canal into four ventricles that remain in continuity with the initial canal as it persists (in a proportionately narrower state) in the spinal cord.

Much as the digestive tube attains greater length and surface area by coiling and developing outpocketings, the embryonic brain develops flexures and folds, that is, the cerebral hemispheres. Just as certain parts of the digestive tract are modified to perform special functions and yet are interdependent, so the brain has developed a number of specialized, interrelated subdivisions. The five major subdivisions of the brain may be used as points of reference in describing the various specialized regions and their interrelationships.

For didactic purposes the brain is generally divided into three regions: *cerebrum* (or cerebral hemispheres), *brain stem,* and *cerebellum* (or cerebellar hemispheres). The brain stem consists of medulla, pons, mesencephalon, and diencephalon.

### ■ What anatomic features of the cerebrum explain its functions?

For the purposes of this discussion the telencephalon will be considered to be composed of cerebral hemispheres, the basal ganglia, and cranial nerves I and II as outgrowths of the brain.

The cerebrum consists of two cerebral hemispheres incompletely separated by a deep, medial longitudinal fissure, at the base of which is the corpus callosum composed of axons interconnecting the two hemispheres anatomically and functionally. The surface of the hemisphere possesses shallow grooves called *sulci* and deep grooves called *fissures.* Of the two major grooves on the lateral surface, the ones beginning near the top and running almost vertically form the *central sulcus of Rolando.* The area anterior to this fissure is called the *frontal lobe;* the area immediately posterior to it is called the *parietal lobe.* The horizontal lateral groove is called the *lateral (sylvian) fissure;* it separates the frontal and parietal lobes above from the *temporal lobe* below. A parieto-occipital fissure, aligned with the lambdoid suture of the skull, separates the posteriorly located *occipital lobe* from the anterior lobes.

The cerebral hemispheres consist of a peripheral *cortex* and a deeper *medulla.* The cortical portion is gray because it consists primarily of cell bodies; the medulla is white because its principal components are myelinated fibers passing to and from the cortex.

Different areas of the cortical gray matter are specialized for the performance of specific functions, for example, the speech area or motor eye field, and are designated as various *Brodmann's areas* by Arabic numerals accorded them by a turn of the century neurologist. For general purposes areas anterior to the central fissure are of a motor nature; those posterior to it are of a sensory nature. For example, sensory fields associated with various parts of the body, for example, foot, knee, chest, or head, can be represented on a "sensory homunculus" projected in relation to the postcentral gyrus (Brodmann's area 3). The part of the cortical gray matter representing the foot is near the corpus callosum; the part representing the head is near the inferior border of the temporal lobe. A comparable "motor homunculus" is represented in the precentral gyrus (area 4).

Three major pathways exist in the cerebral white matter. *Transverse,* or *commissural, fibers* connect one hemisphere to the other, for example, the corpus callosum. In contrast, *association tracts* of various lengths and degrees of complexity connect different Brodmann's areas of the same hemisphere. *Projection tracts* pass to and from the brain stem, becoming part of the corona radiata that is continuous with the internal capsule.

For discussions of the coordinating centers known as the basal ganglia, of the olfactory brain, and of cranial nerves I and II, any standard neurology text may be consulted.

The telencephalon contains the first and second ventricles.

## ■ What are the anatomic and physiologic characteristics of the cranial nerves?

For ease of didactic discussion scientists have identified the 12 pairs of cranial nerves associated with the brain with both Roman numerals, I to XII, rostrocaudally, and with names. Cranial nerves (CN's) I and II, the olfactory and optic nerves, respectively, are actually outgrowths of the brain associated with smell and vision. Some of the CN's, that is, V, VII, VIII, IX, and X, possess extracephalic (outside of the brain) nuclei, which are analogous with the dorsal root ganglia of the spinal nerves. Some, that is, all but I, II, and VIII, possess motor nuclei within the brain, just as the cell bodies of the neurons forming the ventral roots of the spinal nerves are found within the cord's ventral horn.

For a detailed discussion of the location of the nuclei and of the anatomic distribution and the function of the CN's textbooks of anatomy and/or physiology should be consulted to the depths desired.

## ■ What anatomic features of the diencephalon explain its functions?

For the purposes of this discussion the diencephalon will be considered to be composed of the thalamus, hypothalamus, pituitary stalk and associated posterior lobe, and parts of the visual apparatus lying outside of the principal portion of the brain. For further discussion of the pituitary gland texts of anatomy and/or physiology may be consulted. The study of the visual system is out of the realm of discussion of this text.

With the exception of the olfactory nerves, every sensory impulse must synapse in the thalamus before being relayed to the cerebral cortex. Axons leaving the thalamus on their way to the cortex initially become part of the internal capsule, then perforate the corpus callosum and fan out as the corona radiata to become part of the various projection tracts going to specific cerebral sensory areas.

Inferior to the thalamus is the hypothalamus, which is an "emotional center" containing the origin of some of the sympathetic and parasympathetic fibers.

The third ventricle is located in the diencephalon.

## ■ What anatomic features of the mesencephalon explain its functions?

For the purposes of this discussion the mesencephalon, or midbrain, will be considered to consist of the corpora quadragemina and the cerebral peduncles, or crus cerebri.

The term *"corpus quadrigeminum,"* or *tectum,* applies to the four bodies distributed as anterior and posterior pairs on the dorsum of the midbrain. The anterior pair, called *superior colliculi,* or *optic tectum,* is a relay station for receiving impulses derived earlier in the synaptic chain from the retina. This pair subsequently synapses with neurons involved in moving the eyes and head and also helps to regulate the diameter of the pupil. The posterior pair, called the *inferior colliculi,* or *auditory tectum,* forms a relay station for receiving impulses derived earlier in the synaptic chain from the organ of Corti (for hearing).

The ventral aspect of the mesencephalon contains the nuclei of CN's III and IV, several descending pathways, and several ascending pathways.

The third ventricle passes through the mesencephalon as the *aqueduct of Sylvius.*

### ■ What anatomic features of the metencephalon explain its functions?

For the purposes of this discussion the metencephalon will be considered to consist of the pons, cerebellar peduncles, and cerebellum.

The *pons* is divided into a more dorsal *tegmentum* and the more ventral *cerebral crura.* It contains the nuclei of CN's V to VIII. Pathways found in the ventral part are very similar to those encountered rostrally in the midbrain. The existence of a pontine reflex respiratory center was already mentioned in the section on the respiratory system.

Three bilateral pairs of *cerebellar peduncles* are prominent bundles of fibers connecting the cerebellum with the brain stem. The *inferior peduncles,* also called the *restiform bodies,* carry fibers from the spinal cord to the cerebellum. Fibers of the *middle peduncle,* or *brachium pontis,* arise from pontine nuclei and extend to the cerebellum. The *superior peduncle,* or *brachium conjunctivum,* constitutes the main efferent connection of the cerebellum, containing fibers for the thalamus, reticular formation, and red nucleus, the latter being a synaptic relay nucleus for fibers whose destination is the spinal cord.

Although the *cerebellum* receives many afferent fibers for proprioception and stereognosis, it is not involved in conscious perception. Rather it is a coordinator of muscle group actions, timing their contractions to perform smoothly and accurately. Although voluntary movements can proceed without it, such movements are usually clumsy and disorganized. *Cerebellar ataxia,* or *asynergy,* produced by cerebellar dysfunction, results in a lack of motor skills. To a considerable extent, if sufficient time elapses, other brain mechanisms compensate for cerebellar defects.

Unlike the cerebrum, where the right half of the brain has motor control over the left side of the body and vice versa, the coordination of muscle movements on the right side is associated with the right half of the cerebellum.

Both the met- and myelencephalon contribute to the formation of the fourth ventricle.

### ■ What anatomic features of the myelencephalon explain its functions?

The term "myelencephalon" is synonymous with the term *"medulla."* CN's IX to XII are associated with the medulla.

Since the medulla is directly continuous with the spinal cord, many of the descending fibers arising above the medulla continue caudally into the cord, and many of the fiber tracts associated with the cord are represented in the medulla. For example, on the dorsal surface axons of the cord tracts called the *fasciculus gracilis* and *fasciculus cuneatus* synapse in the medullary centers called, respectively, the *clava* and *cuneate tubercle.*

The ventral aspect is characterized by the prominent groups of corticospinal motor fibers forming the pyramids, which cross over in the lower half of the medulla in the *decussation of the pyramids.* As a result, as mentioned previously, the right half of the brain controls the motor functions of the left side of the body.

On the lateral aspect of the medulla, swellings known as the *inferior olivary nuclei* bulge out between the origins of CN's XI and XII. Axons from the perikaryons located here travel via the restiform body to the cerebellum.

The central canal is modified in relation to the met- and myelencephalon to form the fourth ventricle.

## ■ What are some of the major fiber tracts?

### *Pyramidal system*

It was indicated in discussing the anatomic features of the cerebrum (p. 49) that various Brodmann's areas are responsible for the voluntary selection of muscle movements but that area 4 is responsible for their execution, with the entire body being represented by a motor homunculus here. Actions evolving from willed impulses initiated by area 4 are said to be part of the pyramidal system, as compared with those initiated in premotor area 6, considered to be part of the extrapyramidal system.*

As the axons of the pyramidal system descend to striated muscles, two orders of neurons are involved:

| | | |
|---|---|---|
| Upper motor neurons (pyramidal fibers) | To CN nuclei of III to VII and IX to XII | As corticomesencephalic and corticobulbar tracts |
| | To ventral horn cells | As corticospinal tracts |
| Lower motor neurons (peripheral fibers) | From CN nuclei | As CN's |
| | From ventral horn cells | As 31 pairs of spinal nerves |

As in the case of most other nerve tracts, compound names are given to the bundles in which these axons travel, the first name being the site of origin, the second the destination, for example, corticospinal. On leaving the cortex all of the upper motor neurons first interdigitate with the ascending sensory fibers and pass alongside of them in the *internal capsule,* which is the area between the thalamus (medially) and the basal ganglia, or corpus striatum (laterally).

*Corticomesencephalic tract fibers* descend to the levels of the nuclei of CN's associated with the extraocular muscles, that is, III, IV, and VI. Unlike the other upper motor neurons that start from area 4, these neurons have their origins in area 8. During surgery with part of the calvaria removed, stimulation of the right area 8 causes both eyes to turn to the left.

*Corticobulbar tract fibers* (and those of the corticospinal tract as well) start from area 4 but continue (with the corticospinal tract) through the mesencephalic peduncles to the pons and medulla, where the bulbar fibers synapse with the nuclear cells of CN's V to VII and XI to XII. Since CN VIII has no motor output, there is no need for corticobulbar fibers to go to its nucleus.

*Corticospinal tract fibers* constitute what are classically referred to as the *pyramidal (tract) fibers.* While most of them decussate in the medullary pyramids, as indicated previously, some of them remain uncrossed, but in any event, whether they descend in the anterior or lateral funiculus of the cord, they finally synapse with anterior horn cells. The anterior horn cells provide the axons of the ventral (motor) roots of the spinal nerves.

### *Extrapyramidal system*

The term "extrapyramidal system" usually does not allude to "any descending fibers other than those in the pyramidal system," as might well be assumed, for this would include the descending components of the vestibular and cerebellar systems. Rather, clinically the extrapyramidal system refers to the corpus striatum and its associated reticulospinal tract. The *corpus striatum* consists of a caudate nucleus and a lentiform nucleus, the latter in turn being composed of the putamen and the globus pallidus, or pallidum. (By way of relationships, it should be remembered that the internal capsule

*Simultaneous discharges from all parts of the motor cortex produce the movements seen in *epileptic attack,* as compared with a small focus of irritation near one part of the motor area that may precipitate *jacksonian seizures.*

passes between the thalamus and the corpus striatum.) Ignoring the details of the internal circuits, the outflow of impulses from the corpus striatum probably emerges entirely from the pallidum. Those fibers that extend from the pallidum to the subthalamic nuclei split up, some continuing to the red nucleus and some to the *reticular activating system* (RAS), or *reticular activating formation* (RAF).

The RAS controls the state of arousal or sleep and focuses attention. While arousal is a nonspecific phenomenon affected by all sensory inputs, it is characterized by both ascending and descending divisions. The ascending division influences the excitability of the cerebral cortex, cerebellum, and hypothalamus, disinhibiting them and arousing them. The descending division, via the *reticulospinal tract,* makes synapses in the anterior horn, thus influencing the muscle reflexes; it also affects the autonomic nerves.

## ■ What are the functional relationships of the ANS?

The ANS is composed of two subdivisions, the sympathetic and the parasympathetic systems, each of which is characterized by a two-neuron complex composed of preganglionic (first-order) and postganglionic (second-order) neurons. In both sympathetic and parasympathetic systems the preganglionic fibers are myelinated and the postganglionic fibers are nonmyelinated.

### *Sympathetic system*

The sympathetic preganglionic (first-order) neuron has its cell body located in the lateral horn of the gray matter (intermedolateral column) found from spinal nerve levels T1 through L2. The preganglionic axon of any vertebral level, for example, T6, leaves the cord via the ventral root and passes to a local paravertebral sympathetic ganglion. There one of four potential branchings, which will be indicated as types A, B, C, and D, may occur[5]:

Type A: One of the collaterals may synapse in the local *paravertebral ganglion.* The postganglionic fiber, second-order neurons in the case of T6, would possibly join the sixth intercostal nerve initially, then shortly join the corresponding artery.

Type B: A collateral could leave the paravertebral ganglion without synapsing locally and synapse instead in a nearby *collateral ganglion,* for example, the *coeliac ganglion.* In such a case, the postganglionic fiber, as a splanchnic nerve, might go to the tunica muscularis of the gut, causing an inhibition of gastric motility, and/or it might go to a mesenteric artery, potentially causing vasoconstriction.

Type C: Another collateral could proceed down to the next several paravertebral ganglia, potentially synapsing at each of these, then act as in A or B branching.

Type D: After entering the local paravertebral ganglion, for example, at T6, a collateral could turn rostrally to the next several higher paravertebral ganglia, then act as in A or B branching.

As a result of the presence of the ascending and descending fibers from one paravertebral ganglion to another, a *sympathetic chain* is created bilaterally.

In summary, the sympathetic nerves may produce the following phenomena: vasoconstriction, whether the vessel be in smooth muscle or gland; speeding up of the heartbeat; bronchiospasm; uterine contraction; inhibition of gastric motility; and pupillary dilatation.

The neurosecretion at synapses between pre- and postganglionic fibers is ACh. That at the end of the postganglionic fiber is norepinephrine. This provides the basis for referring to the sympathetic nerves as *adrenergic fibers.*

### *Parasympathetic system*

The parasympathetic system is referred to as the *craniosacral* portion of the ANS because it arises in part in association with CN's and in part in the derivatives of spinal nerves S2, S3, and S4. The sites of origin of the cranial preganglionic (first-order) fibers are nuclei located near the nucleus of the CN with which the preganglionic fiber travels for part of its course. At some point along the course of the nerve the main components of the CN separate from the parasympathetic components, and the latter join an autonomic ganglion in order to synapse with the postganglionic component. Ganglia associated with parasympathetic fibers that are temporarily components of, or travelling with, CN's are ciliary ganglion (for the ciliary body muscles and sphincter pupillae of the eye), CN III; submaxillary ganglion (for the sublingual and submaxillary glands), CN VII; sphenopalatine ganglion (for secretions of the lacrimal gland, nose, and paranasal sinuses), CN VIII; optic ganglion (for the parotid gland), CN IX; and Meissner's and Auerbach's plexuses and cardiac nodes (to promote peristalsis of the gut and to slow down the heart), CN X.*

Preganglionic (first-order) fibers of the sacral portion of the parasympathetics, similar to the sympathetic fibers, arise from cell bodies located in the lateral horn—intermedolateral column—of the spinal cord, but at the level of origin of nerves S2, S3, and S4. The preganglionic fibers, again similar to the sympathetic fibers, leave the cord with the ventral root of the spinal nerve. However, they do not go to the sympathetic paravertebral ganglia. Rather, they leave the sacral nerves shortly and join one another to form the *pelvic splanchnic nerves.* These pass to the distal ends of the gastrointestinal tract, where they synapse in Meissner's and Auerbach's plexuses within the gut wall and enhance peristalsis when activated.

The parasympathetic fibers secrete ACh at the end of the pre- and postganglionic fibers. This provides the basis for referring to them as *cholinergic fibers.*

## ■ What are the meninges?

The *meninges* are membranous coverings disposed in three layers around the brain and spinal cord. The most peripheral layer, the *dura mater,* consists of tough, fibrous connective tissue. However, it differs in the cranial cavity and the vertebral canal, being a double layer in the former and a single layer in the latter. In the skull the outer layer constitutes an internal periosteum and stays with the skull when the brain is removed, whereas the inner layer covers the brain. In addition to the numerous branches of the meningeal arteries and veins invested in the dura mater, there are large venous channels known as *venous dural sinuses* that relate in part to the circulation of the cerebrospinal fluid. In the spinal cord an *epidural space* filled with connective tissue exists between the bone and the dura mater. The periosteum of the vertebra forms the outer boundary of the epidural space.

The *pia mater* is adherent to the brain, dipping down between the convolutions as a fine layer of areolar tissue. It is thicker and less vascular in relation to the cord than it is in relation to the brain.

The *arachnoid* is a delicate, fibrous tissue forming a cobweblike network of trabeculae between the dura mater and pia mater. The open spaces between the trabeculae constitute the *subarachnoid space,* which contains blood vessels and cerebrospinal fluid.

## ■ What is cerebrospinal fluid; how does it form and circulate?

*Cerebrospinal fluid (CSF)* is a clear, slightly viscous solution of inorganic salts with traces of dextrose, protein, urea, and other organic substances. Although it normally contains 0 to 6 WBC's/$mm^3$ (counts over 10 WBC's/$mm^3$ are considered as indicating cerebrospinal infection), the presence of RBC's is considered abnormal.

As was indicated in the sections on the telencephalon through myelencephalon, the brain contains four fluid-filled, communicating ventricles, one of which is located in each cerebral hemisphere (the first and second ventricles), one in the diencephalon (the third), and one on the dorsum of the pons and medulla (the fourth). CSF is formed by secretion from capillary-like *choroidal plexuses* on the ventricular walls at a rate sufficient to replace its 120 to 135 ml vol-

*The vagus nerve is composed primarily of sensory fibers (two thirds).

ume about three times daily. To prevent a buildup of pressure above the normal (130 to 150 ml water), it circulates in a definite pattern and then is rejoined with the blood. CSF formed in ventricles I and II flows successively through ventricles III and IV, acquiring additional fluid and draining via foramina into the subarachnoid space. It circulates down and around the spinal cord and through the subarachnoid space around the brain, ultimately passing into and through a number of villi that protrude into the venous dural sinuses. The venous sinuses ultimately join the internal jugular vein.

Obstruction to the normal flow causes increased intracranial pressure, which causes papilledema (swelling at the optic disc), persistent headache, and vomiting. If the condition is present from birth, hydrocephalus results with its typical postnatal enlargement of the head.

While the termination of the cord is at the level of L2, the subarachnoid space extends to the level of about S2. In removing samples of CSF the needle is usually introduced into the subarachnoid space between the third and fourth lumbar vertebrae. Where general anesthesia might not be desirable, caudal blocks may be done, taking advantage of the fact that (relatively large) doses of epidural injections will diffuse into the subarachnoid space when injected into the region of the sacral hiatus.

## NEUROPHYSIOLOGY

### ■ What is meant by membrane potential and how is it maintained?

Although the positive sodium and potassium ions are found both inside and outside of the neuronal membrane, externally the $Na^+$ concentration is high and the potassium ion ($K^+$) concentration is low; inside the cell the situation is reversed. The equilibrium potentials of sodium and potassium are such that during the resting or inactive state the inside of the membrane has a negative charge of 90 mv compared with the outside. (For detailed discussion of these equilibrium potentials any standard physiology text may be consulted.) The neuron is said to exhibit a *membrane potential* of –70 mV. The $Na^+$ and $K^+$, respectively, constantly leak into and out of the cell. Efforts to compensate for this are at least partially accounted for by an active "$Na^+$-$K^+$ pump," in which $Na^+$ is (1) picked up by an enzyme from the inside of the cell, (2) transferred to the outside of the cell, (3) dumped and exchanged for $K^+$, which is (4) transferred to the inside of the cell and dumped in exchange for more $Na^+$, etc. Energy to accomplish this active pumping is derived by the breakdown of ATP to ADP.

### ■ What is meant by action potential and generator potential?

The *nerve impulse,* or *action potential,* is a transient reversal of the resting potential, usually from –70 mV (internally) to +30 mV, a total amplitude of about 100 mV, in which the nerve is said to be *depolarized.* The stimulus for depolarization may be initiated (1) by dendritic receptors, for example, those for touch or pressure; (2) by synapses with other neurons, that is, by release of substances such as ACh; or (3) spontaneously, for example, intrinsic cardiac beat and brain waves of the alpha type. Much research on depolarization has centered on ACh activity, although this is not the transmitter at most synapses. Therefore the second option is usually chosen as the basis for discussing depolarization.

For an action potential to occur the membrane potential must be reduced to a critical level, called the *threshold potential.* The minimum stimulus capable of producing the threshold potential—and in turn an action potential—is called the *threshold stimulus.* Stimuli of greater capacity are referred to as suprathreshold stimuli. The threshold potential for most neurons is usually only 5 to 15 mV less than the resting membrane potential. Achievement of this 5 to 15 mV depolarization is *generated* by several means and is therefore known as a *generator potential.*

The accumulative depolarization, or generator potential, evolves at the axon hillock, or initial segment, where the axon is beginning but does not yet have a myelin sheath. It is affected by (1) strength, (2) duration, and (3) polarity of the stimulus, among other factors. Although thousands of synaptic knobs may end on a single neuron—a phenomenon referred to as *final common pathway*—potentiating its more rapid firing, no one knob, as a rule, can cause an action potential.* Different dendrites of the same neuron, as well as different neurons themselves, have different thresholds, the result being that as stimulus strength is increased, more and more nerves are "fired," or activated, to stimulate multiple final pathways. The result may be both temporal and spatial summation, which ultimately lowers the recipient neuron's generator potential to threshold. (For further discussion a standard textbook of physiology may be consulted.) Actually some neurons release neurohumors, for example, adenosine 3′,5′-cyclic phosphate (cyclic AMP) and γ-aminobutyric acid (GABA), that increase the polarity rather than reverse it, that is, make the inside of the cell even more negative. Such *inhibitory neurons* cause increased permeability to $K^+$ and $Cl^-$ and are said to produce a state of *hyperpolarization* rather than depolarization. ACh and norepinephrine can act as inhibitory or excitatory agents, depending on the nature of the postsynaptic membrane.

## ■ What is meant by the "all-or-none" law?

Regardless of the nature of the stimulus, once sufficient generator potential has been developed to attain the threshold level, an action potential is induced; its shape, magnitude, and duration are the same every time, thus the "all-or-none" law. Within a nerve each neuron is firing independently of the others, according to its individual threshold level. However, once fired the action potential of each neuron in the nerve is basically the same. The response per se gives no indication as to whether the generator potential reached the threshold on the basis of the strength of the stimulus, the frequency of the stimulus, or some other factor.

## ■ What histochemical events occur when the threshold is reached?

When the generator potential reaches threshold, within a fraction of a millisecond the membrane undergoes a change in its permeability to sodium, ions of the latter streaming to the inside at the axon hillock. (The exact relation between reaching threshold and $Na^+$ permeability is not understood.) The ascending phase of the spike potential represents the $Na^+$ inflow. Equally suddenly $Na^+$ reaches its new equilibrium, and the entry of additional ions is shut off, thus this is the apex of the spike. After a brief lag $K^+$ streams out of the cell, returning the membrane voltage to normal. When the spike has returned to 0, the net effect is that the fiber has exchanged equal amounts of $Na^+$ for $K^+$, most of the temporary residual imbalances soon being redressed by the $Na^+$-$K^+$ pump. However, the increased permeability to $K^+$ can continue for some time, causing a hyperpolarization, or positive afterpotential.

## ■ How is the impulse propagated along the axon?

Conduction within the axon is frequently compared with the flow of electrons in a wire. In both the wire and the neuron it is possible for an impulse to produce local changes in potential as ions move short distances internally across the surface of the wire or the membrane and externally produce local currents. In the case of the nerve, when sufficient current flow has been induced, the membrane permeability to $Na^+$ is changed, and the development of a typical action potential is initiated.

Since the strength of the current decreases exponentially as a function of the distance, in nonmyelinated nerves the time required for inducing the depolarization from one area to its adjacent area becomes comparatively significant. Propagation of the impulse here involves sequential depolarization along the entire length of the neuron. In contrast,

*This statement applies primarily to an internuncial neuron having multiple synaptic areas, as compared, for instance, with a myofiber that might be activated by a single nerve ending.

in myelinated nerves, because of the interrupted electrical insulation created by the myelin, conduction jumps along the axon from node to node—a phenomenon called *saltatory conduction*—and is much more rapid. (See discussion of conduction rates of A, B, and C fibers on p. 46.) When anesthestics are applied to the myelin of the internode, they are relatively ineffective at blocking transmission; when applied at the nodes, they are very effective.

### ■ What happens at a synaptic area?

Of the various neurohumors stored in the vesicles at the ends of neuronal arborizations, ACh and the catecholamines have been studied most. Presuming that a proper amount of $Ca^{++}$ is present in the vicinity when the impulse arrives at the arborization's vesicle, the neurohumor, in this case ACh, previously stored in the vesicle is allowed to escape. This diffuses to the receptor site on the postsynaptic membrane, where it may enhance the development of a generator potential in another order of neurons. If the nerve terminal is associated with a muscle, its modified form is termed a *motor end-plate*. ACh released from the end-plate increases the susceptibility of the receptor site to increased ion flow, setting off a wave of depolarization that spreads to the interior of the myofiber via the T tubules.

If ACh were permitted to accumulate at the receptor site, the postsynaptic neuron would remain depolarized. Repolarization is able to occur because (1) some of the ACh is destroyed by the interaction at the receptor site, (2) much of it is destroyed by the enzyme acetylcholinesterase (AChE), (3) some of it diffuses away from the area, and (4) some of it diffuses back into the synaptic vesicle.

### ■ What are the nutritive needs of the nervous system?

It was mentioned earlier that the RQ of the brain is 1.0, indicating that its energy requirements are satisfied completely by carbohydrates. Since neurons do not reproduce after birth, the amount of nucleoprotein and similar substances required for growth from childhood to adulthood is relatively negligible. The need for $O_2$ is indicated by the speed with which unconsciousness results when the carotid arteries are occluded. Additionally serious brain damage results if the lack of $O_2$ continues for more than 6 to 8 minutes. Surgical experience has shown that the 4-minute interval quoted in earlier years is not commonly of serious consequence. Whereas in the adult about 20% of the total $O_2$ utilized by the body is consumed by the nervous system, the amount is even greater in the child, where the brain is proportionately larger.

### ■ How extensive is the blood supply to the brain?

Since the rate of $O_2$ utilization by the nervous system is 10 times that of the rest of the body tissues, it requires a rich blood supply. The epineurium of the spinal nerves contains vessels essential for the nerve's vitality. Accordingly, in nerve grafts it is important to preserve the integrity of the nerve sheaths.

An anterior and two posterior spinal arteries run the length of the spinal cord, lying in close proximity to it and nourishing it. The brain has an especially rich blood supply, receiving the internal carotid arteries plus the vertebral arteries as major sources, the latter uniting to form the basilar artery within the skull. The basilar artery unites with the internal carotid arteries to form the circle of Willis, whose functional integrity may provide important collateral in the event of loss of one of its components.

## Related pharmacology

### ■ How are the receptor sites and associated drugs classified pharmacologically?

It has become customary to refer to all neurons secreting catecholamines (CA's) as *adrenergic* and to all ACh-secreting neurons as *cholinergic*. In brief, adrenergic secretory tissues are as follows:

Neurons of the CNS secreting CA's
Postganglionic sympathetic neurons
Adrenal medulla

plus similar "chromaffin tissue" scattered throughout the body.

By comparison, the following are classified as cholinergic neurons:

Neurons of the CNS secreting ACh

Peripheral (skeletal) motor nerves (The majority of peripheral sensory nerves are not cholinergic.)

Both sympathetic and parasympathetic preganglionic neurons

Postganglionic parasympathetics

Sympathetic postganglionic neurons to sweat glands

Generally speaking, drugs that simulate the activities of the sympathetic nervous system are referred to as *sympathomimetic,* or *adrenergic, drugs* or *agents,* and their receptors are referred to as *adrenergic receptors.* Drugs that simulate the activities of the parasympathetic system are referred to as *parasympathomimetic,* or *cholinergic, drugs* or *agents,* and their receptors are referred to as *cholinergic receptors;* both of these types of receptors are shown in Fig. 2-7. Contrariwise, pharmaceutical agents that interfere with the synthesis or release of the body's adrenergic compounds or destroy them, as well as those that block their receptors, are called *antiadrenergic drugs.* Pharmaceuticals having similar relations to the body's cholinergic compounds are referred to as *anticholinergic drugs.*

Nicotine (and certain other drugs) may replace ACh at both sympathetic and parasympathetic autonomic ganglia and at skeletal myoneural junctions. Such postsynaptic tissues are therefore said to possess *nicotinic receptors.* Muscarine (and certain other drugs) may replace ACh at the synapse between the postganglionic parasympathetic neurons and the tissue with which it, in turn, synapses. The reactor sites for such tissues are referred to as *muscarinic receptors.*

## ■ What is involved in the formation, release, response to, and deactivation of ACh?

The enzyme *choline acetyltransferase,* or *choline acetylase,* is synthesized in the neuronal soma and migrates out the axon to the terminals where ACh is formed and subsequently stored in vesicles as the concentrated ion. On the arrival of an action potential at the terminals, ACh is released from the vesicles and in turn from the neuronal membrane into the synaptic cleft. The process will not occur unless the proper amount of calcium ions ($Ca^{++}$) is present and even then can be inhibited by the presence of magnesium ions ($Mg^{++}$). The freed transmitter is attracted to the receptor, where its acceptance results in an almost instantaneous change in membrane permeability. Sequential to the membrane change is the develop-

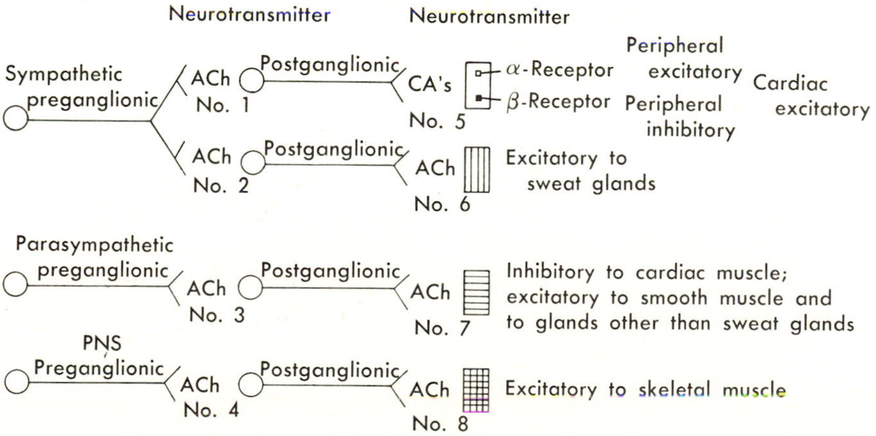


**Fig. 2-7.** Adrenergic and cholinergic receptors.

ment of an action potential in the postsynaptic structure if the synapse is interneuronal, a muscle contraction if the postsynaptic structure is a myofiber, or the release of a secretion if the postsynaptic structure is a gland cell. Within 1 to 2 milliseconds after its release, ACh is removed from the synaptic cleft. This is the result of the following:

1. Destruction of the neurohormone by interaction at the receptor site
2. The conjoined action of the catabolic enzyme AChE, which decomposes ACh
3. The reabsorption of ACh back into the presynaptic terminals for restorage in the vesicles
4. Diffusion away from the area

## ■ What basic pharmacologic principles are needed to understand what is happening at synapses?

Some compounds act only at smooth muscle, ANS ganglia, or skeletal myoneural junctions, whereas ACh acts on all of these. Presumably ACh has a simple structure, enabling it to react with numerous, basically similar receptors without necessarily being equally effective with all of them. It can easily be anticipated that, in view of the vagaries of drug actions, the rational therapeutic use of cholinergic and adrenergic drugs requires some basic knowledge of drug interactions. The review of the basics presented here will incorporate only a few selected examples of some of the commonly used cholinergic and adrenergic drugs. The reader is encouraged to seek additional specific information from comprehensive books on pharmacology.[4-6]

Although drugs produce many reactions within the body, for example, blocking enzyme reactions within various body systems or within invasive, disease-producing microorganisms or osmotic effects, as in the kidneys or in using enemas, in this portion of the chapter, the terms "drugs" and "pharmaceutical agents" will be used in the context of neuropharmacologic reactions. Although topographically applied drugs admittedly have effects on peripheral nerves, didactic discussions of neuropharmacology are usually oriented in relation to synaptic phenomenon, wherein the termination of the presynaptic fiber, the synaptic cleft, and the postsynaptic sites are treated sequentially.

At axonal terminations drugs may facilitate or impede the synthesis, storage, release, and reabsorption of the neurohumor. In the synaptic cleft antiacetylcholinesterase (anti-AChE) agents are clinically effective. However, anticatechol-*O*-methyltransferase (anti-COMT) agents find no striking medical application.

Because of their inherent complex nature, a more lengthy description of receptor reactions is in order.

The receptor is generally conceived of as being responsible only for combination with the drug and not for the subsequent type of response of the postsynaptic tissue. For example, after ACh has combined with the receptor the response in one instance might be contraction of gastrointestinal muscle but in another inhibition of cardiac muscle. However, it is also necessary to rationalize this concept with the realization that at different times two drugs can occupy the same receptor, with drug A having one effect and drug B another. A common interpretation is that the two drugs produced different conformational changes in the receptor.[7] An alternative, partially satisfactory interpretation is that the membrane "pores" of the receptor were blocked by one compound but permitted a postsynaptic reaction with the alternate drug, the postsynaptic response itself being subject to variations depending on various factors, for example, the prior physiologic state of the cell.

If two drugs are essentially equally attractive to the receptor, the law of mass action will prevail, and the agent present in the greatest concentration will "compete" most successfully for the majority of the reactive sites. In line with the discussion just presented, when this competition exists at a cholinergic receptor, the cholinomimetic effects produced by the second drug may be completely or only partially similar to those produced by the ACh, or the second drug may completely block the reactive site, resulting in no postsynaptic reaction.

If the second agent is more powerfully

attracted chemically to the cholinergic receptor, it also may either block the postsynaptic cell, preventing a "normal" reaction, or it may yield a cholinomimetic effect completely or only partially, similar to the situation produced by ACh. Comparable situations exist for pharmaceuticals interacting on adrenergic receptors.

In the event that the drug is introduced intravenously the degree of its success in competing with ACh, or any other drug, will depend on the following: its initial blood serum concentration, the efficiency of diffusion into and away from the receptor site, the relative chemical attractiveness to the receptor, the rapidity with which it is metabolized both within the bloodstream and at the receptor site, whether it is a short or long-acting drug, and other interactions relating to the prior and present state of the reactive area. Obviously despite the ubiquitous nature of ACh, neither it nor any other drug will be acceptable at all receptors.

### ■ What are some drugs whose therapeutic use relates to the synthesis, storage, and release of ACh at nicotinic synapses?

Hemicholinium (HC-3) interferes with the mechanism for transporting choline from the soma to the nerve terminals, effectively inhibiting the production of ACh. Furthermore, it also inhibits choline acetyltransferase. Carbachol (carbamylcholine) was used for treating urinary retention and gastrointestinal spasm until more effective agents were developed. Its current use is primarily as a miotic, relating to its presumed release of ACh at parasympathetic ganglia. Botulinus toxin, the causative agent of certain types of food poisoning, prevents the release of ACh and thus causes respiratory failure. Once the toxin is firmly bound to the receptor, it can no longer be neutralized by antitoxins.

### ■ How are the actions of the AChE's modified and what effects do these have?

Drugs inhibiting the action of AChE's allow the buildup of ACh and its associated increased amount and duration of ACh action, for example, increased activity of organs and tissues receiving parasympathetic innervation, increased skeletal muscle activity, and CNS effects. Such anti-AChE's can be divided into two groups: reversible and irreversible. Reversible agents include the shorter acting (1 to 2 hr) edrophonium (Tensilon) and the longer acting (2 to 8 hr) plant derivative physostigmine and synthetic neostigmine. Because of their toxicity, the nonreversible anti-AChE's find little clinical usage, being limited primarily to the treatment of glaucomas, as with the drug isoflurophate (Floropryl). The nonreversible anti-AChE's find widespread commercial use as insecticides and have considerable potential for use as chemical warfare agents. Patient treatment consists of removing the toxic agent and administering atropine and pralidoxime (2-PAM).

### ■ How are ganglionic blocking agents categorized?

Based on their mode of action, ganglionic blocking drugs are categorized into two classes. In one, the *nondepolarizing agents,* the competing drug occupies the postsynaptic receptor in place of the ACh but has no stimulating effect, a classic example being *hexamethonium.* These drugs act on areas arbitrarily numbered 1 and 2 on Fig. 2-7. The second class, known as *depolarizing agents,* act first to stimulate, then to block the ganglion by causing persistent depolarization. The classic example is *nicotine.* Initially, in light and moderate doses, nicotine is cholinomimetic for gastric mobility, resulting in diarrhea and secretory activity in certain glands (salivary, bronchial, and perhaps gastric), but these effects are followed by depressed activity. In large doses the initial stimulation is very quickly followed by a blockage of transmission. Areas 1, 2, 3, and 8 of Fig. 2-7 are acted on by these depolarizing agents.

### ■ What drug interactions take place at the myoneural junction?

Similar to the ganglionic blocking drugs, pharmaceuticals acting at myoneural junctions may be classified as nondepolarizing and depolarizing. Since the myoneural junction was listed earlier as a nicotinic receptor, it should be noted that, although nicotine produces a depolarizing effect here similar to that at autonomic ganglia, it is much more active on ganglia than on myoneural junctions. Therapeutically the depolarizing compound most frequently used as a surgical adjunct is *succinylcholine chloride* (Anectine). The nonpolarizing drugs *curare* and *flaxedil* (gallamine) also find clinical usage. Because of their histaminic-releasing action, the nondepolarizing blockers, especially *d-tubocurarine,* are not recommended for use in patients with asthma or other diseases producing histamine-like effects.

## ■ What happens at cholinergic muscarinic receptors?

As indicated at the beginning of this discussion (p. 57) muscarine, the *Amanita* mushroom toxin, and muscarine-like compounds compete with ACh at the synapse between the postganglionic parasympathetic neuron and its postsynaptic cell. Both atropine and scopolamine are derived from the African plant belladonna. When the excessive release of ACh by the vagus and pelvic splanchnic (parasympathetic) nerves produces intestinal spasm, when hyperacidity of the gastrointestinal tract is evidenced, in bronchial spasm, and in spasticity of the ureters and bile ducts, *atropine* provides valuable treatment. The atropine derivative *homatropine* is used by ophthalmologists in eye refraction to produce mydriasis.

Because of its depressant effects on the CNS, *scopolamine* is used mainly as a sedative, although it is also used to relieve motion sickness. Both atropine and scopolamine are used to prevent salivation during surgery. They are also used by the neurologist to reduce the tremors and rigidity of parkinsonism. Their pharmacologic effects sometimes persist from 3 to 10 days or more, unless reversed by some means.

*Pilocarpine,* a South American shrub alkaloid, has a potent muscarinic action, but also has some slight nicotinic effects, explaining the slight hypertension observed after its administration. Its use in chronic, simple glaucoma is based on its ability to cause constriction of the iridial and ciliary muscles. It is used subsequent to ophthalmic examination to counteract the effects of atropine.

*Bethanechol chloride* (Urecholine) is a long-acting muscarinic drug used to treat urinary retention and constipation, especially that caused by autonomic-blocking, antihypertensive agents.

## ■ Which of the body's monoamines are important as neurotransmitters, and how may their cycle be described briefly?

The monoamines considered to be neurohumors are an indolamine, 5-hydroxytryptamine (5-HT or serotonin) and a group of three CA's: epinephrine, norepinephrine, and dopamine. The formation of CA's is sequentially related. Technically phenylalanine can be converted to *tyrosine* to start the anabolic process. However, there is so much tyrosine normally available that this step is not ordinarily deemed important within the body. In the soma of the postganglionic sympathetic neuron tyrosine is converted by the enzyme tyrosine hydroxylase to dopa, and dopa is subsequently converted (by another enzyme) to *dopamine* (DA). DA migrates down the axon and enters the storage vesicles where it is changed into *norepinephrine* (NE). In the adrenal gland, first NE is manufactured in the medullary cells and stored in vesicles. It then leaves the granules, is methylated to *epinephrine* (E) in the cytoplasm, then is taken into a different group of vesicles within the cytoplasm, where it is stored until released.

As with cholinergic nerves, the arrival of an action potential in a postganglionic sympathetic neuron terminal results in the release of the neurotransmitter, providing the proper amount of $Ca^{++}$ is present and $Mg^{++}$ does not cause inhibition.

Having been released into the synaptic space, the transmitter is potentially picked up by and activates receptor sites of two types: alpha ($\alpha$) sites, which are excitatory, and beta ($\beta$) sites, which are inhibitory and cardiac excitatory. The postsynaptic cell—smooth muscle or gland cell—may have $\alpha$-

or $\beta$-receptors, or both, although there is usually a preponderance of one type.

The fate of the neurohumor is somewhat similar to the fate of ACh. Part of it is utilized in producing the postsynaptic reaction; part of it diffuses away. Most of it is taken back into the synaptic vesicles for storage, with the cytoplasmic surplus being decomposed by an enzyme stored in the mitochondria, *monoamine oxidase* (MAO). The transfer into the terminals is brought about by an "amine pump." Comparable to the AChE of cholinergic synapses is the compound *catechol-O-methyltransferase* (COMT). The catabolic phenomenon is remembered with the mnemonic "*C*OMT *c*leans up the synapse; *M*AO *m*ops up the intraneuronal surplus CA." However, it is generally held that the process of active reuptake by the pump is of itself adequate to account for removal of NE at the synapse.

A feedback, self-limiting control of NE production has been proposed in which the overproduction of NE inhibits the enzyme tyrosine hydroxylase from converting tyrosine to dopa.

In the medulla of the adrenal gland about 80% of the CA stored in the vesicles is E and about 20% NE. An action potential brought to the medullary cells by a preganglionic sympathetic neuron results in the release of E and/or NE into the bloodstream and the subsequent distribution of these CA's to various receptor sites throughout the body.

### ■ What are some drugs whose actions affect the synthesis, storage, release, reuptake, and destruction of CA's at the synapse?

It was mentioned previously that the rate-limiting enzyme in the formation of CA's was tyrosine hydroxylase, involved in transforming tyrosine to dopa as a presumed, natural feedback mechanism. Pharmacologically $\alpha$-methyl-*p*-tyrosine provides a similar blocking action, thereby ultimately depleting the supply of NE.

Sometimes the normal neurohumor is not stored in the vesicles. This may be accomplished by introducing substrates that are analogues of those normally involved in producing the neurosecretion, producing what are referred to as *"false transmitters,"* with lesser excitatory effects at the receptor than the NE they displace. Examples are $\alpha$-methylmetatyrosine and $\alpha$-methyldopa (Aldomet). In the brain the former of these two drugs reduces brain NE without affecting 5-HT and produces sedation.

The mechanism for active reuptake of CA's into the vesicles after firing is sufficiently nonselective to permit the acceptance as substitutes of sympathomimetics such as *cocaine, imipramine,* and *chlorpromazine.* As a result, NE collects at extracellular sites and/or acts at the receptors. It is by such means that the tricyclic preparations produce their antidepressant, therapeutic effects. In a more indirect manner some drugs, for example, *ephedrine, amphetamine,* and *tyramine,* act by displacing NE from the neuronal cytoplasm, thereby resulting in the NE sustaining transmitter effects on the receptor cells. The rebound phenomenon following amphetamine administration may be the result of a temporary NE depletion. While ephedrine, amphetamine, and tyramine produce brief effects quickly, *guanethidine* is slow to produce more prolonged effects.

Storage of CA's is also blocked by the use of *reserpine,* a product of the plant rauwolfia, lowering the blood pressure and pulse and acting as a tranquilizer, because the NE is destroyed by the mitochondrial MAO's. The reserpine does not block the formation of CA's, just the ability of the vesicle to concentrate and bind the CA's. It acts the same way in relation to 5-HT, again producing sedation, reduced smooth muscle activity, and parasympathetic effects. It is interesting that peripherally reserpine can produce complete adrenergic blockage, whereas in the CNS adrenergic effects can still be elicited following the administration of reserpine.

By inhibiting MAO's, *iproniazid* (Marsilid), the antituberculosis drug, which is the most thoroughly studied MAO inhibitor, causes the supply of NE to increase, thereby acting as an antidepressant.

### ■ What drugs act at adrenergic synapses and receptor sites?

COMT is inhibited by *pyrogallol*. Therefore when the latter is administered, it prolongs the effects of injected CA's, delaying their disappearance from the body.

*Phenylephrine* can combine at both α- and/or β-receptors to produce sympathomimetic effects.

The most potent normal activator of α-receptors is E, being up to 10 times more active than NE and more than 100 times as potent as the synthetic isoproterenol. *Isoproterenol* is the most potent β-activator, being up to 10 times more active than E and more than 100 times as potent as NE.

### ■ What is the neuropharmacologic significance of 5-HT?

Another indoleamine of questionable potential for acting as neurotransmitter in the CNS is 5-HT. Whereas DA and NE cannot pass the blood-brain barrier, 5-HT can. The question concerning to what extent the 5-HT found within the brain is formed there vs the amount transported there from extracranial sites is currently under investigation. As an MAO, 5-HT is also deaminated by MAO's. Being an indoleamine rather than a CA, it is not acted on by COMT. Considerable literature has evolved relative to the possible relation of 5-HT to behavior,[8] for example, schizophrenia. *LSD* is recognized as a 5-HT opponent.

### ■ How do anesthetics work?

Although drugs are used in treating all of the body systems, in this section attention is directed of course to drugs affecting the nervous system. The scope of such drugs would include such major categories as anesthetics, drugs acting as CNS depressants or sedatives, drugs affecting behavior, anticonvulsive drugs, and drugs acting on the ANS and musculoskeletal system.

Anesthesia may be of a permanent or a temporary nature, whether induced intentionally or accidentally or generally or locally. Permanent palliative treatment for pain may be achieved surgically, or where opportune, locally by injection of alcohol, etc. General anesthesia probably works on the reticular activating formation rather than the spinothalamic tracts, affecting both the ascending and descending components.[9] The effect on the descending components is probably responsible for the muscle relaxation seen in deep surgical planes.

While the disadvantages inherent to general anesthesia include the necessity for ongoing attendance by an anesthesiologist, additional equipment, postsurgical recuperative phase requiring an attendant, the risk to cardiac patients, etc., compensatory advantages include the absence of multiple problems associated with patient apprehensiveness and the availability of a wide range of volatile, gaseous, and intravenous agents.

It can be demonstrated in the PNS that anesthesia progressively lowers the height of the action potential, slows the rate of its rise, elevates the firing threshold, slows the speed of impulse conduction, and lengthens the refractory period until the threshold of the nerve is no longer reached; the nerve is blocked, since depolarization no longer occurs. The ability to raise the $Na^+$ permeability and generate an action potential is interfered with.[10]

Good local anesthesia practice demands that the injection be placed near the nerve but not in it. The connective tissue sheaths, the perineurium and, if present, the epineurium, represent the most significant barrier to penetration. Therefore since the roots of the spinal nerves are devoid of perineurium, they provide an excellent site for injection. Once the drug reaches the neurilemma, (high) fat solubility and (low) molecular weight seem to be important attributes in determining penetration rate. Since the nerves are frequently components of neurovascular bundles, when using local anesthetics the drug, in addition to blocking the nerve, usually enters the bloodstream, either by diffusion, especially if a substance such as hyaluronidase (Wydase) is added as an expediter, or by inadvertent intravenous injection.

If local anesthetics do enter the bloodstream, at high levels they act as convulsants; at low levels they exert anticonvulsant effects.

Subsequent to local injection into an extremity, it will be observed clinically that anesthesia progresses gradually proximodistally and that the spatial (temporal) pattern is reversed as the pool of drug injected is gradually diffused away, diluted with tissue fluid, and metabolized. The pattern relates anatomically to the fact that, generally speaking, fibers near the surface of a nerve innervate the proximal portion of the region supplied by the nerve, whereas the deeper fibers innervate the distal portion. Physiologically it relates, according to the fact that, as the anesthetic diffuses from the surface to the center of the nerve, it will attain threshold doses first centrifugally and later centripetally.

## ■ How do pain mechanisms work?

Realizing that not only articles but entire books continue to appear in the literature regarding the nature and control of pain, obviously it would be futile to pretend to attempt an adequate coverage of either aspect of the subject in this discussion.

In both human and animal experiments, work with a conscious individual is complicated by the "prior experience of pain" factor, indicating the potential value of EEG studies on patients in the nonwakeful state. Although the idea of a pain "center" has long since been abandoned, the sensation and its general relation to the RAS, the cerebral cortex, and the hypothalamus remain recognized.

Although pain is commonly produced by stimuli that at weaker intensities evoke other somatic sensations such as warmth or cold on mechanical contact, nonetheless, it seems to be a separate sensation with its own first-order neurons. One type of pain, the "fast" type, is transmitted by the slower components of the delta group of A fibers and is associated with the pricking form of cutaneous pain.

The second, "slow" type of pain is transmitted by some of the peripheral, unmyelinated C fibers and is associated with long-lasting burning sensations, an unbearable quality of suffering, and prolonged after-image following removal of the stimulus. Local drug injection may reduce conduction in the peripheral nerves by only 20% in producing typical anesthesia. However, it is not known what effect the local anesthetic may have on C fibers.

From the periphery, nociceptive stimuli arrive at portions of the spinal cord known as Lissauer's tract and the gelatinous substance and cross over to the contralateral side to ascend in the spinothalamic tract of the ventral half of the lateral funiculi. While some argue as to possible control of pain at this level, the *double-gate theory* of pain control,[4] others seriously debate the point. Palliative control of intractable pain and complete elimination of this form of stress are addressed by the use of drugs, surgery, hypnosis, acupuncture, psychic control, and manipulation; it sometimes remains difficult to make objective evaluations of the relative successes and merits of these various modalities.

Whereas the mode selected for treatment will vary with the practitioner's education and background of experience, such factors as the possible association of the pain with pathologic lesions, the severity and duration of noxious periods, and the patient's age are always of prime importance. When the use of other modalities fails, transection of the anterolateral column of the cord may be indicated to induce hemianesthesia (for pain and temperature control) of the contralateral side. Stereotaxic electrodes may be used to destroy selected regions of the brain with minimum damage to adjacent structures. Last resort procedures involve lesioning part of the thalamus or transecting the fibers linking it to areas 9 to 12 of the frontal lobe.

An excellent summary of clinical manifestations founded in neurologic origins is presented by Gatz.[11]

## REFERENCES

1. Ham, A. W.: Histology, ed. 6, Philadelphia, 1969, J. B. Lippincott Co.

2. Lindsay, N. K., and Birch, J. R.: Thin skin healing, Can. J. Surg. **7**:297-308, 1964.
3. Elliott, H. C.: Textbook of neuroanatomy, ed. 2, Philadelphia, 1969, J. B. Lippincott Co.
4. DiPalma, J. R., editor: Drill's pharmacology in medicine, ed. 4, New York, 1971, McGraw-Hill Book Co.
5. Goodman, L. S., and Gilman, A.: The pharmaceutical basis of therapeutics, ed. 4, New York, 1970, Macmillan Publishing Co., Inc.
6. Carrier, O., Jr.: Pharmacology of the peripheral autonomic nervous system, Chicago, 1972, Year Book Medical Publishers, Inc.
7. Gero, A.: Intimate study of drug action. III. Mechanisms of molecular drug action. In DiPalma, J. R., editor: Drill's pharmacology in medicine, ed. 4, New York, 1971, McGraw-Hill Book Co.
8. Barchas, J., and Usdin, E.: Serotonin and behavior, New York, 1973, Academic Press, Inc.
9. Vandam, L. D.: Uptake and transport of anesthetics and stages of anesthesia. In DiPalma, J. R., editor: Drill's pharmacology in medicine, ed. 4, New York, 1971, McGraw-Hill Book Co.
10. de Jong, R. H.: Physiology and pharmacology of local anesthesia, Springfield, Ill., 1970, Charles C Thomas, Publisher.
11. Gatz, A. J.: Manter's essentials of clinical neuroanatomy and neurophysiology, ed. 3, Philadelphia, 1966, F. A. Davis Co.

## BIBLIOGRAPHY

Deutsch, S., and Vandam, L. D.: General anesthesia. I. Volatile agents. In DiPalma, J. R., editor: Drill's pharmacology in medicine, ed. 4, New York, 1971, McGraw-Hill Book Co.

Elliott, H. C.: Textbook of neuroanatomy, ed. 2, Philadelphia, 1969, J. B. Lippincott Co.

Globus, A., et al.: Effects of differential experience on dendrite spine counts in rat cerebral cortex, J. Comp. Physiol. Psychol. **82**:175-181, 1973.

Goodman, L. C., and Gilman, A.: The pharmaceutical basis of therapeutics, ed. 4, New York, 1970, Macmillan Publishing Co., Inc.

House, E. L., and Pansky, B.: A functional approach to neuroanatomy, New York, 1960, McGraw-Hill Book Co.

Iggo, A.: New specific sensory structures in hairy skin, Acta Neuroveg. **24**:175, 1963.

Melzack, R., and Wall, P. D.: Pain mechanisms: a new theory, Science **150**:971-979, 1965.

Mountcastle, V. B.: Medical physiology, ed. 13, vol. I-II, St. Louis, 1974, The C. V. Mosby Co.

Netter, F. H.: The Ciba collection of medical illustrations, nervous system, vol. 1, Summit, N.J., 1957, Ciba Pharmaceuticals.

Ranson, S. W., and Clark, S. L.: The anatomy of the nervous system: its development and function, ed. 11, Philadelphia, 1974, W. B. Saunders Co.

Slonim, N. B., and Hamilton, L. H.: Respiratory physiology, ed. 2, St. Louis, 1971, The C. V. Mosby Co.

Vander, A. J., Sherman, J. H., and Luciano, D. S.: Human physiology: the mechanisms of body function, New York, 1970, McGraw-Hill Book Co.

# *chapter 3*
# Pharmacology

**DENNIS L. MING**
**KARIN ZENK**

This chapter is designed to provide information on some of the more common problems encountered in critical care and will deal with certain key areas wherein the care of the critically ill patient poses certain pharmacologic questions. It is hoped that the reader will be encouraged to seek further knowledge through the use of the references provided and any number of other excellent publications available.

## CARDIOVASCULAR DRUGS

■ **Are there any precautions that should be taken when using metaraminol in patients who have been treated with reserpine?**

If an indirect-acting sympathomimetic agent such as metaraminol (Aramine) is given to counteract hypotension in a patient taking reserpine, the pressor response is less than expected. If the patient has been taking large doses of reserpine for a long period of time, the vasopressor, that is, metaraminol, may be completely ineffective. This is caused by the amine-blocking and depleting effects of reserpine. The use of levarterenol (Levophed) would produce a better effect because of its direct stimulating properties.

■ **What are some of the drugs used for the treatment of hypertensive crisis?**

Drugs used in the treatment of hypertensive crisis are summarized in Table 3-1.

■ **Since diazoxide will cause retention of sodium and water, should a diuretic be administered concomitantly?**

Because the repeated administration of diazoxide may cause sodium and water retention, a diuretic should be administered to patients receiving multiple doses in order to achieve maximum hypotensive effects, avoid congestive heart failure, and prevent the development of apparent drug resistance. Although thiazide diuretics prevent sodium and water retention, these drugs may be ineffective or may aggravate the condition of the patient with renal impairment. More potent diuretics such as furosemide and ethacrynic acid are more useful because of the increased action on preventing sodium retention and because they do not lower the glomerular filtration rate. This is important when a hypertensive crisis is associated with acute pulmonary edema or renal failure.

■ **Are there any differences in the digoxin tablets made by various manufacturers that could affect the way patients respond to therapy?**

Digoxin is a drug with a very narrow therapeutic index, that is, a very small range between therapeutic and toxic doses; therefore altering the amount of digoxin that is absorbed can be dangerous. Physicians should be aware that either underdigitalization or toxicity may result from changes in the source or even the lot of the digoxin tablet from the manufacturer. If a particular patient is doing well on a particular brand of digoxin, it should be continued. However, if a change occurs in the patient's response to therapy, serum digoxin concentrations should be measured in blood taken 8 hours or more after the last oral maintenance dose. Doses of 0.25 to 0.5 mg daily of a preparation of good bioavailability usually create serum concentra-

**Table 3-1.** Drugs used for hypertensive crisis

| *Drug* | *Onset of action* | *Duration of action* | *Disadvantages* |
|---|---|---|---|
| Diazoxide (Hyperstat), IV | Within 5 min | 12-24 hr | Difficulty in control of blood pressure because of bolus injections |
| Trimethaphan camsylate (Arfonad) | Immediate | About 15 min | Necessary to frequently monitor blood pressure |
| Sodium nitroprusside, IV | Immediate | About 15 min | Necessary to frequently monitor blood pressure and to protect solution from light |
| Pentolinium (Ansolysen), IM | 10-30 min | 4-8 hr | May cause severe hypotension, also has parasympatholytic effects |
| Hydralazine (Apresoline), IV, IM | About 15 min | 2-6 hr | Produces cardiac-stimulating effects |

tions between 0.5 and 2.0 ng/ml. This is usually a good therapeutic range for most patients. Toxicity can occur at serum levels over 2.0 ng/ml.

### ■ What are some of the drugs used in cardiopulmonary arrest?

#### *Sodium bicarbonate*

Sodium bicarbonate is an alkalinizing agent that is used to combat acidosis in cardiopulmonary arrest. Acidosis occurs rapidly in arrest situations caused by lactic acid accumulation. Vasopressor drugs, if necessary, may be ineffective in acidosis.

ADMINISTRATION: From 3.75 to 7.5 g (45 to 90 mEq) contained in 50 to 100 ml is given initially by IV push followed by another 3.75 g every 15 minutes if cardiac arrest persists or recurs. A dose of 500 ml of 5% solution (contains 25 g of sodium bicarbonate) should be given over 60 minutes. Arterial pH should be determined frequently to regulate repeat doses or to indicate infusion by IV drip.

CAUTION: Sodium bicarbonate should not be mixed with epinephrine or calcium salts. Epinephrine will become rapidly deactivated, and calcium carbonate will form if mixed with calcium salts. Excess amounts may cause alkalosis, tetany, or pulmonary edema.

AVAILABILITY: Sodium bicarbonate may be obtained as 3.75 g (44.6 mEq)/50 ml in prefilled syringes.

#### *Lidocaine*

Lidocaine reduces irritability of the heart. It is used in recurrent cardiopulmonary arrest caused by ventricular fibrillation and when the heart resumes sinus or nodal beats with frequent ectopic ventricular beats.

ADMINISTRATION: Lidocaine is administered initially in doses of 1 to 2 mg/kg (usually 50 to 100 mg) by IV push. This is followed by starting an infusion of lidocaine containing 1 g in 250 ml of 5% dextrose in water (4 mg/ml). This is usually administered at the rate of 2 to 4 mg/min (30 to 60 micro drops/min). If an IV push is not given, it will take approximately 8 to 9 minutes to achieve a therapeutic blood level after an infusion of lidocaine is started.

CAUTION: Lidocaine should be withheld if the ventricular rate is less than 60 beats/min or if heart block is present. It will produce hypotension, atrioventricular (AV) block, and CNS stimulation with twitching, fasciculation, and convulsions. The dosage should be reduced in patients with liver and/or renal impairment or congestive heart failure.

AVAILABILITY: Lidocaine is available as 100 mg/10 ml (1%) in prefilled syringes for IV push. As 1 g/25 ml (4%) in prefilled syringes, it must be diluted before use.

#### *Epinephrine*

Epinephrine is an adrenergic agent with alpha (vasoconstrictor) and beta (cardiac-stimulating, peripheral-vasodilating, and smooth muscle–relaxing) effects. In cardiopulmonary arrest epinephrine stimulates an asystolic heart to contract and increases the amplitude of fibrillating ventricular waves. This latter effect may increase the success rate of defibrillation, but it may also increase the tendency toward ventricular fibrillation.

ADMINISTRATION: Epinephrine is administered in doses of 0.5 to 1.0 mg by IV push or intracardiac injection (5 to 10 ml of 1:10,000 solution).

CAUTION: Epinephrine must be used as a 1:10,000 dilution. It may cause tachycardia or ventricular arrhythmias, including fibrillation; it must not be mixed with or injected into the sodium bicarbonate IV line, since up to 60% of epinephrine's activity will be destroyed on contact with sodium bicarbonate.

AVAILABILITY: Epinephrine may be obtained as 10 ml of 1:10,000 solution in prefilled syringes with a 1½-inch needle for IV push or 3½-inch needle for intracardiac injection.

### *Atropine*

Atropine blocks vagus nerve activity (vagolytic and anticholinergic), thus increasing the sinoatrial (SA) and AV nodal activity. It is used in sinus arrest, bradycardia, and AV block.

ADMINISTRATION: Atropine may be given in doses of 0.5 to 1.0 mg by IV push. Frequent smaller doses are preferred if the drug is to be used repeatedly.

CAUTION: Atropine may cause tachycardia, arrhythmias, and occasionally ventricular fibrillation. Urinary obstruction and acute glaucoma may be initiated or worsened.

AVAILABILITY: Atropine is available as 1 mg/10 ml in prefilled syringes.

### *Isoproterenol*

Isoproterenol (Isuprel) is a $\beta$-adrenergic drug that will increase cardiac rate and contraction (at the expense of increased $O_2$ requirement) and cause peripheral vasodilation. It is used in complete heart block with slow ventricular rates and in certain forms of shock.

ADMINISTRATION: Isoproterenol is never given by IV push. A 4 $\mu$g/ml solution is prepared by adding 2 mg of isoproterenol to 500 ml of 5% dextrose in water. Using a micro drop administration set, the preparation is given by IV infusion at a rate of 1 to 4 $\mu$g/min (0.25 to 1 ml/min).

CAUTION: The blood pressure and ECG should be monitored during infusion. The drug should be stopped or the rate of infusion decreased if the blood pressure exceeds 120/60 or if premature ventricular contractions or ventricular tachycardia occurs.

AVAILABILITY: Isoproterenol is available as 2 mg/10 ml in prefilled syringes and as 1 and 5 ml ampules of 1:5000 solution.

### *Calcium*

Calcium ion is necessary for cardiac muscle contractility. It is sometimes administered in cardiopulmonary arrest to strengthen the contractions of the heart. It is a very short-acting drug, but ectopic calcific deposits may occur.

ADMINISTRATION: From 5 to 10 ml of calcium chloride (supplies 6.8 to 13.6 mEq of calcium ion) or 10 to 20 ml of calcium gluconate is administered by IV push (supplies 4.8 to 9.6 mEq of calcium ion). Note that the chloride salt provides almost one and one-half times the calcium ions that the gluconate salt provides.

CAUTION: Calcium chloride is very acid and should be avoided in acidosis; instead, calcium gluconate should be used. Calcium ion can also cause hypotension, and if used in excess, it may be cardiotonic. Intracardiac administration of calcium salts is usually not recommended. Calcium should not be used in digitalis toxicity. Calcium salts will precipitate when in contact with sodium bicarbonate; that is, calcium carbonate is formed and may obstruct the IV line.

AVAILABILITY: Calcium chloride is available as 1 g/10 ml (10%) in prefilled syringes. Calcium gluconate may be obtained in 1 g/10 ml (10%) ampules.

## ■ What are some of the ECG changes resulting from quinidine therapy?

The ECG changes that result from the direct effects of quinidine include a decrease in rate, an increase in the QRS duration, and an increase in Q-T interval. The direct (depressant) effect of the drug on AV conduction is to increase the P-R interval, whereas the antivagal effect, when present, is manifested by a decreased P-R interval.

## ■ What are some of the pharmacokinetic and toxic properties of procainamide?

Similar to quinidine, procainamide (Pronestyl) is well absorbed after oral administration and excreted primarily by the kidneys. About 50% is excreted unchanged. It can be given by IV administration, but it is considerably more depressant than lidocaine when given by this route. The most common side effects of procainamide when used orally are gastrointestinal disturbances such as nausea and vomiting. Flushing, hypotension, and dizziness may occur. Direct cardiac toxicity may occur as with quinidine; this takes the form of decreased contractility, sinus arrest, and conduction impairment. Severe overdosage may cause cardiac arrest or ventricular fibrillation. These properties have relegated procainamide to the role of quinidine substitute when the latter drug is not well tolerated.

## ■ When should digitalis treatment precede quinidine therapy?

Quinidine, when used in the treatment of atrial arrhythmias, may occasionally produce an increased ventricular rate caused by a vagolytic effect. Quinidine therapy should then be preceded by digitalization in the treatment of atrial arrhythmias; digitalization may reduce but does not abolish the possibility of increased ventricular rate.

## ■ What is the role of magnesium in the treatment of cardiac arrhythmias?

In hypomagnesemia both ventricular and supraventricular arrhythmias have been reported. The exact mechanism for the arrhythmias remains speculative but lack of adenosine triphosphate activity as a result of magnesium depletion appears to cause a diastolic leak of potassium from myocardial cells, producing an unstable milieu. A number of studies have shown that magnesium depletion potentiates and promotes digitoxic arrhythmias. Clinical studies have also revealed a higher incidence of hypomagnesemia in patients with digitoxic arrhythmias.

Magnesium was used for digitoxic arrhythmias as early as 1935. Studies, however, have shown that magnesium in doses of 10 ml of 20% $MgSO_4$ is inconsistent and transient in its therapeutic effect, whereas a dosage of 15 to 20 ml of 20% $MgSO_4$ is more consistent in normalizing the rhythm. Arrhythmias not caused by digitalis have also been treated. The results with 10 ml of 20% $MgSO_4$ solutions were also inconsistent, although 20 ml of the 20% solution is more effective.

A safe and effective dose would be 10 ml of 20% $MgSO_4$ given IV over a 60-second period followed by 500 ml of 2% solution given over 6 hours. If magnesium deficiency can be established, a second bottle of 500 ml of 2% $MgSO_4$ can be given during the remainder of the 24-hour period. As much as 70% of the infused magnesium will be excreted if urine production continues, even though the patient is depleted of magnesium.

Toxic effects of magnesium are probably related to serum magnesium levels. Transient symptoms of flushing and increased sensation of heat may occur with the initial IV injection. Prolonged levels above 5 mEq/L should be avoided, since hypotension, bradycardia, and AV blocks are observed in dogs having levels greater than this. Tendon reflexes probably are depressed or abolished when serum levels exceed 6 mEq/L. Respiratory depression, respiratory arrest, and cardiac arrest occur when levels exceed 10 mEq/L.

## ■ What are the disadvantages of subcutaneous administration of heparin?

The subcutaneous administration of heparin is not recommended unless an IV dose cannot be administered and relatively rapid anticoagulation is desired. Local pain, ecchymosis, and hematoma occur on injection. Absorption may be unpredictable and uncontrollable, depending on the patient's condition. Large doses or frequent injections are required. Clotting times must be determined at certain times relative to when the last dose was given. Neutralization with protamine sulfate is difficult and unpredictable. Hemorrhagic complications include hemorrhage into the rectus abdominis muscle, femoral nerve paralysis secondary to a hematoma in or on the iliac muscle, and retroperitoneal hemorrhage.

■ **If a patient receives an overdose of heparin or warfarin, what can be done to control the hemorrhaging?**

*Heparin*

The antedote to heparin is protamine sulfate. It neutralizes heparin by forming a complex that is pharmacologically inert. Protamine is also an anticoagulant and care must be taken to avoid overdosage, since it may cause a continuation of the bleeding. Other side effects of protamine sulfate include hypotension, bradycardia, dyspnea, nausea, vomiting, and lassitude. Protamine is administered by slow IV injection over a 1- to 3-minute period. Generally 1 mg of protamine sulfate will neutralize 100 to 120 units (USP) of heparin. Since heparin blood levels decrease rapidly after IV administration, the dose of protamine sulfate required also rapidly decreases as time elapses following IV administration of heparin. Not more than 50 mg should be given in any 10-minute period.

*Warfarin*

Vitamin $K_1$, also known as phytonadione (Aquamephyton), is the drug of choice for warfarin (Coumadin) overdose. Because of its more rapid, more potent, and more prolonged action, IV administration of phytonadione is preferred to other vitamin K analogues such as menadione in the presence of impending or actual hemorrhage. Following IV administration, the effects of the drug appear within 15 minutes, bleeding is usually controlled within 6 hours, and a normal prothrombin level may be obtained in 12 to 14 hours. Oral administration of the drug generally produces beneficial effects in 6 to 10 hours. It is not effective in reversing the action of heparin. When bleeding is not present or immediately threatening, 2.5 to 10 mg of phytonadione may be administered orally or by IM injection. This dose can be repeated in 12 to 48 hours. When bleeding is present or immediately threatened, 5 to 25 mg of phytonadione may be given by IV injection.

■ **What are some precautions to take when administering digoxin to infants or children?**

The recommended precautions in using digoxin are as follows:

1. Check the dose given. The average total digitalizing dose for infants or children is 0.03 to 0.05 mg/kg body weight. One half of the total digitalizing dose is given (usually by IM administration) to start. If this is enough, the digitalization may be stopped. If further digitalization is needed, one fourth of the digitalizing dose is given in 6 to 8 hours. If necessary, in another 6 to 8 hours, the last one fourth of the digitalizing dose is given. The maintenance dose is calculated as one eighth of the effective amount of digoxin used for digitalization and is given orally every 12 hours. The maintenance dose is started 12 hours after administration of the last digitalizing dose. If the patient has renal or liver disease, a smaller maintenance dose of digoxin or a greater interval between doses will be required.
2. Another person who is knowledgeable in this area should calculate the volume of digoxin to be administered before the drug is given to the patient.
3. During digitalization and changes in digoxin dosage, a lead II rhythm strip is run on the ECG machine. This is most useful at the time of maximum effect of the drug, that is, 1½ to 5 hours after administration.
4. Hypokalemia, hypercalcemia, hypermagnesemia, or hypoxia may predispose the patient to cardiac arrhythmias.
5. Digoxin and diuretic should be discontinued at the first suspicion of toxicity and a physician notified.
6. Cardiac toxicity is usually treated by administration of potassium by IV infusion,

and the ECG should be monitored frequently. If cessation of digoxin and diuretic and administration of potassium does not control arrhythmia, an antiarrhythmic agent such as procainamide may be used.

## ■ What side effects are seen with furosemide therapy?

Furosemide (Lasix) is a rapid-acting diuretic more potent than the thiazide diuretics and therefore more apt to cause severe adverse effects. As with other diuretics, excessive diuresis may cause water and electrolyte depletion that may result in circulatory collapse or vascular thrombosis and embolism, particularly in older patients. Reversible deafness has been seen in patients who have been given high IV doses (over 1 g), especially in the presence of diminished renal function. Therapy with furosemide can lead to hyponatremia and convulsions. An increase in the excretion of potassium, calcium, and magnesium occurs consistently, and the ensuing fall in blood level of these electrolytes can cause cardiac and neuromuscular abnormalities. Also, it has in rare instances precipitated attacks of gout, it interferes with carbohydrate metabolism, and it may produce hyperglycemia and glycosuria.

## ■ How does dopamine exert its action in patients with cardiogenic shock?

Dopamine possesses a variety of useful pharmacologic properties. It functions as an $\alpha$-adrenergic agonist, causing vasoconstriction of peripheral capacitance and resistant vessels; it also is a $\beta$-adrenergic agonist, producing an increase in cardiac rate and an augmentation of myocardial contractility. It also dilates renal and mesenteric vascular beds directly. Recent evidence indicates that dopamine inhibits the renal tubular reabsorption of sodium. Thus dopamine can be used to increase systemic arterial pressure by stimulating the myocardium without compromising renal blood flow and urine output. Dopamine may be the sole drug utilized after volume expansion and therapy with other catecholamines have proved ineffective. In other instances another catecholamine in combination with dopamine may prove efficacious.

Dopamine hydrochloride should be diluted in 5% dextrose and water to a concentration of 800 $\mu$g/ml for IV administration. Infusion is usually begun at a rate of 1 to 2 $\mu$g/kg body weight/min. This dose is increased by 1 to 4 $\mu$g/kg/min every 15 to 30 minutes until an optimal effect is obtained as judged by urine output and systemic arterial pressure. Maintenance doses in surviving patients average approximately 9 $\mu$g/kg/min.

## ■ What are some of the uses for glucagon?

Glucagon has been used in the treatment of insulin-induced hypoglycemia. It may be given by the IV, IM, or subcutaneous route in a dose of 1.0 mg. When it is given subcutaneously for hypoglycemic coma, a return to consciousness should be observed within 20 min; otherwise IV glucose must be administered as soon as possible.

Investigators have shown that small amounts of glucagon released by the pancreas stimulate hepatic glycogenolysis and gluconeogenesis. Large amounts increase adipose tissue lipolysis, stimulate the adrenal medulla to release catecholamines, exert inotropic and chronotropic effects on the myocardium, and stimulate insulin secretion.

Clinical investigations are being conducted to explore the use of glucagon in cardiac disorders as an inotropic and chronotropic agent that may be less productive of cardiac arrhythmias than are $\beta$-adrenergic catecholamines.

## ■ In what conditions would phentolamine be indicated?

Phentolamine (Regitine) is an $\alpha$-adrenergic blocking agent used frequently in the diagnosis of pheochromocytoma. In patients with sustained hypertension the ability of the $\alpha$-adrenergic blocking agents to block circulating catecholamines in smaller doses than are required to block neurally liberated norepinephrine can be utilized.

Phentolamine is also used to prevent the local necrosis that may follow the accidental paravenous injection of norepinephrine during the treatment of shock. The drug is infiltrated locally.

■ **How does morphine work in patients with acute pulmonary edema?**

Morphine is the drug of choice in the treatment of acute pulmonary edema, and its effectiveness is such that it is often described as a specific treatment. The mechanism by which morphine brings about relief is not clear. Its effectiveness is one of several pieces of data suggesting that acute pulmonary edema, which occurs in association with other than cardiac disease, should not be thought of as a consequence of acute left ventricular failure but as a reflexly generated state that can be interrupted by this central depressant. It does help to allay the anxiety that patients with acute pulmonary edema experience. The drug is usually administered by IV push as a dilution of 1 ml of morphine mixed with 9 ml of normal saline solution to give a dilution of 1 mg/ml. This dilution is pushed slowly to avoid acute depression of respiration.

## ANALGESIC AGENTS

■ **In what instances would acetaminophen have advantages over aspirin?**

Acetaminophen (Tylenol) has some of the pharmacologic properties of aspirin, that is, as an analgesic and antipyretic agent. However, it lacks the anti-inflammatory action for which aspirin finds usefulness in the treatment of arthritis. The side effects are also different. Acetaminophen is less likely than aspirin to cause gastrointestinal bleeding and irritation, asthmatic attacks in susceptible patients, drug interactions with oral anticoagulants, adverse effects on platelet function, and, in patients with gout, interference with tubular excretion of uric acid.

■ **How effective is naloxone in comparison with other narcotic antagonists?**

Naloxone (Narcan) is a relatively new addition to the small group of narcotic antagonists. It is available in a 0.4 mg/ml solution for IV, IM, and subcutaneous injection. Similar to the other narcotic antagonists nalorphine (Nalline) and levallorphan (Lorfan), naloxone will also antagonize the respiratory, analgesic, miotic, and most other pharmacologic effects of narcotics such as morphine, meperidine, methadone, and heroin. The important contrast between naloxone and the other antagonists is that naloxone, when not preceded by the administration of a narcotic, will not produce respiratory depression, sedation, analgesia, or miosis, which do occur when nalorphine and levallorphan are administered. It is almost completely free of such effects. Unlike the two other drugs, it can counteract the narcotic-like effects of pentazocine (Talwin). It will not, however, counteract the respiratory depression caused by barbiturates, cocaine, and cannabis. Because of its lack of respiratory depressive effects, it is the drug of choice if the diagnosis of narcotic poisoning is in error, as in barbiturate overdose. If large amounts of narcotics have been taken, naloxone can be given by IV administration as 0.01 mg/kg repeated every 5 minutes if required. Its maximum effect occurs 2 to 3 minutes after IV administration; after IM or subcutaneous administration it occurs after 15 minutes.

■ **Why are medications, specifically analgesics, given to patients preoperatively?**

In order to reduce the patient's anxiety so that the induction and maintenance of anesthesia will be smooth, preanesthetic medications are administered. Some of the broad classifications of drugs used for this purpose are narcotics, anticholinergics, and sedatives.

### *Narcotics*

Narcotic agents are useful for patients who may have pain preoperatively; however, they may cause respiratory depression, hypotension, nausea, vomiting, and constipation. The two most common agents are meperidine (Demerol) and morphine. There is available a fixed-ratio combination of fentanyl, a narcotic, and droperidol, a sedative. This combination, however, has sometimes produced apnea, anoxia, respiratory depression, and death. When pentazocine (Talwin) is used, care must be taken because pentazocine is a narcotic antagonist and may produce problems in unrecognized narcotic addicts, and when narcotics are used during or after surgery, its analgesic effects may be antagonized.

### *Anticholinergics*

Anticholinergic agents are used to control excess respiratory secretions and prevent bradycardia. Examples are atropine and scopolamine.

### *Sedatives*

Sedatives are used to potentiate the CNS-depressing effect of narcotics to achieve the overall desired effect of reducing anxiety for the purpose of easing the induction of anesthesia. Drugs such as barbiturates, diazepam (Valium), and antihistamines such as hydroxyzine (Atarax) and promethazine (Phenergan) have been used. The antihistamines are less likely to cause hypotension or respiratory depression.

## ■ Why is morphine sometimes given by IV injection to children?

The principal reasons for which morphine may be given by the IV route to children are as follows:

1. Morphine exerts an immediate effect on pain and anxiety.
2. It is possible to know promptly what effect has been achieved.
3. There will be no risk of delayed absorption such as could occur with poor peripheral circulation as in shock or with edema of tissue. If circulation is restored, it will then pick up a great deal of drug left in tissue, resulting in an overdose.

In addition to relieving pain and anxiety, morphine may also be used for relief of pulmonary edema in the infant or child with congestive heart failure. When given by IV injection, morphine must be administered slowly over several minutes. The dose in children is 0.1 to 0.2 mg/kg/dose. Overdoses of morphine are treated with a narcotic antagonist such as naloxone at a dose of 0.01 mg/kg/dose administered by IM injection.

## ■ What are some of the drugs currently being used to treat neonatal withdrawal syndrome?

Infants born to mothers who are addicted to drugs are often addicts themselves and have withdrawal symptoms shortly after birth. Paregoric, chlorpromazine, and phenobarbital are used to treat this neonatal withdrawal syndrome. The major advantages of paregoric are oral administration and lack of adverse effects (constipation may be seen with excessive doses). Withdrawal from paregoric can take a long time, since a too rapid lowering of the dose may lead to recurrence of symptoms. Chlorpromazine (Thorazine) is also effective. If symptoms are controlled, the drug is continued for 5 to 10 days. Discontinuance with dosage tapering can often be accomplished in 2 to 3 weeks, but occasionally a 2-month treatment is necessary in severe cases. Phenobarbital may also control neonatal withdrawal symptoms, especially irritability and insomnia. The dose is maintained for 4 to 10 days and tapered off over 1 to 3 weeks. High phenobarbital doses may sedate the infant and prevent adequate fluid and caloric intake.

## ■ What are some of the adverse effects of oxyphenbutazone and phenylbutazone?

Phenylbutazone (Butazolidin) and oxyphenbutazone (Tondearil) are closely related and are used in the treatment of rheumatoid (ankylosing) spondylitis and acute gout after other first-line drugs have failed. Both drugs can produce such adverse effects as aplastic anemia and agranulocytosis. Other harmful effects include ulceration of the esophagus and stomach, hepatitis, nephritis, serum sickness, purpura, and sodium and water retention. Because the toxic effects of these drugs are believed to be more severe in older patients, these two agents should be used cautiously, and particular attention should be paid to salt and water retention leading to edema, congestive heart failure, and hypertension.

## ■ What is the treatment for Lomotil poisoning in children?

Lomotil is an antidiarrheal preparation containing diphenoxylate, a narcotic somewhat similar to meperidine, and atropine. The clinical features of toxicity from accidental ingestion include the anticholinergic syndrome caused by atropine with flushing, hallucinations, hyperpyrexia, lethargy, urinary retention, and tachycardia. At the same time or following the atropine effects, respiratory depression, miosis, lethargy, coma, and death have also occurred as a result of the narcotic effects of diphenoxylate. Treatment includes inducing emesis, unless contraindicated by convulsions, coma, or absence of a gag reflex. Naloxone (Narcan), a narcotic antagonist, in a dose of 0.01 mg/kg should be used. Admission for observation in an intensive care unit for 24 hours following ingestion, regardless of clinical status, should be undertaken, because gastric emptying may be significantly delayed by the drug and the onset of symptoms may be retarded. Magnesium sulfate, 250 mg/kg, may be given orally or by lavage with or following the administration of activated charcoal.

## DRUGS AFFECTING THE RESPIRATORY SYSTEM

### ■ Are antihistamines such as diphenhydramine and chlorpheniramine beneficial in the treatment of asthmatic attacks?

Antihistaminic drugs exert their greatest beneficial effect on nasal allergies. Seasonal hay fever is benefited more than vasomotor rhinitis; however, nasal obstruction and headache caused by edema of the sinus mucosa are often refractory to antihistamine therapy. Diphenhydramine (Benadryl) and chlorpheniramine (Chlor-Trimeton), among others, do not prevent or effectively relieve asthma, which frequently accompanies hay fever. These drugs are usually not effective in treating bronchial asthma and should be used with caution in asthmatic patients because of the atropine-like drying effects of these agents.

### ■ When should corticosteroids be used in the treatment of status asthmaticus?

When an adequate trial or sympathomimetic drugs and aminophylline has failed and the patient received steroids in the preceding year, a dose of corticosteroids may be warranted. However, the most common errors committed in using corticosteroids are (1) using too small a dose during the acute episode and (2) anticipating a quick response when the usual response time is 4 to 6 hours. Tapering the dose is usually not necessary if the total daily steroid course was 5 days or less.

### ■ In the treatment of asthma, are there any differences between isoproterenol and metaproterenol as bronchodilators?

Isoproterenol (Isuprel) was the first of the synthesized $\beta$-receptor stimulants and rapidly became the most commonly used as well as the prototype for future bronchodilators. Most pharmacologists agree that, although isoproterenol is a very rapidly effective bronchodilator, its action is relatively brief and its side effects many; specifically, tachycardia is a problem when another cardiotonic agent such as aminophylline is being administered concomitantly. For this reason the structural formula of isoproterenol was altered to form metaproterenol (Alupent, Metaprel). The resulting agent has greater selectivity for bronchial activity rather than general action on both cardiac and bronchial muscle. Other advantages of metaproterenol are longer duration of action, minimum side effects, no tachyphalaxis, and no paradoxical reactions.

### ■ What precautions should be taken when aminophylline is being administered by the IV route?

The principal cautions to be observed are as follows:

1. Aminophylline should be administered slowly to avoid headaches, fall in blood pressure, and subjective awareness of a forceful heartbeat.
2. When used as a rapid infusion, it should be infused over 20 to 30 minutes to minimize the side effects just mentioned.
3. Adding other drugs to the solution containing aminophylline should be avoided because of the problem of precipitating theophylline crystals.
4. The concomitant administration of cardiotonic agents such as isoproterenol should

be avoided. The doses can be staggered in terms of the times of each administration to avoid any cardiac side effects such as tachycardia.

5. The practitioner should be aware of recent aminophylline treatment to avoid toxicity; for example, the patient may have been given an aminophylline suppository just prior to hospitalization, during which aminophylline is to be administered by the IV route.

■ **Are there any incompatibilities with aminophylline in solution?**

The optimum pH range for stability is above pH 8.0. Crystals of theophylline will deposit below pH 8.0, but probably not unless the concentration is over 40 mg/ml. Therefore this incompatibility is more apt to occur if certain admixtures are made in syringes or small volumes of fluids than if components are added separately to large-volume IV fluids.

■ **What are some of the drugs that should be avoided in the treatment of asthma?**

All respiratory depressants such as narcotics, barbiturates, propoxyphene (Darvon), and tranquilizers and agents that are anticholinergic in activity, thereby drying mucous secretions, should be avoided.

■ **Are there any patients who should not use acetylcysteine?**

*N*-Acetyl-*l*-cysteine (Mucomyst) is effective in thinning extremely viscid tracheobronchial secretions. Its clinical usefulness has been limited because it is difficult to administer and will react with most metals, rubber, and to some extent oxygen. It decreases the viscosity of sputum to a much greater extent than does a saline control solution. However, the drug may increase bronchial secretions independent of its effect on sputum, particularly in patients with bronchial asthma. This effect may lead to serious bronchial obstruction; therefore this agent should not be used in asthmatic patients without concomitant bronchodilator treatment. The drug may also produce stomatitis, rhinorrhea, and hemoptysis.

■ **If an asthmatic child cannot take aminophylline orally, could rectal suppositories be used?**

The absorption of aminophylline from rectal suppositories in children is unpredictable. Serious overdosages have occurred when the drug was administered by this route. If a child cannot take medications orally, the IV route should be used.

■ **What physical measurements should be monitored in treating asthmatic patients with bronchodilators?**

Changes in blood pressure, heart rate, and cardiac rhythm must be carefully and frequently observed to establish the maximum acceptable dose of bronchodilator. Measurements of pulmonary function and pulse rate before and 10 minutes after the initial dose of aerosol are important in assessing the maintenance of a therapeutic effect.

■ **What are the differences between epinephrine hydrochloride and epinephrine solution?**

Acute asthmatic attacks are usually relieved within 3 to 5 minutes after subcutaneous injection of 0.2 to 0.5 mg of epinephrine. Repeated doses can be administered every 15 to 20 minutes. If symptoms occur, massage of the site of injection may produce relief by enhancing absorption of the drug.

For prolonged relief from bronchospasm, usually in chronic asthma, epinephrine in suspension (Sus-phrine) is sometimes used, and a dose of this may produce relief. Epinephrine in suspension provides both rapid and sustained epinephrine activity. The rapid action results from the epinephrine in solution, whereas the sustained activity is caused by the crystalline epinephrine free base in suspension. Prolonged activity has been found to last for as long as 8 to 10 hours, avoiding the need for constant and repeated injection of aqueous epinephrine (1:1000 solution). Caution should be taken to avoid giving epinephrine aqueous solution in addition to the epinephrine in suspension. Additional doses of epinephrine should not be administered within 4 hours of the previous dose.

Whatever drug is chosen, the smallest dose affording relief should be used.

■ **What are some of the drugs used to control respiration?**

The most frequently used drugs are succinylcholine and pancuronium bromide. Neither of these drugs should be mixed with any barbiturate drugs or with diazepam (Valium) in the same syringe or needle because of the possibility of precipitation of either of the latter two drugs.

***Succinylcholine***

Succinylcholine (Anectine) is an ultrashort-acting depolarizing-type muscle relaxant. When a single effective IV dose of the drug is given, muscular relaxation occurs within 1 minute, persists for about 2 minutes, and returns to normal within 8 to 10 minutes. If a paralyzing IM dose is given, the onset of action may be delayed for 2 to 3 minutes. When given by IV drip, a predetermined degree of muscular relaxation can be closely approximated by adjusting the rate of flow of the infusion. The paralysis following the administration if succinylcholine is generally initially selective and usually appears in the following muscles consecutively: levator muscles of the eyelids, muscles of mastication, limb muscles, abdominal muscles, muscles of the glottis, and finally intercostal muscles and the diaphragm.

The IV drip solution containing 1 mg/ml may be administered at a rate of 0.5 to 10 mg/min to obtain the desired amount of relaxation. The amount required will depend on the individual response as well as the degree of relaxation required. The IV dose for infants and children is 1.0 to 2.0 mg/kg body weight.

***Pancuronium bromide***

Pancuronium bromide (Pavulon) is a nondepolarizing neuromuscular blocking agent possessing all of the characteristic pharmacologic actions of the curariform class of drugs on the myoneural junction and is approximately five times as potent as *d*-tubocurarine. The onset and duration of action of pancuronium are dose dependent. With the administration of 0.04 mg/kg the onset of action is usually within 45 seconds, and its peak effect is usually within 4.5 minutes; 90% recovery usually takes place in less than 1 hour. Larger doses, more suitable for endotracheal intubation, such as 0.08 mg/kg have a time of onset of about 30 seconds, and a peak effect within 3 minutes. Pancuronium has little effect on the circulatory system. The most frequently reported observation is a slight rise in pulse rate. It also has no known effect on consciousness, the pain threshold, or cerebration. It is therefore useful as an adjunct to anesthesia to induce skeletal muscle relaxation or to facilitate the management of patients undergoing mechanical ventilation.

In adults the initial IV dosage range is 0.04 to 0.1 mg/kg. Later incremental doses starting at 0.1 mg/kg may be used; however, the higher increments will increase the magnitude and duration of the blockage. Experience in children is insufficient at this time to provide a dosage range.

***d-Tubocurarine***

*d*-Tubocurarine (curare) is used primarily to produce skeletal muscle relaxation during surgery after general anesthesia has been induced. It may be used to increase pulmonary compliance during assisted or controlled respiration and for facilitating endotracheal intubation.

Following the usual single IV dose of *d*-tubocurarine, muscle relaxation occurs rapidly and reaches a maximum within 5 minutes. The duration of paralysis is related to the total dosage and the number of doses administered, subsiding in 20 to 30 minutes.

The initial dose of *d*-tubocurarine as an aid in controlled respiration is 16.5 μg/kg body weight (average 1 mg); subsequent doses should be determined by the requirements and response of the patient.

## ANTISEIZURE MEDICATIONS

■ **Are there any special precautions to follow when diluting diphenylhydantoin for IM or IV use?**

The special diluent for sodium diphenylhydantoin (Dilantin) injection contains propylene glycol, benzyl alcohol, and water and is buffered to pH 10.0 to 12.3 with sodium hydroxide. Reconstituted, clear solution of sodium diphenylhydantoin may be stored at room temperature and should be discarded if haziness or precipitation develops or if the solution is not used within 4 to 6 hours of preparation. Solutions of sodium diphenylhydantoin are not compatible with acid solutions; a precipitate may form if the drug is diluted with dextrose or other acidic solutions.

■ **Are there any problems associated with the IV administration of diphenylhydantoin?**

Following IV administration, shock, hypotension, cardiovascular collapse, respiratory depression, bradycardia, partial or complete heart block, and ventricular fibrillation with resultant precipitation or potentiation of heart failure may occur. Therapy should be discontinued if any of these reactions occur. These effects may be minimized by administering the drug at a rate not to exceed 50 mg/min. Repeated IV use may produce a cumulative effect in decreasing the force of myocardial contractions.

■ **What drug is considered by many as the drug of choice for most cases of status epilepticus in adults and children?**

Diazepam (Valium) given by the IV route is now considered by many as the drug of choice in most cases of status epilepticus. Distinct advantages are its swift effectiveness, sometimes within seconds, and its margin of safety if administered properly as the initial drug. If the patient has already received parenteral barbiturates or other hypnotic agents, blood pressure and respiration should be monitored carefully.

■ **How is diazepam administered safely for status epilepticus in children?**

Valium must be administered slowly at a rate of 1 mg every 1 to 5 minutes up to a total, if necessary, of 5 to 10 mg each session in a child 5 years or older. In infants the dose is 0.2 to 0.5 mg up to a total of 5 mg each session. Because of its relative water insolubility, diazepam may also precipitate when administered by the IV route and hence may occasionally cause thrombophlebitis. Therefore it is important to ensure that the needle does not inadvertently penetrate an artery and that each dose is followed by a thorough flushing of the vein with saline solution.

■ **What is the main disadvantage of diazepam administered by the IV route?**

The swift control of status epilepticus by diazepam can be short lived. It is not unusual that seconds after injection the patient ceases convulsing, only to begin convulsing again. However, a second or third injection may bring lasting relief.

■ **Can paraldehyde be used for status epilepticus in children?**

Some authorities advocate the use of paraldehyde alone or as an adjunct for the treatment of status epilepticus, especially in children. Its volatile mode of excretion and wide margin of safety are indeed points in its favor for use in emergency situations. It can be administered rectally at a dose of 1 ml for each year of age, not to exceed a total of 5 ml regardless of age; this dose may be repeated 1 hour later. Because of its irritative action on the rectal mucosa, a gastric tube should be used if repeated administration is anticipated. Gavage of 2 to 5 ml can be performed at 2- to 4-hour intervals.

■ **What startling reaction can occur when children are given phenothiazines, particularly prochlorperazine?**

The phenothiazines, most commonly prochlorperazine (Compazine), may produce undesirable side effects, not necessarily related to dosage, characterized by the acute onset of contractions of various voluntary muscle groups with torticollis, trismus, opisthotonus, drooling, and swallowing difficulty. These episodes are sometimes called "pseudotetanus" or "extrapyramidal crisis." They may be mistaken for psychotic episodes, postinfectious encephalomyelitis, or tetanus.

■ **What is the antidote for pseudotetanus or extrapyramidal crisis caused by prochlorperazine?**

The extrapyramidal signs are dramatically alleviated within minutes by the slow IV administration of 1 to 5 mg of diphenhydramine (Benadryl)/kg. No other treatment is usually indicated.

■ **What are some of the drugs used to treat alcoholic delirium tremens, and are any more effective than others?**

It is generally considered that symptoms of the different stages or degrees of severity of the alcohol withdrawal syndrome are best treated by replacing alcohol with a drug pharmacologically equivalent to alcohol in its action on the CNS. Alcohol is unsatisfactory because of its short duration of action. There have been a few well-controlled studies using agents such as paraldehyde, chloral hydrate, the barbiturates, diazepam (Valium), and chlordiazepoxide (Librium). Phenothiazines have been used but have been shown to be less effective than the other drugs previously mentioned. Some consultants regard paraldehyde as more effective than chlordiazepoxide in the prevention and control of delirium tremens; however, the odor of paraldehyde may be intolerable to the patients and hospital personnel, and glass syringes are needed if injected, since paraldehyde will react with plastic syringes. It can also cause sterile abscesses at the site of IM injection. Diazepam may possibly be more effective than chlordiazepoxide and may prove to be as effective as paraldehyde in preventing and controlling delirium tremens by the IM or IV routes of administration. However, more well-controlled trials are needed before any conclusive statements can be made about the relative merits of these drugs.

## ANTIBIOTICS

■ **For which antibiotics should the doses and dosing intervals be modified in patients with renal impairment?**

Since most antibiotics are eliminated by the renal route, severely impaired excretion may result in dangerously high concentrations in the blood and tissues unless the interval between doses is greatly increased or the individual doses are decreased in conjunction with careful, frequent monitoring of renal function and blood level. Modifications should be made in the administration of kanamycin, streptomycin, gentamicin, the polymixins, tetracycline, cephaloridine, and vancomycin. Methicillin in high doses has caused renal nephritis and should be used cautiously in patients with renal impairment. The recommendations of the manufacturers for modifying dosages should be followed.

■ **How should gentamicin and kanamycin be administered to a patient with elevated serum creatinine levels?**

Since both of these agents have the potential to cause renal toxicity and hearing loss, the doses should be reduced and the interval between doses increased. Many clinicians have developed nomograms to determine dosages for their patients; however, if the nomograms are unavailable, a simple method to calculate the dosing interval can be used. For example, in using gentamicin for a patient with a serum creatinine level of 3, this value is multiplied by eight to give a rough estimate of the number of hours between each dose:

$$3 \times 8 = 24 \text{ hr}$$

Therefore the dose should be reduced to 1 to 2 mg/kg given every 24 hours.

For kanamycin, if the value of the serum creatinine level is multiplied by nine, this will give a rough estimate of the number of hours between each dose:

$$3 \times 9 = 27 \text{ hr}$$

Therefore the dose should be reduced to 7.5 mg/kg given every 27 hours.

These figures are, again, rough estimates, and efforts should be made to adjust the doses according to available nomograms for each drug. Of course the most ideal way would be to measure the serum concentrations periodically in order to arrive at the proper dose based on renal excretion and blood level data.

**■ Why is probenecid occasionally administered with penicillin?**

Probenecid is a uricosuric agent that decreases the tubular reabsorption of urates. When administered with penicillin or a cephalosporin, it increases the serum concentration of the antibiotic by inhibiting its tubular secretion; it has proved useful when high antibiotic concentrations are needed. The peak serum levels of either oral or parenteral penicillin are elevated 50% to 300%. The duration of activity in the blood is prolonged, and the cerebrospinal fluid level is raised. The disadvantages are that probenecid can cause nausea and vomiting, can be only administered orally, and can cause a rash, which would make it difficult to judge whether the probenecid or the antibiotic is responsible if an allergic reaction should occur. The dose is 0.5 g/6 hr during therapy.

**■ What is the "gray baby syndrome" in relation to the use of chloramphenicol in neonates?**

The gray baby syndrome is fatal chloramphenicol toxicity, which may develop in neonates, especially premature babies, when exposed to excessive doses of this drug. The illness usually begins 2 to 9 days (average 4 days) after treatment is started. Manifestations in the first 24 hours are vomiting, refusal to suck, irregular and rapid respiration, abdominal distention, periods of cyanosis, and passage of loose green stools. All infants are severely ill by the end of the first day and in the next 24 hours develop flaccidity, ashen gray color, and a decrease in temperature. Death occurs in about 40% of the patients, most frequently on the fifth day of life. This toxic effect is thought to be caused by failure of the drug to be detoxified by the liver and inadequate renal excretion of the drug. Children 1 month of age or younger should receive chloramphenicol in a daily dose no larger than 25 mg/kg body weight. After this age daily quantities of up to 50 mg/kg may be given without difficulty. The child should be observed very carefully during treatment and the drug discontinued at the first sign of toxicity.

**■ Are there any advantages to using clindamycin rather than lincomycin?**

Clindamycin is a semisynthetic derivative of lincomycin that is available for use in parenteral and oral form. It has a distinct advantage over lincomycin in its lesser incidence of side effects. The spectrum of action is similar; clindamycin is effective against bacteroides.

**■ What serious systemic reactions could occur when a child is given a pertussis vaccine (alone or as diphtheria-pertussis-tetanus vaccine)?**

Convulsion, severe febrile reaction, or thrombocytopenia are the reactions of greatest consequence.

**■ What type of child is more susceptible to these reactions?**

Children with cerebral damage should not be innoculated with diphtheria-pertussis-tetanus vaccine. In such infants active immunization procedures should be delayed until active cerebral irritation has subsided or until the child has reached 1 year of age. Thereafter single antigens are recommended and pertussis should be administered last. An initial dose of 0.05 or 0.1 ml should be given to test tolerance before the remainder of each dose is administered.

**■ Why are sulfonamides such as sulfisoxazole not administered to neonates?**

Certain factors predispose an infant, especially a premature infant, to the development of kernicterus at lower serum levels of bilirubin. These factors (acidosis, low albumin levels, sulfonamide administration, elevated free fatty acid, etc.) mainly result in decreased albumin-binding capacity for bilirubin. In addition, sulfonamides compete with the glucuronide transferase system, the system in the liver of the infant that changes bilirubin to a soluble form so it may be excreted. A marked increase in kernicterus and death has been reported in premature infants receiving sulfisoxazole (Gantrisin).

■ **With regard to the toxicity of sulfonamides in the newborn infant, is it safe to use topical sulfa creams in treating burns of patients in this age group?**

The manufacturers' literature concerning silver sulfadiazine cream warns that, because sulfonamide therapy is known to increase the possibility of kernicterus, the cream should not be used at term pregnancy, on premature infants, or on newborn infants during the first month of life. The manufacturers have found that in the treatment of burn wounds involving extensive areas of the body the serum sulfa concentration may approach adult therapeutic levels even though the application is topical.

■ **Are there any advantages that cefazolin sodium has over the other injectable cephalosporins?**

Cefazolin is an antibiotic similar to cephalothin and cephaloridine. It is available for IM and IV administration. It does not produce the severe pain associated with IM doses of cephalothin and, unlike cephaloridine, it does not appear to damage the kidneys. The antibacterial spectrum of cefazolin is similar to that of the other cephalosporins, but it is more active against *E. coli* than cephalothin and somewhat more easily inactivated by penicillinase than other cephalosporins. Organisms resistant to cephalothin are generally resistant to cefazolin. For those infections caused by organisms susceptible to both penicillin and cefazolin, penicillin is still the drug of choice and much less costly to administer.

■ **Why is it not advisable to change from ampicillin administered IV to ampicillin therapy using the IM or oral route after several days of treatment of *Haemophilus influenzae* meningitis in a child even though the child is afebrile and seems to be doing well clinically?**

Ampicillin achieves a cerebrospinal fluid (CSF) concentration that is 30% of the simultaneous blood concentration early in the course of the meningitis. Later, as the inflammatory responses subside, the concentration in the CSF may, somewhat surprisingly, fall to 5% of that in blood. Such a dramatic fall might easily reduce the CSF antibiotic concentration to less than that which is antibacterial, a phenomenon that may operate in cases reported as ampicillin failures. As the inflamed meninges heal, less antibiotic can cross into the CSF and thus the last few days of antibiotic treatment are the most critical. Adequate levels of antibiotic can best be assured by using IV therapy throughout the course of treatment.

■ **What are the criteria for discontinuing ampicillin therapy when treating a child who has *Haemophilus influenzae* meningitis?**

A recent review of the diagnosis and treatment of bacterial meningitis suggests the following criteria: (1) therapy should be continued until the patient is afebrile for 5 days and (2) if at that time the spinal fluid contains 50 or less mononuclear leukocytes per milliliter and the protein concentration is less than 50 mg/100 ml, antibiotic therapy is discontinued. In most infants this means 10 to 14 days of antibiotic therapy.

■ **What is one of the most important drugs to administer immediately to a child who has just been diagnosed as having *Haemophilus influenzae* meningitis?**

A child who has just been diagnosed as having *Haemophilus influenzae* meningitis should have ampicillin administered by IV push. Usually the earlier a child is treated, the better the prognosis will be.

■ **What are the different types of penicillin allergy and what is the recommended treatment?**

Penicillin is the drug of choice for many infections. The drug has a low incidence of toxicity, estimated to be 1% to 5% of the courses of penicillin therapy. Allergic reactions are most common in patients with histories of asthma, hay fever, or atopic dermatitis.

The allergic reactions are divided into three categories based on the time of onset of the allergic reaction:

1. Immediate. These reactions generally occur within 20 minutes with symptoms such as urticaria, flushing, and diffuse pruritus. Less commonly the reactions are anaphylactic and are manifested by shock, cardiac arrhythmias, and laryngeal edema, sometimes with wheezing.
2. Accelerated. Accelerated reactions start between 1 and 72 hours after penicillin therapy and are usually urticarial, although other rashes occasionally appear.
3. Late. These reactions begin from days to weeks after the initiation of therapy, usually with urticaria or other rashes.

Ampicillin is more likely to cause rashes than other penicillins; some rashes are the result of true allergy, others are not.

Treatment of penicillin allergy would be to discontinue the medication and, in cases of anaphylaxsis, treat the patient with epinephrine administered by the subcutaneous or IV route. The subcutaneous dose is 0.3 to 0.5 ml of a 1:1000 solution. The IV dose is 0.2 to 0.3 ml diluted in 10 ml of saline solution and injected slowly. IV fluids and plasma expanders should be available to raise the blood pressure.

Care must be taken to avoid the automatic and sometimes routine use of cephalosporins in patients with penicillin allergies, since these series of drugs have been shown to have cross-reactions; that is, certain patients allergic to penicillin have also been allergic to cephalosporins.

## FLUID AND ELECTROLYTE SOLUTIONS

■ **In treating hypernatremic dehydration in children, what fluid and electrolyte solutions should be used and at what rate?**

If dehydration is severe, 20 ml/kg of normal saline solution or Ringer's lactate should be given and repeated once if necessary. To calculate liters of water necessary to restore present serum sodium concentration ($C_p$) to normal, the following formula may be used:

$$\frac{C_p - 140}{140} \times \text{kg body weight} \times 0.6$$

When shock has been corrected, water is given as 5% dextrose and 0.25% normal saline solution at a rate calculated not to lower serum sodium more than 15 mEq/L/day. The state of hydration and serum sodium concentration should be evaluated every 6 hours to determine the end point of IV therapy.

■ **What severe complication could occur if the sodium concentration dropped too rapidly in the treatment of hypernatremic dehydration?**

The rapid correction of hypernatremia and reexpansion of cells can result in convulsions.

■ **What is the program of management of acute dehydration in children in terms of fluids to be administered and rate of administration?**

Treatment is directed toward the restoration of extracellular fluid by infusion of isotonic solution in the following sequence:

1. Immediately give by IV route 20 ml/kg of 0.9% normal saline solution. This may be repeated once.
2. Replace fluids gradually to allow them to be absorbed and not overload the heart. One way in which this may be done is to give one half of the calculated deficit in the first 8 hours and the remainder in the following 16 hours.
3. Do not add potassium to the IV solution until urine flow is established.

■ **Why is it a good idea to include 5% dextrose in all maintenance parenteral fluids?**

All maintenance solutions should contain at least 5% dextrose to reduce the caloric deficit that usually occurs in patients who need parenteral fluid and electrolytes. The use of dextrose also minimizes ketosis and the buildup of "starvation solutes" (urea, phosphate, and other protein breakdown products) that increase the excretory load.

■ **How can acidosis associated with impaired renal function, starvation, or diabetes be corrected?**

Continuous rehydration, which enhances renal perfusion, and, in diabetics, insulin therapy usually suffice to correct acidosis. When the plasma pH is less than 7.2 or carbon dioxide content is less than 10 mEq/L, however, administration of bicarbonate or bicarbonate precursors may be required.

■ **What are the maintenance water requirements intended to supply normal daily requirements to patients who are not taking water orally?**

These requirements are summarized in Table 3-2.

■ **What could be some manifestations of the accidental IV administration of a toxic dose of potassium and how could they be treated?**

The manifestations of hyperkalemia are muscle weakness, tetany, or paresthesias with ascending paralysis. ECG shows elevated T waves, QRS lengthening, and ventricular fibrillation. To treat the patient, if cardiac arrhythmias are present or serum potassium levels are over 8.0 mEq/L, sodium bicarbonate and/or 10% calcium gluconate are given slowly by the IV route. For serum potassium levels over 6.0 mEq/L sodium polystyrene sulfonate (Kayexalate) enemas may be given as necessary. Dialysis is occasionally indicated.

**Table 3-2.** Maintenance water requirements based on surface area

| *Body weight* | | *Surface area* | *Approximate maintenance water (ml/24 hr)* |
|---|---|---|---|
| *kg* | *lb* | | |
| 3 | 6.6 | 0.21 | 300* |
| 6 | 13.2 | 0.30 | 500 |
| 10 | 22.0 | 0.45 | 700 |
| 20 | 44.0 | 0.80 | 1300 |
| 30 | 66.0 | 1.05 | 1700 |
| 40 | 88.0 | 1.30 | 2100 |
| 50 | 110.0 | 1.50 | 2400 |
| 60 | 132.0 | 1.65 | 2600 |
| 70 | 154.0 | 1.75 | 2800 |
| 80 | 176.0 | 1.85 | 3000 |

*Less in the first 2 weeks of life.

■ **When is replacement therapy needed in addition to maintenance therapy with IV fluids?**

Replacement therapy is needed when there is a heavy loss of water and electrolytes, as in severe vomiting, diarrhea, nasogastric suction, or fistulous drainage.

■ **What is the formula for calculating the amount of replacement IV fluid therapy a patient might need?**

A *Medical Letter Review* on parenteral water and electrolyte solutions states that in many instances 70 ml of an electrolyte solution/kg/day in addition to the maintenance water requirements will replace about 70% of the deficit in a 10% dehydrated adult. Thus a 50 kg patient would require 3500 ml of electrolyte solution for replacement plus 2400 ml for maintenance. In order to avoid the consequences of fluid overload, especially in elderly patients and those with renal or cardiovascular disorders, monitoring of the central venous pressure is considered desirable.

■ **A patient's urine output has suddenly dropped; however, measurement of the IV fluids indicates that they have maintained the same rate as when the kidneys were functioning well. Later the patient develops tachycardia, tachypnea, and edema. What is wrong and how could it be corrected?**

The patient is probably fluid overloaded. The manifestations of this complication are the clinical signs of congestive heart failure (tachycardia, tachypnea, hepatomegaly, venous distention, edema, increased weight, weakness, and cardiac gallop). The patient would be treated as for congestive heart failure through the use of oxygen, sedation, diuretics (furosemide), and rarely, digitalis.

**■ For patients in shock or in the absence of clinical improvement after 2 hours of rapid replacement IV therapy, what IV solutions may be indicated?**

Whole blood, plasma, albumin, plasma protein fraction, or dextran may be indicated if the patient is in shock or if no clinical improvement has occurred after 2 hours of rapid replacement. The patient's central venous pressure should not be elevated and pulmonary congestion should not be present if these solutions are used. Albumin and dextran have the advantage of not transmitting serum hepatitis.

**■ What cautions should be observed in administering sodium bicarbonate to a newborn?**

Sodium bicarbonate is administered by the IV and sometimes oral route to newborn infants for correction of acidosis. The formula used to calculate the dose is:

$$NaHCO_3 \text{ (mEq)} = \text{Body weight (kg)} \times \text{Base deficit} \times 0.35$$

Recent data suggest that excessive sodium bicarbonate administration to newborns with or without hypernatremia may place the infant at a higher risk of intracranial hemorrhage. Thus the newborn's sodium intake from all sources should be carefully controlled, and intakes of more than 8 mg/kg body weight/24 hr should be regarded as excessive.

**■ An irritative substance (such as calcium, hypertonic bicarbonate, vinblastine, etc.) is being administered by the IV route to a child, and the solution has leaked into the surrounding tissue, which appears red and swollen and feels hot. How could this be treated?**

Irrigation with saline solution, aspiration, immobilization of the extremity, application of heat pads, and cutaneous application of 0.1% triamcinolone cream with occlusive dressing may allow adequate steroid absorption to decrease local reaction.

**■ A toxic IM dose of a drug has accidentally been administered to a child. What could be done?**

The potential complications of the toxic dose are drug dependent and must be treated as toxic overdose (specific antidotes if available). When IM or subcutaneous routes are used, the procedure involves the following:

1. Use of proximal tourniquet
2. Local irrigation and aspiration with saline solution
3. Local application of ice
4. Administration of subcutaneous epinephrine into injection site, 0.01 ml/kg of 1:1000 solution

**■ What are some of the precautions that should be taken with patients on parenteral hyperalimentation?**

Parenteral hyperalimentation solutions are usually composed of amino acids, dextrose, vitamins, and minerals to provide the necessary caloric and other nutrient requirements to patients with disorders that prevent them from being fed orally. Formulas have been prepared and are available commercially; however, any formulation must be altered to fit the needs of the individual patient.

Because these solutions are hypertonic, they must be infused into large central veins where rapid dilution prevents damage to vessels. Therefore daily catheter care should include dressing removal, skin cleansing with an antiseptic, and restoration of occlusive dressings. Catheters should be immediately removed and cultured for bacteria and fungus if a patient shows signs of sepsis.

A 0.45 $\mu$ in-line final filter should be used to filter the solution and changed every 24 hours or when difficulty is encountered in adjusting the flow rate.

To prevent the accidental infusion of large amounts of fluid, an infusion pump should be used to regulate the flow. Even with the pump frequent checks should be made to verify that the proper rate of infusion is maintained.

It is not advisable to administer antibiotics or other IV medications through the alimentation cannula, since precipitation or other physical or chemical incompatibilities may result, and the chance of bacterial or fungal contamination may also be increased. Drugs that are catabolic such as tetracycline should be avoided if possible, or at least the weight of the patient should be monitored carefully to make sure that a drug interaction is not occurring. Insulin has been added to the solutions with the purpose of increasing the storage of the dextrose; however, insulin has a tendency to adhere to the sides of the IV bottle and to the tubing to an extent of 20% to 40%.

Since the solutions contain large amounts of electrolytes and glucose, dangerous electrolyte imbalances may occur, and frequent determinations of serum electrolyte (especially potassium) levels and glucose concentrations are essential during the first few days of therapy.

Other precautions include watching for fluid overload, especially in small infants, hypophosphatemia, elevation in blood ammonia levels, and acidosis.

Total IV fluid therapy is effective; however, precautions must be taken to ensure safety for the patient. Great care in all phases of the technique should be exercised to reduce the risk of septicemia, etc. This therapy should be carried out by an experienced team and in areas where frequent monitoring of the patient can be provided.

■ **What caution must be observed in correcting hypernatremic dehydration in adult patients?**

Water intoxication must be prevented in the correction of hypernatremic dehydration. Serum sodium concentration should be determined after administration of one half of the calculated water deficit. The volume of water necessary to restore the serum sodium concentration to normal (body water deficit) in adults may be estimated by the following calculations (TBW is total body water):

$$\text{TBW (L)} = 0.6 \times \text{Normal body weight (kg)}$$

$$\frac{\text{Normal serum }(Na^+) \times \text{TBW}}{\text{Measured serum }(Na^+)} = \text{Current TBW}$$

$$\text{Normal TBW} - \text{Current TBW} = \text{Body water deficit}$$

Correction of the salt deficit is best performed gradually with a sodium-free solution. The patient should be observed for improvement in skin turgor and stabilization of blood pressure and central venous pressure.

■ **What is an essential guideline for treatment of dehydration?**

Acute change in weight is directly related to change in fluid volume. Just as the amount of water lost in dehydration equals the weight loss, the amount of water gained in the process of rehydration equals the amount of weight gained by the patient. Weighing the patient daily or twice daily is helpful in assessing the progress of the patient in the treatment of dehydration.

## MISCELLANEOUS DRUGS

■ **What precautions should be taken in changing drug regimens prior to surgery to avoid interactions with anesthetics and/or the surgical procedure?**

Although there are no rigid criteria for the discontinuation of medications prior to surgery, the possible interactions should be considered.

### *Anticoagulants*

Anticoagulants may cause bleeding with spinal, epidural, dental, or other types of regional blocks or with tracheal intubation or other instrumentation. They may also increase bleeding during and after surgery.

### *Antimicrobials*

Tetracyclines predispose to renal insufficiency after methoxyflurane anesthesia. Kanamycin, streptomycin, gentamicin, and neomycin may cause neuromuscular block and apnea and therefore have an additive effect if *d*-tubocurarine or other nondepolarizing neuromuscular blocking agents are used.

### *Cardiovascular drugs*

$\beta$-Adrenergic blockers such as propranolol may add to the myocardial depression of general anesthetics, induce bronchospasm, and prevent adequate circulatory response to blood loss. Despite these hazards, it may sometimes be preferable to continue the drug in certain patients. Digitalis and other cardiac glycosides should as a rule be continued, but the possibility of digitalis intoxication during general anesthesia should be kept in mind. Quinidine, procainamide, and lidocaine may aggravate myocardial depression, impair cardiac conduction, and cause peripheral vasodilation. They may also potentiate neuromuscular blocking agents. Diuretics, especially the thiazides, furosemide, and ethacrynic acid, can lead to hypovolemia, hypotension, alteration in sodium and potassium metabolism, and prolonged paralysis when used together with muscle relaxants. Antihypertensive agents may cause additive hypotensive effects.

*Corticosteroids*

Corticosteroid agents should not be discontinued; sudden withdrawal may cause adrenocortical insufficiency.

*Drugs acting on the nervous system*

Anticonvulsants should not be tapered off in too short a period before surgery because this may result in convulsions, and sudden cessation may lead to status epilepticus. Phenobarbital can add to respiratory depression. Phenothiazines may add to the hypotensive effects of sedatives, narcotics, and general anesthetics.

*Insulin*

Dosage should be reduced at the time of surgery. Some anesthesiologists have withheld insulin until the postoperative period.

■ **Are there any rules that should be followed when different insulins are to be mixed in the same syringe?**

Insulins are mixed primarily to modify their action in customizing the insulin requirements to individual needs. This usually results in an intermediate-acting mixture; however, with commercially available intermediate insulins this is less common. If a mixture is needed, the shorter acting insulin should always be drawn into the syringe first. For example, in mixing regular insulin with protamine zinc insulin, if the protamine zinc insulin is drawn first and then injected into the regular insulin vial, the amount of protamine zinc insulin will gradually change the activity of the regular insulin to that of a longer acting compound. Hence the activity curve for the regular insulin is altered and its actions become unpredictable.

**Table 3-3.** Forms and times of action of insulin

| *Insulin* | *Onset (hr)* | *Peak (hr)* | *Duration (hr)* |
|---|---|---|---|
| Fast-acting preparations | | | |
| Regular insulin (crystalline zinc) | ½-1 | 2-6 | 5-8 |
| Semilente insulin | ½-1 | 3-9 | 12-16 |
| Intermediate-acting preparations | | | |
| Lente insulin | 1-4 | 6-16 | 16-24 |
| NPH insulin | 1-4 | 7-12 | 24-30 |
| Long-acting preparations | | | |
| Ultralente insulin | 4-8 | 10-30 | 34-36 |
| Protamine zinc insulin | 1-8 | 12-24 | 30-36 |

■ **What are the different forms of insulin and their hours of activity?**

Data concerning insulin are summarized in Table 3-3.

■ **What are some of the drugs that are commonly abused, and how effective is either forced diuresis or hemodialysis in treating overdosage of these agents?**

*Meprobamate*

Hemodialysis is effective and appropriate in very severe cases. Good clinical results have also been noted with peritoneal dialysis. Since a small amount of this drug is excreted in the urine and is relatively insoluble in water, forced diuresis may be of little value. The drug is nonionized; therefore pH adjustment of the urine would probably have no effect on excretion.

*Ethchlorvynol*

Hemodialysis and forced diuresis have been successful in removing this drug. Peritoneal dialysis is probably somewhat less effective than forced diuresis. Since the drug is not ionized, there appears to be no reason for alkalinizing the urine.

### *Methyprylon*

This drug is reasonably soluble in water and its excretion should be increased by forced diuresis. Diuresis and peritoneal dialysis are not as effective as hemodialysis.

### *Benzodiazepines*

The benzodiazepines (chlordiazepoxide, diazepam, oxazepam) are strongly bound to tissue protein so that blood levels are very low. Consequently, neither forced diuresis nor dialysis techniques are likely to be of much help in increasing the excretion of these drugs.

### *Phenothiazines*

Chlorpromazine and related psychotropic phenothiazine derivatives are strongly bound to tissue proteins, and the chances of effectively accelerating the metabolism of the absorbed drug appear not to warrant the use of forced diuresis or dialysis techniques.

### *Dibenzazepines*

In relation to the dibenzazepines (imipramine, amitriptyline), as with the phenothiazine derivatives, tissue binding appears to be of such a high degree that dialysis techniques offer little in the way of effective treatment.

### *Barbiturates*

Forced diuresis increases excretion and decreases the duration of coma in patients with long-acting barbiturate intoxication. The removal rate of pentobarbital is increased 20% by osmotic diuresis; phenobarbital removal is doubled. Alkalinization of the urine does not increase the nonionic diffusion of short-acting barbiturates into the urine because the pH of these drugs is above that which can safely be achieved in the urine. Hemodialysis removes barbiturates 10 to 30 times faster than diuresis, depending on the specific drug ingested. The removal of short-acting barbiturates is slower with either method because of protein binding. Barbiturate clearance with diuresis varies from 5 ml/min with short-acting drugs to 17 ml/min with long-acting barbiturates. Hemodialysis is the procedure of choice when renal failure and barbiturate intoxication coexist.

## ■ A patient who has been on chronic steroid therapy is scheduled for surgery. What should be done to prevent adrenal crisis?

Patients who are receiving adrenal steroids currently or who have received adrenal steroids from 4 to 30 days in the past 6 months, or 1 to 3 months during the past year, or 3 months or more anytime in their lives have an unpredictable degree of functional adrenocortical suppression. These patients should be managed as if they have adrenocortical insufficiency. The recommended schedule involves the administration of cortisone acetate in doses of 100 mg IM 12 hours preoperatively, 100 mg in the morning prior to surgery, and 100 mg in the evening postoperatively. The total daily dose can be tapered over several days.

If hypotensive crisis occurs during or following surgery, the patient should be treated with hydrocortisone sodium succinate or phosphate in doses of 100 mg given by the IM or IV route immediately and 100 mg IV infusion every 8 hours for the first day. The same amount is given every 8 hours on the second day, and then the dosage is gradually reduced. The regimen of dose reduction should be judged by clinical status. When the patient can tolerate oral feedings, the drug can be given orally.

## ■ What are the different types of oral hypoglycemic agents?

There are two classes of oral hypoglycemic agents currently used in the treatment of diabetes: the sulfonylureas and the biguanides. The sulfonylureas act by stimulating the release of insulin from the beta cells of the islets of Langerhans.

In the absence of the pancreas or in cases of juvenile diabetes where the pancreas is grossly deficient in its ability to secrete insulin, the sulfonylureas are ineffective. These drugs are of greatest value in the treatment of mild maturity-onset diabetes wherein the pancreas continues to produce insulin.

Examples of these drugs are tolbutamide (Orinase), chlorpropamide (Diabinese), and tolazamide (Tolinase). These drugs differ primarily with respect to their duration of action.

The biguanides, for example, phenformin (DBI), do not activate the release of insulin from the pancreas, nor do they induce hypoglycemia in nondiabetic patients. It appears that phenformin may act by accelerating the intracellular oxidation of glucose, a process that is depressed in the absence of insulin. Phenformin is used alone for the treatment of maturity-onset diabetes and in combination with insulin in juvenile diabetes. Some physicians can achieve better management of diabetes by concurrently using sulfonylureas and phenformin.

## BIBLIOGRAPHY

AMA Department of Drugs: AMA drug evaluation, ed. 2, Acton, Mass., 1973, Publishing Sciences Group, Inc.

American Hospital Formulary Service, Washington, D.C., 1975, American Society of Hospital Pharmacists.

Beckman, H.: Dilemmas in drug therapy, Philadelphia, 1967, W. B. Saunders Co.

Bennett, E. J., et al.: Pancuronium bromide: a double-blind study in children, Anesth. Analg. (Cleve.) **52**:12-18, 1973.

Boeder, E. C., and Dauber, J. H.: Manual of medical therapeutics, ed. 21, Boston, 1974, Little, Brown & Co.

Chui, L.: The review of antiepileptic drugs, The Pharmacy Newsletter, Orange County Medical Center **5**:1-5, May, 1974.

Goodman, L., and Gilman, A.: The pharmacologic basis of therapeutics, New York, 1968, Macmillan Publishing Co., Inc.

Horowitz, K., and Iseri, L. T.: Drugs used in cardiopulmonary arrest, The Pharmacy Newsletter, Orange County Medical Center **4**:2-6, April, 1973.

Hospital formulary monograph on Silvadene Cream (Micronized Silver sulfadiazine), Kansas City, Mo., 1973, Marion Laboratories, Inc.

Iseri, L. T.: Magnesium and cardiac arrhythmias, The Pharmacy Newsletter, Orange County Medical Center **5**:4, March, 1975.

Karliner, J. S.: Dopamine for cardiogenic shock, J.A.M.A. **226**:1217-1218, 1973.

Kempe, C. H., Silver, H., and O'Brien, D.: Current pediatric diagnosis and treatment, Los Altos, Calif., 1972, Lange Medical Publications.

Kempe, C. H.: Immunization update with a word of caution, Drug Therapy, pp. 71-82, 1974.

Khan, W., et al.: Hemophilus influenza type B resistant to ampicillin, a report of two cases, J.A.M.A. **229**:289-300, 1974.

Lasry, J. E., and Glassner, M. L.: Cardiovascular drugs, 1970, The California Heart Association Publication.

Loeb, H. S., et al.: Acute hemodynamic effects of dopamine in patients with shock, Circulation **44**:163-173, 1971.

Lombroso, C. T.: The treatment of status epilepticus, Pediatrics **53**:536-540, 1970.

Melmon, K. L., and Morrelli, H. F.: Clinical pharmacology, basic principles in therapeutics, New York, 1972, Macmillan Publishing Co., Inc.

Meyers, F.: Review of medical pharmacology, Los Altos, Calif., 1972, Lange Medical Publications.

Nadas, A.: Pediatric cardiology, Philadelphia, 1963, W. B. Saunders Co.

Parenteral electrolyte solutions, 1973, Med. Lett. Drugs Ther. Reference Handbook.

Parker, E. A.: Parenteral incompatibilities, Hosp. Pharm. **4**:14-22, 1969.

Pascoe, D., and Grossman, M.: Quick reference to pediatric emergencies, Philadelphia, 1973, J. B. Lippincott Co.

Pierog, S. H., and Ferrara, A.: Approach to the medical care of the sick newborn, St. Louis, 1971, The C. V. Mosby Co.

Randall, R. J.: Diazoxide, The Pharmacy Newsletter, Orange County Medical Center **5**:2-5, Jan., 1974.

Rumack, B. H., and Temple, A. R.: Lomotil poisoning, Pediatrics **53**:495-500, 1974.

Shirkey, H. C.: Pediatric dosage handbook, Washington, D.C., 1971, American Pharmaceutical Association.

Shirkey, H. C.: Pediatric therapy, ed. 5, St. Louis, 1975, The C. V. Mosby Co.

Simon, M., et al.: Hypernatremia, intracranial hemorrhage and sodium bicarbonate administration in neonates, N. Engl. J. Med. **291**:6-10, 1974.

Smith, D. H., et al.: Bacterial meningitis, diagnosis and treatment, a symposium, Pediatrics **52**:586-600, 1973.

Tomeh, M., et al.: Ampicillin-resistant haemophilus influenza type B infection, J.A.M.A. **229**: 295-297, 1974.

Travenol guide to fluid therapy, Deerfield, Ill., 1970, Travenol Laboratories.

Treatment of neonatal withdrawal syndrome, Med. Lett. Drugs Ther. **15**:46-47, 1973.

Visconti, J. A.: The dialysis of drugs, Philips-Roxan Laboratory White Sheet.

*chapter 4*

# Psychiatric aspects of critical care

WILLIAM F. KIELY

The widespread development of special hospital units for the care of the critically ill and injured during the past decade has brought life-saving benefits for thousands of patients. Multiple organ support systems; monitors of cardiovascular, ventilatory, and renal excretory functions; and techniques for the noninvasive measurement of a variety of circulatory, respiratory, and hemodynamic parameters have been of tremendous value in the care of the dangerously ill patient. A benefit to such patients less heralded but of very great importance has been the sharpened focus brought to bear on altered states of consciousness, emotional responsiveness, and behavioral reaction in the critically ill. Responsibility for the lives of such patients has given the staffs of intensive care facilities increased respect for the integrative action of the CNS, on whose reliable function much of the coordinated action of other body systems depends. Skill in the appraisal and evaluation of the cerebrocortical functions of attention, perception, conception, orientation, and memory as well as of attitudes, feelings, and behavioral responses of the person who is ill are becoming part of the comprehensive care approach of the staffs of critical care units. Practitioners have come to the recognition that anxiety on the one hand or apathetic depression on the other is a danger signal interacting with a precarious balance of forces in the severely ill patient.[1]

Physicians, nurses, and other critical care professionals are becoming increasingly aware of the importance of the patient's previous life experience, coping style, and particular strengths or vulnerabilities in the face of stress and are planning treatment strategies to take account of such factors. It becomes increasingly evident that, although the treatment of disease may be highly impersonal and technologized to a very great extent, the care of a patient must be highly personal. The mind-body relationship, or psychosomatic unity, is nowhere more evident than as exhibited by patients in the grip and under the stress of critical illness.

## ■ What is stress?

Stress, which originally was a concept of the physical sciences, has come into the parlance of the life sciences to denote a state in which vital functioning of the organism is threatened either from an internal or an external source. Stress involves a sufficiently potent danger to physical or psychologic well-being as to require extraordinary measures for the maintenance of organized, adaptive function. These failing, stress may lead to disorganized emotional reaction, cognitive function, physical behavior, and physiologic or biochemical response patterns.

## ■ How do physical and psychologic stress differ?

The terms "physical stress," "emotional stress," and "social stress," among similar notions, are often used to denote different sources of threat to organized function. Although all have in common the potential for interfering with integrated organismic function by overtaxing adaptive capacities, they derive from different sources of challenge. In critical care medicine and surgery the stressors are most often multiple, deriving from illness or injury to vital organs or systems, from psychologically threatening challenge to the patient's repertory of adaptive capacities, and from interruptions of social role functions and the imposition of new role functions involving dependency on and trust in the reliability of total strangers.

■ **What are the most important determinants of psychologic stress and of behavioral reaction among the critically ill?**

There is generally a subtle interweaving of a variety of determinants from several sources, including (1) features reflective of the patient's previous life experience and expressive of personal coping style, (2) factors related to the particular variety of illness or injury being experienced, (3) elements reflective of the critical care unit's distinctive environmental impact on the patient, and (4) patterns reactive to aspects of the treatment program imposed on the patient.

■ **What specifically are such person-related factors?**

The manner in which persons experience and cope with the threat posed by illness or injury and how they accept hospitalization and the imposed sick role will to an important degree reflect their previous life experience in dealing with crisis. If the patient has successfully mastered similar hazards in the past, there is less likelihood that the experience will be overwhelming, because the patient knows what to expect and how to deal with such challenges. Under such circumstances the psychologic threat is likely to be manageable and not spill over into disorganized arousal patterns of emotional, cognitive, behavioral, or psychophysiologic reaction. Coping style with the present challenge will generally reflect personality characteristics typical of that individual's previous manner of functioning, but often in an accented form; for example, the individual may be taciturn, cranky, self-willed, emotionally labile, or depressive. The patient brings to this crisis situation habitual attitudes toward and modes of dealing with novelty and the unfamiliar, dependency, authority figures, and passivity—the hallmarks of the sick role in critical care facilitities. The effect of such adaptive psychologic problems on the patient's current nexus of family relationships—with spouse, parents, and children—and in turn the reactive influence of such family members—particularly their own capacity to cope adaptively—have effects on the patient, and sometimes on the intensive care staff, that may bear importantly on the success or failure of treatment.[2] Previously unrecognized or compensated chronic cerebral insufficiency —related to age, cerebral vascular disease, or previous brain damage—is often thrown into acute decompensation by a sudden change in customary surroundings, particularly if there are deficits in function of the important orienting senses of vision and hearing.[3] Delusional misinterpretation of time, place, and person as well as hallucinatory excitement is sometimes induced in the elderly patient by such minimum degrees of sensory deprivation. In sum, the patient's age, level of cerebral competence, characteristic personality style, emotional state, and nexus of interpersonal relationships all may contribute to the illness experience and determine the reaction to it.[4]

■ **What are some of the disease-related factors?**

The frequency of occurrence of critical care psychiatric syndromes varies considerably with the type of illness and differs in prevalence in the several types of intensive care facilities. The concept of a critical care unit psychiatric syndrome developed originally out of reports of a high incidence of delirium (40% to 70%) following open-heart surgery.[5] Some observers believed that this syndrome, developing typically between the third and fifth postoperative day, reflected the influence of the intensive care unit's environmental impact on the patient. A combination of sleep deprivation, sensory monotony, and loss of a sense of time passage and of a day-night cycle were felt to be major contributing factors to the loss of reality sense.[6] Postcardiotomy delirium has subsequently been found to be highly correlated with neurologic deficit and organically determined cognitive dysfunction[7] perhaps related to the duration of exposure to cardiopulmonary bypass, microemboli originating in the heart, duration of hypothermia, and depth and duration of anesthesia. Significant differences in the incidence of psychiatric disturbances following lung surgery are noted in comparison to open-heart surgery. It would appear that the incidence of such syndromes in well-organized coronary care units is considerably less than that noted in postcardiotomy recovery rooms.[8] Intensive care units treating a wide spectrum of critically ill and injured patients, including the seriously burned, will number among their patients a majority who may suffer from renal, cardiac, or pulmonary failure, serious septic or hypovolemic shock, considerable anemia, fever, and toxemia. Such disease-related elements very probably account for the significantly different incidence of delirium and other psychiatric disorders among such patients as compared to the generally much more physically intact acute coronary patient or even many postcardiotomy patients.

### ■ How may the critical care unit's environment affect the patient's coping with illness?

The introduction of critical care facilities has served, among other consequences, to focus attention on the psychobiologic effects of the kinds, variety, and quantity of sensory input that such environments bring to bear on persons who are ill. Reference has already been made to the effect, especially on the elderly, that transfer to such an unfamiliar environment may have. The usual design of critical care units results in windowless, austere, multi-bed rooms with a variety of monitors, respirators, and other bedside equipment whose meaning and purpose to a marginally rational and critically ill patient may be ambiguous at best. Too often the patient lies prone, movement impeded by intubation of some or all of the body orifices, experiencing the persistent stress of pain or discomfort, and with perceptual faculties dulled or impaired by sedatives, tranquilizers, and/or hypnotic analgesics. The compounding influences of azotemia, anoxemia, hypercapnia, and hypovolemic or septic shock may further complicate the task for the patient of making meaningful and purposeful sense of this entire spectrum of input.

In some measure and to variable degrees in the course of treatment of such critical illness there are likely to be elements of (1) sensory underload or deprivation, (2) some periods of sensory overload, (3) much sensory monotony, (4) erratic and interrupted sleep patterns, (5) social isolation, (6) unfamiliarity with the human and situational environment, and (7) prolonged immobilization. Each of these factors has been shown experimentally to be capable of contributing to clouding of consciousness, perceptual distortion, behavioral confusion, and sometimes to frankly delusional and hallucinatory experiences.[9] A number of observers have pointed to the role of reduced or destructured sensory input in the production of delirium such as occurs after eye surgery,[10] with the use of tank-type respirators,[11] and with placement in intensive care units.[12] The passivity and immobilization may reduce very considerably the level of kinesthetic and proprioceptive feedback from muscles and joints on which the midbrain reticular formation and hypothalamus depend to sustain adaptive alertness and orientation in the overlying cerebral cortex.[13] Under such conditions vital subcortical reciprocal balance between arousal and withdrawal systems may break down, resulting in the delivery to the interpretative neocortex of a depatterned, meaningless volley of signals to which cognitive sense is difficult for the patient to assign.[14]

### ■ What are the neurobiologic bases for the wide spectrum of emotional, behavioral, and psychophysiologic reaction patterns encountered in crisis care of the ill or injured?

Hess,[15] as early as 1925, pointed out that an animal's reaction to environmental challenge is importantly reflective of the influence of subcortical centers that coordinate autonomic, somatic, and psychic functions. He suggested that these centers were organized through reciprocally balanced systems, which he termed *ergotropic* and *trophotropic.* Highly integrated neural functions of the type underlying the cognitive process, generally considered reflective of cortical activity, are under the modulating influence of these primitive, tonically active subcortical systems. All perceptual stimuli, whether of exteroceptive or interoceptive source, as well as memory and logical thought sequences reveal the shaping influence of these balanced systems. Their anatomic basis, physiologic interconnections, and neurochemical transmitters are distinguishable and separable.[16] Their influence is identifiable across the entire continuum of consciousness from sleep to the heights of ecstasy physiologically[13] and from stupor to catatonic excitement psychopathologically.[14]

The ergotropic system integrates functions that prepare the individual for positive action. It is characterized by alerting, arousal, excitement, increased skeletal muscle tone and sympathetic nervous activity, and the release of catabolic hormones. The trophotropic system, on the other hand, integrates systems that promote withdrawal and conservation of energy: raising the stimulus barrier to perceptual input, decreasing skeletal muscle tone, increasing parasympathetic nervous function, and circulating anabolic hormones. A developing body of data indicates that the biogenic amines norepinephrine and dopamine are neurotransmitters for the ergotropic system, whereas 5-hydroxytryptamine (serotonin) and acetylcholine play similar roles for the trophotropic system.[17]

## ■ Are there relatively consistent physiologic principles that underlie the operation of these reciprocally opposed systems?

Yes, a few basic principles play a primary role in the operation of this quite complex psychobiologic process and underlie the resultant patterns of behavior. First, the two systems stand in mutually reciprocal relationship and share tonic, enduring, and balanced physiologic activity. With increasing degrees of activation of the ergotropic "go" (approach) system there is a corresponding degree of inhibition of the trophotropic "no go" (avoidance) system; the converse is also true.

Second, when either system is stimulated, the reactivity of both systems is altered, affecting their state of readiness, set, or tuning,[18] so to speak. In moderate states of activation, or tuning, the reactivity of the various anatomic and physiologic components of the affecting system is heightened, whereas that of the reciprocal system is correspondingly reduced. Thus in situations of moderate, but not extreme, challenge or threat the "go" system expresses itself cortically through alerting, or vigilance; autonomically in a sympathetic stimulation; and behaviorally in a state of muscular readiness. At the same time the reactivity of the several components of the "no go" system is correspondingly suppressed.

Third, at maximum stimulation reciprocal balance between systems breaks down and both discharge simultaneously. A clinical example is the state of anxiety wherein a variety of psychic, skeletal muscular, and visceral disturbances reflect such simultaneous discharge of opposing systems. Flooding of the cerebral cortex by afferents from both systems may be experienced as dread; weak knees may coexist with tremulous hands; and sweating, tachycardia, and hypertension may coexist with nausea, vomiting, and bowel or bladder hyperactivity.

## ■ What are the most common varieties of psychiatric syndromes encountered in critical care units?

The most common syndromes encountered in critical care units are schematically characterized in Table 4-1. They may range from the occasionally encountered overwhelming fear reaction, accompanied by a paralyzing sense of helplessness in which the behavioral-avoidance grip of the "no go" system is evident, through more adaptive but sometimes physiologically stressful states of restless tension. In these polar opposite states of tuning, or adaptation, reciprocal suppression of the opposing system is maintained. At higher degrees of CNS arousal maladaptive, sustained anxiety is encountered with simultaneous discharge to varying degrees of both

**Table 4-1.** Neurobiology of psychiatric syndromes

| *State of tuning* | *Clinical example* | *Pharmacologic intervention* | *Site of action* |
|---|---|---|---|
| Trophotropic dominance | Acute fear | Benzodiazepine agent (Librium, Valium, Serax, Tranxene) | Limbic forebrain and midbrain serotonergic suppressor sites |
| Ergotropic dominance | Sustained tension | Benzodiazepine agent (Librium, Valium, Serax, Tranxene) | Limbic forebrain and midbrain serotonergic suppressor sites |
| Simultaneous "T" and "E" discharge | Anxiety | Benzodiazepine agent (Librium, Valium, Serax, Tranxene) | Limbic forebrain and midbrain serotonergic suppressor sites |
| | Agitated depression | Benzodiazepine agent (Librium, Valium, Serax, Tranxene) | Limbic forebrain and midbrain serotonergic suppressor sites |
| | Acute schizophreniform stress reaction | Butyrophenone (Haldol) | Neostriatal and mesolimbic dopamine receptor sites |
| | Acute delirium | Butyrophenone (Haldol) | Neostriatal and mesolimbic dopamine receptor sites |
| | | Benzodiazepine agent (Librium, Valium, Serax, Tranxene) | Limbic forebrain and midbrain serotonergic suppressor sites |

"go" and "no go" systems as noted psychically, viscerally, and in skeletal muscle groups.

At still higher degrees of stimulation, anxious or agitated depression reactive to the stress of crisis may be encountered. One sometimes sees examples of acute schizophreniform psychotic disintegration with thought disorder, delusions, or hallucinations maintained in the context of clear consciousness and without loss of orientation or memory function. Especially where elements of cardiac, pulmonary, renal failure, or circulatory shock complicates the clinical course of the illness, and particularly in the middle-aged or elderly, one frequently encounters delirium, that is, a state of cerebral insufficiency with impairment of some or all of such cognitive functions as attention, perception, conception, logical sequence, orientation, and memory. Some degree of clouding of consciousness not uncommonly punctuated by lucid intervals, is characteristic of this state. The affect of the delirious patient may vary from apathy to irritable restlessness, and the autonomically modulated visceral concomitants may follow a corresponding spectrum.

### ■ What principles ought to be followed in the choice of psychoactive drugs for treatment of this spectrum of psychiatric disorders?

Based on the neurobiologic principle of balance, the disturbance of which is accompanied by psychopathology and often by very undesirable psychophysiologic visceral and behavioral concomitants in critically ill patients, the goal in the use of psychoactive drugs should be the restoration of physiologic reciprocity between opposing ergotropic and trophotropic systems, a situation wherein clarity of cognitive function, smoothness of visceral autonomic activity, and overall behavioral control may be recovered.

Table 4-2 summarizes a fairly reliable approach to the use of a modest number of drugs whose dosage range, site of principal CNS action, and expectable effects are fairly clear. Efficacy is claimed for literally scores of psychoactive drugs produced under a wide variety of trade names, too numerous for the average clinician to develop personal experience with. A wise course, particularly for the physician treating acute, life-threatening ill-

**Table 4-2.** Psychoactive drugs for the critically ill and effective dosage ranges

| Drug class | Generic name | Trade name | Daily adult dose range (mg)* | |
|---|---|---|---|---|
| | | | High | Moderate |
| Benzodiazepines | Chlordiazepoxide | Librium | 150-300 | 75-150 |
| | Diazepam | Valium | 30-60 | 15-30 |
| | Oxazepam | Serax | 75-120 | 45-75 |
| | Clorazepate | Tranxene | 45-90 | 25-45 |
| Butyrophenone | Haloperidol | Haldol | 15-60 | 6-15 |

*Reduce by one half for IM use.

nesses of limited duration, is to master the use of a small group of drugs of antianxiety, antipsychotic, and antidepressant classes and to know their actions and interactions, their modes of administration, dosage ranges, and potential side effects.

## ■ What antianxiety drugs are most useful for critical care patients?

As antianxiety agents, the benzodiazepines are preferable to the meprobamate group, being available in both oral and parenteral form, which the latter are not; likewise the benzodiazepines are preferable to the barbiturates in not significantly depressing cerebrocortical functions in dosage ranges wherein tranquilizing is achievable. The four available benzodiazepines, chlordiazepoxide (Librium), diazepam (Valium), oxazepam (Serax), and clorazepate (Tranxene), are essentially identical except for dose and duration of action, chlordiazepoxide being the longest acting and oxazepam the shortest acting of the group. All rank with the moderate- or long-acting barbiturates, such as phenobarbital, in duration of action. Although oxazepam is an active metabolite of diazepam, poorer bowel absorption necessitates a larger dose. There is pharmacologic evidence to suggest that the antianxiety effects of the benzodiazepines are the result of action in limbic forebrain and limbic midbrain areas rather than on the reticular formation, an important site of barbiturate and nonbarbiturate sedative-hypnotic action. The interruption of serotonergic neurotransmission in limbic suppressor sites appears to block the avoidance (trophotropic) side of approach-avoidance conflict and in so doing reduces fear and tension, permitting more physiologic balance between opposing "go" and "no go" systems.[19]

## ■ How may depression be managed among the critically ill?

The kinds of depressive syndromes encountered in critically ill patients are generally reactive to or concomitants of the overwhelming illness being treated and more often than not are associated with considerable reactive anxiety or agitation. Since the clearest indication for the use of tricyclic antidepressants is in retarded, endogenous, or psychotic depressions, and since an average of 2 to 3 weeks is generally required for clear-cut efficacy to become apparent from the use of these drugs, they are best avoided in critically ill patients. One of the benzodiazepine group of antianxiety agents is often of some use in depressed patients with prominent symptoms of tension, anxiety, or somatic complaints. Controlled trials indicate that antianxiety drugs may be useful in these types of depression.[20] Because of the danger of inhibition of monoamine oxidase (MAO) in critically ill patients, many of whom might require vasopressor circulatory support or sympathomimetic bronchodilator inhalation aerosols, the use of MAO inhibitors is best avoided in the care of the critically ill.

## ■ What are the most desirable antipsychotic drugs for the seriously ill or injured patient?

At present the most widely used antipsychotic agents are of the phenothiazine class, with chlorpromazine (Thorazine) the most thoroughly studied member of the class. In comparison to trifluoperazine (Stelazine) or fluphenazine (Prolixin, Permitil), it is of lower potency and has greater sedative effect. The potential of phenothiazines, particularly chlorpromazine, to block $\alpha$-adrenergic vasopressor receptor sites and to intensify the vasodilating and other $\beta$-adrenergic effects of epinephrine together with other autonomic side effects makes this class of drug less desirable for use in the seriously ill patient than the newer butyrophenone compound haloperidol (Haldol). This agent is rapidly and completely absorbed from the gastrointestinal tract and is available in injectable form as well. It causes little autonomic nervous system receptor blockage and has no adverse interactions with digitalis, diuretics, or other cardiovascular drugs. For the elderly, for those with cardiovascular disease, and for the deliriously excited patient it may be the drug of choice where psychotic behavior and confusion require drug treatment.[21]

### ■ What elements in the critical care treatment program itself bear scrutiny with respect to their psychologic effects on the patient?

Considerations such as those outlined in this chapter should call attention once more, amid a medical technology revolution, to man as the proper measure of relevance for invention. And meaning is the measure by which a man unifies and integrates the world as individually perceived. This refers to the personal significance of the information input for the receiver. How the individual interprets the somatic and visceral sensory input together with the environmental surroundings is of crucial importance for emotional, psychophysiologic, and behavioral response patterns. Where sensory input is dulled by drugs or disease consequences (anoxemia, azotemia, etc.), or made monotonous by immobilization, fixed lighting, and acoustic input, the additive influence of CNS habituation further isolates and deprives the interpretive cortex of variety and novelty. The net result is diminished meaningfulness of perceptual input, detachment, disengagement from the environmental surroundings, and hypnagogic or dreamlike uprooting from time and place, leading toward outright delusional and hallucinatory experience. Such isolation from the environment deprives the patient of the meaningful information ordinarily depended on to make sensible interpretation of an experience. If the patient cannot organize the input in meaningful terms in relation to past experience, the situation may become chaotic psychologically, the visceral concomitants of this disorganization may sometimes be dangerous (cardiac rate, rhythm, blood pressure, etc.), and the reactive behavior may call for restraints or further sedation, sometimes with additional consequences in terms of sensory deprivation.

### ■ How might supportive treatment be provided in critical care units to best take into account the psychosocial needs of the patient?

Certain practical therapeutic measures suggest themselves as having both preventive and corrective value for such psychiatric syndromes:

1. Of prime importance preventively, as well as practically, in the presence of beginning mental decompensation is the fact and utilization of the potential of a trusting, confident, caring practitioner-patient relationship.[22] The sense of isolation and helplessness in a potentially hostile environment and the overwhelming feeling of powerlessness accompanying this situation can be devastating for many patients. A number of persons who have been interviewed in depth following harrowing periods of critical care unit experience have testified to the power of trust and hope in tiding them through the experience. The degree of trust and magical power attributed to their physicians appeared proportional to the length of and overall quality of the relationship antedating the critical illness.

2. As a corollary of the point just mentioned, although it is not the rule to anticipate the admission to critical care units for those acutely medically ill, it is possible to anticipate or plan such care for elective surgical patients, as in the case of cardiac, pul-

monary, or other major surgical problems. Time spent familiarizing the patient with the broad plan of postoperative care, a visit to the intensive care unit with some explanation of the purpose and the life-supportive power of much of the technologic equipment, and a personal meeting with some of the key nursing and medical staff who will be responsible for the patient's welfare can increase the patient's understanding of and trust in the place and persons in whose care his or her life is to be placed.

3. During the course of critical care periodic physical examination for signs of deteriorating function and mental examination in terms of level of attention, concentration, and time orientation will allow early application of corrective therapy.

4. Overdependency on monitoring and telemetric equipment at the expense of regular, reassuring, and supportive personal contact with the patient by critical care personnel should be avoided.

5. All procedures should be explained to the patient in simple, clear terms. Movement should be as unrestrained as is consistent with the disease under treatment; the patient should be engaged, as much as possible, in the actions of grooming, eating, drinking, and toileting.

6. Where possible, the patient should be surrounded by personally familiar bedside objects, for example, clock, radio, or family photos, and should be allowed brief visits by the family.

7. Oversedation and excessive use of narcotic analgesics should be avoided, with alertness for the paradoxical responses to such medications that are occasionally seen, especially in the young or the elderly. The benzodiazepines or butyrophenone, which depress cortical functions much less than subcortical ones, are in general preferable to narcotics or barbiturates and can be utilized to lower the required dosages of the latter where indicated.

## SUMMARY

Our overall view is that many, if not most, patients meet the challenge of acute, severe illness or injury with admirable equanimity and fortitude. The physical setting of the critical care unit itself, forbidding as it appears to the uninitiated even among medical and nursing staff assigned to duty elsewhere in the hospital, need not be unduly stressful to the patient if the human concern, interest, and caring attitude of the critical care staff in whose hands his or her life and welfare have been placed can be sensed. The humanizing element of person-to-person contact is capable of rapidly desensitizing the patient to the alarm, fear, or bewilderment that strikes the visitor to such intensive care units. An understanding of basic neurobiologic and psychologic principles in constructing a medical and nursing care program for the critically ill is fundamental to improving the quality of the experience for the patient and may well contribute significantly to lowered mortality risk for certain types of illness or injury.

## REFERENCES

1. Kiely, W. F.: Psychiatric aspects of critical care, Crit. Care Med. **2**:139-142, 1974.
2. Kiely, W. F.: Coping with severe illness, Adv. Psychosom. Med. **8**:105-118, 1972.
3. Engel, G. L., and Romano, J.: Delirium, a syndrome of cerebral insufficiency, J. Chronic Dis. **9**:260-276, 1959.
4. Lipowski, Z. J.: Physical illness, the individual, and the coping processes, Psychiatry Med. **1**:91-96, 1970.
5. Blachly, P. H., and Starr, A.: Post-cardiotomy delirium, Am. J. Psychiatry **121**: 371, 1964.
6. Kornfeld, D. S., Zimberg, S., and Malm, J.: Psychiatric complications of open-heart surgery, N. Engl. J. Med. **273**:282-287, 1965.
7. Gilman, S.: Cerebral disorders after open-heart operations, N. Engl. J. Med. **272**:489-494, 1965.
8. Hackett, T. P., Cassem, N. H., and Wishnie, H. A.: Coronary-care unit: appraisal of its psychologic hazards, N. Engl. J. Med. **279**: 1365-1367, 1968.
9. Freedman, S. J., Grunebaum, H. V., and Greenblatt, M.: Perceptual and cognitive changes in sensory deprivation. In Solomon, P., et al., editors: Sensory deprivation, Cambridge, Mass., 1961, Harvard University Press.
10. Weisman, A. D., and Hackett, T. P.: Psychosis after eye surgery, N. Engl. J. Med. **258**:1284-1287, 1958.

11. Leiderman, P. H., et al.: Sensory deprivation: clinical aspects, Arch. Intern. Med. **101**:389-393, 1958.
12. McKegney, F. P.: The intensive-care syndrome, Conn. Med. **30**:633-636, 1966.
13. Gellhorn, E., and Kiely, W. F.: Mystical states of consciousness: neurophysiological and clinical aspects, J. Nerv. Ment. Dis. **154**: 399-405, 1972.
14. Gellhorn, E., and Kiely, W. F.: Autonomic nervous system in psychiatric disorder. In Mendels, J., editor: Biological psychiatry, New York, 1973, John Wiley & Sons, Inc.
15. Hess, W. R.: The functional organization of the diencephalon, New York, 1958, Grune & Stratton, Inc.
16. Gellhorn, E.: Principles of autonomic-somatic integrations, Minneapolis, 1967, University of Minnesota Press.
17. Kety, S.: Brain amines and affective disorders. In Ho, B. T., and McIsaac, W. M., editors: Brain chemistry in mental diseases, New York, 1971, Plenum Publishing Corporation.
18. Gellhorn, E.: Further studies on the physiology and pathophysiology of tuning of the central nervous system, Psychosomatics **10**: 94-104, 1969.
19. Wise, C. D., Berger, B. D., and Stein, L.: Benzodiazepines: anxiety-reducing activity by reduction of serotonin turnover in brain, Science **177**:180-183, 1972.
20. Raskin, A., Schulterbrandt, J. G., Reatig, N., Crook, T. H., and Odle, D.: Depression subtypes and responses to phenelzine, diazepam, and placebo, Arch. Gen. Psychiatry **30**:66-75, 1974.
21. Appleton, W. S., and Davis, J. M.: Practical clinical psychopharmacology, New York, 1973, Medcom Press.
22. Holland, J., Sgroi, S. M., Marivit, S. J., and Solkoff, N.: The ICU syndrome: fact or fancy, Psychiatry Med. **4**:241-249, 1973.

*chapter 5*

# Prehospital emergency care

JOYCE CARNES
EUGENE NAGEL
DONNA A. ZSCHOCHE

One of the most outstanding recent advances in emergency care has been the delivery of emergency treatment to the ill and injured at the scene of the incident and during transportation to an emergency facility. In prior times many persons involved in an accident or medical emergency received inadequate medical care. They were merely placed in an emergency vehicle and transported to the nearest hospital with little attempt made to stabilize their condition or to prevent further complications.[1, 2] The patient was usually referred to as the victim, and in most situations this was precisely the situation; the patient was a victim not only of the emergency situation, but also of inadequate treatment and handling.

Emergency care, as one of the newest critical care specialties, is defined as a practice of definitive initial care with the major emphasis on triage and stabilization. If we consider critical care medicine as divided into three levels, it may help to define emergency prehospital medicine more clearly. The three areas are intensive care (IC), emergency department care (EDC), and prehospital emergency care (EC). All represent levels of critical care practice. They differ in terms of diagnostic information available, treatment modalities available, and time allowable in which to apply these already limited skills.

The development of prehospital emergency care had its origins in the physician's house call, American Red Cross first aid, and military medicine. The concept of emergency care extending to *medical* care and not just lay-administered first aid, began with medical corpsmen, pharmacist mates, and specially trained paramedics who delivered critical care in the field. By 1963 Day[3] had evolved a method of continuous monitoring and early definitive treatment for the high-risk coronary patient. It was an easy step for Pantridge in Belfast, Ireland,[4] Lareng in Toulouse, France,[5] and the Russians to take these methods into the field. Thus mobile coronary care was added to Day's original in-hospital method. The physician-directed unit idea was brought to the United States by Grace[6] (New York) and Warren (Ohio). Nagel[7] and Lareng[5] first experimented with telemetry, and it was their idea that technicians could be directed in emergency care procedures by hospital-based physicians using special communication facilities.

Emergency medical systems (EMS) are being developed to deliver immediate critical care to the scene of an incident. Paramedical personnel specializing in prehospital care in a mobile intensive care unit equipped with basic and advanced life-support equipment, working through a communication system with a physician or critical care nurse based at the hospital, can provide vital life-support assistance to stabilize a patient prior to transport to a hospital. The main objective of this chapter is to outline the steps in evaluating and treating the critically ill patient before arriving at the hospital. Both basic treatment and treatment that can be provided via the mobile intensive care unit will be discussed. A complete discussion would be an entire book, so this discussion will serve to highlight examples of what can now be done in prehospital care for the more common disorders.

## THE PREHOSPITAL ARENA

### ■ What are the components of the prehospital care system?

The developing critical care systems vary in different localities, but the basic components include personnel specifically trained in providing critical care in the prehospital environment, equipment and medications, a vehicle for transportation, and a communication system linking the unit with a base medical facility. However, this unit is not fully developed in many areas of the United States, and prehospital critical care varies in what can be accomplished, depending on the availability and development of each of the components.

### ■ How does a prehospital team function typically?

Regardless of the location or situation, the goal of the prehospital team is to reach the scene of the incident quickly, to stabilize the patient's condition at the scene, and to transport the patient safely to an appropriate medical facility for definitive care.

### ■ What are the limitations of the prehospital care system?

The medical or surgical emergencies that are treated in the field are limited. There are limitations on the availability of equipment and personnel, but even when a well-equipped advanced life-support unit is available, not every condition can or should be treated in the field. The goal of the prehospital system is to stabilize, not to provide more extensive definitive care. Laboratory, x-ray, and other diagnostic facilities are not available. A physician may be available via a communications system, but not usually at the scene. Those conditions that can await medical treatment without danger to the patient before transportation to a hospital need not be treated at the scene. Certain other conditions require diagnostic information or treatment modalities not available at the scene, such as surgical intervention, and the patient must be transported to a facility where these procedures can be carried out. The prehospital personnel in communication with the base facility must evaluate the situation and make a decision as to urgency, ability to treat, and where and when to transport the patient to the base facility.

Conditions at the scene of an incident are rarely as ordered as they are in the hospital setting. The patient, instead of being on a gurney in a well-equipped room, may be in a very inconvenient position in a closet-like room or pinned in a vehicle. Crowds of overeager bystanders or hysterical friends and relatives may hamper rescue operations. Sterile conditions are not obtainable when the patient is lying beside the road in the mud, and lighting is seldom adequate. Frequently not every type of supply and equipment is available, so treatment must be altered to accomplish the most that is possible by improvising with what is at hand. The medical person who is confident with almost any situation in the hospital may not be familiar with field conditions or function as well in the field and may be at a loss as to what to do.

### ■ How does prehospital care differ in rural areas vs the urban environment?

The urban system for providing critical prehospital care has every advantage over the rural system: minimal distance to travel, multiple hospitals, opportunity for personnel to maintain their level of experience, good communications, more tax dollars available, and nearby training opportunities; the list could go on. These factors should highlight the difficulties in providing minimal or near-adequate care in the rural setting. Because of the distances involved in the rural environment, there is delay in reaching the critically ill patient, and if his or her condition cannot be completely stabilized at the scene, there is the factor of the miles and critical time separating the scene of the injury or illness from a medical facility. The paradox is apparent. The low incidence of calls, large distances, and long times involved make critical care more important to a successful outcome in the rural area, but much more difficult to provide. It is a realm of volunteer personnel, multiple-use personnel, and making good use of what is available. It is therefore surprising to find examples throughout the country of rural systems offering a surprisingly high quality of emergency care. The need for more such systems is obvious.

## ON-THE-SCENE EVALUATION

### ■ What should be included in the initial evaluation of patients in the field?

The emergency on-the-scene examination is carried out according to priorities, with life-threatening conditions being treated as soon as they are recognized, instead of performing the complete physical examination as is done in an elective in-hospital or office setting. There are certain situations in which the patient must be removed from a dangerous or potentially dangerous situation, such as fire or contact with a live electric wire, before evaluation for the critical "ABC's" (airway, breathing, and circulation) may be carried out. Otherwise, the lives of the victim and the rescuer would be threatened. Other than this, an orderly evaluation for an open airway, presence of adequate respiration, and a pulse should be made in *all* patients and deficiencies corrected before taking time to obtain a history or continue the physical examination. Adequacy of these basic, life-sustaining functions may seem apparent in the alert, minimally ill or injured patient, but additional efforts must be made to assure these functions when there is any doubt. It is inexcusable to focus on dressing and splinting an open fracture while the patient is becoming hypoxic from a totally obstructed airway.

Subsequent examination will depend on the situation. It may not be necessary or even appropriate to perform a complete examination in the field. For many conditions the examination is limited to the involved systems, but in the case of generalized trauma such as occurs in a vehicle accident or fall an abbreviated but comprehensive examination should be carried out. After assuring the ABC's, the rescuer must determine whether there is any serious bleeding, either external or internal, and when present, take measures to control this condition before proceeding. After these urgent conditions are evaluated, a "head-to-toe" examination is made. At the scene of an accident it is usually not practical or appropriate to completely undress a patient to perform this examination. Part of the examination will involve palpating through clothing, determining the most serious problems, and waiting until the patient arrives in the emergency room for a more thorough examination. When conditions indicate, however, the examination in the field will demand removal of clothing to permit treatment of the affected part.

In all cases the examination is pointed toward the detection of potentially life-threatening conditions. The order of the examination may vary with different examiners, but the following basics should be included after the previously mentioned problems have been treated:

1. State of consciousness and general appearance
2. Inspection of the chest for symmetric movements and presence of fractures and, where appropriate, checking for percussion tone and presence of clear breath sounds bilaterally to determine presence of a pneumothorax or flail chest.
3. Examination of the face and scalp for lacerations and contusions with possible bleeding or underlying fractures
4. Observation of the pupils for equality and reaction to light, denoting CNS damage; noting this may be important as a baseline for future examination
5. Gentle palpation along the cervical spine for the presence of tenderness or deformity (accomplished without moving the patient's neck), indicating fractures; examination for shift of the trachea from the midline
6. Inspection and palpation of the abdomen for possible trauma to organs or

vessels (In the field it usually is not practical to auscultate for bowel sounds.)

7. Stressing the pelvis to determine the presence of fractures and possible source of shock
8. Observation and palpation of the extremities for soft tissue injuries and fractures and determination of gross sensory and motor function to determine possible spinal cord damage; where any indication of vascular compromise, pulses to be checked
9. Examination of the back for spine fractures and soft tissue injuries (When no neurologic deficit exists but there is suspicion of spine injury, the spine can be gently palpated with the examiner's fingers without moving the patient, and if a neurologic deficit is present, further examination in the field may not be indicated.)

In the critically ill patient the examination will necessarily be even more abbreviated and limited to the most serious problems.

### ■ What type of history should be obtained in the field?

The history is usually obtained in conjunction with the examination rather than waiting to complete a history before beginning the examination. The status of the patient will determine how much time can be devoted to history taking. If the patient is in cardiac arrest or has sustained severe injury, immediate treatment takes priority. However, in most cases a quick history can be obtained that will aid in evaluating the the patient's condition. This history will not be unlike that which would be obtained in the emergency room, although more abbreviated. Occasionally there will be family or bystanders available only at the scene who may have information that would be valuable if transmitted to the medical personnel at the hospital. Information regarding a description of the incident, past medical history, current medications, and recent changes in the health or behavior of the patient should be elicited from these persons, especially if the patient is unconscious or confused.

Careful observation at the scene can provide important information. For example, at the scene of a vehicle accident, findings that may be important include the following:

1. Location of the patient. Was the person thrown from the vehicle, and if so, where did he or she land? These data may be an index of the severity of impact. Was the patient a pedestrian? Did the patient remain in the vehicle, and if so, as the driver or as a passenger in the front or back seat?

2. Indications of impact. A broken windshield may indicate possible head injury, and a bent or bloody dashboard gives evidence of head, trunk, or extremity injury. A bent steering wheel implicates chest injury with possible rib fractures, pneumothorax, flail chest, hemothorax, or cardiac contusion.

3. Seat belts. Were seat belts being worn, and if so, what type? If the patient is still strapped in, was the seat belt in proper position over the pelvis? Or was it over the abdomen? Some injuries are found more commonly when a seat belt is worn.[8-10] Noting that a seat belt was worn, particularly if it was improperly applied and the accident was severe, and reporting that information to the emergency room personnel may alert them to injuries that otherwise might not be considered.

## AIRWAY AND VENTILATION

### ■ How is airway obstruction recognized?

The airway may be obstructed by secretions, vomitus, foreign bodies, or soft tissue. Obstruction may range from partial obstruction with minimal ventilatory effect to total occlusion that, if not corrected, will lead invariably to cardiac arrest and death. Signs of obstruction may be obvious, but they may be so subtle as to be missed unless a conscious effort is made to look for them. Partial obstruction is indicated by stridor or snoring sounds. Suprasternal, supraclavicular, or intercostal (especially in children) retractions may be present along with labored breathing and use of accessory muscles. In severe obstruction there will be cyanosis, and with developing hypoxia, agitation. Finally, there will be loss of consciousness. A person found unconscious may appear to be sleeping, whereas actually the person is not breathing at all. If movement of air is not felt from the nose or mouth, immediate action must be taken.

## ■ How is the airway opened?

Unless foreign body obstruction of the airway is present, an open airway can usually be attained by proper positioning of the head and neck. Obstruction of the airway in the unconscious person commonly occurs when the tongue falls back into the pharynx. Hyperextension of the neck will elevate the tongue, thereby opening the airway. An oropharyngeal airway can then be inserted, with caution being taken not to force the tongue back into the throat with the insertion. An alternate method to extension of the neck is elevation of the mandible. When vomitus or secretions are present, they are removed by suction or with the examiner's finger, if suction is not immediately available.

## ■ How can the airway be opened when a cervical spine injury is suspected?

When an unstable cervical spine injury is present, movement of the neck may cause cervical cord compression with permanent damage. Therefore when there is any suspicion of cervical spine injury, every effort must be made not to move the neck. If there is airway obstruction, the airway can usually be opened by first stabilizing the head through placing one hand on either side of the patient's head and then displacing the mandible forward by pushing against the angles of the mandible with each index finger. If this is not effective, an attempt should be made to insert an oropharyngeal or nasopharyngeal airway without moving the neck. If there is still life-threatening obstruction, a decision must be made either to perform a cricothyrotomy or to take the risk involved in extending the neck slightly more until an airway is obtained and then stabilizing the neck in that position.

## ■ What else can be done to elevate soft tissue that is obstructing the airway?

Fractures of the mandible may lead to loss of support of the tongue and tissues of the oropharynx with consequent airway obstruction. In many cases this obstruction can be relieved by grasping the tongue and pulling it forward. Better traction can be obtained with a 4 × 4 inch gauze or cloth.

## ■ What should be done to remove a foreign body from the airway?

A foreign body that is totally obstructing the airway must be removed or the airway otherwise opened immediately if the patient is to survive with salvageable cerebral status. It does little good to perform closed chest massage if no oxygen is reaching the lungs. Initial attempts to ventilate a patient who is properly positioned will usually reveal obstruction when it is present. The obstruction will be felt as resistance, and the chest will not rise when positive pressure is applied.

Persons have been known to aspirate astonishingly large pieces of meat.[11] These usually lodge at the vocal cords, and phonation is prevented. The victim may grasp at the throat, become cyanotic, and then collapse (the typical "cafe coronary"). Foreign body aspiration should be a prime consideration when someone suddenly collapses while eating.

The "Heimlich maneuver" as developed by Dr. Henry J. Heimlich, Director of Surgery at Jewish Hospital in Cincinnati, Ohio, is a simple first-aid maneuver that may be used in dealing with "cafe coronaries." There is some residual air trapped in the lungs when a foreign body is aspirated. The Heimlich method advocates applying quick upward pressure against the victim's abdomen below the rib cage. The foreign body is thereby expelled from the larynx.

This maneuver was developed as an alternative to emergency tracheostomy and especially as a first-aid technique that laymen can use. Some complications from the procedure have been reported, but this technique may be life saving.[12, 13]

The foreign object can sometimes be removed by sweeping the index finger or the index and middle fingers deeply across the back of the throat. If a laryngoscope is at hand, and if there are personnel trained in its use, the foreign body can usually be removed under direct visualization. If the preceding measures fail, the object may be dislodged by turning the patient on the side and delivering sharp blows with the heel of the hand between the victim's shoulder blades. The small child with persistent upper airway obstruction can be inverted over the rescuer's arm while the blows are delivered. As a last resort, cricothyrotomy may be required in an adult patient.[14]

## ■ What should be done in the field for a child who has partial obstruction of the lower airway?

It is not uncommon for a child to aspirate a small object (for example, a peanut or a small plastic toy) through the larynx and into one of the main stem bronchi, most often on the right. Respiratory difficulty may be present, and there may even be audible wheezing. It is important at this point to determine that there is air exchange to one lung by noting movement of air through the nose or mouth, observing the chest for appropriate movement with respiration and the absence of suprasternal, supraclavicular, or intercostal retractions, and auscultating for breath sounds. If there is ventilation to one side, oxygen should be administered, and the patient should then be transported to a facility where a definitive procedure can be accomplished under controlled conditions. Attempts to dislodge an object that is only partially obstructing the airway may result in its being moved to the upper airway, where it may cause complete obstruction.

## ■ What is an esophageal obturator airway?

The esophageal obturator airway is a relatively new concept in emergency care (Fig. 5-1). It is especially well suited to field situations, as no direct visualization of the vocal cords is necessary for its insertion, and it requires less skill to insert than an endotracheal tube. Its use at this time is limited to adult patients without a gag reflex. It consists of an endotracheal-like tube mounted through a face mask. The tube is cuffed and has a closed end. There are multiple openings in the upper third of the tube at the level of the pharynx. The tube is inserted into the

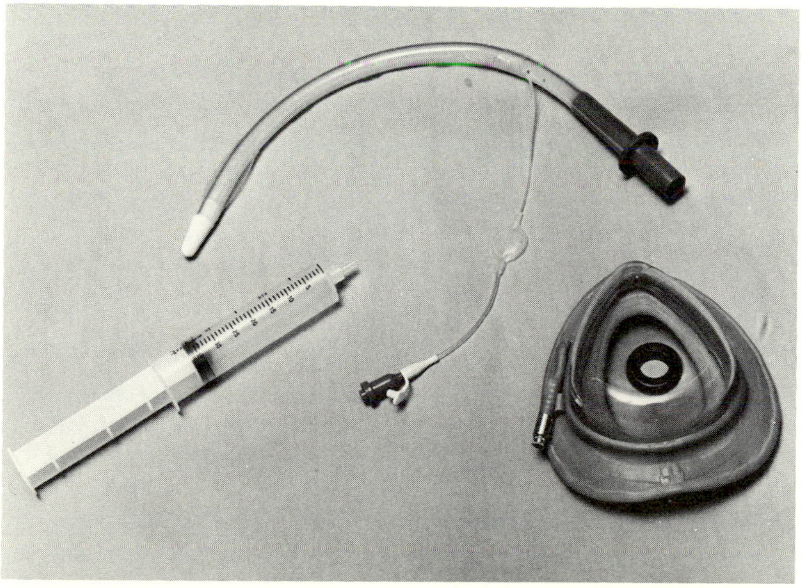

**Fig. 5-1.** Esophageal Airway. (Courtesy DynaMed Inc., Leucadia, Calif.)

esophagus, and once its position there is confirmed by seeing the chest rise and by listening for breath sounds, the cuff is inflated with 35 cc of air, thus occluding the esophagus distally. A tight seal is made with the mask against the patient's face, and air or oxygen is delivered through the tube and enters the oropharynx via the multiple openings. Since the esophagus is blocked and the seal of the mask prevents escape of air, the air will enter the trachea. The esophageal airway has been used to successfully ventilate numerous patients in the field. In addition to providing adequate ventilation, this device, by blocking off the esophagus, also tends to prevent gastric distention and regurgitation during resuscitation.

Frequently regurgitation of stomach contents occurs when the esophageal airway is removed, and it is imperative that suction be available and that the patient be positioned properly before its removal so that aspiration does not occur. When an endotracheal tube becomes available, it can be inserted under direct vision and the esophageal airway removed after the trachea is protected. However, adequate ventilation via the esophageal airway cannot be provided when the mask is not firmly in place, and the usual precautions must be taken to assure adequate oxygenation during the transition between the two forms of ventilation.

### ■ When is a cricothyrotomy indicated?

In some instances the airway may not be opened by the usual methods, and the obstruction may be complete enough to cause hypoxia, leading to serious deterioration or death, before the patient can be transported to the hospital. A foreign body may wedge between the vocal cords and instruments will not be available to extract it, or severe facial trauma may prevent access to the airway via the nose or mouth. In dire circumstances such as these, immediate access to the airway below the obstruction must be made. Even in skilled hands and under optimum circumstances, a tracheostomy may require several minutes to complete, and by the time the previously outlined methods have been attempted, little if any time remains. A cricothyrotomy will provide the fastest access to the trachea. The cricothyroid membrane is located just below the thyroid cartilage (the most prominent cartilage or "Adam's apple"). There is little overlying tissue in this area and less chance of bothersome bleeding. The opening can be maintained by insertion of an object that will not be aspirated.[15, 16]

An alternative to the cricothyrotomy that may be more adaptable to use by unskilled persons at the scene of an incident is needle puncture of the cricothyroid membrane.[17] This needle is then attached to high-flow oxygen. It must be understood that this is a stopgap method and that the patient must be transported as quickly as possible to a facility where a more adequate airway can be established. The flow of oxygen to the lungs must be carefully monitored so that large intrapulmonary pressures are not produced, particularly in the case of apneic patients, and provision made for exhalation.

## CIRCULATORY INADEQUACY

It has been estimated that 1 million people suffer heart attacks in the United States each year. Of the 650,000 people who die each year as a result of ischemic heart disease, over half die outside the hospital. Many of these deaths can be prevented if proper action is taken immediately at the scene of collapse and if equipment and skilled personnel are available soon thereafter to stabilize the patient's condition prior to transport to the hospital. It was for this reason that mobile intensive care units (MICU's) were first put into use, and many patients have since been resuscitated at the scene of cardiac arrest.

### ■ How is cardiac arrest treated at the scene?

No special equipment is needed to diagnose cardiac arrest. It is recognized by absence of a pulse in the large arteries (carotid or femoral) in an unconscious patient. If the cardiac arrest is reliably known to have been present for more than 10 minutes without cardiopulmonary resuscitation (CPR), irreversible cerebral damage is likely to be severe, and resuscitative efforts are usually not begun. However, if there is any question as to the duration of the arrest, the patient should be given the benefit of the doubt and CPR started. Exceptions to the 10-minute time limit are infants suffering cardiac arrest and individuals with hypothermia, each of whom may survive with less severe neurologic deficit.

CPR should be started as soon as the diagnosis of cardiac arrest is made (except as stated previously) so that oxygen can begin to be provided to the brain while equipment and resuscitative medications are being made available. The victim must be in a supine position on an unyielding surface in order for effective cardiac output to be produced from external chest compression. The patient who is sitting in a chair or stadium seat or lying on a stairway or a very soft mattress must first be moved to the closest firm surface, usually the floor. When an advanced life-support unit is available, resuscitative procedures, including defibrillation, ventilation via esophageal or endotracheal airway, administration of cardiotonic and antiarrhythmic medications, and continuous cardiac monitoring, can be carried out at the scene under voice communication with a physician or certified mobile intensive care nurse at the base hospital. In some systems the cardiac rhythm can be observed by the base hospital personnel via telemetry. Within the boundaries of an emergency medical service, the patient in cardiac arrest receives not only basic life support, but also definitive therapy. The condition is stabilized at the scene before transport, and medical care is given during transport to the hospital. Pneumatic assist devices may be useful adjuncts in the provision of CPR both on the scene and during transport.

In certain situations it will be impossible to stabilize the patient's condition in the field. If advanced life-support units are not available or if the rescue team has been at the scene for approximately 30 minutes and no response to therapy is noted, the patient may need to be transported to an emergency facility where additional treatment can be obtained. Procedures such as open-chest cardiac massage, insertion of pacemaker wires, or venous cutdown are best performed in the hospital setting.

For more detailed information on cardiopulmonary resuscitation the reader is referred to the latest standards established by the American Heart Association and the National Academy of Sciences–National Research Council. Information can be obtained from the local chapter of the American Heart Association.

## TRAUMATIC INJURY

### ■ How is bleeding controlled in the field?

Almost all external bleeding can be stopped by direct pressure over the wound. A sterile compress is not always readily available at the scene of an accident, and if bleeding is profuse, pressure can be applied with the closest clean cloth or even with the bare hand if necessary. After bleeding is slowed by manual or digital pressure, a pressure dressing may have to be applied to some wounds in order to maintain hemostasis during transport to the hospital.

If direct pressure is not effective or if the rescuer cannot apply direct pressure to the wound, as may be the case with a patient trapped in a vehicle, applying pressure to a major artery proximal to the wound may diminish the flow of blood. If neither direct nor proximal pressure control bleeding, a tourniquet may be necessary. Adverse effects from tourniquets include compressive nerve damage from a too-narrow band, ischemic limb damage, and possible loss of the limb. The tourniquet should be used only when the threat to life from blood loss justifies possible loss of the limb. It should be applied as distally as possible and tightly enough to stop all arterial flow. Once applied it should not be loosened until the patient is in the hospital. The time when the tourniquet was applied should be noted and that information transmitted to the emergency room with the patient.

The use of hemostats in the field is not recommended because visualization of the bleeding vessels is usually not adequate. Probing around inside a wound can cause further damage, and a hemostat mistakenly clamped on a nerve can cause irreversible damage. Only physicians thoroughly familiar with the anatomy involved and with surgical techniques should attempt hemostasis with hemostats in the field.

### ■ How is severe bleeding with shock managed in the field?

Control of bleeding is the top priority in the treatment of hemorrhage. If there is severe bleeding from internal injury that cannot be stopped, it may be necessary to transport the patient to a hospital immediately, with other treatment being instituted en route. Oxygen should be administered to augment the diminished oxygen-carrying capacity of the blood. If there are no fractures of the lower extremities, elevating the legs will provide increased venous return to the heart. If IV fluids are available, one or preferably two lines are established using large-bore needles, and rapid volume replacement is begun using various ionic or colloid solutions such as Ringer's lactate solution, albumin, dextrose in saline solution, or dextran.

### ■ What is done to an impaled object?

A not uncommon occurrence in the field is to find a patient who has been stabbed with an object such as a knife, ice pick, or pencil or who is impaled through the trunk, extremity, or even head with a sharp object as the result of a vehicle accident. In almost all instances the impaled object should be left in place, since removal could release tamponade of a bleeding source or could conceivably cause additional injury in the process of extraction. The protruding portion of the object should be stabilized with a bulky dressing to prevent it from moving during transport, with consequent further damage.

### ■ How is chest injury evaluated and treated in the field?

First, observation is made for adequacy and difficulty of respiration, including whether the airway is open. Immediately life-threatening conditions from chest injury include flail chest, open pneumothorax, tension pneumothorax, massive hemothorax, and cardiac tamponade.

#### *Flail chest*

A flail chest occurs when several ribs are fractured in more than one place, producing a segment of chest wall that moves in the opposite direction from the remainder of the chest wall with inspiration and expiration, that is, "paradoxical movement." If the segment is large enough, there may be severe respiratory embarrassment that will not await treatment until the patient arrives at the hospital. Presence of a flail chest is suspected when there is blunt trauma to the chest such as impact with a steering wheel. In the field initial treatment of the flail chest includes oxygen therapy, placing a hand on the flail segment to decrease the paradoxical movement, stabilizing the segment with sand bags, or placing the patient so that the flail segment is down.

#### *Open pneumothorax*

An open pneumothorax is recognized by hearing a sucking sound as air is drawn in through the open wound. The wound must be covered immediately with the nearest clean object or even with the hand to prevent further respiratory compromise. At the scene there may not be time to find a sterile dressing initially. When the dressing is applied in the field, it should not be completely occlusive, as there is danger of tension pneumothorax developing. The dressing should allow air to exit if increasing intrapleural pressure develops.

#### *Tension pneumothorax*

A tension pneumothorax develops when a flap of tissue allows air to flow into the pleural space with inspiration but closes over the opening to prevent escape of air on expiration. Air and pressure increase in the pleural space, progressively compressing the opposite lung and impairing venous return to the heart. Positive pressure breathing may convert a simple pneumothorax into a tension pneumothorax, and with the increasing use of positive pressure breathing in the field, we can expect to have an increasing incidence of tension pneumothorax. Special care should be taken to repeatedly examine the patient with chest trauma who is on positive pressure breathing to assure that necessary steps are taken if this condition develops at the scene or during transport. This same precaution should be taken in a patient undergoing CPR, as a pneumothorax may be sustained from a rib fracture or attempted intracardiac injection. When severe respiratory distress develops with clinical signs of tension pneumothorax, and if time to the nearest hospital is more than a few minutes, insertion of a large-bore needle into the involved side may be a life-saving procedure.

### *Massive hemothorax*

Little can be done at the scene to correct massive intrathoracic bleeding; this is one of the situations in which immediate transportation to the nearest emergency hospital should be instituted. Even when a MICU is on the scene, if severe shock caused by hemothorax is present, transport should begin immediately, with venipuncture and administration of IV fluid instituted en route.

### *Cardiac tamponade*

Cardiac tamponade is best managed in the hospital setting, but in grave circumstances relief of severe symptoms can be achieved by pericardiocentesis performed by persons trained in this technique.

## ■ What can be done at the scene for a patient with abdominal trauma?

Abdominal trauma can be subdivided into penetrating and nonpenetrating injuries. It is important to know the mechanism of injury and to convey that information to physicians at the hospital. In nonpenetrating trauma the source and type of impact (for example, steering wheel, seat belt, or fall) should be considered. For penetrating wounds both the type and trajectory should be determined. A description of the inflicting agent of a stab wound (knife, ice pick, scissors, bottle glass, etc.) will be helpful. Was the blade 2 or 10 inches long? If at all possible, the object should be brought to the hospital with the patient. The type of gunshot wound, caliber, and approximate distance from the patient when the gun was fired should be included. The abdominal wound from a penetrating injury should be covered with a sterile dressing, and if viscera are exposed, it is especially important that the dressing be moist.

Physical examination at the scene is limited. In addition to observation of the wound, in cases of penetrating trauma palpation may reveal tenderness or guarding, but auscultation is not useful for several reasons:

1. With the typical noise and confusion at this kind of incident, it is difficult to hear even loud bowel sounds, and listening for several minutes is wasting valuable time.
2. Early in the situation, bowel sounds may not be diminished, even in the presence of intestinal injury.
3. The presence or absence of bowel sounds does not change prehospital treatment.

Regardless of the etiology of the trauma, the only immediate life-threatening problem in abdominal injury at the scene is hemorrhage, and therefore, as with chest wounds, when severe shock is present as a result of intra-abdominal bleeding, it is of prime importance to transport the victim to a hospital where surgical intervention can take place without delay. Rapid IV volume replacement, when available, can be initiated en route.

## ■ Is there anything that can be done at the scene of an accident to control intra-abdominal or pelvic bleeding?

A recent advance in this field is the pneumatic compression garment[18] that is similar in some respects to the pilot's G suit (Fig. 5-2). It encases each leg separately, as well as covering the pelvis and abdomen to the rib cage. In cases where there is hypotension and/or trauma to the abdomen, pelvis, or lower extremities suspected, the garment is applied and inflated until the vital signs are restored or the maximum pressure is obtained (2 psi or 107 mm Hg). The garment tends to produce three desirable results:

1. Reduction in hemorrhage in the area of

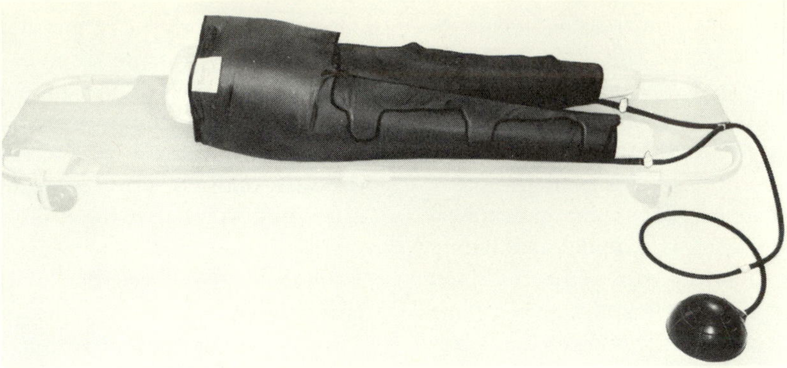

**Fig. 5-2.** Mast Trousers. (Courtesy David Clark, Inc., Worcester, Mass.)

application, including major intra-abdominal bleeding
2. Autotransfusion from lower to upper part of the body, including brain and heart
3. Limitation of effective circulation to upper body, tending to correct hypovolemia in cases of hemorrhagic shock

The garment is a major new weapon in the treatment of the severely traumatized individual in the field.

## ■ How is a head injury treated at the scene?

Other than stopping bleeding from scalp lacerations, little can be done to treat a head injury in the field. Ventilation and circulation are supported. If the patient is in shock, a source other than the head injury is almost always present, and the shock is treated as it usually would be. Concomitant injury to the cervical spine should be considered, and the neck should be splinted during transport. If there will be a delay in arrival at the hospital, the physician stationed there may order steroids to be administered en route but most treatment must await arrival at the hospital.

## ■ How should an extremity fracture be treated prior to transport?

Movement of fracture fragments can lead to injury to vessels, nerves, and adjacent muscles. Stabilizing the fracture site will prevent this injury and will also improve patient comfort. Before splinting, any open wounds should be covered with a dressing. There are many methods for stabilizing fractures, and the type of splint will depend on the site of the fracture and the splinting devices that are available. In most cases the fracture is splinted as it is found, although when there is severe deformity, it may be necessary to apply gentle traction to straighten the extremity in order to fit the patient on a gurney and into the ambulance. If the patient is still in a vehicle, the suspected fracture is splinted prior to removal of the patient. The only exception is when there is danger of fire or heavy traffic that might endanger the rescuer and victim.[19]

Cardboard splints are commonly used for upper arm and lower leg fractures. Cotton batting can be placed around the extremity to prevent movement of the limb in the splint, but before placing the batting, any wounds should be covered with a dressing to keep the batting from sticking to the wound. The cardboard splints come in various sizes and store readily (Fig. 5-3).

Another type of extremity splint is the vacuum splint. This splint consists of a pliable plastic bag filled with small polystyrene plastic balls. The splint is placed around the fracture site, and suction is then applied to a connecting tube. When the air is removed, the splint becomes hard and maintains the fracture in its original deformity.

Air splints consist of a pliable plastic tube that is fitted around the extremity. Air is then

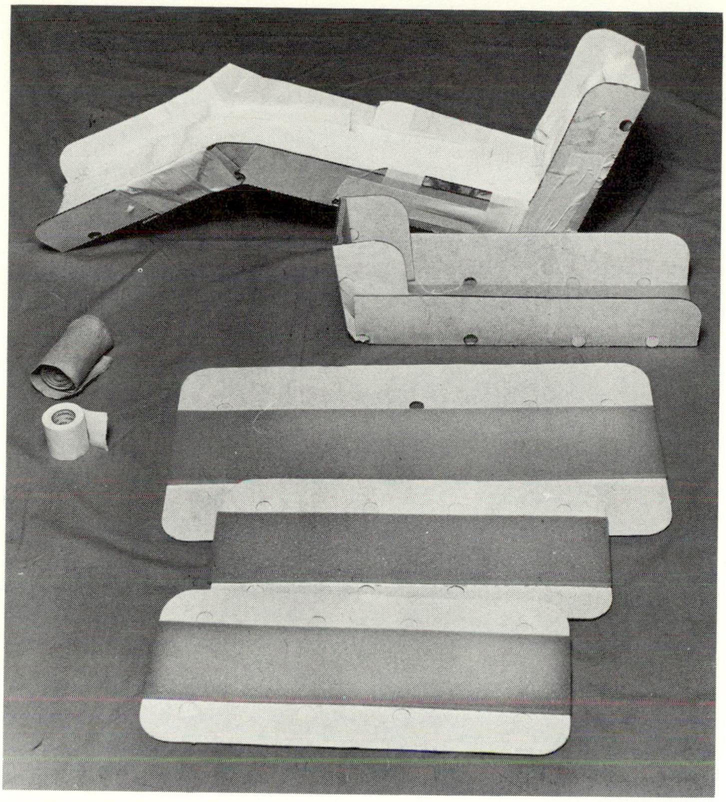

**Fig. 5-3.** Cardboard splints.

blown into the tube. This device is used mainly for nondisplaced distal leg and wrist fractures.

Upper extremity and shoulder fractures or dislocations are stabilized by applying a sling or sling and swath. Hand fractures generally do not require splinting during transport.

Femur fractures are readily stabilized by using a half-ring splint such as the Thomas splint or Hare Traction Splint (Fig. 5-4). This device stabilizes the fracture through the use of traction and provides marked improvement with regard to pain. The splint can be left in place throughout evaluation in the emergency room; if possible, there should be an extra traction splint available in the emergency department to be interchangeable with that of the ambulance so that a busy ambulance is not delayed in returning to service.

When already prepared splints are not available, splints can be improvised from a variety of common objects such as folded newspapers or boards.

### ■ What can be done to stabilize a suspected spine fracture?

Because of the possibility of spinal cord damage from spine injuries, it is essential that any suspected back or neck injury be stabilized as early as possible. When a patient is still in an automobile, the affected area is splinted prior to removing the patient from the vehicle. A short spine board is placed behind the patient's back, and the patient's head and trunk are strapped to the board using cloth strips or tape. If this equipment is not available and there is a suspected neck injury, one rescuer applies traction to the patient's head to maintain the neck in neutral position during extrication procedures. The patient is transported on a backboard, preferably one that is radiolucent so that the patient need not be removed from that surface

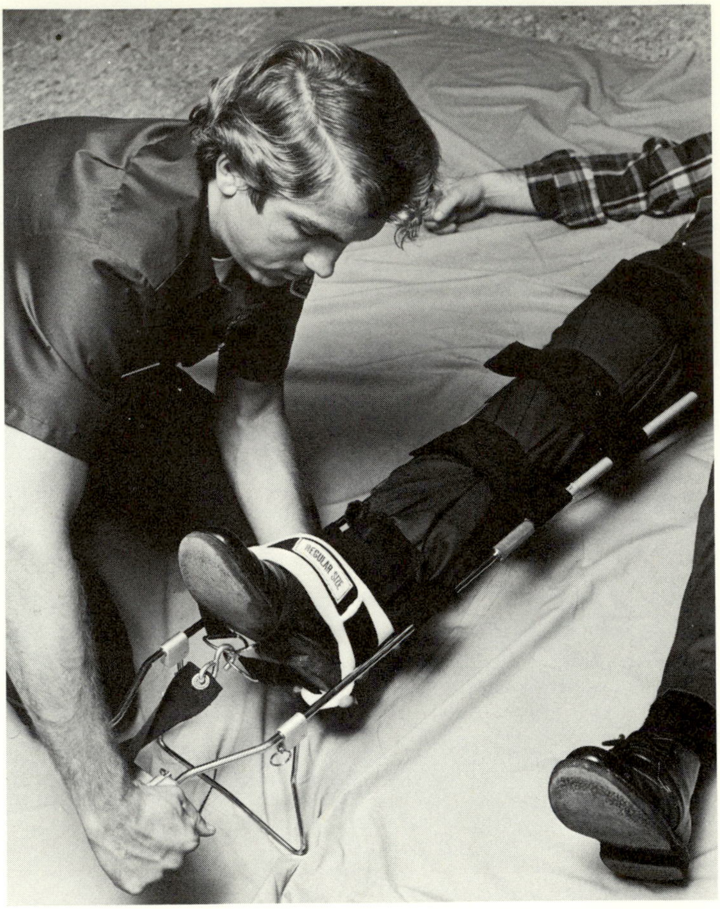

**Fig. 5-4.** Hare Traction Splint. (Courtesy DynaMed Inc., Leucadia, Calif.)

during x-ray examination. In some other instances a soft cervical collar will be used. When it is available, cervical traction can be maintained by applying a chin strap and attaching this to weights. When necessary, a cervical collar can be improvised from folded newspapers.

### ■ When are narcotic analgesics used in the field?

There are very few indications for narcotics such as morphine in prehospital care. Analgesics are contraindicated in most cases of trauma for several reasons:

1. Respiratory depression may result with consequent hypoxia and hypercapnia. This is especially true in persons who already have a respiratory deficit, which may not be readily apparent. Agitated behavior may be caused by hypoxia or hypovolemia rather than by pain, and administration of morphine sulfate may lead to respiratory arrest.

2. Developing symptoms of injury, such as intra-abdominal injuries or head injuries, can be masked, leading to delayed diagnosis and treatment of serious conditions after the patient arrives at the hospital.

3. Morphine sulfate's respiratory depressant effect can lead to hypercapnia with consequent cerebral vasodilatation and exacerbation of the cerebral edema of head injury.

4. Morphine sulfate also causes peripheral vasodilatation. This usually does not cause a drop in blood pressure in the normal supine person, but in a person in shock with compensatory vasoconstriction, this vasodilating

effect may lead to decreased central perfusion.

Morphine sulfate is administered under the direction of a physician in cases of myocardial infarction and pulmonary edema, and it may be indicated in some instances where extrication is required, but in the vast majority of cases narcotic analgesics should not be given until the patient is in the hospital and has been examined by a physician. When given as an analgesic, as in cases of severe burns and extreme pain, it is vital to have IV lines available and to monitor vital signs and respirations.

## ■ How is a burned patient managed in the field?

An extensive burn almost invariably elicits a sense of panic, if not in the patient, at least in the rescuer who has not dealt with burned patients before. It is important for the rescuer to remain calm. Although the burn wound may look like the patient's most imminent problem, it is often not. As is true with treating other emergency patients, the burned patient is approached according to priority needs. In order to provide the best treatment, the patient must first be removed from the source of the burn.

Respiratory, circulatory, and bleeding problems can all be more immediately life-threatening than the burn wound itself, and they should be evaluated before attention is turned to the burn.

Presence of an open airway and adequate respiration are assessed immediately. If the patient was in an enclosed-space fire, airway damage or inhalation of toxic fumes such as carbon monoxide is considered. Because respiratory distress from burns to the airway may not develop until several hours or days after the damage occurs, any patient with suspected inhalation injury should be transported to the hospital for evaluation and observation. Oxygen is administered at the scene and en route in cases of toxic fume inhalation or suspected pulmonary damage.

Immediately after assuring an open airway and breathing, attention is turned to the presence of a pulse. Hypoxia from the inhalation of toxic fumes or electric shock may produce lethal dysrhythmias. If there is no pulse, CPR is started at once.

In cases where there is any chance of additional trauma, examination for the presence of bleeding is made and the bleeding is brought under control. Shock present within an hour after the burn occurs is usually not directly caused by the burn, and other sources such as external or internal blood loss should be sought.

When a burn is associated with a vehicle accident or if the victim has fallen from a height in escaping from the fire, the possible existence of a fracture is investigated. Fractures are stabilized even if it means applying a splint over burned skin, but if possible, a clean dressing or sheet is first applied over the burn. Cotton batting to pad the splint should not be placed directly in contact with the burned tissue.

Burned clothing is removed from the patient, since the clothing may retain heat and increase the depth of the burn. Cold water or ice water application to the burn wound is being recommended by many experts. However, an extensive burn should *not* be packed in ice for long periods of time, since hypothermia and damage can result. No creams or ointments are applied at the scene; the burn is covered with a wet or dry clean sheet. If there will be more than a 30-minute delay before arrival at a hospital, an IV line is established and Ringer's lactate solution is administered en route for patients with burns covering greater than 20% of the body. As a general rule, analgesics are not used in the field for the reasons outlined on pp. 108-109. If there are no complicating conditions, the burned patient does not need to be transported at an unsafe speed. A detailed discussion of burn treatment is found in Chapter 21.

## ■ How is a chemical burn treated?

The principle of first removing the patient from the source of burning is especially true for chemical burns. The offending chemical is copiously irrigated with the most readily available source of water. With rare exceptions, there should be no delay to obtain a special agent for cleansing. All clothing, including underwear, that is permeated with the chemical must be removed if the skin is to be adequately cleansed.

## COMMON MEDICAL EMERGENCIES

### ■ How is a suspected myocardial infarction treated in the field?

A lethal cardiac dysrhythmia may occur early in the course of a myocardial infarction, and therefore it is important that a cardiac care unit be made available to the patient as soon as possible. In many communities this is best provided by an MICU. An IV line is established, using low-flow 5% dextrose in water, as a "life line" to be used to administer medications, and continuous cardiac monitoring is established. Morphine sulfate is administered by the IV route to relieve pain, and oxygen may be administered. Some experts recommend the routine administration of lidocaine.[20, 21] The patient is then transported to the hospital while continuous cardiac monitoring is maintained. If a dysrhythmia develops during this time, it can be treated with the medications and supplies available in the MICU.

### ■ How is the patient with diabetes managed in the field?

The treatment of the patient with uncontrolled diabetes begins in the field. In the unconscious or confused diabetic taking either oral agents or insulin hypoglycemia is a strong consideration, and because hypoglycemia can lead to permanent brain damage, this is one of the problems that can and should be treated in the field. One or more tubes of blood are drawn, and then glucose is given orally if the patient is awake; if the patient is unconscious, 50 to 100 ml of 50% dextrose in water is given by IV administration. For a patient in diabetic coma immediacy of treatment is not as critical as is true when there is severe hypoglycemia.

### ■ How is congestive heart failure treated?

The seriousness of congestive heart failure can vary from a mild problem that can await a visit to the doctor's office to an immediately life-threatening problem that cannot wait even the few minutes' ride in the ambulance to the emergency room. In the former instance no treatment is indicated in the field, but in the latter case treatment is initiated with oxygen; a sitting position and extremity tourniquets are utilized to trap blood in the extremities. Administration of morphine sulfate and furosemide (Lasix) may also be used when available and ordered by the physician at the base hospital.

### ■ How is a patient with severe asthma treated in the field?

When an advanced life-support unit is available, much can be offered the critically ill asthmatic patient in the field when the severity of the disease would endanger life if treatment waited until arrival at the hospital. The patient usually feels best in a sitting position and is allowed to remain in that position during transport. Oxygen is administered, and epinephrine or aminophylline is given, along with 5% dextrose in water solution, intravenously. Sedatives or narcotics are not used in the patient with severe respiratory distress. It is sometimes difficult to distinguish between "simple" allergic asthma and wheezing associated with congestive heart failure or chronic obstructive pulmonary disease, and the treatment varies among these entities. It is important to try to distinguish among them by past medical history and physical examination.

### ■ What is done for the comatose patient at the scene?

The initial evaluation of a comatose patient does not differ from evaluation of any other patient. The ABC's are first evaluated and treated. It is after this that the cause of the coma is considered. However, diagnostic information is very limited in the field, and the etiology of unconsciousness is therefore difficult to determine. Even when the etiology of coma is known, treatment in the field is limited, and in the majority of cases the patient must be transported to a hospital for further diagnosis and treatment. If the patient is diabetic, hypoglycemia is a likely etiology; this is treated at the scene. In addition, where narcotic overdose is a possibility, naloxone (Narcan) is given.

**■ How is anaphylaxis treated in the field?**

Anaphylactic reaction can be brought on by a variety of causes outside the hospital. Many persons with an anaphylactic reaction will not survive transport to a hospital. Ventilatory support is provided with high-flow oxygen, and epinephrine is administered. Benadryl and steroids may also be given at the scene or en route to the hospital.

**■ How is the patient with seizures treated in the field?**

As in all situations, priority for treatment must be directed to ventilation and circulation. (It is not uncommon for a patient in cardiac arrest to manifest seizure activity.) Care is taken that the patient not inflict self-injury during the seizure. To prevent biting of the tongue, a guard may be inserted between the teeth, if this is done before the teeth become clenched or if there is chewing activity that allows insertion, but when the teeth are clamped tightly together, it is difficult to insert the guard, and by forcing the guard into the mouth more damage may be done. The administration of oxygen may be indicated if the patient is cyanotic or if the seizure is prolonged. Ventilation of a patient who is actively undergoing a seizure with teeth clenched may not be possible, and usually ventilation will resume spontaneously in a few seconds.

Most seizures will terminate within a few minutes and no treatment other than airway support will be needed, although, under the order of a physician, medications may be given as prophylaxis against additional seizures during transport. If a seizure lasts longer than 5 minutes, IV medication is usually administered by paramedical personnel at the scene and under the direction of a physician. The shorter acting agent diazepam is usually favored, so that the patient may more quickly recover at the emergency department and be more definitively evaluated and treated.

**■ What is the on-the-scene treatment of near drowning?**

Artificial ventilation is started as soon as feasible, even before the victim is removed from the water. External cardiac compression is not effective in the water but should be started as soon as the pulseless patient is on a nonyielding surface. If there is distention of the stomach, which interferes with effective ventilation, this can be relieved by turning the victim to the prone position and lifting the body around the abdomen to compress the stomach. High-flow oxygen is administered at the earliest possibility. The lethal injury usually resulting from near drowning is tissue hypoxia, and administration of good ventilation with 100% oxygen is the major form of therapy.

Almost all near drowning victims are acidotic,[22] and an initial dose of sodium bicarbonate should be administered at the scene or en route to the hospital.

**■ How is a patient with suspected drug overdose treated in the field?**

If a patient has ingested an overdose of medications or a noncaustic poison recently and is still awake, emesis can be induced at the scene, especially if the distance to the hospital is considerable. If the patient is comatose, respiration is supported, and it may even be necessary to administer fluids and vasopressors en route if the patient is in shock. It is important to prevent aspiration during transport, and the patient should be suctioned frequently and transported lying on the side, so that if vomiting occurs, the vomitus will not be aspirated.

When a young patient is found comatose with shallow respirations and pinpoint pupils, heroin overdose should be a strong consideration, especially when needle tracks are present or injection materials are nearby. (In late stages, after hypoxia has developed, pupils may be dilated.) Ventilation is of primary importance when there is respiratory depression or apnea; intubation is usually not necessary. A patient with narcotic overdose can be maintained for a long period of time with only artificial ventilation, but because it is sometimes difficult to provide artificial ventilation during transport, a narcotic antagonist such as naloxone (Narcan) is given when it is available. When coma is caused by narcotic overdose, a narcotic antagonist brings striking reversal of both respiratory depression and coma. Commonly the patient will suddenly become very alert and refuse to go to the hospital. However, because the action of naloxone may be shorter than the action of the narcotic, the patient may subsequently develop deepening coma again and should be urged to go to the hospital for observation. Hypoglycemia has been found in some patients with narcotic overdose, and infusion of 50 ml of 50% glucose in water may be indicated. When there is continued cyanosis after reversal of the overdose, pulmonary edema or aspiration is likely, and the administration of high-flow oxygen and immediate transport are indicated.

## REFERENCES

1. National Academy of Sciences–National Research Council, Committee on Trauma and Committee on Shock, Division of Medical Sciences: Accidental death and disability: the neglected disease of modern society, Washington, D.C., 1966, U.S. Government Printing Office.
2. Frey, C. F., Huelke, D. F., and Gikas, P. W.: Resuscitation and survival in motor vehicle accidents, J. Trauma **9**:292-310, 1969.
3. Day, W.: Acute coronary care—a five-year report, Am. J. Cardiol. **21**:2152, 1968.
4. Pantridge, J. F., and Geddes, J. S.: Mobile intensive care unit in the management of myocardial infarction, Lancet **2**:271-273, 1967.
5. Larent, L., et al.: L'intervention du médecin dans la relève et le transport des grands blessés et malades par l'électronique, La Presse Méd. **75**:1539, 1967.
6. Grace, W. J.: The mobile coronary care unit and the intermediate coronary care unit in the total systems approach to coronary care, Chest **58**:363, 1970.
7. Nagel, E. L., Hirschman, J. C., Nussenfeld, S. R., Rankin, D., and Lumblad, E.: Telemetry-medical command in coronary and other mobile emergency care systems J.A.M.A. **214**:332-338, 1970.
8. Williams, J. S., and Kirkpatrick, J. R.: The nature of seat belt injuries, J. Trauma **11**: 207-218, 1971.
9. Smith, W. S., and Kaufer, H.: Patterns and mechanisms of lumbar injuries associated with lap seat belts, J. Bone Joint Surg. **51A**: 239-254, 1969.
10. Huelke, D. F., and Snyder, R. G.: Seat belt injuries: the need for accuracy in reporting of cases, J. Trauma **15**:20-23, 1975.
11. Haugen, R. K.: The cafe coronary. Sudden deaths in restaurants, J.A.M.A. **186**:142-143, 1963.
12. Editorial: Simple method relieves "cafe coronary," J.A.M.A. **229**:746, 1974.
13. Heimlich, H. J.: A life saving maneuver to prevent food-choking, J.A.M.A. **234**:398-401, 1975.
14. American Heart Association and National Academy of Sciences–National Research Council: Standards for cardiopulmonary resuscitation (CPR) and emergency cardiac care (ECC) J.A.M.A. **227**(suppl.):833-868, 1974.
15. Nicholas, T. H., and Rumer, G. F.: Emergency airway—a plan of action, J.A.M.A. **174**:1930-1935, 1960.
16. Ruhe, D. S., Williams, G. V., and Proud, G. O.: Emergency airway by cricothyroid puncture or tracheotomy: a comparative study of methods and instruments, Trans. Am. Acad. Ophthalmol. Otolaryngol. **64**: 182-203, 1960.
17. Pascoe, D., and Grossman, M.: Quick reference to pediatric emergencies, Philadelphia, 1973, J. B. Lippincott Co.
18. Kaplan, B. C., et al.: The military antishock trouser in civilian pre-hospital emergency care, J. Trauma **13**:843-848, 1973.
19. Kossuth, L. C.: The removal of injured personnel from wrecked vehicles, J. Trauma **5**: 703-708, 1965.
20. Lie, K. I. et al.: Lidocaine in the prevention of primary ventricular fibrillation. A double-blind, randomized study of 212 consecutive patients, N. Engl. J. Med. **291**:1324, 1974.
21. Valentine, P. A. et al.: Lidocaine in the prevention of sudden death in the pre-hospital phase of acute infarction. A double-blind study, N. Engl. J. Med. **291**:291, 1974.
22. Modell, J. H., Davis, J. H., Giammona, S. T., Moya, F., and Mann, J. B.: Blood gas and electrolyte changes in human near-drowning victims, J.A.M.A. **203**:337-343, 1968.

## BIBLIOGRAPHY


Adgey, A. A. J., and Pantridge, J. F.: Symposium on arteriosclerotic heart disease: the prehospital phase of treatment for myocardial infarction, Geriatrics **2**:273-275, 1967.

Adgey, A. A. J., et al.: Management of ventricular fibrillation outside hospital, Lancet **1**:1169, 1969.

American Academy of Orthopaedic Surgeons, Committee on Injuries: Emergency care and transportation of the sick and injured, Menasha, Wis., 1971, George Banta Publishing Co.

American College of Surgeons, Committee on Trauma: Emergency care of the sick and injured, Philadelphia, 1966, W. B. Saunders Co.

Anderson, G. J., Knoebel, S. B., and Fisch, C.: Continuous prehospitalization monitoring of cardiac rhythm, Am. Heart J. **82**:642-646, 1971.

Artz, C. P.: Severe burns: current concepts of specialized care, Mod. Med. April 30, 1973.

Ballinger, W. F., II, Rutherford, R. B., and Zuidema, G. D., editors: The management of trauma, Philadelphia, 1973, W. B. Saunders Co.

Barber, J. M., et al.: Mobile coronary care, Lancet **2**:133-134, 1972.

Baum, R. S., Alvarez, R., and Cobb, L. A.: Mechanisms of out-of-hospital sudden cardiac death and their prognostic significance, Circulation **43**(suppl. 4):40, 1973.

Bondurani, S.: Problems of the pre-hospital phase of acute myocardial infarction, Am. J. Cardiol. **24**:612-616, 1969.

Boswick, J. A., Jr.: Guide to initial management of burns, 1973 revision, Committee on Trauma, American College of Surgeons.

Boswick, J. A., Jr., and Pandyo, N. J.: Emergency care of the burned patient, Surg. Clin. North Am. **52**:115-123, 1972.

Burnette, W. E.: The AMA Commission on Emergency Medical Services and the Emergency Medical Technician, Chicago.

Chamberlain, D. A., et al.: Mobile coronary care provided by ambulance personnel, Br. Heart J. **35**:550, 1972.

Chan, D., Kraus, J. F., and Riggins, R. S.: Patterns of multiple fracture in accidental injury, J. Trauma **13**:1075, 1973.

Chazov, E. J., Ruda, Y. A., and Trubetskoy, A. V.: Early coronary care, G. Ital. Cardiol. **1**: 497-505, 1971.

Cobb, L. A., Conn, R. D., and Samson, W. E.: Prehospital coronary care: the role of a rapid response mobile intensive coronary care system, Circulation **43**(suppl. 2):139, 1971.

Crampton, R. S., et al.: Reduction of community mortality from coronary artery disease by the community-wide emergency cardiac care system, Circulation **48**(suppl. 4):94, 1973.

Crampton, R. S., Miles, J. R., Jr., Gascho, J. A., Aldrich R. F., and Stillerman, R.: Amelioration of prehospital and ambulance death rates from coronary artery disease by prehospital emergency cardiac care, J. Am. Coll. Emergency Physicians, vol. 4, No. 1, 1975.

Dewar, H. A., and Floyd, M.: Deaths from ischaemic heart disease outside hospital and experience with a mobile resuscitation unit, Br. Heart J. **31**:389, 1969.

Dixon, T. C.: Cardiac arrest: experience and results in emergency treatment outside the operating theatre, Med. J. Aust. **1**:754-759, 1970.

Duberstein, J. L., and Kaufman, D. M.: A clinical study of an epidemic of heroin intoxication and heroin-induced pulmonary edema, Am. J. Med. **51**:704, 1971.

Franklin, W.: Treatment of severe asthma, N. Engl. J. Med. **290**:1469, 1974.

Freeark, R. J.: Penetrating wounds of the abdomen, N. Engl. J. Med. **291**:185, 1974.

Frey, C. F., Trollope, M., Harpster, W., and Snyder, R.: A fifteen year experience with automotive hepatic trauma, J. Trauma **13**: 1039, 1973.

Gearty, G. F., et al.: Pre-hospital coronary care service, Br. Med. J. **3**:33-35, 1974.

Goldberg, A. H.: Cardiopulmonary arrest, N. Engl. J. Med. **290**:381, 1974.

Goldstein, S., and Moss, A., editors: Symposium on the pre-hospital phase of acute myocardial infraction, Am. J. Cardiol. **24**:609-611, 1969.

Goldstein, S., Moss, A. J., and Greene, W.: Sudden death in acute myocardial infarction. Relationship to factors affecting delay in hospitalization, Arch. Intern. Med. **129**:720, 1972.

Grace, W. J., and Chadbourn, J. A.: The mobile coronary care unit, Dis. Chest **55**:452, 1969.

Grace, W. J.: Prehospital care and transport in acute myocardial infarction, Chest **63**:469, 1973.

Hackett, T. P.: Factors contributing to the delay in responding to the signs and symptoms of acute myocardial infarct, Am. J. Cardiol. **14**: 551, 1969.

Howard, F. M., Seybold, M. E., and Reiher, J.: The treatment of recurrent convulsions with intravenous injection of diazepam, Med. Clin. North Am. **52**:977-987, 1968.

Hunt, T. K.: Triage, Ariz. Med. **26**:139, 1969.

Kernohan, R. J., and McGucken, R. B.: Mobile intensive care in myocardial infarction, Br. Med. J. **3**:178-180, 1968.

Kossuth, L. C.: Vehicle accidents: immediate care to back injuries, J. Trauma **6**:582, 1966.

Kossuth, L. C.: The extrication of victims from the accident, Ariz. Med. **26**:128, 1969.

Lambrew, C. T., Scharchman, W. L., and Cannon, T. H.: Emergency medical transport systems: use of ECG telemetry, Chest **63**:477-482, 1973.

Lewis, A. J., Ailshire, G., and Criley, J. M.: Pre-hospital cardiac care in a paramedical mobile intensive care unit, Calif. Med. **117**:1-8, 1972.

Lewis, R. P., Warren, J. V.: Factors determining mortality in the pre-hospital phase of acute myocardial infarction, Am. J. Cardiol. **33**:152, 1974.

Liberthson, R. R., Nagel, E. L. Hirschman, J. C., and Nussenfeld, S. R.: Prehospital ventricular defibrillation. Prognosis and follow-up course, N. Engl. J. Med. **291**:317, 1974.

Lown, B., Klein, M. D., and Hershberg, P. I.: Coronary and precoronary care, Am. J. Med. **46**:705-724, 1969.

Moss, A. J.: Delay in hospitalization during the acute coronary period, Am. J. Cardiol. **24**:659, 1969.

Nagel, E. L.: Recommendations of the international symposium, mobile intensive care units and advance emergency care delivery systems, Mainz, Germany, Sept. 24-27, 1973.

Nagel, E. L., et al.: Telemetry—medical command in coronary and other mobile emergency care systems, J.A.M.A. **214**:332-338, 1970.

Pantridge, J. F.: Mobile coronary care, Chest **58**:229, 1970.

Pantridge, J. F., and Adgey, A. A. J.: Pre-hospital coronary care. The mobile coronary care unit, Am. J. Cardiol. **24**:666-673, 1969.

Ramirez, A., and Abelmann, W. H.: Cardiac decompensation, N. Engl. J. Med. **290**:499, 1974.

Robin, E. D., Cross, C. E., and Zelis, R.: Pulmonary edema. 2. N. Engl. J. Med. **288**:292, 1973.

Rosati, M. C., et al.: Community hospital mobile coronary care unit, N.Y. State J. Med. **70**: 2462-2465, 1970.

Rose, L. B., and Press, E.: Cardiac defibrillation by ambulance attendants, J.A.M.A. **219**:63-68, 1972.

Shires, G. T., and Jones, R. C.: Initial management of the severely injured patient, J.A.M.A. **213**:1872, 1970.

Uhley, H. N.: Electrocardiographic telemetry from ambulances: a practical approach to mobile coronary care units, Am. Heart J. **80**:838-842, 1970.

Waller, J. A., Gettinger, C. E., and Weiner, M. A.: Implementing rural emergency health service systems, J. Am. Coll. Emergency Physicians **3**:151, 1974.

*chapter 6*

# In-hospital emergency care

**TERESA L. ROMANO**
**DAVID R. BOYD**

The Industrial Revolution began the mechanization of our society; with the greater use of machines there has been an increase in the number of serious injuries from vocational and recreational activities. In 1972 the National Safety Council reported 11 million injuries from all types of accidents. Wage losses, medical expenses, and insurance administrative costs resulting from trauma totaled $13.5 billion. The estimated overall cost of this pandemic is over $30 billion annually. In the United States there are about 100,000 civilian accidental deaths annually, of which one half are the result of vehicular accidents. The one-millionth traffic fatality occurred in 1951 and, if the present rate continues, the two-millionth victim will die by 1976. Accidents are currently the third most common cause of death in the United States, the accidental death rate being only slightly less than those of cardiovascular disease and cancer. Trauma is the leading cause of death in individuals under 40 years of age.[1] There are over 15 million injuries to children under 14 years of age annually, and of these 16,000 are fatal. Trauma is the commonest cause of death in children, the peak incidence occurring in children from 2 to 3 years of age. One third of all hospital admissions, approximately 2 million a year, are the result of accidents. In one study pediatric patients accounted for 47% of all emergency room visits, and of these one fourth were treated for trauma.[2]

The continually increasing incidence and magnitude of serious injuries resulting from high-speed transportation, complex industrial equipment, civil disturbances, and unpredictable mass catastrophes necessitates a reevaluation and reeducation concerning the priorities and techniques of trauma patient care. Changing patterns of traumatic injuries of all types and newer developments in the surgical subspecialties and biomedical disciplines have been responsible for major progress in the field of trauma management.

Trauma care is team care. The functions of the team begin in the prehospital phase and may appropriately be performed by specialized physicians, nurses, and allied health professionals such as emergency medical technicians or paramedics. This chapter elucidates some of the key aspects of resuscitation and initial treatment of the injured patient to be carried out in the emergency department, with emphasis on the team concept.

## ■ What are the priorities in the emergency management of the trauma patient?

The outcome after severe trauma depends on two basic factors: availability of initial medical care and adequacy of early therapeutic measures. The first objective in examining an injured person is the preservation of life. Resuscitation and proper evaluation of life-endangering injuries are critical to survival. Injudicious or inadequate emergency management can result in unnecessary fatality or permanent disability. When dealing with acute trauma, it is impossible to separate diagnostic and therapeutic measures. Resuscitation is not dependent on an etiologic diagnosis. Airway obstruction, shock, and cardiorespiratory failure often must be treated without knowledge of the precipitating cause of these disorders. Once the patient's functions are stable, rapid and thorough evaluation of the cause of these derangements is in order. Patients with complex, multiple-system injuries often require the skills of many specialists. In these cases it is essential that one practitioner assume the role of the patient's primary physician. This person remains in charge during the entire course of the illness and coordinates the efforts of other consultants utilizing established priorities. This team concept is carried through the operative and acute posttraumatic period. When the patient can be safely managed by one specialist, the individual is then released to that practitioner's care. Patients may need to be moved to a more distant facility or to other remote areas in the hospital, such as the x-ray department, for additional evaluation and treatment. During this period they should be continuously observed by a physician, nurse, or highly qualified emergency medical technician. Once stabilized, the patient can be moved to the intensive care unit for additional monitoring or to the operating room, as indicated. Also, transportation to distant specialty centers can be safely performed when the patient is fully resuscitated.

### ■ What are the factors leading to airway obstruction in the injured patient and what are the essential steps in establishing and maintaining an adequate airway?

Patients with depressed consciousness from intoxication, cerebral injury, or shock have a high risk of aspiration of blood, food, vomitus, and dentures. Insertion of an oropharyngeal airway after aspiration and removal of any foreign bodies are the first considerations. The patient must be observed closely and suctioning performed frequently. The patient must not lie unattended flat on the back or be restrained in this position. A semiprone position is more satisfactory. Two common causes of upper airway obstruction are bleeding of and edema of the mouth, tongue, posterior pharyngeal wall, and epiglottis. Penetrating wounds of these parts are particularly dangerous. Cervical spine injuries producing vertebral subluxation and retropharyngeal hematoma can also compromise the upper airway. Severe maxillofacial trauma with obliteration of the nasal passage will contribute to these problems. Respiratory distress with stridor, a contusion of the neck, and a history of steering wheel injury may indicate the presence of a fractured larynx or trachea. Endotracheal intubation will be unsuccessful in such a case, and emergency tracheostomy is necessary. A patient exhibiting only abdominal breathing may have a cervical vertebral dislocation and spinal cord injury. Any manipulation before stabilizing the neck may complete a partial transection of the spinal cord. Vascular injuries in the neck producing hematomas may compress the airway and require intubation. Patients must be examined for evidence of sucking chest wounds, flail chest, tension pneumothorax, hemothorax, simple pneumothorax, or contused lungs. Airway obstruction (suction and intubation) and respiratory insufficiency (oxygen and positive pressure ventilation) must be relieved. Patients who are combative because of hypoxia can be intubated by using a rapidly acting neuromuscular depolarizing agent. Primary tracheostomy is almost never indicated today, except for patients with major upper airway obstruction from severe facial trauma, massive soft tissue trauma, or cervical vertebral dislocation. Although tracheostomy is relatively easy in a nonemergency situation, it is extremely risky in patients who are restless and agitated from hypoxia. Primary endotracheal intubation followed by controlled tracheostomy is the safest approach.

### ■ What can cause cardiac arrest in trauma?

Severe hypoxia and profound metabolic acidosis are probably the most common causes of cardiac arrest associated with trauma. In addition, direct trauma to the heart may cause cardiac tamponade or cardiac arrest. In rare cases a fatal arrhythmia may be triggered by indirect trauma. Standard cardiac arrest procedures must be instituted immediately if arrest occurs. Mouth-to-mouth resuscitation must be employed immediately, followed by endotracheal intubation. Closed chest massage is preferred and is effective except when the chest wall is unstable, as in flail chest. In such cases, emergency thoracotomy and manual cardiac compression may be necessary. Ventilation with an Ambu (manual ventilator) bag and oxygen are provided while cardiac compression is carried out. Metabolic acidosis is corrected with the IV administration of sodium bicarbonate. Initial and periodic arterial blood gas and pH analyses are essential. ECG monitoring is mandatory. Cardiac defibrillation may be needed, since an hypoxic and acidotic heart is prone to arrhythmias, fibrillation, and asystole.

## ■ What are the acceptable methods of hemorrhage control in the injured patient?

Direct manual pressure over the bleeding site can control most external hemorrhage. Continued gentle pressure is often all that is necessary until the patient is taken to the operating room, where vascular repair may be necessary. There is no place for the application of tourniquets or clamping and ligation of bleeding vessels, as further injury may ensue. The possibility of loss of blood within the body cavities must be evaluated; thoracentesis and paracentesis will help establish the diagnosis of such hemorrhage.

## ■ How can blood loss be assessed and appropriate volume replacement and treatment be determined?

Once hemostasis has been obtained, blood volume must be restored. Major blood loss must be replaced by blood. The magnitude of blood loss can be estimated by clinical observation. Keen observation of physiologic signs and an accurate assessment of all potential injuries can provide a working basis for initiating shock therapy and blood replacement. The severity of traumatic hemorrhage can be effectively graded or categorized into minor (I), moderate (II), major (III), and massive (IV) for initial assessment and to anticipate immediate treatments.[3] Subsequent patient improvement or failure of an adequate treatment response can be measured and reassessed in relationship to these shock-hemorrhage categories.

### *Minor blood loss*

The normal circulating blood volume in a 150-pound (70 kg) adult is approximately 5 L. Small injuries with minor (grade I) blood loss of less than 10% to 15% (500 to 750 ml) may cause no apparent physiologic changes. This type of hemorrhage may be caused by blood donation, a laceration, or bleeding into a distal extremity fracture site. The treatment is simply control of further hemorrhage and blood replacement by crystalloid solution (Table 6-1 shown on p. 118).

### *Moderate blood loss*

A moderate (grade II) hemorrhagic loss of 15% to 30% of the circulating blood volume (750 to 1500 ml) should be well compensated for in most individuals who are otherwise healthy. The injured patient with this degree of injury should demonstrate many of the visible signs of physiologic compensation (Table 6-1, grade II): cool skin, slight tachycardia (110 beats/min), tachypnea (24 respirations/min), a fall in pulse pressure, and possibly a small decrease in systolic blood pressure. These effects are caused by significant injuries such as ruptured spleen or a major femoral shaft fracture. Treatment is by hemorrhage control and the rapid infusion of blood substitutes, that is, crystalloid and colloid solutions (plasma or albumin). Oxygen should be administered by mask. If hemorrhage is controlled, blood replacement will not be required, and the infusion of 2 to 3 L of crystalloid and colloid solutions will suffice.

### *Major blood loss*

Major (Table 6-1, grade III) hemorrhage with a loss of 30% to 45% of the effective circulating blood volume (1500 to 2250 ml) will cause marked physiologic decompensation. This classic "shock" patient has cold, clammy skin, is restless, and exhibits tachycardia (120 beats/min), tachypnea (32 respirations/min), and hypotension (less than 80

**Table 6-1.** Classification and treatment of hemorrhagic shock*

| Grade | Clinical findings | Etiology | | Treatment |
|---|---|---|---|---|
| | | *External loss* | *Internal loss* | |
| I—minor blood loss, 10%-15% of blood volume (500-750 ml) | Well compensated; dizziness; tachycardia (100 beats/min) | Blood donation; laceration | Hematoma; extremity fracture; hemothorax | Control of hemorrhage; crystalloid infusion |
| II—moderate blood loss, 15%-30% of blood volume (750-1500 ml) | Partial compensation; cool, sweating skin; thirst, anxiety; tachycardia (110 beats/min); tachypnea (24 respirations/min); slight hypotension (90-100 mm Hg); decrease in pulse pressure | Major laceration | Visceral injury (for example, spleen rupture); fractured femur | Control of hemorrhage; crystalloid and colloid infusion; oxygen administration; evaluation of obscure bleeding |
| III—major blood loss, 30%-45% of blood volume (1500-2250 ml) | Decompensation; pale, cold, clammy skin; restless, agitation; tachycardia (120 beats/min); tachypnea (32 respirations/min); hypotension (80 mm Hg); oliguria (30 ml/hr); metabolic acidosis | Vascular injury | Visceral injuries (for example, liver rupture); pelvic fracture | Control of hemorrhage; crystalloid, colloid, and blood infusion; oxygen and bicarbonate administration; physiologic monitoring |
| IV—severe blood loss, 45% of blood volume (over 2250 ml) | "In extremis"—marked pallor, cyanosis; semiconscious; tachycardia (over 120 beats/min); respiratory distress; profound hypotension (60 mm Hg); anuria; metabolic acidosis | Traumatic amputation | Vascular (for example, aortic rupture); multiple injuries | Control of hemorrhage; oxygen administration; blood, colloid, and crystalloid infusion; bicarbonate administration; cardiac monitoring; antibiotics |

*Modified from Boyd, D. R.: S. Afr. J. Surg. **11**:163-175, 1973.

mm Hg); oliguria and a marked metabolic acidosis will also be present.

Obvious points of external loss from a major vessel or severe internal injuries (lacerated liver or pelvic fractures) should be the suspected lesions. Whole blood replacement for resuscitation must be included in addition to those measures just discussed. Bicarbonate ($NaHCO_3$) must be administered to combat the metabolic acidosis of shock, and these patients will need to have repeated physiologic monitoring of systolic blood pressure and central venous pressure (CVP), urinary output, hematocrit, and arterial blood gas concentrations. The seriously ill patient can be effectively resuscitated if therapy is appropriate to a sound diagnosis, a correct interpretation of the physiologic derangements, and those pathophysiologic signs that are readily detectable by the astute clinician.

### *Massive blood loss*

Massive (Table 6-1, grade IV) blood loss is a catastrophic situation wherein the extent of loss (over 45%) has gone uncorrected and the patient is first seen in extremis. The physiologic compensatory mechanisms have failed, and many have developed pathologic characteristics and are effecting further detriment to the patient.

The patient may be cyanotic with marked pallor, have a severe and irregular tachycardia, experience respiratory distress, exhibit marked hypotension (less than 50 mm Hg), and have complete anuria. Patients with catastrophic losses of over 45% of their effective circulating blood volume are severely prostrated, hypoxic, and unresponsive. These patients, if not vigorously resuscitated, will progress to cardiopulmonary arrest.

Massive trauma and shock are associated with decreased function of the reticuloendothelial system, so that during the early posttraumatic period the ability of the body to clear bacteria from the circulation is depressed. Prophylactic antibiotic therapy may be indicated in these circumstances.

Multiple severe trauma will cause these effects, but more importantly such injuries and even lesser trauma can deteriorate to this state if hemorrhage is not initially controlled and physiologic therapy is not correctly administered. These patients, unfortunately, often represent a "systems failure" or a "patient management failure," wherein the proper trauma care was not given early enough to prevent this deteriorated state.

## ■ What are important considerations in blood volume replacement in shock?

For initial volume replacement infusion of moderate volumes of a buffered saline solution (Ringer's lactate) is satisfactory. It is necessary to replace approximately two to three times as much of this crystalloid solution as the estimated amount of blood lost. The oxygen-carrying capacity of hemoglobin is diminished by the hemodilution. It is safe in most patients without previous cardiovascular disease to maintain the hematocrit at 30% to 35%. There has been considerable argument about the equilibration period for blood after hemorrhage. The hematocrit determination has certain limitations during acute changes, but serial measurements provide valuable information about hypovolemic shock. No other parameter, including blood volume determinations, has proved to be more helpful during this acute period.[4] The management of shock is facilitated by repeated observations of blood pressure, heart rate, respiratory rate, skin temperature, CVP, and urinary output. An increase in systolic blood pressure and a decrease in pulse and respiratory rates herald successful resuscitation. A return of normal skin temperature and urinary output and improved state of consciousness attests to the restoration of adequate tissue perfusion.

## ■ How is the CVP used in the patient in shock?

CVP monitoring is one of the most significant advances in the management of shock patients. An IV catheter is inserted into the superior vena cava. A venous blood sample is taken for type, cross match, blood counts, and biochemical tests, and an infusion of Ringer's lactate solution is started. The CVP is monitored intermittently through the catheter in the superior vena cava using a simple water manometer. The pressure readings are not a measure of "blood volume"; instead, they reflect a dynamic state between the adequacy of the venous return and the pumping action of the right ventricle. Absolute values are not as important as relative changes observed over periods of time. Typically in hypovolemic shock the CVP is below the normal values of 4 to 8 cm of saline solution. With adequate volume replacement a rise in CVP and systolic blood pressure is observed. A persistently low CVP after adequate volume replacement should stimulate a search for occult bleeding. Blood losses into fracture sites, especially the major long bones or pelvis, occult rupture of the liver or spleen, and collections in silent areas such as the pleural cavity and the retroperitoneal space must be considered. An elevated CVP and low systemic blood pressure suggests a pericardial tamponade, myocardial infarction, or acute congestive heart failure. Changes in the quality of the heart tones, cardiac rhythm, ECG findings, and the response to volume loading are helpful in this diagnostic dilemma.

All patients with blood loss, chest injury, or major trauma should have a CVP catheter inserted and serial measurements taken.

■ **What are the advantages and disadvantages of the commonly employed volume replacement fluids?**

The use of crystalloid solutions in initial volume replacement has become an acceptable clinical practice. Normal saline solution (0.9% NaCl) and buffered salt solutions (Ringer's lactate) are inexpensive, stable in storage, readily available, free of immediate reactions, and do not require any special matching prior to use. There are theoretical advantages to using the buffered salt solutions, and they are preferred even though they contain a small (28 mEq/L) amount of lactate. This small amount of lactate is inconsequential when compared to the massive amounts of lactate produced by the body during shock. As the circulation is restored, the lactate is readily converted by the liver to bicarbonate and excreted as carbon dioxide by the lungs. Noncolloid salt solutions rapidly diffuse out of the circulation to the extravascular extracellular space, so that two and one-half to four times the amount of blood lost must be infused as crystalloid solutions to restore the blood volume.

The effects of dilution on the hemoglobin and plasma protein concentrations are factors limiting the use of crystalloid solutions. It is desirable to maintain the hematocrit above 30% and the total protein in excess of 6 g/100 ml. At these values the oxygen-carrying capacity and oncotic pressure of the blood will protect against further hypoxia and tissue edema. There is no place for salt-free crystalloid solutions (dextrose in water) in primary resuscitation. When given in the early posttraumatic state, the water is retained because of the action of antidiuretic hormone, and hypo-osmolality results.

### *Albumin*

A 6% solution of human serum albumin is readily available and free from risk of hepatitis. Albumin is a highly effective plasma expander and has other advantages, one of which is that this protein is easily metabolized and spares body muscle proteins from catabolism.

### *Plasma*

Plasma stored for 6 months at 30° C under ultraviolet radiation still can transmit serum hepatitis. Type-specific single units of plasma may be given after simple screening cross match, although isosensitization may still occur. Plasma may be given without cross matching and is an excellent blood volume expander that may be safely used when the hematocrit is above 30%. Its use also may be considered when plasma losses are anticipated, as in burns, peritonitis, and pancreatitis.

### *Dextrans*

Both clinical dextran (average molecular weight 70,000) and low viscosity dextran (mean molecular weight 40,000) are effective plasma expanders. They are inexpensive and relatively free of serious reactions. Besides the obvious intravascular expansion of the circulating blood volume, there is an added beneficial effect of these agents, since they decrease blood viscosity and improve microcirculatory flow. Decreased sludging, or the breaking up of erythrocyte aggregations, is a suggested mechanism for the observed improved general and intraorgan (liver, kidney, and gastrointestinal) blood flow. Use of these agents may affect coagulation mechanisms both by dilution and by their viscosity-reducing properties. The use of dextrans should be limited if there are large soft tissue injuries or if an operation that will involve retroperitoneal dissection is anticipated. In any circumstance, no more than 1000 ml should be given in a 24-hour period. In addition, dextran may interfere with proper type and cross matching and should never be given before an accurate type and cross match have been obtained.

### *Blood transfusions*

Major losses of whole blood must be replaced by blood to maintain a hematocrit level above 30%. A need for unmatched universal donor (O negative) blood is uncommon, as most patients can be adequately supported initially by one of the blood substitutes mentioned previously. An increase in heart and respiratory rates, cardiac output, and tissue oxygen extraction are the major mechanisms employed to compensate for the loss of erythrocytes in hemorrhage and during the dilutional phase of volume restoration. Untoward reactions of blood transfusions are major and minor blood group incompatibilities, isosensitization, serum hepatitis, and occasionally the transmission of bacteria or their metabolic by-products. Banked blood becomes progressively more acidotic and hyperkalemic, and there is a rapid loss of many coagulation factors. Massive rapid transfusions (over 20 pints) are associated with a high incidence of reactions. Frozen blood, now becoming more readily available, has numerous advantages. Acid citrate is not necessary as a preservative, alleviating the problems of low calcium concentrations and acidotic pH found in banked blood. Oxygen-carrying capacity of the blood is also better maintained. In addition, frozen blood can be stored for at least 2 years without breakdown of red blood cells and resultant accumulation of potassium. Most important, there is a marked reduction in the incidence of hepatitis.

### ■ What drugs are commonly needed in treating the injured patient?

In shock decreased tissue blood flow and oxygenation lead to anaerobic glycolysis. Excess lactic and pyruvic acids are produced and enter the circulation. The metabolism of these organic acids by the liver is depressed, and metabolic acidosis supervenes.

Sodium bicarbonate (5%) is an extracellular buffer effective in combating this acidosis and is available in 500 ml bottles. Rapid changes in blood pH may be induced and cause cardiac arrhythmias, so that patients receiving rapid infusions of buffers must be monitored by continuous ECG's.

Maintenance of adequate urinary output (over 30 ml/hr) is a prime aim in the management of shock and major trauma. In shock sympathetic compensatory mechanisms cause a decrease in renocortical blood flow and a marked elevation of circulating antidiuretic hormone (ADH), promoting increased water reabsorption from the distal tubule. Effective circulating plasma volume is thus conserved. When hypovolemia is inadequately treated, or when circulating tissue debris (hemoglobin and myoglobin) is filtered but not cleared from the tubules because of decreased urine flow, renal shutdown may result. Osmotic or chemical diuretics in addition to volume replacement should be employed early when renal function is precarious or when frank failure is suspected. Mannitol, a monosaccharide that is filtered but not reabsorbed by the kidney, induces an obligate excretion of filtered water that helps maintain renal tubular flow and patency. Up to 100 ml of 20% mannitol solution may be infused rapidly, and the infusion may be repeated within the next hour if diuresis is not established. Mannitol also acts as a plasma expander; the CVP must be monitored during therapy. If no response is obtained to mannitol, ethacrynic acid (50 mg) or furosemide (10 to 20 mg) may be given. These agents also may be repeated within 1 to 2 hours. The effectiveness of diuretic agents is dependent on an adequate circulating blood volume. Neither approach (osmotic or chemical) will be effective in hypovolemia.

Should a urinary output be initiated, an attempt should be made to maintain the hourly volume at over 60 ml/hr. Urine specific gravity, which is simple to measure, or urine osmolality, determined by the freezing point depression method, is a guide to the efficacy of therapy and helps in estimating the functional status of the kidneys. A high urine specific gravity (over 1.025) or osmolality (700 mOsm/kg) indicates persistent hypovolemia; a low specific gravity (under 1.010) or osmolality (150 mOsm/kg) may mean overinfusion. An isosmotic value (specific gravity 1.010 or osmolality 300 mOsm/kg) may represent the effect of diuretics or be the first sign of loss of concentrating function and impending tubular failure. Further fluid or diuretic therapy may be chosen intelligently by comparing serial serum and urine osmolality measurements. Mannitol and chemical diuretics can be given intermittently each 6 to 8 hours as necessary to maintain adequate urine flow.

Release of endogenous catecholamines is maximal after major trauma and hemorrhage. The adrenal medulla secretes large quantities of norepinephrine, causing increased arteriolar tone, increased peripheral resistance, and diminished flow in the vascular beds of the skin and viscera. Administration of vasoconstrictor agents only augments this pathophysiologic state, causing further cellular hypoxia, anaerobic glycolysis, and lactic acid production. The basic defect in traumatic and hemorrhagic shock is a blood volume deficit. Therapy must be directed toward correction of this primary defect. Vasoconstrictors may be helpful in other conditions associated with disturbances in vascular reactivity, for example, neurogenic, cardiac, septic, or anaphylactic shock. Norepinephrine (Levophed), 1 ampule (0.4 mg). or metaraminol (Aramine), 10 ml vial (100 mg), may be given in 1000 ml of crystalloid solution initially infused at a rate of 1 ml/min and titrated to produce a systolic blood pressure of 100 mm Hg. It is mandatory that hypovolemia be entirely ruled out as the cause of hypotension prior to administration of any vasoconstricting agent.

Theoretically the use of drugs to block the intensive sympathetic vasoconstriction observed in shock would allow blood flow to return to previously ischemic, hypoxic, and acidotic tissues. Prior to administering vasodilating agents, blood volume must be restored and volume repletion continued concomitantly with administration of the drug. Without these precautions the patient may develop total peripheral collapse, for as tissue beds are opened up pharmacologically there must be adequate circulating volume available to fill the expanded system. Of the clinically available vasodilating drugs, chlorpromazine (Thorazine) given by the IV route every 2 to 3 hours (5 to 15 mg) will produce an appreciable change in tissue perfusion, at least in terms of skin temperature and color.

In most cases of traumatic shock one is dealing with an otherwise normal myocardium that has become hypoxic. Digitalization is not usually needed, since heart function will improve with successful treatment of the blood volume deficit. However, older patients who may have underlying primary myocardial disease, patients who develop a very rapid tachycardia that persists after volume replacement, and certainly those patients who develop cardiac failure or exhibit a high CVP with a low systemic blood pressure are candidates for digitalis therapy. The serum potassium concentration must be measured before giving digitalis. The rapidly acting cardiac drugs lanatoside C (Cedilanid) and digoxin are preferred. Contraindications to digitalization include the presence of conduction abnormalities (partial or complete heart block) and irritability of the myocardium (ventricular ectopic beats or ventricular tachycardia).

Isoproterenol (Isuprel) has both inotropic and chronotropic effects on the heart, that is, it increases both contractility and heart rate. Isoproterenol also stimulates $\beta$-receptor sites in peripheral muscle beds, causing vasodilation and improved flow to these tissues. The total effect is a decreased blood pressure and peripheral resistance and an increased cardiac output. A serious drawback to the use of isoproterenol is that many patients develop a tachycardia (over 140 beats/min) and administration of the drug must be decreased or discontinued.

## ■ How much sodium bicarbonate is necessary to reverse the acidosis of shock?

After major blood loss and shock, tissue anoxia results in an increased concentration of lactic acid in the blood. Accumulation of hydrogen ion causes a fall in blood pH. Usually there is an attempt to compensate for this by increased ventilation, permitting excretion of hydrogen ion from carbonic acid (as water and carbon dioxide). In a typically severe case the arterial blood pH is 7.30 or below, and the $P_{CO_2}$ is 28 or below. Using standard nomograms (Sigaard-Andersen), the degree of metabolic acidosis is expressed as a base deficit (–10 to –20 mEq/L) (Figs. 6-1 and 6-2). For adequate replacement the

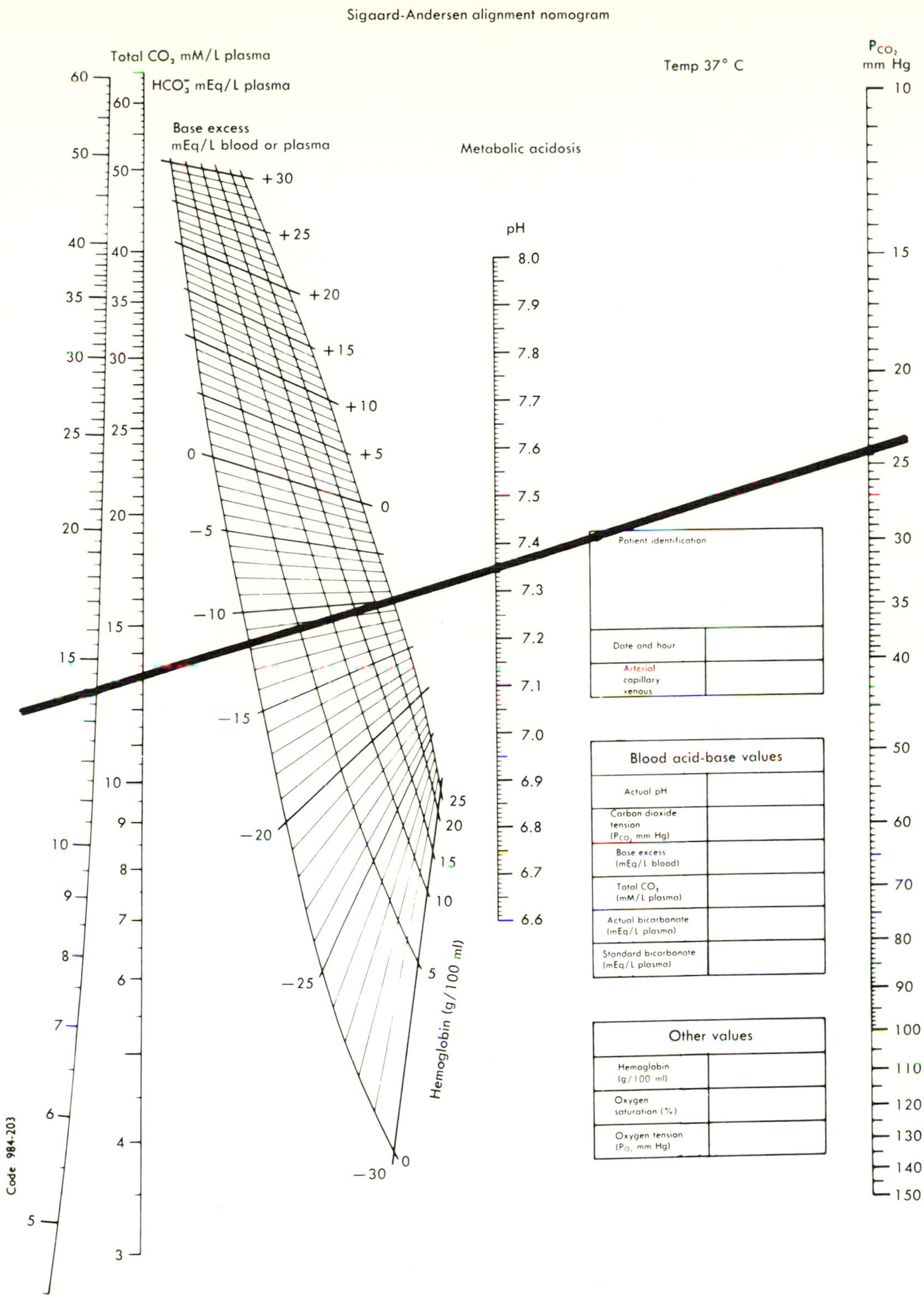


**Fig. 6-1.** This blood gas and pH nomogram uses two known (measured) variables, arterial $CO_2$ tension ($P_{CO_2}$) (far right column) and arterial acidity (pH) (middle column), to determine a third derived variable, the base deficit or base excess, in milliequivalents per liter of blood (middle hatched area). Base changes are affected slightly by hemoglobin levels, hence grid to account for possible effects of hemoglobin in any clinical setting. Alignment of this shock patient's $P_{CO_2}$ (24 mm Hg) and pH (7.35) results in base deficit of 11 mEq/L (read as –11 at 15 g/100 ml of red blood cell hemoglobin).

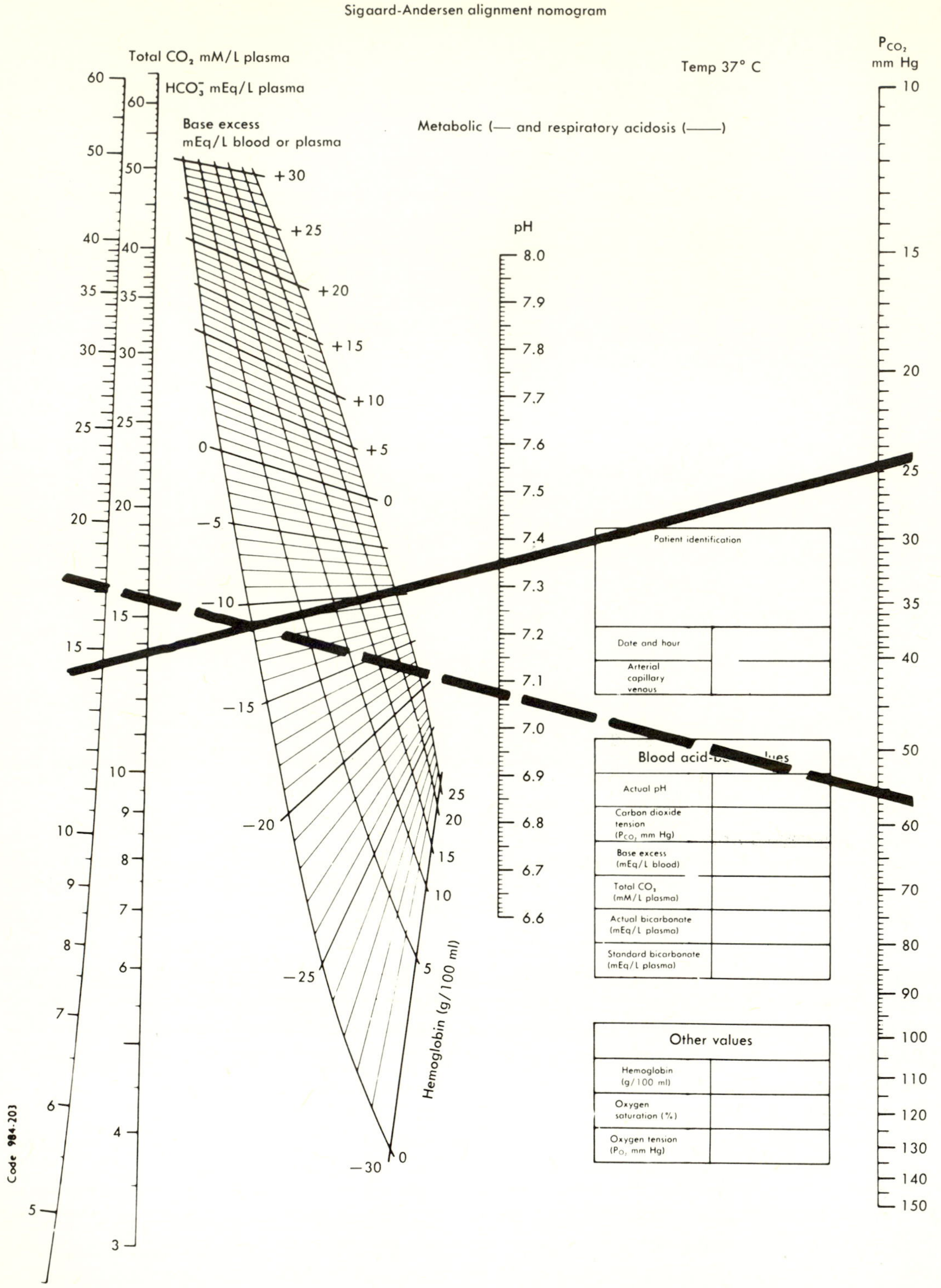


**Fig. 6-2.** When respiratory compensatory mechanism is impeded by failure of ventilation, $CO_2$ retention occurs, as is shown by hatched lines ($P_{CO_2}$ 55 mm Hg). At the same time, base deficit infers that metabolic or lactic acidosis has not worsened. Patient's arterial blood pH is brought down to 7.06, very near absolute lethal level.

milliequivalent of bicarbonate needed is equal to the base deficit (milliequivalents per liter) multiplied by body weight in kilograms by the bicarbonate space factor of 0.30, as in the following formula[5]:

$$\text{Bicarbonate (mEq)} = \text{Base deficit (mEq/L)} \times \text{Body weight (kg)} \times 0.30$$

**■ Besides obvious external hemorrhage, what are the possible etiologies of shock in the trauma patient?**

Blood loss from fractures, especially of the long bones or pelvis, occult rupture of the liver or spleen, and collections of blood in "silent areas" such as the pleural cavity and the retroperitoneal space must be considered. Blood loss into tissues around fracture sites may be deceptive. A fracture of the femoral shaft may cause the loss of 2 to 4 pints of blood, but a pelvic fracture may result in the loss of 10 or more pints. Hematuria, hemoptysis, bloody nasogastric suction, or rectal bleeding are other possible sources of blood loss. Most injuries causally related to shock are either obvious on careful inspection or can be diagnosed by simple measures. Paracentesis, thoracentesis, intravenous pyelography (IVP), and endoscopy will indicate most occult bleeding sites. Inability to restore blood pressure and circulating volume in an acutely traumatized patient by adequate blood volume replacement indicates that a source of uncontrolled hemorrhage is present. Continuing major hemorrhage is seen commonly in liver, retroperitoneal, and vascular injuries. Further attempts to stabilize the circulation in such cases will be unsuccessful and may cause the death of the patient. Patients with such injuries often must be taken to the operating room in shock and exploratory procedures performed for direct access to the sources of bleeding.

**■ What are the steps to take following resuscitation of the injured patient?**

After successful resuscitation the critically ill trauma patient must be continually evaluated for the possible deterioration of any vital function. The assessment includes careful observation of the level of consciousness, spontaneous motion of the extremities, chest excursion, abdominal habitus, and injured regions. A total clinical evaluation is performed. All patients are disrobed and totally examined, including a complete physical examination. Deformities or asymmetry of body parts, lacerations, and contusions demand special attention. A rapid assessment of the extent of injuries is performed by gentle but firm palpation of all body parts, especially those areas where injuries are suspected. Palpation of the scalp, facial bones, trachea, and vertebral column as well as gentle compression of the thorax, ribs, pelvis, and extremities will expose hidden fractures and dislocations and lead to intelligent and precise requests for x-ray films to be taken. Local tenderness, crepitation of subcutaneous air, and grating of bony parts will suggest a diagnosis. The chest is auscultated for signs of pleural collapse, rub, and effusion. Changes in heart tones and the occurrence of murmurs in the chest or over extremities will be diagnostic of vascular injuries. A careful abdominal examination for peritoneal irritation and distension is mandatory. Rectal and pelvic examination are routinely performed. Checking palpable pulse, temperature, and neuromuscular tone of all extremities is necessary.

This initial rapid physical examination must be followed by an in-depth evaluation of each regional anatomic area and its relevant physiologic systems. Those with obvious injuries will be carefully scrutinized. This must not divert the examiner to concentrate only on the most apparent injuries, but a continual search for the less obvious hidden occult injuries must complete the examination.

A patient with multiple injuries from an automobile accident will require such a rapid and repeated examination. Much information about this patient can be obtained by simple observation. One can observe cranial, facial, and laryngeal injuries. This observation, along with the respiratory noises caused by blood and aspirated materials, is enough to appraise initially the adequacy of the upper airway. High-pitched and rattling breath sounds will dictate the obvious necessary first resuscitative steps.

A quick appraisal of the state of consciousness, arousal, and pupillary reflexes will afford an advantage in evaluating the frequency, depth, and adequacy of spontaneous ventilatory efforts. Thoracic contusions, bony irregularities, open wounds, asymmetric paradoxical movements, or lack of intercostal muscle activity will provide adequate information for instituting the proper life-saving measures.

Hemorrhage may be obvious, as from a forearm laceration. However, unexplained shock may be caused by an occult injury, and blood loss may be occurring into the pleural space (hemoperitoneum) or into the soft tissues around fractures or major burn sites.

Obvious external rotation and shortening of a leg provides the necessary preliminary diagnosis; a lesser priority of care is assigned to this situation, although the injured limb is positioned to prevent unnecessary further injury. Simple identification, dressing, and splinting of all soft tissue and extremity injuries of scalp, forearm, and leg is all that is necessary at this initial stage. To attempt more definitive care at this junction would probably give less than optimum results and may detract the practitioner from other and possibly less obvious critical injuries. This initial evaluation and care can and should be performed at the accident scene or in the emergency department prior to transportation of the patient. At this time as much information as possible is obtained from clinical examination and interviewing. All critical information must be gained as soon as possible.

The patient must be observed in an emergency department or trauma care hospital. The airway should be established and maintained by the passage of an endotracheal tube. This is the most direct and sure way and should be among the skills of every practitioner, nurse and physician alike. In many communities rescue emergency medical technicians are becoming skilled in this and other life-saving techniques.

Additional information can be readily obtained at this time. Clinical findings must be reevaluated and recorded in order to recognize treatment progress or clinical deterioration. Repeated examination should be performed by the same individual or a team of trauma specialists so that reliable and correct management decisions can be made. It is essential that all critical parameters (blood pressure, CVP, pulse, urinary output, and physical findings) be recorded sequentially to detect early pathophysiologic trends.

## ■ What essential facts from the history should be obtained?

As thorough a history as possible is obtained, including health status before the injury, factors causing the accident, and conditions at the scene of the accident. Previous medical problems, allergies, medications, or diseases (for example, coronary disease or hemophilia) must be ascertained. Since this information may be critical to survival, it must be sought from any source possible.

## ■ What laboratory and diagnostic tests are indicated in the emergency trauma patient?

An aggressive diagnostic approach to the trauma patient is necessary for proper evaluation. The decision as to how many x-ray films to order is based on the clinical situation and status of the patient. X-ray films take valuable time and are performed under conditions that are not ideal for continuous observation. Often a few routine views are adequate. The unconscious patient is more difficult to evaluate and may require additional studies. Single views of possible fractures and dislocations and standard views of chest and abdomen are obtained. Special studies such as tomograms of facial fractures can be obtained later. The IVP, cystogram, and arteriography are often useful. The patient with traumatic hematuria from any cause and with suspected renal trauma must have an IVP. To identify injuries to the bladder, pelvic fractures are evaluated by cystography, visualizing the full and empty bladder in the standard and lateral views.

Arteriography is particularly useful when circulation in an extremity is impaired, in abdominal and chest trauma, and in closed head injuries. There is no significant morbidity from these studies, and they are often of great value. An incidental excretory nephrourogram is obtained 15 minutes after the arteriogram.

Paracentesis is helpful for the rapid evaluation of intra-abdominal injuries. If fluid is obtained, it is tested for bile and examined microscopically for white and red blood cells; a portion is sent for determination of amylase concentration. If no fluid is obtained, a plastic catheter may be inserted through the lower abdominal area in the midline and 300 ml of peritoneal dialysis solution slowly infused.[6] The fluid is then aspirated after 5 minutes and tested. A positive tap is a definitive indication for laparotomy.[7] A negative tap cannot be considered evidence of the absence of intra-abdominal injury.

Thoracentesis may be employed for the rapid evaluation of the patient with a possible chest injury. Blood and air, especially if under pressure, are immediate indications for establishment of tube drainage even prior to taking x-ray films. These findings prompt investigation for other underlying visceral injuries.

Direct laryngoscopy and bronchoscopy are performed when injury of the upper airway, trachea, and major bronchi are suspected. Proctoscopy is done in all suspected rectal injuries prior to operation.

Since the introduction of ultrasonic techniques by Leksell,[8] the usefulness of echoencephalography in acute head injuries has been established. Rapid and repeatable examinations are of great value, especially in children. Repeated echoencephalograms and neurologic examinations are effective and reliable ways to observe head trauma patients safely.

Routinely ordered biochemical tests include serial serum and urine amylase determinations, especially in those patients with abdominal injuries caused by a blunt force. A high amylase concentration suggests major injury to the pancreas. Complete blood counts are serially performed. Changes in hematocrit reflect the status of the circulating red cell mass. Leukocyte counts are elevated in those patients with visceral injuries, especially when serosal irritation is present. Determination of osmolality by freezing point depression is useful in the monitoring of fluid and electrolyte problems and in defining the status of renal function after severe injury.[9] It is also more useful than measurements of the specific gravity of the urine.

## ■ How are fractures and soft tissue injuries best handled in the emergency trauma patient?

Gross fractures of an extremity are easily identified by simple inspection and palpation. Grossly deformed limbs should be gently returned to an anatomic position and then adequately immobilized. Pneumatic and Thomas splints should be available in every ambulance and emergency department. Proper care will prevent a closed fracture from becoming an open one. The presence of distal pulses before and after manipulation of a deformed extremity should also be noted. Many times it is not possible to treat soft tissue wounds at the time of injury because other important visceral injuries require attention. In these situations it is best to elevate the wounded part, provide hemostasis by compression, and dress the area to protect it against further injury and contamination. Tetanus prophylaxis and antibiotics must be given. When definitive therapy of a soft tissue wound is to be carried out, it is necessary to provide suitable anesthesia, clean the wounds and surrounding area, remove all foreign matter, debride, repair injured tissues, close the wound if indicated, apply an absorptive bulky dressing, and immobilize and elevate the injured part.

## ■ What are significant pathophysiologic events of critical injury?

### *Shock*

***Decreased venous return.*** The common denominator pathophysiologically basic to all forms of shock is a decrease in venous return. The circulating blood volume is deficient and has either been lost externally or is held out in the body periphery and cannot be effectively redistributed by the heart. Consequently, a decreased venous return is the first defect observed in shock. The CVP is a convenient bedside monitor of this physiologic function.

***Decreased cardiac output.*** Decreased venous return is followed by a decrease in cardiac output, which is normally about 5 L/min. This decreased pumping action is one of the causes of poor circulation in peripheral tissues in the shock state. The cardiac output can be measured accurately electronically by a dye dilution technique. A rough measure of the adequacy of the cardiac output can be quantified clinically by evaluating the systolic blood pressure and the systolic pulse pressure. This important parameter can also be estimated at the bedside by carefully palpating the femoral or radial pulses for rate, rhythm, strength, and fullness. With some practice a good clinician can become quite expert at estimating this important central cardiac function at the bedside.

***Arteriolar constriction.*** A decreased cardiac output stimulates arteriolar vasoconstriction. This arteriolar compensatory mechanism attempts to restrict blood flow in nonvital areas and to make the available blood volume go further. This is a normal physiologic response. However, if sustained for extended time periods, it will create a pathologic condition. The intense vasoconstriction seen in the shock patient is first observed in the skin as it becomes cold, clammy, and loses color, and later may be identified in other organs as a decrease in urinary output or a loss of consciousness. As blood volume is restored, these pathologic events should be reversed, and the changes in these areas can be used as an index of successful treatment.

***Decreased tissue perfusion.*** During these compensatory processes there is a decreased tissue perfusion that will subsequently affect all vascular beds. By this mechanism blood is diverted initially away from the skin and muscle and later from the liver and kidneys so that blood flow will be maintained through the vital organs (heart and brain). This decreased blood flow to the muscle beds, skin, and then kidneys results in a decreased skin temperature, decreased muscle motion, decreased urinary output, decreased liver function, and intermediary metabolism. In each organ this diminished blood flow has its specific effects while, in addition, contributing to a developing metabolic acidosis and lactic acid production and accumulation.

***Hypoxia and anaerobic glycolysis.*** Decreased perfusion leads to tissue hypoxia because oxygen and nutrients do not enter the tissues. Cellular metabolism in these tissues then converts to an anaerobic form of glycolysis (hypoxic carbohydrate metabolism). This is a complex process, but essentially glucose is metabolized without efficient consumption of oxygen. In this type of metabolism there is only a small amount of energy produced and the vital energy is generated in a less efficient manner. Under these circumstances energy is produced in much smaller amounts and at a greater cost to the patient. This shift in glucose metabolism from a normal aerobic (oxygen-consuming) to an anaerobic state is a normal compensatory mechanism that is useful in moderate exercise, but when this situation exists for prolonged periods, the patient will deplete existing energy stores necessary for essential cellular work functions.

***Lactic acidosis.*** In the anaerobic glycolytic pathway glucose is not broken down to carbon dioxide and water but to lactic acid. This organic acid is produced normally in exercise, and these circulating lactates are readily metabolized in the healthy body if there is normal muscle and liver perfusion. In the pathologic shock state lactic acid and other metabolic acids accumulate and cause a myriad of problems. These acids decrease the tissue and blood pH and may in themselves be considered a biologic toxin at high levels.

Blood pH can now be easily measured along with oxygen and carbon dioxide tensions in millimeters of mercury. Blood lactates can also be measured, but the time required to do so precludes this parameter from being an emergency department tool. From the pH–blood gas nomogram the base deficit can be extrapolated and used as a fairly accurate indicator of the magnitude of the existing metabolic acidosis. This should be made available for patient management decisions in the emergency department.

***Respiratory alkalosis.*** Early in shock a compensatory respiratory alkalosis occurs in response to changes in blood pH and the lactic acidosis. Shock patients compensate by breathing heavily and blow off carbon dioxide in order to raise the blood pH and to lessen the effects of the metabolic acidosis. Another early sign of shock is hyperventilation caused both by tissue hypoxia and acidosis. As shock patients hyperventilate to improve their oxygen intake, they concomitantly eliminate the metabolite carbonic acid ($H_2CO_3$) as volatile carbon dioxide ($CO_2$). This compensatory hyperventilation may become impeded by muscular fatigue or by any cause of mechanical ventilatory dysfunction; this is rapidly associated with $CO_2$ retention and respiratory acidosis. This final insult will further increase hypoxia and worsen the metabolic acidosis, and the patient will die as a result of the drastic reduction in blood pH ($pH < 6.9$).

The shock syndrome with its diminished venous return, lowered cardiac output, increased peripheral resistance (arteriolar vasoconstriction), decreased tissue perfusion, metabolic acidosis, and respiratory alkalosis can be observed and measured during the emergency period. A sound knowledge of the pathophysiologic sequelae of shock and skills in interpreting certain critical parameters will result in better shock management and patient survival in these true emergencies.

### *Ventilatory insufficiency*

Pulmonary dysfunction can be caused by direct injury or can be secondary to nonthoracic trauma. Improvements in the treatment of shock, methods of blood procurement and replacement, prevention of renal failure, and control of overwhelming clostridial and other bacterial infections have produced a new form of posttraumatic sequelae in certain patients. Many of these patients develop an insidious and progressive pulmonary insufficiency. This syndrome, which probably has many different etiologic mechanisms, is becoming more readily recognized as a potential hazard to all patients who have had major trauma or surgery. The syndrome has been described by many eponyms that usually relate to the apparent precipitating cause (for example, shock lung, postperfusion lung, congestive atelectasis, or posttraumatic pulmonary insufficiency). The ability to distinguish these entities by clinical comparisons or experimental models has not yet been developed. Similarities in the progression of clinical events and postmortem analysis suggest a common pathophysiologic basis and probably represent the limited nature by which the pulmonary parenchyma is able to react to trauma of varying types.

The commonly associated conditions responsible for the development of this clinical problem have been direct injury, fluid overload, and embolization of microthrombi of fat, fibrin, and cellular debris from peripheral sources. Also, circulating catecholamines, histamine, serotonin, fatty acids, and the vasoactive polypeptides, especially bradykinin, have been implicated because of their known effects on vascular permeability and bronchospasm.

The complex interrelationship of extravascular fluid movements with the lung has received considerable attention. Alterations of pulmonary surfactant production can occur after a wide variety of pathologic conditions, including those that affect the alveolar lining cells, as occurs after aspiration and transudation of fluid into the lung parenchyma. Pulmonary surfactant is a complex phospholipid that is essential for the physiologic stability of the air-liquid phase in each alveolus. The pathologic effects of oxygen toxicity may be caused by direct injury to the alveolar cells that produce this important surface-active agent. Other conditions that are known to be detrimental to the lung include shock, systemic and pulmonary sepsis, prolonged cardiopulmonary bypass, and disseminated intravascular coagulation.

### ■ What are the clinical features of pulmonary insufficiency?

All patients with a major surgical stress develop some degree of pulmonary impairment and may progress, if not adequately supported, to terminal respiratory failure.

The initial phase, which occurs immediately after injury, is characterized by cardiovascular stabilization; after being adequately resuscitated the patient may go on to develop a high cardiac output and lowered peripheral resistance. There is usually associated mild hypoxemia ($P_{aO_2}$ = 70 to 80 mm Hg), hypocapnia, and hyperventilation. Patients usually show arterial alkalosis, primarily respiratory, and have an adequate oxyhemoglobin saturation level. A patient may improve at this point, at which time these pathophysiologic changes will subside. A satisfactory outcome depends on many factors, including the magnitude of injury, the necessity of extensive resuscitative measures with colloid-poor crystalloid solutions or stored blood, and the length and nature of the surgical intervention.

For reasons not well understood, many patients progress insidiously to a phase of greater pulmonary difficulties. Some of these patients appear surprisingly well at this time but on closer examination will show increased ventilatory effort with tachypnea and shallow breathing. These patients are usually not very cyanotic, and they may even show a rosy complexion. The skin is warm and pink, because the peripheral vessels are dilated and oxygen is less readily released from hemoglobin in the alkalotic state (Bohr effect). The pulse rate is elevated and the cardiac output will remain high. Blood gas concentrations will deteriorate with a fall in arterial oxygen tensions ($P_{aO_2}$ = 60 mm Hg). Hypocapnia persists ($P_{aCO_2}$ = 24 to 30 mm Hg). The alkalosis is now caused by a combination of both metabolic and respiratory components (pH = 7.58, base excess +12 mEq). At this point patients are working harder to breathe, are less able to extract oxygen from the air and, despite increased cardiac action and tissue flow, are less able to release oxygen at the cell level for normal metabolic processes. These patients will soon require some form of enhanced oxygen delivery, including assisted ventilatory support. Those patients who are adequately evaluated, monitored, and sustained during this period can and should survive.

Without intensive management at this point and because of still poorly understood reasons, some patients go on through a phase of progressive pulmonary insufficiency when normal arterial oxygen tensions cannot be maintained even while on assisted ventilation. Carbon dioxide excretion becomes impossible, cellular oxidative metabolism is diminished, and cardiac or respiratory arrest is inevitable. Terminally, blood lactic acid levels rise and the arterial pH falls as hypoxic blood is sluggishly and poorly distributed through the systemic and pulmonary circulatory systems.

### ■ What are the essential steps in the evaluation of thoracic trauma?

Chest trauma may result from penetrating or blunt injury of the chest or its contained viscera. An initial assessment of airway patency is essential. The patient should be observed for signs of obstruction such as stridor, retraction, or wheezing. An evaluation should be made with regard to the possibilities of obstruction from fractures of mandible, maxilla, larynx, or trachea; aspiration of blood; or obstruction by a foreign body. An oral airway and frequent suctioning may be necessary to keep the upper airway patent. As stated previously, endotracheal intubation is preferable to tracheostomy as an initial means of bypassing upper airway obstruction.

Next the adequacy of ventilation must be assessed. This should be done by physical examination and supported by determination of arterial blood gases. The patient should be observed for cyanosis or gasping respiration. Restlessness alone may indicate beginning hypoxia. An examination should be made for failure of chest expansion and for flail or paradoxical motion. Auscultation and percussion of both sides of the thorax should be performed to evaluate the possibilities of pneumothorax and/or hemothorax.

Cyanosis or gasping respiration in a patient who does not have airway obstruction, hemothorax, or pneumothorax means that insufficient oxygen is being absorbed across the alveolar membrane. The cause may be lung contusion, intra-alveolar hemorrhage, or pulmonary edema. Positive pressure ventilation with oxygen enrichment is indicated.

The possibility of respiratory failure must be considered. In massive trauma and shock this may pass undetected while attention is focused on the emergency situation and adequate resuscitation. Fast, shallow respiration may occur early after trauma but may disappear as muscular fatigue progresses. Acute respiratory failure may result from massive atelectasis, lung contusion, simple pneumothorax, hemothorax, tension pneumothorax, flail chest, pneumonia, pulmonary embolism, hemoptysis, or aspiration. Chest tube insertion coupled with positive pressure ventilatory support may be necessary.

### ■ What are the consequences of flail chest?

Flail chest develops when several ribs are fractured on both sides of the point of impact, leaving a portion of the rib cage unstable. Fracture of the sternum in several places may also result in flail chest.

The unsupported chest wall segment behaves in paradoxical fashion, sucking in during inspiration (negative intrapleural pressure) and blowing out during expiration, preventing full lung expansion and adequate oxygen exchange. The lung under the flail segment becomes progressively atelectatic. During expiration end-expired air leaving the unaffected lung is drawn into the affected lung. This to-and-fro movement results in an increase in the dead space and a decrease in arterial oxygen saturation. The failure of the lungs to fill and empty synchronously causes the mediastinum to swing back and forth. This compromises venous return with a resultant decrease in cardiac output. The abnormal movements of the chest wall and the accompanying pain impair effective coughing and result in retention of secretions.

### ■ What is the treatment of flail chest?

Stabilization of the flail segment can be accomplished most effectively by tracheostomy and mechanical volume ventilator support. Less commonly, operative internal fixation of fracture segments with internal wires and plates may be employed when there are multiple fractures of the sternum, a large rib flail segment, or bilateral injury to the thoracic cage.

In the emergency period an endotracheal tube may be used, followed later by tracheostomy. Anywhere from 1 to 4 weeks under this treatment regime, or until paradoxical motion of the chest has decreased and the patient is able to maintain arterial oxygen saturation without ventilatory support, will be necessary. Ventilatory support must be provided by a mechanical ventilator capable of delivering sufficient volume at whatever pressures are necessary to ventilate the lungs. The patient's pH, $P_{O_2}$, and $P_{CO_2}$ must be evaluated frequently. Ventilatory defects secondary to direct lung injury may further affect adequacy of ventilation. The patient can be weaned gradually from the ventilator with close observation of the arterial blood gas concentrations.

Towel clips or hooks passed around the flail segment with the application of external traction is an ineffective method of stabilization and should not be used.

### ■ What are the pathologic consequences of hemothorax and pneumothorax and the appropriate clinical intervention?

Pneumothorax, the accumulation of air in the pleural cavity, can result from both penetrating and nonpenetrating chest injuries. In pneumothorax air is sucked into the pleural space by negative intrapleural pressure during inspiration, gradually accumulating and compromising effective ventilation. Clinically the patient may present with diminished or absent breath sounds on the injured side, asymmetry of chest expansion, and subcutaneous emphysema. All major forms of traumatic pneumothorax are treated definitively by insertion of a chest tube connected to underwater seal drainage or to suction. Minimal (under 30%) pneumothorax may be treated conservatively and will reabsorb spontaneously.

A condition warranting immediate attention in order to prevent rapid deterioration and death is tension pneumothorax. Usually associated with fractured ribs, or less commonly with penetrating injuries such as stab wounds, tension pneumothorax results from the accumulation of air under tension in the pleural space. Unlike pneumothorax, where air enters and leaves the pleural sac with inspiration and expiration, a "valvelike" effect occurs in tension pneumothorax that prevents the release of air and increases pressure in the sac with each inspiration. As pressure builds, the mediastinum is pushed to the contralateral side with progressive impairment of venous return and ventilatory exchange.[10] The clinical picture is severe respiratory distress, cyanosis, and distended neck veins. Breath sounds are absent on the affected side, and tympany is present on percussion. If not recognized and treated immediately by needle aspiration, the patient will experience respiratory arrest. Needle aspiration will bring immediate dramatic results and of course should be followed by definitive thoracostomy and water-seal drainage.

Hemothorax is an accumulation of fluid or blood in the pleural cavity. Laceration of vessels of the chest wall, of intrathoracic great vessels, or of the heart may lead to hemothorax with hypovolemic shock, compression of lung, hypoxemia, and hypercapnia. The clinical picture is similar to pneumothorax. Restoration of blood volume by fluid or blood administration and removal of blood from the pleural cavity should be carried out immediately and simultaneously.

Major hemothorax is drained with a chest tube and suction. The chest tube should be placed in a dependent position, the best location being through the sixth or seventh intercostal space in the midaxillary line, directing the tube posterior to the lung.

Hemothorax may require emergency thoracotomy and operative control of the bleeding source under specific clinical circumstances, for instance, if there is a large clotted hemothorax with a shift in the mediastinum that does not improve on tube drainage, if measured blood loss from the chest tube continues at a rate greater than 250 ml/hr after the first 2 hours, or if the blood loss persists for more than 6 hours.

### ■ What is cardiac tamponade and what are the necessary steps for resuscitation?

Cardiac tamponade is an accumulation of blood in the closed pericardial sac, most commonly caused by a small wound in the heart. As blood is trapped within the inelastic pericardium, blood flow to and from the heart is impeded, resulting eventually in shock and finally cardiac arrest. This cardiogenic shock can occur within several minutes to several hours, depending on the amount of blood accumulated, but may become life-threatening at a volume of as little as 150 ml.

A small puncture wound anywhere on the chest or upper abdomen should arouse suspicion of cardiac tamponade. Characteristic features include muffled or distant heart sounds, a falling blood pressure, and most importantly, a rising venous pressure. It is essential for this reason that all patients with chest or upper abdominal trauma have a CVP catheter inserted and monitored closely.

Once the diagnosis is made, treatment must be initiated immediately. Needle pericardiocentesis (aspiration) is the initial treatment. The removal of as little as 15 to 20 ml of blood may be sufficient to revive the patient. Pericardiocentesis is accomplished using a No. 21 spinal needle attached to a three-way metal stopcock. A 50 ml syringe is placed on one outlet of the stopcock and the chest lead of a standard ECG monitor is attached to the remaining outlet. The monitor is set to lead II and is closely watched while the practitioner inserts the needle just lateral to the xiphoid process at a 45-degree angle inward and upward (Larrey's point).

An ECG tracing of large ventricular QRS complexes indicates that the needle has traversed the pericardial sac and made contact with the ventricular wall (Fig. 6-3). The needle is then withdrawn slightly with continued aspiration. Any fluid or blood aspirated is from the pericardial cavity. This aspiration may cause relief of symptoms but may only be considered a temporary treatment. The patient must be observed continuously, with the anticipation of subsequent aspiration and possible surgery. The CVP, pulse, and blood pressure must be checked

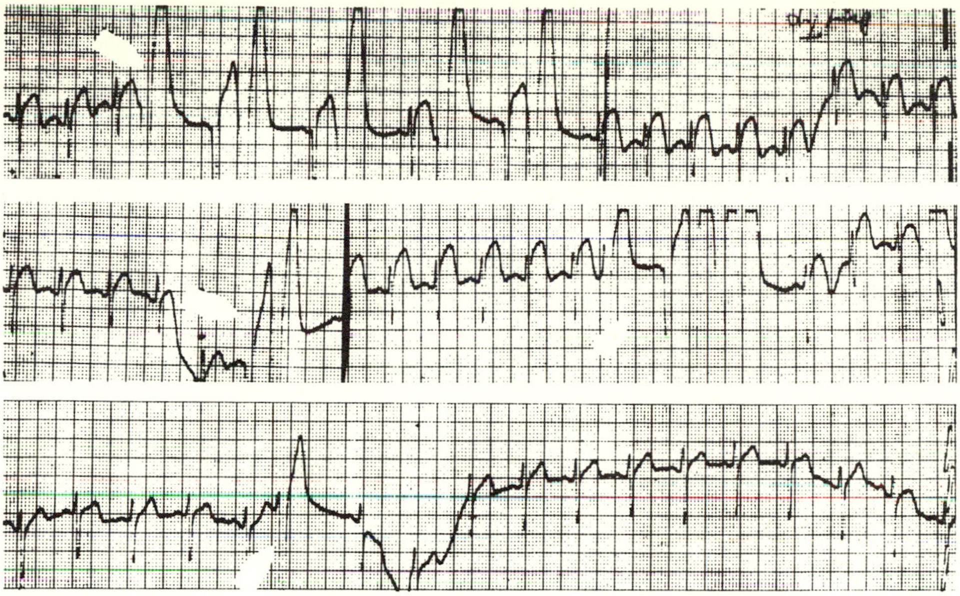

**Fig. 6-3.** Pericardiocentesis using ECG control. Note large ventricular waves and absence of P waves, denoting ventricular contact and intrapericardial position of needle.

every 15 to 30 minutes because of the possibility of recurrence of tamponade. Continued or massive bleeding will indicate the need for operative intervention.

## ■ What are other less obvious consequences of thoracic trauma?

Contusions of the lung, heart, and other thoracic viscera are common sequelae of blunt chest trauma. Contusion of the heart is manifest by ECG changes in epicardial injury or myocardial ischemia. Contusion of the lung reveals itself as an area of increased density in the chest x-ray film, appearing 12 to 72 hours after injury. Areas of lung contusion are associated with hemorrhage; cavitation of the damaged area may occur later.

Tracheal or bronchial rupture or laceration produces pneumomediastinum or pneumothorax. Tension pneumothorax occurs occasionally. Mediastinitis and compression of the trachea are the chief complications. The presence of subcutaneous emphysema, especially in the neck, may indicate the possibility of a serious airway injury. Bronchoscopy may establish the diagnosis. Tracheostomy is used to control respiration, to remove secretions, and to prevent further leakage of air from the high intratracheal pressures that occur with coughing or a Valsalva maneuver. Chest tubes should be inserted if pneumothorax is present. If the volume of air leaking is large, operative repair of the tracheal or bronchial laceration should be done as soon as the patient's general condition permits.

Rupture of the diaphragm is seen after blunt trauma to either the chest or abdomen. The torn diaphragm is totally ineffective and no longer provides a barrier between the thorax and the abdomen. The respiratory impairment caused by diaphragmatic ruptures is very similar to that seen in flail chest. During inspiration (increased negative intrathoracic pressure) abdominal viscera are drawn into the chest, preventing normal inflation of the lung, which then becomes atelectatic. During expiration the involved lung becomes partially filled by the gases being released from the other lung. Compromise of circulation caused by shift of the mediastinum and arterial oxygen unsaturation as a result of shunting are the consequences. A ruptured diaphragm must always be repaired operatively.

Blunt chest trauma, especially of the deceleration type, may lead to aortic injury. The most common point of rupture is just distal to the origin of the left subclavian artery. A widened mediastinum seen on an upright posteroanterior chest x-ray film indicates the possibility of a ruptured aorta and demands diagnostic aortography that, if positive, warrants emergency thoracotomy with cardiopulmonary bypass.

## SUMMARY AND CONCLUSIONS

The approach to the multiple injury patient is resuscitative, diagnostic, and finally therapeutic. Airway and ventilatory adequacy are essential to maintenance of resuscitative effort, and subtle respiratory insufficiency can best be detected by measuring the pH and arterial blood gas concentrations. Treatment of hypovolemia and shock should always include adequate volume replacement and only the judicious use of drugs such as mannitol, vasodilators, dextrans, isoproterenol, and digitalis to improve and maintain tissue perfusion after adequate volume replacement has been assured.

Diagnostic evaluation should be limited to necessary procedures and performed with a minimum of delay and patient manipulation. Abdominal trauma resulting in rupture of solid organs (liver and spleen) and/or retroperitoneal vascular injury can only be managed by operative intervention. Physical findings, paracentesis, and evaluation of vital signs will give indications for surgery. All of the resuscitative measures discussed must be performed to adequately prepare such a patient for operative intervention. The team approach to the multiple injury patient is essential to accomplishment of these aims.

## REFERENCES

1. National Academy of Sciences–National Research Council, Committee on Trauma and Committee on Shock, Division of Medical Sciences: Accidental death and disability: the neglected disease of modern society, Washington, D.C., 1966, U.S. Government Printing Office.
2. Izant, R. J., Jr., and Hubay, C. A.: The annual injury of 15,000,000 children: a limited study of childhood accidental injury and death, J. Trauma **6:**65-74, 1966.
3. Boyd, D. R.: A systems approach to improve trauma patient care, S. Afr. J. Surg. **11:**163-175, 1973.
4. McLean, L. D.: What's new in surgery shock and metabolism? Surg. Gynecol. Obstet. **126:**299-301, 1968.
5. Shoemaker, W. C., et al.: Sequential oxygen hemodynamic events after trauma to the unanesthetized patient, Surg. Gynecol. Obstet. **132:**1033-1038, 1971.
6. Gumpert, J. L., Froderman, S. E., and Mercho, J. P.: Diagnostic peritoneal lavage in blunt abdominal trauma, Ann. Surg. **165:**70-72, 1967.
7. Gertner, H. R., Jr., et al.: Evaluation of the management of vehicular fatalities secondary to abdominal injury, J. Trauma **12:** 425-431, 1972.
8. Leksell, L.: Echoencephalography. II. Midline echo from the pineal body as an index of pineal displacement, Acta Chir. Scand. **115:**225, 1958.
9. Boyd, D. R., and Mansberger, A. R., Jr.: Serum water and osmolal changes in hemorrhagic shock: an experimental and clinical study, Am. Surg. **34:**744-749, 1968.
10. Ballinger, W. F., II, Rutherford, R. B., and Zuidema, G. D.: The management of trauma, Philadelphia, 1968, W. B. Saunders Co.

# chapter 7

# Electrocardiographic changes

ALLAN PRIBBLE
THOMAS A. PRESTON

## ELECTROPHYSIOLOGY

ECG changes in critically ill patients result from a wide variety of metabolic, pharmacologic, ischemic, and inflammatory influences. Changes in heart rhythm, in QRS, T, and P complexes, and in S-T and Q-T segments are commonly seen in the intensive care unit, both as a result of disease and from therapeutic intervention. Arrhythmias may compromise cardiac function but are even more important as clinical signals of underlying metabolic or hemodynamic changes. Alterations of the Q-T and S-T segments and of the various wave forms do not interfere with cardiac function but may provide clues to underlying metabolic problems.

Before discussing specific problems a brief review of the electrophysiology of cardiac electrical activity and its relation to rhythm and conduction is necessary. General mechanisms that alter these electrophysiologic events and their ECG implications will be explained.

### ■ How is cardiac electrical activity generated?

Cardiac electrical activity is generated by the movement of charged particles—sodium ($Na^+$) and potassium ($K^+$) ions—across cell membranes. Fig. 7-1 relates the sequence of these events in a single cell to the electrical forces recorded on the surface ECG.

#### *Depolarization (phase 0)*

An electrical stimulus conducted to the cell membrane causes the resting potential to move toward 0 mv (become less negative). When the transmembrane potential reaches the threshold potential (approximately −70 mv), a sudden change in membrane permeability allows instantaneous movement of positively charged $Na^+$ into the cell. This sudden inrush of positively charged particles changes the intracellular potential to nearly +20 mv.

As the wave of depolarization spreads through the heart muscle, the action potentials generated are recorded on the ECG as the QRS complex. Although depolarization of a single cell requires only 1 millisecond, sequential depolarization of the entire ventricular muscle mass requires 0.06 to 0.12 second.

#### *Depolarized state (phases 1 and 2)*

Following depolarization, the transmembrane potential quickly decreases to 0 (phase 1) and establishes a new steady state (phase 2). Normally no change in transmembrane potential is recorded during phase 2 so the ECG is recorded as a baseline potential, the S-T segment.

#### *Repolarization (phase 3)*

Return to the original resting state requires repolarization (phase 3) of the cell membrane, which begins after a brief pause (S-T interval) in the depolarized state. Repolarization is equal in electrical magnitude to depolarization but occurs more slowly. For this reason the ECG manifestation of repolarization, the T wave, is longer in duration than the QRS complex of depolariza-

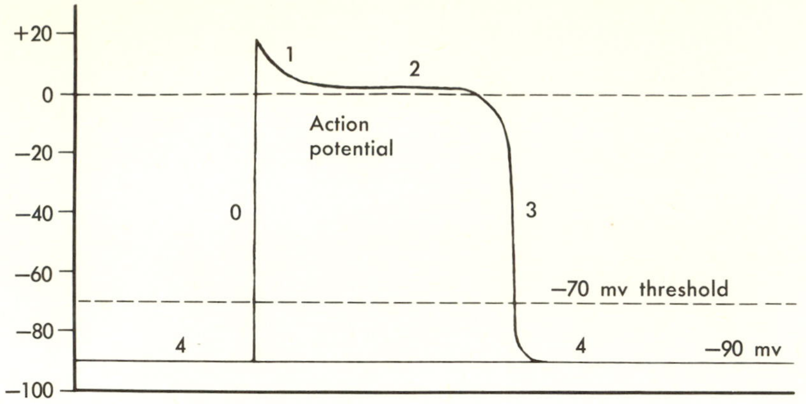


**Fig. 7-1.** Cardiac cell membrane potential.

tion. During repolarization $K^+$ flows out of the cell, causing inscription of the T wave. When repolarization is complete, ionic steady state is achieved, with the transmembrane potential at −90 mv.

### *Baseline potential (phase 4)*

During diastole (phase 4) the muscle cell membrane is fully polarized with a transmembrane potential of −90 mv, the inside of the cell being negative in relation to the outside. Intracellular $K^+$ concentration is 30 times higher than extracellular concentration, and extracellular $Na^+$ concentration is 10 times higher than intracellular concentration. Net ionic motion is prevented by the cell membrane, so that no current is generated, and the ECG is recorded as a baseline potential.

## ■ What function does cardiac electrical activity serve?

Cardiac electrical activity regulates the timing of cardiac contraction and the synchronization between atrial and ventricular contractions. Three major types of heart tissue participate in cardiac electrical activity: pacemaker, or automatic, tissue, conduction tissue, and myocardium. Pacemaker, or automatic, cells originate the electrical impulses that begin muscular contraction. Normally the dominant pacemaker area is the sinoatrial (SA) node, which depolarizes rhythmically approximately 80 times/min. Pacemaker cells in the atrioventricular (AV) junctional area have a slower intrinsic rate of 40 to 60 beats/min. Conduction cells rapidly transfer electrical impulses from pacemaker sites to myocardium. Myocardial contraction is initiated by depolarization of myocardial cell membranes. Only myocardial electrical activity is visible in the surface ECG, because its bulk is relatively much greater than that of the conducting and pacemaking tissue. Although the cells of each of these tissues have distinctive electrical characteristics and functions, the basic sequence of depolarization and repolarization described in Fig. 7-1 is common to all.

## ■ How do pacemaker cells initiate impulses?

Pacemaker cells are called automatic cells because they depolarize spontaneously. Fig. 7-2 illustrates the basic characteristic of automatic cells; that is, the presence of slow, spontaneous depolarization during phase 4. When this slow diastolic depolarization reaches threshold, spontaneous depolarization occurs. An external current applied during diastolic depolarization can cause the automatic cell to depolarize before it reaches threshold spontaneously. In this way pacemaker cells of the SA node, with rapid diastolic depolarization, dominate other automatic cells by depolarizing them before they reach threshold spontaneously. If the SA cells

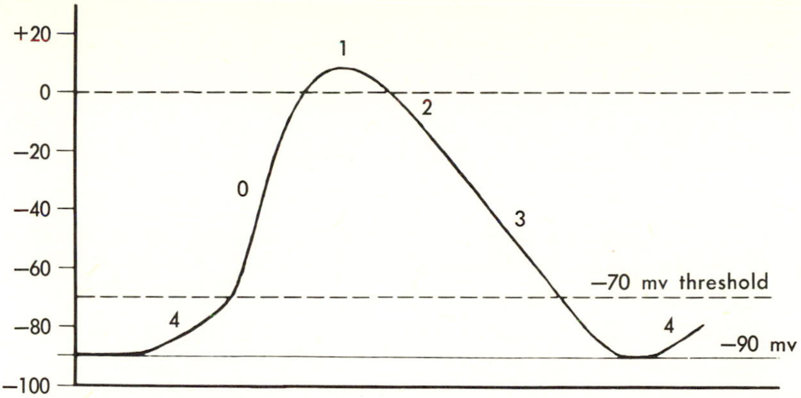


**Fig. 7-2.** Spontaneous but slow depolarization during phase IV allows cell membrane to reach threshold for depolarization and to generate spontaneous action potential. Pacemaker cells depolarize more slowly than Purkinje and muscle cells, and resulting action potential is of lower amplitude.

fail to depolarize, the next fastest depolarizing cells, located in the atrium or AV node, "escape" the dominance of the SA node and assume pacemaking duties at their slower intrinsic rates. Safety valve automatic cells in the ventricular conducting system can initiate contractions at a rate of approximately 40 times/min if AV conduction fails (complete heart block).

## ■ What ECG changes correlate with changes in phases of the action potential?

Decreased rate of rise of the action potential (phase 0) results in slowed conduction that can be manifested by widened P and QRS complexes, AV block, and fascicular or bundle branch block.

Phase 2 corresponds to the S-T interval, and therefore shortening (during digitalis therapy) or prolongation (in response to hypocalcemia) of phase 2 is reflected in the duration of the S-T segment. Since the duration of the Q-T interval is more conveniently measurable, phase 2 changes are expressed as shortening or prolongation of the Q-T interval. Damage to the cell membrane may render it incapable of normal regulation of ionic flow during the normally isoelectric phase 2, resulting in a "current of injury" reflected by elevation or depression of the S-T segment (see Fig. 7-18).

Rapid repolarization during phase 3 is represented by the T wave. Prolongation of phase 3 (caused by hypokalemia) causes lower amplitude and longer duration of the T waves.

Phase 3 terminates with a period of supernormal excitability that coincides with the U wave. Hypokalemia exaggerates the prominence of the U wave by prolonging phase 3.

## ■ How do arrhythmias result from alterations of action potential characteristics?

Stimuli that increase the rate of diastolic depolarization (phase 4 of automatic cells) can result in the appearance of ectopic beats from the atria, junctional area, or ventricles. Prolongation of repolarization (phase 3) or of depolarization (phase 0) provides special circumstances favoring the development of reentry circuits that are manifested as repetitive tachycardias (atrial or ventricular tachycardia) and as isolated extrasystoles.

## ■ How do metabolic abnormalities influence cellular electrical activity?

Since cellular electrical impulses are generated by ionic movement across the cell membrane, alterations in ionic activity and in the membrane itself can alter the shape and duration of the action potential.

Certain electrolyte abnormalities exert specific and identifiable effects on the ECG through alterations of the action potential

(Table 7-1). Many drugs, particularly antiarrhythmic agents, alter phases of the cellular action potential and result in changes in the ECG (Table 7-2).

Automaticity (spontaneous phase 4 depolarization) can be increased by many stimuli, such as hyperadrenergic states, hypoxemia, acidosis, and alkalosis. Acidosis and alkalosis may influence cellular electrical activity only indirectly by causing hyperkalemia and hypokalemia, respectively. Hyperkalemia and certain antiarrhythmic drugs are particularly important causes of slowed conduction, because they decrease the rate of rise and the amplitude of phase 0.

## Common metabolic problems

Major illness, trauma, and the postoperative state are almost invariably attended by metabolic abnormalities. The combination of hypoxemia and respiratory alkalosis, with or without metabolic acidosis, occurs in more than 60% of postsurgical patients and is common during acute myocardial infarction, shock, and other trauma.

Endogenous serum catecholamines, which

**Table 7-1.** Influence of serum potassium and calcium abnormalities on the ECG

| *Serum electrolyte abnormality* | *Effect on action potential* | *Effect on ECG* |
|---|---|---|
| Hypokalemia | Prolonged phase 3, shortened phase 2 | Prolonged low-amplitude T wave and prominent U wave with normal Q-T interval |
| | Increased rate of spontaneous (phase 4) depolarization | Ectopic beats |
| Hyperkalemia | Decreased slope phase 0 | Slowed conduction with intra-atrial, AV, and intraventricular block |
| | Shortened phases 2 and 3 | High-amplitude "peaked" T waves |
| Hypocalcemia | Prolonged phase 2 | Prolonged Q-T interval |
| Hypercalcemia | Shortened phase 2 | Shortened Q-T interval |

**Table 7-2.** Commonly used medications and ECG changes

| | *Serum level* | |
|---|---|---|
| *Preparation* | *Therapeutic* | *Toxic* |
| Anti-arrhythmic drugs | | |
| Quinidine, procainamide | QRS complex prolonged up to 25%, prolonged Q-T interval, depressed S-T segment, low-amplitude or inverted T wave, prominent U wave | QRS complex prolonged 25% to 50%, AV block, SA block, asystole |
| Diphenylhydantoin, lidocaine | Shortened P-R and Q-T intervals | AV block |
| Propranolol | Slowed AV conduction and sinus rate | Sinus bradycardia, AV block |
| Digitalis | S-T segment depressed, short Q-T interval, T wave changes | Arrhythmias, AV block |
| Mood changers | | |
| Phenothiazines | Shortened P-R interval, prolonged Q-T interval, flattened and notched T waves | Arrhythmias, including ventricular fibrillation |
| Tricyclic amines | Prolonged Q-T and P-R intervals, prolonged QRS and P complexes | Ventricular and supraventricular arrhythmias, AV block |
| Catecholamines | Sinus tachycardia, shortened P-R interval | Subendocardial infarction pattern, supraventricular and ventricular arrhythmias |

are potent stimuli to automaticity, are elevated in many illnesses, especially acute myocardial infarction, congestive heart failure, and shock.

Abnormalities of serum electrolytes, particularly serum potassium and calcium, accompany many illnesses, either as primary illness-related problems or as consequences of therapy. Many therapeutic agents, including bronchodilator and pressor catecholamines, anesthetic agents, digitalis and other cardioactive drugs, and even tranquilizers, have direct or indirect effects on the ECG. Intelligent interpretation of arrhythmias, conduction abnormalities, and changes in ECG complexes and intervals in the critically ill patient requires an understanding of these basic facts.

The following case histories illustrate ways in which metabolic derangements can complicate the care and alter the ECG's of critically ill patients.

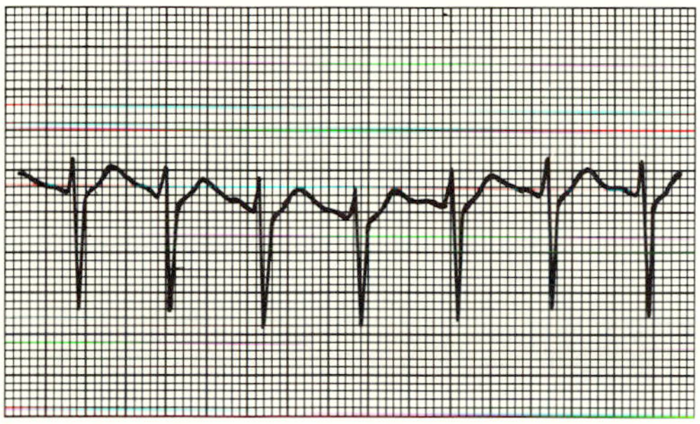

**Fig. 7-3.** Sinus tachycardia at 125 beats/min with Q-T interval at 0.36 second.

- **Fig. 7-3 is an ECG monitor strip from a 21-year-old female with aspiration pneumonia following spontaneous ventricular fibrillation. What is abnormal, what phase of the action potential is implicated, and what is the metabolic cause of the abnormality?**

Referral to Table 7-3 reveals that the Q-T interval is prolonged for a heart rate of 125 beats/min in a female. Prolongation of the Q-T interval means that repolarization,

**Table 7-3.** Upper limits of the normal Q-T interval

| *Heart rate (beats/min)* | *Men and children (sec)* | *Women (sec)* | *Heart rate (beats/min)* | *Men and children (sec)* | *Women (sec)* |
|---|---|---|---|---|---|
| 40 | 0.49 | 0.59 | 70 | 0.40 | 0.40 |
| 43 | 0.48 | 0.49 | 75 | 0.38 | 0.39 |
| 46 | 0.47 | 0.48 | 80 | 0.37 | 0.38 |
| 48 | 0.46 | 0.47 | 86 | 0.36 | 0.37 |
| 50 | 0.45 | 0.46 | 92 | 0.35 | 0.36 |
| 52 | 0.44 | 0.46 | 100 | 0.34 | 0.35 |
| 54 | 0.44 | 0.45 | 109 | 0.33 | 0.33 |
| 57 | 0.43 | 0.44 | 120 | 0.31 | 0.32 |
| 60 | 0.42 | 0.43 | 133 | 0.29 | 0.30 |
| 63 | 0.41 | 0.42 | 150 | 0.27 | 0.28 |
| 66 | 0.40 | 0.41 | 172 | 0.25 | 0.26 |

**Table 7-4.** Upper limits of normal P-R interval

| *Heart rate (beats/min)* | *Adults* | | *Children* | | |
|---|---|---|---|---|---|
| | *Large (sec)* | *Small (sec)* | *14-17 yr (sec)* | *7-13 yr (sec)* | *1½-6 yr (sec)* |
| Below 70 | 0.21 | 0.20 | 0.19 | 0.18 | 0.16 |
| 71-90 | 0.20 | 0.19 | 0.18 | 0.17 | 0.165 |
| 91-110 | 0.19 | 0.18 | 0.17 | 0.16 | 0.155 |
| 111-130 | 0.18 | 0.17 | 0.16 | 0.15 | 0.145 |
| Above 130 | 0.17 | 0.16 | 0.15 | 0.14 | 0.135 |

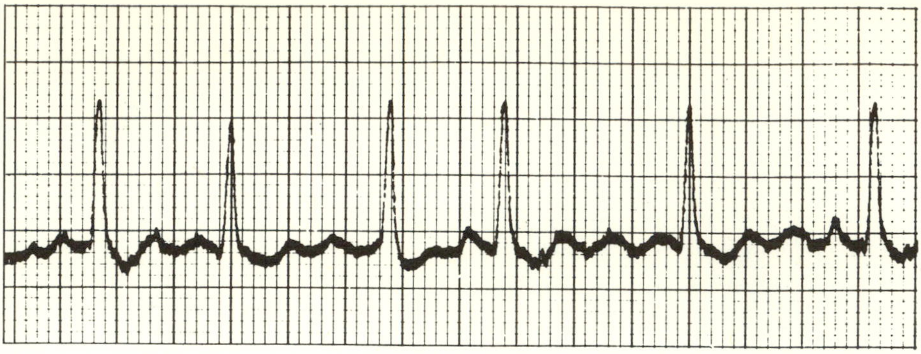

**Fig. 7-4**

(phases 2 and/or 3 of the action potential) is prolonged. Blood gas analysis revealed a $P_{O_2}$ of 55 mm Hg. When normal oxygenation was restored, the Q-T interval returned to normal.

■ **During therapy for bacterial pneumonia with mild respiratory failure, the patient's pulse rate suddenly became rapid and irregular. The rhythm strip shown in Fig. 7-4 was obtained. What does it show, and what are the clinical and electrophysiologic implications?**

This rhythm strip demonstrates atrial fibrillation with a ventricular rate varying from 100 to 150 beats/min. (See later discussion of arrhythmias.)

The development of arrhythmias in respiratory failure often results from increased automaticity, that is, more rapid rate of diastolic (phase 4) depolarization of ectopic pacemakers caused by metabolic abnormalities. Blood gas analysis of this patient revealed moderate hypoxemia and respiratory alkalosis from overventilation. The combination of hypoxemia and respiratory alkalosis is particularly arrhythmogenic and is a common metabolic problem in the critically ill patient.

■ **The ECG shown in Fig. 7-5 was recorded after diuretic therapy for acute pulmonary edema had caused a 6 L diuresis over a period of 8 hours. What abnormalities are present, and what action potential abnormalities do they represent?**

This ECG implicates prolongation of phase 3 of the action potential manifested by prolonged, low-amplitude T waves and prominent U waves. Rapid diuresis frequently causes rapid loss of body potassium stores, resulting in significant hypokalemia. Replacement of potassium quickly corrected these abnormalities.

■ **During the initial evaluation of a patient in diabetic ketoacidosis, the ECG shown in Fig. 7-6 was obtained. What does it illustrate?**

This ECG reflects the characteristic high-amplitude, peaked T waves of early hyperkalemia caused by shortening of phases 2 and 3 of the action potential.

Administration of insulin and appropriate IV fluids rapidly corrected this potentially dangerous situation. Fig. 7-7 graphically illustrates the progressive changes associated with increasing serum potassium levels, culminating in ventricular fibrillation or asystole. Recognition of hyperkalemia from the ECG can alert the critical care worker to a life-threatening danger for the patient.

■ **During treatment with IV aminophylline for acute asthma, the rhythm strip shown in Fig. 7-8 was obtained from a 24-year-old male. What may be seen?**

A normal sequence of electrical activity is followed by a ventricular ectopic beat. (See discussion of arrhythmia analysis.) This patient was mildly hypoxemic and was receiv-

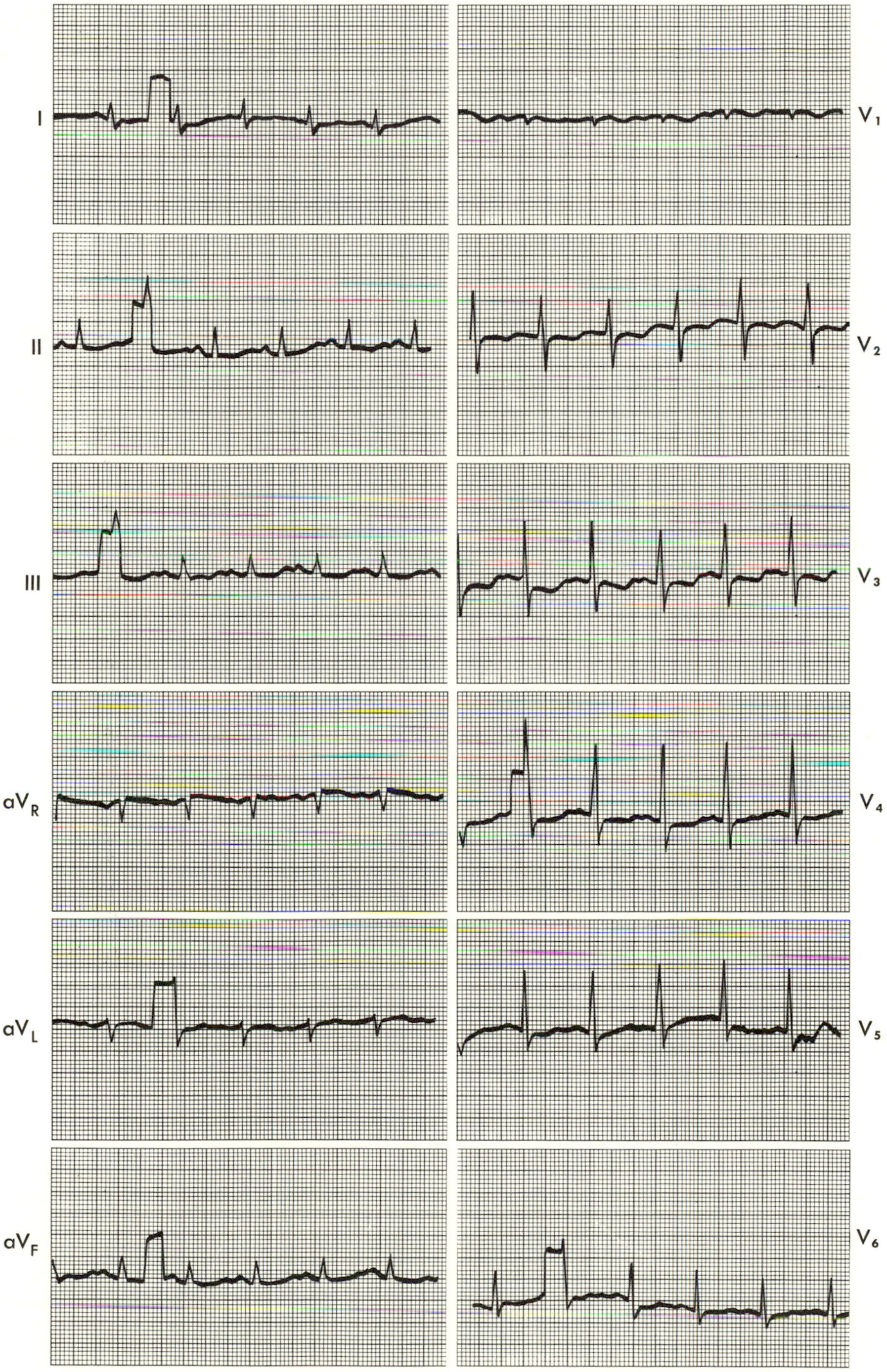


**Fig. 7-5**

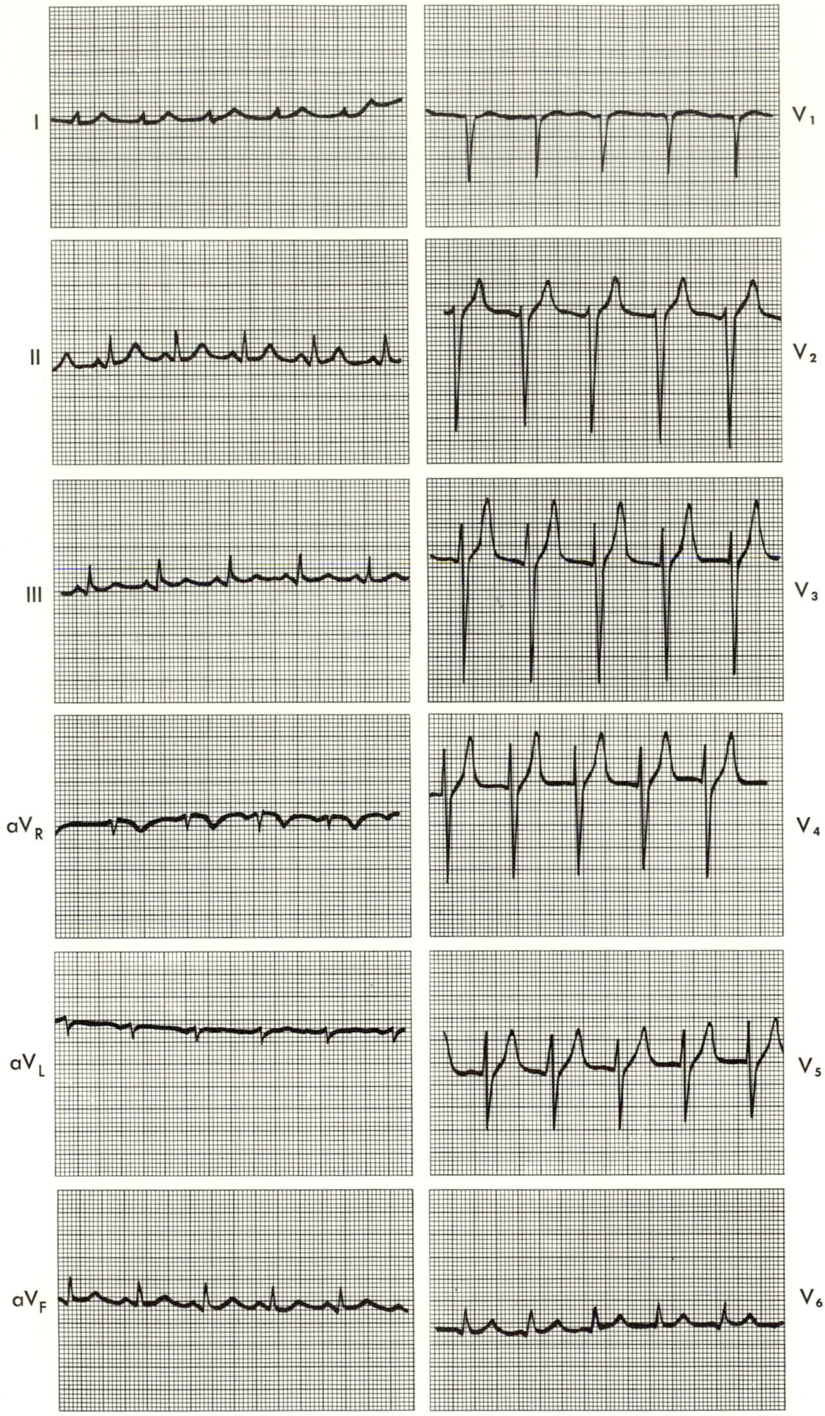


**Fig. 7-6**

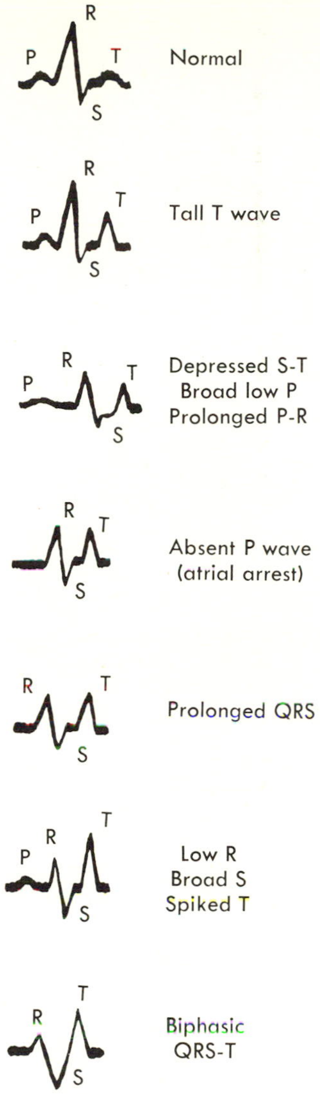


**Fig. 7-7.** QRS-T changes at progressively increasing serum potassium levels.

ing the catecholamine aminophylline, thus being subjected to two potent stimuli of phase 4 depolarization. Careful monitoring and cautious dose reduction allowed the continued use of aminophylline without progression to a more serious arrhythmia.

■ **During dialysis for acute renal failure a routine ECG (Fig. 7-9) was obtained. What abnormalities are present, and what is their significance?**

This ECG demonstrates marked prolongation of the Q-T interval consistent with increased duration of phases 2 and/or 3 of the action potential. Determination of serum electrolyte concentrations demonstrated hypocalcemia, a frequent abnormality during renal failure.

## ARRHYTHMIAS

■ **When are arrhythmias dangerous?**

Arrhythmias are dangerous if they reduce cardiac output or if they predispose to ventricular fibrillation.

Rapid supraventricular tachycardias can reduce cardiac output by limiting diastolic filling time. Elderly patients may experience significant decreases in cardiac output at ventricular rates above 150 beats/min. The absence of coordinated atrial contraction, as with atrial fibrillation or ventricular tachycardia, also impairs ventricular filling and can decrease cardiac output. When the atrial contribution to ventricular filling is lost, rapid heart rates that limit diastolic filling time are particularly deleterious to cardiac output.

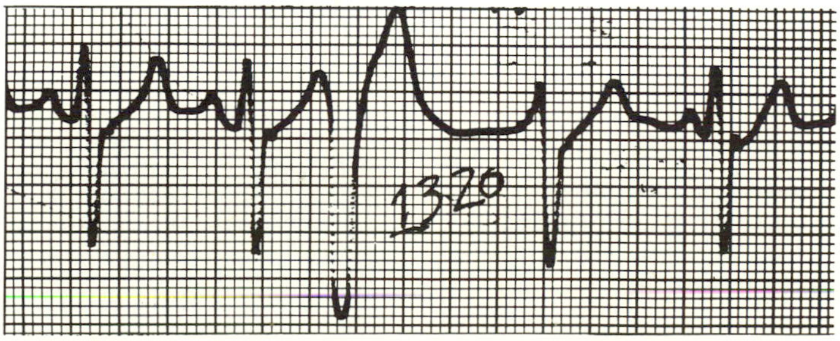


**Fig. 7-8**

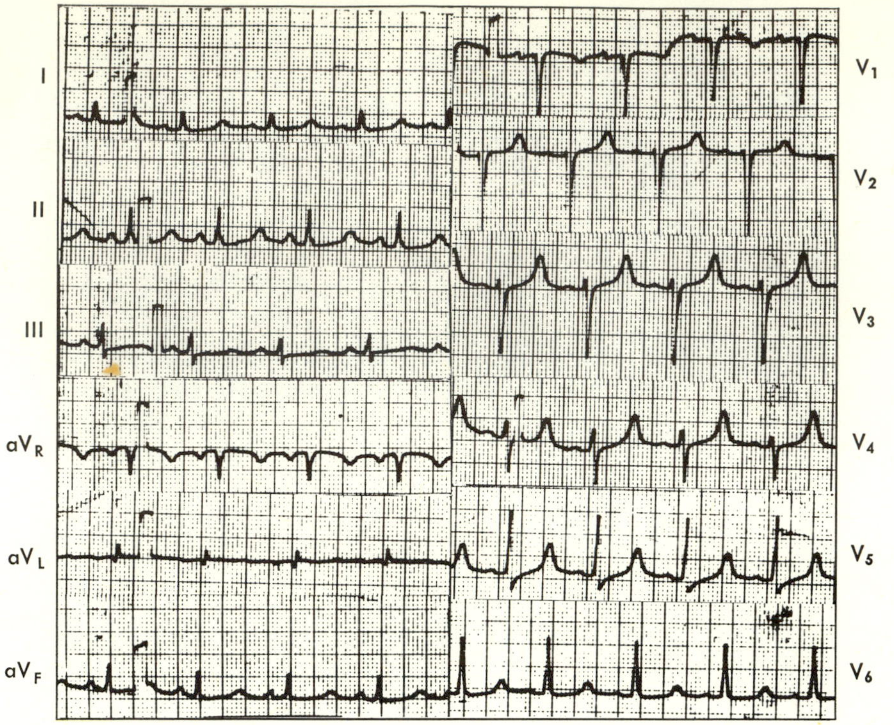


Fig. 7-9

Premature contractions force the ventricle to eject blood before adequate diastolic filling has occurred, thus limiting stroke volume. Cardiac output can be reduced by premature contractions when they are very frequent.

Progression to ventricular fibrillation is the major danger of any ventricular arrhythmia during acute myocardial infarction and acute respiratory failure. Certain types of ventricular arrhythmias are traditionally considered to be signs of advanced heart disease and predictive of subsequent sudden cardiac death. Fig. 7-10 illustrates these phenomena.

## ■ What is the clinical approach to arrhythmia interpretation?

Interpretation of the clinical significance of arrhythmias includes the following:

1. Assessment of the hemodynamic impact. Does the patient exhibit signs of inadequate cardiac output?
2. Assessment of prognostic significance. Will this arrhythmia predispose to a more serious one such as ventricular fibrillation?
3. Assessment of the reason for its appearance. What underlying hemodynamic or metabolic changes prompted its appearance?
4. Assessment of the relationship of digitalis therapy to the arrhythmia. The possibility of digitalis toxicity is enhanced in critical care situations and is an important and frequent cause of arrhythmias.
5. Diagnosis of the specific type of arrhythmia. Recognition is necessary in evaluating the overall significance of the condition.

## ■ How are arrhythmias diagnosed using the ECG?

Most of the commonly observed arrhythmias can be rapidly diagnosed by using the following five simple checkpoints:

1. Ventricular rate. Ventricular rates above 150 beats/min are commonly associated with

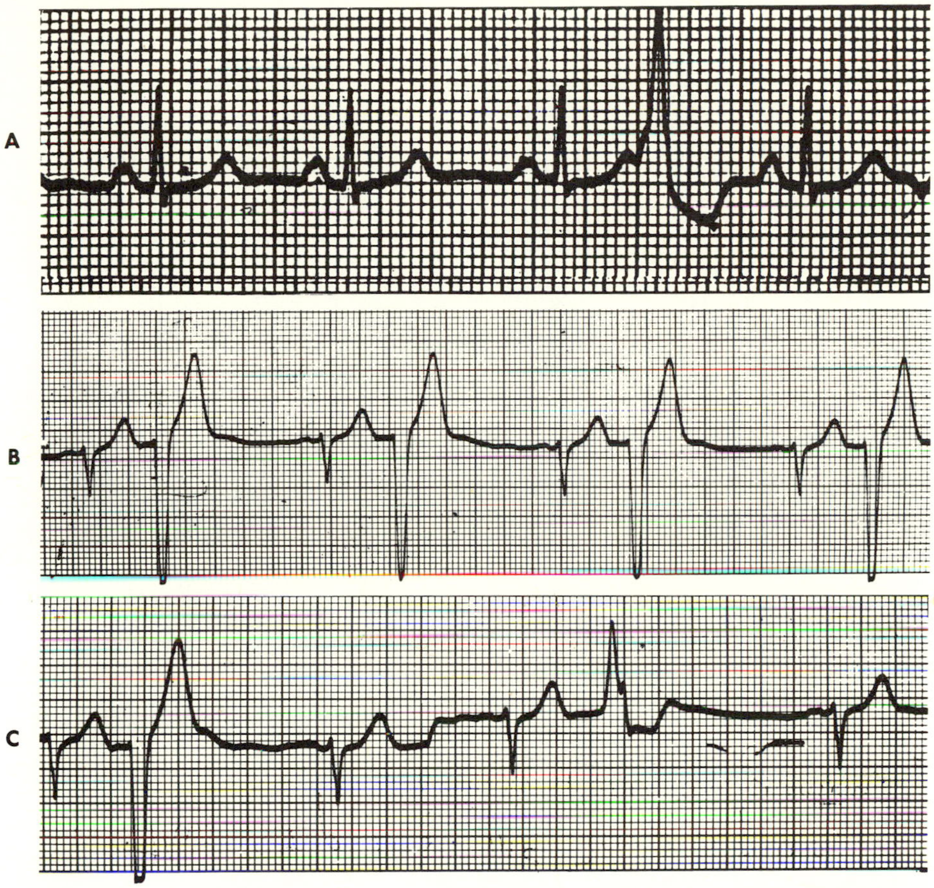

*Continued.*

**Fig. 7-10.** Ventricular ectopic beats more complex than unifocal premature beats. During acute myocardial ischemia these abnormal beats may rapidly progress to ventricular fibrillation. When seen during routine evaluation of asymptomatic individuals, they correlate with subsequent sudden cardiac death. **A,** "R-on-T" phenomenon. The T wave following the third QRS complex is interrupted by a premature ventricular QRS complex. **B,** Ventricular bigeminy. Each normal QRS complex is followed at a consistent interval by a premature ventricular beat. The abnormal beats are identical in form and thus presumably originate from the same focus. **C,** Multifocal ventricular premature beats. Two abnormal premature ventricular complexes are seen. Both the QRS forms and the coupling intervals are different, suggesting two different foci of origin. **D,** Ventricular tachycardia. A premature ventricular beat is followed by four ventricular beats at a rate of approximately 150 beats/min. This arrhythmia is nearly always indicative of serious underlying heart disease. **E,** Repetitive premature ventricular beats. Two premature ventricular complexes, possibly from different foci, occur without intervening normal complexes. **F,** Ventricular fibrillation. There is total absence of definable QRS complexes. This random, disorganized electrical activity reflects totally disorganized ventricular muscle activity. During ventricular fibrillation there is essentially no blood flow, and instantaneous loss of consciousness ensues.

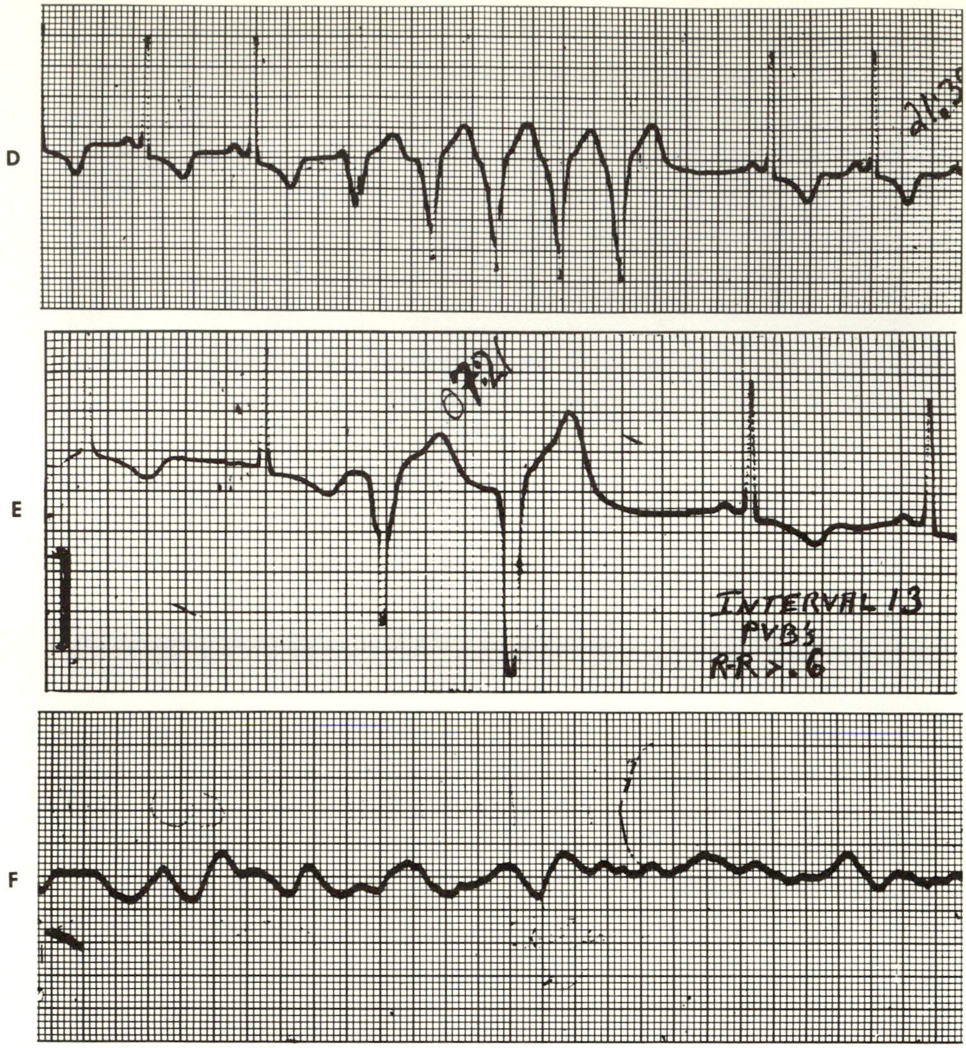


**Fig. 7-10, cont'd.** For legend see p. 145.

paroxysmal supraventricular tachycardia, atrial flutter or fibrillation, or ventricular tachycardia. Ventricular rates below 50 beats/min suggest sinus bradycardia, junctional escape rhythm, or complete heart block with idioventricular rhythm.

2. Ventricular rhythm. Ventricular response to supraventricular arrhythmias may be regular or irregular. Totally irregular ventricular response is found with atrial fibrillation and chaotic atrial tachycardia, as well as with random unifocal and multifocal atrial and ventricular ectopic beats. Group beating, or repetitions of a series of irregular beats, characterizes the Wenckebach phenomenon, trigeminy, and bigeminy.

3. QRS analysis. QRS analysis helps determine whether the arrhythmia is ventricular or supraventricular. Normal-width (less than 0.12 second) QRS complexes always denote an atrial or junctional (supraventricular) focus. Arrhythmias of ventricular origin always have wide (0.12 second or more) QRS complexes. Aberrant conduction of supraventricular impulses frequently causes wide QRS complexes, leading to confusion with ventricular arrhythmias.

4. P wave analysis is crucial to identifica-

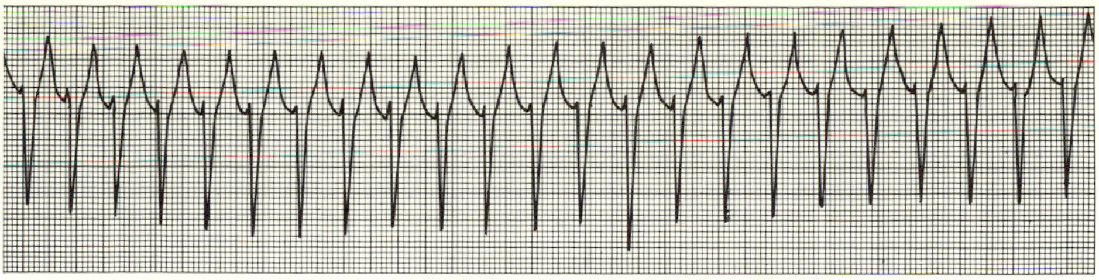

**Fig. 7-11**

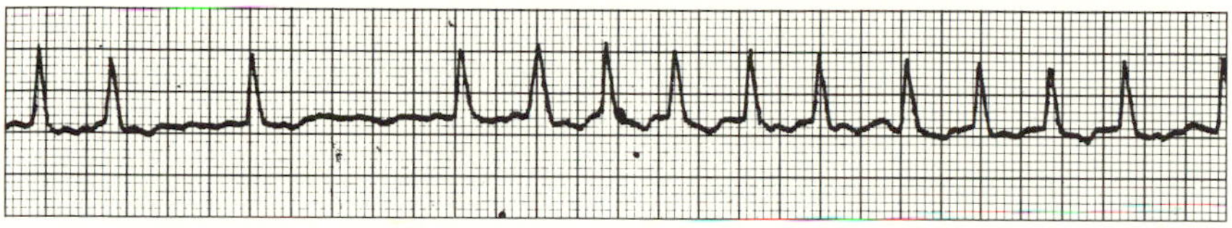

**Fig. 7-12.** From Conover, M. H.: Cardiac arrhythmias, St. Louis, 1974, The C. V. Mosby Co.

tion of supraventricular arrhythmias. If P waves are not visible in the 12-lead ECG, then esophageal, right atrial, or Lewis leads should be employed to identify them. Carotid sinus massage may slow a rapid ventricular rate enough to expose atrial activity otherwise obscured by QRS complexes.

5. Observation of the onset and termination of sustained tachycardias can yield valuable diagnostic information. Supraventricular tachycardias are nearly always initiated by a premature supraventricular beat with an abnormal P wave. Ventricular arrhythmias are not preceded by ectopic P waves. Following termination of a supraventricular arrhythmia, there is a period of sinus pause, or abnormal P waves, occurring before resumption of normal sinus rhythm. Ventricular tachycardias may be followed by a full compensatory pause.

### ■ Is the arrhythmia shown in Fig. 7-11 supraventricular or ventricular?

The ventricular rate is 175 beats/min, immediately placing the arrhythmia in the category with paroxysmal supraventricular tachycardia, atrial flutter or fibrillation, or ventricular tachycardia. Because the QRS complexes are normal in duration, this is a supraventricular tachycardia. The rate and regular rhythm make this paroxysmal atrial tachycardia.

### ■ What commonly encountered arrhythmia is shown in Fig. 7-12?

The ventricular rate of approximately 130 beats/min is not specific for any particular arrhythmia, but the normal QRS duration identifies a supraventricular origin. In this case the rhythm is the leading indicator of the arrhythmia, as it is totally irregular and therefore must indicate atrial fibrillation. Multifocal or chaotic atrial tachycardia could also give an irregular rhythm, but no definite P waves are seen, affirming that this is atrial fibrillation.

### ■ What is perhaps the most commonly misdiagnosed serious arrhythmia?

Since the QRS complexes are normal in duration, the arrhythmia shown in Fig. 7-13 is of supraventricular origin, and the possible diagnoses based on the rate of 130 beats/min are sinus tachycardia, paroxysmal supraventricular tachycardia, and atrial flutter. Careful inspection reveals that what appears to be a terminal positive QRS deflection is actually a P wave. Atrial flutter with 2:1 conduction frequently presents this way, with every other P wave (flutter wave) hidden or

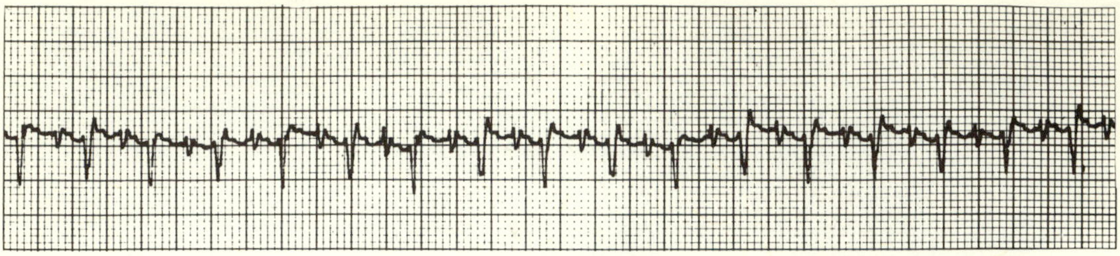

Fig. 7-13

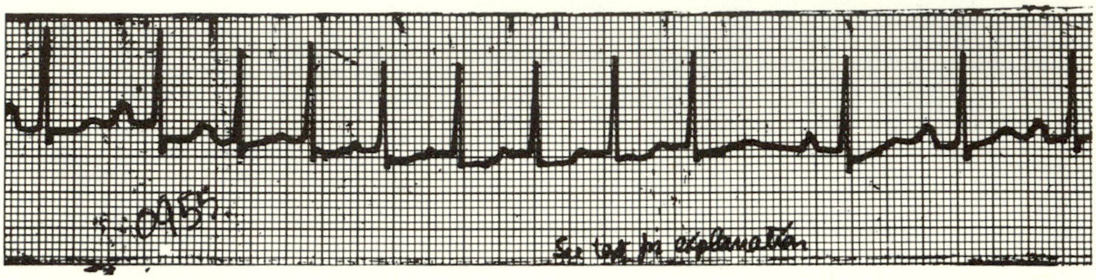


Fig. 7-14

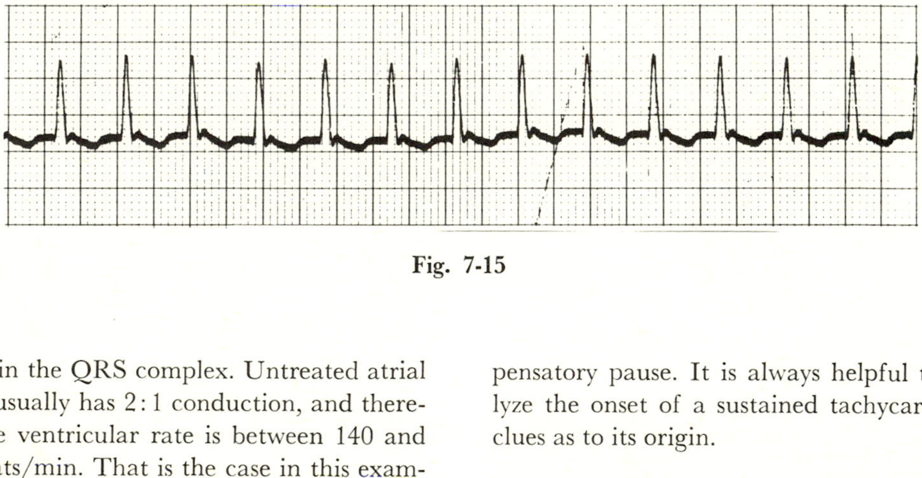

Fig. 7-15

buried in the QRS complex. Untreated atrial flutter usually has 2:1 conduction, and therefore the ventricular rate is between 140 and 160 beats/min. That is the case in this example, and the diagnosis is confirmed by gentle carotid sinus massage, increasing the block at the AV node and unmasking a series of two or more consecutive flutter waves, by which the diagnosis can be made.

■ **What is the mechanism of the onset of the arrhythmia shown in Fig. 7-14?**

In this case the tachycardia was initiated by an atrial ectopic beat (sixth complex from left) followed by a supraventricular tachycardia. After termination of the arrhythmia sinus rhythm resumes without a full compensatory pause. It is always helpful to analyze the onset of a sustained tachycardia for clues as to its origin.

■ **What might cause a relatively long pause in the P wave?**

P wave analysis could show an absence of one P wave at a time when it should have occurred. The P wave terminating the long pause would occur at the expected time; thus the arrhythmia would consist of one missed atrial depolarization and one QRS complex. Had a P wave occurred during the pause, but with no QRS complex following it, the diagnosis would have been AV block; with no atrial activity occurring, it is an SA node block. The block may be in the tissue

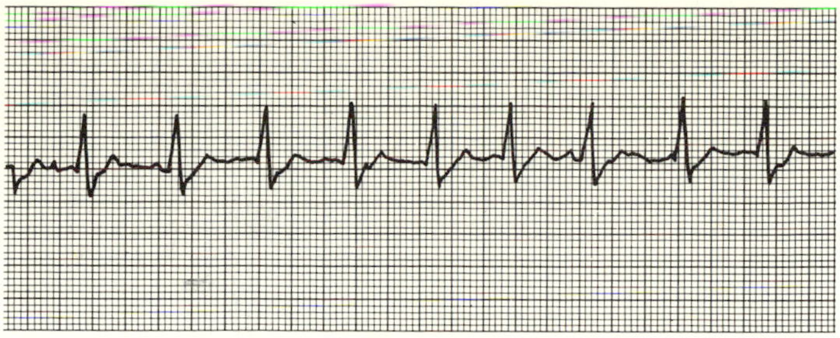

Fig. 7-16

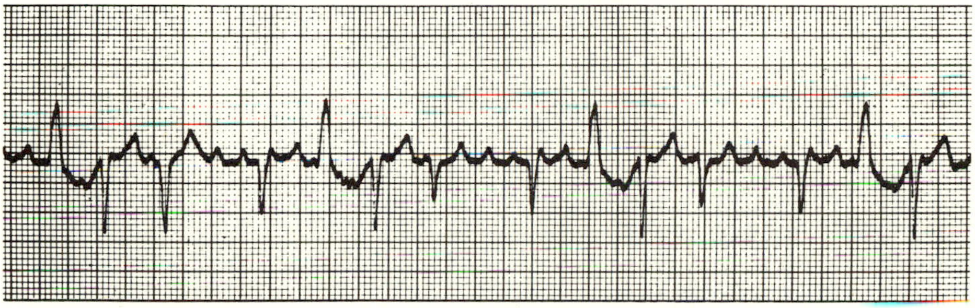

Fig. 7-17

surrounding the SA node, thus preventing escape of the impulse into the atria.

■ **Are the atria and ventricles associated or dissociated in Fig. 7-15?**

In this example there is one P wave with every QRS complex, and a constant relationship exists between them. Therefore there is association between the ventricles and atria; in this example, however, the P waves follow the QRS complexes rather than preceding them. This is typical of an AV junctional rhythm. The diagnosis is based on the occurrence of the P wave after each QRS complex and on an abnormal P wave configuration, representing retrograde conduction from the AV junction through the atria.

■ **On the basis of the QRS configuration, what are the two possible reasons for the arrhythmia illustrated in Fig. 7-16?**

With large, wide QRS complexes this is either ventricular tachycardia or a supraventricular tachycardia with aberrant conduction (intraventricular conduction defect). In this case the presence of P waves occurring at a different rate and unassociated with the QRS complexes confirms that this is ventricular tachycardia. With a supraventricular tachycardia there would be a 1:1 relationship between the P waves and the QRS complexes.

■ **What is the nature of the wide, abnormal-looking QRS complexes in Fig. 7-17?**

This is an example of aberrant conduction of supraventricular impulses. The abnormal beats are conducted with a right bundle branch block configuration. In most patients the right bundle branch remains refractory slightly longer than the left bundle branch, resulting in a brief period during which a premature supraventricular impulse conducted through the ventricles travels through the left bundle branch but is blocked at the right bundle branch. This results in a QRS complex with a right bundle branch block configuration. Occasionally the phenomenon occurs with left bundle branch block, but in the majority of cases the aberrant conduction is of the right bundle branch variety.

Three general rules help to identify aberrant conduction:

1. If a P wave precedes the anomalous QRS complex, it is probably supraventricular.
2. The period during which aberrant conduction can occur is at the end of the refractory period following the previous impulse. Therefore a beat that comes at a relatively short interval following a beat that was preceded by a relatively long interval is likely to undergo aberrant conduction. The general rule favoring aberrant conduction is a short R-R interval following a longer R-R interval.
3. In most cases, aberrant conduction is of the right bundle branch block variety.

## HEART DISEASE

### ■ What ECG changes are caused by coronary artery disease?

Heart damage from coronary arteriosclerosis is caused by obstruction to coronary blood flow leading to myocardial hypoxia. Three degrees of hypoxic damage are associated with specific ECG changes. *Ischemia* refers to reversible myocardial damage leading to altered repolarization. Deep, symmetric T wave inversion is the ECG sign of epicardial ischemia, and a large, peaked T wave is the sign of subendocardial ischemia. *Injury* is a more severe form of damage, in which cell membrane abnormalities result in a *current of injury* that displaces the normally isoelectric S-T segment. This electric current is registered as elevation or depression of the S-T segment. Subendocardial injury causes S-T segment depression, and subepicardial or transmural injury causes S-T segment elevation. Areas of injury can recover or proceed to infarction. *Infarction* is irreversible death of myocardium leading to absence of normal electrical forces and is manifested by a negative initial QRS deflection called the *Q wave.* Q wave duration must be 0.04 second or greater to correlate significantly with infarction. (Many normal individuals have initially negative QRS deflections of 0.02-second duration in left ventricular leads that represent septal depolarization.)

Coronary artery disease is clinically manifested as myocardial infarction, which causes ECG changes in 80% to 90% of incidents, and as angina pectoris, which is associated with less frequent and less specific changes.

### ■ What ECG changes result from acute myocardial infarction?

Myocardial infarction can be *transmural,* that is involving at least the outer two-thirds of the ventricular wall, or *subendocardial,* that is, limited to the inner one third or endocardial surface of the ventricular wall.

Acute transmural infarction causes the appearance of the Q wave. An accompanying S-T segment elevation (epicardial injury) and T wave inversion (epicardial ischemia) indicate that the event is probably recent.

### ■ Why does a Q wave result from transmural infarction?

Dead tissue is unable to generate a depolarization current; it is electrically silent. Leads monitoring the depolarization current from an infarcted area will record an initial negative deflection caused by depolarization of the opposite heart wall. The Q wave is the ECG sine qua non of transmural infarction and represents dead tissue.

### ■ Why are S-T segment and T wave changes present?

Surrounding the infarction area is a zone of injury and around that a zone of ischemia. Since transmural infarction involves the epicardial surface of the heart, epicardial injury occurs and an elevated S-T segment results. S-T segment elevation usually resolves within a few days and therefore is considered necessary for ECG diagnosis of *acute* myocardial infarction.

Symmetrically inverted T waves indicate the presence of an ischemic zone of altered repolarization. Transmural myocardial infarction usually causes epicardial ischemia as well as injury, and therefore T wave inversion is usually present at some time during the event.

Fig. 7-18 schematically illustrates typical S-T segment and T wave changes.

Infarction of the subendocardial layer, which includes the inner third of the ventricular wall, causes only S-T segment and T wave changes. Healthy tissue in the overlying epicardium is still capable of generating a normal QRS complex and no Q waves appear. However, the ischemia and injury associated with the infarction are manifested by the S-T segment and T wave changes. S-T segment depression reflects endocardial injury, contrasting with the S-T segment elevation of epicardial injury normally seen in transmural infarction. Deep symmetric T wave inversion occurs if the endocardial ischemia extends to the epicardial surface.

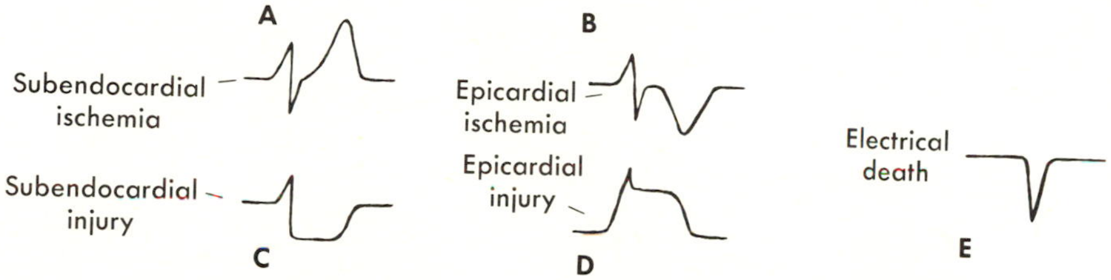


**Fig. 7-18.** Schematic ECG forms of ischemic events. **A,** Tall T waves of subendocardial ischemia. **B,** Inverted coved T waves of epicardial ischemia. **C,** RST segment depression of subendocardial injury. **D,** RST segment elevation of epicardial injury. **E,** QS wave of electrical death.

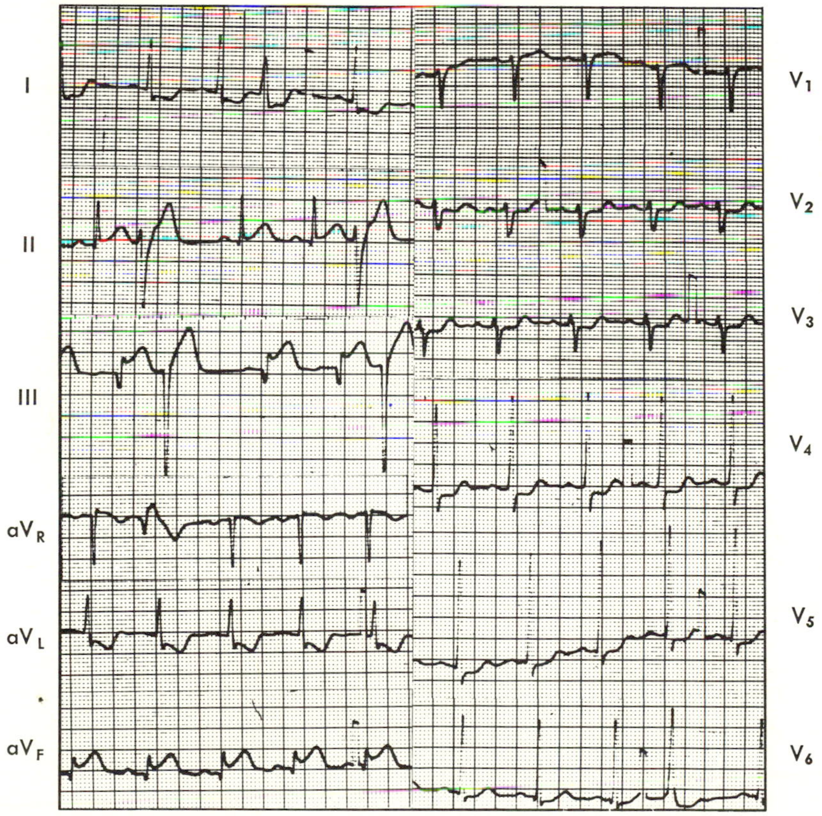


**Fig. 7-19**

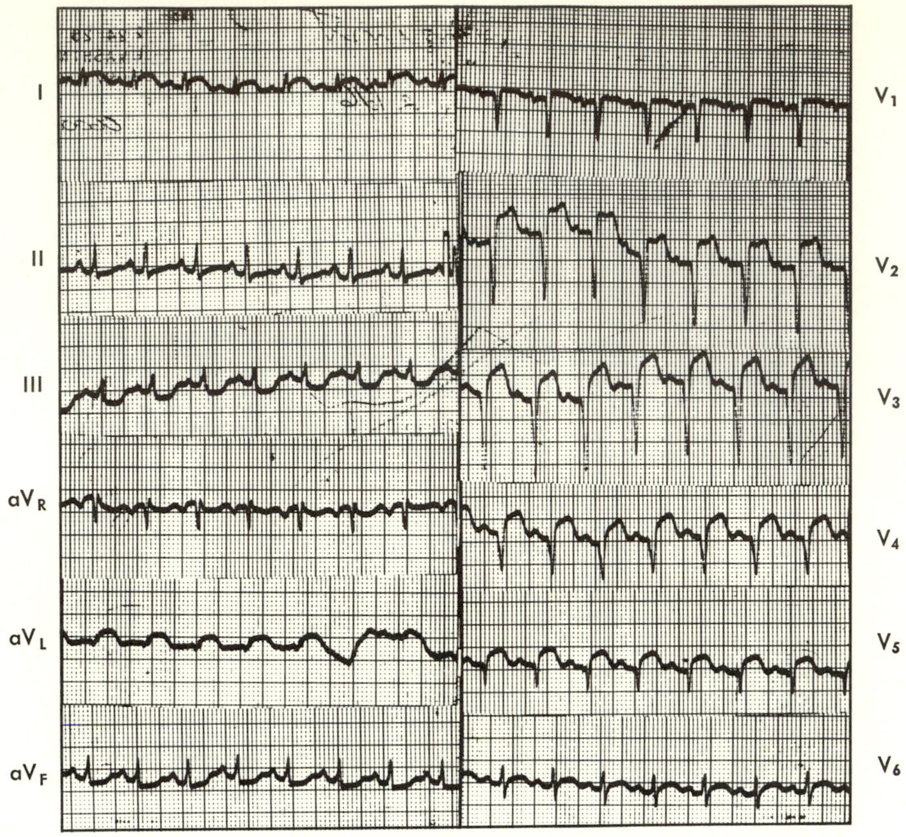


Fig. 7-20

■ **The ECG shown in Fig. 7-19 was taken after the patient had been resuscitated from ventricular fibrillation. What is the diagnosis?**

Compared with a prior normal ECG, this one demonstrates the recent appearance of 0.04-second duration Q waves in lead III, plus S-T segment elevation in leads that monitor the inferior or diaphragmatic surface of the heart—II, III, and $aV_F$. Reciprocal S-T segment depression appears in leads I and $aV_L$. The pattern is typical of acute diaphragmatic (inferior) transmural myocardial infarction. Premature ventricular contractions are also present, and with acute myocardial infarction, might lead to ventricular fibrillation.

■ **Shortly after a 58-year-old man developed crushing precordial chest pain and severe weakness, the ECG shown in Fig. 7-20 was obtained. What abnormalities are present, and what is the location of the infarction?**

Leads I, $aV_L$ and $V_1$ through $V_6$ exhibit striking S-T segment elevation, and reciprocal S-T segment depression is found in leads II, III, and $aV_F$. The absence of initial R waves, that is, the presence of Q waves, in precordial leads $V_2$ through $V_4$ designates this as an anterolateral myocardial infarction. T wave inversion has not yet developed.

■ **What are the earliest ECG findings of acute myocardial infarction?**

Fig. 7-21 displays precordial leads from a patient whose myocardial infarction developed in the hospital. The tracing in Fig. 7-21, *A,* is the normal admission record. In the tracing in Fig. 7-21, *B,* there is a dra-

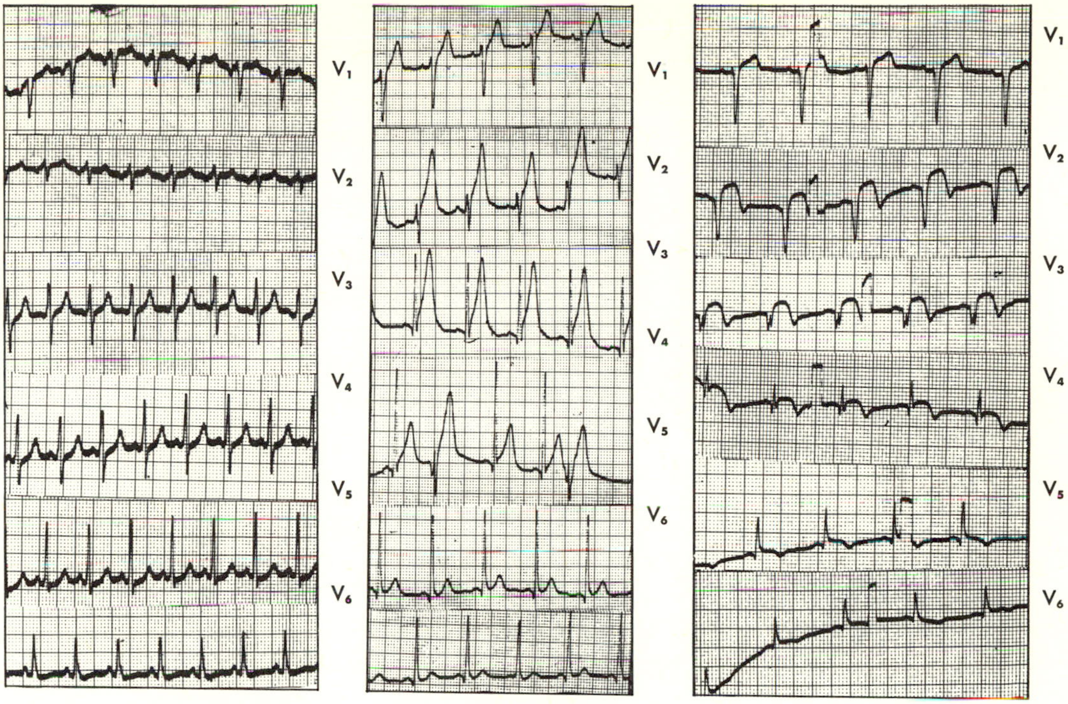


**Fig. 7-21**

matic increase in T wave amplitude associated with S-T segment elevation in leads $V_1$ through $V_3$ and reciprocal depression in leads $V_4$ through $V_6$. One day later, 0.04-second Q waves appear in leads $V_2$ through $V_4$, with S-T segment elevation and T-wave inversion in leads $V_2$ through $V_6$.

Initial epicardial injury (S-T segment elevation) and endocardial ischemia (tall, peaked T waves) characterize the "hyperacute" myocardial infarction. Within hours or days the more familiar Q waves of transmural infarction and T wave inversion of accompanying epicardial ischemia evolve.

### ■ How long does the ECG remain changed after an acute myocardial infarction?

S-T segment changes can disappear within hours or may persist for days. S-T segment elevation present months after an infarction may signal the presence of a ventricular aneurysm. T waves may remain inverted for months, and Q waves usually remain permanently. Q waves may regress or disappear after months or years as the myocardial scar contracts and decreases in size.

### ■ How does the ECG localize infarctions anatomically?

Areas of infarction are localized by determining which leads display pathologic Q

**Table 7-5.** ECG localization of infarction

| *Anatomic type of infarction* | *ECG leads affected* |
|---|---|
| Inferior (diaphragmatic) | II, III, $aV_F$ |
| Anteroseptal | $V_1$-$V_3$ |
| Anterior | $V_2$-$V_4$ |
| Anterolateral | I, $aV_L$, $V_4$-$V_6$ |
| Apical | $V_3$, $V_4$ |
| Posterior* | $V_1$, $V_2$ |

*The truly posterior infarct is sensed only reciprocally by $V_1$, since there are no leads over the back. If an esophageal lead is used, Q waves, S-T segment elevation, and T wave inversion are found—the reciprocal changes of which are reflected in $V_1$ as a broad (0.04-second) R wave, S-T segment depression, and upright T waves.

waves. Leads II, III, and $aV_F$ best display changes from the inferior surface of the heart, whereas the anterior and lateral walls of the left ventrical are monitored by I, $aV_L$ and $V_2$ through $V_6$. Lead $V_1$, over the right ventricle, senses changes in the posterior left ventricular surface. Table 7-5 lists anatomic sites of infarcts relative to the ECG leads in which Q waves appear.

### ■ What ECG changes accompany angina pectoris?

Three syndromes of angina pectoris exist, and all three can be associated with ECG changes. Approximately 50% of the episodes of stress-induced angina pectoris result in subendocardial injury with S-T segment depression. Specific criteria have been developed to separate the stress-induced subendocardial injury pattern of S-T segment depression caused by coronary disease from that caused by metabolic and nonspecific changes. Reliable correlation with the presence of coronary disease requires that the S-T segment be depressed at least 1 mm below the baseline (P-R interval) for at least 0.06 second after the junction point between the QRS complex and the S-T segment is written (Fig. 7-22).

Preinfarction angina is clinically a more severe form of angina pectoris with a high rate of progression to myocardial infarction. ECG changes of typical angina pectoris are often observed in this syndrome. Prinzmetal, or "variant," angina pectoris is a syndrome of angina occurring at rest associated with S-T segment elevation.

### ■ What other problems cause S-T segment depression?

Many nonspecific metabolic and inflammatory processes cause S-T segment depression. These can create confusion by imitating subendocardial "injury." Adherence to the criteria described previously for stress-induced injury patterns will usually resolve the confusion.

Common causes of S-T segment depression not associated with subendocardial injury in critically ill patients include the following:

1. Digitalis therapy can cause a smoothly "scooped-out" concave S-T segment depression (Fig. 7-23).
2. Hyperventilation can cause mild S-T segment depression and T wave inversion.
3. Rapid heart rates can result in artifactual depression of the initial part of the S-T segment (Fig. 7-24).

### ■ What cardiac problems other than coronary artery disease cause ECG changes?

Myocarditis, endocarditis, and pericarditis are encountered in critically ill patients either as primary problems or as complications of other diseases.

Myocarditis and endocarditis are relatively uncommon diseases and cause nonspecific S-T segment and T wave changes. Myocarditis with acute rheumatic fever often

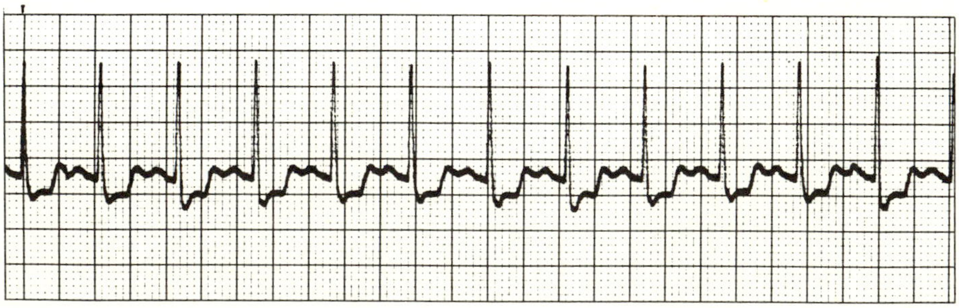

**Fig. 7-22.** S-T segment remains depressed more than 1 mm below baseline (P-R or T-P interval) 0.06 second after the "J" point is inscribed. This pattern correlates with underlying coronary artery disease.

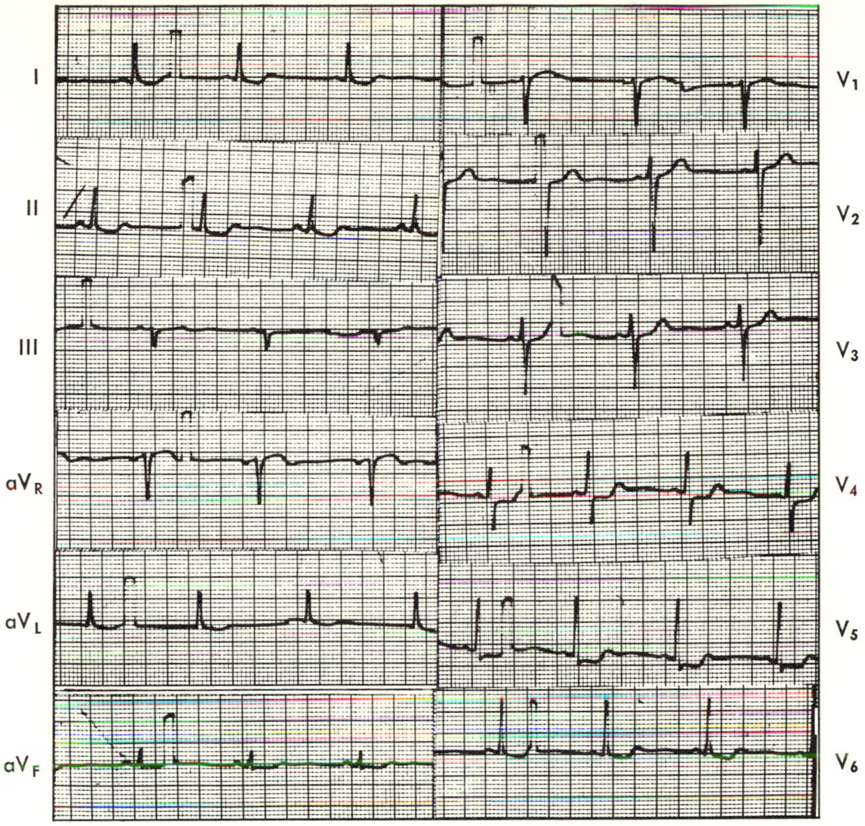


**Fig. 7-23.** Digitalis causes a nearly unique smoothly "scooped" depression of the initial part of the S-T segment.

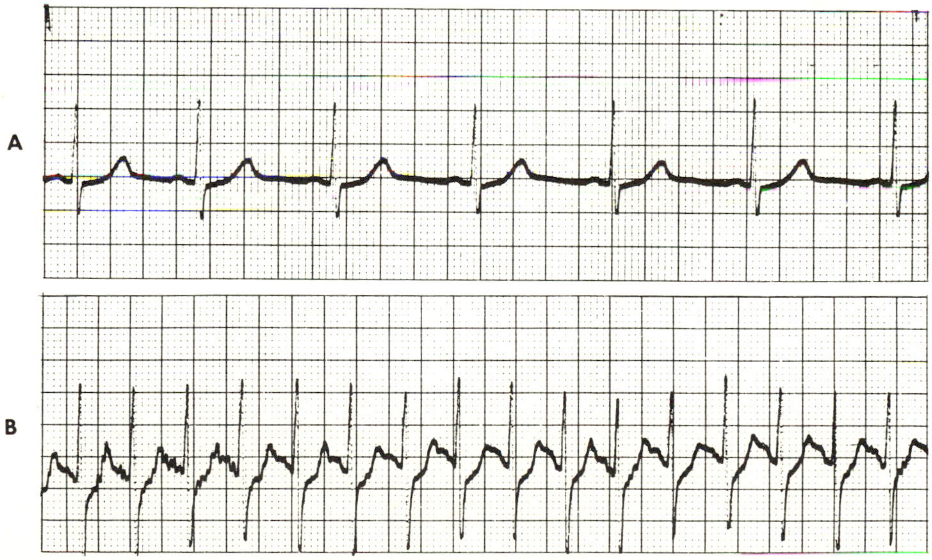


**Fig. 7-24.** Depression of S-T segment for less than 0.06 second is commonly seen in healthy persons when the heart rate increases.

causes transient first-degree AV block with P-R interval prolongation. Vegetations from endocarditis can embolize to a coronary artery and causes acute myocardial infarction with associated ECG changes.

Pericarditis is a common clinical event associated with specific ECG changes. Pericarditis complicates hemodialysis for renal failure, chest trauma, open-heart surgery, pulmonary embolism, disseminated bacterial or fungal infections, metastatic malignancies, collagen-vascular diseases, and allergic reactions to drugs. "Idiopathic" pericarditis can occur spontaneously in healthy individuals and often creates confusion with myocardial infarction.

■ **Both pericarditis and myocardial infarction can complicate hemodialysis for renal failure. How can the ECG help distinguish acute pericarditis from acute myocardial infarction?**

Acute pericarditis and acute myocardial infarction both cause epicardial injury leading to S-T segment elevation in the left ventricular leads. Myocardial infarction, however, is a focal event involving one discrete area of the heart, whereas pericarditis often involves the entire surface of the left ventricle. Consequently, pericarditis classically causes S-T segment elevation in nearly all left ventricular leads, whereas infarction involves only a few. Reciprocal S-T segment depression occurs in leads opposite those reflecting a myocardial infarction but is usually absent in pericarditis because all leads are recording epicardial injury.

Pericarditis also causes a progression of changes differing from that of acute myo-

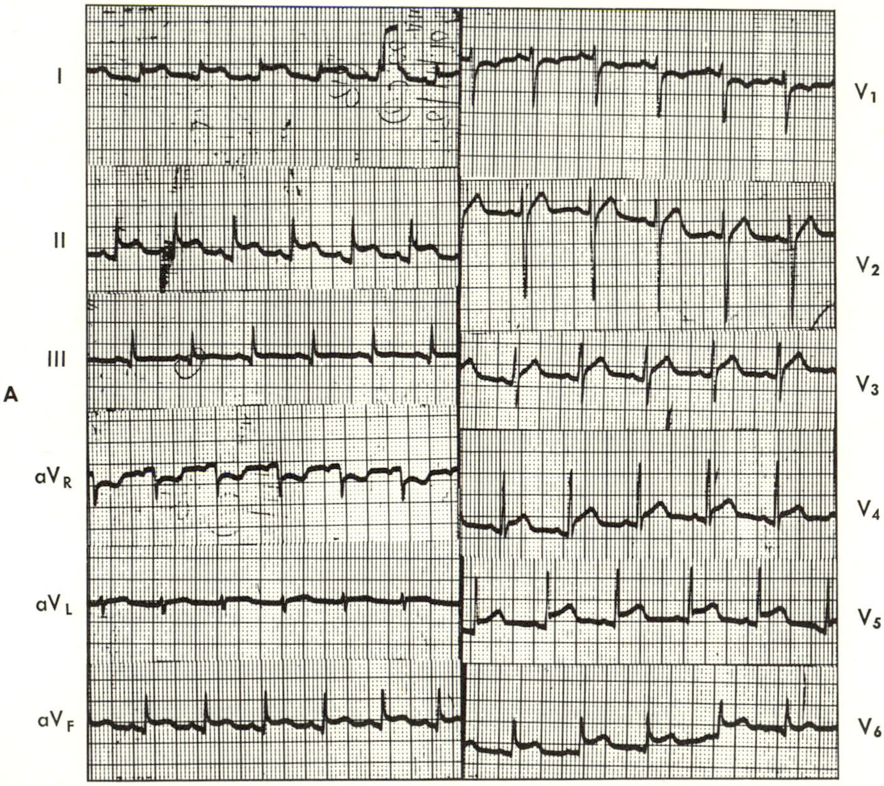


**Fig 7-25.** Acute pericarditis. Tracing in **A** demonstrates striking S-T segment elevation in limb leads I, II, III, and $aV_F$ and in all precordial leads except $V_1$. Reciprocal S-T segment depression is apparent in leads $aV_R$ and $V_1$, the "right ventricular" leads. Tracing in **B** documents return of S-T segment to baseline and development of T wave inversion in leads I, $aV_L$, and $V_2$ through $V_6$.

cardial infarction (Fig. 7-25). The sequential ECG changes of pericarditis are as follows:

1. Diffuse S-T segment elevation
2. Return of S-T segment to baseline potentials
3. Inversion of T waves
4. Return of T waves to normal

Q waves do not evolve in pericarditis. S-T segment elevation and T wave inversion usually do not occur simultaneously in pericarditis but often do in myocardial infarction. Unfortunately 75% of patients with pericarditis display nonspecific ECG changes because of the limited extent of the inflammation or simply because one or more of the typical sequential changes was missed or did not occur. These patients may have only mild S-T segment and T wave changes.

Arrhythmias of all kinds frequently complicate pericarditis but those of ventricular origin do not lead to ventricular fibrillation, in contrast to the situation in acute myocardial infarction.

## ■ What ECG changes occur in patients following open-heart surgery?

Open-heart surgery patients represent an increasingly numerous population in the critical care unit. In addition to the metabolic and pharmacologic influences common to all patients during recovery from major surgery, special cardiac problems are observed.

Pericardiectomy is a necessary maneuver for exposing the heart and results in pericarditis, manifested by appropriate ECG changes, during healing.

Acute myocardial infarction occurs in up to 15% of coronary artery bypass operations and presents with Q waves with or without S-T segment and T wave changes.

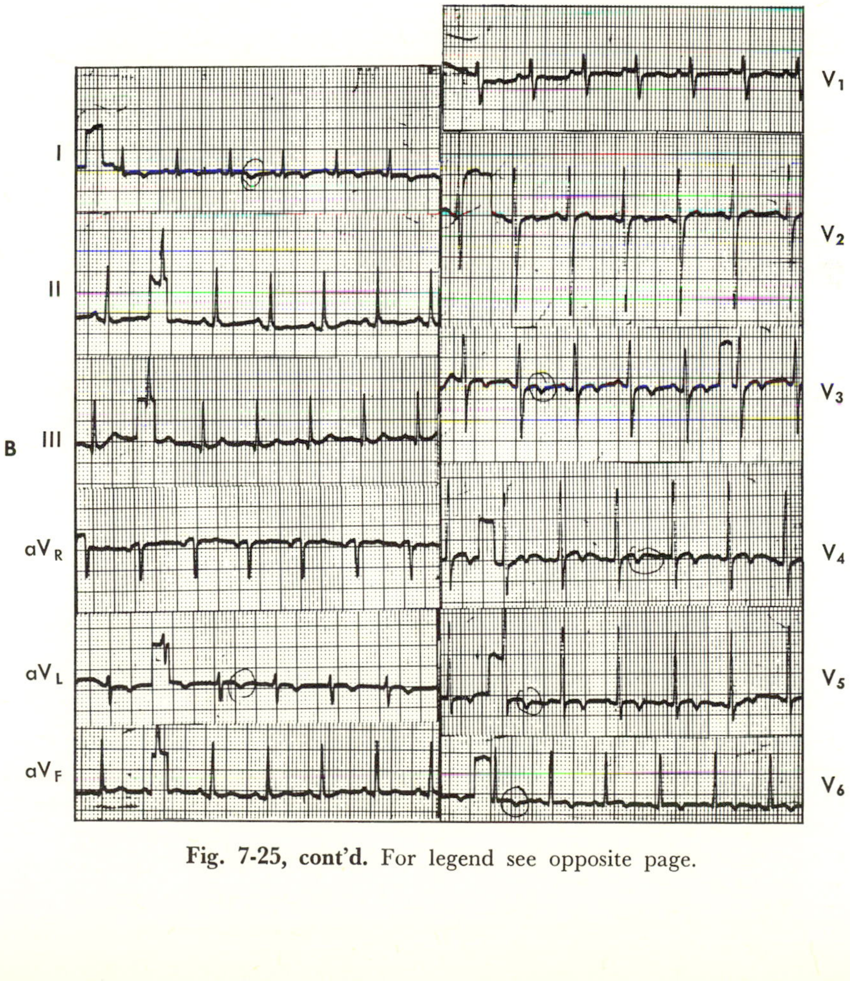


**Fig. 7-25, cont'd.** For legend see opposite page.

Arrhythmias are the most frequent ECG abnormalities after heart surgery. Although any type of arrhythmia may complicate this situation, some general rules are useful:

1. Supraventricular arrhythmias commonly complicate mitral valve surgery, particularly when atrial dilatation is present.
2. Complex ventricular arrhythmias (other than unifocal premature ventricular contractions [PVC's]) occurring after coronary artery bypass procedures should be treated with the same vigor as those complicating acute myocardial infarction; ventricular tachycardia or fibrillation in the postoperative coronary artery bypass patient is associated with 50% mortality.

## ECG CHANGES AND PULMONARY DISEASE

### ■ How does respiratory failure alter the ECG?

Arrhythmias and alterations of the ECG wave forms and intervals frequently accompany respiratory failure.

Most of the ECG effects of acute and chronic respiratory failure result from the metabolic and hemodynamic effects of hypoxemia. Hypoxemia with or without hypercapnia is an invariable result of respiratory failure. Besides its metabolic effects on automaticity and repolarization, hypoxemia causes pulmonary hypertension by stimulating the vasoconstriction of pulmonary arterioles. Pulmonary hypertension can cause acute right atrial and ventricular dilatation,

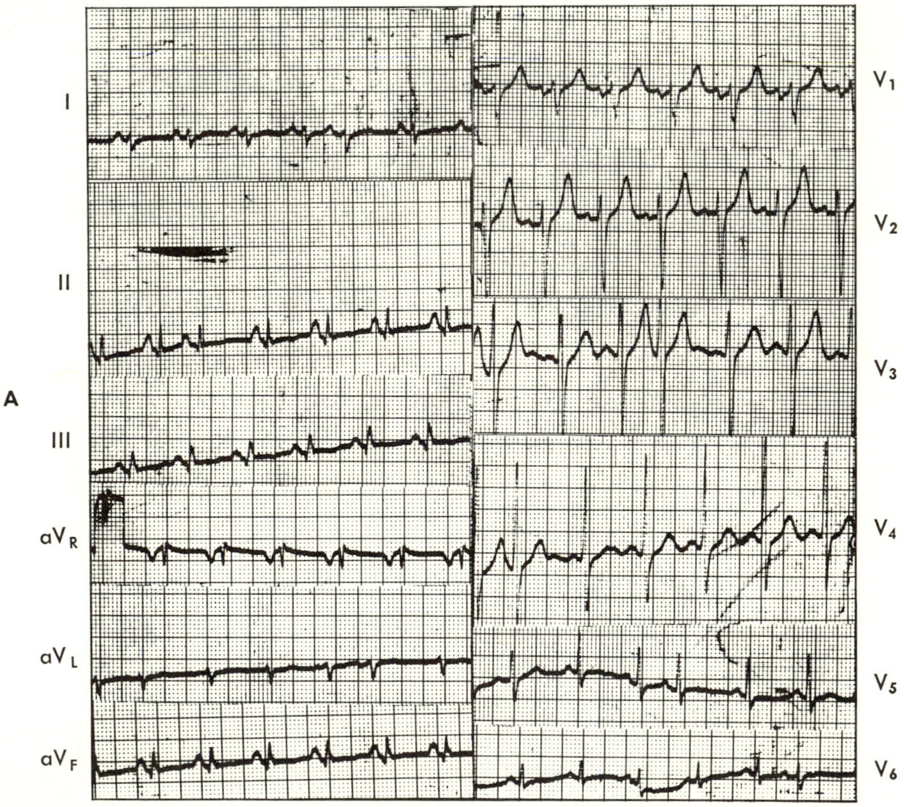


**Fig. 7-26.** ECG in **A** shows frontal plane axis of 100 degrees, incomplete right bundle branch block, and P waves 3.5 mm high in lead II with P wave axis at 60 degrees. Occasional PAC's are noted. Changes could represent acute pulmonary hypertension or chronic cor pulmonale. Comparison with previous ECG, **B,** demonstrates that rightward axis shift, abnormal P waves, and incomplete right bundle branch block are all recent changes. Pulmonary angiography confirmed acute pulmonary embolism.

and if sustained, will eventually cause right atrial and ventricular hypertrophy.

Arrhythmias can also be stimulated by the use of $\beta$-adrenergic bronchodilators in hypoxemic patients, by overventilation with respirators, causing respiratory alkalosis, and by hypercapnia. Endotracheal suction frequently induces arrhythmias, both by transient hypoxemia from interrupted ventilation and by vagal stimulation.

## ■ Do acute and chronic respiratory failure differ in their ECG effects?

Arrhythmias are frequent in both acute and chronic respiratory failure. The major ECG difference between the two is the development of right atrial and right ventricular hypertrophy with chronic respiratory failure. Chronic hypoxemia causes sustained pulmonary hypertension and results in right ventricular hypertrophy (eventually causing right atrial hypertrophy), which in the absence of left ventricular disease is called cor pulmonale. Acute hypoxemia occuring in an otherwise healthy person, such as when respiratory arrest results from barbiturate overdose, may cause arrhythmias and Q-T interval prolongation but does not usually cause P wave or QRS complex alterations. Acute pulmonary embolism is associated with ECG changes thought to represent the effects of sudden acute pulmonary hypertension (Fig. 7-26), as demonstrated by the following example.

Thirty-six hours after an abdominal hysterectomy a 47-year-old patient experienced the sudden onset of pleurisy and dyspnea and was found to be wheezing and hypotensive. An emergency chest x-ray film demonstrated right lower lobe atelectasis, arterial oxygen tension was 55 mm Hg, and the ECG shown in Fig. 7-26, *A,* was obtained

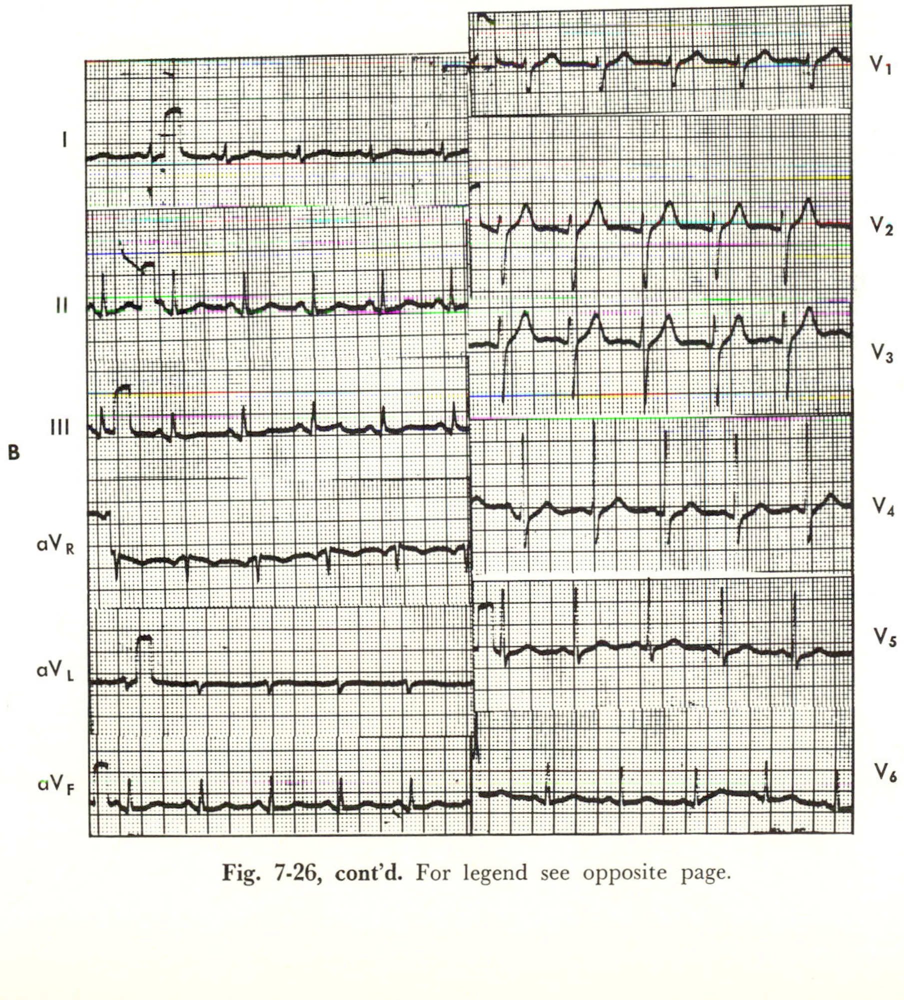


**Fig. 7-26, cont'd.** For legend see opposite page.

for comparison with the preoperative ECG (Fig. 7-26, *B*).

Large, acute pulmonary embolism causes sudden pulmonary hypertension, which may force dilatation of the right atrium and ventricle. This sudden dilatation may be observed electrocardiographically as P pulmonale, transient right bundle branch block (complete or incomplete), a rightward and posterior shift of the mean QRS axis, clockwise rotation with QS or rS complexes in leads $V_1$ to $V_4$, and S-T segment deviation and T wave inversion in right precordial and inferior limb leads. P pulmonale is manifested by P waves at least 2.5 mm high in leads II, III and $aV_F$, denoting inferior shift of the P wave vector. QRS vector alterations can result in the $S_1$, $S_2$, $S_3$, or $S_1Q_3$ patterns in the limb leads. Chest leads may demonstrate smaller amplitude R waves in leads $V_1$ to $V_5$ as the QRS axis shifts posteriorly.

Acute cor pulmonale of pulmonary embolism can resemble diaphragmatic myocardial infarction if the $S_1Q_{III}$ pattern occurs (Fig. 7-27). Lack of appropriate S-T segment changes and failure of Q waves to develop in other inferior leads (II, $aV_F$) are helpful differential clues.

Rarely, S-T segment elevation and T wave inversion in lead $V_2$ may occur, simulating anterior myocardial infarction. Lack of Q wave development and rapid resolution of this pattern help exclude anterior myocardial infarction as a diagnosis.

Arrhythmias can complicate major pul-

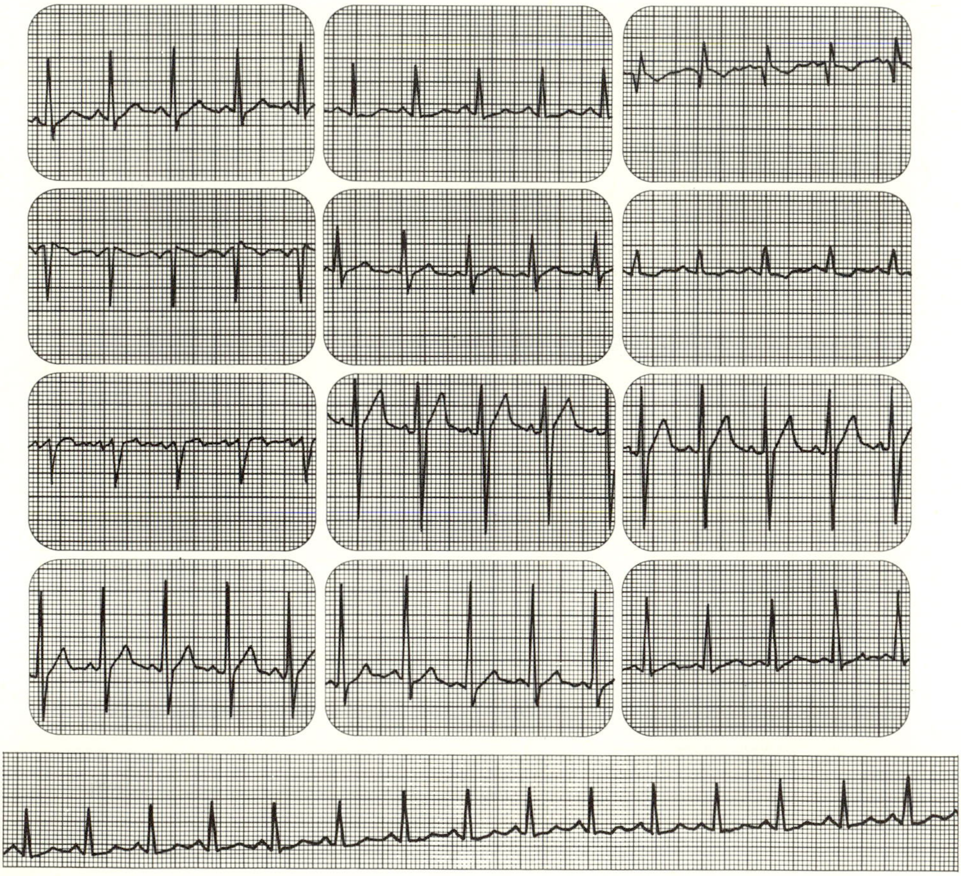

**Fig. 7-27.** Sudden development of "$S_1$,Q3" pattern in acute pulmonary embolism can cause initial confusion with acute myocardial infarction.

**Table 7-6.** ECG changes with major pulmonary embolism*

| *ECG changes* | *Percentage of patients affected* |
|---|---|
| Nonspecific S-T segment changes | 41 |
| Nonspecific T wave changes | 42 |
| "Acute cor pulmonale" (one or more of the following: $S_1Q_3T_3$ or right bundle branch block or P pulmonale or RAD) | 26 |
| Low voltage | 6 |
| Normal ECG | 6 |
| Left axis deviation | 7 |
| Right axis deviation | 7 |

*Applies to patients not having had prior cardiac or pulmonary disease.

monary embolism, especially when underlying heart disease is present, but they are usually of no clinical significance.

Although these "classic" ECG changes are helpful when they occur, most large pulmonary emboli cause nonspecific changes, and medium-sized and smaller emboli usually cause no changes. ECG changes in patients experiencing major acute pulmonary embolism who did not have prior cardiac or pulmonary disease are listed in Table 7-6. These changes are transient and usually disappear within 2 weeks.

Acute ECG changes have also been described with large (30% to 100%) spontaneous pneumothorax. This syndrome of sudden pleurisy, dyspnea, and apprehension clinically mimics acute pulmonary embolism

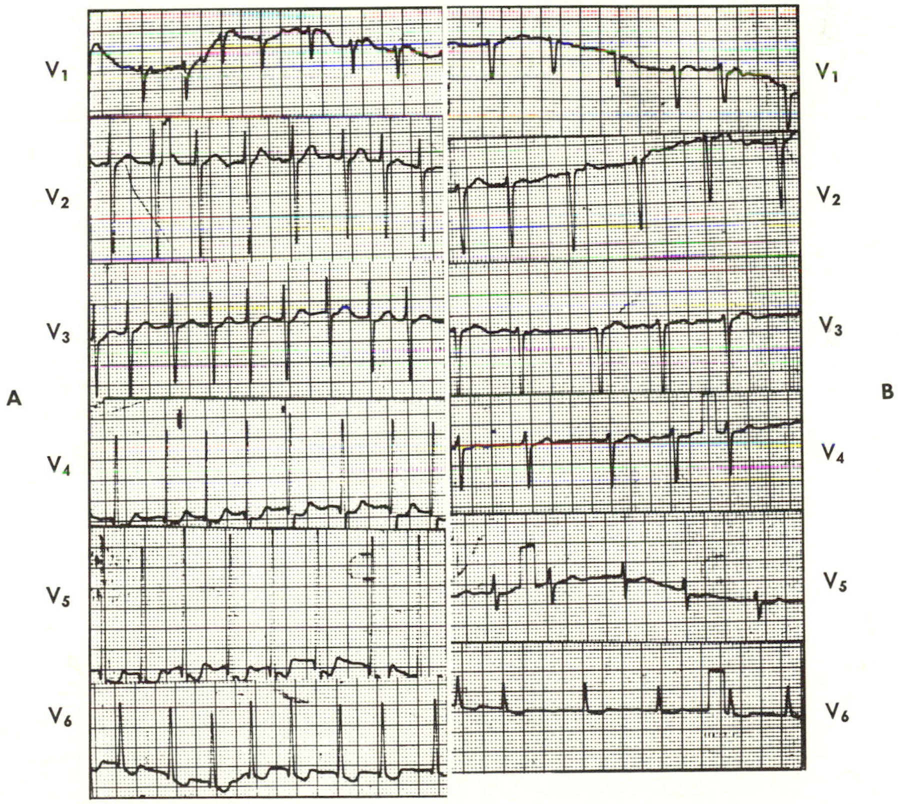


**Fig. 7-28.** Tracing in **A** represents chest leads of admission ECG from a patient with fever and pleural effusion. Shortly after diagnostic thoracentesis he complained of severe shortness of breath, and tracing in **B** was obtained. Significant posterior shift in QRS axis has caused much reduced amplitude of precordial R waves. Chest x-ray film demonstrates large left pneumothorax.

and acute myocardial infarction. Since ECG changes accompany all these entities, care must be given to interpretation of these changes in arriving at a correct diagnosis. Spontaneous and induced pneumothorax can cause a rightward shift in the mean frontal QRS axis, diminution of the precordial R wave voltage, decreased QRS amplitude, and precordial T wave inversion (Fig. 7-28). Since these changes can also accompany acute pulmonary embolism, differentiation of these two entities requires a chest roentgenogram. Acute transmural myocardial infarction is easily differentiated when Q waves and S-T segment elevation are present. Subendocardial infarction manifested only by inverted precordial T waves does not cause a rightward shift of the frontal plane axis or a decrease in precordial R wave and QRS amplitude.

### ■ What are the ECG changes of chronic pulmonary disease?

Two factors influence the ECG in patients with chronic pulmonary disease: (1) hyperinflation of the chest and (2) hypertrophy of the right atrium and ventricle.

Chest hyperinflation increases the distance between the heart and the chest leads and can result in low-amplitude QRS complexes in these leads.

Right atrial hypertrophy is reflected by tall (greater than 2.5 mm) P waves in leads II, III, and $aV_F$, and a P wave axis greater than 75 degrees in the frontal plane. Right ventricular hypertrophy is manifested in lead

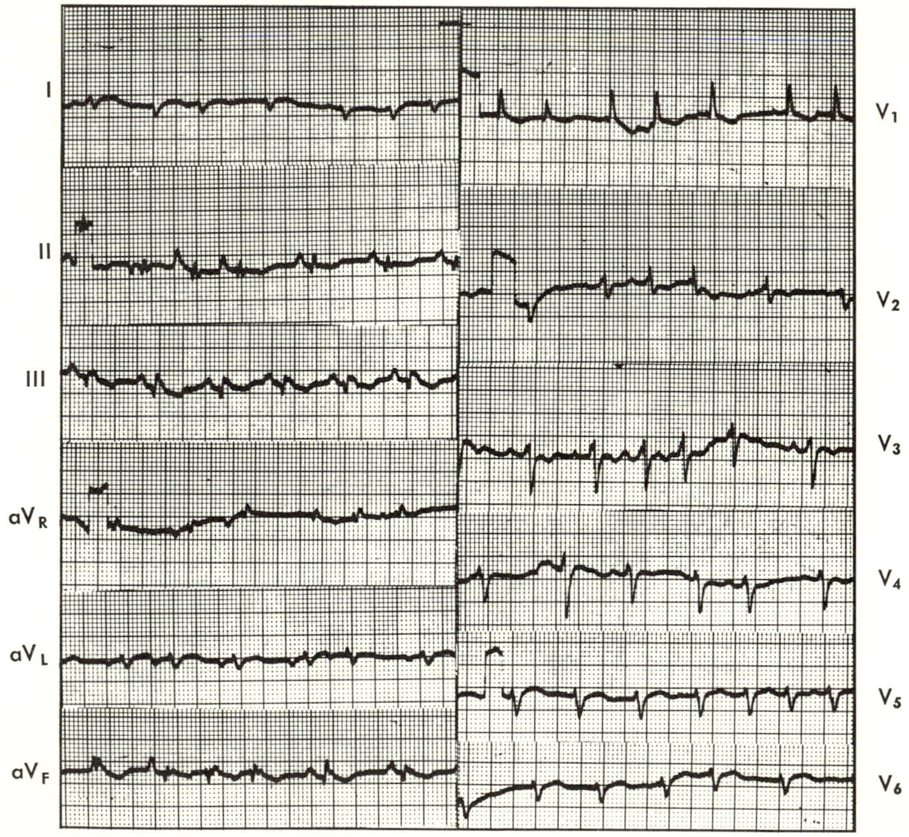


**Fig. 7-29.** Right axis deviation, low QRS amplitude, and P pulmonale are visible in frontal plane leads. Incomplete right bundle branch block and posterior QRS axis are present in chest leads. Sinus arrhythmia and frequent premature atrial contractions are also demonstrated.

$V_1$ by a dominant (greater than 7 mm) R wave in lead $V_1$, with an R:S ratio greater than 1. Because the increased muscle mass of the hypertrophied right heart requires more time to depolarize and generates more electrical force, the QRS axis may be shifted toward the right and anteriorly. Prolongation of depolarization prolongs the terminal QRS complex, resulting in an S wave of greater than 0.02-second duration in leads I, II, and III (the $S_1S_2S_3$ pattern) and/or "incomplete right bundle branch block" with normal QRS duration and an rsR′ pattern in lead $V_1$. Fig. 7-29 demonstrates some of these changes. Unfortunately cor pulmonale usually causes only nonspecific changes in the S-T segment and T wave and remains difficult to detect.

■ **Ventricular and supraventricular arrhythmias of variable severity can be detected in more than 80% of patients with chronic stable pulmonary disease. What arrhythmias complicate acute respiratory failure?**

Both ventricular and supraventricular arrhythmias occur during acute respiratory failure. Supraventricular arrhythmias other than premature atrial contractions are seen in nearly 50% of these patients. Any supraventricular arrhythmia can occur, but chaotic or multifocal atrial tachycardia and paroxysmal atrial tachycardia are the most common arrhythmias.

Ventricular arrhythmias more complex than PVC's are common and include ventricular bigeminy, tachycardia, and fibrillation. Ventricular fibrillation is reported to occur in up to 25% of patients with acute respiratory failure. Ventricular arrhythmias carry grim prognostic implications for the patient, probably because they reflect severe underlying pulmonary disease. Nearly 70% of patients having acute respiratory failure who develop PVC's die during that hospitalization.

Table 7-7 lists the arrhythmias developing during acute respiratory failure in one study.

**Table 7-7.** Arrhythmias during acute respiratory failure in 70 patients*

| *Arrhythmia* | *No. of patients affected* |
|---|---|
| Sinus tachycardia | 43 |
| Sinus brachycardia | 2 |
| Sinus arrhythmia | 3 |
| Ectopic atrial pacemaker | 9 |
| Wandering atrial pacemaker | 5 |
| Atrial tachycardia | 11 |
| Atrial flutter | 7 |
| Atrial fibrillation | 6 |
| MAT | 12 |
| AV junctional arrhythmia | 5 |
| Ventricular bigeminy | 5 |
| AV dissociation | 4 |
| Idioventricular rhythm | 4 |
| Ventricular tachycardia | 4 |
| Ventricular fibrillation | 15 |

*Most patients experienced more than one arrhythmia.

■ **How should arrhythmias be treated during acute respiratory failure?**

Treatment for arrhythmias during respiratory failure is based on correction of hypoxemia and other metabolic abnormalities and discontinuance of $\beta$-adrenergic bronchodilators if possible. If these drugs must be used, careful monitoring is essential. The following example illustrates a common occurrence in the critical care unit.

During treatment for an episode of acute respiratory failure a patient developed the rapid, irregular supraventricular arrhythmia shown in Fig. 7-30, *A*, after receiving an aminophylline suppository. It appears to be atrial fibrillation. An alert consultant recorded P waves from a transvenous right atrial electrode in order to document the diagnosis and presented the rhythm strip shown in Fig. 7-30, *B*. The right atrial recording shows P waves of variable configuration with a variable P-R interval and a ventricular rate above 120 beats/min, thus satisfying the diagnostic criteria for multifocal (chaotic) atrial tachycardia (MAT).

This arrhythmia mimics atrial fibrillation when the surface ECG does not record recognizable P waves. Treatment of MAT with digitalis, a drug normally recommended

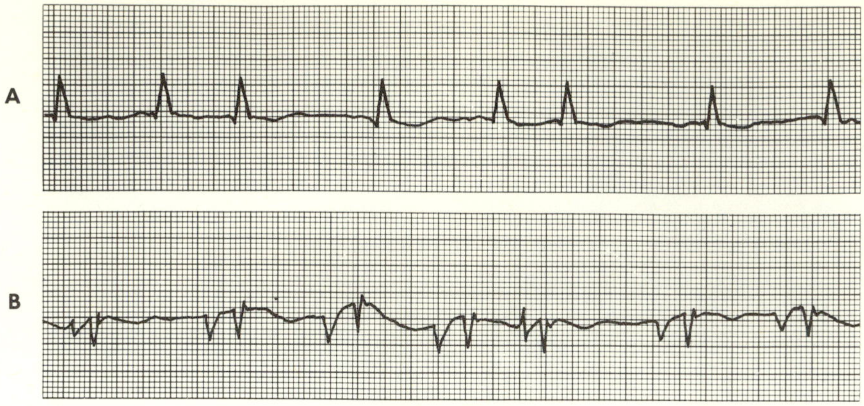


**Fig. 7-30.** Tracing in **A** reveals irregular supraventricular arrhythmia mimicking atrial fibrillation. Tracing in **B,** from an intra-atrial lead, clearly demonstrates definite P waves of variable configuration preceding each QRS complex.

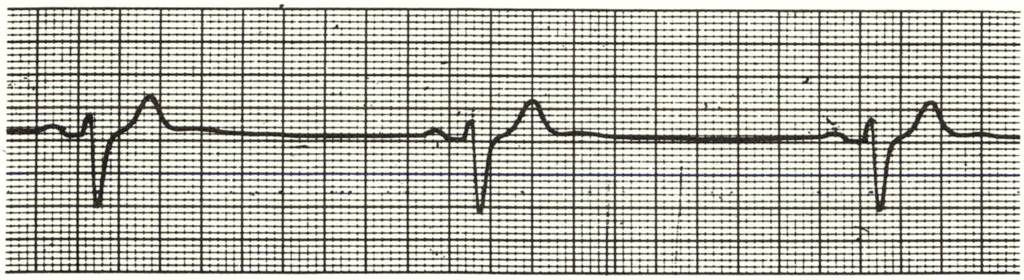

**Fig. 7-31.** Rhythm strip from respirator-dependent patient.

to slow AV conduction in atrial fibrillation, is usually not helpful, because this arrhythmia is associated with advanced pulmonary disease and its attendant metabolic abnormalities. In addition, patients with pulmonary insufficiency are highly susceptible to digitalis toxicity.

Similar to PVC's in respiratory failure, MAT is associated with a poor prognosis because of its association with severe underlying pulmonary disease. Fortunately this arrhythmia is transient and usually does not cause serious hemodynamic deficiencies. Correction of the underlying pulmonary abnormalities is the best therapeutic approach.

## MISCELLANEOUS ELECTROGRAPHIC ABNORMALITIES—CASE HISTORIES

### Case 1. Respiratory arrest

A 38-year-old male with acute ascending paralysis (Guillain-Barré syndrome) was being monitored while completely dependent on a respirator for ventilation. An alert practitioner noted a sudden change in the ECG monitor pattern and obtained the rhythm strip shown in Fig. 7-31.

Sinus bradycardia was diagnosed because each normal QRS complex was preceded by a normal P wave and the rate was 32 beats/min.

Acute hypercapnia, particularly in the presence of hypoxemia, causes intense vagal stimulation, which can result in sinus bradycardia or arrest. This patient had become separated from the respirator when a connecting tube broke. Rapid restoration of ventilation restored sinus rhythm by lowering the arterial $P_{CO_2}$ and improving oxygenation.

### Case 2. Hypothermia

A 45-year-old male chronic alcoholic was found unconscious in a city park. On admission his rectal temperature was less than

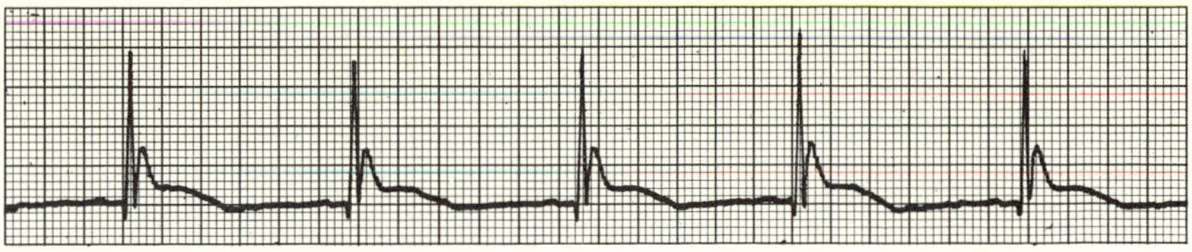

**Fig. 7-32.** ECG from patient with hypothermia. (From Conover, M. H.: Cardiac arrhythmias, St. Louis, 1974, The C. V. Mosby Co.)

**Table 7-8.** ECG effects of hypothermia

| *Temperature (°C)* | *ECG results* | *Physiologic abnormality* |
|---|---|---|
| 35-37 | Sinus bradycardia | Increased vagal tone, cooling of SA node |
| 30-35 | Prolongation of P-R interval, QRS complex, Q-T interval | Slowing of depolarization and repolarization |
| 27-30 | Ventricular arrhythmias | ?Myocardial ischemia |
| 25 | "Osborn wave"—positive deflection of terminal 0.04 sec of QRS complex | Unknown |

30° C and the ECG shown in Fig. 7-32 was recorded.

Hypothermia has both reflex and direct effects on cardiac automaticity and conduction. Induction of hypothermia, such as for cardiac surgery, is relatively arrhythmia free, but rewarming can be hazardous. During rewarming the core temperature, including that of the heart, lags behind the peripheral temperature. As the peripheral temperature increases, peripheral oxygen demand increases, but if the heart is still hypothermic, cardiac output cannot increase adequately to meet this demand. Both peripheral and myocardial hypoxia can result, and ventricular fibrillation may ensue. Slow rewarming with careful cardiac monitoring will help to avoid this complication.

Table 7-8 lists the effects of hypothermia on the ECG.

Sinus bradycardia and an abnormal deflection of the terminal QRS complex (Osborn wave) suggest hypothermia. Marked slowing of repolarization is reflected by the low-amplitude T waves and Q-T interval prolongation.

## Case 3. Tricyclic amine overdose

A 44-year-old female was found comatose after telephoning a friend that she had just taken a bottle of "tranquilizers." Shortly after admission she suffered a grand mal seizure. The rhythm strips shown in Fig. 7-33 were obtained.

The initial postictal tracing demonstrates markedly prolonged intraventricular conduction followed by development of wide-complex tachycardia. This combination of coma, grand mal seizures, and arrhythmias is characteristic of tricyclic amine overdoses. These commonly used antidepressants slow depolarization and thus slow intra-atrial, AV, and intraventricular conduction. Supraventricular and ventricular arrhythmias commonly occur and may progress to ventricular fibrillation. Treatment with diphenylhydantoin successfully reversed the ECG abnormalities of this patient.

## Case 4. Subarachnoid hemorrhage

The ECG shown in Fig. 7-34 was obtained from a 49-year-old female admitted to the intensive care unit because of sudden onset of severe headache followed by a rapid loss of consciousness and the development of acute pulmonary edema.

This ECG demonstrates striking T wave inversion and minor S-T segment depression consistent with subendocardial injury and epicardial ischemia, but no Q waves are apparent. This pattern is consistent with sub-

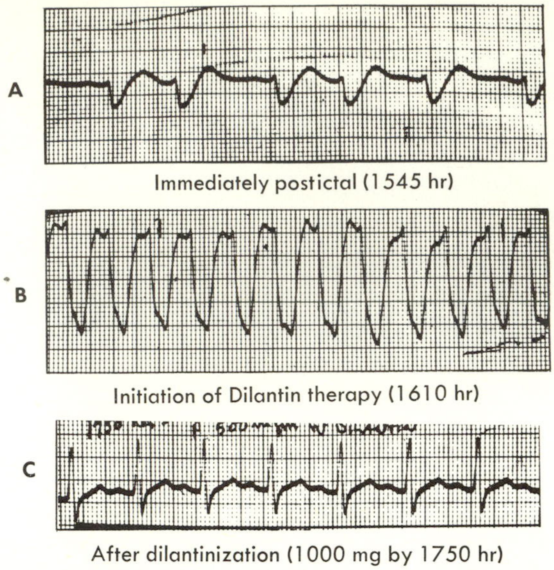


**Fig. 7-33. A,** Abnormal intraventricular conduction followed by ventricular tachycardia, **B. C,** Dilantin therapy corrected both conduction defect and arrhythmia.

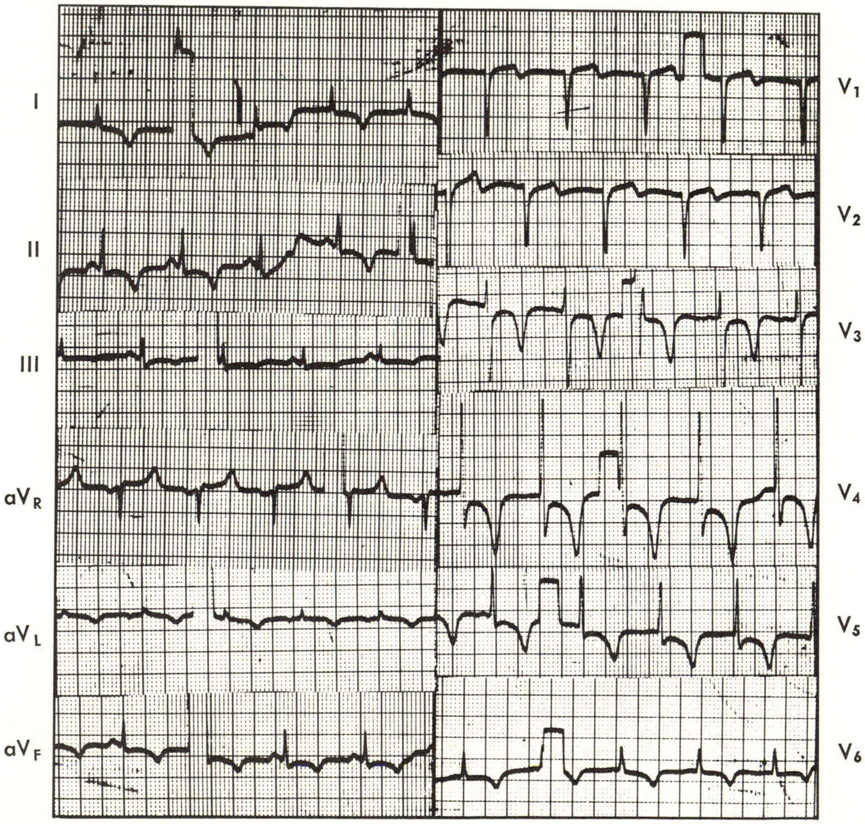


**Fig. 7-34.** Striking T wave inversion in a patient with acute subarachnoid hemorrhage.

endocardial infarction. A diagnosis of subarachnoid hemorrhage was documented by lumbar puncture and arteriograms.

ECG changes associated with subarachnoid hemorrhage are transient and reflect spotty subendocardial and intramural myocardial necrosis. S-T segment and T wave changes reflecting subendocardial infarction are most commonly seen, but the Q waves of transmural infarction are also occasionally observed. In many instances only Q-T interval prolongation or arrhythmias occur. A sudden increase of serum catecholamine levels is thought to be the reason for myocardial necrosis in these patients.

Although subarachnoid hemorrhage is the most common neurologic cause of ECG changes, they are also seen with status epilepticus, intracranial mass lesions, meningitis, cerebral infarction, and diagnostic procedures, including pneumoencephalography. Similar ECG changes have been reported following carotid endarterectomy.

## SUMMARY

Cardiac electrical activity recorded by the ECG is generated by ionic motion across the myocardial cell membrane. Ionic motion and the membrane itself are altered by changes in the metabolic environment. Critically ill patients experience frequent and varied metabolic, inflammatory, and hemodynamic abnormalities that can alter the ECG. Many therapeutic maneuvers and pharmacologic agents can also alter the ECG. Intelligent interpretation of the ECG of the critically ill patient requires thorough knowledge of the extent and meaning of these changes.

## BIBLIOGRAPHY

Ayres, S. M., and Grace, W. J.: Inappropriate ventilation and hypoxemia as causes of cardiac arrhythmias, Am. J. Med. **46**:495-505, 1969.

Bellet, S.: Essentials of cardiac arrhythmias, Philadelphia, 1972, W. B. Saunders Co.

Bhargava, R. K.: Cor pulmonale, Mount Kisco, N. Y., 1973, Futura Publishing Co., Inc.

Hoffman, B. F., and Cranefield, P. F.: The physiological basis of cardiac arrhythmias, Am. J. Med. **37**:670-684, 1964.

Hudson, L. D., Kurt, T. L., Petty, T. L., and Genton, E.: Arrhythmias associated with acute respiratory failure in patients with chronic airway obstruction, Chest **63**:661-665, 1973.

Lipman, B. S., Massie, E., and Kleiger, R. E.: Clinical scalar electrocardiography, Chicago, 1972, Year Book Medical Publishers, Inc.

*chapter 8*

# Clinical management of common cardiac abnormalities*

ROBERT E. INGHAM
THEODORE B. BERNDT
DONALD C. HARRISON

Abnormalities of the heart and great blood vessels frequently produce emergencies that necessitate the admission of a patient to a critical care unit. The large number of conditions that may be present and their diagnosis and management can be discussed only briefly in this chapter; therefore those syndromes that occur most commonly have been selected for emphasis. In each instance the syndrome is defined, its diagnosis outlined, classic examples presented, and the prognosis discussed. The following specific syndromes are presented:

- Cardiac arrhythmias
- Congestive heart failure and pulmonary edema
- Cardiogenic shock in acute myocardial infarction
- Acute valvular lesions
- Acute pericarditis
- Acute myocarditis
- Infective endocarditis
- Dissecting aneurysm of the aorta

## CARDIAC ARRHYTHMIAS

### ■ What is a cardiac arrhythmia?

An arrhythmia is an alteration of the formation or conduction of an electrical impulse so that the rate of a portion of the heartbeat is abnormally fast or abnormally slow, or the rhythm is irregular. In the normal heart an impulse originates in the sinoatrial (SA) node, and from there the impulse spreads throughout the right and left atria, eventually reaching the atrioventricular (AV) node. After spending some time traversing the AV node the impulse emerges to be conducted through the bundle of His to the right and left bundle branches. These main bundle branches arborize throughout the myocardium. This normal conduction sequence is represented in Fig. 8-1. If a sinus impulse results in a heart rate slower or faster than normal, if an impulse arises from some location other than the SA node, or if a normal impulse is conducted through the heart in an abnormal fashion, an arrhythmia results.

### ■ What is the clinical importance of cardiac arrhythmias?

The appearance of an arrhythmia has little significance in itself, but it must be considered in relation to the clinical situation it accompanies. Sinus bradycardia in a 65-year-old male is a very different situation from sinus bradycardia in a 22-year-old distance runner. Similarly, paroxysmal supraventricular tachycardia in an 18-year-old female has a different significance from such a tachycardia occurring in a 48-year-old male with severe aortic stenosis. The approach to take and the degree of significance to be attached to an arrhythmia may be determined by answers to the following questions:

1. What is the nature of the arrhythmia?
2. What are the hemodynamic effects of the arrhythmia, as manifested by men-

*Supported by NIH Grants No. HL-5866 and HL-15833-01.

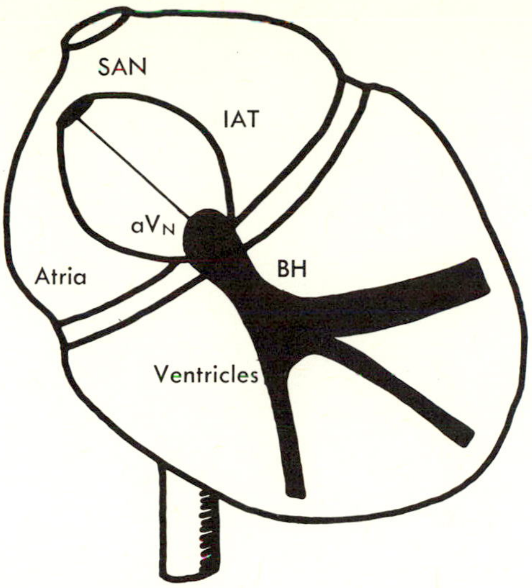


**Fig. 8-1.** Normal conduction sequence. *SAN,* sinoatrial node; *IAT,* intra-atrial tracts; *AVN,* atrioventricular node; *BH,* bundle of His.

**Table 8-1.** Common arrhythmias (with usual rates in the absence of treatment)*

| *Arrhythmia* | *Atrial rate (beats/min)* | *Ventricular rate (beats/min)* | *Rhythm* |
|---|---|---|---|
| Sick sinus syndrome—brady-tachy syndrome | 40-60, 100-200 | 40-60, 100-200 | Regular |
| Atrial flutter | 250-350 | 75-150 | Regular with constant block, irregular with varying block |
| Atrial fibrillation | 300-500 | 140-175 | Grossly irregular |
| Paroxysmal supraventricular (atrial) tachycardia | 150-250 | 150-250 | Regular |
| AV junctional tachycardia | 100-180 (retrograde depolarization of atria) | 100-180 | Regular |
| Ventricular tachycardia | Variable (AV dissociation) | 150-200+ | Regular (usually slightly irregular) |
| Sinus bradycardia | 40-60 | 40-60 | Regular |
| Escape rhythms† | | | |
| AV junctional rhythm | Variable | 40-60 | Regular |
| Idioventricular rhythm | Variable | 30-40 | Regular |

*From Coltart, D. J., and Harrison, D. C.: Primary Care 1:123, 1974.
†The term "escape rhythms" refers to those rhythms originating in lower centers when SA rhythmicity is depressed or when marked AV block occurs.

tal status and renal, respiratory, and myocardial function?

3. What is the prognosis of the arrhythmia in this patient?
4. Will the patient be symptomatically or physiologically improved with therapy for this arrhythmia?

In attempting to answer each of these questions in an individual clinical situation, the relative importance of any arrhythmia to a patient's general condition will become clearer.

Table 8-1 summarizes the common arrhythmias that may be encountered in a critically ill patient. Table 8-2 summarizes the common antiarrhythmic medications used in the therapy of these conditions.

**Table 8-2.** Commonly used antiarrhythmic drugs: pharmacologic principles*

| *Drug* | *Therapeutic range* | *Dosage* | *Elimination* | *Absorption* | | | *Toxic reactions* |
|---|---|---|---|---|---|---|---|
| | | | | *Orally* | *IV* | *IM* | |
| Quinidine | 2-8 μg/ml | 400 mg 4 times daily | Renal, decreased in alkaline urine | Maximum effect 1-3 hr, duration 6-8 hr | | Maximum effect 30-90 min | Cinchonism, nausea, vomiting, diarrhea |
| Procainamide | 4-8 μg/ml | 6 mg/kg every 3 hr IV, 100 mg/5 min until 1 g given | 60% excreted by kidney | Maximum effect 15-60 min | Maximum effect 5-10 min | | Agranulocytosis, lupuslike syndrome |
| Propranolol | 20-120 ng/ml | 20-80 mg 4 times daily orally, 0.15 mg/kg IV | Hepatic metabolism | Maximum effect 1-2 hr | Maximum effect 10-30 min | | Respiratory, hypoglycemia |
| Lidocaine | 1-6 μg/ml | 20-60 μg/kg/min | Hepatic metabolism | | Maximum effect 2-5 min | Maximum effect 30 min | Muscle fasciculation, drowsiness, convulsions |
| Diphenylhydantoin | 10-20 μg/ml | 0.5-0.6 g daily orally, 100 mg every 15 min IV | Hepatic metabolism | Maximum effect 8-12 hr | Maximum effect 30-60 min | | Nystagmus, lethargy, ataxia |

*From Coltart, D. J., and Harrison, D. C.: Primary Care **1**:123, 1974.

## ■ What are the important tachycardias?

### *Paroxysmal supraventricular (atrial) tachycardia*

Common causes of paroxysmal supraventricular tachycardia (PSVT) in the ill patient include digitalis intoxication, rheumatic heart disease, acute myocardial infarction, pulmonary embolism, and chronic obstructive pulmonary disease. PSVT also occurs relatively frequently in persons with the preexcitation syndrome and may occur in otherwise normal people. The ECG's of patients with PSVT show an atrial rate generally between 150 to 250 beats/min, although faster or slower rates may occur. During the tachycardia P waves are difficult to identify, and conduction through the ventricles may be in an aberrant fashion. The ventricular response depends on the degree of AV block, but is frequently 1:1, with a ventricular response equal to the atrial rate. Various degrees of AV block will exist when there is excessive digitalis present (Fig. 8-2).

Episodes of PSVT may precipitate angina pectoris, myocardial infarction, syncope, or frank congestive heart failure with pulmonary edema or shock and, as such, require urgent measures. Electrical cardioversion at 50 to 200 watt-seconds is the treatment of choice in any situation requiring emergency measures, although if digitalis intoxication is the probable cause, other therapy should be attempted first. Carotid sinus massage, edrophonium (Tensilon) given as 10 mg by the IV route, Valsalva's maneuver, or pressor agents such as methoxamine (if there are no contraindications to pressor agents) may be attempted individually. Digitalis is a preferred therapy if the patient has not been taking the drug. If digitalis intoxication is the probable cause, digitalis should be discontinued and blood drawn for a serum digitalis level determination. Diphenylhydantoin may be useful if digitalis intoxication is suspected, and if the serum potassium level is low, IV fluids containing

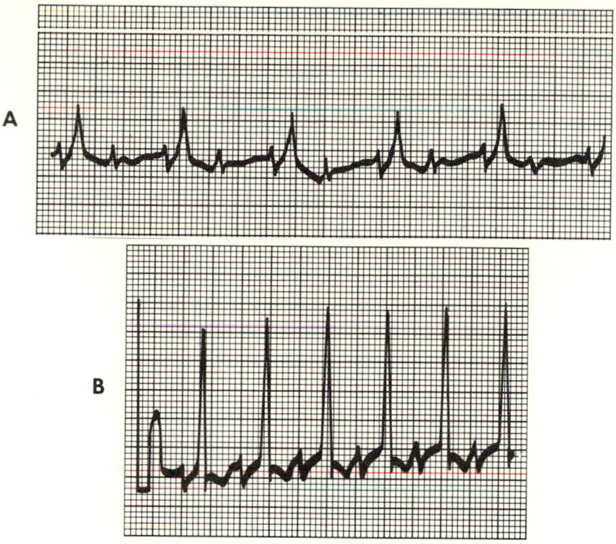

**Fig. 8-2. A,** Paroxysmal atrial tachycardia with block. **B,** Sinus tachycardia. Serum digoxin level was in toxic range when the ECG in **A** was taken but had dropped to therapeutic levels on trace in **B.**

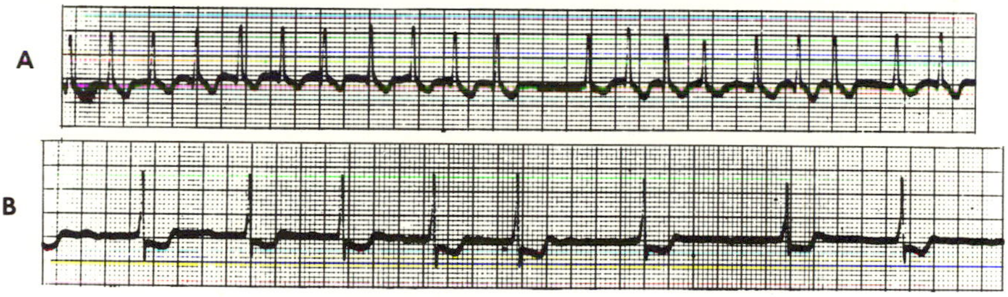

**Fig. 8-3. A,** Untreated atrial fibrillation with rapid ventricular response. **B,** Atrial fibrillation well treated with digoxin. Ventricular response is slow and irregular. Atrial fibrillatory waves can be seen.

potassium chloride should be administered. Propranolol has proved useful in slowing and breaking episodes of PSVT.

Patients may find recurrent episodes of PSVT very incapacitating, and in such a situation chronic medical therapy may be required. Digitalis is useful if PSVT is not caused by digitalis intoxication. Other medications that may be tried on a chronic basis are propranolol, quinidine sulfate, procainamide, reserpine, and guanethidine. The patient should also be advised to stop smoking and to eliminate caffeine and other stimulants. It should be emphasized that PSVT in and of itself is not an indication for chronic medical therapy, but when there is evidence of hemodynamic compromise, as often occurs when other abnormal cardiovascular conditions exist, it should be treated aggressively.

### *Atrial fibrillation*

Atrial fibrillation is a common arrhythmia that can be associated with a number of conditions such as rheumatic heart disease, pericarditis, hyperthyroidism, ischemic heart disease, hypertension, or chronic obstructive pulmonary disease. The ECG of a patient in atrial fibrillation shows total disorganization of atrial activity, which is represented by fibrillary waves along the baseline (Fig. 8-3). The ventricular response to this chaotic atrial activity is irregularly irregular, and the rate can span the range from slow to very fast. The loss of atrial contraction may be an important contributing factor to a low cardiac output state, and when combined with a rapid ventricular response, there may be a serious hemodynamic compromise that requires urgent therapy.

When a patient has atrial fibrillation, the goals of therapy must be determined; that is, would the patient be significantly improved by returning to sinus rhythm, or would the patient be improved simply by slowing the ventricular response to allow better diastolic filling of the ventricles? If the goal of therapy is sinus rhythm and the patient has not received digitalis, the treatment of choice is electrical cardioversion. The acutely ill patient who has atrial fibrillation and who exhibits shock, pulmonary edema, or other signs of cardiac decompensation should have electrical cardioversion without delay. When a patient has chronic atrial fibrillation and is not significantly compromised by the arrhythmia, then there is more time for medical therapy, and control of the ventricular response can be the primary goal of therapy. Digitalis is the drug of choice because it slows conduction through the AV node, thereby allowing fewer of the atrial impulses that constantly bombard the AV node to gain entrance to ventricular conducting tissues. The result is a slowing of the ventricular rate. Propranolol is also a useful agent in slowing the ventricular rate. Quinidine sulfate, in combination with digitalis, has previously been used in an attempt to "medically cardiovert" a patient from atrial fibrillation to normal sinus rhythm; however, episodes of ventricular fibrillation have been reported, and this is not a recommended procedure.

### *Atrial flutter*

The causes of atrial flutter are much the same as those of atrial fibrillation. The ECG features of atrial flutter include an undulating, wavy baseline with regular flutter waves at a rate commonly between 250 and 350 waves/min (Fig. 8-4). The ventricular rate is some fraction of the atrial rate, usually one half, one fourth, or one third, expressed as 2:1, 4:1, and 3:1 AV block, respectively, and is typically very regular. There may be confusion between atrial flutter with 2:1 block, PSVT, and atrial fibrillation, because each may have similar ventricular responses. Carotid sinus massage, Valsalva's maneuver, or edrophonium may slow the ventricular response sufficiently to allow characterization of the atrial mechanism. Atrial flutter can be a source of difficulty to the patient when there is no AV block (a 1:1 atrial-ventricular response) or only 2:1 AV block, so that the ventricular response is very rapid. The treatment of atrial flutter is much the same as that of atrial fibrillation and requires a clinical judgment as to the urgency of the situation. If the rapid rate is compromising the hemodynamic status of the patient, then electrical cardioversion is the treatment of choice. This can usually be accomplished at low energies (25 to 100 watt-seconds). If more time is available, digitalis will produce AV block and slow the ventricular rate to

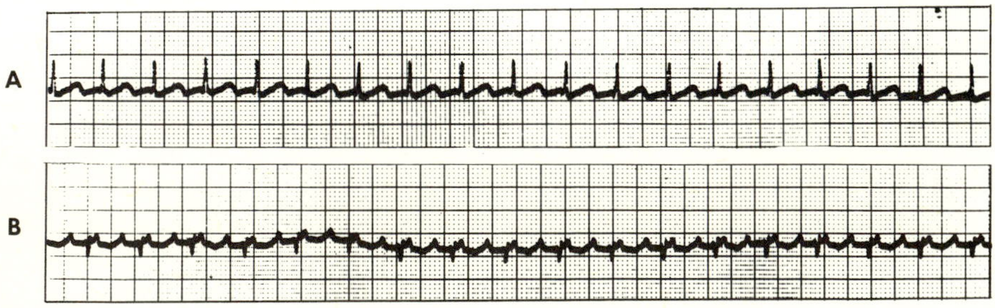


**Fig. 8-4.** Atrial flutter. **A,** Lead II. **B,** Lead $V_1$. Leads in this combination best show flutter waves as characteristic undulations with no isoelectric interval.

a level that is better tolerated. Propranolol may also produce AV blockage and thereby slow the ventricular rate. Not infrequently the result of such medical therapy is atrial fibrillation.

### *Sick sinus syndrome—"brady-tachy syndrome"*

The sick sinus syndrome falls in the general category of a "brady-tachy syndrome," a term that describes episodes of sinus bradycardia interrupted by bursts of supraventricular tachycardia that are not necessarily sinus in origin. In the brady-tachy syndrome, the tachycardia episodes may be PSVT, atrial flutter, rapid atrial fibrillation, or sinus (in which case the term "sick sinus syndrome" is applied). The brady-tachy syndrome is characterized by episodes of very fast heart rate alternating with very slow heart rate, and the patient may develop symptoms from either of these aberrations. The sinus P waves are characteristically normal but are very irregular. Either syndrome may be a result of ischemic heart disease or generalized cardiomyopathy, or it may also occur without other evidence of cardiovascular disease. The dilemma in therapy for these patients comes in treating episodes of tachycardia with medications that may be detrimental during the phase of bradycardia. Therapy is therefore aimed at minimizing the bradycardia with a transvenous pacemaker and treating the tachycardia episodes with such medications as digitalis, propranolol, quinidine sulfate, and procainamide. It should be noted that there is significant incidence of disease of other portions of the conducting system of the heart in patients with sick sinus syndrome, or brady-tachy syndrome, giving added importance to the need for a pacemaker before medical therapy is undertaken.

### *Ventricular tachycardia*

Ventricular tachycardia is defined as three or more consecutive ventricular ectopic beats. Paroxysms of such beats may begin with an appropriately timed ventricular premature contraction that falls in the vulnerable period of a sinus beat and can then initiate a repetitive response of ventricular tachycardia. An irritable ventricular focus can also initiate a series of impulses at a rapid rate and produce ventricular tachy-

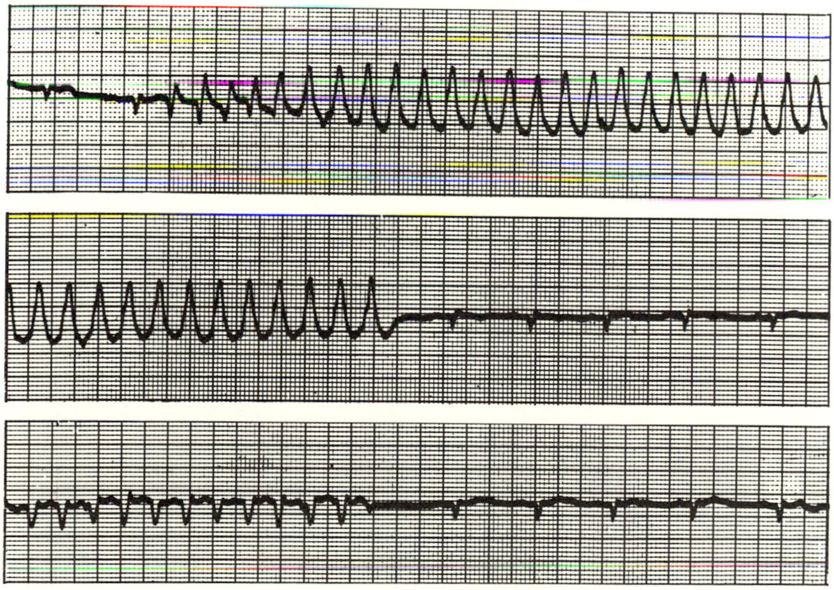

**Fig. 8-5.** Ventricular tachycardia followed by nodal tachycardia.

cardia. Such repetitive episodes are most common in diseased hearts and cause a severe compromise of the hemodynamic status of the patient because of a disorganized ventricular depolarization and lack of effective stroke volume. Common settings for ventricular tachycardia are acute myocardial infarction, cardiomyopathy, and digitalis intoxication. The ECG features of ventricular tachycardia include broad bizarre-appearing ventricular complexes, usually at a rate of over 100 beats/min (Fig. 8-5). If untreated, ventricular tachycardia frequently degenerates into ventricular fibrillation. Electrical counter shock is the treatment of choice, and lidocaine may be given in an attempt to suppress ectopic activity after conversion has been completed. If lidocaine fails to suppress subsequent runs of ventricular tachycardia or frequent ventricular ectopic beats, then procainamide by slow IV injection may be attempted. Other medications that could be considered are quinidine sulfate, diphenylhydantoin, potassium chloride (especially if the serum potassium level is low), and propranolol. Occasionally cardiac pacing has been successful in overdrive suppression of the ventricular focus. All other potentially reversible conditions that may predispose to ventricular tachycardia, such as hypoxia, acidosis, and hypotension, should be treated.

*Ventricular fibrillation*

Ventricular fibrillation constitutes a cardiac emergency, and immediate therapy with electrical defibrillation should be undertaken at 400 watt-seconds. Cardiopulmonary resuscitation should be instituted, and simultaneous attention should be given to correcting situations that may cause ventricular fibrillation, such as ventricular ectopy, shock, hypoxia, bradycardia, and digitalis intoxication. Rapid ECG recognition of ventricular fibrillation is mandatory; the ECG exhibits a waving baseline without evidence of ventricular depolarization (Fig. 8-6).

## ■ What are the important bradycardias?

*Sinus bradycardia*

Sinus bradycardia has already been mentioned as a component of the sick sinus or brady-tachy syndrome (Fig. 8-7). It may also be a normal response in the physically fit. When sinus bradycardia appears to compromise hemodynamic status, as is most commonly the case in older patients with some degree of coronary artery disease, it warrants therapy with a permanent cardiac pacemaker.

*Heart block*

Heart block is an abnormality in the conduction of sinus beats to the ventricles. The most common site for such an abnormality

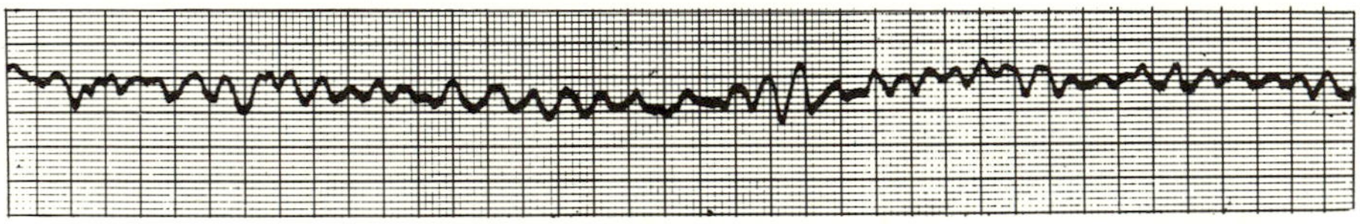

**Fig. 8-6.** Ventricular fibrillation.

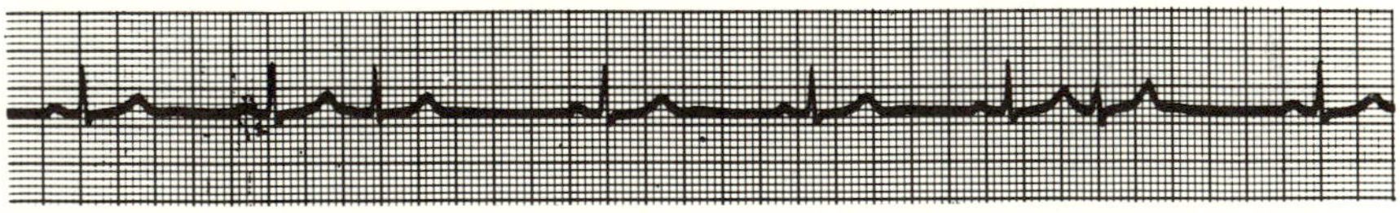

**Fig. 8-7.** Sinus bradycardia with atrial extrasystoles.

is in the AV node, and the conduction disturbance may be of several types. First-degree heart block consists simply of a prolongation of the P-R interval to greater than 0.20 second and rarely requires therapy. Second-degree heart block is a condition wherein some, but not all, sinus impulses are transmitted to the ventricles. Mobitz type I second-degree heart block (Wenckebach's phenomenon) is characterized by progressive prolongation of the P-R interval in successive sinus beats, with subsequent block of a sinus beat (Fig. 8-8). The net effect is a "grouping" of QRS complexes on the surface ECG and varying P-R intervals. Common causes of Wenckebach's phenomenon include digitalis intoxication, increased vagal tone, and inferior myocardial infarction. Wenckebach's phenomenon rarely causes hemodynamic compromise, and hence rarely does the arrhythmia itself require treatment.

Another type of second-degree heart block is termed Mobitz type II and is characterized by the occasional lack of propagation of sinus beats through the AV junctional area to the ventricle. The patient is in sinus rhythm with regular P waves, but occasional P waves are not followed by a QRS complex. Mobitz type II heart block itself does not require therapy unless the dropped beats are so frequent as to result in a bradycardia that is a source of difficulty for the patient. Atropine or isoproterenol may result in lessening of the degree of the block, but pacing may be required to restore an adequate ventricular rate. The major importance in recognizing Mobitz type II heart block is that it commonly progresses to third-degree heart block and severe bradycardia with frequent hemodynamic compromise. This progression occurs most often in conjunction with acute myocardial infarction of the anterior wall or a cardiomyopathy.

When third-degree (complete) heart block is present, there is a slow ventricular rate from a junctional or ventricular pacemaker (less than 60 beats/min), and there is frequently a lack of response of this low rate to various physiologic stresses. Therapy in the form of a pacemaker is usually required. Complete heart block is identified on the ECG by a lack of relationship between P waves and QRS complexes (Fig. 8-9). Patients with either ischemic heart disease or cardiomyopathy are generally less able to tolerate this slower-than-physiologic heart rate, and therapy is required more urgently. Isoproterenol given by IV drip may temporarily increase the heart rate to levels better tolerated by the patient, but this requires close monitoring because a ventricular rhythm may degenerate into ventricular tachycardia or fibrillation. Temporary transvenous pacemakers also increase the heart rate in complete heart block. Temporary pacing is accomplished by inserting a unipolar or bipolar electrode percutaneously into a peripheral vein (usually subclavian or in-

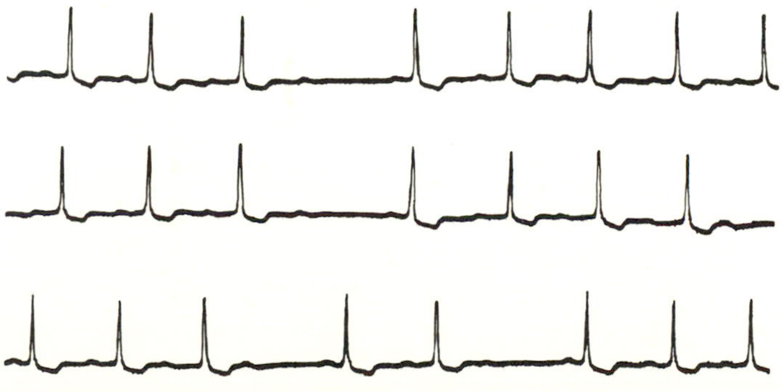

**Fig. 8-8.** Mobitz type I (Wenckebach) second-degree AV block. Note progressive prolongation of P-R interval until no ventricular response follows a P wave. Cycle is then reset.

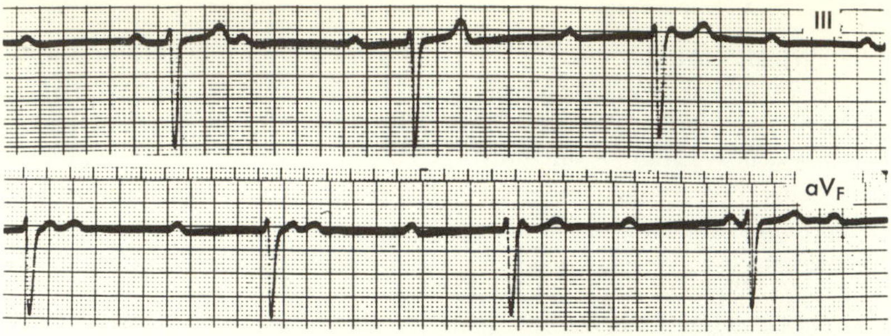


**Fig. 8-9.** Complete heart block. Note absence of any association between P waves and QRS complexes.

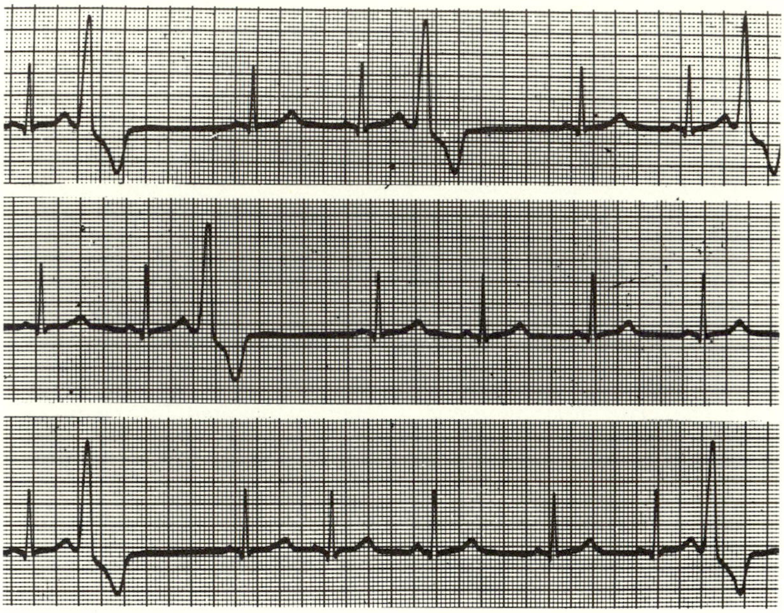

**Fig. 8-10.** Ventricular premature beats with compensatory pauses.

ternal jugular) and positioning it in the right ventricle under fluoroscopic and ECG monitoring. A pacemaker is then attached to this electrode and ventricular pacing instituted.

## ■ What is an "ectopic" rhythm?

An ectopic beat is one that originates outside of the usual site of impulse formation, which is located in the SA node; this beat may originate in the conduction system, the ventricle, atria, or elsewhere.

Ventricular premature beats (VPB's) are ectopic beats that originate in the ventricle and produce broad, bizarre QRS complexes and T waves that are markedly different from the patient's sinus QRS complexes and T waves (Fig. 8-10). VPB's may occur in otherwise normal people, or they can be caused by myocardial ischemia, hypoxia, digitalis intoxication, pulmonary emboli, ventricular aneurysm, or hypotension. They may also be parasystolic in origin, or they may be related to a sinus bradycardia.

The hemodynamic effect of VPB's relates to the following: (1) the duration of time after the preceding sinus beat that allows for ventricular filling and (2) the degree of disorganization of ventricular contraction as a result of an abnormal sequence of ventricular depolarization. If the ventricles are not allowed to fill, as occurs with an early VPB, or if there is a large degree of asynchrony in the depolarization of the ventricles so that there is ineffective ventricular contraction, frequent VPB's may cause hypotension, pulmonary vascular congestion, and other signs of low cardiac output. An additional situation that demands attention even in the absence of hemodynamic compromise is when VPB's occur on the peak or early downsloping portion of the T wave (R-on-T phenomenon). These VPB's fall in the vulnerable period of ventricular repolarization and are associated with ventricular tachycardia and fibrillation.

VPB's that are multifocal, that is, that have a number of broad bizarre configurations in any given ECG lead, are also considered malignant and predispose to ventricular tachycardia and fibrillation. VPB's in conjunction with myocardial ischemia or infarction should be observed closely, and if the frequency is greater than 3 VPB's/min, they should be treated.

Given these situations that demand therapy for VPB's, the first step is to diligently search for reversible underlying causes. If this is not successful in eliminating the VPB's, medical therapy should be instituted. Useful drugs include a lidocaine bolus followed by a drip infusion of lidocaine, procainamide, or quinidine sulfate; Table 8-2 offers a guide to the therapeutic blood levels of the most useful antiarrhythmic preparations. If frequent VPB's occur in the setting of sinus bradycardia, ventricular pacing may serve to suppress the irritable ventricular focus.

## CONGESTIVE HEART FAILURE AND PULMONARY EDEMA

### ■ What is congestive heart failure and associated pulmonary edema?

Congestive heart failure is a clinical state in which the heart is unable to maintain an adequate cardiac output in relation to the venous return and tissue metabolic needs at that particular moment. Symptoms result from the secondary inadequate tissue perfusion and organ congestion. Pulmonary edema is the acute accumulation of fluid within the pulmonary interstitial spaces and alveoli, usually caused by severe left heart failure.

Myocardial infarction occurs as an acute insult to the heart often associated with severe two- or three-vessel coronary artery disease. Scars from an old myocardial infarction may also be present. Furthermore, reflex mechanisms from the acute myocardial injury, reaction to the severe pain, and drugs used to control symptoms or arrhythmias may further compromise the normal circulation.

Recently the hemodynamics of congestive heart failure and pulmonary edema associated with acute myocardial infarction have been defined. Cardiac output is usually maintained, and total peripheral resistance is not significantly increased. Heart rate is increased and stroke volume index and stroke work index are significantly decreased, whereas left ventricular filling pressure is increased. On rare occasions, usually in association with inferior wall myocardial infarction, there may be a predominance of right ventricular damage and right ventricular failure. With an acute myocardial infarction the left ventricle also appears to become "stiffer," with altered compliance that may last several days. When the high left ventricular filling pressure is transmitted to the lungs and the pulmonary capillary hydrostatic pressure exceeds the oncotic pressure, fluid exudes into the intra-alveolar and interstitial space. Secondary right ventricular failure may follow and other hormonal homeostatic mechanisms are set in motion, causing further fluid retention.

Depending on the criteria used, some form of heart failure occurs in 23% to 71% of patients hospitalized with acute myocardial infarction. Severe congestive heart failure or pulmonary edema occurs in only about 12% of patients hospitalized with acute myocardial infarction. The incidence of congestive heart failure appears to be greater with anterior wall myocardial infarction and to increase with age and with a history of previous myocardial infarction. In some cases congestive heart failure or pulmonary edema may be the presenting manifestation of a recent myocardial infarction. At other times an acute arrhythmia such as rapid atrial fibrillation may precipitate pulmonary edema in patients with acute myocardial infarction.

### ■ What are the signs and symptoms of congestive heart failure?

The signs, symptoms, and abnormal laboratory studies in congestive heart failure reflect organ dysfunction secondary to poor perfusion and fluid congestion. Dyspnea and orthopnea are common. Paroxysmal nocturnal dyspnea may occur with intermittent left ventricular dysfunction. Right upper quadrant pain from liver congestion, with or without ascites, and peripheral edema occur with progressive heart failure as fluid is retained.

Physical examination usually reveals a sinus tachycardia with or without a complicating arrhythmia contributing to the congestive heart failure. A ventricular filling sound ($S_3$) is usually heard, as may be an $S_4$. An $S_3$, however, may occur without ventricular decompensation, especially when there is associated mitral regurgitation. Jugular venous distention may be present in cases of right ventricular congestive heart failure or after a right ventricular myocardial infarction. Inspiratory rales are usually heard over the lung fields.

Chest x-ray films show pulmonary venous distention, loss of definition of pulmonary vessels, pulmonary clouding, prominent septal lines, pleural effusions, increased diameter of the right pulmonary artery, and almost invariably some increase in cardiac size. Pulmonary edema is recognized when excessive intra-alveolar fluid accumulation produces a characteristic butterfly-shaped pattern in the pulmonary vascular markings.

The clinical signs of congestive heart failure often correlate poorly with roentgenographic findings and hemodynamics. Furthermore, chest x-ray films often show subtle changes of congestive heart failure (interstitial edema, pulmonary venous congestion) before overt clinical signs of congestive heart failure develop. Similarly, clinical signs of congestive heart failure may resolve before the roentgenographic signs. Generally there is some correlation between the left ventricular filling pressure and the degree of congestive heart failure noted on chest films.

Arterial hypoxemia is common following an acute myocardial infarction, and the degree generally correlates with the severity of left ventricular dysfunction. This is secondary to pulmonary arteriovenous shunting, and its degree generally correlates with the pulmonary artery diastolic pressure.

The myocardial damage from the acute myocardial infarction, the altered ventricular geometry from areas of akinesia and dyskinesia, the mitral regurgitation secondary to loss of integrity of the mitral valve apparatus, the metabolic acidosis secondary to poor tissue perfusion, the arterial hypoxia from pulmonary arteriovenous shunting, in addition to complicating arrhythmias, and the use of drugs that may further suppress the heart all contribute to congestive heart failure with acute myocardial infarction.

The prognosis of congestive heart failure with acute myocardial infarction is variable. Mortality rates range from 8% to 44% and correlate with the degree of congestive heart failure. Very high left ventricular filling pressures and a low cardiac work level indicate a poor prognosis.

### ■ What is the usual therapy for acute myocardial infarction?

Bed rest, oxygen, pain relief, sedation, and correction of metabolic abnormalities should be instituted in these patients. Hemodynamically significant arrhythmias and significant hypertension should receive prompt attention. Since the incidence of pulmonary emboli is higher with congestive heart failure, many advocate short-term anticoagulation therapy in this clinical setting. Mild congestive heart failure—rales, apical $S_3$, early interstitial edema on chest x-ray films—often respond to diuretics such as furosemide administered by the IV route. Potassium losses and severe hypovolemia must be avoided. The administration of digitalis to patients with acute myocardial infarction is controversial. There is some evidence that hearts suffering recent myocardial infarction do not respond to digitalization with increased inotropism and that myocardial injury may actually increase when digitalis is given. Furthermore, the toxic threshold to digitalis decreases in animals having recent myocardial infarction. Many practitioners, however, have noted generally good clinical response to digitalis in patients with congestive heart failure from an acute myocardial infarction. They therefore advocate cautious IV digitalization when there are signs and symptoms of significant congestive heart failure that has not responded to salt restriction and diuretics. Blood levels of the digitalis preparation should be monitored.

### ■ What measures may be taken to relieve pulmonary edema?

Pulmonary edema is an emergency condition and requires prompt attention. Patients with pulmonary edema are usually extremely anxious and suddenly develop dyspnea and cough productive of frothy sputum; they literally drown in their own secretions. Treatment requires a rapid reduction of the left ventricular filling pressure. This is accomplished by IV morphine sulfate, which causes venous pooling and relieves anxiety; rapid-acting and potent diuretics such as IV furosemide; phlebotomies; and the use of oxygen. Cautious use of digitalis, especially with PSVT's, may be beneficial. Intermittent positive pressure breathing will often improve the arterial oxygen saturation.

Usually these measures will relieve the signs and symptoms of congestive heart failure and pulmonary edema. However, not uncommonly these patients progress to further ventricular dysfunction manifested by a shock state.

## CARDIOGENIC SHOCK IN ACUTE MYOCARDIAL INFARCTION

### ■ What is cardiogenic shock in acute myocardial infarction?

General concepts regarding shock are presented in detail in Chapter 26. Thus only a brief consideration of the pathophysiology, diagnosis, and therapy of cardiogenic shock in acute myocardial infarction will be presented here.

Shock may be defined as a critical fall in capillary perfusion that reduces oxygen delivery to levels below the tissues' nutritional requirements to maintain cellular viability. This may be caused by inadequate venous return to the heart, inadequate ejection of blood from one of the cardiac chambers, or an abnormality of the peripheral circulation so that the capillary beds receive inadequate circulation. In cardiogenic shock secondary to myocardial infarction the problem is usually major with irreversible damage to the left ventricle, which is unable to eject enough blood. In a few cases there may be an inadequate response of the peripheral systemic resistance in the face of a relatively normal cardiac output. Severe coronary artery disease with two- or three-vessel involvement is common, especially in the case of the left coronary artery that has suffered recent damage involving at least 40% of the left ventricle. Anteroseptal wall infarction and surrounding areas of borderline viability are noted. There may be an associated interventricular septal perforation and/or papillary muscle dysfunction and/or rupture. Hemodynamics usually show a diminished cardiac output with increased total peripheral resistance, increased left ventricular filling pressures, a diminished ejection fraction and stroke volume, and increased sympathetic nervous tone. The mean aortic pressure is reduced, further impairing coronary blood flow. Metabolic acidosis and compensatory hyperventilation follow inadequate tissue perfusion. This is reflected by elevated blood lactate levels and arterial blood gases that show hypocapnia initially and acidosis and hypoxia as the shock state progresses. These metabolic changes further suppress already critically depressed myocardial function.

Recognition of the clinical state of shock involves signs and symptoms reflecting poor tissue and organ perfusion and increased sympathetic tone modified by associated factors such as fever and arrhythmias. The clinical setting is usually a recent myocardial infarction (0 to 5 days old). There may be persistent or recurrent major arrhythmias and/or chest pain. The heart rate is rapid and the blood pressure is low, usually less than 90 mm Hg systolic. Ausculatory brachial blood pressure determinations may be inaccurate estimators of the central aortic pressure when there is peripheral vascular constriction, and intra-arterial pressures may be required. The skin is cool and clammy. The peripheral pulses are small or absent. Mentation is altered with states of agitation, restlessness, confusion, and somnolence. Heart examination may reveal a diffuse point of maximal impulse (PMI) with secondary impulses, an $S_3$ or $S_4$, and murmurs of an interventricular septal defect or mitral regurgitation from papillary muscle dysfunction or rupture. Urine flow is diminished (less than 20 ml/hr) with high specific gravity and osmolality in the early phase.

It is important to emphasize that the shock syndrome associated with recent myocardial infarction is not uniformly caused by pump failure secondary to myocardial necrosis. The following lists other etiologies of the shock syndrome that may occur in conjunction with myocardial infarction.

*Shock with myocardial infarction: other considerations*

- Arrhythmias—marked tachycardias or bradycardias
- Iatrogenic causes
  - Analgesics
  - Sedatives
  - Diuretics—hypovolemia
  - Other drugs—antiarrhythmic drugs and propranolol
- Other cardiopulmonary causes
  - Cardiac tamponade
  - Pulmonary embolism
  - Aortic dissecting aneurysm

The appropriate diagnosis and therapy of these alternatives may correct the shock state and prevent further myocardial necrosis and death. These causes should be excluded in any person with shock and myocardial infarction.

The aim of therapy is to restore tissue perfusion as soon as possible and minimize further cardiac damage. Appropriate therapy requires continuous monitoring of the cardiac rhythm and central venous pressure. If possible, pulmonary artery and intra-arterial blood pressures should be monitored with a Swan-Ganz catheter in the pulmonary artery and with a brachial artery or femoral artery catheter. Urine output, total fluid balance, electrolytes, and arterial blood gases should be measured frequently. If hypovolemia is present as manifested by a decreased central venous pressure and/or pulmonary artery wedge pressure, appropriate fluid should be administered so that left ventricular filling pressure is in the optimum range of 14 to 18 mm Hg. Hypoxia and hypercapnia should be treated with oxygen and, if required, endotracheal intubation with positive pressure ventilation. Sodium bicarbonate may be required to correct acidosis, but volume overloading should be avoided.

Various drugs that raise cardiac output, heart rate, and peripheral resistance or redistribute blood flow have been utilized in the treatment of cardiogenic shock. This is usually accomplished at the expense of increased myocardial oxygen consumption and possible extension of myocardial injury. Norepinephrine increases total peripheral resistance and arterial blood pressure. Metaraminol causes similar changes. Isoproterenol increases cardiac output and heart rate and decreases total peripheral resistance with little change in blood pressure. Dopamine increases cardiac output and arterial blood pressure with fewer chronotropic effects than isoproterenol. Digitalis has little inotropic effect on an acutely infarcted heart and probably should be avoided unless there are associated arrhythmias or signs of overt congestive heart failure. The role of glucagon and corticosteroids in cardiogenic shock remains controversial. More recently the use of left ventricular afterload reduction by nitroprusside in cardiogenic shock has shown some encouraging results. Despite the use of all these measures, the mortality for shock caused by acute myocardial infarction continues to be in the range of 80% to 100%. During the last few years coronary artery bypass grafting and infarctectomy have been tried in this clinical setting, usually with disappointing results. Surgical correction of a ruptured papillary muscle or repair of a ruptured interventricular septum may, however, be lifesaving.

Because of the continuing high mortality of cardiogenic shock in acute myocardial infarction, various devices coming under the heading of assisted circulation have been used when other medical measures fail. Basically these are devices that increase tissue perfusion without increasing myocardial oxygen demands. Of these, the intra-aortic balloon pump has received the greatest clinical trial. The effect these devices have on mortality remains uncertain. They may buy time and allow studies so that the patient may eventually reach surgery.

## ACUTE VALVULAR LESIONS

The left side of the heart, being the systemic, high-pressure system, is subjected to much greater forces than the right side, low-pressure system. Abnormalities of valvular structures of the left side therefore have a greater impact on the efficiency with which the heart performs than do abnormalities of valves of the right side. Two valvular lesions, acute mitral insufficiency and severe aortic stenosis, are most likely to produce an acute illness in a cardiac patient. Other valvular diseases tend to follow a protracted course over several years marked by progressive symptoms, and the patient is less likely to seek medical aid for an acute illness.

### ■ What is the etiology of acute mitral insufficiency?

The rupture of chordae tendineae results in a flail mitral leaflet that is free to prolapse into the left atrium. This may occur in conjunction with chronic mitral regurgitation secondary to rheumatic heart disease, or it may result in an acute form from infective endocarditis. Less common causes of ruptured chordae include traumatic blows to the chest, myxomatous degeneration of valve structures, or simply nonspecific thinning and stretching of chordae. The amount of regurgitation produced depends on the extent of mitral leaflet tethered by the ruptured chorda; rupture of small chordae close to the leaflet produces less regurgitation than does rupture of large chordae close to the papillary muscle.

If mitral regurgitation suddenly develops in a patient who has coronary artery disease or has recently had myocardial infarction, it is most likely caused by papillary muscle dysfunction or rupture of a papillary muscle. These muscles are particularly susceptible to ischemic injury and abnormal function can produce varying degrees of mitral regurgitation. Rupture of a papillary muscle represents the most severe form of this spectrum and commonly occurs in a very dramatic fashion in association with recent infarction. The patient becomes acutely ill with intractable congestive heart failure and often dies within 24 hours. The combination of acute severe mitral regurgitation and an infarcted ischemic myocardium apparently dictates the patient's fate rather than either of these factors alone.

### ■ What treatment is recommended for acute mitral insufficiency?

Digitalis glycosides are often useful when severe mitral regurgitation is present and serve to help the ventricle pump more efficiently as well as to control the PSVT's that are frequently present. Potent diuretics such as furosemide or ethacrynic acid also help relieve pulmonary congestion. If the patient is in shock, pressor agents are of little benefit and will most likely cause increased mitral regurgitation. Significant advances have been made recently in the use of afterload-reducing agents such as nitroprusside and hydralazine when shock is associated with the acute mitral regurgitation. These agents appear to decrease the regurgitant fraction and increase the forward cardiac output as a result of reducing afterload. If afterload reduction is attempted, adequate measures must be taken to monitor arterial pressure (preferably with an intra-arterial line), central venous or pulmonary artery pressure, urine flow, and heart rhythm. It should become apparent early in the course whether medicine alone will stabilize the patient's condition. Surgical replacement of the mitral valve should not be delayed for the patient who does not respond to medical therapy.

In an effort to assess the risks of surgery, patients with severe mitral regurgitation should undergo hemodynamic evaluation and left ventricular angiography. The angiogram will help quantitate the degree of mitral regurgitation as well as general myocardial dysfunction. The greater the degree of myocardial abnormalities, the greater is the risk of surgery and the less likely is the possibility that mitral valve replacement alone will alter the patient's course.

■ **What factors should be considered in the diagnosis of end-stage aortic stenosis?**

When a patient with aortic stenosis complains of angina-like chest pain, episodes of faintness or symptoms of heart failure such as shortness of breath or orthopnea, it is likely that a severe degree of stenosis has developed. These symptoms may signal a rapid deterioration in the patient's condition and survival is usually limited to less than 3 to 4 years after the onset of these symptoms. Congestive heart failure appears to be the most ominous sign and generally heralds a rapidly deteriorating condition developing over a period of 2 to 3 years.

There are several indications on physical examination that there is severe stenosis. If the stenosis is severe, the crescendo-decrescendo murmur tends to peak late in systole. The second heart sound may be diminished or even absent. Fourth heart sounds are most common with severe degrees of aortic stenosis, and a third heart sound is indicative of some degree of left ventricular failure in older patients with aortic stenosis. Evidence of left ventricular hypertrophy on the ECG is often present when lesions are severe, and the chest x-ray film commonly reveals calcium in the aortic valve. If a patient with stenosis complains of ominous symptoms or has these physical findings, cardiac catheterization should be undertaken without delay in an effort to assess the severity of the aortic disease. Coronary angiography should be performed in anyone with signs or symptoms of ischemia, even though this may occur without coronary artery disease. It has been our general practice to perform coronary angiography in any patient undergoing aortic valve replacement for aortic stenosis, even if symptoms of angina are not present.

■ **In the management of end-stage aortic stenosis, what modalities should be considered?**

Acute decompensation in severe aortic stenosis may take the form of pulmonary edema, shock, or syncope. Arrhythmias, especially atrial fibrillation, are poorly tolerated in patients with thick, hypertrophied, noncompliant left ventricles and should be managed in a critical care unit. If the patient is hypotensive, inotropic agents such as isoproterenol should be administered promptly. Digitalis glycosides may be administered. If pulmonary edema is present, rotating tourniquets and opiates should be utilized, but a vigorous diuresis is to be avoided. Time should not be lost in medical therapy that is not promptly effective. The patient should undergo cardiac catheterization as soon as possible, and a decision should be made regarding valve replacement. Although the risks of aortic valve replacement in the acutely ill patient are considerable, the risks of ongoing medical management are greater, and many reports of successful acute aortic valve replacement are available.

## ACUTE PERICARDITIS

■ **What is acute pericarditis?**

Acute pericarditis is an inflammatory process involving the visceral and parietal pericardium, usually with associated fluid accumulation in the pericardial sac.

The following is a list of some of the well-recognized etiologies of acute pericarditis.

*Etiology of acute pericarditis*

Connective tissue disorders—rheumatoid arthritis, acute rheumatic fever, disseminated lupus erythematosus

Infections
- Viruses—coxsackie B virus, echovirus, influenza
- Bacterial infections
- Fungi—histoplasmosis

Neoplasm—especially lung and breast

Uremia

Radiation—to the chest
Drugs—procainamide, hydralazine
Postmyocardial infarction syndrome (Dressler's syndrome)
Postthoracotomy
Traumatic—penetrating and nonpenetrating injuries to the chest
Iatrogenic—cardiac catheterization, central venous pressure lines
Idiopathic

Many infectious agents that cause myocarditis may also cause pericarditis, often during the same illness. In the United States the most common etiologies of acute pericarditis are probably viruses and uremia. In many cases no cause can be identified.

### ■ What are the signs and symptoms of acute pericarditis?

The signs and symptoms are those of the primary systemic illness and the inflammatory process of the pericardium. Often a viral upper respiratory infection has occurred in the preceding week. Complaints may be restricted to those of the systemic illness such as fever, arthralgia, myalgia, fatigue, or symptoms of uremia. Usually there is substernal chest pain radiating to the neck and left arm that increases on sudden turning of the thorax, deep inspiration, or lying flat on the back and is relieved by sitting forward. Physical examination will often show tachycardia, fever, a pericardial friction rub that may have from one to three components, distended neck veins, and a diffuse PMI if there is significant pericardial fluid. With pericardial tamponade a paradoxical pulse (greater than 8 mm Hg drop in systolic pressure during quiet inspiration) and on occasion inspiratory neck vein distention (Kussmaul's sign) will be found.

The ECG will usually demonstrate generalized S-T segment elevation followed by T wave inversion. Low voltage and electrical alternans (of the P wave and QRS complexes) can be seen if there is significant pericardial fluid accumulation. The chest x-ray film is often normal. There may be an associated pleural effusion and pulmonary infiltrate and cardiomegaly if significant pericardial fluid accumulates or associated myocarditis is present. Radioisotope and contrast studies will often demonstrate an increased pericardial space. Currently the best technique to demonstrate pericardial fluid accumulation is echocardiography. Fig. 8-11 shows the records of a typical case of acute pericarditis with large accumulation of pericardial fluid.

An etiologic diagnosis will depend on a complete medical evaluation and appropriate stains and cultures of various body fluids, including pericardial fluid. Serologic studies may also be of aid.

### ■ What treatment modalities are indicated?

Treatment is directed at the underlying systemic illness and the relief of symptoms caused by the pericardial inflammatory process. Bed rest with the head of the bed elevated 30 to 45 degrees is recommended.

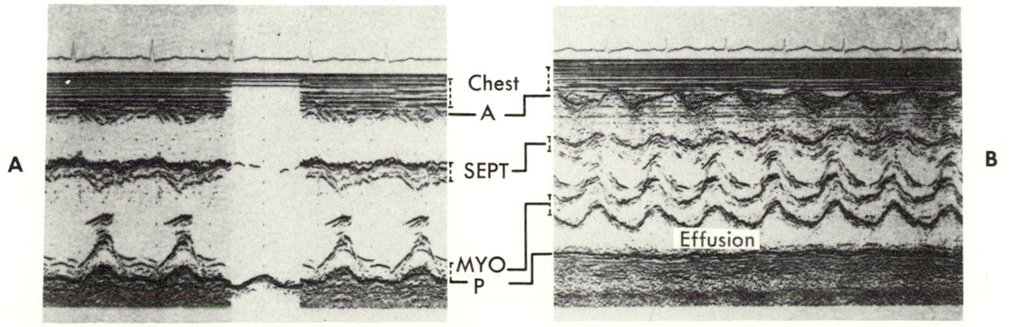


**Fig. 8-11. A,** Normal echocardiogram. **B,** Echocardiogram depicting pericardial effusion. *A,* Anterior heart wall; *SEPT,* interventricular septum; *MYO,* myocardium of posterior left ventricle; *P,* pericardium. Space between left ventricular myocardium and pericardium represents pericardial effusion.

Fever and pain should be relieved with aspirin. Indomethacin is also beneficial. In some cases stronger analgesics will be required. If symptoms persist and are severe, and bacterial, fungal, and tuberculous etiologies have been excluded, adrenal steroids may give dramatic symptomatic results in idiopathic, postradiation, postmyocardial infarction, and postthoracotomy pericarditis. If a bacterial, fungal, or tuberculous agent has been identified, appropriate therapy for the infection should be started immediately. Uremic pericarditis usually responds to hemodialysis and lupus erythematosis is susceptible to steroids and/or antimetabolite preparations.

In a small percent of patients with pericardial inflammation or injury pericardial tamponade results secondary to rapid fluid accumulation in the pericardial sac. Usually this is marked by rapidly progressive cardiorespiratory distress and classically by a rising central venous pressure, a falling arterial blood pressure, and a small, quiet heart. The primary problem is resistance to cardiac filling secondary to increased intrapericardial pressure. On physical examination there is a low blood pressure with a reduced pulse pressure and increased paradoxical pulse, with or without a positive Kussmaul's sign, tachycardia, high central venous pressure, and a quiet precordium with distant heart sounds. An ECG may show generally low voltage and/or total electrical alternans. Cardiomegaly may or may not be present on chest x-ray films. Echocardiography provides more specific diagnostic information. The final diagnosis and treatment requires immediate needle aspiration of the pericardial fluid, usually with dramatic results. If pericardial fluid rapidly reaccumulates further consideration must be given to a pericardiectomy or repair of an associated cardiac lesion. If facilities for a pericardial tap and/or further cardiac surgery are not immediately available, temporary support may be given by providing optimum filling pressures (maintaining a central venous pressure in the range of 14 to 18 ml $H_2O$) and by the use of inotropic agents such as isoproterenol that augment left ventricular emptying.

## ACUTE MYOCARDITIS

### ■ What is acute myocarditis?

Myocarditis may be defined as an inflammatory process involving the myocardium. Many bacteria, viruses, rickettsia, fungi, and parasites may cause the syndrome. Acute myocarditis can occur with exposure to certain toxic agents, radiation therapy to the chest, and coronary vasculitis. However, the leading causes are the postviral syndromes that occur following infection with many viral agents. The incidence and agent involved vary with age, location, and criteria used to describe the disease. In some cases the myocarditis may be secondary to a vasculitis or an immunologic phenomenon following an infection. Myocarditis may occur in 10% to 25% of patients with diphtheria, usually during the second week of illness. The diphtheria toxin disturbs cellular metabolism. Typhoid fever may be associated with peripheral vascular collapse and myocarditis, usually in the second or third week of illness. A $\beta$-streptococcus infection may of course be followed in 3 weeks by a pancarditis involving the myocardium. Meningococcemia, especially fatal cases, may involve an interstitial myocarditis and associated circulatory collapse. Any case of endocarditis can include small infarctions, microabscesses, and myofiber swelling. Other less common bacterial causes may be found on pp. 185-186. Rickettsial infections such as Rocky Mountain spotted fever and Q-fever may cause myocarditis. In the United States coxsackie B virus and influenza virus have been the best documented etiologic agents of clinical myocarditis. Often, however, no specific etiologic agent can be identified by bacteriologic, serologic, or fluorescent techniques.

Pathologically the heart is usually large and flabby. Microscopically there may be areas of focal hemorrhage, interstitial edema, myocardial degeneration and necrosis, a mononuclear or polymorphonuclear cellular infiltrate, small abscesses, areas of vasculitis, gumma, or tuberculous nodules, depending on the agent involved. In many cases an inflammatory process also involves the endocardium and/or pericardium. Mural thrombi can often be seen in both ventricles.

Clinical recognition involves signs and symptoms reflecting the primary infectious process with its unique features, inadequate cardiac output, and associated congestive heart failure. Often there are associated signs and symptoms of an inflammatory process of the endocardium and/or pericardium. There may have been previous upper respiratory or enteric symptoms. Typically the patients complain of dyspnea, fatigue, palpitations, and chest discomfort. On physical examination there may be fever, hypotension, tachycardia, an enlarged heart with a diffuse PMI, distended neck veins, soft heart sounds with an associated $S_3$ and/or $S_4$, murmurs of tricuspid and/or mitral regurgitation, and other symptoms of congestive heart failure. A pericardial friction rub is often heard. The ECG will often show diffuse ST-T wave changes, occasional QRS abnormalities, various degrees of heart block, and all the known types of atrial and ventricular arrhythmias. Final diagnosis depends on appropriate cultures and serologic tests. The entire course may conclude in sudden death, systemic or pulmonary emboli, severe heart failure, partial resolution with a persisting chronic congestive cardiomyopathy, or total and complete recovery.

Appropriate treatment requires an early etiologic diagnosis so that appropriate antibacterial, antirickettsial, or antifungal agents or antitoxin are utilized. Bed rest, oxygen, salt restriction, ECG monitoring, and control of fever are essential, since there is experimental evidence that hypoxia and exercise can enhance viral myocarditis in animals. Hemodynamically significant arrhythmias should be treated with antiarrhythmic agents, although these drugs should be used with caution in such patients so as to prevent further myocardial depression. Heart failure should be treated with diuretics and digitalis, although increased sensitivity to digitalis in myocarditis requires the use of lower doses. Patients should receive anticoagulants if there have been any systemic or pulmonary emboli; however, vigilance should be applied to avoid any development of hemopericardium. The use of steroids and other anti-inflammatory agents in rheumatic myocarditis or vasculitis appears to be of significant benefit. The role of steroids in acute viral or idiopathic myocarditis is controversial. Other inflammatory reducing agents such as aspirin, indomethacin, and cytotoxin may be indicated. The preventive role of immunization and vaccination should always be emphasized.

## INFECTIVE ENDOCARDITIS

### ■ What is infective endocarditis?

Infective endocarditis is a bacterial, fungal, or possibly viral infection of cardiac structures that destroys or damages these structures and makes them incompetent. Virtually any bacteria or fungus can cause endocarditis, but some organisms are more common than others and can infect heart valves, frequently accompany congenital defects, or contaminate prosthetic materials placed at the time of heart surgery. The organisms invade the tissues, resulting in inflammatory and immunologic reactions that then destroy these tissues. Holes in valve cusps and leaflets, ruptured chordae, myocarditis, myocardial abscesses, or communications between chambers may develop. The mass of organisms, fibrin, collagen, and debris as they collect and organize on a valve or prosthetic structure can impede the motion of a valve, rendering it stenotic or incompetent. As a result, there are a number of possible ways the heart may exhibit infection.

Endocarditis also produces a classic but atypical syndrome involving practically every system in the body. Neurologic, hematologic, renal, musculoskeletal, peripheral vascular, and integumentary manifestations of infective endocarditis may all appear. With such a variety of possible systemic manifestations it is not uncommon for a patient to be treated for a number of the peripheral manifestations of infective endocarditis rather than to have the primary process itself discovered or even considered.

### ■ What is the differentiation between "acute" or "subacute" infective endocarditis?

Endocarditis may be either acute or subacute. The term "acute infective endocarditis" is applied to the disease in patients who do not survive for an arbitrary length of time, usually 6 to 8 weeks, while the term "subacute infective endocarditis" refers to the disease in patients who experience a longer and more indolent course. This distinction originated in the preantibiotic era when the natural course of the disease could be observed unaltered by the administration of antibiotics. Acute infective endocarditis affects and destroys cardiac structures before more chronic manifestations can develop, whereas in subacute infective endocarditis there is more time for immunologic and inflammatory factors to evolve the full-blown, classic syndrome. Certain organisms such as staphylococcus and pneumococcus are more commonly associated with the acute form of the disease, whereas less virulent organisms such as *Streptococcus viridans,* fungi (particularly *Candida*), or enterococcus usually cause subacute endocarditis. The rapid appearance of extensive damage such as acute aortic regurgitation or tricuspid regurgitation in a setting suggestive of endocarditis, signals the probability that a more virulent process exists. This classification is useful in characterizing the tempo of an episode of endocarditis, but it is not useful in dictating early management of a given patient. Pragmatically each case of endocarditis should be considered to be "potentially acute" and deserves prompt attention.

## ■ What factors should be considered in the diagnosis of endocarditis?

Fever is the most common presenting symptom of a patient with infective endocarditis, and fever in a person with acquired valvular abnormalities or congenital heart disease should always signal the possibility of an infectious cardiac process. Although rheumatic heart disease is still the most common underlying cardiac abnormality, the relative incidence of other abnormalities such as mitral valve prolapse or calcific or atheromatous lesions of the aortic or mitral valves has been increasing in frequency. The incidence of infective endocarditis in normal hearts has increased recently as well, particularly in conjunction with heroin abuse or chronic hemodialysis when IV manipulations are common or in the patient taking immunosuppressive agents. Therefore any fever even without cardiac abnormality suggests the possibility of endocarditis. The absence of fever does not, however, rule out a cardiac infection, particularly in aged or uremic patients. The previous empiric use of antibiotics is also a common disguise for a fever.

The most significant laboratory tests pinpointing the diagnosis of infective endocarditis are positive blood cultures. One positive blood culture does not determine the diagnosis, but its occurrence should stimulate further blood cultures and suggest the possibility of infectious endocarditis. Some organisms such as diphtheroids or *Staphylococcus albus* are common contaminants in routine blood cultures, but the practitioner should also be aware that these organisms have been implicated in infectious endocarditis as well and should not totally dismiss them as contaminants.

Generally five to six blood cultures, appropriately obtained under strict conditions of asepsis, will be sufficient to recover an organism if endocarditis is present. The timing of the cultures may be important. Blood obtained just prior to a temperature elevation is likely to be most productive, but as a temperature rise may not be anticipated, the next best yield will be obtained as the fever rises. A volume of 10 ml of venous blood obtained after thoroughly cleansing and sterilizing the venipuncture site should be planted in both aerobic and anaerobic culture medium. Cultures are frequently negative when infection is present on the right side of the heart, if antibiotics have been administered, or if the responsible organism, such as a rickettsia, simply will not grow on the culture media.

## ■ What therapeutic approach is recommended in the management of endocarditis?

Adequate therapy for infective endocarditis requires characterization of the causative organisms. Once this information is available from the microbiology laboratory, the most logical course of therapy is often clear. It may be reasonable to delay therapy until these antibiotic sensitivities are determined, particularly if the clinical course appears to be that of a subacute infection, that is, symptoms have been present for some time. If the symptoms of acute endocarditis are present, that is, the patient appears acutely ill, has had symptoms for a relatively short period of time, and does not have any murmurs or has murmurs of tricuspid or pulmonic insufficiency, and bacteremia with a virulent organism may possibly be present, no time should be lost in instituting therapy on a presumptive basis. If staphylococcus is suspected to be the causative agent, the regimen should include large doses of a penicillinase-resistant semisynthetic penicillin. The initial regimen should cover the most likely organisms against each serum dilution. A serum dilution of 1:8 that impedes multiplication of the organism is considered effective therapy.

The duration of recommended therapy has been somewhat empiric, and it is generally accepted that at least 4 weeks of therapy are required. Although there is no statistical evidence, some practitioners prefer to prolong treatment for 6 weeks. There is the theoretical consideration that with the broad spectrum of coverage gained by high doses of antibiotics and with a longer treatment period, there will be some predisposition to superinfection.

### ■ What factors should be considered during the follow-up evaluation of the patient?

Signs of early or increasing heart failure must be carefully sought. Heart failure may be caused by myocarditis but more often is a result of progressive valvular destruction or disruption of the valvular mechanism by vegetation. Such valvular disturbances are usually marked by murmurs that may change as valvular damage increases. The heart size and contour on chest x-ray films is important in demonstrating cardiac enlargement, which may result from either congestive heart failure or insufficiency of aortic or mitral valves. The appearance of a pericardial friction rub indicates the possibility of the extension of infection, particularly in acute bacterial endocarditis, through cardiac structures to involve pericardial surfaces. Such an extension can rapidly develop into purulent pericarditis or pericardial tamponade, and the echocardiogram is a sensitive tool for early detection of accumulating pericardial fluid. Jugular venous pulse waves, as visualized at the bedside and recorded on the phonocardiogram, may be of importance in evaluating competence of the tricuspid valve in the presence of endocarditis of the right side. The evolution of new infiltrates in the lung fields associated with supposedly adequate antibiotic therapy of endocarditis of the right side points toward an ongoing infectious valvular process. ECG's should be obtained occasionally, as the evolution of new conduction defects support an ongoing infectious process.

### ■ Under what circumstances would aggressive surgical intervention be indicated, and what complications might be anticipated?

Progressive and intractable cardiac failure as a result of infective endocarditis destroying valve mechanisms is the most common indication for surgery, and congestive heart failure secondary to mitral regurgitation is the most common lesion.

Valve surgery in patients with infective endocarditis is associated with a high mortality rate that must be contrasted to the 100% fatality rate of progressive cardiac failure if surgery is not performed. Failure can also result from rupture of the interventricular septum and can require surgical repair. When one course of antibiotic therapy has not eradicated the infection, a second course should be attempted; little is gained, however, by trying a third or fourth course, and surgical excision should be considered. Such a situation is most common with fungal infections of valves on the right side. The resistant nature of fungal endocarditis and the very toxic nature of the therapeutic regimens required for treatment raise the issue of surgery whenever endocarditis caused by a fungus is documented.

With the abundance of prosthetic materials placed in the heart during cardiac surgery over the past decade, the significance of positive blood cultures in the setting of these prostheses has become a frequent issue. Positive blood cultures in the early postoperative period (less than 25 days), considering the many complicating factors and modes of entrance to the bloodstream available in the surgical patient, are generally not regarded as indicative of infection of prosthetic material. Bacteremia occurring more than 25 days after surgery has more significance, and should suggest the probability of infected prosthetic materials. There is a high incidence of fungal (particularly *Candida*) antibiotic-resistant gram-negative organisms (*Staphylococcus epidermitis* and *Staphylococcus aureus*) in the postoperative patient. In view of the very poor results in treating infections of prosthetic materials by medications alone and the bizarre nature of the organisms usually involved, time should not be wasted in attempting repeated courses of antibiotics; early surgery is the preferable course of action.

## DISSECTING ANEURYSM OF THE AORTA

### ■ What is a dissecting aneurysm of the aorta?

Dissecting aneurysm of the aorta is a cleavage of the layers of the aortic wall by blood and hematoma that gains access through a tear in the intima of the aorta. The dissection may spread both proximal and distal to the initial tear. Dissection occurs in people who are hypertensive but may occur in Marfan's syndrome or when there has been trauma to the chest. The danger involved in a dissecting aneurysm is rupture of the aorta and most often occurs into the pericardial sac with acute tamponade and death. A dissection may also occlude any of the major branches of the aorta with subsequent ischemia or infarction of end-organs. Dissecting aneurysm of the aorta is a medical-surgical emergency and requires prompt aggressive therapy with close monitoring.

### ■ On what basis is the diagnosis made?

The most frequent presenting symptom of a patient with a dissecting aneurysm is commonly described as a "ripping" or "tearing" chest pain located in the substernal region or in the interscapular area. It commonly radiates down the back as the hematoma dissects along the aortic wall. Shortness of breath, orthopnea, or symptoms of frank pulmonary edema result from involvement of the aortic root and resultant aortic regurgitation. Shock as a result of leakage into a body cavity or the pericardium with tamponade may occur. Signs of occlusions of major branches of the aorta such as stroke or bowel ischemia are seen.

The impressive chest pain suggests a myocardial infarction. However, the ECG in uncomplicated dissections is normal, and when myocardial infarction is eliminated after normal enzymes and no ischemic patterns appear on the ECG, a dissecting aneurysm should be suspected.

Physical examination is not very helpful in diagnosing a dissecting aneurysm. Pressure differentials in the arms, pulseless lower extremities, signs of pericardial effusion or tamponade, and shock are all relatively nonspecific, but when seen together are highly suggestive of a dissecting aneurysm. Chest roentgenograms classically demonstrate a wide mediastinum that is the result of dilation of the ascending aorta, descending aorta, or both. The heart may be enlarged and bottle shaped if pericardial fluid is present.

The definitive diagnosis of a dissection is made by aortography, and this should be undertaken as soon as possible after the diagnosis is suspected. The study should define the intimal tear, the extent of the aneurysm, and any occluded blood vessels to aid in the surgical corrections.

### ■ What treatment may be considered when the presence of a dissecting aneurysm is suspected?

The initial therapy of any patient exhibiting the signs of a dissection, that is, hypertension and severe chest or back pain, should consist of immediate blood pressure control with the goal of maintaining a systolic blood pressure of 100 to 120 mm Hg. The medication useful in achieving this is trimethaphan (Arfonad) in combination with propranolol (Inderal). Propranolol will decrease the force with which blood is ejected from the heart. Pain must be controlled, and opiates are required in most cases. Urine flow, state of mentation, blood pressure (preferable with an arterial line), and central venous or pulmonary artery pressure should all be monitored.

After the diagnosis has been confirmed and adequate blood pressure control achieved, a decision regarding surgery must be made. Generally surgery is the therapy of choice when the aneurysm originates in the ascending portion of the aorta. Aneurysms from this location are associated with a higher risk of death and occlusion of major vessels than aneurysms from the descending portion of the aorta. Medical therapy as outlined may be attempted for aneurysms occurring in the descending aorta, but any signs of progression such as ongoing pain or leakage should be indications for surgery.

## ■ What is the prognosis?

The percentage of survival from a dissecting aneurysm of the descending aorta has been reported to be about 70% in patients medically treated and at least 75% when a combination of medical and surgical therapy is applied to an ascending aortic aneurysm. Aortic valve replacement is often required if there is severe aortic regurgitation. The basic pathologic process of cystic medial necrosis is obviously still present in a patient who has recovered from the acute stages of a dissecting aneurysm. Continued blood pressure control and diminution of the force with which blood is ejected from the left ventricle (dp/dt) are therefore imperative. Reserpine and propranolol are probably the best medications for these purposes. Blood pressure should be monitored with the patient in a supine position and should be less than 130 systolic. Chest x-ray films should be followed routinely for further discrete dilatations. Any report by the patient of renewed pain or symptoms referable to new major arterial branch occlusions indicates an ongoing dissection process, and surgical therapy is warranted.

## BIBLIOGRAPHY


### Arrhythmias

Coltart, D. J., and Harrison, D. C.: Office management of arrhythmias, Primary Care **1**:123, 1974.

Marriott, H. J. L., and Myerberg, R. J.: Recognition and treatment of cardiac arrhythmias and conduction disturbances. In Hurst, J. W., and Logue, R. B., editors: The heart, New York, 1970, McGraw-Hill Book Co.

### Congestive heart failure and pulmonary edema

Karliner, J. S., and Braunwald, E.: Present status of digitalis treatment of acute myocardial infarction, Circulation **45**:169-180, 1972.

Lassers, B. W., George, M., Auderton, J. L., Higgins, M. R., and Philip, T.: Left ventricular failure in acute myocardial infarction, Am. J. Cardiol. **25**:511-522, 1970.

Ramo, B. W., Myers, N., Wallace, A. G., Starmer, F., Clark, D. O., and Whalen, R. E.: Hemodynamic findings in 123 patients with acute myocardial infarction on admission, Circulation **42**:567-577, 1970.

Wolk, M. J., Scheidt, S., and Killip, T.: Heart failure complicating acute myocardial infarction, Circulation **45**:225-238, 1972.

### Cardiogenic shock in acute myocardial infarction

Haddy, F. J.: Pathophysiology and therapy of the shock of myocardial infarction, Ann. Intern. Med. **73**:809-827, 1970.

Page, D. L., Caulfield, J. B., Kastor, J. A., DeSanctis, R. W., and Sanders, C. A.: Myocardial changes associated with cardiogenic shock, N. Engl. J. Med. **285**:133-137, 1971.

Perlroth, M. G., and Harrison, D. C.: Medical therapy for shock in acute myocardial infarction. In Yu, P. N., and Goodwin, J. F., editors: Progress in cardiology, Philadelphia, 1973, Lea & Febiger.

Scheidt, S., et al.: Intra-aortic balloon counterpulsation in cardiogenic shock, N. Engl. J. Med. **288**:979-984, 1973.

Shubin, H., and Weil, M. H.: Practical considerations in management of shock complicating acute myocardial infarction. A summary of current practice, Am. J. Cardiol. **26**:603-608, 1970.

### Acute valvular lesions

Cobbs, B. W.: Clinical recognition and medical management of rheumatic heart disease and other acquired valvular disease. In Hurst,

J. W., and Logue, R. B., editors: The heart, New York, 1970, McGraw-Hill Book Co.

**Acute pericarditis**

Connolly, D. C., and Burchell, H. G.: Pericarditis: a ten-year survey, Am. J. Cardiol. **7**:7-14, 1961.

Fowler, N. O., and Manitsas, G. T.: Infectious pericarditis, Prog. Cardiovasc. Dis. **16**:323-336, 1973.

Grist, N. R., and Bell, E. J.: Coxsackie viruses and the heart, Am. Heart J. **77**:295-300, 1969 (editorial).

Shabetai, R., Fowler, N. O., and Guntheroth, W. G.: Hemodynamics of cardiac tamponade and constrictive pericarditis, Am. J. Cardiol. **26**:480-489, 1970.

Spodick, D. H.: Differential diagnosis of acute pericarditis, Prog. Cardiovasc. Dis. **14**:192-209, 1971.

**Acute myocarditis**

Abelmann, W. H.: Virus and the heart, Circulation **44**:950-956, 1971.

Abelmann, W. H.: Viral myocarditis and its sequelae, Annu. Rev. Med. **24**:145-152, 1973.

Gardiner, A. J. S., and Short, D.: Four faces of acute myopericarditis, Br. Heart J. **35**:433-442, 1973.

Gerzen, P., Granath, A., Holmgren, B., and Zetterquist, S.: Acute myocarditis, a follow up study, Br. Heart J. **34**:575-583, 1972.

Wenger, N. K.: Infectious myocarditis, Cardiovasc. Clin. **4**:167-185, 1972.

**Infective endocarditis**

Weinstein, L., and Schlesinger, J.: Treatment of infective endocarditis, Prog. Cardiovasc. Dis. **16**:275, 1973.

**Dissecting aneurysm of the aorta**

Daily, P. O., et al.: Management of acute aortic dissection, Ann. Thorac. Surg. **10**:237, 1970.

Wheat, M. W., Jr.: Treatment of dissecting aneurysms, Prog. Cardiovasc. Dis. **16**:87, 1973.

*chapter 9*

# Clinical management of cardiac medical emergencies

HOWARD N. ALLEN

An emergency can be defined as a sudden condition or state of affairs calling for immediate action. The term "cardiac emergency" obviously implies that such a condition involves the heart. The definition of an emergency can be further amplified to include those conditions that threaten life but are potentially correctable with prompt therapeutic intervention. Since these conditions require immediate action and since therapy is predicated on the establishment of a correct diagnosis, it is important to make a prompt and correct diagnosis. An understanding of the pathophysiology of the existing condition is also essential to rationally manage the patient's problem. It is thus important for the practitioner to be aware of the clinical features of the various cardiac emergencies, to have some understanding of the pathophysiology of these conditions, and to be able to act in an appropriate manner based on this knowledge.

Conditions that can be considered cardiac emergencies include cardiac arrest, other serious dysrhythmias, acute pulmonary edema, cardiogenic shock, cardiac tamponade, pulmonary embolism, and infective endocarditis.

Since space does not allow for an adequate discussion of cardiac arrest, the reader is referred to the *Standards for Cardiopulmonary Resuscitation (CPR) and Emergency Cardiac Care (ECC)*,[1] a publication stating the recommendations of a national conference cosponsored by the American Heart Association and National Academy of Sciences–National Research Council.

Chest pain is a symptom that is common to several of the cardiac emergencies and frequently is the immediate symptom for which a patient seeks medical care in an emergency facility. A detailed discussion relative to the evaluation of a patient with chest pain is therefore included in this chapter.

The management of acute myocardial infarction will not be covered separately. However, the diagnosis and management of serious complications of acute myocardial infarction including acute pulmonary edema and cardiogenic shock will be reviewed in detail.

Since Chapter 7 deals with ECG changes involved in critical illness, the discussion of dysrhythmias in this chapter will be limited primarily to a review of the general principles involved in the management of dysrythmias.

The format for each of the cardiac emergencies covered in this chapter will include discussion of (1) definition of the condition, (2) clinical features, (3) the various causes for each condition, (4) a summary of the diagnostic features of the entity, and (5) management.

## ACUTE PULMONARY EDEMA

### ■ What is pulmonary edema?

Acute pulmonary edema is a condition resulting from the transudation or shift in fluid from the intravascular compartment first to the interstitial and later to the alveolar spaces in the lungs with resultant impairment of (1) ventilation and (2) diffusion of oxygen ($O_2$) from the alveoli into the capillaries.

■ **What are the clinical features of acute pulmonary edema?**

The symptoms include dyspnea, orthopnea, and frequently a sensation of chest tightness. Physical examination usually reveals the patient to be in respiratory distress. The patient may be cyanotic with cool, clammy skin and may have a cough productive of pink frothy sputum. There is usually sinus tachycardia or an inappropriate rhythm and an increased respiratory rate. Examination of the lungs usually reveals rales and wheezes. If there is associated right heart failure, the venous pressure will be elevated and neck veins distended, the liver will be enlarged, and dependent edema will be present. Cardiac examination may be difficult because of the noisy respiration and the difficulty in properly positioning the patient for a detailed examination of the heart. However, third and fourth heart sounds may be heard and the pulmonic component of the second heart sound may be increased in intensity. In addition, the findings of the underlying cardiac condition may be noted.

■ **What does the ECG reveal?**

The ECG may reveal sinus tachycardia or other dysrhythmia, as well as findings consistent with the basic underlying cardiac disease such as acute or old myocardial infarction, ventricular hypertrophy, and/or atrial enlargement.

■ **What are the chest x-ray findings in this condition?**

The chest x-ray film usually reveals cardiomegaly, increased prominence of the upper lobe veins, pulmonary vascular blurring, haziness of the hilar regions, and possibly pleural effusion.[2]

■ **What are the causes of pulmonary edema?**

Pulmonary edema is usually the result of an increase in pulmonary capillary pressure, altered pulmonary capillary permeability, or decreased oncotic pressure. An increase in pulmonary capillary pressure can occur in any condition that results in an elevation of the left ventricular diastolic pressure or wherein there is obstruction across the mitral valve, as occurs in mitral stenosis, with resultant increase in left atrial pressure without elevation in left ventricular diastolic pressure. Pulmonary edema can thus be seen in (1) arteriosclerotic heart disease associated with myocardial necrosis and/or fibrosis, papillary muscle dysfunction, perforation of the ventricular septum, or ruptured papillary muscle; (2) rheumatic heart disease with mitral and/or aortic valve disease; (3) hypertensive cardiovascular disease; and (4) cardiomyopathies. Altered pulmonary capillary permeability can be caused by uremia, radiation pneumonia, aspiration pneumonia, smoke inhalation, and inhaled toxic agents such as phosgene. Decreased oncotic pressure occurs with hypoalbuminemia caused by hepatic or renal disease, protein-losing enteropathy, or malnutrition. Pulmonary edema may also occur secondary to CNS lesions or the effects of high altitude.

■ **What are the precipitating factors resulting in pulmonary edema?**

In evaluating and managing a patient with pulmonary edema the factors responsible for aggravation of an underlying stable condition resulting in the development of pulmonary edema should be considered. These factors include dysrhythmias, recent history of excessive salt and/or fluid intake, failure to take medications as prescribed, an acute infection, impaired renal function, acute injury to cardiac muscle, infective endocarditis, severe hypertension, pulmonary emboli, and emotional crisis.

■ **On what is the diagnosis based?**

The diagnosis is generally obvious from the history and physical examination, as previously noted. If wheezing as a result of bronchospasm is the predominant finding on examination of the lungs, acute pulmonary edema must be differentiated from bronchial asthma, which characteristically presents with wheezing. Generally the antecedent history and other findings of heart failure will help to differentiate these two conditions.

■ **What is included in the management of a patient with this condition?**

The patient should be allowed to sit up, either in a chair or with the feet dangling from the side of the bed. This will decrease venous return to the heart. Since the patient is usually hypoxemic, $O_2$ should be administered. This can be achieved with an $O_2$ mask delivering $O_2$ at a flow rate of 6 to 8 L/min, giving an inspired $O_2$ concentration of approximately 40%. The application of rotating tourniquets will decrease venous return to the heart. The presence of peripheral vascular disease is a relative contraindication to the use of rotating tourniquets.

Morphine sulfate should be administered; this is best given by the IV route in a dose of 8 to 15 mg. The heart rate, blood pressure, and respiratory rate should be monitored during the IV administration of this drug, which has a peripheral vasodilating effect and decreases the patient's anxiety.

A rapidly acting diuretic such as furosemide can be administered; usually an initial dose of 40 to 80 mg given by the IV route slowly is adequate. The mechanism of action of furosemide in relieving pulmonary edema is related to an increase in systemic and pulmonary venous capacitance rather than to its diuretic effect.[3]

If the patient does not respond to these measures, intermittent positive pressure breathing can be utilized. This results in a decrease in venous return to the right side of the heart because of the increased intrathoracic pressure and also results in a shift of fluid from the alveolar spaces to the pulmonary capillaries because of an increase in intra-alveolar pressure.

A phlebotomy to remove 300 to 500 ml of blood may occasionally be required, providing the patient is not anemic. If bronchospasm is a prominent feature as manifested by wheezing, aminophylline can be given by the IV route slowly at a rate of 25 mg/min with a total dose of 250 mg. Digitalis preparations are not generally necessary in the initial treatment of acute pulmonary edema unless there is an associated supraventricular tachyarrhythmia such as atrial tachycardia, flutter, or fibrillation.

If appropriate monitoring capabilities are available to follow the pulmonary capillary wedge and systemic intra-arterial pressures, afterload-reducing agents such as nitroprusside may be utilized, especially if the patient is hypertensive or has mitral insufficiency. Precipitating factors should be sought and treated appropriately, including correction of dysrhythmias and control of infection.

## CARDIOGENIC SHOCK

■ **What is cardiogenic shock?**

Shock can be defined as a clinical state in which there is usually a marked decrease in the systemic arterial blood pressure associated with manifestations of diminished perfusion of the various organs. There are a number of causes of shock, including the following: (1) impairment of cardiac function, which produces cardiogenic shock; (2) decreased effective circulating blood volume, which produces hypovolemic shock; and (3) infection, which produces septic shock. The discussion in this section will be limited to cardiogenic shock.

■ **What are the clinical features of this condition?**

The patient may complain of marked weakness, shortness of breath, anorexia, nausea, and/or vomiting. Physical examination will reveal a sinus tachycardia or an inappropriate rhythm. The blood pressure will usually be low, with the systolic arterial pressure less than 80 mm Hg. The respiratory rate is usually increased. The skin is usually cool, clammy, and pale with peripheral cyanosis. The patient may be restless, lethargic, confused, or comatose. Cardiac examination will reveal findings related to the basic underlying cardiac disease. The abdomen may be distended with diminished or absent bowel sounds. The peripheral pulses will be markedly diminished in amplitude.

■ **What are the causes of cardiogenic shock?**

Cardiogenic shock results from marked impairment of left ventricular function. The most common cause is acute myocardial infarction. This may be the result of extensive damage to heart muscle (usually greater than 40% of left ventricular muscle mass)[4] or may result from perforation of the interventricular septum, papillary muscle dysfunction, or rupture of a papillary muscle. Other forms of cardiac disease can result in cardiogenic shock when the disease has progressed to a point at which there is marked impairment of left ventricular function. Even though a patient may have known cardiac disease, it is still important to exclude other causes of shock. Hypovolemia is not an infrequent cause of shock in cardiac patients. In addition, a dysrhythmia can result in shock in a patient with cardiac disease, and correction of the dysrhythmia can result in resolution of the shock state.

## ■ On what is the diagnosis based?

The presence of the shock state is usually apparent by the typical signs of cardiogenic shock as observed on clinical evaluation of the patient. The urine output will be noted to be low, less than 20 ml/hr. Hemodynamic measurements will reveal elevated left ventricular filling pressure and diminished cardiac output.

## ■ What is included in the management of a patient with this condition?

The cardiac rhythm should be evaluated. If there is a dysrhythmia that may be partly or wholly responsible for a low cardiac output, appropriate antiarrhythmic therapy should be instituted. In the case of a supraventricular tachyarrhythmia, direct-current cardioversion is preferred. In the case of a bradyarrhythmia, artificial cardiac pacing may be required. Venous blood should be obtained for electrolyte and serum enzyme determination. Arterial blood should be obtained for blood gas determination. Hypoxemia should be treated with $O_2$ and adequate ventilation. Acidosis should be treated with adequate ventilation and sodium bicarbonate. It may be necessary to assist the patient's breathing with a ventilator.

The urine output should be monitored; an indwelling catheter is usually necessary. Ideally, the left ventricular filling pressure, intra-arterial pressure, and cardiac output should be continuously monitored. Monitoring of central venous pressure alone will not provide adequate information to manage the patient in cardiogenic shock.[5]

Estimation of left ventricular filling pressure can be obtained by use of a Swan-Ganz flow-directed balloon-tipped catheter.[6] This catheter can be inserted relatively rapidly at the bedside with minimum risk and without the need for fluoroscopy. Either pulmonary artery pressure (with balloon deflated) or occluded pulmonary artery pressure (with balloon inflated) can be obtained. Multipurpose flow-directed balloon-tipped catheters are available that can be used not only for monitoring pulmonary artery pressure, but also for monitoring right atrial pressure, determining cardiac output by the thermodilution technique, obtaining intra-atrial and intraventricular electrograms, and performing artificial pacing.[7]

If the left ventricular filling pressure is low, that is, less than 15 mm Hg, IV fluids should be administered until an optimum filling pressure of 15 to 18 mm Hg is attained.[8] A significant number of patients in shock associated with acute myocardial infarction may be hypovolemic. These patients have a good prognosis when treated appropriately with fluid administration.[9]

If the left ventricular filling pressure is elevated as indicated by an elevated pulmonary artery diastolic or pulmonary capillary wedge pressure, afterload reduction has been found to be quite effective.[10] Initially sodium nitroprusside is infused by the IV route with careful monitoring of pulmonary capillary wedge and systemic intra-arterial pressures, as well as determination of cardiac output. The infusion rate of sodium nitroprusside is increased until the left ventricular filling pressure is in the optimum range, that is, between 15 to 18 mm Hg. At this level there is usually an increase in the cardiac output without significant decrease in the systemic arterial pressure and frequently an increase in arterial pressure.

If the intra-arterial pressure is very low at the onset, adrenergic agents such as dopamine or norepinephrine may be useful in elevating the blood pressure to levels that will provide adequate coronary and cerebral blood flow. It has been shown that digitalis is of little value in the management of cardiogenic shock secondary to acute myocardial infarction.[11] Isoproterenol, although it may initially result in improvement of cardiac output, may actually be responsible for further myocardial necrosis in the patient with an acute myocardial infarction.

Mechanical circulatory assistance by one of the various methods available,[12] such as intra-aortic balloon pumping, may be required if standard medical therapy is ineffective. If there is an acute mechanical problem, such as perforation of the interventricular septum or rupture of a papillary muscle, in association with acute myocardial infarction, early surgical intervention may be indicated.

## CARDIAC TAMPONADE

### ■ What is cardiac tamponade?

Cardiac tamponade is a condition resulting from the accumulation of fluid in the pericardial space with a resultant rise in the intrapericardial pressure, which then results in marked impairment of ventricular diastolic filling. The clinical syndrome is characterized by a rising venous pressure, a falling arterial pressure, features of a low cardiac output, and usually a quiet heart. The amount of fluid accumulating within the pericardial space necessary to result in tamponade depends on the rate at which the fluid accumulates. The accumulation of fluid in the pericardial space is called pericardial effusion, and a rapidly developing effusion of 200 to 300 ml may produce tamponade. On the other hand, if the effusion develops slowly, greater than 1000 ml of fluid may not produce the clinical syndrome of cardiac tamponade.

### ■ What are the clinical features of this condition?

This condition should be suspected in any patient who has prominent neck veins, decreasing systemic arterial blood pressure with a low pulse pressure, exaggerated respiratory variation in the arterial pulse, and low cardiac output.

The symptoms also include weakness, dyspnea, and orthopnea. The patient usually feels more comfortable sitting up and leaning forward, because this shifts the fluid anteriorly and inferiorly, relieving the pressure on the bronchi and lungs. The physical signs include (1) sinus tachycardia or possibly supraventricular tachycardia, (2) elevated venous pressure with distended neck veins, (3) decreased systemic arterial pressure with a low pulse pressure, (4) pulsus paradoxus, and (5) possibly diminished intensity of the heart sounds. Pulsus paradoxus is an exaggeration of the normal slight inspiratory decrease in the systemic arterial systolic blood pressure. In cardiac tamponade the examiner will note an obvious diminution in amplitude or disappearance of the systemic arterial pulse during inspiration. The magnitude of this change can be determined by taking the patient's blood pressure as follows: The blood pressure cuff is inflated and then slowly deflated until the level at which the Korotkoff sounds are first heard is reached. It will be noted that at this level Korotkoff sounds are not heard with every cardiac cycle and are noted only during expiration. The blood pressure cuff is further deflated until a level is reached where the Korotkoff sounds are heard during all cardiac cycles. This level is noted. The difference in the levels of blood pressure at which Korotkoff sounds are first heard but not with every cardiac cycle and at which Korotkoff sounds are heard during all cardiac cycles indicates the magnitude of the pulsus paradoxus or exaggeration of respiratory variation in the arterial pulse.

### ■ What are the ECG findings in cardiac tamponade?

Characteristically the ECG will reveal diminution in voltage, and electrical alternans may be noted. Electrical alternans is the alternate variation in amplitude of the QRS complex. Total electrical alternans implies alternation of the P, QRS, and T complexes and is virtually diagnostic of cardiac tamponade.

### ■ What information does the chest x-ray examination yield?

The chest x-ray film usually reveals an enlarged cardiac silhouette with the lung fields being clear.

### ■ What are the causes of cardiac tamponade?

The causes of cardiac tamponade include those conditions affecting the pericardium that can result in a pericardial effusion of sufficient magnitude to restrict ventricular diastolic filling. These conditions include (1) trauma, either direct or indirect; (2) neoplastic disease involving the pericardium, either primary or metastatic; (3) rupture of the heart or great vessels; (4) uremic pericarditis; (5) postmyocardial infarction syndrome; (6) postthoracotomy syndrome; (7) radiation pericarditis; (8) infections involving the pericardium; (9) anticoagulants administered in the presence of pericarditis; (10) idiopathic pericarditis; and (11) pericarditis secondary to connective tissue diseases.

### ■ How can the diagnosis be confirmed?

The safest and probably most reliable method is echocardiography. With this technique the presence of an effusion can be confirmed by noting a space between the epicardial and pericardial layers. The procedure can be done at the bedside without moving the patient, can be completed in a relatively short period of time, and is noninvasive. Other techniques that can be used to demonstrate the presence of a pericardial effusion include (1) radioisotope cardiac scanning, which involves the IV injection of a radioactive substance such as radioactive iodinated serum albumin and scanning over the heart to demonstrate the greater-than-normal distance between the cardiac blood pool (intracardiac chambers) and the boundaries of the cardiac silhouette noted on the chest x-ray film; (2) the obtaining of a chest x-ray film following the injection of carbon dioxide ($CO_2$) through a central venous catheter with the patient lying in the left lateral position to demonstrate an increased distance between the $CO_2$ gas bubble and the lung; and (3) angiocardiography, which involves the obtaining of x-ray films immediately following the injection of contrast material into the right atrium to demonstrate an increased distance between the boundaries of the cardiac silhouette and the contrast material.

### ■ What is the treatment for cardiac tamponade?

The immediate management of pericardial tamponade is to perform a pericardiocentesis, which involves the insertion of a long needle into the pericardial space in order to aspirate fluid. (I prefer to initially use the subxiphoid approach for this procedure.) The equipment necessary to perform this procedure includes the following: (1) an appropriately grounded electrocardiograph machine; (2) a skin preparation tray equipped with local anesthetic; (3) a pericardiocentesis tray, including an appropriate needle and sterile wire with alligator clips; (4) appropriate specimen containers; and (5) a defibrillator.

The patient is elevated to 45 degrees and the needle is inserted between the xiphisternum and left costal border at a 45-degree angle to the frontal and sagittal planes of the chest and abdomen. The needle is thus directed superiorly and toward the left shoulder. The position of the needle, as it is advanced, is monitored electrocardiographically by connecting the metal hub of the needle to the V lead of the ECG by means of a wire with alligator clips. The ECG is observed for the development of an injury current, that is, S-T segment elevation, which indicates that the needle is touching the epicardium. Generally when there is a large pericardial effusion, the operator will note a popping sensation as the pericardium is punctured, and fluid will be aspirated before the needle comes in contact with the epicardium. A 6-inch 20-gauge indwelling needle catheter is very convenient, since this allows for advancement of the catheter into the pericardial space and removal of the needle with advancement of the catheter once fluid is aspirated. Trauma to the heart by a sharp needle is thus avoided during the aspiration of fluid. It is generally best to remove as much fluid as possible and hopefully prevent the redevelopment of tamponade.

The fluid obtained should be appropriately analyzed, particularly if the underlying cause is not obvious. The gross appearance of the fluid should be noted, cell counts and protein determination should be obtained, cytologic examination should be performed, and the fluid should be sent for appropriate cultures. The underlying cause should be treated in order to prevent recurrence of effusion. If cardiac tamponade recurs, creation of a pericardial window or pericardiectomy may be necessary.

## ACUTE PULMONARY EMBOLISM

### ■ What is pulmonary embolism?

Pulmonary embolism is a condition in which a thrombus or portion of a thrombus migrates from one part of the body, usually from the lower extremities but occasionally from the pelvic veins, right atrium, or right ventricle, to a pulmonary artery, where occlusion of this vessel results. Pulmonary embolism can also result secondary to migration of fat, air, tumor, or vegetation.

### ■ What are the clinical features of this condition?

The patient usually complains of acute shortness of breath. In addition, retrosternal pressure pain similar to that seen in acute myocardial infarction may be present. Other symptoms include cough and wheezing. When pulmonary infarction has occurred, pleuritic-type chest pain may be present, and there may be associated hemoptysis. Additional symptoms include nausea, vomiting, and dizziness.

The physical findings include sinus tachycardia or possibly a supraventricular tachyarrhythmia, tachypnea, anxiety, and restlessness. Cyanosis is often present. If the pulmonary embolus involves a major pulmonary artery, right heart failure will be evident, with the presence of distended neck veins indicative of elevated jugular venous pressure, a left parasternal lift, third and/or fourth heart sounds of right-sided origin, and possibly wide splitting of the second heart sound. The pulmonic component of the second heart sound is usually not accentuated in acute pulmonary embolism, but it may be increased in intensity with recurrent pulmonary embolism.

When pulmonary infarction has occurred, examination of the lungs may reveal decreased excursion, dullness to percussion, a pleural friction rub, and rales over the involved area. If the embolus is massive, the patient will be hypotensive or may be in shock; the physical findings previously described for cardiogenic shock will then be apparent.

### ■ What are the ECG findings in acute pulmonary embolism?

The ECG may reveal sinus tachycardia or a supraventricular tachyarrhythmia, T wave inversion in the right precordial leads, an $S_1Q_3$ pattern, a QRS axis shift to the right, right bundle branch block, tall, peaked P waves in leads II, III, and $aV_F$, and ST-T abnormalities compatible with subendocardial ischemia.

### ■ What are the chest x-ray findings?

The chest x-ray film frequently does not reveal any abnormalities. The abnormalities that may be seen include a decrease in the vascular markings over the involved portion of the lung, elevation of the diaphragm on the affected side, pulmonary infiltration, and pleural effusion.

### ■ What are the predisposing factors to pulmonary embolism?

Pulmonary embolism is seen most often in patients who have been confined to bed for a prolonged period of time. Conditions with which pulmonary embolism most frequently occurs include acute myocardial infarction, chronic congestive heart failure, stroke, postsurgery complications, fractures of the lower extremity, particularly the hip, and malignancy. Pulmonary embolism can also occur following sitting for a prolonged period of time in a cramped position.

■ **On what basis can the diagnosis be established?**

Pulmonary embolism should be suspected when the clinical features described previously are noted. Blood gas analysis will almost always reveal an arterial $P_{O_2}$ of less than 80 mm. The serum lactic dehydrogenase (LDH) enzyme level is frequently elevated. A lung scan will reveal decreased or absent perfusion in the involved area.[13] The concentration of fibrin split products in the blood is frequently increased.[14]

However, the most definitive method for confirming the diagnosis of pulmonary embolism is pulmonary angiography. This involves right heart catheterization and the injection of contrast material into the main pulmonary artery. In the presence of pulmonary embolism the contrast material will be noted to come to a dead end at the site of obstruction, or filling defects may be noted in the involved vessels.

■ **What is the treatment for acute pulmonary embolism?**

Treatment is directed at prevention of further embolization. This is achieved by administering anticoagulant medications, preferably heparin, to the patient. Heparin can be administered as a continuous infusion following an initial loading dose or can be given by IV push doses at regular intervals. If there is a minor embolism without hypotension or shock, 7500 to 10,000 units should be administered every 4 to 6 hours for 7 days. A Lee-White clotting time or partial thromboplastin time should be determined 1 hour prior to the next anticipated dose. If the patient's condition is stable, the changeover to an oral anticoagulant such as warfarin can begin on the fifth day.

If the embolism is massive with hypotension and shock, initially 12,000 to 15,000 units should be administered by the IV route, and then 10,000 to 15,000 units should be given by IV administration every 4 hours until the patient's condition is stable. The dose can then be decreased to 7500 to 10,000 units given by the IV route every 4 to 6 hours for 7 to 10 days.[15] Appropriate analgesia should be administered for pain.

If the patient is hypotensive or in cardiogenic shock, appropriate therapy is indicated, including the use of digitalis, vasopressors, and administration of $O_2$. Fibrinolytic therapy utilizing urokinase has been evaluated for the treatment of acute pulmonary embolism, but the results have not warranted its general use.

On rare occasions, if the patient continues to deteriorate despite adequate medical management, a pulmonary embolectomy may have to be performed. If the patient is having recurrent pulmonary emboli despite adequate heparinization or if anticoagulation is contraindicated, vena cava interruption should be performed. This can either be done by ligation or plication of the inferior vena cava just below the renal veins or through the use of an umbrella device positioned in the inferior vena cava transvenously.

■ **What precautions should be taken in the management of a patient with this condition?**

The patient should be observed for possible signs of hemorrhage, including retroperitoneal hemorrhage, which may cause the patient to complain of back pain. If this develops, further heparin administration should be withheld until an assessment of the situation can be made. Other sites of bleeding can include the gastrointestinal and the genitourinary tracts. The development of pulmonary embolism may be prevented by early ambulation, elevation of the legs in order to prevent venous stasis, and use of elastic stockings or bandages in those patients who are at risk for developing pulmonary embolism. Intramuscular injections should be avoided or given with caution to the patient who is taking anticoagulant medication.

## INFECTIVE ENDOCARDITIS

■ **What is infective endocarditis?**

Infective endocarditis is an inflammatory alteration of the inner lining of the heart. This inflammatory process most frequently involves the valvular endocardium. This inflammation can be secondary to infectious and noninfectious processes. The latter includes rheumatic endocarditis and the endocarditis associated with systemic lupus erythematosus. The term "infective endocarditis" implies that a microorganism is the cause of the inflammation, with bacteria most frequently being responsible for this condition. Previously infective endocarditis was subdivided into acute and subacute bacterial endocarditis. However, the term "infective endocarditis" is now preferred.

### ■ What are the clinical features?

The clinical features may be secondary to (1) the general effects of the infection, (2) emboli, and (3) the effects of the infection on the heart. The general symptoms include fever, chills, diaphoresis, headache, weakness, easy fatigability, anorexia, and weight loss. The embolic manifestations include petechiae involving the skin and conjunctiva. In addition, vertical hemorrhagic streaks may be noted in the skin underneath the nails. These are referred to as splinter hemorrhages and are not specific for infective endocarditis, being seen under other circumstances, particularly following trauma to the nail bed. Hematuria, usually microscopic but occasionally gross, may be noted, and the spleen is frequently enlarged. Symptoms resembling those of meningitis or encephalitis may occur, and clubbing of the fingers occurs frequently.

If there is embolization involving a large vessel to an extremity, there may be sudden pain, loss of function, coldness, pallor, or cyanosis in that extremity. Joint pains are frequently seen. Examination of the heart may reveal a murmur not previously present or changing characteristics of a murmur. Manifestations of heart failure may develop secondary to (1) insufficiency of a valve as a result of destruction from the infective process, (2) myocarditis, or (3) myocardial infarction as a result of coronary embolization.

### ■ What causes infective endocarditis?

Infective endocarditis can result from a number of bacterial or fungal infections involving the heart. Some of the more commonly found bacteria include *Streptococcus viridans, Staphylococcus aureus,* microaerophilic streptococcus, enterococcus, $\beta$-hemolytic streptococcus, and nonhemolytic streptococcus. Fungal endocarditis is relatively infrequent, with *Candida* being most commonly found.[16] Patients with preexisting cardiac valvular disease or shunts such as a ventricular septal defect and patent ductus arteriosus are predisposed to the development of endocarditis. In addition, patients with intracardiac prostheses, including prosthetic heart valves, are also predisposed.

### ■ On what is the diagnosis based?

The diagnosis is based on obtaining positive blood cultures. Therefore whenever a diagnosis of infective endocarditis is suspected, blood cultures should be obtained. Generally no more than five or six sets are necessary to establish the diagnosis. Negative blood cultures may occur in documented cases of endocarditis. This generally results from improper technique either in obtaining or in culturing the blood or from absence of the microorganisms in the blood at the moment of collecting the sample, possibly as a result of the patient previously receiving antibiotics.

### ■ What is the treatment of infective endocarditis?

The treatment depends on the establishment of an etiologic diagnosis from cultures of the blood with the administration of an antibiotic or antibiotics to which the organism is sensitive. Generally the antibiotic should be administered parenterally for a 4- to 6-week period. Orally administered antibiotics may be irregularly absorbed, particularly in individuals who are quite ill. Repeat blood cultures should be obtained, particularly if the patient is not improving. In order to determine the effectiveness of the antibiotic, it is often very helpful to measure the antibacterial activity of the patient's serum against the organism recovered from the blood.[17] It may be necessary to perform cardiac surgery if the patient's condition is deteriorating despite adequate medical therapy. Surgery has been performed primarily for heart failure but has also been done to control the infection.

**■ What circumstances predispose an individual to infective endocarditis?**

In those individuals who have cardiac deformities such as abnormalities of heart valves, the following circumstances may result in a bacteremia that will then result in endocarditis: (1) dental procedures, (2) intestinal procedures, (3) urologic instrumentation, (4) vaginal procedures, (5) boils, and (6) use of unsterile equipment by narcotic addicts.

**■ What can be done to prevent the development of this condition?**

Those patients who have congenital or acquired cardiac lesions should receive appropriate antibiotic prophylaxis immediately prior to and for 12 to 24 hours following any unsterile surgical procedure. This includes dental work, urologic instrumentation, vaginal or intestinal procedures, and bronchoscopy.

## DYSRHYTHMIAS

**■ What are some of the prerequisites in managing cardiac dysrhythmias?**

It is important that the dysrhythmia be identified precisely, since appropriate treatment depends on establishment of the proper diagnosis. There should be some knowledge of the natural history of the dysrhythmia. For example, if a patient has been in atrial fibrillation for a number of years, there is little point in attempting to revert the rhythm to a sinus rhythm. There should be some understanding of the mechanism of the dysrhythmia, since this will aid in selecting appropriate drugs. The critical care team should (1) have a reasonable understanding of the pharmacology of the antiarrhythmic drugs, (2) know whether intervention will beneficially alter the course, and (3) determine whether therapy has a reasonable probability of success without prohibitive side effects.

**■ What are the causes of dysrhythmias in the critical care unit?**

There are both cardiac and noncardiac causes for dysrhythmias. The noncardiac causes include the following: (1) electrolyte imbalance, that is, hypokalemia or hyperkalemia or, much less often, hypocalcemia or hypercalcemia; (2) acid-base imbalance, that is, metabolic or respiratory acidosis or metabolic or respiratory alkalosis; (3) hypoxemia; and (4) digitalis toxicity, which may be related to excessive dosage, impaired renal excretion, or enhanced sensitivity secondary to electrolyte imbalance (hypokalemia, hypercalcemia, or hypomagnesemia), acid-base imbalance (alkalosis or acidosis), or hypoxemia. Cardiac causes of dysrhythmias include congestive heart failure, acute myocardial infarction, pulmonary embolism, and pericarditis. It is important that the critical care team review the clinical setting in which the dysrhythmia is occurring in order to correct any predisposing factors. Not infrequently by resolution of the aforementioned predisposing factors, the use of antiarrhythmic drugs can be avoided.

**■ When is it necessary to treat dysrhythmias?**

Dysrhythmias should be treated when they are responsible for hemodynamic deterioration or when they may predispose to a more serious dysrhythmia. If the patient is essentially asymptomatic and hemodynamically stable, and the dysrhythmia is not known to predispose to more serious dysrhythmias, it is not essential that specific antiarrhythmic drug therapy be instituted.

**■ Are all dysrhythmias treated with antiarrhythmic drugs?**

Since there are a number of factors that can predispose to the development of dysrhythmias, it is important that these factors be treated. Serum electrolyte determinations should be made, and if the patient is hypokalemic, potassium should be administered either orally or by IV infusion. If the patient is hyperkalemic, further potassium administration should be withheld and potassium-retaining diuretics should be avoided. Exchange resins such as sodium polystyrene (Kayexalate) that remove potassium from the gastrointestinal tract may be administered either orally or by rectal enema.

In situations where there is acute or chronic renal failure, either peritoneal or hemodialysis may be needed in order to remove potassium from the body. In acute situations where it is important to rapidly lower the serum potassium, the IV administration of sodium bicarbonate is preferred. An IV infusion of glucose and insulin will also lower the serum potassium.

Calcium can also be administered by the IV route to counteract the effects of hyperkalemia on the heart. However, if the patient is taking digitalis, calcium should be administered cautiously.

Arterial blood gas determinations should be obtained. If the patient is hypoxemic, oxygen should be administered and adequate ventilation should be ensured. Acidosis should be corrected by appropriate ventilation if it is respiratory in origin and by administration of sodium bicarbonate for metabolic acidosis.

If digitalis toxicity is suspected, further administration of digitalis should be discontinued. Determination of blood levels of the digitalis preparation may be very helpful in determining the presence of digitalis toxicity. In addition to withholding digitalis, those factors that may predispose to digitalis toxicity should be treated. Patients with bradyarrhythmias, particularly AV block, will frequently require artificial cardiac pacing.

### ■ What are the major uses of antiarrhythmic drugs?

Drugs used to treat dysrhythmias include the digitalis preparations, quinidine, procainamide, propranolol, diphenylhydantoin, lidocaine, atropine, and isoproterenol. Digitalis preparations are most effective in the treatment of supraventricular tachyarrhythmias. The administration of digitalis will slow the ventricular rate in the presence of atrial fibrillation or atrial flutter and may revert atrial tachycardia to a normal sinus rhythm. Quinidine and procainamide are effective against both supraventricular and ventricular dysrhythmias. Propranolol is most effective in the treatment of digitalis-induced dysrhythmias, but it can also be used in the treatment of supraventricular tachyarrhythmias and premature ventricular complexes.

Diphenylhydantoin is most effective in the treatment of digitalis-induced dysrhythmias, but it can also be used to treat nondigitalis-related ventricular dysrhythmias. Lidocaine is most effective in the treatment of ventricular dysrhythmias and has little effectiveness in the management of atrial dysrhythmias. Atropine is the agent that should be initially used in the treatment of sinus bradycardia. If atropine is ineffective, isoproterenol may be infused in small doses. Isoproterenol may also be given to increase the ventricular rate in a patient with advanced AV block until a pacing catheter can be inserted.

It is important that antiarrhythmic drugs be administered in proper doses and at appropriate intervals. If there is any question relative to whether the patient is receiving adequate amounts of a given drug or may have manifestations of drug toxicity, blood levels should be determined.[18]

## CHEST PAIN

### ■ What are some of the causes of chest pain?

Chest pain may be secondary to disease involving either thoracic or extrathoracic structures. The origins of the thoracic causes of chest pain include the following: (1) cardiac, resulting from a discrepancy between myocardial oxygen supply and demand and manifested as angina pectoris, acute coronary insufficiency, myocardial infarction, or secondary to pericarditis; (2) pulmonary, secondary to pulmonary embolism, pulmonary infarction, pneumothorax, pneumonia, or pleuritis; (3) esophageal, secondary to esophagitis, cardiospasm, esophageal neoplasm, esophageal rupture, or diffuse esophageal spasm; (4) aortic, as a result of dissection; (5) mediastinal, as a result of mediastinitis; or (6) chest wall, including manifestations of thoracic spine disease, fractured rib, intercostal neuritis, myositis, costochondritis, and herpes zoster. Pain may be referred to the chest as a result of diseases involving extrathoracic structures, including the following: (1) cervical spine disease, (2) peptic ulcer, (3) cholecystitis, (4) pancreatitis, or (5) splenic flexure syndrome. There may be no organic disease to account for the pain, and it may then be of psychogenic origin secondary to neurocirculatory asthenia and/or hyperventilation.

**■ How can the various causes of chest pain be differentiated?**

It is important to characterize the chest pain by asking the patient the following questions: (1) Where is the pain located or where was it first noted? (2) Where does the pain radiate? (3) What is the character of the pain, that is, is it dull, sharp, pressurelike, constricting, burning, etc.? (4) Did the pain reach its maximum intensity suddenly or gradually? (5) Does anything relieve the pain? (6) Does anything aggravate the pain? (7) Is the pain persistent or is it intermittent? (8) How long did the pain last? (9) Has similar pain ever been present? (10) Are there any symptoms associated with the pain, including shortness of breath, diaphoresis, weakness, palpitations, light-headedness, fever, cough, paresthesias in the extremities, anorexia, nausea, or vomiting? It is also important to note the associated physical and laboratory findings.

**■ Which of the features just mentioned are characteristic of the various causes of chest pain?**

*Cardiac pain*

***Angina pectoris.*** The pain is usually *located* retrosternally with frequent *radiation* into the neck and left arm. The pain is usually *precipitated* by exertion, eating, or emotional upset and is *relieved* by rest and/or nitroglycerin; the pain does not usually *last* for more than a few minutes.

***Acute coronary insufficiency.*** The pain is similar to that of angina pectoris in location and radiation and may be *precipitated* by exertion, eating, or emotional upset or may occur at rest. It is *not* immediately *relieved* by nitroglycerin or rest and may *last* for an hour or longer. It must thus be distinguished from the pain of acute myocardial infarction.

***Acute myocardial infarction.*** The pain is usually retrosternal in *location* and frequently *radiates* to the neck and/or left arm or both arms. The pain is usually pressurelike or constricting in *character* and is usually more severe than the pain of angina pectoris. The pain is not necessarily *precipitated* by the patient's activity, and it is *not relieved* by nitroglycerin or rest. There may be *associated* weakness, shortness of breath, diaphoresis, nausea, and light-headedness. Serum cardiac enzyme determinations and ECG's are necessary to distinguish the pain of acute coronary insufficiency from that of acute myocardial infarction.

***Pericarditis.*** The pain is usually *not precipitated* by exertion, is usually sharp in *character,* is *located* retrosternally or over the left anterior chest, and may *radiate* to the neck and shoulders. The pain is usually *relieved* by sitting up and becomes more intense when lying in the supine position. The pain may be *aggravated* by inspiration, coughing, or swallowing. Fever may be *associated* with the pain. *Physical examination* usually reveals a pericardial friction rub.

*Pulmonary pain*

***Pulmonary embolism.*** The pain of a large pulmonary embolus may be similar in *location* and *character* to that associated with coronary insufficiency. There is usually *associated* weakness and shortness of breath. *Physical examination* will reveal findings of right heart failure, including prominence of the jugular veins, enlarged right ventricle, and third and/or fourth heart sounds of right-sided origin.

***Pulmonary infarction.*** The pain of pulmonary infarction is usually *located* laterally over the chest wall. It is sharp in *character* and is *aggravated* by inspiration or coughing. There may be *associated* fever and hemoptysis. *Physical examination* may reveal dullness to percussion, decreased breath sounds, and a pleural friction rub over the involved area.

***Pneumothorax.*** The pain is usually sharp in *character,* reaches its *maximum intensity* at the onset, and is usually *associated* with shortness of breath. *Physical examination* will reveal increased resonance to percussion and diminished breath sounds over the involved area. If there is a large pneumothorax, the patient will appear very apprehensive, and there will be an associated tachycardia.

***Pneumonia.*** The pain is usually *located* laterally over the chest wall, is sharp in *character,* is *aggravated* by inspiration or coughing, and may be *associated* with fever and a productive cough. *Physical examination* may reveal dullness to percussion and rales over the involved area.

***Pleuritis.*** The pain is usually *located* laterally over the chest wall, is sharp in *character,* and is *aggravated* by inspiration and coughing. On *physical examination* a pleural friction rub may be heard, and if there is an associated pleural effusion, there may be dullness and decreased breath sounds over the involved area.

### *Esophageal pain*

***Esophagitis.*** The pain is usually *located* over the lower retrosternal region and may *radiate* up into the throat. The pain is usually described as burning in *character,* is usually *aggravated* by lying in a supine position, and is *relieved* by sitting up and/or ingesting antacids. There may be *associated* regurgitation of gastric contents into the mouth and/or a peculiar taste.

### *Aortic pain*

***Dissecting aneurysm.*** The location of the pain depends on the origin of the dissection. If the dessection originates in the ascending aorta (type I or II), the pain is usually located retrosternally. If the dissection originates in the descending aorta (type III), the pain is usually located in the back over the interscapular region. Recurrences of pain may be *located* in the back or abdomen. The pain generally reaches its *maximum intensity* at the onset and may be sharp or tearing in *character. Physical examination* may reveal unequal or absent pulses in the extremities or neck. *Chest x-ray films* may reveal widening of the mediastinum. On *physical examination* an early diastolic murmur of aortic insufficiency that was not previously present may be heard.

### *Chest wall pain*

***Thoracic spine disease.*** The pain may be *located* in the back at the involved vertebral level and *radiate* around the chest. It may be *aggravated* by change in position. *Physical examination* will reveal tenderness over the involved vertebrae.

***Fractured rib.*** The pain is *located* in the area of the fracture, is usually sharp in *character,* and is *aggravated* by inspiration. *Physical examination* will reveal tenderness over the involved area and crepitation may be noted on auscultation.

***Myositis.*** The pain may occur following physical activity involving the affected muscle. The pain is *localized* over the involved muscle and is *aggravated* by movement.

***Costochondritis (Tietze's syndrome).*** The pain is *localized* over the involved costochondral junction. The second through fourth costochondral junctions are most commonly involved. *Physical examination* will reveal exquisite tenderness over the involved costochondral junction.

***Herpes zoster.*** The pain is *located* at the involved dermatomic level. It is usually sharp or burning in *character.* The typical skin lesions will subsequently appear.

### *Chest pain not originating from the thorax—referred pain*

***Cervical spine disease.*** The pain is usually *aggravated* by movement of the head and neck. *Physical examination* may reveal localized tenderness over the involved vertebrae or disc level and pain and/or limitation of neck motion.

***Disease involving abdominal organs.*** The pain may occur with the symptoms usually seen in these disease processes, and *physical examination* will usually reveal tenderness over the involved organ.

### *Psychogenic causes*

If the history and physical examination fail to reveal any apparent organic cause of the chest pain, nonorganic causes should be considered.

***Hyperventilation syndrome.*** The pain is usually periapical in *location,* and the patient is usually somewhat nondescript about its *character*. The pain is generally not *precipitated* by exertion. The patient frequently notes *associated symptoms* including lightheadedness, shortness of breath, paresthesias in the hands and possibly around the mouth, dryness of the mouth, and palpitations.

## REFERENCES

1. Standards for cardiopulmonary resuscitation (CPR) and emergency cardiac care (ECC), J.A.M.A. **227**(suppl.):833-868, 1974.
2. McHugh, T. J., Forrester, J. S., Adler, L., Zion, D., and Swan, H. J. C.: Pulmonary vascular congestion in acute myocardial infarction: hemodynamic and radiologic correlations, Ann. Intern. Med. **76**:29-33, 1972.
3. Dikshit, K., Vyden, J. K., Forrester, J. S., Chatterjee, K., Prakash, R., and Swan, H. J. C.: Renal and extrarenal hemodynamic effects of furosemide in congestive heart failure after acute myocardial infarction, N. Engl. J. Med. **288**:1087-1090, 1973.
4. Page, D. L., Caulfield, J. B., Kastor, J. A., DeSanctis, R. W., and Sanders, C. A.: Myocardial changes associated with cardiogenic shock, N. Engl. J. Med. **285**:133, 1971.
5. Forrester, J. S., Diamond, G., McHugh, T. J., and Swan, H. J. C.: Filling pressures in the right and left sides of the heart in acute myocardial infarction. A reappraisal of central venous pressure monitoring, N. Engl. J. Med. **285**:190-193, 1971.
6. Swan, H. J. C., Ganz, W., Forrester, J., Marcus, H., Diamond, G., and Chonette, D.: Catheterization of the heart in man with use of a flow-directed balloon-tipped catheter, N. Engl. J. Med. **283**:447-451, 1970.
7. Swan, H. J. C., and Ganz, W.: Use of balloon flotation catheters in critically ill patients, Surg. Clin. North Am. **55**:501, 1975.
8. Crexells, C., Chatterjee, K., Forrester, J. S., Dikshit, K., and Swan, H. J. C.: Optimum level of filling pressure in the left side of the heart in acute myocardial infarction, N. Engl. J. Med. **289**:1263-1266, 1973.
9. Allen, H. N., Danzig, R., and Swan, H. J. C.: Incidence and significance of relative hypovolemia as a cause of shock associated with acute myocardial infarction, Circulation **36**:II-50, 1967.
10. Chatterjee, K., and Swan, H. J. C.: Vasodilator therapy in acute myocardial infarction, Mod. Concepts Cardiovasc. Dis. **43**: 119-124, 1974.
11. Bezdek, W., Forrester, J., Chatterjee, K., Ganz, W., Parmley, W., and Swan, H. J. C.: Myocardial metabolic effect of ouabain in acute myocardial infarction, Circulation **46**: II-113, 1972.
12. Resnekov, L.: Mechanical assistance for the failing heart, Mod. Concepts Cardiovasc. Dis. **43**:81-85, 1974.
13. Szucs, M. M., Brooks, H. L., Grossman, W., Banas, J. S., Meister, S. G., Dexter, L., and Dalen, J. E.: Diagnostic sensitivity of laboratory findings in acute pulmonary embolism, Ann. Intern. Med. **74**:161-166, 1971.
14. Rickman, F. D., Handin, R., Howe, J. P., Alpert, J. S., Dexter, L., and Dalen, J. E.: Fibrin split products in acute pulmonary embolism, Ann. Intern. Med. **79**:664-668, 1973.
15. Crane, C.: The treatment of pulmonary embolism. In Dalen, J. E., editor: Pulmonary embolism, New York, 1973, Medcom Press.
16. Weinstein, L., and Rubin, R. H.: Infective endocarditis—1973, Prog. Cardiovasc. Dis. **16**:239-274, 1973.
17. Weinstein, L., and Schlesinger, J.: Treatment of infective endocarditis—1973, Prog. Cardiovasc. Dis. **16**:275-302, 1973.
18. Atkinson, A. J.: Clinical use of blood levels of cardiac drugs, Mod. Concepts Cardiovasc. Dis. **42**:1-4, 1973.

*chapter 10*

# Preoperative care of the adult cardiac surgical patient

ROBERT A. STEEDMAN

It was not unusual in the mid-1950's to read medical publications relating to the cardiac surgical patient and to note that the mortalities occurring subsequent to this surgery centered around the fiftieth percentile. Now, 20 years later, large university centers and community hospital cardiac teams are striving in many areas of cardiac surgery to decrease the mortality rate below 1%.

Intraoperative technical advances and the refinements of surgical skills have aided markedly in decreasing mortality in this group of patients. However, the progressive sophistication and medical regimentation of the preoperative, operative, and postoperative care teams have played a major role in the rapid *decline* of *mortality* and *morbidity*. This team sophistication entails the continual and progressive education of all members as well as the concentration toward even the minute practical details that are so often of critical significance. This chapter will deal with these minute details of critical care and is intended as a review for all members of the critical care team.

## INDICATIONS FOR SURGERY

### ■ Which conditions generally require cardiac surgery in adults?

*Congenital defects*

The majority of significant cardiac birth defects require surgery during infancy or childhood as a critical necessity for the prevention of complications. However, some of these disorders are undiagnosed for one reason or another until early or occasionally even late adult life. Surgery for congenital defects is usually undertaken early in life to prevent the development of endocarditis, reversed shunting, irreversible pulmonary hypertension, cardiac decompensation, peripheral embolic phenomena, or even cerebrovascular accidents. Examples of the congenital defects requiring prompt surgery include *patent ductus arteriosus, coarctation of the aorta, ventricular septal defects, atrial septal defects* (with or without partial anomalies of the pulmonary venous return), *aortic stenosis,* varying types of *pulmonary artery stenosis, coronary artery anomalies,* and various *anomalies of the aortic arch.*

In some institutions the mere presence of certain congenital cardiac defects indicates surgical correction; these defects include *patent ductus arteriosus, atrial* and *ventricular septal defects, coarctation of the aorta, anomalies of venous return,* and other miscellaneous anomalies.

Contraindications to the performance of surgery on the adult patient with cardiac anomalies include the presence of irreversible pulmonary hypertension and right-to-left shunting, especially when the patient has polycythemia or is cyanotic. Simple closure alone of certain defects or shunts should not be performed when these anomalies are compensating for defects in which the pulmonary blood flow is decreased, such as in tricuspid atresia, tetralogy of Fallot, and pulmonary atresia. In adult life certain other associated disease processes not infrequently contraindicate surgical intervention. The ultimate decision as to which individuals should or should not undergo surgery for congenital lesions is based on the final analysis of each individual case.

### *Acquired valvular defects*

The group of acquired valvular defects includes mitral, aortic, and tricuspid valve stenosis and/or insufficiency, most commonly resulting from rheumtaic endocarditis. Acquired pulmonary valvular stenosis and insufficiency caused by rheumatic endocarditis occasionally requires surgical treatment. Recently in the literature numerous cases of *Pseudomonas* endocarditis of the pulmonary valve have been reported to occur in the addict using IV drugs; this defect eventually requires surgery.

### *Adhesive pericarditis or calcification of the pericardium with pericardial constriction*

These cases can occur after inflammatory pericarditis or traumatic hemopericardium and frequently require extensive pericardiectomy.

### *Conditions developing from coronary artery disease*

These indications are becoming more standardized; however, there are still many diversified opinions as to the specific indications for surgical intervention. Cases in which there is little question as to the need for surgery include patients with crescendo angina or angina uncontrollable by medications associated with a major obstructive lesion in the left coronary artery system as proved by catheterization. Other indications include intractable angina in any patient with severe obstruction in multiple vessels, repeated myocardial infarctions, refractory ventricular irritability, ventricular aneurysms with congestive failure or unstable arrhythmias, postinfarction ruptured chorda tendineae and progressive refractory failure, and postinfarction intractable cardiogenic shock. Much controversy centers today around the patient in the younger age group who has suffered a *single* myocardial infarction or who has *controllable angina* with a flow-limiting stenotic lesion in one of the major coronary arteries. The commercial airline pilot or executive presents an even greater problem. Any such patient is a candidate for a cardiac workup, and if a major block (70% or greater) is demonstrated by arteriography in the left main or left anterior descending coronary artery proximal to the first perforating branch, coronary bypass surgery should be performed.

### *Traumatic cardiac lesions*

Depending on the location of the cardiac surgical center, cardiac injuries from knife wounds, bullet wounds, or blunt chest trauma account for a respectable volume of injuries leading to surgery. The majority of the stab wounds of the heart require intervention for cardiac tamponade and hemorrhage and involve simple closure of the chamber lacerations. Occasionally coronary artery bypass to a transected or partially transected coronary artery is also necessary.

Blunt chest trauma with rupture of one of the four major chambers of the heart usually causes immediate death; however, with better paramedic facilities and faster cardiac surgical team efforts, it is possible to institute surgical therapy and to repair the ruptured cardiac chamber. Rupture of the various heart valves and chorda tendineae and/or papillary muscles can now be successfully repaired.

Probably the most common of the vascular blunt trauma injuries requiring surgery is *traumatic dissection of the aorta.* The unquestionable indications for surgery in these injuries include the presence of cardiac tamponade, refractory failure, or cardiac shock (refractory); however, in most situations the diagnosis itself is an indication for surgery.

## PREPARATIONS FOR SURGERY

■ **What methods are used to emotionally and psychologically prepare the patient and the family?**

The patient should develop confidence in the cardiac surgical team; this can be done in several ways. Usually the patient has been referred by a physician who knows the capabilities of the cardiac team, and this knowledge should reassure the patient. In addition, the patient has usually met someone in the community who has had a similar surgical procedure. Frequently the patient hears encouraging comments from the nursing staff as to the results of the operating team.

All of the foregoing situations are important and beneficial. However, direct exposure to a patient who has had a similar operation is one of the most satisfactory methods of decreasing the patient's anxiety or apprehension. A patient who has undergone the surgery 3 to 5 days previously is often pleased to discuss the surgery with the surgical candidate.

A member of the *Mended Hearts Association* should be invited to meet the patient and family during the preoperative period. The Mended Hearts Association is composed of county, state, and national chapters of individuals who have previously undergone cardiac surgery. The organization was formed explicitly for the purpose of providing service to individuals who are about to undergo similar operations. The group's function is to help one another after surgery or to help any patient who might have postoperative financial, emotional, or even medical difficulties. One or more representatives of the organization should be invited to meet with the patient, at which time the patient may seek answers to questions related to the coming surgery. All members of the association have been schooled in the techniques of visitation and are careful not to increase the patient's apprehension by the visit.

It is recommended that the operating surgeon and/or other members of the critical care team meet preoperatively with the patient and the family to explain the procedure and to answer any questions. In addition, nursing members of the *cardiac intensive care unit* should meet the patient prior to surgery and conduct a tour of the critical care unit. The patient should be acquainted with the various monitoring devices, endotracheal intubation, and positive breathing equipment and techniques. A detailed explanation relative to the multiple procedures necessary during the coming stay in the unit should be provided.

The anesthesiologist should meet with the patient, usually the night before surgery, to reemphasize certain procedures such as use of IV lines and the probable use of endotracheal respiratory assistance postoperatively.

A valuable adjunct to the cardiac surgery team effort is the incorporation of a liaison practitioner or nurse who would be available at any time to answer questions from the patient or the family. This person should have completed an apprenticeship through the preoperative, operative, and postoperative phases and would be expected to make multiple daily pre- and postoperative visits. This clinician should attend a portion of the cardiac surgery and should serve as a valuable communication link between the operating room and the waiting family and as a major communication vector between the operating surgeon and the hospital critical care unit staff during the postoperative period.

All of the preceding modes of introducing the patient to the surgical procedure have produced marked beneficial insight in our patients undergoing preparation for surgery. However, in recent years there has been an increasing tendency to overinform the interested public with regard to cardiac surgery. This has included the presentation on television of actual operating room visualizations of cardiac surgeries in progress; these have been detailed to the point of even showing near-catastrophic occurrences in surgery such as bleeding problems, delayed defibrillation in fibrillated hearts, and other complications. This public participation, so to speak, has created great apprehension, especially among patients who visualize television documentary dramas immediately prior to their own surgery. In attempting to ease the patient's apprehension by providing information about the surgical procedure, it is possible that the patient is becoming too deeply involved in a situation for which he is unprepared.

### ■ What type of room is ideal for the intended cardiac surgical patient?

The patient probably understands his own personality best; therefore if he specifically desires a private room and it is possible, such accommodations should be provided. It is generally better for patients to be in a semiprivate room with a relatively well room partner, preferably not a patient undergoing surgery performed by the same surgeon. Short-term exposure to patients with similar doctors is good, but long-term exposure is not always advantageous.

Selection of the patient's room is of extreme importance and should be considered carefully by the staff. For example, placing a smoking patient with a cardiac surgical candidate is a poor selection; an extremely hyperactive or uncooperative patient is a poor room companion; a patient who has an incurable disease or a condition with a poor general outlook is also a poor companion. It is extremely important to obtain a room companion for the cardiac surgical patient who will allow plenty of rest, not cause undue anxiety, and not be critical of the operating team or the hospital.

### ■ What medications should be used for preoperative showers and how often should they be used?

Many hospitals still utilize hexachlorophene solutions (pHisoHex) for the preoperative showers. However, because of its wide use in commercial preparations, proof that *Pseudomonas* can grow on the periphery of hexachlorophene containers, desensitization of many bacteria to this preparation, and reports of allergic reactions in infants, we now use preparations of povidone-iodine (Betadine).*

Patients are usually admitted 3 days before surgery and are given a Betadine shower at least once daily, including the morning of surgery.

If the patient has been scheduled for cardiac surgery prior to being discharged after catheterization, an attempt should be made to administer at least two preoperative showers.

If the patient has recently undergone cardiac catheterization or any other surgical procedure, local scrubbing of the anticipated surgical areas are utilized instead of full-body showers.

### ■ What diets are recommended for the patient admitted for cardiac surgery?

If the patient has been admitted for myocardial revascularization procedures such as aorto-coronary-saphenous vein or internal mammary artery bypass and has not had congestive failure or diet restrictions for other conditions such as diabetes or gouty arthritis, a patient-select regular diet is recommended. The food is more palatable, nutrition is maintained during the period of expected apprehension, and for the short period of 2 to 3 days no complications should develop.

If the patient was admitted for valvular surgery, has received digitalis preparations and diuretics, and has been maintained on a low salt diet, then a similar or even more stringent diet should be continued until surgery. This patient will not be disturbed at this restriction because this is probably similar to the preadmission diet.

Overweight patients should be allowed to select their diet, as they probably have been on a weight control regimen for a period of time prior to the operation unless the surgery is urgent; even then the 2 or 3 days prior to surgery will not add any more hazard in contrast to the mental anguish and apprehension produced by calorie restriction.

### ■ How often should the patient be weighed preoperatively?

It is our policy to weigh the patient daily, both on the standing and bed scales. This gives a correlation between the two scales and introduces the patient to bed-scale weighing, which will be the method of weighing in the immediate postoperative period. This is necessary in routine postoperative cases and especially for patients who are undergoing rapid diuresis or "drying out."

---

*Occasional blister formation has occurred when tape is placed over Betadine preparation solutions that were not washed off prior to the application of dressings.

### ■ Should respiratory therapy be utilized routinely, even for the patient who does not have pulmonary disease or problems?

It is essential for the cardiac surgical patient to be introduced to inhalation therapy techniques prior to the postoperative period. This preoperative instruction entails two or three visits from personnel of the respiratory therapy department to establish the pulmonary modalities in preparation for the immediate postoperative period. If the patient is not educated preoperatively, apprehension and air swallowing may result, producing gastric distention, diaphragm elevation, basilar atelectasis, and possibly even regurgitation and aspiration.

The patient should be instructed in postural drainage and percussive postural therapy, either by respiratory or physiotherapy department personnel or by the bedside critical care practitioner.

The preoperative therapy for the patient with pulmonary disease includes an extremely diligent regimen and frequent treatments with intermittent positive pressure breathing, often using one of the mucolytic agents to loosen secretions, followed two or three times a day with percussive postural drainage. The secretions obtained are cultured so that appropriate antibiotic therapy can be instituted preoperatively or be ready for postoperative use. Bronchodilators are only selectively utilized, as they may produce arrhythmias in patients with ischemic or sensitive myocardium.

Better therapeutic results can be obtained if the patient has refrained from smoking during the several weeks before the surgery. However, some benefit is obtained even if smoking has been suspended for the 3 to 7 days preceding the surgical procedure. This often requires some form of tranquilization; we prefer diazepam (Valium), 2 mg, given four times a day.

The specific and usual orders for respiratory therapy would include the following:

1. Administer 0.5 ml of 20% acetylcysteine (Mucomyst) with 3 ml saline solution.
2. In patients with bronchospasm or demonstrated improvement of pulmonary functions with bronchodilators, add 0.25 ml of Bronkosol (preferred) or 4 drops of isoproterenol (Isuprel) to the combination just mentioned.
3. For the patient with nonallergic history who becomes anorexic or nauseous with acetylcysteine, substitute 100,000 units of pancreatic dornase (Dornavac) for acetylcysteine.
4. Use postural drainage either two or four times a day, especially following the early morning and late evening treatments. Any local lung areas to be drained are specified in the orders (for example, left lower lobe or right middle lobe).

In addition, the patient is instructed in the use of the Bartlett incentive spirometer.

### ■ What preoperative precautions are taken against the development of infection?

It is recommended that patients be placed on sterile linen from the time they enter the hospital and instructed in appropriate hygienic and modified aseptic room procedures. These procedures are enforced more with the infection-prone (diabetic) patient or patients who will receive prosthetic devices.

Preoperative cultures are obtained on the day of admission from the sputum, skin, blood, and urine. Positive pathogenic cultures have been obtained in 2% to 3% of surgical patients. Positive yields have occurred in each of the mentioned culture sites, including pathogenic *Staphylococcus* from the sputum and skin, *Serratia marcescens* in the blood, and various gram-negative organisms in the urine. Positive cultures and indications of sensitivities frequently are identified the day of or the day following surgery and treatment may be initiated immediately.

The utilization of preoperative antibiotics has been a point of controversy for many years; however, there is general agreement that prophylactic antibiotics should be used in the patient who is destined to have valve surgery, especially if insertion of a prosthetic valve replacement is anticipated. The antibiotic regimen has varied almost semiannually with the introduction and advent of newer synthetic penicillins and newer antibiotics for gram-negative organisms. Each cardiac team seems to have its own preoperative, operative, and postoperative antibiotic regimen; therefore this will not be discussed in detail here.

The adjunctive use of IM procaine penicillin and streptomycin is recommended 24 hours, 12 hours, and 2 hours prior to surgery, even for myocardial revascularization procedures, and 4 g of Keflin should be placed in the pump preparation at the time of surgery. The utilization of cephalosporins in numerous patients with a history of pencillin allergy has demonstrated no evidence of cross sensitivity in our cases.

**■ What surgical preparation is ordered for the cardiac surgical patient, when is the best time for it to be performed, and who should do it?**

In most patients the entire chest, both axillae, the abdomen, the pubic area, and the groin are prepared before surgery. In cases where the saphenous vein is to be harvested, the preparation is extended to the toes, totally circumscribing the legs. In cases in which other than midsternotomy incisions are used, the side of the chest is prepared similar to preparation for thoracotomy and is specifically described by the operating surgeon, who should be contacted if there are any questions.

There remains controversy as to the ideal time to prepare the patient because of reports suggesting that if the patient is prepared too early prior to surgery, there is the potential for instigating infection in abrasion sites and hair follicles. We also believe that if prepared too early, for example, the day or evening before surgery, the patient may have increased apprehension and anxiety; however, this time schedule is occasionally necessary because of personnel reasons.

Immediately after the surgical preparation the patient should have a Betadine shower as well as on the morning of surgery. It is recommended that the patient be prepared the morning of surgery before going to the amphitheater.

The individual performing the preparation must be professionally oriented; unfortunately it is not uncommon in some hospitals to assign this responsibility to the least experienced member of the surgical team. As a result the patient may appear to require a blood transfusion or develop additional anxieties as a direct consequence of an inappropriate comment or attitude demonstrated by the individual in attendance. Occasionally patients are inadequately prepared for the surgical procedure, creating complications for the waiting surgeon or assistant who finds the patient is incompletely shaved after having already undergone the surgical scrubbing or partial draping.

**■ Who should obtain the surgical consent for operation, and how should it be worded?**

Today with the more practical approach of enthusiastic introduction of the patient to the preoperative, operative, and postoperative phases by the surgeon, anethesiologist, Mended Hearts representatives, critical care practitioners, and a cardiac team liaison person, the patient can be more than duly informed of the procedures to be performed. It is recommended that the operating surgeon make note, on the surgeon's order sheet, of the specific wording to be used and note that the patient has been informed, following which it is appropriate for another critical care team member to actually obtain the patient's signature on the consent-for-operation form.

**■ Should the patient be confronted with the legally recommended fully informed consent form?**

This question, we believe, fits into the category of the aforementioned overly dramatized television exposure for the patient. Preparation and presentation to the cardiac surgical patient of a complete informed consent form inclusive of all the minor and major problems or complications and their associated implications could require nearly 3 days of the patient's awake hours and still create confusion or the feeling of not being fully informed. It is not uncommon today in certain subspecialty fields (such as vascular radiology) for practitioners to approach the patient with a most vivid and extensive informed consent form, resulting in a number of patients refusing the crucial procedure recommended. The patients become confused when told of the multiple (however improbable) sequelae that can occur, and it has now been demonstrated that a practitioner can be held liable for complications occurring as a result of a diagnostic or therapeutic procedure not having been performed (for example, the patient was prevented from having the procedure by being frightened or improperly influenced).

We attempt to establish a general agreement and understanding with the patient that the procedure selected is best, and there is the possibility of complications despite the fact that they are not expected. If the complication potentials are higher in a specific patient and if the discussion of these potential complications might endanger the patient's successful outcome in surgery, these factors are usually discussed at length with the members of the family.*

## ■ Is preoperative bowel control necessary?

The majority of patients are allowed oral intake between 12 and 36 hours after the operative procedure; therefore complete evacuation of the bowel contents is not necessary. Patients should receive bisacodyl (Dulcolax) suppositories for two nights preceding surgery, and if this is not successful, a rectal sodium biphosphate (Fleet) enema should be utilized for evacuation of the sigmoid and descending colon the evening before surgery. If the patient has a history of chronic constipation, oral cathartics and/or stool softeners are utilized from admission throughout the preoperative period.

*It has become a cold and treacherous professional community when in some circumstances a surgeon is prompted and even advised to possibly sacrifice the patient's successful mental and/or physical outcome to prevent injudicial legal morbidity or assassination. At this time there are several states in the process of dropping all malpractice coverage for physicians because of unrelenting legal opportunists.

## ■ What medications should be discontinued on admission?

The routine use of a preadmission brochure or mimeographed instruction sheet designed to inform the patient to bring all present medications to the hospital on admission is an important policy. These medications are further verified by the admission medication checkoff sheet obtained by the admitting ward or unit.

The specific times for discontinuing certain medications prior to surgery vary; however, it is recommended that certain medications be discontinued.

### *Anticoagulants*

Anticoagulants such as warfarin (Coumadin) or dicoumarol (Dicumarol) (and occasionally dipyridamole [Persantine]) are discontinued 2½ to 3 days prior to surgery, depending on the admission prothrombin, bleeding, clotting, and partial thromboplastin times. The reason for discontinuing these drugs is evident as an unnecessary nuisance, causing possibly even life-endangering bleeding during the preliminary and early phases of the operation. The timing and discontinuance of anticoagulants in some cases are varied according to individual patient needs. Long-term or chronic use of acetylsalicylic acid (aspirin) products or phenylbutazone (Butazolidin) can also produce bleeding problems postopeartively.

### *Digitalis preparations*

Digoxin (Lanoxin), digitoxin, etc. are discontinued 3 days prior to the surgical procedure unless the patient is absolutely dependent on them (for example, if the patient has severe congestive heart failure). The period of 2½ to 3 days is an adequate time for discontinuance in the faster acting and rapidly excreted forms of digitalis. The major reason for discontinuing digitalis preparations is to prevent cardiac irritability and arrhythmias, which are especially prone to occur in the overly digitalized patient during and after pump perfusion. Pump perfusion alters the extra- and intracellular concentrations of potassium, which, in conjunction with large digitalis stores, can produce these dangerous arrhythmias. Some authors have advocated the evaluation of patients preoperatively with the injection of 2 ml of meralluride theophylline (Mercuhydrin), and if a diuresis of 3 to 4 pounds of fluid occurs within a short period of time, they believe the patient should be given digitalis preoperatively or maintained on digitalis. We have used this technique in thoracic surgical candidates rather than in cardiac surgical candidates. Publications have indicated increased cardiac irritability associated with the use of digitalis preoperatively in younger thoracic and cardiac surgical patients.[1]

### *Diuretics*

Diuertics such as furosemide (Lasix) and ethacrynic acid are preferably discontinued 3 days prior to surgery to prevent an increased loss of potassium. If maintenance of an extremely dry weight is necessary, these drugs can be continued but with careful daily monitoring of the serum potassium concentration. Restriction of sodium intake is preferred over use of excessive diuretics in the immediate preoperative period. The reason for discontinuing these medications is again the concern of cardiac irritability in the digitalized and even nondigitalized patients with hypokalemia.

### *Antihypertensive agents*

Preparations such as guanethidine sulfate (Ismelin), reserpine (Serpasil), and methyldopa (Aldomet) are discontinued at least 3 days prior to surgery, as they can produce severe induction and operative and postoperative hypotension. These drugs produce their hypotensive effects by facilitating a decrease in circulating catecholamine (epinephrine and norepinephrine) concentrations.

### *Tranquilizers*

Certain tranquilizers such as the phenothiazine derivatives (Thorazine, Stelazine, Compazine, and Combid) can also decrease circulating catecholamine concentrations and produce profound hypotension at various stages of the operation. We now use diazepam (Valium) for control of preoperative anxiety and apprehension and have observed no operative or postoperative complications. Diazepam dosages range from 2 mg four times a day to 10 mg four times a day, but we have been successful in the majority of the patients with only 2 mg four times a day. This can usually be given until the night preceding surgery.

### *Antidiabetic preparations*

Antidiabetic drugs and oral hypoglycemic agents such as tolbutamide (Orinase), chlorpropamide (Diabinese), or phenformin hydrochloride (DBI) should be discontinued 24 hours preoperatively. Subcutaneous or IV regular insulin should not be given later than 12 hours preceding surgery, and long-acting insulins should not be utilized after the patient's admission to the hospital. Better control can be maintained using a sliding scale with regular insulin. Discontinuing these drugs at the recommended times prevents their optimum effects from occurring in the immediate preoperative or operative phase, at which time moderate hypoglycemia may produce severe hypotension with all its complications (myocardial infarction, stroke, etc.).

### *Propranolol*

Propranolol (Inderal) is usually discontinued a minimum of 3 days prior to surgery; it is my practice, if the patient's condition can be appropriately controlled, to withhold its use for as long as 7 days prior to surgery. There are articles in the recent literature that claim that this drug can be continued as late as 24 hours preoperatively. This drug has $\beta$-adrenergic blocking properties and has demonstrated blockage of both chronotropic and inotropic actions of such drugs as isoproterenol (Isuprel), epinephrine, and norepinephrine. During anesthesia and after pump perfusion it can produce severe depression of myocardial contractility, cardiac failure with asystole, and death. Some cardiac teams still insist on the discontinuance of this drug at least 3 weeks before surgery.

#### *Phenoxybenzamine*

Phenoxybenzamine (Dibenzyline) is used infrequently today but has effects similar to propranolol.

• • •

For many patients who have been on multiple medications prior to admission to the hospital it is frequently safer to consider which drugs can be safely continued rather than which drugs should be discontinued.

### ■ Are there medications that should be continued and, if so, why?

#### *Potassium*

Potassium supplementation is continued or instituted until the night before surgery. Potassium is given in some form of palatable liquid in dosages of 10 to 30 mEq three or four times a day. In most cases any excess dose will be excreted by the kidneys. The reason, prevention of hypokalemia, has previously been discussed.

#### *Other preparations*

Some anemic patients continue to take oral iron supplements until the night before surgery. Diabetic patients continue to take insulin until approximately 12 hours before the operative procedure. Patients with severe regurgitant esophagitis or gastric hypersecretion are maintained on antacids or coating agents such as Gelusil or Gaviscon Foamtabs until the night before surgery. Continuation of diazepam (Valium) when necessary has been mentioned.

Many incipient complications have been averted by the diligent evaluation of the patient's preoperative medication by the admitting practitioner.

### ■ When and how are premedications given?

Premedication orders are specifically tailored to each patient and are based on the anesthesiologist's evaluation of the patient's disease, physical findings, and laboratory data. A sedative is usually given the evening preceding surgery. An analgesic agent is given in conjunction with an agent to decrease mucous secretion and block vasovagal responses approximately 45 minutes to 1 hour prior to surgery. It is important to administer this premedication early so as to make the patient relaxed and possibly sleepy for the trip to the amphitheater and to prevent complications in performing endotracheal intubation and induction.

One of the conditions that has markedly improved in most hospitals is the competent but relaxed approach used in giving patients the premedication. In the past it has not been uncommon for the staffing to be less than ideal on the 11 P.M. to 7 A.M. shift when the majority of premedications are required. The premedicating personnel have been disproportionately busy at this time. It is important that the staff appear relaxed and efficient in administering the premedication, even though this may entail giving one premedication, smiling, appearing relaxed, and then leaving the room and running down the hall to administer the next premedication injection. If the staff appears rushed or flustered, the patient may assume that this is a reflection of the surgical encounter to follow.

### ■ How detailed should the bedside practitioner's preoperative evaluation of the patient be?

The purpose of publications and texts on intensive care includes stimulation to increase the knowledge of all concerned; therefore I believe that in addition to the principal practitioner's overall evaluation of the patient, the critical care team members should also make their own evaluations. It is of definite advantage to team and patient alike for each team member to perform the following:

1. Read and be acquainted with the patient's history and physical condition on admission.

2. Evaluate the returning laboratory results and be sure the principal practitioner is aware of abnormal reports.

3. Appropriately determine the vital signs, with special care to include both apical and radial pulses. (The bedside practitioner may be the first to pick up an essential variation in peripheral pulses.)

4. Always take the blood pressure in both arms, as it is not uncommon in the patient with advanced atherosclerosis to have a partial block of one subclavian or innominate vessel, with a difference of 10 and possibly even 40 mm Hg between the two determinations. This can be a salient factor in monitoring in the operative and postoperative period. It can also be significant in patients previously undergoing catheterization through upper extremity vessels.

5. Evaluate preoperative pulses. All practitioners should know how to find and evaluate the carotid, brachial, radial, ulnar, femoral, popliteal, posterior tibial, and dorsalis pedis pulses. These should be evaluated before surgery and recorded on the chart as to their intensity (as absent, weak, or strong, or 0, 1+, or 2+, or occasionally 0, 1+, 2+, 3+, or 4+). This evaluation and record can aid in the detection of arterial clots or peripheral dissection and initiate prompt successful intervention. The patient often can also be saved an unnecessary return to surgery by the notation of certain pulses being absent preoperatively. These recordings serve to confirm the principal practitioner's findings.

6. A most important adjunct to the overall preoperative evaluation of the surgical patient is the "complete look" procedure. Many times when patients are examined in the office, in an examining room, or in the hospital their gowns will be brought down to the groin or their trousers will be brought up from the feet, possibly missing or avoiding an area between the limits of the clothing. Occasionally in sitting up in bed or turning over, small areas of the back or the back of the head are missed. In attempting close scrutiny during the examination, a gross asymmetry of body structure can be missed. However, if the patient is evaluated at a distance completely unclothed from the front, back, and side, major factors might be noticed that could even preclude the indication for surgery or could avoid complications at the time of surgery; for example, a large squamous cell tumor of the skin or a metastatic growth, a pulsatile mass in one of the peripheral vessels, a large local varicosity with a thrombus, a local or disseminated area of pyoderma or possibly even an ecchymotic area suggesting coagulation problems may suggest other modes of therapy. For individuals who might be embarrassed during this examination, it frequently can be accomplished during the routine weighing procedures, which are performed with the patient nude or in scanty undergarments. In this day of medicolegal infringements any bruises, contusions, or gross deformities should be noticed and recorded before surgical intervention.

## ■ What preoperative laboratory work is necessary for the cardiac surgical patient and why?

With the sophisticated patient monitoring systems, computerized laboratory tests, and increasing numbers of patients in critical care units, it becomes the responsibility of each and every member of the team to evaluate all laboratory work. The majority of laboratories today have a mechanism for bringing to the attention of the supervising personnel those laboratory tests that are abnormal (separate columns, encircling, or recording in differently colored inks). Emphasis is placed in the laboratory on notifying the appropriate critical care personnel of any grossly abnormal laboratory results.

The following are the baseline laboratory tests ordered for preoperative cardiac surgical patients:

1. A routine complete blood count is done to determine if the patient is anemic, has an abnormal platelet count, or exhibits signs of infection or other blood disorders.

2. Urinalysis should be performed primarily to demonstrate any spill of protein or sugar or any signs of tissue breakdown as demonstrated by the presence of acetone. In addition, it is important to note any casts or abnormal pus cells, which might suggest a tendency toward renal failure or postoperative infection.

3. Fasting blood sugar levels are measured routinely to rule out the need for further diabetic workup. In proved diabetic patients

they are measured at least daily in correlation with the urine sugar evaluation performed four times each day as a baseline for control. In diabetic patients a fasting blood sugar level is determined the morning of surgery because marked hypoglycemia can be associated with hypotension, gastric hypersecretion, and other complications in the operative and postoperative period.

4. Blood urea nitrogen (BUN) concentrations are obtained as a preliminary evaluation of renal function and also as a baseline indication of dehydration or possible gastrointestinal bleeding.

5. Serum creatinine levels are a better baseline determination of renal function, and if elevated, prompt a more thorough evaluation, including creatinine clearance, intravenous pyelogram, and urologic consultation. When the creatinine and BUN levels are above normal, dosages of certain nephrotoxic antibiotics such as gentamicin sulfate are lowered accordingly.

6. The VDRL serology test is performed on admission in a majority of hospitals as routine. (However, because of certain administrative and financial dictums associated with state and federal health plans, ECG's and chest x-ray films [even in certain age groups] cannot be routine admission requirements.)

7. Electrolyte determination is performed routinely. Sodium and chloride levels are measured initially to establish sodium loss and/or water retention, and if abnormal, correlation must be made with the patient's physical findings and appropriate balances established. Potassium levels are extremely important in the preoperative phase, as numerous patients take potassium-eliminating medications, and the increased arrhythmias and ventricular irritability associated with digitalis preparations and hypokalemia are well known. Occasionally in patients with chronic renal infection hyperkalemic states can herald a major incipient problem prior to surgery.

Calcium and phosphorus concentrations are obtained for baseline studies and occasionally may indict parathyroid abnormalities, metabolic bone disorders, or possibly disseminated malignant disease.

Serum magnesium studies were infrequently obtained prior to the past 10 years; however, it is not uncommon for individuals who have been on starvation diets, undergoing the long-term use of IV fluids, and occasionally after surgical procedures to have lower magnesium levels. Low levels of circulating magnesium have been suggested in the past as causative of severe mental confusion and occasionally convulsive episodes, especially in patients with chronic brain disease or a previous history of ethanolism.

8. Arterial blood gas measurements should be obtained in conjunction with pulmonary function studies and are important adjuncts to rule out hypoxemia, hypercapnia, and *both* respiratory and metabolic derangements. *With the frequency of utilization of this modality, every graduating critical care practitioner should be able to interpret blood gas evaluations.* Critical care personnel must ensure that arterial puncture is not made in femoral vessels in patients with poor leg pulses or questionable peripherovascular insufficiency. The radial artery, which might be used for the arterial cannulation at the time of surgery, should only be used as a last resort for blood samples. Appropriate hemostatic techniques must be utilized when blood gases are drawn, especially in the patient who has been on anticoagulant therapy. It is important that pressure be maintained directly over the puncture site for a minimum of 10 minutes after obtaining a sample and that a modified pressure dressing then be applied. Pressure dressings over the wrists are composed of a small sterile 2 × 2 inch folded pledget, rolled so that it is approximately 1 cm in height, and applied firmly with tape, being sure that the tape does not totally encircle the wrist (complications have occurred with totally encircling constrictive dressings on the extremities). If the blood gas measurement must be obtained in the groin, this pressure dressing is applied using tincture of benzoin spray on the medial aspect of the thigh just below the pelvis and above the iliac crest; when dry, tape is applied well under the

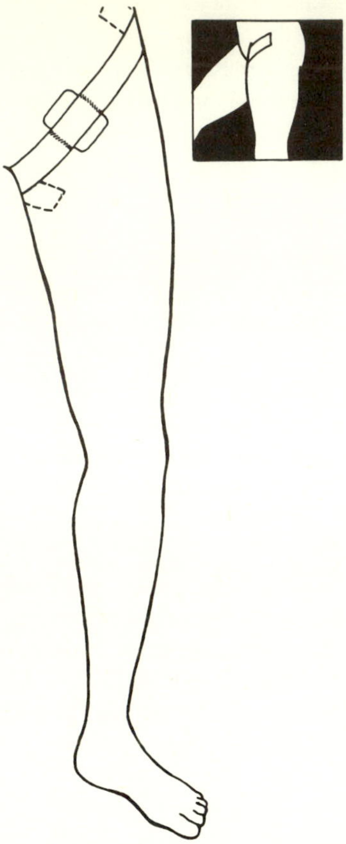

**Fig. 10-1.** Pressure dressing for femoral artery puncture sites.

medial aspect of the thigh and stretched across to the iliac crest, firmly fixing a ¾-inch wad of sterile dressing over the arterial puncture site (Fig. 10-1). *These dressings are left on no longer than 2 hours and then removed.* If this prodedure is followed, there is seldom any extravasation found at surgery.

9. Baseline coagulation screens are routine and include bleeding and clotting time tests performed using one of the accepted methods, partial thromboplastin and prothrombin time tests, fibrinogen level determinations, platelet counts, euglobulin lysis tests, and clot retraction evaluations.

10. The ECG is obtained on admission and compared by the cardiologist with previous ECG's. If the patient has not had previous ECG's in the admitting hospital, attempts are made to obtain previous recent ECG's. The ECG is repeated just prior to surgery and compared with the previous interpretation, which is recorded on the chart. A major change in the cardiac rhythm, development of ischemia, or possibly even a silent infarct has been known to occur in the time elapsing between admission and surgery.

11. Cardiac enzyme levels are also measured. If the patient has daily or crescendo-type angina, daily enzyme levels are obtained to eliminate the possibility of acute infarction, which could precipitate immediate surgery or postponement. If the patient's condition is relatively stable and angina does not occur at rest, enzyme levels are measured on admission and on the day preceding surgery. The basic cardiac enzymes usually determined include glutamic-oxaloacetic transaminase (SGOT), glutamic-pyruvic transaminase (SGPT), creatine phosphokinase (CPK), lactic dehydrogenase (LDH), and $\alpha$-hydroxybutyric dehydrogenase ($\alpha$-HBD). The use of CPK and LDH isoenzymes may be indicated to determine if recent myocardial damage is present (Chapter 12).

12. Posteroanterior and lateral chest x-ray films are obtained at the time of admission regardless of the time of the last film because a small pneumothorax, pulmonary infiltrate, or signs of failure might have recently developed. If this is the first admission for the patient, special roentgenograms are obtained with and without barium in the esophagus to establish enlargement of the various cardiac chambers.

13. A liver profile includes the prothrombin time test, which reflects hepatic parenchymal function, SGOT and SGPT determinations, which are raised in parenchymal injury, alkaline phosphatase determination, the value of which is elevated with intraductal or postductal obstruction, and bilirubin level determination, the value of which is elevated in biliary obstruction and conditions in which red blood cells are broken down or destroyed. If any of the foregoing tests reveal elevated values, a sulfobromophthalein (Bromsulfthalein, BSP) test is performed, especially in individuals who drink excessively,

## PREOPERATIVE CARDIAC SURGERY ORDERS

1. On admission of the patient to the ward, call primary practitioner regarding these orders.
2. Diet: ______________________________
3. Privileges: ______________________________
4. Record vital signs on admission and once each shift. (Record blood pressure in both arms.)
5. Check all pulses and record.
6. Administer Betadine showers daily each morning and evening and the morning of surgery.
7. Have all previous charts and records on the ward.
8. Have on the ward all medications that the patient has been taking within the past 3 weeks and record.
9. The following medications are to be discontinued: warfarin (Coumadin), digitalis (digoxin, digitoxin, etc.), diuretics, propranolol, quinidine, phenothiazines (Thorazine, Stelazine, Compazine, Combid, etc.), and antihypertensive agents.
10. The following medications are to be continued: potassium (Kaon elixir), 3 drams four times a day (may substitute equal milliequivalents of other preparations); diazepam (Valium), 2 mg three times a day and at bedtime (as needed only); pentobarbital (Nembutal), 100 mg at bedtime as needed for sleeping, may repeat one time; nitroglycerin, ______ grain (at bedside) as needed for chest pain; isosorbide dinitrate (Sorbitrate, Isordil), ______ mg, ______; antibiotics (if valve surgery) ______.
11. The following laboratory tests may be started first day after admission if patient is admitted after 4 P.M.: complete blood count, urinalysis, VDRL, and SMA-12; electrolyte determinations, BUN test, and creatinine level measurement; SGOT, SGPT, LDH, $\alpha$-HBD, and CPK tests; ECG and posteroanterior and lateral chest x-ray films (upright); and cardiac surgery coagulation screening; including platelet count, fibrinogen index (FI), prothrombin time, partial thromboplastin time, activated clotting time, and Lee-White bleeding and clotting times.

**FIRST DAY AFTER ADMISSION** Day (          )

1. Perform EEG.
2. Evaluate complete pulmonary function with arterial blood gas determinations. (If done within previous 4 weeks and records available, perform pulmonary function screening test only.)
3. Introduce the patient to respiratory therapy personnel and equipment and give instructions regarding procedures and use.
4. Perform intermittent positive pressure breathing (IPPB) therapy four times a day using 20 cm $H_2O$ pressure for 10 minutes. Utilize mouthpiece or mask with ______ nebulization.
5. Perform postural drainage following morning and evening IPPB treatments (with) (without) percussion. Concentrate on ______ lobe or segments.
6. Type and cross match 8 units of blood for surgery.
7. Obtain culture and evaluate sensitivity of blood, sputum, skin, and urine.
8. If the patient is constipated, give standardized senna concentrate (Senokot granules) 2 drams at bedtime or a laxative of the patient's choice. If no results, give bisacodyl (Dulcolax) suppository at bedtime, and if still no results, call physician.
9. Mended Hearts representatives may visit the patient. Critical care department should be notified of the patient's admission.
10. If valve surgery is to be performed, continue antibiotics as ordered on admission.

**SECOND DAY AFTER ADMISSION** (day before surgery?) Day (          )

1. Repeat cardiac enzyme determinations and ECG.
2. Obtain consent for photograph.

*Continued.*

**PREOPERATIVE CARDIAC SURGERY ORDERS—cont'd**

3. Arrange wording of surgical consent to read as follows: ______________________________
______________________________________________________________
______________________________________________________________
4. Perform the cardiac surgery preparation on entire trunk, including both axillae, abdomen, pubic area to toes, *completely* around legs, and all around forearms to fingers.
5. Administer procaine penicillin, 600,000 units, and streptomycin, 0.5 g by the IM route at 6 A.M., 6 P.M., and 6 A.M. the day of surgery. *If the patient is allergic to penicillin,* administer cephalothin (Keflin), 0.5 g, by the IM route at 6 A.M., 6 P.M., and 6 A.M. the morning of surgery.
6. If valve surgery is to be performed, continue antibiotics as ordered on admission.
7. Administer bisacodyl (Dulcolax) suppository at bedtime. If no results, give sodium biphosphate (Fleet) enema; if no results, call physician.
8. Check all pulses and record. If any are different from admission, call physician.
9. If the patient develops severe chest pain, call physician.
10. Take all x-ray films, charts, cineangiography, and the cineangiograph to surgery with patient.
11. The patient is allowed no oral intake after midnight.
12. Give medication at bedtime and on call as per anesthesiologist.

who have a history of hepatitis, or who have been subjected to hepatotoxic anesthetics such as halothane. If any of these tests are abnormal, it is essential for the anesthesiologist and cardiac team to avoid potentially hepatotoxic agents.

14. Pulmonary function is evaluated. As previously mentioned, the patient is introduced to the pulmonary therapist, and if history or laboratory and physical findings suggest pulmonary disease, it is essential to obtain a complete evaluation of pulmonary function, including vital capacity, lung volume, expiratory flow rate, forced expiratory volume ($FEV_1$, $FEV_3$), and maximum ventilatory volume (MVV or MBC). Consideration of total pulmonary function should also include determination of arterial gas concentrations, as previously mentioned. Some laboratories include measurement of dynamic arterial gases (arterial gas levels during various activities). Very young patients or those without any pulmonary problems are subjected simply to a pulmonary function screening test.

15. The EEG is performed as a baseline to determine if there are any irregularities preoperatively and for comparison with any postoperative studies. This is also medicolegally wise.

• • •

The boxed material on pp. 217-218 is a typical example of the preoperative orders for each patient admitted for cardiac surgery.

## ■ What procedure should be followed once the patient is en route to surgery?

First of all, the patient should be allowed a short visit from the family the morning of cardiac surgery.

Ideally the individual responsible for the transport of the patient should give the impression of being in control and fully aware of the patient's surgery to be performed. It can be extremely upsetting for a patient to hear an orderly or pickup team arrive at the ward and ask the ward practitioners, "Where is the heart?" or "Where is Mr. What's his name?" or mispronounce the name. The poor patient could be fearful of arriving in the wrong amphitheater and undergoing another patient's surgery. Such considerations may sound trivial; however, when discussing the hospital stay with patients, *these* are examples of what is remembered most about the surgery, as well as the feelings of insecurity or anxiety these thoughts produced.

The patient should be transported to the operating room, hopefully, well covered and warm and securely strapped to the gurney. Ideally opearting amphitheaters should have anterooms so that it would be unnecessary for a patient to remain on a gurney in the hallway (possibly listening to nonprofessional chatter or observing other patients en route to other operating rooms). The cardiac patient especially should be privileged an escort or a constant attendant until the anesthesiologist is present.

## REFERENCE

1. Juler, G. L., Stemmer, E. A., and Connolly, J. E.: Complications of prophylactic digitalization in thoracic surgery patients, J. Thorac. Cardiovasc. Surg. **58**:352-360, 1969.

*chapter 11*

# Operative care of the adult cardiac surgical patient

ROBERT A. STEEDMAN

Following transportation of the patient to the operating room or to an induction room, anesthetics should be administered and monitoring devices inserted by the anesthesia department personnel. If there is difficulty in the percutaneous establishment of the monitoring equipment, the surgical staff should be solicited for appropriate surgical (cutdown) insertion of the required devices. In many hospitals such procedures are performed in the operating room under anesthesia or, in "poor risk" patients, insertion of monitoring catheters as well as femoral artery and vein cannulation for temporary bypass may be performed under local anesthesia prior to the patient's induction. This is especially true in patients undergoing surgery for massive pulmonary embolization.

## ANESTHESIA

In articles concerning the care of the cardiac surgical patient the role of the anesthesiologist is frequently underplayed. His or her role is most important during the operative phase in maintaining the confidence of the patient before induction and establishing stable vital signs during surgery, utilizing a combination of muscle relaxants, anesthetic agents, and pain medications. The anesthesiologist must guarantee that the patient does not receive any toxic insult to the cardiac, pulmonary, renal, CNS, or hepatic systems and therefore has a very tedious but extremely major role in the care of the cardiac surgical patient.

## MONITORING

### ■ What vessel is used for arterial monitoring?

An attempt is usually first made with a percutaneous puncture using one of the large-bore plastic-sleeve needles; once the artery is entered, the sharply pointed needle is removed, and the noncutting plastic sleeve is manipulated for 3 to 4 cm up the radial artery. It is stabilized to the skin with suture to prevent pullout (Fig. 11-1).

If the percutaneous method is not successful or not facilitated easily, a small transverse incision is used, the vessel is isolated, the needle and cannula are inserted without incising the artery, and recannulation and preservation of the artery after removal is improved. Special notches are carved in the plastic hub of the needle to which sutures are secured. If the radial arteries cannot be utilized, a cutdown can be performed over the ulnar artery.

If there are no radial pulses, prior to the ulnar artery cutdown the patient is evaluated with the Allen test to be sure that there is adequate collateral circulation; this test is performed by compressing both the ulnar and radial arteries while the patient repeatedly makes a fist to establish claudication in the hand (pale blanching and tingling) and then either the radial or the ulnar artery is released. If the palm fails to blush after the release of either one of these arteries, this suggests decreased vascular supply to the palmar arch from that vessel and the remaining vessel should probably not be used.

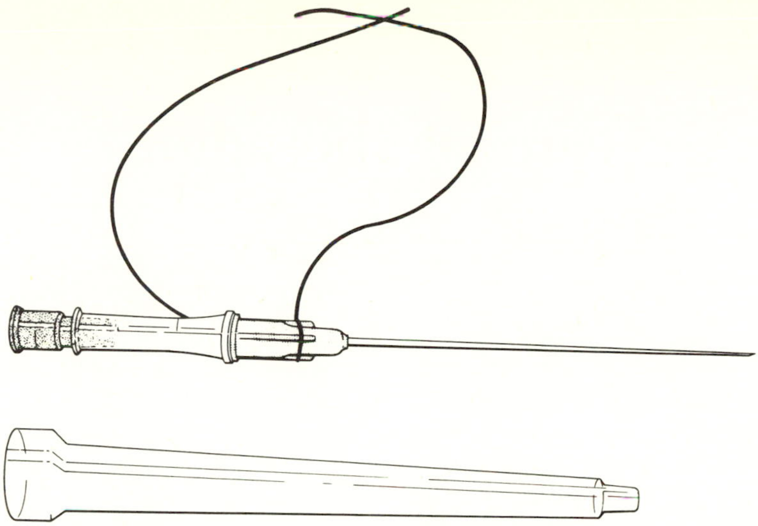

**Fig. 11-1.** Intra-arterial monitor needle with stabilizing sutures.

In the literature it is extremely rare for digit or hand loss to complicate use of these arteries; however, there have been local areas of necrosis reported. Occasionally these areas of necrosis are caused by frequent irrigation or partial blockage of collaterals from the plastic cannula. There have, however, been recent verbal communications of digit loss from harvesting the radial artery for use in aortocoronary artery bypass.

### ■ What other vessels can be utilized for arterial monitoring?

The nonperfused femoral artery can be used by means of a percutaneous puncture or direct cutdown isolation.

At the Massachusetts General Hospital a small transverse incision is made in the antecubital space (at the time of isolating the basilic and cephalic veins for central venous pressure monitoring and venous infusion) with isolation of the brachial artery for arterial monitoring; no complications have been reported. In experienced hands this appears to be a good technique.

A modification of a technique described by Hegeman, Rappaport, and Berger[1] involves the use of the superficial temporal artery. This artery has been used in young adults and children who are burn victims with no accessible extremity arteries. This artery can be interrupted without consequence, the scar can be hidden later by normal sideburn growth in males and usual hairdos in females. The only drawback is the occasional cannulation in a tortuous thin-walled artery.

When the aorta is to be clamped in cases of resection or surgical repair of dissection, it becomes necessary to have an upper extremity (preferably the right) and a lower extremity arterial monitor, so the left heart bypass apparatus can be adjusted to prevent brain and upper extremity hypertension but maintain abdominal visceral perfusion.

### ■ What complications can occur as a result of the insertion of arterial monitors?

In the radial artery small dissections of the intima can occur when attempting to thread the plastic cannula; this causes thrombosis, but if the occlusion is very distal and the ulnar artery is open, there will be no major complications.

Either by misjudgment or error, medications can be injected into this cannula and cause severe spasm and thrombosis with resultant skin slough. No medications other than heparinized solutions should be given in arterial lines.

Overenthusiastic irrigations in wrist arteries can produce necrosis and local skin slough.

With femoral artery monitoring, peripheral clots, embolized atheroma, intimal dissection, posterior wall perforations, hematomas, and hemorrhage can occur and occasionally require surgical correction. Some investigators are more skilled than others at performing this procedure.

In the hands of those who use the brachial artery routinely morbidity is probably extremely low; however, because of reports of complicating thrombosis resulting in partial limb loss occurring in young patients monitored by this method, its use is avoided.

The cannulation and monitoring procedure that best fits the situation and is most successful in the critical care team's experience should be used.

### ■ What are the reasons for using arterial monitors?

Accurate cuff pressures are extremely difficult to obtain during perfusion when the nonpulsatile mean pressures range between 50 and 70 mm Hg. The arterial monitor decreases the frequent need of wrapping a cuff around the arm when there might be multiple infusion lines in that arm. It also provides a withdrawal line for arterial gas determination, electrolyte levels, and other blood tests during the critical operative and postoperative period.

### ■ Can the pressures vary from arm to arm?

There can be variances as high as 30 to 40 mm Hg between the right and left arm if subclavian stenosis from atherosclerosis or brachial artery narrowing from heart catheterization exists; again, this is a valid indication for determining blood pressures in both arms (possibly even simultaneously) as well as evaluating and reporting the quality of each pulse in the preoperative period.

### ■ What techniques are utilized and what is the purpose of central venous pressure monitors?

Any major peripheral vein that will allow manipulation of a catheter into the central venous system (right atrium and superior or inferior vena cava) will usually suffice for central venous pressure monitoring. This can be performed through the external or internal jugular or subclavian veins by percutaneous puncture, through the basilic or cephalic veins percutaneously or by cutdown, or via a branch of the greater saphenous vein.

The cephalic or basilic veins, with attempted manipulation of the catheter into the subclavian, innominate, and finally into the superior vena cava, may be used, but frequently the catheter cannot be passed beyond the peripheral valves or deviates into the veins of the neck or head.

Many anesthesiologists have become skilled at performing percutaneous punctures of the subclavian or internal jugular veins, but problems with hematoma, pneumothorax, and complicating infections have been reported.

Occasionally the external jugular system can be approached by the anesthesiologist through the use of a percutaneous puncture and manipulation of the cannula down into the superior vena cava (similar to passing a transvenous permanent or temporary electrode), but this procedure is more often successful with a cutdown approach. The purpose of the central venous pressure monitor is to establish a guide for fluid replacement to indirectly assess ventricular function. It is more accurate in assessing the need for fluid replacement than it is for monitoring overhydration. There are multiple reports wherein the central venous pressure monitor reflected overhydration, but a left atrial cannula demonstrated hypovolemia; occasionally the opposite has also occurred.

### ■ What other methods of measurement of hydration and cardiac function or left ventricular function are available?

Some institutions routinely utilize a left atrial cannula. This can be placed in the left atrium at surgery by manipulating a plastic catheter through a No. 20- or 18-gauge needle and removing the needle, leaving the catheter in place and stabilized by a small pursestring suture. Problems with this technique include dislodgement of the catheter during the operative and immediate postoperative period, and where the catheter is brought out a separate puncture site in the anterior chest wall, it can become kinked or plugged. Despite these problems, use of the left atrial cannula is a more accurate means of evaluating left ventricular function and hydration.

When there is dire need of better left ventricular and left atrial assessment, a Swan-Ganz pulmonary artery catheter with an inflatable small balloon tip can be floated from a peripheral vein through the right atrium and right ventricle into the pulmonary artery. The catheter can be manipulated into a peripheral pulmonary artery branch and wedged; this "wedge pressure" reflects the left atrial pressure. It is most often positioned by a cardiologist via a right antecubital vein, but other veins can be used.

Urinary output is a prime reflection of cardiac output and renal perfusion. A catheter is placed aseptically after the other monitor lines have been stabilized. When personnel other than surgeons place these catheters, it is of utmost importance that free-flowing urine be obtained before inflation of the balloon and that the accurate positioning of the catheter be confirmed. If these measures are not followed, creation of a false channel or intraurethral inflation of the balloon can produce a critical situation.

Another parameter of appropriate perfusion during use of the pump is the body temperature, and rectal and esophageal temperature probes are placed prior to induction. These are essential in patients requiring systemic cooling and rewarming.

## THE OPERATION

### ■ What scrub and preparation technique is utilized?

For most cardiac operations today, especially the revascularization procedures, the patient is scrubbed from the chin down to and including the toes. I utilize a 10-minute Betadine surgical soap scrub followed by drying, application of the Betadine preparation solution, and redrying. The standard techniques of working away from the incision sites to the periphery are followed.

### ■ Are there any special adhesive coverings utilized?

Most institutions today use various forms of plastic drapes over the intended incision sites; these drapes serve a twofold purpose: they decrease incision contamination from surrounding skin areas, and they are nonconductable, thus preventing possible skin burns.

### ■ How often is the electrical cautery used and are there any special precautions to be taken?

The electrical cautery apparatus is utilized in the majority of open-heart surgeries performed on the West Coast and more frequently now even on the East Coast.

Most surgeons will not utilize this apparatus if a temporary or permanent pacemaker is in place for fear of electrical mishaps associated with either intraventricular or epicardial electrodes.

Special nonconductive containers for the individual electrocoagulation units are essential so that patients and/or personnel are not burned or shocked with an exposed primary or secondary unit. Hand-operated units are preferred so that both surgeon and assistant can utilize a unit independently and replace a unit into a separate nonconductive container.

### ■ What incisions are utilized for cardiac surgery?

The most commonly used incision is the midsternotomy, especially for myocardial revascularization procedures, many of the valve procedures, and most of the adult congenital defect repairs.

Occasionally for the closed-approach valve techniques a right or left inframammary incision is used for cosmetic reasons and technical convenience.

For surgery involving the descending aorta (coarctation, aneurysm, dissection, etc.) the posterior lateral thoracotomy incision is used, frequently requiring two separate intercostal entrances (for example, at the fourth and seventh intercostal junctions).

Transsternal and thoracoabdominal incisions are only used in exceptionally difficult exposure cases, and the parasternal approach is used for local pericardiectomy, placements of temporary epicardial electrodes, and occasionally evacuation of pericardial tamponade.

■ **Which incisions are least painful and less difficult to care for postoperatively?**

The incisions that are least painful, most stable, and easiest to care for are as follows in respective order: midsternotomy, parasternal, subxiphoid, inframammary, transternal, posterior lateral thoractomy, and the troublesome and frequently complicated thoracoabdominal incision.

■ **What precautionary measures are taken prior to making the skin incision?**

Usually 1 or 2 units of blood are in the room prior to splitting the sternum in case any undue bleeding is encountered. It is recommended that 1 or 2 units of the patient's own blood be withdrawn prior to surgery and readministered at the completion of the "pump," or cardiopulmonary bypass apparatus, procedures. This blood will have the patient's own clotting elements, will definitely be compatible, and will not be heparinized. Of course, this preoperative withdrawal of blood is not performed in patients with an unstable myocardium.

The pump technician should be in the room and ready in the event immediate perfusion is necessary.

■ **What are the routine steps in the cannulation procedure?**

The sternotomy incision is completed and electrocoagulation is utilized to control bleeding. Bone wax is applied to control oozing from the divided sternum. The pericardium is carefully cleared of the pleura, thymus, and fatty tissue, taking care not to injure the innominate vein. The pericardium is then opened while a groin incision is made simultaneously for isolation of the common femoral artery with either a single long vertical or multiple small transverse incisions to harvest the saphenous vein. Frequently the saphenous veins from the ankle to the knee are used, as the caliber of the vessel is more proportionate to that of the coronary arteries.

After the pericardium is opened and retracted with stay sutures, two pursestring sutures are placed into the right atrium, and the patient is given heparin. *The anticoagulation dose is usually 3 mg of heparin/kg of body weight.* This heparin dosage and the vial from which it was obtained is *always confirmed* by the anesthesiologist or surgeon; it must be administered by the anesthesiologist via a guaranteed open vein or by the surgeon directly into the right atrium.

Approximately 3 minutes after heparin infusion through the previously placed atrial pursestring sutures, one cannula is placed in the superior and the other in the inferior vena cava. For procedures that do not require absolute total bypass, a single cannula in the atrium can be used, but in cases wherein an absolutely dry field and total emptying of the heart is necessary, the use of two caval cannulas with caval encircling tapes or clamps is preferred.

The femoral artery cannula is then placed, care being taken not to create an intimal flap, and pump lines are connected to the cannulas with careful scrutiny and evacuation of all air bubbles from the arterial lines.

■ **What other methods of arterial cannulation for pump perfusion are available?**

Arterial return can be established through the use of aortic cannulation through a double pursestring suture with the tip directed downstream and away from the head vessels. Also, the femoral route is still used, even though the danger of dissection is somewhat higher than with the aortic technique. The danger of CNS involvement with injection of air and flow and pressure problems in the major vessels supplying the brain is more likely with the aortic route. When femoral artery obstruction or severe atherosclerotic disease is noted at surgery or proved to be present by previous arteriography, the aortic route is used.

■ **What is the pump and how does it work?**

The pump, or cardiopulmonary bypass apparatus, is the mechanical substitute for the heart and lungs. There are a variety of models used, but I will describe only one.

The mechanism of action consists of draining unoxygenated blood by gravity from the atrial cannulas to a reservoir and oxygenator where the blood is filmed over or through thin sheets of plastic and exposed to high concentrations of bubbled or inflow oxygen. The blood, now oxygenated, is pumped back to the femoral cannula by means of a rotating modular roller head. The revolving rollers partially occlude or compress the plastic tubes containing the oxygenated blood and force it back to the body through the arterial cannula.

## ■ With what are the pump and oxygenator primed?

Most oxygenators used today are plastic disposable units initially prepared or primed (filled) with either crystalloid solutions, all blood, all electrolyte solutions, or a combination of these solutions. The all blood solution was the most common prime until approximately 10 years ago, when conversion began toward the use of more crystalloid solutions. In some institutions only 5% dextrose and water is utilized.

When low blood or nonblood primes are initially pumped into the patient, the patient's hemoglobin level and hematocrit are diluted. The hemoglobin content is usually maintained between 7 and 10 g under average circumstances, probably decreasing rouleaux formation of blood cells and preventing sludging and peripheral clotting problems. However, whole blood primes possibly cause fewer postoperative and postperfusion bleeding difficulties and decrease respiratory complications.

Those mechanisms utilizing nonblood primes frequently add protein (in the form of albumin) and therapeutic doses of mannitol as a prophylactic measure against renal shutdown.

The recommended prime solution for a 70 kg (154 lb) male is 2 L of electrolyte replacement solution (Plasma-Lyte), 50 mg of heparin (25 mg/L of diluent), 200 ml of 25% albumin, 500 ml of 10% mannitol (Osmitrol), and four g of cephalothin (Keflin). (Two grams of lincomycin [Lincocin] are added if the patient is allergic to penicillin.) Blood may be added if the hemodilution effect lowers the hemoglobin content below 7 g/100 ml, and corticosteroids are added only if indicated. The hemodilution occasionally appears to initially lower the mean pressure to around 50 mm Hg for about 10 minutes, but this can be immediately counteracted by a minimum IV dose of phenylephrine hydrochloride (Neo-Synephrine).

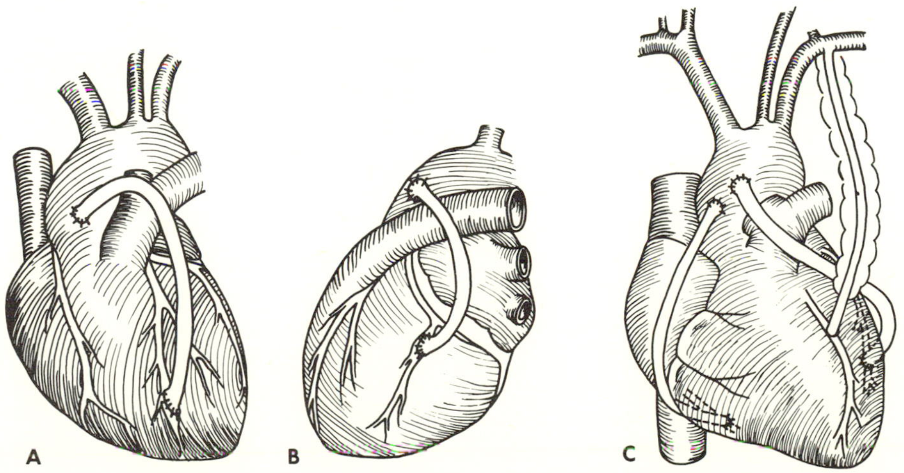


**Fig. 11-2.** Coronary artery revascularization. **A,** Left anterior descending saphenous vein bypass. **B,** Aortocoronary saphenous vein bypass. **C,** Internal mammary artery, left anterior descending coronary artery bypass in conjunction with saphenous vein bypasses to right and circumflex coronary arteries.

■ **What are the specific techniques utilized in revascularization?**

The patient's cardiac functions are usually maintained by the bypass apparatus and stabilized (occasionally, however, the right coronary artery bypass procedure can be performed without using the pump), and the coronary vessel is isolated and opened beyond the obstruction or stenosis with a 0.5 to 1.0 cm vertical slit. Determination of anterograde and retrograde flow is completed. Cannulation can be performed proximally and distally with special sizing probes (1.0 to 2.5 mm). The saphenous vein (which has been harvested and prepared to avoid leakage) is reversed and anastomosed distally to the coronary artery with very fine (6-0 or 7-0) nonabsorbable (Prolene) suture. This distal anastomosis frequently requires fibrillation of the heart or aortic cross clamping. In some cases the left internal mammary artery is dissected from the chest wall and anastomosed to the left anterior descending coronary artery as an in situ end-to-side graft. When all the distal anastomoses are completed, the heart is defibrillated, a partial occluding clamp is placed on the aorta, and the proximal vein anastomoses are completed. The proximal anastomoses (Fig. 11-2) can be performed with the use of the bypass apparatus.

■ **How is the heparin dosage determined during the pump run and how is it reversed at completion?**

If the total time of the pump run is 1 hour or less, the total amount of heparin used is the same as the initial heparinizing dose (3 mg/kg of body weight); however, if the time extends beyond 1 hour, then one half the original anticoagulating dose is given at the end of the second hour and one fourth of the dose is given each following half hour. Hopefully the pump time will be less than 2 hours. Activated clotting, partial thromboplastin, prothrombin, and Lee-White bleeding and clotting times can be monitored to determine the dosages of heparin while the pump is in use or the amount of protamine sulfate to be used for heparin neutralization at the completion of the procedure.

The total reversing dose of *protamine sulfate* is usually 1.5 mg/mg of heparin that has been given for anticoagulation; the development of small clots with decreased oozing is usually evident within minutes after the administration of protamine sulfate. If this does not occur, an additional 50 mg of protamine sulfate is given while coagulation studies are obtained.

■ **Are there any precautions to be taken with the administration of protamine sulfate?**

Rapid IV administration of protamine sulfate has been known to cause hypotension, and sensitivity to IV administration has been demonstrated in some patients; therefore protamine sulfate is given by slow micro drop administration over a period of 10 to 15 minutes so that any hypotensive episodes can be recognized and corrected.

■ **What are vents and how are they utilized?**

After the patient's cardiac functions have been transferred to the bypass apparatus, a small plastic cannula is inserted into the apex of the left ventricle through a pursestring suture and connected to lines that return to the pump. This *left ventricular vent* drains blood back to the pump and prevents overdistention of the left ventricle during aortic cross clamping or fibrillation. Its secondary purpose is to aspirate air that might accumulate in the left ventricle and prevent embolization once the heart again begins to beat.

Many practitioners now recommend venting with a cannula manipulated through a pursestring suture in the superior pulmonary vein into the left atrium. This prevents left ventricular distention by draining blood from the left atrium before it empties into the ventricle.

A cannula developed by Dr. Floyd Loop at the Cleveland Clinic can be introduced through the superior pulmonary vein and manipulated through the mitral valve into the left ventricle, thus eliminating the need for ventriculotomy.

Both left atrial and left ventricular vents are recommended to ensure maximum decompression when bypass surgery is being performed on a patient who has recently experienced infarction (within 2 to 6 hours) and when aortic cross clamping and fibrillation are to be avoided.

■ **Are there any complications that can occur from the use of these vents?**

It is not uncommon for the superior pulmonary vein or the left ventricle to tear with removal of the vent; this can lead to very troublesome operative and postoperative bleeding. Occasionally extensive repair with a Teflon pledget support is necessary for the left ventricle, superior pulmonary vein, or atrium. Extensive left ventricular repairs can affect myocardial function postoperatively.

■ **At what temperature is the cardiac patient maintained, and how is this controlled?**

During cardiac procedures in which only short-term clamping of the aorta or ventricular fibrillation is used normothermic temperatures can be maintained; however, when the ischemic periods experienced by the myocardium are expected to extend beyond 30 minutes, the patient's temperature is cooled to 28° to 30° C, because this allows the myocardium to tolerate decreased perfusion for longer periods of time. In some cases of congenital cardiac surgery (especially in infants and children) deep hypothermia can be used (10° to 20° C), which allows total body perfusion to be suspended for periods of as much as 1 hour. Localized cooling of the heart can be accomplished by packing it in iced slush.

Cooling and warming are accomplished by use of an oxygenating system with an integral heat exchange; however, most of these commercial products do not warm the patient as rapidly as is desired by most surgeons.

■ **What technique can be used to prevent air embolization?**

Air bubbles are carefully manipulated out of all arterial lines prior to beginning the perfusion process in the patient. The left ventricular vent, when used, prevents air accumulation in the left ventricle; prior to removal of this vent the left ventricle is elevated to allow the air to rise to the highest point. If a vent has not been utilized, the ventricular apex is raised and decompressed with an 18-gauge needle.

During the perfusion run some pulmonary positive pressure is maintained at all times; just prior to removal of vents and cannulas the lungs are hyperinflated with applied pressures of 35 to 40 cm, and the left atrial appendage is manipulated so that air will flow toward the elevated left ventricular apex.

During all these procedures the patient remains with the head down or in a modified Trendelenburg position so that air bubbles passing the aortic valve will be trapped in the aortic root, and an 18-gauge needle is used to vent the air from the aorta. During mitral valve and congenital septal defect surgery an aortic "tack" may be sutured directly to the aorta for continual venting during the cardiac procedure and when the patient is released from the pump. This technique was developed by Laurence K. Groves of the Cleveland Clinic.

■ **When are pacemaker wires inserted?**

Pacing wires are sutured to the atrium and myocardium, or myocardium alone, whenever there appears to be increased risk of heart block or any other arrhythmia involving poor cardiac output. These temporary wires can be easily removed in the postoperative period.

When heart block was present prior to the surgery requiring a temporary pacemaker, permanent suture electrodes are placed at the completion of surgery using either General Electric suture electrodes or Medtronics sutureless corkscrew electrodes.

■ **How many chest tubes are utilized, why are they used, and where are they placed?**

If only the mediastinum or pericardium has been violated, two No. 36 argyle plastic chest tubes are sufficient to drain the pericardium, one placed in an anterograde and the other in a retrograde position with regard to the heart for evacuation of blood and clots. When the pleura has been violated on either the left or right side, chest tubes also are placed to evacuate air and allow reexpansion of the lung. The specific placement of the tubes varies with each practitioner. In cases where the pleura has not been violated, some individuals place both chest tubes in a position anterior to the heart; others place one chest tube in an anterior position and the other in a posterior position, hoping to prevent the development of cardiac tamponade.

If either chest cavity has been entered, one chest tube is usually placed in the area of the costovertebral groove to drain blood spilled over from the mediastinum and also to evacuate air. If there is any question of lung perforation, a second tube can be placed near the apex of the lung to ensure air evacuation. In cases where both pleural cavities are entered, it is not uncommon to use as many as four tubes, and when four chest tubes are necessary, I prefer not to connect them all to the same suction apparatus if maximum efficient suction and drainage is to be obtained.

## ■ What parameters are measured during the operative procedure?

Arterial pressures and pulse wave contours are monitored continuously during the procedure as well as the central venous or left atrial pressure.

Arterial gas determinations should be obtained at least every 10 to 15 minutes to maintain expected gas tensions. The levels strived for are as follows: $P_{O_2}$ of 100 to 150 mm Hg, $P_{CO_2}$ of 32 to 40 mm Hg, pH of 7.35 to 7.45, $O_2$ concentration of 95% to 99%, and a base excess near zero.

The serum potassium levels are obtained every 15 to 30 minutes because, as previously mentioned, hypokalemia can lead to serious arrhythmias, and hyperkalemia can prevent return of ventricular contractility.

The hemoglobin and hematocrit levels are evaluated every 15 to 30 minutes to main-

| Urine | $P_{CO_2}$ | $P_{O_2}$ | pH | $O_2$ saturation | $HCO_3^-$ | Hematocrit | Potassium | Time |
|---|---|---|---|---|---|---|---|---|
| 15 ml | 41 | 120 | 7.39 | 98% | 29 | 43 CVP 16 | 5.1 | 8 AM |
| 30 ml | 39 | 104 | 7.41 | 97% | 31 | | | 8.30 AM |
| | | | | On bypass | | → | → | ~~9 AM~~ |
| 100 ml | 33 | 140 | 7.48 | 99% | 24 | 32 | 4.6 | |
| 60 ml | 39 | 160 | 7.43 | 99% | 32 | 29 | 4.0 | 9:30 AM |
| 54 ml | 35 | 130 | 7.46 | 97% | 26 | 27 | 3.7 | 10:00 AM |
| | | | | Aorta cross-clamp | → On | | → | 10:10 AM |
| | | | | Aorta cross-clamp | → Off | | → | 10:24 AM |
| 75 ml | 39 | 170 | 7.43 | 98% | 27 | 29 CVP 12 | 3.1 | 10:30 AM |
| | | | | Off bypass | | → | → | 10:30 AM |
| 100 ml | 33 | 130 | 7.49 | 97% | 24 | 35 | 4.0 | 11.00 AM |
| 25 ml | 39 | 100 | 7.43 | 96% | 27 | 37 | 4.4 | 11:15 AM |
| | | | | To critical care | | → | → | 11:15 AM |
| | | | | | | | | |
| | | | | | | | | |
| | | | | | | | | |
| | | | | | | | | |

**Fig. 11-3.** Intraoperative flow board.

tain hemodilution with a hemoglobin concentration between 7 and 10 g and a hematocrit between 22% and 30% until the pump run is completed, when additional blood is added to obtain more normal levels.

Urinary output is measured every 15 minutes and used as an indication of adequate renal perfusion or possible impending renal shutdown. During perfusion outputs greater than 100 ml/hr are desired, and color concentration is noted to evaluate the amount of red blood cell hemolysis. When moderate hemolysis is evident by a pink or reddened urine, a higher urinary output is induced to protect against renal failure; with the higher output the serum potassium levels must be carefully observed.

All of these parameters should be recorded on an intraoperative flow board (Fig. 11-3) so that the condition of the patient can be evaluated by members of the operating team at any time.

### ■ What are the common intraoperative arrhythmias?

Intraoperative arrhythmias associated with ventricular irritability during periods of myocardial ischemia or immediately after defibrillation are frequently seen and consist of premature ventricular beats (PVB's) and ventricular tachycardia.

Atrial ectopic beats occur often during the period of atrial cannulation, but usually cease spontaneously after manipulation. Atrial fibrillation and flutter occur occasionally after the patient is released from the bypass apparatus, but these can usually be electrically converted during surgery. Sinus bradycardia as a vasovagal or vagovagal response during induction or postperfusion periods with varying degrees of heart block can also occur.

Control of these arrhythmias in the intraoperative period is similar to control in the coronary care units, for example, intravenous lidocaine (Xylocaine) is used for ventricular arrhythmias and ectopic beats; the cautious administration of potassium is employed in hypokalemic-associated ventricular arrhythmias; atropine is utilized in the treatment of severe sinus bradycardia associated with vasovagal or vagovagal response; and occasionally isoproterenol hydrochloride (Isuprel) is used for the hypotensive nonvolume-depleted bradycardia patient.

### ■ How are episodes of intraoperative hypotension and hypertension controlled?

Hypotension during bypass procedures occurs with imbalance of arterial perfusion and venous return and is frequently associated with hypovolemia. Marked angulation of the atrial cannulas can decrease venous return, but on recognition this is easily corrected. Dampening of the arterial monitor cannulas can give false low readings, and simple irrigation of the peripheral arterial line will rapidly correct this pseudohypotension.

Mild periods of hypotension associated with high cardiac output or the suggestion of collapse of peripheral vascular resistance can be controlled with small doses of phenylephrine hydrochloride (Neo-Synephrine), phenylephrine, norepinephrine, or, for short periods of time, metaraminol (Aramine).

Persistent periods of hypotension after multiple attempts to terminate the use of the bypass apparatus may require drug assistance. When adequate volume is demonstrated by a normal or elevated central venous or left atrial pressure, isoproterenol (Isuprel) is administered using a titrated micro drop infusion. Elevation of the blood pressure without tachycardia is the desired effect and the reason for drug titration. Isoproterenol has the advantage of producing an inotropic effect on the heart without constricting the peripheral arterial bed.

The use of drug combinations has been reported in the literature concerning the treatment of hypotension with varying results; these preparations include combinations of epinephrine and isoproterenol, isoproterenol and glucagon, or glucagon or epinephrine solutions alone.

Dopamine (Intropin) has been shown to be very effective in these situations without causing peripheral vascular constriction, uncontrollable tachycardias, or renal complications.

Uncontrollable postoperative hypotension or low cardiac output occasionally requires more radical measures or cardiac assistance. The most common cardiac assistance device used today is the intra-aortic balloon developed as a result of the work of Dr. Adrian Kantrowitz. These apparatuses can be a major asset to the postoperative low cardiac output patient; however, they are not without potential hazards or complications.

Hypertension during the period immediately before using the pump can be extremely hazardous and can cause intracerebral complications or increase the potential for aortic dissection or vascular tears during cannulation or when instituting perfusion. This can usually be controlled by the anesthesiologist in maintaining appropriate depths of anesthesia, by the temporary use of halothane (Fluothane) gas, or with frequent doses of IV morphine sulfate.

In situations where the peripheral arterial bed appears to be constricted as evidenced by severe pallor, lack of capillary blanching, and bluish mottling of the skin, 1 or 2 mg of slowly administered IV chlorpromazine (Thorazine) can be given and repeated as necessary.

If the hypertension occurs during the pumping period, IV chlorpromazine or the sublingual or IV use of one of the nitrate preparations is recommended; titration with IV nitrous prusside (Nipride 100 mg in 1000 ml 5% dextrose in water) can be used.

The patient with postoperative refractory hypertension may require treatment with one of the peripheral vasodilating drugs such as trimethaphan camsylate (Arfonad). This requires very diligent second-by-second bedside monitoring and can be most hazardous to the patient if the appropriate monitoring is not utilized. It is recommended only when other means of control are unsuccessful or for patients with labile aortic vascular repairs.

■ **How is the sternum closed after it has been divided surgically?**

The sternum is reapproximated with No. 22 or No. 24 heavy stainless steel wire brought up through the sternum on each side with the use of a sternal awl. The awl looks like a large hand-driven needle or ice pick with a hole in the tip. The wire is placed through the tip and brought up through the sternum on each side, tightly twisted, and cut off so that a length of approximately ¾ cm remains. The end of this twisted wire is then bent flush with the sternum and the muscle and fascia are approximated over the wire.

Approximately 5% of patients will have some irritation from the sternal wires requiring removal at a later date; this relatively simple procedure can be done under local anesthesia.

Patients should be advised after their surgery not to receive any deep heat treatment (such as microthermy or diathermy) over the area with the sternal wires as this can cause discomfort and tissue damage. The patient should be informed that the sternum has been closed with wires so their presence on future chest x-ray films will not cause him or his attorney to hear that multiple pieces of hardware were left in his chest.

Another technique for closing the sternum utilizes a heavy nonabsorbable plastic suture circumscribing the sternum, with care taken not to injure the internal mammary artery and vein.

There are special stainless steel wire kits with wedged-on needles that can be utilized in closing a thin sternum; however, these are more difficult to pass through a thick sternum.

## TRANSPORT OF THE PATIENT

■ **What specific measures are necessary prior to the transport of the patient from the operating room to the critical care unit?**

Chest tubes, central venous pressure lines, and arterial lines are sutured to the patient during insertion to prevent pullout. The arterial and venous lines are disconnected from the monitors and for transport are connected to large heparinized syringes with three-way stopcocks.

The chest tubes are secured to the skin

with tincture of benzoin and tape. All chest tube connections are taped to prevent any leakage or disconnection during the transfer procedure.

The Emerson suction apparatus is unplugged from its electric energy source or the Pleurovac is disconnected from wall suction, but the tubes are still connected to "underwater seal." *At no time are the chest tubes clamped for transfer.* There still appears to be a major misconception in many hospitals that chest tubes should be clamped during transfer.

The patient is connected to a portable bedside or gurney monitor so the ECG can be observed continually during the transport process.

Oxygen apparatus and an Ambu bag are also connected to the transfer apparatus. A modified shock cart is utilized for the transfer of the patient from the operating room to the critical care unit.

Prior to beginning transport, arterial gas, potassium level, hemoglobin, hematocrit, vital sign, and central venous pressure readings are obtained to establish that the patient's condition is stable.

In the majority of patients the endotracheal tube should be left in place, and the patient should be ventilated with an Ambu bag and 100% oxygen. Transport should be swiftly and carefully accomplished, with at least five members of the cardiac team accompanying the patient during the transfer; this should include the anesthesiologist, at least one surgeon, an operating room practitioner to manage the chest suction device, and two other individuals to assist with the battery-powered defibrillation equipment and to precede the group in order to clear any obstacles between the operating room and the critical care unit.

The family should be escorted to a private waiting room to prevent any undue apprehension associated with seeing the patient en route with multiple tubes and IV bottles, as well as the professional entourage.

Approximately 20 to 30 minutes prior to completion of the operative procedure and again when the patient is being prepared for transfer, the critical care unit personnel should be notified so that appropriate preparation for the patient's arrival can be carried out.

**■ How many practitioners should be in attendance in the unit when the patient arrives?**

A 2:1 or more nursing care ratio is recommended during the initial phases of postcardiac surgery care.

## REFERENCE

1. Hegeman, C. O., Rappaport, I., and Berger, W. J.: Superficial temporal artery cannulation, Arch. Surg. **99**:619-623, 1969.

*chapter 12*

# Postoperative care of the adult cardiac surgical patient

ROBERT A. STEEDMAN

Once the patient has been appropriately placed in the unit, members of the transporting team should step back, remaining prepared to assist if necessary, and observe until all appears stable. Then the postoperative team will take over the patient's care. Needless to say, the patient's overall recuperation from this point on should be primarily the responsibility of the highly skilled critical care unit personnel. The basic routine orders are given in the boxed material on pp. 233-235.

## ■ What items are attended to on the arrival of the patient?

First, attention should be given to providing ventilation and establishing a clear airway. The bedside practitioner and inhalation therapist immediately suction the endotracheal tube, connect the patient to the ventilating apparatus with 100% oxygen, and obtain an arterial gas measurement. Once the first blood gas measurement has been obtained (usually within a period of 5 minutes or less), the tidal volume, respiratory rate, and oxygen concentrations are adjusted appropriately. The original respiratory adjustments are made on the recommendations of the anesthesiologist and surgeon and are based on the patient's needs in surgery. Ventilation adjustments are made every 10 minutes until satisfactory control and gas measurements are obtained. Desired gas concentrations consist of a $P_{O_2}$ from 100 to 130 mm Hg, a $P_{CO_2}$ from 35 to 40 mm Hg, a pH from 7.35 to 7.45, and a relatively normal base excess.

Connection of the ECG and arterial and venous monitor lines is performed simultaneously or immediately following establishment of the airway.

Continuous pressure infusion of heparinized saline solution is started in both the arterial and the venous lines to prevent clotting. With the equipment now available this requires less than 250 to 400 ml of solution in a 24-hour period. The solution is prepared with a maximum of 5000 units of heparin/L of saline solution, but in some institutions the heparin added is as little as 1000 units/L or as much as 10,000 units/L. The amount of heparin utilized depends on the proficiency of the constant infusion devices.

Attention is given to the chest tubes and urinary catheters, and drainage is ensured.

## ■ Who is responsible for the primary care of the patient in the critical care unit?

The operating surgeon or assistant is primarily responsible for all decisions and usually stays with the patient until conditions are stable or until the endotracheal tube has been removed.

It is the responsibility of the critical care staff to know how to contact the surgeon or assistant at any time, and it is imperative that the staff and the hospital telephone operator be able to immediately contact the cardiologist, anesthesiologist, and pump tech-

## POSTOPERATIVE CARDIAC SURGERY ORDERS

### MEDICATIONS

1. Follow routine cardiac (coronary) care orders and medications.
2. Morphine sulfate. Mix 30 mg in 30 ml saline solution. Give 1 to 5 mg (or ml) every hour as needed for pain or respiratory control.
3. Cephalothin (Keflin). Give 1.5 g by IV route (PB) every 6 hours. If the patient is allergic or if valve surgery was performed, contact principal practitioner.
4. Acetylsalicylic acid. Give 20 grains rectally for rectal temperature above 101° F. If no results after 2 hours, repeat; if still no results, initiate treatment by cooling blanket and notify principal practitioner.
5. If the patient is allergic to acetylsalcylic acid, give acetaminophen (Tylenol), 20 grains, rectally, in place of acetylsalicylic acid.
6. Use hyperthermia treatment if rectal temperature is below 97° F. Use hypothermia treatment if there is a persistent rectal temperature above 101° F.

### RESPIRATORY THERAPY

1. Connect the patient to the MA-I volume respirator set at tidal volume as directed by the anesthesiologist or surgeon to administer 100% $O_2$ until the results of the first blood gas analysis are obtained (approximately 10 to 15 minutes).
2. Give routine endotracheal tube care, with irrigation (using 3 to 5 ml saline solution) and suction every 30 minutes or more often as needed. Sigh patient every 15 to 30 minutes (hand or machine).
3. Perform deep breathing and cough routine every 30 minutes of the patient's waking hours when the endotracheal tube is removed.
4. Administer $O_2$ by rebreathing mask at 4 to 6 L after endotracheal tube is removed. Titrate $P_{O_2}$ at 75 to 100 mm Hg and $P_{CO_2}$ at 35 to 45 mm Hg.
5. Perform intermittent positive pressure breathing (IPPB) with MA-I volume respirator or pressure respirator set at 20 cm pressure every 2 hours from 6 A.M. to 12 P.M. and every 3 hours from midnight to 6 A.M., using 20 ml acetylcysteine (Mucomyst) and 3 ml saline solution. After 24 hours, check for new IPPB orders.
6. Administer ultrasonic nebulization as needed to control thick secretions 10 minutes prior to IPPB therapy.
7. Turn the patient every 2 hours side to side. If lateral thoracotomy and pulmonary resection were performed, do not turn on unoperated side.
8. Connect chest tubes to 20 cm suction. Milk and strip tubes every 10 minutes or as needed for 4 hours, then every hour or as needed.
9. If the chest drainage measured over 400 ml total in first 4 hours, or if more than 150 ml drains in any 1 hour, contact principal practitioner.
10. Perform nasotracheal suction as indicated by poor cough, preferably after sedation.

### FLUIDS AND MONITORS

1. Give 1 L 5% dextrose in water every 12 hours (or a total of 2000 ml/24 hr), with 30 mEq of potassium chloride/L. Recheck this order after first electrolyte determination is made.
2. Keep central venous pressure (CVP) line open with administration of heparinized saline solution. If more than 500 ml is required in 24 hours, contact principal practitioner.
3. Keep arterial line open with heparinized saline solution and Travenol administration bag. If more than 500 ml is required in 24 hours, contact principal practitioner.
4. Give 1 unit whole fresh blood for each 500 ml chest drainage during first 24 hours.
5. Attach Foley catheter to overside drainage and obtain hourly measurements.
6. Connect ECG, CVP, arterial, pulmonary artery pressure (PAP), and left atrial pressure (LAP) monitors.

*Continued.*

## POSTOPERATIVE CARDIAC SURGERY ORDERS—cont'd

### VITAL SIGNS AND MONITORS

1. Check vital signs every 5 to 10 minutes during the first 2 hours; then if stable, check every 15 minutes for 4 hours, and if stable, every 30 minutes.
2. Notify principal practitioner if:

   Blood pressure above ________ or below ________ mm Hg
   Pulse above ________ or below ________ /min
   Respirations above ________ or below ________ /min
   Temperature above ________ or below ________ F
   CVP above ________ or below ________ cm $H_2O$ or mm Hg
   LAP above ________ or below ________ mm Hg
   PAP above ________ or below ________ mm Hg
   Wedge pressure above ________ or below ________ mm Hg
   Urinary output above ________ or below ________ ml/hr

   ECG abnormal
3. Perform neurologic check at least every 2 hours for the first 12 hours.
4. Evaluate pulse every hour for 12 hours, then every 4 hours.

### LABORATORY DATA

1. Check arterial gas concentrations 10 minutes after the patient is connected to MA-I volume respirator (or mask), then as needed under direction of principal practitioner until condition is stable.
2. Obtain hemoglobin and hematocrit determinations on arrival in unit. Repeat every 4 hours for 8 hours (or as needed), then check each morning before 7 A.M. for 5 days.
3. Evaluate electrolytes, blood urea nitrogen (BUN), and creatinine on arrival. Repeat in 8 hours or as needed, then in the morning before 7 A.M. for 5 days.
4. Obtain chest x-ray film 15 minutes after arrival in unit. Repeat in 8 hours, then daily before 7 A.M. until chest tube is out, and then as ordered.
5. Measure specific gravity and protein, sugar, and acetone concentrations in urine every 8 hours.
6. Obtain ECG daily for 5 days.
7. Evaluate cardiac enzymes on the third, fifth, and seventh postoperative days.
8. Check calcium, magnesium, and phosphorus levels on second postoperative day.
9. Complete postoperative cardiac surgery coagulation panel on arrival in unit.
10. Perform culture and sensitivity test of endotracheal tube secretions on removal of endotracheal tube.

### DIET

Give nothing orally for 24 hours, then allow the patient the full liquid bland diet for 12 hours. If this is well tolerated, progress to the soft select diet for 36 hours and then the select diet.

### OTHER

1. Elevate the head of bed 30 degrees. The upright position (if tolerated) is used for x-ray examination or eating.
2. Obtain daily weight measurements, using bed scales until tubes are out, then, if tolerated, using the standing scales.
3. Use elastic wraps from toes to groin. Rewrap as needed when wraps become loose or bind in popliteal space.
4. When possible, place antithromboembolic stockings (TED's) over elastic wraps.
5. Do not allow bending of bed or pillows under popliteal areas.
6. With nasogastric tube, if in place, perform low intermittent (gomco) suction. Irrigate every 2 hours with 30 ml gastrolyte solution.
7. Record *all* intake and output, including diaphoresis estimate, bowel elimination, vomitus, nasogastric output, all irrigations that do not return, and drainage from dressings.

**POSTOPERATIVE CARDIAC SURGERY ORDERS—cont'd**

**DRESSING AND WOUND CARE**

1. Clean all Foley, IV, and monitor line entrances daily or as needed, and apply antibiotic ointment.
2. If there is progressive drainage in dressings, call principal practitioner.
3. After practitioner performs first dressing removal, cleanse daily with Betadine and sterile saline solution, drying and reapplying dry sterile dressing until orders are received to leave open. Then cleanse and dry three times a day. If the patient is allergic to Betadine, use 3% hydrogen peroxide.

nician and to set in progress the recall of the complete team.

### ■ How much information does the critical care team need to have regarding the patient's surgery?

The unit staff is entitled to know all of the particulars of the procedures performed, and if necessary, diagram illustrations should be utilized for adequate explanation. The staff should be informed of any possible or potential complications that are expected by the surgeon so that pertinent signs and symptoms will be promptly recognized.

If there are any questions as to where certain monitors, tubes, or drains are located, this should be clarified immediately on the patient's arrival in the unit. Although this may seem rather basic, various cardiac teams place and connect monitoring devices and tubes differently. Those who have seen cases in which oxygen was connected to the nasogastric tube and suction to the nasal cannula can attest to the importance of the need for the proper identification of tubes, drains, catheters, etc.

### ■ What other immediate laboratory work is obtained?

When the first arterial gas determination is made, blood is drawn to evaluate hemoglobin concentrations, hematocrit, electrolyte levels, and, in diabetics, blood sugar levels.

If the patient has bled excessively and there is the possibility of coagulation defects, a coagulation screening test is obtained early, as there are certain portions of this test that require moderate time for completion. This test includes platelet counts, prothrombin, bleeding, and clotting times, fibrinogen levels, and evaluation for fibrin split products.

### ■ How often are the patient's vital signs checked and what are considered normal values?

When the patient first returns to the unit, the vital signs should be checked every 1 to 3 minutes until the patient's condition is stabilized, even though the patient may be connected to arterial pressure lines giving readouts and pressure curves. When the electrical readouts are stable, the vital signs can be checked every 5 minutes; however, monitor readouts of the arterial pressure, central venous pressure (CVP), and ECG are visualized continually.

The critical care unit staff is encouraged to evaluate the preoperative chart and anesthesia record in order to know what vital signs are expected with this patient; however, it is most helpful if the operating surgeon writes in the orders the vital sign parameters expected and what deviations merit notification. This is usually written in the manner shown in the boxed material on p. 234.

Although such detail may seem unnecessary, it is extremely important that certain patients not become hypertensive; others who have been chronically hypertensive might exhibit pressures that are normal for most but are inadequate for perfusion of their vital organs. Slower or more rapid heart rates and lower or higher than normal CVP's *are expected* in some patients; thus preliminary written communication can prompt necessary or eliminate unnecessary calls.

### ■ How important are minimum variations of normal vital signs?

Today it is easy for practitioners to disregard the simple standard evaluations of vital signs because of the sophisticated techniques of monitoring and the numerous laboratory determinations available. But the proper evaluation of vital signs correlated with physical findings can often yield a diagnosis more readily than the finest monitoring equipment or the most advanced laboratory tests.

A falling blood pressure below normal can be a reflection of pain and apprehension, CNS depression caused by oversedation, low output associated with varying arrhythmias, drug-induced peripheral vasodilatation, hypovolemia and impending shock, or low cardiac output for any one of many reasons (poor contractility as a result of infarction, cardiac tamponade, myocardial depression caused by medications, etc.).

Blood pressure elevation can be a sign of peripheral vasoconstriction, pain and apprehension, hypercapnia, CNS insult, or overzealous use of inotropic drugs.

Increases in pulse rate can be associated with hypovolemia, atrial or ventricular irritability, pain and apprehension, sepsis, or the use of any one of many medications.

Slowing of the pulse to under 60 can signify CNS involvement or partial or complete heart block, or it can reflect cardiac response to certain medications such as digitalis, procainamide hydrochloride (Pronestyl) or propranolol.

Temperature elevation in the very early postoperative period most often indicates some degree of atelectasis, but in the later postoperative phase this can be the result of wound or cavity infection, pulmonary embolization, certain medications, blood reactions, or even damage to the CNS. Persistent subnormal temperatures frequently occur when cooling procedures have been used during surgery, but they can also be indicative of CNS injuries, adrenal insufficiency, or early nonseptic shock.

Respiratory rates increase with pain, apprehension, fever, metabolic acidosis, and any form of sepsis.

Depressed respiration can occur with oversedation, extremely painful chest or abdominal incisions, and not infrequently as a result of certain anesthetic respiratory center depressants such as fentanyl-droperidol combinations (Innovar).

Marked variations of the aberrant vital signs just discussed can occur with any metabolic acid-base imbalances and should stimulate a methodical investigation. Careful observation of vital signs by critical care staff can frequently yield information relating to an established trend or an impending problem and allow correction before the reception of a computer analysis or laboratory test returns.

For example, if the pulse rate is slowed to around 50 beats/min without ECG evidence of heart block, the systolic blood pressure is above 170 mm Hg, and the temperature is subnormal, one could look immediately at the possible causes for these variances and come up with the probable etiology. The bradycardia could be caused from drug depression of the heart rate; however, if this is true, the blood pressure should not be elevated. The blood pressure can be elevated in cases of carbon dioxide retention (hypercapnia), but if this were true, the pulse rate should be more rapid. If sepsis or pain is the cause of the increased blood pressure, then again a rapid heart rate should be expected. Thus with the subnormal temperature one would suspect an overmedication effect (digitalization, etc.) or, more likely, CNS injury.

### ■ What volume of urine output is expected?

In most shock units the basic minimum of urine output per hour considered adequate to eliminate body waste and demonstrate perfusion of the kidneys averages around 20 ml/hr. For this reason most urine outputs are measured every hour for at least the first 24 to 36 hours postoperatively.

It is not uncommon for patients in the immediate postoperative period to produce large urine volumes as a result of IV colloid, blood, and other fluids coadministered with mannitol or furosemide (Lasix) during surgery.

Occasionally urinary outputs in the range of 13 to 15 ml/hr will be seen after mitral valve surgery, and yet the patient demonstrates no other signs of perfusion deficit or evidence of low cardiac output, and when given small doses of diuretic the urinary output increases respectively. This has been suspected to be the result of a pressure receptor in the left atrial wall that can stimulate the increased production of antidiuretic hormone. The left atrium is distended and tense in severe mitral valvular regurgitation or stenosis, but after correction of the stenosis or insufficiency the pressure is decreased and the body response can be similar to that in hypovolemia, with retention of fluids in an attempt to increase circulating volume. After the body has adjusted to the lower atrial pressures and the initial stress of surgery, there can be a diuretic phase occurring from 36 to 96 hours postoperatively.

Increased urinary outputs obtained on the second to fourth day after surgery are also not uncommon. This postoperative diuretic phase is associated with the reentry of the interstitial and other third-space fluids into the circulating volume and their subsequent elimination through the urinary system. In the past many practitioners attempted to replace this diuresis volume and encountered understandable overhydration complications; thus carefully titrated fluid replacement should be emphasized. The most important facet in this phase is to maintain a constant evaluation of the *electrolyte concentrations* in order that appropriate replacement may be undertaken.

Another important evaluation of the urine includes measurement of the amount of discoloration associated with hemolysis from the bypass procedure. This can result in a urine color comparable to a "vin rosé" and hopefully not a "Burgundy red" wine. If this discoloration occurs but does not begin to clear within a couple of hours after the operative procedure, there is the possibility of frank bleeding from the urinary system. This can be elevated and correlated with plasma and urine hemoglobin levels and microscopic evaluation of the urine for red blood cells.

The specific gravity of the urine is determined every 1 to 2 hours and aids in evaluating hydration, diuresis, renal function, and antidiuretic hormone activity. Sugar, acetone, and protein determinations are routinely obtained as for any intensive care surgical patient.

## ■ Which specific pulses should be evaluated and why?

Critical care practitioners as well as general ward personnel should be able to evaluate most of the major pulses in the body (Fig. 12-1). Radial and ulnar pulses are most accessible, easily palpated, and most familiar to bedside practitioners. It is extremely important to evaluate the upper extremity pulses when any aortic arch surgery has been performed or when catheters have been utilized previously. With experience this will provide a means of obtaining a palpatory blood pressure in individuals in whom it is difficult to place the cuff and where correlation with the monitors is necessary. These pulses, as well as the others to be described, should all be evaluated shortly after the patient arrives in the unit. Again, it should be stressed that occasionally the blood pressure palpated in the radial or ulnar artery can be lower in one arm than in the other if there is any proximal obstruction (subclavian artery stenosis or brachial artery narrowing from catheterization). These pulses can be absent or nonpalpable as a result of previous arteriotomies or use of monitoring catheters.

Femoral pulses are more often evaluated today; the importance of determining differences of intensity of one pulse as compared to the other is stressed. It is difficult, however, to palpate these pulses through the dressings or after groin incisions have been utilized for perfusion or harvesting of veins, but with simple, careful pressure this can be done without causing the patient too much discomfort. If there is any question as to the integrity of the lower extremity as demon-

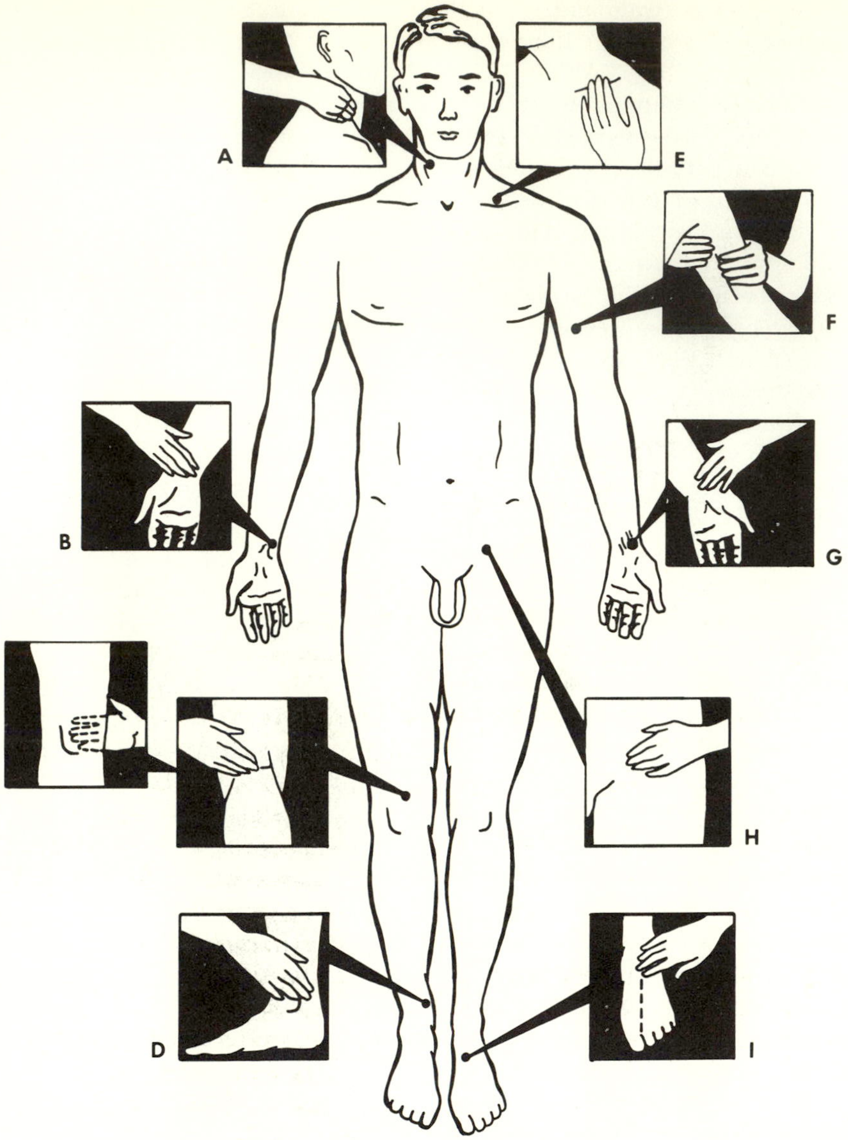


**Fig. 12-1.** Location of pulses. *A,* carotid; *B,* ulnar; *C,* popliteal; *D,* posterior tibial; *E,* subclavian; *F,* high brachial; *G,* radial; *H,* femoral; *I,* dorsalis pedis.

strated by color, pallor, blotchiness, pain, or motor function, the ability to simply determine the presence of a pulse is important, as well as to compare the intensity of an existing pulse to that recorded preoperatively.

The popliteal pulse reflects patency of the superficial femoral artery. Palpating this pulse requires experience and multiple rehearsals in the normal patient. It is best palpated by placing the right hand behind the popliteal space approaching from the medial aspect with the leg relaxed and in a normal anatomic position or minimally rotated externally; then gentle compressive pressure is applied until a pulse is obtained. Another technique is to compress the popliteal space with either one or both hands until resistance is noted from the fascial and bony structures and then to release the pressure slowly until a palpable pulse is noted. The right hand is utilized for evaluating the right popliteal pulse and the left hand is usually used to document the left popliteal pulse. Again, practice and experience are recommended for evaluation of these pulses.

The dorsalis pedis pulse is the pulse of the lower extremity and has been recently emphasized. It is the superficial continuation of the anterior tibial artery and is best located near the instep of the foot extending between the area of the second tarsometatarsal junction and coursing toward the interphalangeal web between the large and the second toe. A decrease or absence of this pulse frequently signifies an obstruction of the femoral artery or one or all of its branches.

The posterior tibial artery is best palpated by placing the fingers just posterior to the medial malleolus; it is somewhat more difficult to palpate than the dorsalis pedis pulse and again requires pressure to be applied until resistance from bone and fascia is encountered and then slowly released until the pulse is noted. In patients with increased fat pads, edema of the lower extremities, or any body structural abnormality, this pulse becomes very difficult to palpate. It reflects the status of the posterior tibial artery and/or more proximal vessels.

Careful evaluation of all of these pulses, but especially the last two described, is most important in the immediate postoperative phase, especially when the patient has been perfused through or is being monitored from one of the femoral arteries. Subsequent decrease or disappearance of these pulses without a drop in blood pressure can signify a possible remedial vascular obstruction, but a delay in detection can cause loss of limb or life. It is not uncommon for the pedal and tibial pulses to be present and the popliteal pulses to be weak or absent as a result of long-term obstruction of the superficial femoral artery and excellent collateralization from the deep femoral artery.

The practitioner should also be acquainted with the subclavian and brachial artery pulsations, as these can be used for evaluation when there are dressings or infusion lines at the wrists.

Occasionally palpated and noted by practitioners is a pulse located just anterior and slightly distal to the external or lateral malleolus. This pulse is palpable only 5% to 10% of the time, and it is called the external malleolar artery pulse. It is produced by a branch of the anterior tibial artery but can be dominantly formed from branches of the peroneal, the posterior tibial, or the anterior tibial artery singly or in combination. It is often present when the dorsalis pedis pulse is congenitally absent or small or in cases of long-term obstruction.

Carotid pulses should be easily located not only by professional personnel, but also by lay persons working in the hospital environment. It is well known that youth organizations such as the Brownies, Girl Scouts, Cub Scouts, and Boy Scouts are becoming well versed in the techniques of cardiopulmonary resuscitation and are aware of the presence of the femoral and carotid pulses. Disappearance of the carotid pulse after surgery can be associated with a major catastrophe such as cardiac arrest, aortic arch dissection, or acute occlusion of the common carotid vessels. Practitioners must be well aware of this pulsation point for use in the assessment of cardiopulmonary resuscitation measures. The carotid pulse is best located halfway between the clavicle and the base of the jaw (angle of the jaw) just anterior to the prominent sternocleidomastoid muscle.

It is highly recommended that ward, critical care, and operating room personnel become accustomed to evaluating these pulses on all patients admitted, so that when their evaluation is of critical necessity, these persons are prepared for the task.

## ■ How are the chest tubes managed postoperatively?

In transport and during most phases of postoperative care the chest tubes *are not clamped,* because if there is an air leak in one or the other part of the chest cavity and the tubes are clamped, no exit is available for the air, thus causing progressive collapse of the lung on the involved side with creation of tension pneumothorax. Eventually alteration of the cardiac output, arrhythmias, and death can occur. In addition, if the chest tubes are clamped for any period of time, the evacuation of blood or clots is impeded and could precipitate cardiac tamponade. Chest tubes should be clamped only when evaluation for leaks is necessary and when changing the chest suction bottles.

Once the patient has arrived from the operating room, the chest tubes should be evaluated to ensure that they are in an underwater trap (underwater seal). Suction should be applied at a pressure of 60 cm $H_2O$ for 15 to 20 seconds and then reduced to 20 cm $H_2O$.

There are multiple apparatuses utilized for applying suction to the chest tubes. The *Emerson* suction apparatus (Fig. 12-2), which operates by means of two large bottles connected to a suction machine that is portable and electrically powered, is quite easy to assemble and the fluid levels are easily visualized close up or at a distance. Suction can be increased or decreased continuously or intermittently with simple valve control. The *Pleur-evac* self-contained suction apparatus (Fig. 12-3) connects directly to wall suction and does not require any electricity for function. However, the maximum amount of suction is determined by the fluid levels in the various containers and cannot be altered without changing these volumes. The Pleur-evac apparatus is a disposable unit constructed so it can be placed at any level without fear of fluid backing up into the chest tubes.

The chest drainage is measured when the patient first arrives in the unit and at least every 5 minutes for the first few hours or until output has markedly decreased or is stable. After that period evaluations every 15 minutes are adequate (Fig. 12-4).

The chest tubes should be milked or

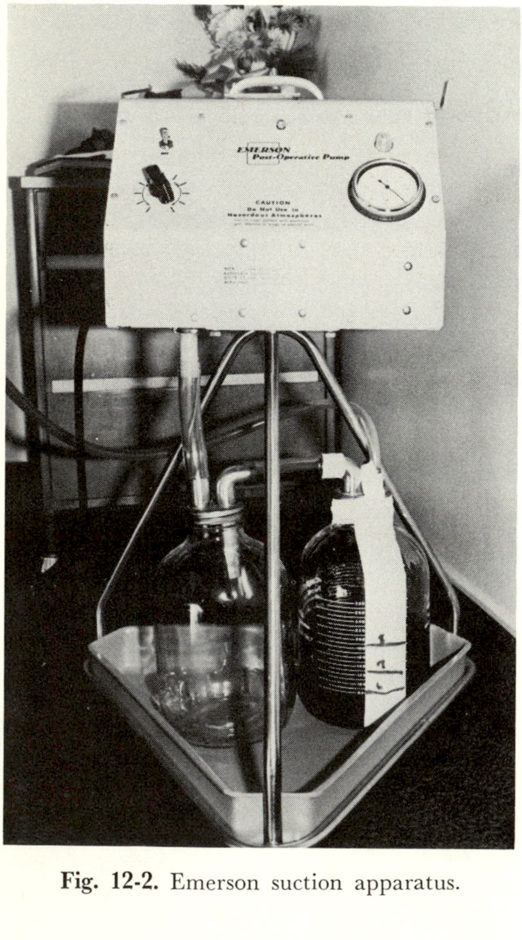


**Fig. 12-2.** Emerson suction apparatus.

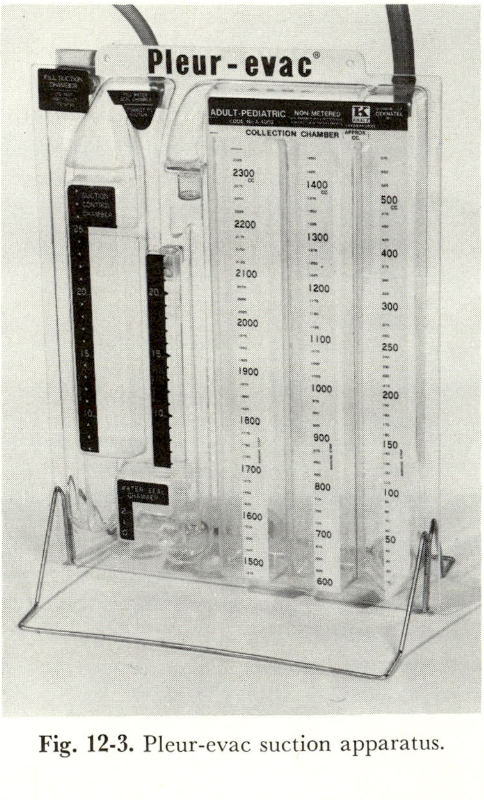


**Fig. 12-3.** Pleur-evac suction apparatus.

stripped whenever there are clots visible or whenever the tubes are completely free (suggesting that there might be intrathoracic clots). They should be stripped at least every 5 to 10 minutes for the first 2 hours, then the frequency should be decreased to not less than once every 30 minutes (Fig. 12-5).

Inspection of the continuity of the chest tubes to the connection with the suction bottles or disposable units should be performed frequently, as it is not uncommon for kinks or twists to develop and prevent needed drainage. Careful scrutiny of bulky chest dressings and chest films may be necessary to recognize kinks or twists at the chest wall or in the thoracic cavity.

Usually the chest tubes are stabilized in the operating room with nonabsorbable sutures and external dressings, but the critical care unit personnel must *ensure* this *stability* with additional tape and benzoin if necessary. All connections should be enforced with *nonporous* tape to prevent leakage.

The chest drainage is measured by using the standard attached scale on the bottles or chest apparatus or using a scale prepared by the critical care unit personnel (Fig. 12-4).

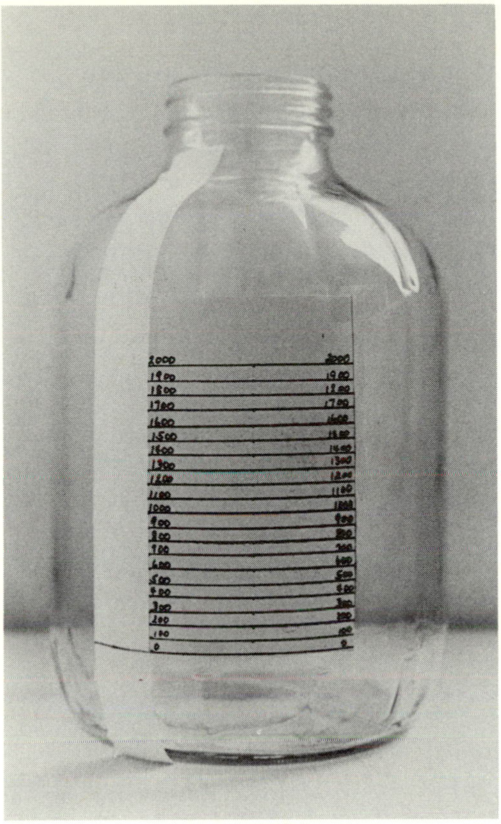

**Fig. 12-4.** Bottle used to measure chest drainage.

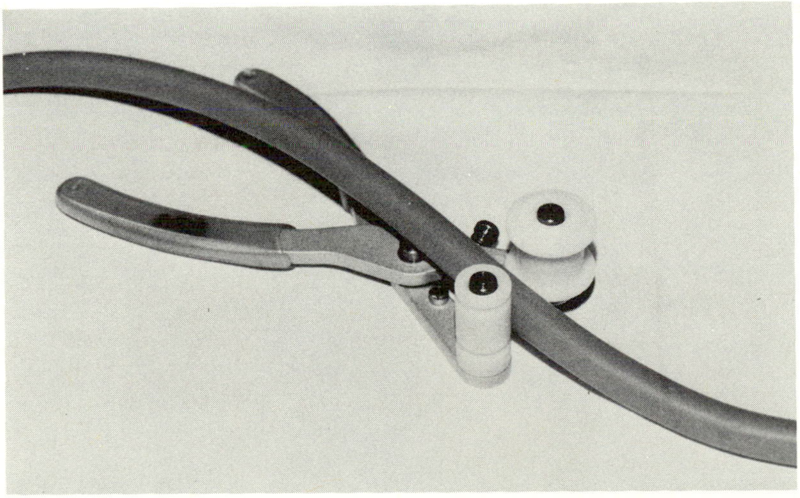

**Fig. 12-5.** Pilling's tube stripper. Hand tube stripper is designed for effectively milking tubes and conserving effort. (Courtesy Pilling Co., Los Angeles, Calif.)

Two chest tube clamps are kept with the suction apparatus for each tube exiting from the patient; if plastic tubes are placed, rubber or plastic covers on the jaws of these clamps should not be used. Again, the chest tubes are clamped only when examining for air leakage or when changing the suction apparatus.

## ■ What is the significance of bubbling or nonbubbling in the chest tubes?

Bubbling in the chest drainage bottles on suction suggests an air leak. The source can be the lung, the stab wound for the chest tubes, a nonairtight connection, or a crack or perforation in the drainage tubes.

Early lack of bubbling simply signifies that

A

B

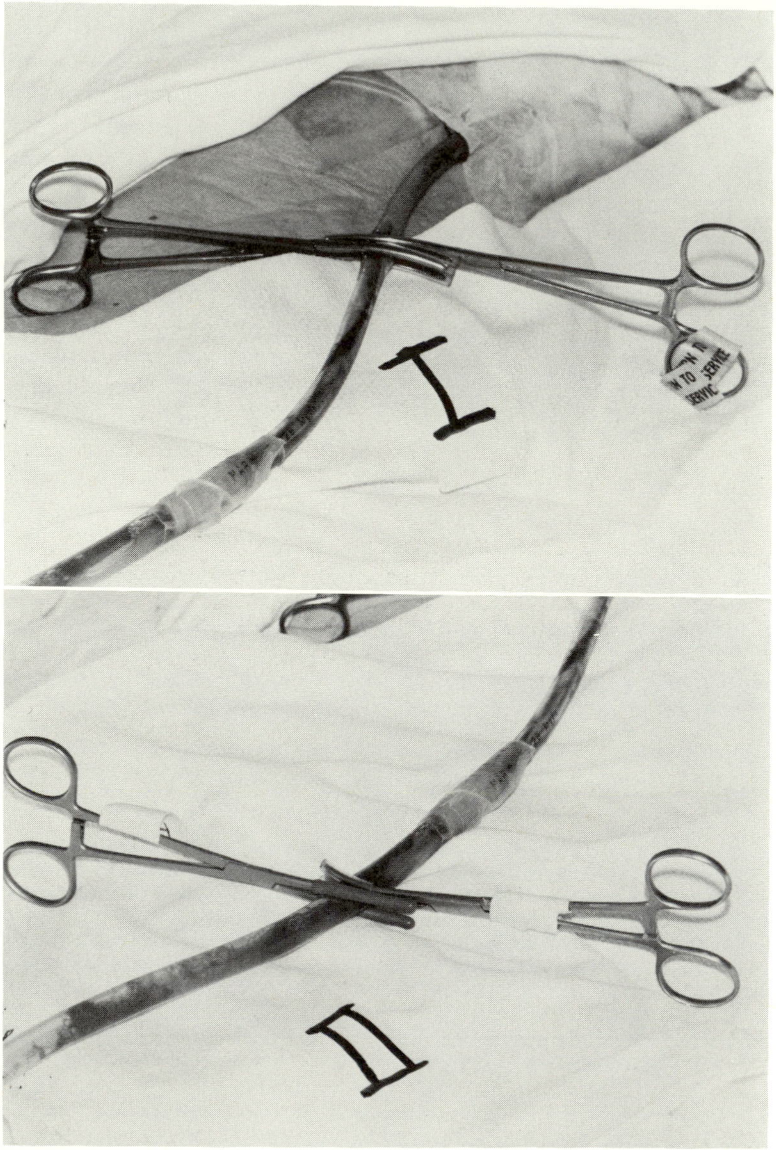


**Fig. 12-6.** Clamping of tubes. **A,** Tubes clamped adjacent to chest. **B,** Clamp placed beyond first connection. **C,** Tubes clamped above chest suction bottle. **D,** Composite of **A, B,** and **C.**

no pleural or lung violation occurred during the procedure and an airtight continuity of all tubes and connections exists. If some air leakage is expected by the surgeon or if bubbling abruptly stops, the tubes must be evaluated for *plugging clots.*

Any acute increase or decrease in bubbling should be reported immediately to the surgeon.

### ■ How are the chest tubes checked for leakage?

When a moderate amount of bubbling occurs in the chest bottles, a single clamping procedure can be performed for detection of air leaks. It is necessary to place *two* clamps across plastic tubes to adequately seal against leakage. These clamps should be placed at 180-degree angles from one an-

C

D

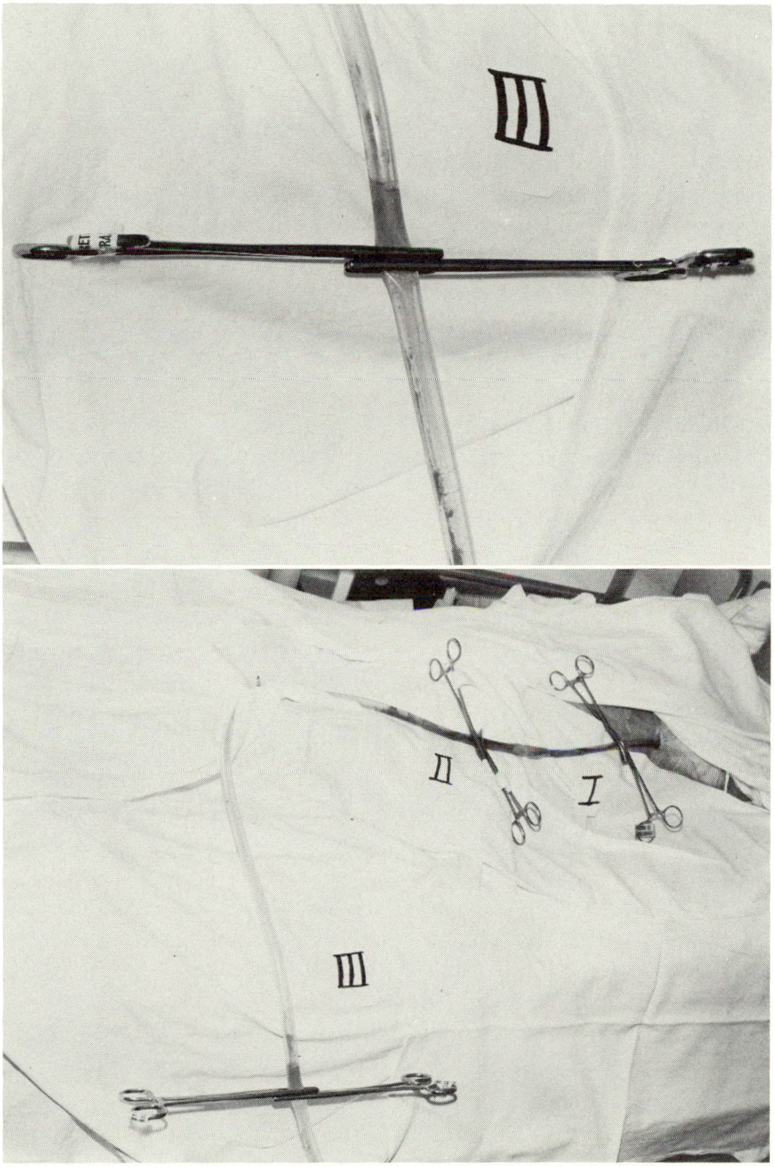


**Fig. 12-6, cont'd.** For legend see opposite page.

other, as demonstrated in Fig. 12-6. The tubes are first clamped just outside the chest cavity, and if bubbling decreases markedly or stops, the leakage is probably from the thoracic cavity. If bubbling continues, it suggests that the leakage is more distal, and the second clamping is performed just above the level where the tube is connected to the suction bottle; if bubbling stops at this time, it confirms a leak between the chest cavity and the bottles. The clamps can then be progressively reclamped proximally until the exact area of leakage is located. Bubbling continuing with this lowest clamping usually signifies the lack of an airtight seal at the tube-bottle connection. Critical care practitioners should be aware of this technique and should also be able to quickly set up a complete chest suction apparatus and tray for emergency tube thoracostomy.

## ■ When are the chest tubes removed and how?

When there are no further clots and minimum drainage, when bubbling has ceased, or when the chest tubes are plugged and the chest appears stable on x-ray film, the chest tubes are removed. In most cardiac cases this occurs between the first and third postoperative days.

Removal of the chest tubes usually requires one or two assistants, depending on the technique utilized. It is recommended that two assistants be available when there are two or more tubes and only one when a single tube is present.

The dressings are removed, any stabilizing sutures are cut, the chest wall around the chest tubes is sprayed with tincture of benzoin, and an encircling pursestring suture around the chest tube incision site (previously placed at surgery) is held taut. The chest suction is increased to 60 cm $H_2O$ (to hopefully suck back any air that might start to enter the chest cavity), and a double thickness 4 × 4 inch gauze sponge that has been partially divided is utilized to compress the skin around the chest tube to be removed. The tube is quickly withdrawn as the pursestring suture is cinched. The ties are completed, the redundant strands of the suture are cut, and firm tape is applied over the 4 × 4 inch gauze sponge that is being applied compressively to ensure against leakage.

If the tubes are connected to Y suction, the tubes are clamped prior to removal so that air entering the removed tube will not simply bypass the Y and go into the chest cavity through the remaining tube. The second and third tubes are removed in a similar manner, and the patient is reassured that the acute discomfort will be relieved within 1 or 2 minutes.

There is a great variance between practitioners as to whether or not the tubes are removed when the patient is inhaling or exhaling. Some utilize sterile petrolatum (Vaseline) gauze under the 4 × 4 inch gauze to seal the wound; however, petrolatum gauze can slip and allow a loss of purchase of skin and air can reenter.

## ■ How often does pneumothorax occur during chest tube removal and how is it treated?

Minimum pneumothorax occurs after removal of the chest tubes in approximately 3% to 4% of patients, and even then it is usually so minimal (<5%) that it does not require tube replacement.

After chest tube removal a chest x-ray film is immediately obtained; if a small pneumothorax is present, the patient is observed very carefully for any respiratory distress or change in vital signs, and a repeat chest x-ray film is obtained in 1 hour. If the chest appears to be stable over that hour period, another chest x-ray film is obtained in approximately 8 hours, and then a daily chest x-ray film is ordered. Simple pneumothorax, if not accompanied by an air leak, will resolve at a rate of 1% to 3% a day if under 10% and if the patient's condition is stable with no other complications.

If the pneumothorax produced by chest tube removal is 10% to 20% or more and the patient has a suspected air leak, borderline pulmonary functions, or CNS involvement, tube replacement and underwater seal should be instituted immediately.

■ **How is the arterial pressure monitored and what apparatus is utilized?**

The patient is monitored in the postoperative period by use of the intra-arterial line placed during surgery. This artery cannula is connected to an electronic measuring system by a transducer. The transducer is a small intricate electromanometer or electronic pressure sensor that converts mechanical pressure into electrical impulses that can be read on the bedside monitor by either an appropriately standardized and scaled arterial pulse wave or by direct readout (digital or sweep gauge).

Setting up and connecting this arterial pressure line with the transducer and monitor is one of the most intricate procedures performed in the immediate postoperative period and should be done only by a person experienced with this system, as it is not uncommon for the transducer to become flooded with blood or to leak. This apparatus is a vital measuring device used to assess the patient's cardiovascular status and must be accurate and functional at all times.

A quality electronic intra-arterial monitor and pressure transducer should be utilized. A pressure infuser with an intraflow filter irrigating device should be connected to the arterial line.

The saline solution in the 500 ml bag is heparinized with as much as 2500 units of aqueous heparin, because of the small volume of solution now required to irrigate the arterial line over a 24-hour period (seldom over 250 ml). Some units use a smaller concentration of heparin, but a larger volume of irrigating solution.

A major reason for utilizing arterial pressure lines, transducers, and electrical monitoring has been to reduce and eliminate the cuff errors found in patients with pressures below 90 mm Hg, as well as for the convenience and in order to observe the pulse pressure wave form.

■ **What complications or specific problems can be expected with the use of arterial monitors?**

Despite the excellent results obtained with electrical arterial monitoring devices, it cannot be overemphasized that this is an artificial unit that can fail and give inaccurate results and must be standardized and correlated frequently with cuff pressures.

Problems with plugging of the arterial line are prevented by frequent and appropriate irrigation. Small clots can be dislodged by forceful irrigation or by reinserting the metal stylet into the cannula, but these procedures can cause peripheral small artery occlusions. Troublesome bleeding around the incision site or the percutaneous puncture site can occur but is most often controlled by simple pressure and then a firm dressing (but the tape should encircle the wrist). The main pressure should be applied directly at the entrance site of the catheter. Whenever pressure dressings are applied, the area must be observed frequently for continued excessive bleeding or blanched ischemic areas indicating impending necrosis. The cannula and pressure tracings must be checked frequently to ensure continued intra-arterial positioning. Arterial cannula dislodgment occurs occasionally in very active or agitated patients, and the simple application of continued pressure over the site for 7 to 10 minutes is the recommended procedure followed by placement of a pressure dressing.

Any of the minor problems or complications just discussed might occur and indicate the need for notification of the principal practitioner.

Accurate records should be kept of the amount of blood withdrawn or discarded each time samples are obtained for the evaluation of arterial gases or electrolytes, as this can contribute to the continual hemoglobin concentration and hematocrit drop in a patient requiring frequent determinations. This blood in critical cases can be immediately readministered to the patient, but otherwise this is not recommended. Also, the lines from the patient to the withdrawing syringe can be shortened, therefore decreasing the amount of withdrawn blood to be discarded.

In withdrawing samples for coagulation screens or for bleeding and clotting studies, the blood should be obtained from a separate vein puncture or a source not potentially contaminated with heparin, as this can give abnormal results and prolong recovery.

Arterial cannulas are removed between the first and third days, depending on the stability of the patient's condition. On removal, all stabilizing sutures are cut and carefully removed, and the cannula is withdrawn, with steady pressure being applied directly over the percutaneous or incision puncture sites. This pressure is applied for a minimum of 7 to 10 minutes followed by placement of a nonencircling pressure dressing.

### ■ What is normal for CVP readings and what does this reflect?

The CVP line is placed in one of the peripheral veins and manipulated up toward the inferior or superior vena cava or right atrium. CVP is a fair reflection of the competency of the pumping mechanism of the heart and a guide to blood volume replacement. The normal values are from 6 to 15 cm $H_2O$.

A line is connected from the patient through one of the usual CVP measuring devices or is connected to a transducer and subsequently to a sophisticated electrical monitor with either digital or calibrated CVP wave readout. It is wise to connect to a manual CVP measuring device in addition to the transducer monitor, as this low pressure system reliability is labile and requires frequent checks.

Fluid is infused in the CVP line continually by slow drip, again with a pressure bag apparatus or with an electrically controlled Ivac fluid administration unit. Because of the usual higher doses of fluid given through the CVP catheter, the solution is heparinized with only 1000 units of heparin/500 ml of fluid. With the larger volumes of fluid given through the CVP line, if larger doses of heparin were used in the irrigation solution, bleeding problems could occur. CVP and atrial pressure measurements should be conducted with the patient supine and the zero point located at the midpoint of the right atrium, usually considered the midaxillary line or half the distance between the front and back of the chest. CVP should be measured with the patient on and off the respirator, and fluctuating and mean pressures not associated with respiration should be noted.

Most practitioners want to be notified whenever the CVP exceeds the 15 to 20 cm $H_2O$ mark or drops below 4 cm $H_2O$.

The complications or problems with CVP lines are similar to those of arterial lines, with bleeding around the puncture or incision site (especially after removal), intermittent plugging of the line, or dampened readings as a result of clot formation at the tip of the cannula. Inappropriate measurements are reflected by low pressure variations on inspiration and expiration and may signify a kinked, bent, partially plugged, or even misplaced line. The CVP line can inadvertently follow an alternate route and end up in the venous tributaries of the neck or leg during initial placement in surgery. When placed in deep veins, these lines are easily stabilized with an encircling stitch around the vein branch in which it has been placed, and on removal of the catheter, steady, even tension is applied to prevent fracture of the line with possible dislodgment and pulmonary embolization of the plastic remnant. All of these lines or cannulas should be carefully inspected on removal, and it is recommended that only radiopaque CVP lines be used so correct placement and, if necessary, embolization sites can be determined by x-ray examination.

CVP line removal also requires the application of pressure until the "ooze" has stopped. Where the CVP line has been placed in the arm, it is quite simple to apply a minor pressure dressing; however, when the CVP line has been placed in the groin, it not uncommonly requires a groin pressure dressing as previously described (Chapter 10 and Fig. 10-1).

### ■ What is the left atrial pressure and how does it differ from the CVP?

The left atrial pressure (LAP) line is placed by suturing a small cannula into the left atrium and bringing it out through a separate stab incision in the chest wall. The line can be cared for and the pressure monitored in a manner similar to that described for the CVP line.

LAP is a more accurate assessment of the circulating volume and the functional capacity of the left ventricle to handle volume load, with normal measurements ranging from 8 to 18 cm $H_2O$. Of consequence are readings below 5 cm $H_2O$ and those above 25 cm $H_2O$. When pressures approach 30 cm $H_2O$, signs of pulmonary edema are not infrequently seen; these will almost always be manifest with pressures above 35 cm $H_2O$.

Accidental dislodgment of the cannula requires the simple application of pressure over the percutaneous or stab wound site. The same problems occur with this line as with the CVP line except that it is somewhat more difficult to maintain in place during the immediate closing of the chest and mediastinum. Atrial tears, inability of removal, or arterial embolization of the catheter are conceivable complications.

The LAP line is in the left side of the heart, and with irrigating procedures the introduction of small amounts of air or clot can result in complications from arterial embolizations to the coronary arteries, brain, or peripheral vessels.

The use of this catheter in some institutions has also been described postoperatively for dye injections and x-ray visualization of the mitral valve or its replacement, as well as for evaluation of cardiac output by injection of indicator dyes. This usually requires a somewhat larger cannula than is required for simple LAP monitoring.

## ■ What is the Swan-Ganz catheter and how is it used with reference to the CVP and arterial pressures?

The Swan-Ganz catheter is a No. 5 or 7 French balloon-tipped catheter used for measuring the pulmonary artery pressure (PAP) as well as the pulmonary artery wedge pressure. The direct measurement of the PAP can be obtained and reflects left heart function, which may indicate intrapulmonary congestion and/or blockage.

The pulmonary artery wedge pressure is obtained by advancing the catheter into one of the peripheral branches of the pulmonary artery and inflating the balloon tip for a reflection of the LAP. Pulmonary artery gas concentrations can also be obtained from this cannula for comparison with the arterial gas concentrations. Since these are *venous* gases, they should never be confused with arterial blood gas concentrations.

The Swan-Ganz catheter is usually inserted into either the basilic or cephalic vein at the elbow (other veins can be utilized when necessary) and floated by means of the balloon tip through the major veins into the right atrium and then by the tricuspid valve into the right ventricles (similar to the pathway of a transvenous electrode). It is then carefully manipulated out into the pulmonary artery. The determination of catheter tip position when placed in the operating room and in the ward is on the basis of visualized pressure tracings on the connected monitor during manipulation. It can then be advanced into a peripheral pulmonary artery branch, wedged appropriately with the balloon partially inflated, and thus give a wedge pressure tracing. Deflation of the balloon, depending on the placement of the catheter, can give a PAP measurement. Again, its placement is determined on the oscilloscope or monitoring device by the pressure waves and tracings. The normal values obtained are shown in Table 12-1.

**Table 12-1.** Normal values for right ventricle, pulmonary artery, and pulmonary artery wedge pressure*

| | *Normal values (mm Hg)* Average | *Normal values (mm Hg)* Range |
|---|---|---|
| Right ventricle pressure | | |
| Peak systolic | 25 | 17-32 |
| End diastolic | 4 | 1-7 |
| Pulmonary artery pressure | | |
| Mean | 15 | 9-19 |
| Peak systolic | 25 | 17-32 |
| End diastolic | 9 | 4-13 |
| Pulmonary artery wedge pressure | | |
| Mean | 9 | 4.5-13 |

*Modified from Yang, S. S., Bentivoglio, L. G., Maranhao, V., and Goldberg, H.: Cardiac catheterization data to hemodynamic parameters, Philadelphia, 1972, F. A. Davis Co.

The care of this catheter requires irrigation and continuous infusion with solutions similar to those used with a venous line. Complications include catheter plugging, dampening, perforation of the pulmonary artery or its branches, and thrombosis of a peripheral vein. This catheter can bend back on itself, withdraw into the right ventricle, or occasionally even entwine and form an intracardiac knot. Another infrequent but possible complication includes rupture of the balloon with dissemination of small fragments into the pulmonary vascular tree.

The Swan-Ganz catheter is placed by the cardiologist when physiologic cardiac measurements are required, and the procedure of removal is similar to that used with CVP lines.

The original discouragement with the use of this cannula was associated with the intricate mechanism necessary to maintain patency and obtain readings; however, these procedures have been simplified in the past few years. Experienced maintenance and critical care personnel must be available in the hospital or on an immediate "on call" basis for any problems that might arise with the intricate monitoring setups. Responsibility rests with the critical care unit practitioner and electrical engineer to maintain appropriate function. Critical care personnel must learn by repetitive practical experience how to handle the original setting up and any problems that might arise. Reference protocols must be readily available and spelled out in great but simplified detail, for if these systems fail and cannot be restored to normal function, the patient's life could be in jeopardy.

## ■ What routine laboratory work is obtained?

Electrolyte determinations should be made immediately after the patient arrives; if normal, these are thereafter obtained daily, with the exception of potassium. If there are any arrhythmia problems, if there is moderate urinary output, or if the original potassium concentration was abnormal, repeat potassium levels are obtained every 4 hours until the level is stable, and then daily thereafter.

In cases where the use of a nephrotoxic drug such as gentamicin sulfate (Garamycin) is necessary, the blood urea nitrogen (BUN) and creatinine tests are also run daily. If the levels of these substances increase at any time, the use of the nephrotoxic drug is decreased or discontinued.

Hemoglobin and hematocrit levels are obtained initially, then every 4 to 6 hours until they are relatively stable, and then daily.

Arterial gas concentrations are obtained as needed to titrate the patient's initial respiratory needs, but once the patient's pulmonary status is stable and the arterial cannula is removed, arterial gas evaluations are not usually necessary. If the need again arises, the opposite radial, brachial, or femoral artery can be used. Whenever an arterial gas measurement is obtained, pressure is applied over the puncture sites and a pressure dressing placed for a period of 1 to 2 hours.

## ■ What abnormal laboratory tests are of major concern?

Potassium is the cation of major concern, because hypokalemia can lead to dangerous arrhythmias, especially with concomitant digitalis administration. When arrhythmias persist even in the presence of low normal potassium concentrations, the patient will be given a continuous IV drip solution containing potassium, as it has been well documented that in the immediate postoperative period the patient can have high serum potassium levels with low intracellular potassium concentrations. Hyperkalemia occurs less often, but when recognized, no potassium supplements are given; if renal failure is suggested, a means of decreasing the levels can be instituted.

The sodium levels can drop with excessive diuresis, moderate diaphoresis, or when salt replacement is withheld. Daily and continuous decrease in the serum sodium concentration is seen in the patient who retains water, but most clinicians are not concerned until the sodium level drops below 125 mEq/L, and then careful replacement and/or diuresis is needed. A regular full diet appears to be the single most important factor in rebalancing electrolyte concentrations; thus it is necessary to place the patient on a full oral regimen as soon as it is safe.

The chloride concentration can drop with the overzealous administration of nonelectrolyte solutions and also with excessive nasogastric suction. This can be replaced with a number of the commercial IV solutions available, but cessation of suction and institution of oral intake are again essential.

The BUN and creatinine levels are of major concern when elevated in a patient who is not bleeding or dehydrated, especially if nephrotoxic agents are being administered or if any abnormalities of urinary output are present. If these two factors progressively increase with increasing potassium levels or poor response to diuresis, a nephrologist should be consulted for evaluation of early renal failure.

Blood is not administered after the second postoperative day if the patient appears to be stable and if the hemoglobin concentration and hematocrit stay above 10 g/100 ml and 30%, respectively. If these measurements continue to drop without evidence of retained fluids or overhydration, blood is administered in the form of packed cells (to decrease the incidence of hepatitis and prevent added volume load). The point at which blood is added is arbitrary, and in some patients with specific religious convictions blood and blood derivatives are refused. It is not uncommon to see the condition of these individuals finally stabilize with a hemoglobin concentration of 6 or 7 g/100 ml and a hematocrit of 18% to 21%. This leaves the attending practitioner uneasy, as these low levels narrow the time available for any successful emergency resuscitation when the oxygen-carrying capacity is markedly decreased. Total body healing is probably slower and resistance to infection poorer with low red cell and hemoglobin counts. On reviewing the cases occurring in volume in some institutions, the nonuse of blood probably carries a higher morbidity and mortality among cardiac patients.

### ■ What additional laboratory tests are performed and why?

Daily cardiac enzyme tests are performed starting on the first or second postoperative day, even though it is common for most of these values to be elevated in the immediate postoperative period. This is especially true when vents and pursestring sutures have been placed in the left ventricle. If the concentrations of these enzymes remain markedly elevated over the fifth to seventh days with abnormal ECG's, infarction is considered, and if established, the patient is treated as for acute myocardial infarction with extended care in the unit. The cardiac enzymes can be elevated in conditions other than acute myocardial infarction; therefore the combinations, times, and duration of elevations are important in substantiating postoperatve infarction. The serum glutamic-oxaloacetic transaminase (SGOT), hydroxybutyric dehydrogenase (HBD), and lactic dehydrogenase (LDH) levels are all usually elevated in myocardial infarction at varying times, but they are also frequently elevated in acute liver damage such as hepatitis, hepatic drug injury, and even passive congestion. They are even moderately elevated in other muscle cell damage situations such as burns, crushing injuries, and IM injections. They can all be elevated in ischemia or infarction of the kidney, spleen, or bowel. The HBD and LDH levels can be moderately elevated even when red blood cell hemolysis occurs as a result of using the pump, but this is not usually true of the SGOT level. The creatinine phosphokinase (CPK) concentration, on the other hand, is elevated more in acute muscle injury (as in acute myocardial infarction), but also in dermatomyositis and muscular dystrophy. With computations of times, degree, and combination of elevations a fairly substantial determination of infarction can be established. More specific assessment of myocardial damage can be made with the use of the CPK and LDH *isoenzymes*. Isoenzymes are multiple molecular forms of a particular enzyme that differ in certain physiochemical properties such as electrophoretic mobility. The organ specificity of the various isoenzymes allows detection of myocardial damage even in the presence of active disease in other organs.

Daily albumin and globulin studies are occasionally run starting on the second postoperative day, when the hemoglobin and hematocrit levels continue to drop in association with a blanket lowering of the electrolyte, BUN, and creatinine levels with normal or low specific gravity. Usually after the second postoperative day the albumin and globulin levels remain stable (if whole blood or albumin has not been administered recently) and can be used as an indication of the patient's hydration. Evaluation of all these factors along with the daily weight of the patient can decrease the unnecessary administration of more electrolyte solutions or blood and possibly fluid restriction or diuresis.

ECG's are run daily; there is, however, the need for more emphasis on ECG interpretation.

Daily chest x-ray films are usually obtained until the patient leaves the critical care unit to evaluate adequacy of chest drainage and rule out any residual atelectasis, fluid, or pneumothorax. During endotracheal intubation a major value of the chest x-ray film is to establish tube placement and ensure against blockage of a mainstem bronchus. Chest x-ray film evaluation by all critical care members is encouraged, and immediate reading by the surgeon or radiologist with written interpretation is imperative and is the responsibilty of the nursing personnel.

Calcium, phosphorus, and magnesium levels are obtained on the fourth or fifth day and appropriate administration performed when low levels are found. If there is any suggestion of parathyroid disease or malnutrition, these studies are obtained sooner and repeated more frequently.

## POSTOPERATIVE VENTILATION

In the past 10 years better mechanical respirators, frequent use of arterial gas determinations, and coordination of intensive care nursing and respiratory therapy teams have influenced the marked decrease in postoperative morbidity and mortality.

### ■ Who is responsible for the respiratory care of the patient?

The primary responsibility still rests with the operating surgeon, but there are times when this responsibility may be shared with the cardiologist and/or the pulmonary internist.

Equally as important in the coordinated care of the patient's pulmonary needs are nursing and respiratory services. With the continued subspecialization and training of respiratory therapists, minor conflicts occasionally develop as to the areas of responsibility. Regardless of designated duties of subspecialty departments, the unit practitioner is the overseer of all aspects of the patient's care, and if the mechanical manipulation and management of the respiratory assistance devices are under the auspices of the respiratory therapy department, the nursing staff must be aware of any changes of the inhalation modalities, gas concentrations, or volumes. The unit practitioner *must* be familiar with the respiratory equipment, and it is the responsibility of the respiratory therapy department as well as the nursing supervisors to guarantee familiarity with each apparatus used. I recommend the continued education of respiratory and nursing personnel in an integrated, coordinated program.

### ■ What are some of the specifics regarding the use of endotracheal tubes?

Endotracheal tubes are usually left in place after the operative procedure until the patient is fully responsive and able to appropriately cough on demand. The purpose of the endotracheal tube is to establish a means for adequate assisted or controlled respiration in the sedated patient during the immediate postoperative period when a decreased effort in breathing and a lower workload for the heart are sought.

Endotracheal tubes are usually equipped with adaptors that easily and quickly fit the majority of mechanical respirators, but there must be an absolute *guarantee* that all connectors will appropriately connect. It is essential to have equipment with universal connectors.

Immediately on reaching the unit, the patient is suctioned, the airway cleared, then connection is made to a mechanical respirator after ventilation with an oxygen-supplied Ambu bag operated by the anesthesiologist is discontinued.

The endotracheal tube should be suctioned and cleared of secretions on an "as needed" basis and at least every half hour, even if retained secretions are not suspected. Suction should not be applied for more than 25 to 30 seconds at a time. This is the average time a healthy person can comfortably hold the breath.

A sterile catheter is utilized each and every time the patient is suctioned, and sterile gloves are worn. Respiratory precautions are used in any patient who has had a prosthetic valve placed.

A chest x-ray film should be obtained using a portable machine after arrival in the unit in order to evaluate expansion of the lung, detect the presence of atelectasis, and determine placement of the endotracheal tube. Interpretation of the x-ray film may be shared with the entire critical care team. Once the x-ray film has been obtained and the postitioning of the endotracheal tube appears to be satisfactory, appropriate restabilization of the tube is accomplished.

The mechanically ventilated patient's oxygen administration should be titrated according to the results of serial blood gas measurements. Chest auscultation should be utilized by critical care personnel as the patient's ventilatory status is evaluated. Visual observation of the patient cannot be overemphasized, since decreased chest excursion may indicate inadequate ventilation.

### ■ What can be done to help the patient tolerate the endotracheal tube?

During the trip from the operating room to the unit the patient is often manually hyperventilated, which decreases carbon dioxide and any hypercapnic drive toward spontaneous respiration. In addition, any low metabolic pH is corrected in the last few minutes of the operation with IV sodium bicarbonate, and this decreases respiratory drive from metabolic acidosis. The 100% $O_2$ used until the first blood gas determinations are obtained decreases the hypoxemic drive to respiration. If all these measures are not adequate to prevent the patient from fighting the respirator or to allow spontaneous control, then the IV use of morphine sulfate is advantageous. The usual dose of IV morphine sulfate is 3 to 5 mg (1/20 to 1/12 grain) initially, followed by 1 to 3 mg/hr as needed to decrease agitation from the endotracheal tube. IV morphine sulfate used in this manner usually does not exhibit myocardial depressive action and usually alleviates pain without severely depressing normal respiration.

Intubated patients may need extra relaxation for respiratory control, and *d*-tubocurarine, gallamine triethiodide, and/or succinylcholine (Anectine) can be utilized in a repeated dosage or by titrated continuous IV drip. With the use of these paralyzing agents the patient must be under absolutely constant observation by the unit practitioners, as accidental disconnection can result in respiratory fatality.

Occasionally the IV administration of 5 to 10 mg of diazepam (Valium) may be useful in readjusting respiratory control or assistance. However, as in the use of all such drugs, careful and slow administration must be used, and at the same time the patient must be observed carefully for any hypotensive episodes.

### ■ What medications are used with respirator nebulizers?

Often only simple saline nebulization is used, but in patients with thick, difficult-to-suction secretions mucolytic agents are added every 4 to 6 hours. Acetylcysteine (Mucomyst), 0.25 to 0.5 ml, is mixed with 3 ml of saline solution, but once excessive secretions are obtained, the mucolytic agents are stopped. Another mucolytic agent is pancreatic dornase (Dornavac), usually given in dosages of 100,000 units every 4 to 6 hours.

Nausea can occur with use of acetylcysteine, especially in patients who cannot usually tolerate the odor of hard-boiled eggs, and an occasional case of bronchospasm may be attributed to an allergic response to a specific mucolytic agent, that is, pancreatic dornase.

Isoetharine-phenylephrine (Bronkosol-2) and isoproterenol (Isuprel) combinations are usually avoided in the immediate postoperative period unless absolutely necessary (for bronchospastic problems, etc.), as they can potentiate cardiac arrhythmias. When absolutely necessary, they are used in minute dosages, such as 4 to 10 drops mixed with 3 to 4 ml of saline solution.

Nebulized antibiotics are not rewarding, are possibly associated with complications (such as allergies and resistance of bacteria), and are seldom used.

### ■ Why is endotracheal intubation preferred over tracheostomy in cardiac surgical patients?

The endotracheal tube placed during the operative procedure can simply be left in place in the immediate postoperative period, whereas the continuity of tracheal secretions from a tracheostomy into the mediastinum (midsternotomy incisions, etc.) is subject to the dangers of infection, mediastinitis, sternal disruption, and even death.

An endotracheal tube can be more easily manipulated with respect to placement in the trachea and can safely be left in place for a period of 36 hours or less, but seldom over 3 to 4 days.

If prolonged ventilation becomes necessary or if there are mechanical reasons why nasotracheal or oral tracheal intubation cannot be instituted or continued, tracheostomy becomes a necessity. After multiple days of endotracheal intubation, complications such as late tracheal stenosis, erosion with hemorrhage, and inappropriate cord function are more apt to occur. During endotracheal intubation the patient cannot talk, and thus valuable communication is prevented.

Bilateral cord paralysis following aortic arch and thoracic aortic surgeries have been reported, and in such cases tracheostomy also becomes a necessity. It can be said that tracheostomy is usually performed as a last resort or when the endotracheal tube has been utilized beyond its safe period.

### ■ What complications can occur during the routine care of endotracheal tubes and how are they controlled?

The irritation and agitation of the patient produced by the endotracheal tube has previously been described, and this is usually controlled with appropriate sedation and relaxation.

Occasionally thick mucous secretions will partially occlude the end of the endotracheal tube; this manifests the need for increased ventilation volumes and is evidenced by difficulty in passing the suction catheters. Total obstruction of the end of the endotracheal tube can occur, causing cyanosis, severe agitation, and inability to breathe or obtain ventilation. The lack of chest excursion, the inability to pass the suctioning catheter, and severe patient distress command the immediate removal of the endotracheal tube. If an error has been made and the tube is not blocked, the tube can be replaced or the patient can be ventilated by mask and oral airway until help arrives. Occlusion of the end of the endotracheal tube has occurred with overinflation of a balloon cuff, producing similar findings; simple deflation of the cuff will usually remedy the situation.

Displacement of the endotracheal tube below the carina into one of the major bronchi can easily occur and result in obstruction of the remaining bronchus and total atelectasis of that lung. The endotracheal tube should be marked with india ink or at the lip level after the first x-ray film is taken, so that advancement can be recognized. Failure of chest excursion to occur or evidence of decreased breath sounds on one side is suggestive, but x-ray films provide confirmative proof.

Active bleeding can occur as a result of irritation of the endotracheal tube and repeated suctioning. This bleeding requires repeated irrigation of the endotracheal tube with saline solution followed by frequent suctioning; evaluation and supervision by the principal practitioner is paramount.

The majority of the complications resulting from the use of the endotracheal tube can be eliminated by alertness and frequent evaluation of the patient's respiratory status by the entire team, especially the nursing and respiratory team members.

### ■ When is the endotracheal tube removed and are there any special techniques to follow?

Extubation is performed at some time within the first 12 hours after surgery, but the time of removal depends on the patient's alertness and the overall general respiratory status as confirmed by arterial gas determinations. When possible, it is best to extubate the patient before 8:00 P.M. so that if minor problems develop they will not develop during the 11:00 P.M. to 7:00 A.M. shift.

The T tube connection, an apparatus for the patient to breathe humidified oxygen off the respirator at concentrations of 40% or 70%, is connected to the patient, and after 10 to 15 minutes an arterial gas determination is obtained. If blood gas concentrations are adequate and the patient is fully awake, the cuff is deflated and the endotracheal tube is removed after the tube and posterior pharynx have been suctioned. This is performed when the patient is exhaling to prevent inhalation of any mucus plugs connected to or in the end of the tube. A large mucus accumulation in the posterior pharynx or trachea is almost always present and must be immediately suctioned or coughed out. It is wise to have tissues ready.

A firm-fitting facial or rebreathing mask is then placed on the patient to deliver oxygen at the same concentration that was used with the T connection. After 10 minutes an additional arterial gas determination is obtained. From this point the patient undergoes titration with arterial gases until stable and until the right concentrations of oxygen and humidity are being used to maintain an arterial $P_{O_2}$ of 80 to 95 mm Hg, a $P_{CO_2}$ of 35 to 40 mm Hg, a pH of 7.35 to 7.45, and an oxygen saturation near 90%. If there is any question of agitation or unavoidable hypoventilation, the patient is reintubated. It is much better to reintubate within a short time after extubation than to wait until the patient is having respiratory difficulties (possibly at 2:00 to 3:00 A.M.).

### ■ What are the ventilation and respiratory care recommendations once the endotracheal tube has been removed?

If the patient's respiratory drive (excursion) is poor using the tight-fitting mask (30% to 40% $O_2$), a rebreathing mask is substituted with similar $O_2$ concentration but with the patient's own exhaled $CO_2$ and moisture. Humidified oxygen is used to prevent drying of secretions.

Instructions are given to frequently breathe deeply and cough at least every 30 to 60 minutes. For this the patient is placed in an upright sitting position utilizing folded pillows. An alternate method would be to have the patient stand while an intensive care staff member provides support to splint or brace the anterior chest wall, decreasing pain and allowing a better cough.

Inhalation therapy treatments using either the mask or the oral tube are administered every 2 hours for the first 12 to 18 hours after removal of the endotracheal tube. The frequency is reduced to every 4 hours or four times a day, depending on the x-ray findings, patient cooperation, and arterial gas concentrations.

Patients who cough poorly, show evidence of retained secretions, and have difficulty in cooperating or utilizing inhalation therapy properly may require appropriate nasotracheal suction. This can be performed in various ways; however, it is recommended that a sterile catheter be carefully passed through the nose and down to the glottic area. The patient's tongue is grasped with a clean sponge and pulled forward. The patient is then asked to inhale, and as he does so, the tube is gently passed down to or beyond the cords, which most often stimulates a cough. Occasionally the tube can actually be passed into the tracheal or bronchial area

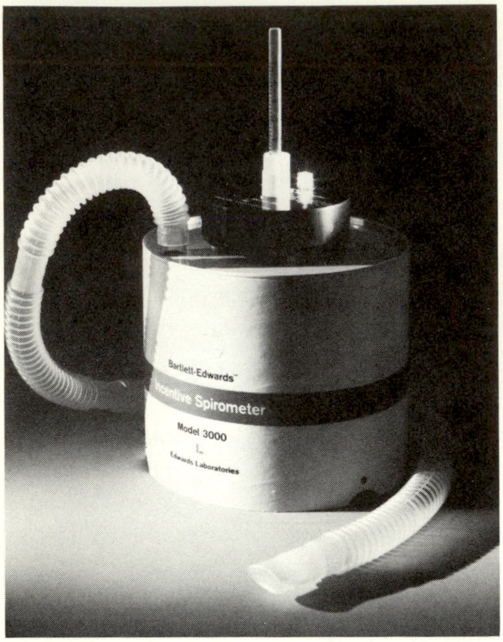

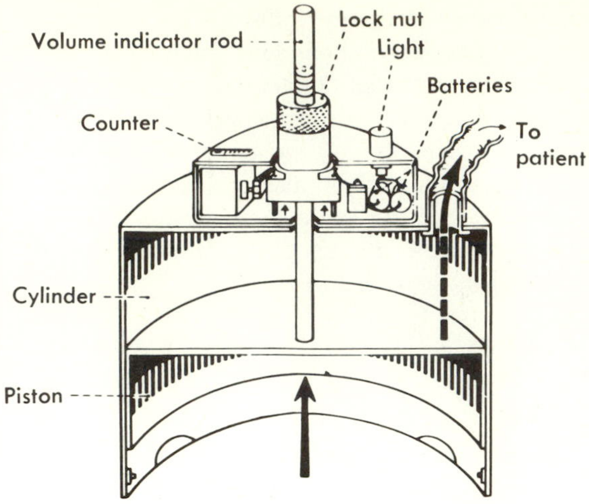


**Fig. 12-7.** Bartlett-Edwards incentive spirometer.

with aspiration of heavy mucus secretions. The points of pulling out the tongue and having the patient take a deep breath are essential to placement of the tube. Turning the head opposite to the bronchus to be aspirated has been recommended in many articles; however, probably more important is manipulation of the tip of the catheter toward the bronchus to be aspirated.

It is extremely difficult to utilize nasotracheal suction in patients with accentuated gag and vomit reflexes, and it may become necessary to loosen secretions by instituting careful but definitive postural drainage techniques. Patients with sternotomy incisions can tolerate these procedures surprisingly well.

An additional pulmonary modality is the Bartlett-Edwards incentive spirometer.* This apparatus is constructed in such a way as to stimulate the patient to take progressively increased deep breaths and thus inflate any small areas of local or patchy atelectasis. It is both a prophylactic and a therapeutic mechanism. It stimulates the patient to improve by providing a challenge. It is relatively simple to operate and appears to have very productive results (Fig. 12-7).

Personnel in respiratory, cardiac, and general intensive care units today should be as versatile and learned in the interpretation of arterial gas measurements as in understanding ECG's electrolyte determinations, vital signs, and blood counts.

## GENERAL POSTOPERATIVE EVALUATIONS

Monitors, laboratory work, and computerized analysis are all very important assests in patient care; however, general physical evaluation of a patient is essential to an uneventful postoperative recovery.

### ■ What can be determined on simple visual and palpatory evaluation?

The patient's color is frequently a guide to the progress being made. Marked pallor associated with unstable vital signs may indicate the need for repeat hemoglobin and hematocrit determinations to establish the presence of bleeding or hidden hemorrhage. Pallor may be attributed to peripheral vaso-

*Edwards Laboratories, Division of American Hospital Supply Corporation, Santa Ana, Calif.

constriction and suggest poor tissue perfusion, indicating the need for a peripheral vasodilating drug. Cyanosis can indicate poor ventilation, major arteriovenous shunting associated with massive pulmonary embolization, or simply be a reflection of the patient's being cold with vascular pooling or sludging.

Palpable coolness with moist diaphoresis can indicate drug reaction or hypovolemic, neurogenic, or cardiogenic shock, whereas coolness without diaphoresis may be caused by the inappropriate warming of the patient after surgical procedure pump cooling. Palpable warmth with diaphoresis associated with hypotension and tachycardia suggests infection or septic shock.

The appearance of urticaria and shaking chills with fever can indicate a blood incompatibility or drug allergy.

A simple look can reveal drainage areas from the chest incision, monitoring sites, or chest tube stab wound. Acquired paraphimosis resulting from retracted foreskin at the time of the initial urinary catheterization in surgery could cause major complications if not recognized in the operating room or intensive care unit. A simple look may result in a major salvage, a happy patient, and no litigation.

Observation (looking, touching, feeling, and palpation) of the patient is stressed so as to avoid missing a correctable problem that could lead to the patient's death. Basic situations can occur such as separation of an arterial line from the patient's wrist under the sheets, disconnection of a chest tube either at the chest tube or the bottle site, or moderate drainage into the dressings.

Visual notes and recordings should be made of any change of consistency of the chest drainage, such as progression from nonclotting bright red blood to clotting darker blood or conversion to serous fluid. In the period following surgeries performed for severe trauma chest tube drainage may reveal discolored secretions or bubbling only after the patient eats, suggesting rupture of the esophagus.

### ■ How often should the patient be weighed, what is the weighing procedure, and what is the value of daily weight records?

Weighings are completed either once or twice daily with bed scales in the immediate postoperative period. Preoperative bed scale weights are obtained for appropriate comparison. If the patient's weight varies over 2 pounds, this suggests a variance of 1 L of fluid. A gain of 4 pounds or more correlated with peripheral edema, pleural effusion, conjunctival edema (chemosis), or auscultation of fine rales in the lung fields signifies moderate overhydration or fluid retention. After the patient has most of the equipment involved in intensive care, such as monitoring lines and chest tubes, removed, the daily weight can also be measured on the standing scale, but always at the same time of day and with the patient wearing the same clothing.

### ■ What simple evaluations can be utilized to evaluate neurologic status?

In the immediate postoperative period it is essential to determine the patient's level of consciousness and whether or not all extremities can be moved successfully. In addition, the pupillary responses and equalities are determined, as well as the ability to cooperate. Any variations could indicate major stroke or minor brain injury associated with embolization of fine particulate matter or air during the pump run.

Agitation, restlessness, and convulsive-like activity can reflect CNS damage from any of the previously mentioned causes or can possibly indicate drug toxicity. In the later stages of the postoperative period agitation, confusion, and psychotic behavior occur and can be associated with sleep deprivation, protein and electrolyte imbalances, or low serum or magnesium either alone or in conjunction with preoperative anxiety, drug or alcohol dependency, or preexisting organic brain involvement.

It is becoming more common for the family or nursing staff to recognize irregular behavior suggestive of symptoms of minor withdrawal from alcohol. The critical care unit staff should notify the principal practitioner initially so that appropriate evaluation and possible therapy can be instituted.

■ **What outputs should be measured, listed, and recorded in easy-to-read form?**

Urinary output should be appropriately recorded whenever a urinary catheter is in place; however, it is also most important to record output when the catheter is removed. If the patient is incontinent, estimated guesses as to the amount of urine lost in the sheets is essential.

Notation should also be made of moderate diaphoresis, as a patient who perspires profusely or who has an elevated temperature can lose as much as 100 ml for each degree elevation in temperature over a 24-hour period. Thus patients who are undergoing diaphoresis and who are moderately febrile (up to 103° to 104° F) can lose from 500 to 1000 ml of low-concentration salt solution each day.

Each *individual* chest tube drainage should be recorded; as previously emphasized, the consistency of the drainage should be noted.

Any vomitus or nasogastric suction aspiration must be recorded accurately and should be replaced with electrolyte solutions similar in composition to gastric contents.

A close approximation in milliliters should be listed of liquid or diarrheal bowel movements; the former terminology of minimal, medium-sized or large should not be used.

■ **What intakes should or should not be listed?**

On arrival in the unit records should be made of all fluids if they are to be maintained. When many units of blood or fluid are required, a numbering system (written on each bottle) facilitates better record keeping.

Intakes should not only include the volume of fluid given in each IV infusion, but also the consistency of that fluid, such as 5% dextrose in water, 0.45N saline solution, albumin, plasma, or blood. Trade name solutions such as Isolyte M and Gastrolyte solution should also be listed.

Any irrigation fluid that is utilized and not returned, such as for urinary catheters, endotracheal tubes, or venous lines, should be represented in a separate column or area on the intake and output record sheet.

The fluids utilized to keep the arterial and venous pressure lines open must also be listed. Ice chips and water sips should be recorded accurately, as complications caused by excessive ingestion of ice chips can occur in both young and old postoperative or post-trauma patients.

All oral intake, even semisolids, must be listed with estimated liquid content, especially in labile cardiac failure patients.

## Dressings and incision care

■ **What special care is utilized for dressings?**

Separate dressings are recommended for the sternotomy incision and the chest tube wound; thus when the chest tubes are milked in the immediate postoperative period and removed on the second or third postoperative day, the sternotomy incision is not disturbed or contaminated.

The dressings applied are usually nonadhesive (such as Telfa) with a thin coating of antibiotic ointment (Bacitracin or Neosporin). Gauze impregnated with nitrofurazone (Furacin) is no longer used because of previous experiences with allergic dermatitis. All monitor areas and chest tube sites are also covered with antibiotic dressing. There is questionable value as to the placement of an antibiotic ointment on the skin at the time of the original dressing; however, it appears to enhance the psychologic security of the intensive care practitioners.

Dressings are removed the second or third postoperative day or sooner if they have become saturated with drainage. Incision sites are then cleansed daily with hydrogen peroxide or with Betadine solution and completely dried; a lighter sterile dressing is reapplied or the incisions are left open to the air. If no bleeding occurs after the dressings are removed on the second or third day, natural lines of defense and resistance have been established, and the incisions can be safely left open to the air.

If Betadine is used for preoperative showering and surgical preparation but not washed off well after the surgical procedure, tincture of benzoin and tape application can produce blistering.

Any suspicious drainage is cultured immediately and abnormal discolorations or odors are immediately reported to the principal practitioner.

## Diet and oral hygiene

■ **When is the patient allowed liquids or food by mouth, and what diet is appropriate in the immediate postoperative period? Can oral hygiene be instituted immediately on arrival at the unit; if not, why not?**

It is recommended that postoperative patients be given absolutely nothing orally for 18 to 24 hours for the following reasons:

1. The patient given ice chips in the immediate postoperative period sucks on the chips. This is accompanied by a moderate amount of air swallowing, which accumulates air and distends the stomach, elevating the diaphragm and possibly producing basilar atelectasis and increasing the tendency to vomit.
2. Techniques for oral hygiene such as astringent rinses of the mouth and lemon and glycerin on the lips, aside from possibly nauseating the patient, cause licking of the lips and, again, swallowing air.

Gastric distention is one of the most, if not the most, common postoperative complications of cardiac surgery. With the use of nasogastric tubes and/or the absolute prohibition of oral intake it is believed that the incidence of postoperative atelectasis and aspiration pneumonia is decreased.

Start of the postoperative diet is not recommended for 36 hours (sooner only if bowel sounds and flatus develop); this diet consists of a full liquid bland regimen, including gelatin (Jello), custard, cooked Cream of Rice cereal with milk, and very liquid boiled eggs. The majority of these items do not stimulate increased gastric secretion and create less gastric irritation than most of the clear liquids, such as tea, apple juice, cider, or the clear but salty and frequently spicy hospital bouillon broths.

Bronchial aspiration in the immediate postoperative period can be of critical consequence to any patient, but especially to a borderline cardiac surgical patient. Many of the clear liquids previously mentioned (and occasionally the patient may receive coffee with this order) cause increased gastric and hydrochloric acid secretions, which, when aspirated into the lungs, can produce serious pneumonitis. These gastric juices seem to be neutralized by the full liquid bland substances.

Patients with cardiac decompensation or those who require no salt, are diabetic, or are following low calorie or other special diets can be replaced on these diets after an 18- to 24-hour trial on this liquid bland or "super soft" diet.

## Intravenous fluids (fluid and electrolyte management)

■ **Which IV solutions are administered and what are the limitations imposed during the immediate postoperative period?**

Between 1500 and 2000 ml of 5% dextrose in water is given during the first 24 hours to most patients, but younger patients without pre- or immediately postoperative cardiac decompensation or renal problems are administered half of this volume as 5% dextrose in a 0.45N saline solution.

Acute blood loss as determined from the chest output, pulse wave configuration, arterial pressures, CVP, and/or atrial pressures, hemoglobin determination, and hematocrit is replaced by whole blood if the patient demonstrates no volume overload or cardiac decompensation. Rapidity of replacement depends on the monitoring factors and clinical manifestations. Except in crisis situations I prefer not to administer blood using the hand pumps, as this can predispose to air embolization and increase fractionization of the red blood cells and platelets. The Travenol pressure administering devices allow a steady rapid inflow of blood with less damage.

■ **What electrolyte imbalances most frequently occur in the postoperative cardiac surgical patient?**

### *Hypokalemia*

Low serum potassium level is the most frequently encountered electrolyte abnormality occurring after cardiac bypass. It is associated with the diuretic regimens and inadequate potassium replacement before surgery. The hemodilution effect from cardiopulmonary bypass and diuresis that occurs during the surgical procedure with the use of mannitol or other diuretics further lowers the serum potassium. Since hypokalemia associated with digitalis administration predisposes to dangerous arrhythmias, when low serum potassium levels are noted, IV administration is started immediately. It should be stressed that the bottle should be well marked, or "flagged," when high concentrations of potassium are used.

In moderate depletion or when hypokalemia is suspected as the cause of troublesome arrhythmias, as much as 40 and sometimes 60 mEq of potassium can be placed in 250 ml of fluid and given over a 90-minute period; however, if allowed to infuse at a more rapid rate, cardiac standstill or asystole can occur. Some reports have stressed never administering more than 20 mEq of potassium over a 1-hour period; however, when life-endangering arrhythmias are present, potassium should be given in these larger concentrations, with constant bedside attention to the specific IV solution. It should also be given through a large vein, preferably via the CVP line and never via the arterial line.

### *Hyperkalemia*

Hyperkalemia is seen occasionally on the second or third postoperative day as the result of overzealous IV administration. Occasionally a marked laboratory error occurs when laboratory personnel mistakenly draw a blood sample from a vein above an infusion line administering potassium solution. Abnormally high levels of serum potassium are found in hemolyzed serum and after the administration of numerous units of old stored blood. If levels above 5.5 mEq/L are obtained, added potassium administration is stopped and potassium levels are measured frequently. If true serum potassium levels reach 6 mEq/L or greater, hypertonic glucose and insulin solutions can be administered to drive the potassium to an intracellular position. However, if there are signs on the ECG of hyperkalemia, this is not a recommended procedure, as it is probably better to maintain the high level of potassium in the serum rather than drive it to an intracellular position. Frequent diuresis with IV furosemide (Lasix) can be utilized to facilitate potassium excretion; in acute situations 1 g of IV calcium chloride can be slowly administered to help counteract the effects of the hyperkalemia. If the potassium level continues to rise, exchange resins may be given by enema or peritoneal dialysis or hemodialysis may be required. Frequent potassium monitoring during these procedures must be utilized. If, in association with the hyperkalemia, there is increased BUN or creatinine levels, a nephrologist should be consulted.

### *Hypernatremia*

Hypernatremia is usually not a problem for the postoperative patient; however, hyponatremia occurs and is most often caused by previous preoperative salt restriction, loss with diuretics, dilutional effects from the cardiopulmonary bypass, and use of nonsaline fluids during recovery. Administration of salt for excessive diuresis is not usually necessary until the sodium levels drop below 125 mEq/L. The most successful mechanism of reestablishing normal sodium balance once gastrointestinal function is reestablished is by instituting oral feedings. However, when nondiluted hyponatremia persists with levels below 120 mEq/L, the administration of normal saline solution and occasionally hypertonic salt solutions is necessary.

### *Hypocalcemia*

Hypocalcemia is encountered with dilution, administration of large volumes of acid citrate dextrose blood, and occasionally in patients with hyperventilation. This can easily be corrected with direct IV infusion of 10 ml of a

10% solution of calcium chloride (1 g) given over a 10-minute time span.

### *Hypercalcemia*

Hypercalcemia is seldom seen but can occur in previously unrecognized malignant conditions and other metabolic disorders. When present, it can be treated with low calcium diet, slow infusion of sodium and potassium phosphate mixtures, corticosteroids, or administration of mithramycin, a calcium-reducing antibiotic. Peritoneal dialysis has also been used in severe cases of hypercalcemia.

### *Hypomagnesemia*

Magnesium deficiency may be noted in patients who have been on long-term administration of IV fluids or are nutritionally depleted; this condition is more common in the cachectic or alcohol-dependent patient. It has been noted that the signs and symptoms of hypocalcemia and hypokalemia can be accentuated with low magnesium levels. Depletion can be treated by IM injection of a 50% solution (1 g) or by slow IV infusion of 500 mg of magnesium sulfate.

## Body positions, wraps, and early postoperative activities

As teams have become more experienced, it has been interesting to note progressive change in the orders for body positions, certain wraps, and activities allowed.

### ■ What body position is preferred for the postoperative cardiac surgical patient?

Sternotomy and also thoracotomy patients obtain more relief from pain when in a low Fowler position as compared to being perfectly flat. This allows the diaphragm to drop for better respiration, decreases fluid return to the heart, seems to allay some apprehension, and is an aid in preventing cerebral edema.

The legs are usually kept extended and straight; under no circumstances is the lower end of the bed bent under the patient's knees, as this contributes to venous stasis in the popliteal veins and potentiates phlebothrombosis and pulmonary embolization.

Commencing 2 to 3 hours after the surgical procedure, the patient should be allowed to turn onto the right or left side if the chest tubes do not impede the turn. All monitor or IV lines are protected against bends or twists. Turning from side to side benefits pulmonary function, prevents pulmonary stasis, and improves lung drainage; it also helps establish better drainage of fluid from the pericardial and thoracic cavities. During the first 2 days the patient is turned every 2 to 3 waking hours.

During the first oral feedings the patient is placed in an upright position; this usually decreases the tendency toward regurgitation and thus aspiration.

When arterial bypass lines have been used in the lower extremities or saphenous veins have been harvested, the legs are wrapped from toes to groin with elastic bandages. When a single long incision has been used for procuring the saphenous vein, a Penrose drain is left in a subcutaneous position for 24 to 48 hours and necessitates frequent dressing changes. Occasionally antiembolic stockings are placed from the toes to the groin over the Ace wraps; when the drains have been removed and there is no need for the wraps, thromboembolic stockings alone are used.

The patient's activities are quite limited for the first 12 to 18 hours after the surgical procedure with simple turning from side to side, slight increases or decreases in the semi-Fowler position, and upright positions allowed occasionally for the chest x-ray films taken by the portable unit. However, the day (24 to 36 hours) after surgery, the patient is allowed to sit upright for intake of fluids or semisolids (as previously described) and is encouraged to use a footboard for flexion and extension of the toes in order to maintain calf activity for better venous return from the legs.

During the period between 24 and 48 hours after surgery the patient is positioned upright on the bedside with the legs semiextended (to prevent binding in the popliteal space). This is performed three to four times on the second postoperative day.

Depending on the progress made, by the

second or third postoperative day the chest tubes and urinary catheter have been removed, most monitoring and IV fluid devices have been discontinued, and the patient is allowed to sit in a chair at the bedside, again with the legs extended. Getting the patient out of bed and into the chair satisfies the activity requirement for patient and personnel, especially when recommended three to four times daily for 15- to 30-minute intervals.

The third or fourth postoperative day the patient is allowed ambulation with assistance. It is recommended that those individuals assisting the patient be strong enough to hold the patient in case he becomes weak. *It is essential that the patient be walked and not dragged,* for studies are conclusive that venous return from the legs is much less in the patient who is upright and motionless than that of a patient even lying in bed. It is common to see patients supposedly being ambulated by very strong aides or physiotherapy technicians with the patient's feet hardly ever touching the floor, or if they touch, they are limply dragging. The purpose of early ambulation is to increase arteriole circulation, improve venous drainage, and retrain muscle groups.

Activity is progressive from this point, depending on the patient's cardiac enzyme levels, ECG, chest x-ray film, other laboratory data, and response to the first simple ambulation. By the sixth or seventh postoperative day, when the patient is usually ready for discharge, the staff members have prepared him for usual home activities such as caring for himself in the bathroom and getting into and manipulating from bed status to sitting in a chair, on a couch, or at a dining table.

When the patient is discharged, it is recommended that home activities be similar to the last hospital day activities.

■ **What specific recommendations are made for body positioning at home, activities, and leg wraps?**

The patient is advised that it is preferable to sleep alone or with a simple pillow separation from his or her bed partner for 5 to 7 days in order to avoid irritating the multiple tender incisions.

An incline pillow can usually be obtained at one of the various department stores or medical supply houses and consists of sponge rubber. This allows the patient to sleep at a 15- to 20-degree incline and frequently avoids the need for a surgical bed.

Instructions are given to avoid any heavy lifting and not to indulge in any active walking or strenuous exercise.

Because of late pulmonary embolic phenomena that occur too often after discharge, strict adherence to the use of antiembolic stockings *whenever* upright, in sitting positions, or ambulating is forcefully recommended for at least 3 weeks. The patient at home, as in the hospital, is to avoid crossing the legs, exerting any pressure on or bending in the popliteal space, or assuming any position where the legs just hang without activity. Activities that are allowed are walking (slowly), sitting (moving the legs and ankles), or lying supine rather than simply standing in one position. But in all cases, the support or antiembolic stockings (leotard type preferred over groin length) should be worn.

## Medication, routes of administration, and precautions

Because of the frequent acute crises that can occur in critical care units, a very broad variety of medications must be immediately available, and mixtures and dosages must be committed to memory. It is paramount for all personnel, but especially critical care practitioners, to be familiar with the dosage of the common drugs used in critical care and to frequently be reacquainted with the indications, contraindications, methods of preparation, and techniques of administration.

■ **What special precautions should be taken with respect to the dosages and administration of medications?**

All units should have accessible and easy-to-read lists of the most commonly used medications, the various effects, and the modes of administration.

The administration of antibiotics is usually preempted by an evaluation of the patient's record as well as repeated questioning of the patient regarding any allergies. Infrequently used antibiotics are rechecked as to routes of administration, because these change intermittently (for example, in the use of chloramphenicol [Chloromycetin]). Certain antibiotics (gentamicin and kanamycin) are nephrotoxic and must be given in dosages determined by the BUN, creatinine, and creatinine clearance levels, and others (certain tetracyclines) should not be given to individuals who have jaundice or a history of severe hepatic disease. Some antibiotics are restricted to absolute emergency situations because of depressing or altering effects on certain white blood cells. A point to remember is that most IM antibiotics should be placed *deep* in the muscle for better absorption and to prevent subcutaneous accumulations, fat necrosis, or abscess.

The administration and mixing of certain solutions such as lidocaine, isoproterenol (Isuprel), metaraminol (Aramine), levarterenol (Levophed), and now dopamine (Intropin), as well as digoxin (Lanoxin), lanatoside (Cedilanid), procainamide (Pronestyl), quinidine, and sodium bicarbonate, should be committed to memory and nearly automatic.

The administration of blood can be associated with multiple problems. In order to prevent such problems, blood should be administered following Ringer's lactate or saline solution rather than after dextrose and water. It should be warmed, if possible, to room temperature to prevent chills and to prevent cold agglutinin reactions. Multiple micropulmonary emboli can be prevented with special microfilters to eliminate the large blood platelet aggregates so often present in stored blood. It is uncommon today to have incompatible blood administered to a patient; however, the blood should be quadruply checked: first, by asking the patient's name; second, by verifying the armband of the patient; third, by comparing the patient and donor blood types; and fourth, by rechecking all of these factors with another person. If a blood reaction develops, appropriate measures such as discontinuing the blood infusion and notifying the principal practitioner should be carried out. A urine sample and another blood sample should be sent to the laboratory for retyping and cross matching. The patient should be closely observed for further signs of blood reaction.

The techniques of the IV use of analgesics such as meperidine hydrochloride (Demerol), 10 to 25 mg/hr, and IV morphine sulfate, 1 to 5 mg every 30 to 60 minutes, should be well known to all critical care unit personnel.

IV paralyzing agents such as succinylcholine (Anectine) and *d*-tubocurarine are used for intubation procedures and respiratory control. All critical care personnel should be familiar with these agents and capable of monitoring patients undergoing such therapy.

Any time large doses of IV potassium are being given, the lines should be set up so that rapid administration greater than 60 mEq/hr cannot possibly occur and cause cardiac standstill. IV calcium chloride (usually 500 to 1000 mg) should be given over a 5- to 10-minute period and never into a line containing acid citrate dextrose blood, as it will precipitate coagulation. Magnesium can be given by the IV route for slower pickup with less danger of acute side effects. When concentrated electrolytes are given by the IV route, the CVP lines are preferred, as many of these solutions cause chemical phlebitis.

IV heparin can be given by "piggy back," push, or (less preferred) diluted in large volumes of fluid. When given by subcutaneous injection, a short (½ inch) No. 25- or 26-gauge needle should be used and the heparin injected in folded fat but never into muscle or subfascia, because this is how large complicating hematomas occur.

Protamine sulfate is required at times to reverse additional heparin effects, but it can produce marked hypotension when given rapidly. It should be diluted and administered over a 10- to 20-minute period.

Chlorpromazine (Thorazine), as well as other phenothiazine agents, can also be responsible for moderate hypotension, especially when given by the IV route. Chlorpromazine is often administered by IV route to correct peripheral vasoconstriction with resultant hypertension and poor perfusion. When needed in the immediate postoperative period, 1 to 2 mg are diluted in 5 to 10 ml of saline solution and administered over a period of 2 to 3 minutes, with repeat doses (up to 10 mg) given as needed. Severe hypotension can occur when larger doses are given in labile postoperative patients.

The reader is encouraged to pursue more in-depth information through independent study and the use of reference material.

*chapter 13*

# Postoperative complications in the adult cardiac surgical patient

ROBERT A. STEEDMAN

Multiple potentially critical complications can occur in the immediate postoperative period. Prior to the era of critical care units, postoperative mortality rates were high. Early recognition and prompt therapeutic intervention in the minor phases can prevent progression to the major phase with its high toll of life.

## CARDIAC COMPLICATIONS

### Postoperative bleeding

■ **What factors indicate excessive postoperative bleeding and how is it recognized?**

Increased output in the chest bottle drainage with volumes in excess of 100 ml/hr for more than 5 hours should stimulate concern, but it is not uncommon during the first 1 to 5 hours for this amount of accumulated blood and fluid to drain. If this rate continues for the first 24 hours (a loss of 2400 ml or 5 units of blood) or if there is no trend toward decreasing output after 5 to 6 hours, reexploration is recommended.

Any patient who demonstrates blood loss between 150 and 300 ml/hr for more than 4 hours is also a candidate for urgent reexploration procedures.

The signs of cardiovascular instability associated with this bleeding include the following:

1. Tachycardia (rates of 100 to 130 beats/min) that responds to administration of any fluid volume and/or blood
2. Labile blood pressure, the hypotensive aspects of which also respond to the administration of blood or other fluid
3. An adequate pulse or pressure wave despite hypotension and tachycardia
4. Continually dropping central venous pressure (CVP) or left atrial pressure (LAP) that also responds favorably to fluid administration
5. Labile vital signs associated with the intended or accidental use of the "tilt" test, evidenced when simple elevation of the patient's torso for the purpose of taking a portable chest x-ray film or administering respiratory therapy is followed by a moderate to marked drop in blood pressure, the temporary decrease in pulse rate proceeding to a compensation tachycardia and frequently associated with moderate pallor, agitation, and diaphoresis

These findings, in conjunction with dropping hemoglobin and hematocrit levels, indicate blood loss out of proportion with blood replacement and are not usually present unless a deficit of 500 to 1000 ml exists.

Hemoglobin and hematocrit determinations are of value in determining the amount of blood loss, but they should never be taken as the primary or single factor determining need for replacement. The hemoglobin and hematocrit levels in the first few hours postoperatively can be falsely high and not adequately reflect the total blood loss; with hemodilution they can even be falsely low. However, if a patient in the immediate postoperative period presents evidence of deterioration by the signs previously mentioned, the hemoglobin and hematocrit determinations can be of critical importance, especially if very low (hematocrit below 25% and hemoglobin below 7 g/100 ml) during this period of false high readings (especially if hemodilution is not suspected).

Any sudden volume increase in chest drainage over a short period of time after surgery is indicative of major hemorrhage. For example, if the chest tubes have been draining a stable amount (for example, 35 to 50 ml/hr), and then shortly after moving the patient or milking the chest tubes, an output of 200 to 500 ml/hr occurs in a matter of 5 to 30 minutes, activation of a new bleeding site or disruption of a suture line must be considered, and rapid evaluation for surgical intervention must be made.

A sudden decrease or cessation of chest tube output may also herald a problem of serious consequence, as continued bleeding without evacuation of the blood can produce pericardial tamponade or compressive hemothorax with complications of mediastinal shift.

Certain anatomic, physiologic, and technical factors associated with some patients or their surgery predispose to bleeding problems. The patients more prone to postoperative hemorrhage are those with preexisting pericarditis or pleuritis requiring more adhesion division and dissection, those having repeat cardiac operations (again through adhesions and scar), patients requiring multiple bypasses (each additional suture line increasing the potential of another bleeding site), patients with anatomically deep vessels in which isolation precludes deep dissection in fatty and muscular tissue, and any patient with generally poor vascular tissue (caused by generalized debility, ischemia, and advanced atherosclerosis in the aorta and coronary vessels). Incidental minute tears and fragmentation of the tissues with simple suturing, or removal of the atrial or ventricular vents or aortic perfusion cannulas are much more common in debilitated patients, those requiring adhesion, or those undergoing a repeat surgery. When the patient arrives in the unit, these factors are still very fresh in the surgeon's mind, and the postoperative team should be alerted to expect increased bleeding.

### ■ What nontechnical factors can be involved in postoperative bleeding?

Patients who preoperatively demonstrate abnormal clotting studies or present a history of clotting problems with simple tooth extraction and minor cuts and bruises should be evaluated preoperatively by a hematologist so that appropriate measures can be instituted preoperatively and postoperatively to replace clotting factors or prepare for postoperative control.

Any heart-lung apparatus basically damages the red blood cells and insults the clotting mechanisms in the blood. Clotting mechanisms are altered as a result of general protein denaturation, destruction of platelets, and activation of certain fibrinolysis. The longer the pump is run, the more likely it is that these factors will occur.

Either inadequate neutralization of the heparin or "heparin rebound" can be responsible for postoperative bleeding. Heparin used in surgery is reversed with 1 to 1.5 mg of protamine sulfate for each milligram of heparin utilized. At the time of closure the anticipated clots from neutralization of the heparin are usually evident, but occasionally as the skin is being closed moderate general ooze is evidenced, suggesting that the heparin effect is still present. When this occurs, activated clotting time or Lee-White clotting and bleeding and partial thromboplastin times are obtained; if altered, additional protamine sulfate is administered, often with dramatic results. The careful and slow administration of protamine sulfate has been mentioned.

The patient with excessive oozing and blood loss during surgery has received multiple units of acid citrate dextrose (ACD) blood; if this blood has been stored for over 3 to 5 days, it is deficient in all clotting factors. The added ACD anticoagulant binds the calcium needed for coagulation, and when multiple units are administered, functional calcium is depleted in the patient's own blood. Thus 1 g of calcium chloride is administered slowly in a nonblood line for every rapid 3 units of ACD blood used.

Circulating fibrinolysins can be demonstrated with bedside tests and by failure of clot formation or evidence of lysis of the clot after it is formed. It is a less common form of coagulopathy; however, at one time in various institutions it was considered to contribute to postoperative bleeding to the extent that an antifibrinolysin agent, ε-aminocaproic acid (Amicar), was administered routinely during or on completion of every pump perfusion. It is now used only if fibrinolytic activity is suspected or evident.

Bleeding associated with chronic liver disease and/or superimposed acute hepatic insult can occur and not infrequently results in death.

### ■ What measures are utilized to evaluate the cause of the bleeding?

Most surgeons, when an early bleeding problem is recognized, order the coagulation screening test, which, as previously mentioned, includes evaluation of platelet count, prothrombin time, partial thromboplastin time, thrombin time, fibrinogen assay, Ivy bleeding time, activated clotting time, Lee-White clotting time, euglobulin clot lysis, clot retraction studies, and fibrin split products.

While waiting for the laboratory returns, it is frequently advantageous for the surgeon to place 3 to 5 ml of the patient's blood into two or three nonheparinized tubes and set them at the bedside. The first of these three tubes can be used to determine if any clot forms, and if it forms, the time required for formation and the integrity of the clot can be noted. Certain other bedside evaluations can be performed with the administration of fresh blood, fibrinogen, platelets, or protamine sulfate to the nonclotting blood to see if a good clot is obtained. If the original blood specimen clots without additives but within minutes undergoes lysis, fibrinolysin activity is suggested. These bedside tests are unsophisticated, but frequently will give some information as to cause.

Equally as important is evaluation of the patient's incision, the chest tubes, and venous puncture sites to see if any clotting or lack of clotting is present.

### ■ How are the various causes of postoperative bleeding managed?

Mechanical causes of postoperative hemorrhage are best handled prophylactically at the time of surgery with appropriate hemostatic suture control and, if necessary, with the use of Teflon pledgets placed for reinforcement of suture lines on the atria, aorta, or ventricle. Diligent electrocoagulation is used on all potential bleeding areas such as the pericardial edges, superior mediastinal areas, substernal musculature, and perichondrial and periosteal edges. Bone wax is used on the divided sternal edges, and all areas are evaluated when the patient's blood pressure is at normal levels. The incidence of reoperation for hemorrhage may be decreased with the use of sponge (Gelfoam) pledgets soaked in thrombin and placed over various oozing operative sites.

The majority of the coagulopathies can be treated with the initial administration of very fresh whole blood. As previously discussed, the technique of withdrawing 1 or 2 units of the patient's own blood (thus with his own clotting factors) and readministering this at the completion of the pump procedure and after protamine sulfate has been given is useful in this respect. During the early phases of cardiac surgery only fresh whole blood should be used; this should be typed and cross matched the evening before or the morning of surgery; however, this is not always feasible.

When severe bleeding problems occur and appear refractory to customary treatment, one of the best modes of therapy for patient salvage is administering multiple units of fresh whole blood (having been obtained within 30 to 90 minutes prior to administration). Regardless of the tedious, time-consuming procedure needed for obtaining fresh whole blood from donors, the efficacy of its use cannot be disregarded.

Fibrinolysis problems can usually be treated effectively with IV ε-aminocaproic acid (Amicar). The patient is usually given

5 g over a 30- to 60-minute period; this is followed by 1 g hourly for the subsequent 4 to 5 hours. Some improvement should be noted after 2 to 3 hours of therapy, and if it is not evident, complete reevaluation with a new coagulation screening test should be performed. Fibrinolysis and intravascular coagulation can occur simultaneously and may require the use of heparin in addition to an antifibrinolysin agent.

Heparin effect is not uncommonly seen in the immediate postoperative period as "heparin rebound." This can usually be determined by the activated clotting time, the partial thromboplastin time, and in cases of moderate overheparinization or inadequate reversal, the prothrombin time can frequently be very low. Slow administration of and titration with protamine sulfate usually reverses all these abnormal tests.

Thrombocytopenia can be detected by microevaluation and platelet counts. When the counts are below 70,000, the situation should be corrected by giving fresh platelet packs; usually a minimum of 4 to 8 packs is necessary with frequent reassessment. Platelet counts are usually difficult to obtain after 3:00 P.M., but when the need for them is suspected, they should be ordered immediately.

In cases where numerous units of ACD blood have been administered or when hypocalcemia is evident, calcium chloride is given, but never in a line containing blood. It is probably true that adequate calcium can be mobilized from the patient's own bones to supplement the needed calcium. However, this takes time, and frequently in cases of heavy bleeding, time is of the essence.

## ■ What is DIC and how is it treated?

The letters "DIC" refer to a syndrome with many titles such as "consumption coagulopathy," "diffuse intravascular clotting," "disseminated intravascular clotting," "intravascular coagulation syndrome," and "disseminated intravascular coagulopathy." A simple explanation would be to tag DIC as a syndrome in which excessive coagulation occurs in the peripheral capillaries and occasionally the precapillary arterioles and postcapillary venules, thus blocking these end vessels and producing decreased tissue perfusion and increased arteriovenous shunting. The extensive peripheral coagulation pulls necessary clotting factors from the plasma, basically reducing it to serum, and thus normal hemostasis can no longer be maintained. Uncontrollable hemorrhage begins and can be visualized from simple needle punctures, incision sites, or from the respiratory, gastrointestinal, genitourinary, and integumentary areas, among other regions. Conditions predisposing to the development of this syndrome include traumatic perfusions (long-term pump runs with excessive suctioning of blood); preoperative, operative, or postoperative hypotension or shock syndromes; infection; severe acidosis and other metabolic imbalances; and severe drug or blood transfusion reactions. In its severe and advanced stages generalized poor tissue perfusion with severe hypoxia, acidosis, hepatic and renal failure, subcutaneous ecchymoses and hemorrhage, and digital and extremity gangrene can occur.

DIC is best identified by appropriate evaluation of the coagulation screening test, although it is occasionally difficult to differentiate from primary fibrinolysis. The laboratory findings in DIC include prolonged prothrombin, partial thromboplastin, and thrombin times. The platelet count and fibrinogen and antithrombin factor III levels are low, and the euglobulin lysis time is shortened or decreased. The levels of fibrin degradation products, or *fibrin split products,* are *elevated;* this is one of the most significant of all the tests mentioned in differentiating DIC from the other coagulopathies. In comparing DIC and primary fibrinolysis, it should be noted that in both conditions the thrombin time is prolonged and the fibrinogen level is low (usually much lower in DIC). Thrombocytopenia can be present in both after a pump run, but the platelet count is lower in DIC than in primary fibrinolysis. The euglobulin lysis time is abnormally short in both conditions, but reduction is much greater in primary fibrinolysis.

The primary *treatment* of this syndrome

is *heparin* administration. The heparin is administered in an attempt to stop the microscopic thrombosis; since heparin exerts antithrombin activity, it hopefully neutralizes free circulating thrombin. Its other anticoagulant principles are even more important in the treatment of this disease. Heparin should be administered by the IV route and frequently given in therapeutic doses with the initial amount sufficient to induce total anticoagulation in the patient (similar to undergoing cardiopulmonary bypass procedures). The therapeutic administration sometimes requires dosages as high as 20,000 units every 2 hours; however, in cases where both renal and hepatic impairment are present, heparin dosage must be markedly decreased, as the heparin half-life is prolonged. (Heparin is eliminated by renal excretion, and heparinase is produced by the liver.)

Needless to say, once uncontrollable bleeding problems are encountered, recruitment of the hematopathologist and/or the hematologist is essential, with immediate investigation into the possibilities of obtaining fresh whole blood.

Occasionally reexploration procedures are necessary when the patient exhibits signs of mechanical bleeding or when the available blood is extremely limited. Patients with rare blood types and those who through their religious beliefs (Jehovah's Witnesses) refuse blood or blood derivatives cannot be treated with long waiting or procrastination when bleeding continues and must be returned to the operating room for mechanical hemostasis.

### ■ What are the complications involved in transfusion of whole blood or blood components, and how are they treated?

Hepatitis can occur from 3 to 20 weeks after the administration of blood, and the incidence increases with the number of units of blood transfused. Renal shutdown can occur any time from the initial transfusion until 7 days later. Allergic reactions with urticaria most often occur within hours after a transfusion, as do febrile reactions with chills and fever.

Those symptoms that can occur in the acute stages of transfusion reactions include chills, fever, urticaria, pruritus, tachycardia, chest pain, dyspnea, nausea and vomiting, back pain, hematuria, and icterus.

When a reaction is suspected, the transfusion should be immediately stopped, and all factors on the blood bag or bottle should be rerecorded and the following steps taken:

1. Return the unit of blood to the blood bank for re-cross matching and retyping with the patient's original clot and with a recently obtained sample.
2. Send a specimen of anticoagulated blood for determination of plasma hemoglobin.
3. Send a sample of urine for hemoglobin determination.
4. Institute therapy with chlorpheniramine maleate (Chlor-Trimeton) or diphenhydramine hydrochloride (Benadryl), and if the allergic reactions involve bronchospasm or signs of angina or ankle edema, the use of epinephrine compounds as well as aminophylline and possibly even hydrocortisone or dexamethasone may be necessary.

In cases where moderate hemolytic reaction is suspected as a result of moderate increase in the plasma and urine hemoglobin, the administration of an osmotic diuretic such as mannitol or the use of furosemide (Lasix) is indicated to prevent pigment deposition in the renal tubules with possible anuria. Sodium bicarbonate can be given in acidotic reactions and aids in creating an alkaline urine in which hemoglobin precipitates less freely. Severe bleeding problems may ensue; these can be a manifestation of DIC. If renal shutdown is a reality, care must be instituted, as discussed later in this chapter and in Chapter 15.

## Low cardiac output syndrome and hypotension

In the immediate postoperative period the low cardiac output condition can develop; this is characterized by low arterial pressure with normally elevated CVP or atrial pressure, cool and possibly cyanotic skin and extremities, a narrowing pulse pressure with tachycardia, poor to nonobtainable peripheral pulses, changes in the sensorium, and suppression of urine formation. Thus a condition exists wherein the central pump mechanism (left ventricular action) for one reason or another is inadequate to maintain appropriate tissue perfusion and satisfy metabolic body requirements.

■ **What are the etiologies to be considered when the hypotension or low cardiac output syndromes occur?**

In all categories of cardiac surgery a mechanical problem such as cardiac tamponade must always be initially considered. In cases of repair of cardiac defects incomplete repair of that defect and/or residual aortic, subaortic, pulmonary valvular, or infundibular stenosis, or disruption of a surgical repair must also be considered.

When valves have been replaced, the possibility of breakdown and leakage around the prosthetic valve must be excluded, and consideration should be made regarding various types of obstruction to inflow and outflow associated with the replaced valves, such as simple clot obstruction of the valve, surgical mishaps (such as sutures impeding appropriate function of the disk or ball components), or placement of a valve cage that is too large for a small ventricle.

Possible additional causes are left atrial thrombosis, pulmonary embolization, pulmonary atelectasis, or severe pulmonary hypertension.

Multiple nonmechanical causes of low cardiac output exist and include the following:

1. Myocardial insult may result from anoxia during the time of surgery such as aortic valve replacement or myocardial revascularization with long periods of cardiac arrest and inadequate coronary perfusion or cooling.

2. Low cardiac output may occur in cases wherein left or right ventriculotomies are performed with resultant repair or in which left ventricular vent tears occur and require extensive suture and pledget reconstruction or support.

3. Some patients who develop this syndrome are prone to myocardial insult; they are usually older or have had chronic strain on the myocardium from cardiac valvular disease, coronary artery obstructive disease with years of poor myocardial perfusion, or associated myocardiopathies of one type or another.

4. Various arrhythmias can produce low output; these include tachycardias, atrial fibrillation or flutter (which does not allow adequate atrial filling or emptying), bradycardia, and certain types of heart block.

5. Other causes include metabolic acidosis or occasionally even respiratory alkalosis, electrolyte imbalances with hyperkalemia, hypocalcemia, and arrhythmias associated with hypokalemia.

6. Numerous drugs can be associated with decreased myocardial contractility in the postoperative period; some of these have been previously mentioned, such as propranolol, large doses of barbiturates, large doses of morphine derivatives, and multiple antiarrhythmic agents.

■ **What is the treatment for low cardiac output syndrome?**

If the etiology of the syndrome is mechanical, return to surgery is necessary for appropriate repair of the mechanical defect (evacuation of clots in pericardial tamponade, completion of the repair for aortic or pulmonary stenosis, and rerepair of any suture line disruptions).

In conditions where electrolyte depletion is suspected, calcium and potassium can be replaced as previously mentioned. In hyperkalemia diuretics, exchange resins (oral or rectal), or the other methods of lowering potassium can be used.

Respiratory alkalosis can simply be corrected with attention to proper respiratory mechanics; metabolic acidosis can be frequently corrected by the instillation of sodium bicarbonate by IV push or infusion of a 5% bicarbonate solution.

The treatment of the various arrhythmias has been described elsewhere in this text, but emphasis should be placed on the critical care practitioner's responsibility for understanding causes such as infarction anoxia, ischemia, or hypokalemia.

The use of certain inotropic agents after adequate hydration or volume replacement is the most common mode of therapy for this syndrome, and the drug most frequently used is isoproterenol (Isuprel) titrated until the inotropic effect is evidenced. This drug works moderately well in patients appropriately hydrated and when the cardiac rate is below 70 beats/min. In hypovolemia its use can aggravate the hypotension, and when the heart is irritable or tachycardia persists, it can precipitate critical arrhythmias. Metaraminol (Aramine) can be used in a concentration of 100 to 300 mg in 500 ml of solution and titrated to the desired pressure; however, sustained use has been indicted as causing constrictive ischemia to the kidneys with irreversible renal damage. Phenylephrine (Neo-Synephrine) can be utilized intermittently as a direct IV bolus or in intermittent piggyback solutions; however, refractory reactions to this drug occur in a very short period of time. Other drugs used alone or in combination have been epinephrine, epinephrine and isoproterenol, isoproterenol and glucagon, and epinephrine and glucagon.

Combinations of the previously mentioned inotropic and vasoconstricting drugs with peripheral vasodilating drugs such as phenoxybenzamine (Dibenzyline) or chlorpromazine (Thorazine) have been described. I have seen marked reduction in the systolic blood pressure with very minimum amounts of these vasodilating drugs even in hypotensive states, and I use them with a maximum of caution.

As a last resort it may be necessary to rely on levarterenol (Levophed), which is a very potent vasoconstricting agent and is known to cause decreased peripheral perfusion and to predispose to renal failure, especially when used in high concentrations or for long periods of time. This drug also can be used in combination with one of the peripheral vasodilating agents, but I limit its use.

A relatively new drug is dopamine hydrochloride (Intropin). This drug is a naturally occurring catecholamine precursor of norepinephrine that exerts an inotropic effect on the myocardium to effect an increased cardiac output. It is most commonly used by adding 5 ml or 200 mg to 250 or 500 ml of any one of the commonly used solutions (5% dextrose in water, 5% dextrose and 0.45N saline solution, etc.). These dilutions yield a final concentration for administration of 800 μg/ml (200 mg in 250 ml dilution) or 400 μg/ml (200 mg in 500 ml). In most of my patients the increase in cardiac output has paralleled an increase in urine output and has occurred without the nuisance of tachycardia during short-term use. Recent articles have reported that long-term and increased dosage use where 50 μg/min is necessary for relatively long periods of time result in annoying tachycardia. Other reports have also been promising as to the combined usage of dopamine hydrochloride and isoproterenol, with smaller concentrations of each.

The use of steroids in massive doses (10, 000 to 20,000 mg of hydrocortisone, 3000 mg of methylprednisone, and 300 to 400 mg of dexamethasone) has been reported in cases of low cardiac output syndrome, and during the past 10 years numerous articles have appeared regarding this technique. It is common to see the effects of peripheral vasodilatation (warm skin, improved color, etc.), but often these effects are associated with a further drop (10 to 30 mm) in systemic pressure and usually without any significant major improvement in the patient's overall outcome. I have since ceased the use of this regimen.

All sophisticated modes of monitoring and measuring are necessary at this time of low cardiac output and an extremely diligent search for the specific etiology of this life-endangering condition is continued. LAP, pulmonary, and wedge pressure measurements are invaluable in this condition.

### ■ What are cardiac assistance devices and when are they used?

Certain devices have been developed to decrease cardiac workload and support mean aortic pressure. The use of these instruments is usually restricted to cases wherein all conventional measures have resulted in failure and the patient is otherwise destined to die.

The most commonly used apparatus today, the counterpulsation or diastolic augmentation device, consists of an intra-aortic balloon that is usually inserted through the femoral artery and then connected to a helium-filled inflating device. Once inserted and connected, the balloon is coordinately inflated during diastole and deflated during systole. This apparatus reportedly reduces the myocardial oxygen demand, decreases cardiac work, and increases coronary flow when it raises the diastolic aortic pressure during inflation. The balloon is usually passed through a Dacron graft connected to the femoral artery and positioned in the thoracic aorta just distal to the left subclavian artery. It can be placed preferably in surgery or when necessary in the unit.

■ **Are there any problems associated with the use of the intra-aortic balloon?**

The use of this apparatus requires heparin anticoagulation and/or use of dextran and carries the usual inherent complications of any anticoagulation and/or intravascular foreign body. Manipulation of the catheter beyond the aortoiliac junction is often very difficult, and loss of the lower extremity has occurred with difficult placement and long-term use. Difficult placement has required more extensive retroperitoneal dissection for common iliac or lower abdominal placement with bleeding and infection problems. If the balloon migrates or is malpositioned, it can occlude the major vessels to the arm or head with limb loss or death.

■ **Can this apparatus be used at an earlier time rather than as a last resort?**

Investigators have recently developed the means of earlier detection in cases that will require such support, and it is possible that the judicial use earlier will increase survival in these specific patients.

■ **Are there any other support devices?**

For very short-term intervals (3 to 10 hours) some of the partial cardiac bypass procedures can be used, but the continual need for heparin creates problems. Encouraging are the results of a left ventricular bypass apparatus devised by Wakabayashi and Connolly, which, because of simple construction and a nonthrombogenic polyurethane-polyvinyl graphite coating, requires no heparin and has been used as an assistance for as long as 8 days.

## Pericardial tamponade

Increased collection of blood and/or clots in the pericardium with impedance of ventricular expansion and contraction, pressure compression of the atria, and tight constriction of the venae cavae impedes cardiac filling and output and produces the characteristic pericardial tamponade syndrome. The potential salvage of the patient depends on prompt recognition.

■ **What are the factors leading to pericardial tamponade?**

Any surgical intervention that has resulted in moderate bleeding without appropriate drainage or evacuation of blood and clots predisposes to tamponade. A typical condition is one in which moderate to massive bleeding has been occurring, with an acute cessation of the bleeding once the coagulopathy or bleeding problem has been controlled, resulting in rapid deterioration or development of low cardiac output.

The CVP continues to rise rapidly, the arterial systemic pressure drops with a noticeable decrease in the pulse pressure (pressure difference between the systolic and diastolic levels), cyanosis of the head and neck develops with evident venous distention of the neck and arm veins, and the patient is severely apprehensive and anxious. Auscultation of the heart reveals distant cardiac sounds, and paradoxical pulse is usually present.

Paradoxical pulse is described as an abnormal inspiratory fall in systolic blood pressure, a normal fall being 6 and 10 mm. A drop in the systolic blood pressure during inspiration of greater than 10 mm Hg is considered accentuated or paradoxical. It is detected by inflating a cuff pressure to a level greater than the expected systolic pressure, having the patient slightly accentuate the depth of respiration, and as the cuff pressure is slowly released, auscultating the blood pressure on expiration and then on inspiration. The difference between expiration and the re-pickup during inspiration, if greater than 10 mm Hg, is considered paradoxical.

### ■ How is pericardial tamponade treated?

Giving an inotropic drug such as isoproterenol (Isuprel), epinephrine, or dopamine will frequently increase the systolic pressure without change in the CVP and is probably indicative of pericardial tamponade. However, if the findings just discussed regarding CVP and paradoxical pulse are found, there is need for a diagnostic pericardiocentesis. If positive, or even suggestive, the patient should be immediately returned to surgery for pericardial evacuation.

It is necessary in these cases to do as much as possible of the evacuation procedure under local anesthesia, as deep anesthesia before evacuation frequently produces more hypotension. The large-bore pericardiocentesis needle should be left in the pericardial space for continued evacuation during the preparation and initial surgical procedure to maintain decompression of the pericardial chamber. Once the pericardium is opened, there is usually an explosive evacuation of blood and clots with immediate improvement of the patient's cardiodynamic situation.

In two instances I have observed patients with some but not all of the indicative findings of pericardial tamponade, that is, without evidence of markedly elevated CVP and without extensive widening of the mediastinum but very labile CVP and mean arterial pressures. In these two instances the patients were returned to surgery, and localized clot obstruction of the left atrium was found. Immediately on evacuation of this large left atrium–compressing clot, there was dramatic improvement in the cardiac status. Others have reported similar instances of local chamber tamponade.

## Cardiac arrhythmias

The arrhythmias occurring in the postoperative cardiac surgical patient are recognized by alarm tapes, reevaluated by replay systems, and generally diagnosed and treated similar to the arrhythmias occurring under other conditions; their diagnosis and specific care has been outlined in other chapters in this text. Today it is a constant effort for the family practitioner specializing in areas other than cardiology or internal medicine to keep up with the critical care staff with regard to knowledge of the interpretation, treatment, and consequences of the varying arrhythmias.

### ■ What arrhythmias occur in the postoperative cardiac surgical patient and how are they managed?

Sinus tachycardia is common in the immediate postoperative period and frequently is a response to hypovolemia, metabolic alterations, pain and apprehension, dehydration, myocardial irritability caused by anoxia, hypercapnia, or medications. It is most frequently treated by caring for the underlying cause: analgesia for pain, administration of adequate fluids for dehydration, decreasing or eliminating certain tachycardia-promoting drugs, appropriate respiratory control with arterial gas titration, etc. Occasionally sinus tachycardia requires digitalization, but before this is instituted digoxin levels are obtained to ensure that the tachycardia is not a sign of digitalis toxicity. In later postoperative periods if tachycardia persists, occasionally propranolol hydrochloride (Inderal) is utilized, but only in otherwise very stable patients.

Premature ventricular beats (PVB's) commonly occur at some phase in the postoperative period and should precipitate special attention, as they are frequently precursors of ventricular tachycardia and possibly ventricular fibrillation. Again, conditions such as anoxia, hypokalemia (especially when digitalis is being given), myocardial ischemia, and acid-base imbalances are frequently causative factors, but if PVB's continue once the suspected cause is corrected (such as administration of potassium in hypokalemic states) and occur more often than three to five times each minute, an IV bolus (25 to

100 mg) of lidocaine (Xylocaine) is given. At the same time a continuous lidocaine drip should be started and titrated to control the ectopic beats. Precaution is used to avoid lidocaine toxicity manifested by seizures and other CNS abnormalities and occasional suppression of myocardial contractility.

Patients with known preoperative ventricular ectopic beats are prophylactically given 350 mg of procainamide (Pronestyl) orally every 4 hours at the time of admission and continued on this dosage by IV route postoperatively until oral medications can be reinstituted. The 350 mg is then given orally every 4 hours until it can be decreased to 500 mg every 6 hours.

Diphenylhydantoin (Dilantin) can be given by either IV or IM route in individuals sensitive to lidocaine and can be the drug of choice when the ectopic beats are associated with digitalis toxicity. Diphenylhydantoin is administered by the IV route in 100 mg increments for a total initial dose of 300 to 500 mg followed by 100 to 200 mg given by the IM or IV route every 6 hours for maintenance, with conversion to oral dosage when feasible.

Quinidine can be utilized in IM doses of 200 to 600 mg every 6 hours and 100 to 400 mg in slow titrated piggyback IV drips every 6 hours; however, there have been potential complications with the use of IV quinidine, and this drug is used only after exhaustion of other methods.

Propranolol (Inderal) has also been recommended for control of both atrial and ventricular ectopic beats, but because of its hypotensive potentials, its use is limited to the completely stable postoperative patient.

Atrial and occasionally ventricular pacing can be utilized to override ectopic beats by suppression if pacing wires were left in place at the time of surgery. This occasionally requires rates well over 100 beats/min, and the taxation of the myocardium must be considered.

Ventricular tachycardia is a frequent precursor of ventricular fibrillation and is treated in a manner similar to PVB's; however, when nonrelenting ventricular tachycardia persists, electrical conversion (cardioversion) is indicated.

Ventricular fibrillation, unless converted immediately or assisted by cardiopulmonary compression and ventilation, is associated with imminent death. The early treatment of the often preceding PVB's or ventricular tachycardia is a hopefully preventive measure against the development of ventricular fibrillation, but once it occurs, appropriate measures against cardiopulmonary arrest are instituted and when conversion is completed, preventive measures are reinstituted.

Supraventricular arrhythmias, such as atrial fibrillation and flutter, can be associated with very rapid ventricular response and can be caused by poor atrial contractions, with ventricular filling and cardiac output often decreased. If the patient has not previously been treated with digitalis, this is the treatment of choice, but if conversion is unsuccessful in the face of adequate digitalization, electrical conversion may be indicated. When this arrhythmia develops in surgery with the heart exposed, electrical conversion is attempted at that time. Cardioversion requires relatively low voltage and can frequently be accomplished on the ward or in the emergency room with use of IV diazepam (Valium). The treatment of atrial flutter when associated with low cardiac output is similar to that of atrial fibrillation. Propranolol is occasionally used when vital signs are stable, but before using this drug surgeons usually prefer arrhythmia control to be fully in the hands of the cardiologist.

Paroxysmal atrial tachycardia (PAT), when diagnosed, is first treated with attempts at carotid sinus massage, eyeball pressure, and various Valsalva maneuvers. When not associated with heart block and in a nondigitalized patient, refractory PAT's are treated with rapid digitalization. If the PAT is associated with block and potassium depletion is present, potassium should be replaced; if still refractory, diphenylhydantoin (Dilantin) therapy should be instituted.

Premature atrial contractions (PAC's) are

not uncommon in postoperative patients and are more frequent in association with valvular surgery; if not treated, atrial fibrillation or flutter will often develop. Recommended treatment is IM or oral (if the patient is able) quinidine, with 200 mg (300 mg orally) given every 6 hours.

Atrioventricular (AV) dissociation may be noted at the time of surgery in the repair of ostium primum, endocardial cushion, or ventricular septal defects. It can also occur during aortic and tricuspid valve replacement. If the block occurs at the time of surgery, it is more likely that permanent pacemaking modes will be required postoperatively. Temporary or permanent pacemaker wires can be inserted at surgery. AV dissociation and heart block not infrequently occur following mitral valve surgery. However, this is usually temporary and may be associated with digitalis toxicity and hypokalemia and may respond to potassium replacement and cessation of digitalis administration. Slow nodal rhythms (45 to 60 beats/min) may be managed by use of isoproterenol, atropine, or if temporary pacemaker wires are in place, atrial or ventricular pacing.

## Cardiac arrest

The treatment of true cardiopulmonary arrest or ventricular fibrillation with apnea is a topic that could require volumes for complete discussion. However, certain basics will be mentioned. A marked contribution to the increased survival rate in cardiac surgical patients has resulted from prompt recognition of ventricular fibrillation and other life-endangering arrhythmias with appropriate conversion. The rapid institution of cardiopulmonary resuscitation in those individuals refractory to defibrillatory measures has also contributed to salvage rates. *All* practitioners, regardless of their specific areas of specialty, should be capable of appropriate cardiopulmonary resuscitation as a single rescuer or as a member of a full resuscitation team. The reader is referred to the American Heart Association reference material related to proper cardiopulmonary resuscitation techniques.

### ■ What are some of the basic considerations with respect to cardiopulmonary resuscitation?

The recognition of cardiac arrest is more easily expedited in the critical care unit where the patient is still connected to the monitoring and signaling devices. If the recognized condition is ventricular fibrillation, often simple defibrillation is adequate to restore appropriate cardiac function; however, if the heart is refractory to fibrillation, immediate cardiac compression and ventilation are instituted. Initially the patient should be ventilated, after clearing the airway, with 3 to 5 full breaths, cardiac compression should be instituted until a solid object can be placed under the chest, and the resuscitation team should be summoned. If the patient was not previously utilizing endotracheal or tracheal respiratory assistance, mouth-to-mouth or manual bag ventilation should be used with the appropriate airways until all the necessary equipment for endotracheal intubation, including an individual capable of performing the intubation, are present. A frequent mistake made by inexperienced personnel is to use critical resuscitation time in attempting intubation when the patient can be appropriately ventilated with a manual breathing bag and airway. Infusion lines are established as resuscitation is in progress.

All medications and equipment necessary for cardiopulmonary resuscitation and the potential minor complications that can occur should be present on the emergency cart. In addition to the usual items, this should include cutdown trays, large needles in case a tension pneumothorax must be decompressed, rib spreaders, material for simple tube thoracostomy, tracheostomy tray, suction apparatus, equipment for CVP line placement, materials for an arterial line, and monitoring equipment. The more commonly used medications such as epinephrine, sodium bicarbonate, lidocaine, calcium chloride, digitalis preparations, isoproterenol (Isuprel), metaraminol (Aramine), levarterenol (Levophed), diphenylhydantoin (Dilantin), morphine sulfate, and succinylcholine (Anectine) should be close at hand, preferably in prefilled syringes.

Extension of the neck to ensure a patent airway, 1½- to 2-inch compression of the sternum 60 to 80 times a minute, interposed with ventilation between the fifth and sixth compression, continual evaluation of the femoral and/or carotid pulses to check the effect of compression, blood gas measurements, and sodium bicarbonate administration should be carried out simultaneously.

When cardiac standstill is evident, intracardiac injection of 5 to 10 ml of a 1:10,000 concentration of epinephrine may be performed rapidly, with reinstitution of cardiac compression. If ventricular fibrillation occurs, defibrillation is utilized, and if unsuccessful and accompanied by a weak fibrillation pattern, 500 to 1000 mg of intracardiac calcium chloride (5 to 10 ml of a 10% solution) is given. These techniques are repeated until adequate cardiac output is established. Defibrillation is accomplished using 100 to 400 watt-seconds, usually starting at the lower levels. Electrode paste should be used to prevent burning and to ensure adequate contact. If the blood pressure is established but is too low for adequate perfusion, the various modes previously described for low cardiac output syndrome are instituted. Chest x-ray films should be obtained periodically to rule out pneumothorax resulting from intracardiac injections and forceful ventilation and to pursue evidence of possible aspiration or a misplaced endotracheal tube.

If external cardial compression is unsuccessful as determined by the arterial monitor or lack of palpable carotid and femoral pulses, an incision is made in the fourth or fifth left intercostal space (if the previous operative incision is not as accommodating), and open cardiac massage is employed. If the pericardium for some reason has not previously been violated, it should be opened at a point located anteriorly to the phrenic nerve. A chest tray prepared for minor surgery with rib spreaders should be on the emergency cart or readily available. Open massage procedures are more often necessary in emphysema patients, patients with immobile chests, and when the pericardium has been widely opened for the cardiac surgery.

Once adequate circulation is reestablished, it is necessary that a complete reevaluation be carried out; all laboratory studies—electrolyte evaluation, blood gas determination, digoxin level, hemoglobin concentration, hematocrit, ECG, and chest x-ray films—should be reevaluated postoperatively. All appropriate measures should be taken to avoid recurrence of the cardiac arrest.

It is recommended that the use of analgesics and muscle relaxants be discontinued in the operating room so that the patient will be relatively alert on arrival in the unit. Sedation can be instituted once the status of the CNS is known.

## Peripherovascular complications

Because of the usual generalized atherosclerosis in a large number of adult cardiac and especially coronary surgery patients, peripheral arterial occlusions in perfused and even nonperfused vessels can occur with relative frequency.

### ■ What are the signs and symptoms indicative of peripheral vessel obstruction?

Coldness, pallor, blotchy discoloration, loss of pulses with delayed venous and capillary refilling, and paresthesias and pain during activity or rest of an extremity are indicative of acute arterial obstruction. Evidence of these signs in one extremity and not in any others is even more conclusive of local arterial obstruction.

If signs of arterial obstruction appear in both lower extremities, this may indicate embolic or thrombolic blockage of the aortoiliac bifurcation or even a distal aortic dissection. Once this diagnosis is highly suspected or established, immediate surgical intervention is necessary, as the prognosis is frequently related to the efficacy and speed with which successful surgical intervention and correction are employed.

Occasionally a severely ischemic and swollen leg is indicative of the anterior tibial compartment syndrome resulting from anoxia and edema after femoral artery perfusion;

this requires femoral artery embolectomy, reconstruction, or even multiple compartment fasciotomies for complete restoration of circulation and prevention of limb loss.

### ■ What venous problems can occur during the postoperative phase?

Phlebothrombosis or thrombophlebitis of the lower extremities is the most common venous complication occurring in the postoperative cardiac patient. It is usually well treated prophylactically with adequate hydration in the preoperative, operative, and postoperative phases, compressive wraps or antiembolic stockings placed in the operating room or on arrival in the intensive care unit, and the adequate use of a footboard for continual foot and leg activity. Frequent removal and reapplication of thromboembolic stockings or wraps periodically or as necessary combined with appropriate progressive activities and mobilization have previously been described. Phlebothrombosis and thrombophlebitis can occur in the upper extremities as a result of the use of irritating IV medications, and I have encountered three instances of total occlusion of the subclavian-axillary venous drainage of the upper extremity with typical phlegmasia cerulea dolens (severe purplish edematous and painful extremity) that required immediate surgical intervention and evacuation of clots by Fogarty catheter thromboembolectomy and irrigation with heparinized saline solution.

In cases of phlebothrombosis or thrombophlebitis of the lower extremities surgery is almost never indicated (unless phlegmasia cerulea dolens occurs), and as soon as it is safe, heparin therapy and/or low molecular weight dextran administration is started. Phenylbutazone (Butazolidin) is useful as an adjunctive drug in thrombophlebitis, but when used in combination with dextran or other anticoagulant-like drugs, bleeding complications can occur. Other side effects possible with this drug prevent its usage by many practitioners. If there are contraindications to the utilization of heparin and the patient has exhibited pulmonary emboli, if pulmonary emboli have occurred while the patient has been undergoing anticoagulation therapy, or if there is evidence of septic pulmonary embolization, surgical interruption of the inferior vena cava is imperative.

## Pulmonary embolization

Although not common, most cases with small but symptomatic pulmonary emboli have been noted in patients whose vein was harvested below the knee and in patients where internal mammary artery implantation alone was used with only simple groin dissection for arterial perfusion.

### ■ How is pulmonary embolization in the immediate postoperative period recognized?

In the responsive or conscious patient the rapid development of dyspnea associated with cyanosis, pleuritic-type chest pain, tachycardia, initial onset of mild hypotension followed by normal or elevated blood pressure, signs and symptoms of bronchospasm, hemoptysis, apprehension, and hypoxia (evidenced by arterial blood concentrations) either alone or in combination is highly indicative of pulmonary emboli. Later findings include signs of pulmonary hypertension as manifested by findings on auscultation, x-ray films, and ECG or in combination with pleural friction rub, x-ray evidence of peripheral infiltrates, or hypovascularity with or without pleural effusion.

### ■ How are pulmonary emboli treated?

If the diagnosis is fully established and it is safe to do so, heparin anticoagulation is instituted. Heparin is the only drug of choice for the first 7 to 10 days, and its administration by IV route is preferred. The therapeutic anticoagulation levels are evaluated by activated clotting time, partial thromboplastin time, and Lee-White bleeding and clotting time studies.

As previously mentioned, surgical intervention is recommended only in cases where recurrent embolization occurs under anticoagulation, when anticoagulation is contraindicated, or if septic embolization is suspected. Pulmonary embolectomy is seldom indicated and reserved only for those patients exhibiting a course of continual deterioration despite nonsurgical treatment. Although this patient presents a poor surgical risk, utilization of the partial bypass instituted prior to diagnostic pulmonary arteriography and preceding anesthesia induction for removal of the pulmonary embolus increases the chance for survival.

## PULMONARY COMPLICATIONS

Strict attention to preoperative, operative, and postoperative pulmonary care provides the greatest means for decreasing the increased respiratory morbidity and/or mortality seen among cardiac surgery patients in the postoperative period.

### ■ What prophylactic measures are taken to decrease pulmonary complications?

Depending on the history and physical examinations, inclusive of chest x-ray films and baseline pulmonary function, a patient may appropriately be assessed preoperatively as to total pulmonary function, including arterial gas concentrations. If there is any question of emphysema, bronchitis, asthma, bronchiectasis, airway obstruction, or pulmonary insufficiency with chronic or potential infection, the patient is preventively treated with an intensive prophylactic and therapeutic regimen, as previously mentioned.

These therapeutic modalities utilized preoperatively include preoperative education with respiratory assistance devices (intermittent positive pressure breathing and incentive spirometry), adequate utilization of mucolytic agents, humidification and bronchodilators as indicated, the use of postural and/or percussive postural drainage, and in cases where there is the suspicion of preoperative infection, appropriate therapy with antibiotics.

As previously mentioned, preoperative sputum cultures are obtained regardless of the history or findings so that appropriate therapy can be instituted in the immediate postoperative period if signs of pulmonary infection are present.

Abstinence from smoking and/or isolation from smoke-filled rooms at least in the immediate preoperative period (hopefully for weeks or months preoperatively) is urged.

The education of the patient in appropriate and productive postoperative deep breathing and coughing exercises is stressed.

### ■ What important measures are utilized during surgery to prevent postoperative pulmonary complications?

During pump perfusion and especially during long pump runs proteins are probably denatured and the physiologic characteristics of surfactant are altered, therefore making the cardiopulmonary bypass patient prone to atelectasis. When surfactant is altered or decreased, any partial or total collapse of the lung or alveoli can be associated with troublesome postoperative atelectasis. It is standard policy to apply varying intermittent pressures of inflation before, during, and after perfusion.

Antibiotics are added to the pump or given intravenously, and although their primary purpose is to prevent any mediastinal or cardiac infection from the skin or other sources, this probably adds prophylaxis to pulmonary infection.

In cases with extenuating circumstances that require longer than usual pump runs, excessive transfusion of blood, and maintenance of somewhat lower than optimum mean pressures on the pump, additional precautionary measures are taken, including the use of Swank microfilters for blood (to prevent platelet aggregate pulmonary emboli) and the occasional use of IV or pump steroids to hopefully prevent perfusion ("pump") lung.

Every precaution should be taken to prevent regurgitation and aspiration of gastric contents. The high acid content of the gastric secretions, when brought in contact with the pulmonary mucosa, can predispose to overwhelming and diffuse aspiration pneumonia. If at any time during the operative or postoperative period aspiration is suspected, bronchoscopy and bronchial irrigation using a sodium bicarbonate and steroid solution is employed along with the administration of systemic corticosteroids and antibiotics. Today this complication occurs rarely because of the adequate use of nasogastric suctioning, appropriate inflations of the endotracheal tube cuffs, and decrease in overenthusiastic tendencies to feed or give the patient oral intake before the gastrointestinal tract has returned to normal function.

### ■ What specific complications can occur in the postoperative period and how are they prevented?

Atelectasis is a patchy, segmental lobar or total airless collapse of a lung, usually as a result of proximal bronchial obstruction from retained thick secretions, obstructing tubes, or aspirated material. It is usually accompanied by temperature elevations to 102° to 104° F, increases in pulse and respiratory rates, and evidence of AV shunting by the arterial gases, and it is confirmed by decreased breath sounds and excursions on the involved side and x-ray evidence of increased densities.

When major atelectasis occurs, mediastinal shift toward the affected side and frequently elevation of the diaphragm are evident on the chest x-ray film. Atelectasis appears to be the most common postoperative complication; by strict interpretation of the x-ray films, this appears in some form in at least 50% of the postoperative cases in which the pump was used. Frequently the only sign is visualization on the x-ray film of minimum infiltration or discoid atelectasis in the basilar segments. This is probably associated with the decreased surfactant, vascular congestion, and decreased ventilation of these areas during bypass.

The recommended therapy for this minimum or more involved atelectasis is frequent tracheobronchial suction, administration of adequate volume for ventilation, frequent use of the sigh mechanisms on the respirator, and when possible, constant positive end-expiratory pressure (PEEP) to maintain inflation of all areas and segments of the lung. Stimulation of deep breathing and coughing (using pillow supports over the incision for splinting) and appropriate use of humidification, mucolytic agents, and if not contraindicated, bronchodilators are also necessary adjuncts to both the treatment and the prevention of atelectasis.

Adequate use of pain medication prior to suctioning, pulmonary therapy, and coughing exercises enables the patient to obtain full respiratory excursions and produce better coughs. Postoperative complications are decreased with the use of the midsternotomy incision in contrast to the other chest incisions, because its solid bone-to-bone closure produces less pain in the postoperative period and use of this incision usually avoids entering either thoracic cavity. One of the most painful of all chest incisions is the posterolateral approach, with the anterolateral, the anterior inframammary, and the parasternal mediastinal incisions being progressively less painful.

Pneumothorax occurs in a small percentage of cases where pleural violation was not suspected and is usually recognized on the routine postoperative chest x-ray films. When first noticed, repeat x-ray films are obtained to ensure against progression, and if significant increase is present, immediate tube thoracostomy with underwater seal drainage is essential. Evaluation of chest excursion and auscultation combined with percussion lead to early recognition of this entity. Whenever ventilatory problems occur without other positive findings, pneumothorax should be suspected. A high index of suspicion should be maintained after any intracardiac injections following cardiopulmonary resuscitation procedures.

Pleural effusion associated with blood or serous accumulation in one chest cavity or the other occurs to some degree in a fair percentage of patients. If respiratory embarrassment develops with abnormal arterial blood gas concentrations or if the fluid increases, therapeutic aspiration and/or tube thoracostomy should be instituted.

Bronchial aspiration occurs infrequently today, but if moderate aspiration is visualized, it is recommended that the endotracheal tube be irrigated, while the patient is frequently turned, with a combination of saline solution, bicarbonate solution, and steroids.

The mixture should contain sodium bicarbonate in a concentration of 2.3% to 2.5%. If irrigation is inadequate, bronchoscopy with therapeutic aspiration and irrigation with similar solution is indicated, followed by the use of steroids. The incidence of this complication can be lessened by the judicious use of the nasogastric tube and avoidance of the overzealous use of ice chips and other oral intake before gastrointestinal tract activity is established.

Inadequate ventilation is identified by visual and auscultation evaluation combined with frequent blood gas assessment. Causes of inadequate ventilation include inappropriately low volumes, decreased oxygen concentrations, lack of adequate humidification, poor use of end-expiratory pressures, improper placement of the endotracheal tube, and all previously mentioned factors such as atelectasis, pneumothorax, hemothorax, and hydrothorax, as well as endotracheal and airway resistance associated with a too-small tube or nonaspirated secretions. In patients whose ventilatory studies are not adequate after the third or fourth day using endotracheal intubation, a tracheostomy should be instituted for better toileting and prevention of ventilatory cuff and endotracheal tube problems.

Infection can also occur as the result of inadequate ventilation, inappropriate suctioning, and general inability to eliminate pulmonary secretions, as well as from aspiration and atelectasis occurring after using the pump. Once infection occurs, a very enthusiastic regimen must be employed, including sputum cultures and sensitivity tests, more vigorous pulmonary modalities, and appropriate antibiotic therapy. I have found a somewhat increased incidence of infection resulting from many of the gram-negative organisms, especially *Serratia marcescens,* after the prophylactic use of cephalosporins. Certain otherwise nonpathogenic bacteria can become opportunists when prophylactic antibiotics are used. When pulmonary infection occurs in a patient taking more than adequate doses of antibiotics, gentamicin sulfate and/or carbenicillin are frequently added to the antibiotic regimen. When marked atelectasis occurs on either the left or right side as a result of retained secretions and does not clear within a 6- to 8-hour period or respiratory efficiency is decreased, bronchoscopy with therapeutic aspiration and irrigation is rapidly instituted to prevent progressive pulmonary infection and/or abscess.

Perfusion ("pump") lung is a condition exhibited by progressive patchy atelectasis and worsening hypoxia and in late stages is associated with hypercapnia, acidosis, and severe hypoxemia. The characteristics of this entity closely parallel those of posttraumatic pulmonary insufficiency, and unless reversal is enacted in the early phases, death frequently ensues. It is often mandatory to treat this condition with continuous ventilatory support utilizing the mode of PEEP, corticosteroids, and all the previously mentioned pulmonary modalities.

## RENAL COMPLICATIONS

Postoperative acute renal failure is a dreaded complication and is not infrequently encountered following cardiopulmonary bypass. Once fully developed, it carries an overall mortality of over 40%. The precipitating factors seem to be preexisting chronic renal disease or continual insult associated with the cardiac condition requiring surgery. This, in addition to possible decreased perfusion of the kidneys during bypass or associated hypotensive episodes or physiologic renal vasoconstriction from drugs, can precipitate the condition. The accumulation of serum and urine hemoglobin after moderate red blood cell destruction during bypass procedures in association with the previously mentioned factors predispose to the development of renal failure. The shifting of body fluids with functional dehydration has also been suggested as a definite precursor to renal failure in bypass patients.

■ **What modes of therapy can be utilized in the prophylactic treatment of acute renal failure?**

When possible, maintenance of adequate hydration in the preoperative, operative, and postoperative periods with balanced electrolyte solutions is recommended. The hydration levels can be monitored by the amount of urinary output, the CVP, and the atrial pressure in the immediate postoperative period.

The use of high perfusion rates and flows during bypass with use of an osmotic diuretic such as mannitol is prophylactic, especially in cases where plasma and urine hemoglobin levels are elevated.

Preoperative microscopic evaluation of the urine for casts and inflammatory cells with cultures and sensitivity tests for infections followed by appropriate urologic consultation when abnormal can help prevent the acute renal problem.

## ■ What factors or signs suggest the development of acute renal failure?

When urinary output is low in the postoperative period (below 20 ml/hr), it usually is a reflection of low cardiac output or dehydration, but it can be an early indication of renal failure. However, occasionally relatively static or high flows of urine can be present but with fixed low specific gravities; this can also be a manifestation of early renal failure.

The progressive elevation of the blood urea nitrogen (BUN) and serum creatinine and the continued decrease in urinary output despite adequate hydration with elevation in serum potassium levels and microscopic urinary pigments usually confirm the suspected diagnosis.

## ■ What findings differentiate between renal failure, low cardiac output, and dehydration as the cause of decreased urine output?

The rapid influx of 500 to 1000 ml of fluid (in a patient whose cardiodynamics can tolerate this) over a 2- to 3-hour period will usually establish whether or not a patient is dehydrated. If the urinary output increases with this measure, the patient is probably dehydrated or hypovolemic.

If overall cardiac output appears low and hypotension is present, the use of one of the inotropic agents that does not cause peripheral constriction in the renal capillary beds will usually elevate the blood pressure, and if urinary output increases, the decreased urinary flow was probably associated with low cardiac output.

When the preceding two measures fail along with increased doses of diuretics (in refractory cases doses as high as 200 mg of furosemide [Lasix] have been used in bolus form), the assumption of acute renal failure is probably confirmed.

## ■ How is acute renal failure managed?

When the diagnosis is highly likely and no response to the previously described measures has occurred, a nephrologist joins the team, takes over the management of fluids, and recommends dosages of drugs excreted by or toxic to the kidney.

When the potassium and BUN levels cannot adequately be controlled by restriction of potassium and protein intake, exchange resins (administered through the rectum or nasogastric tube) are necessary, and if these are ineffective, peritoneal dialysis and/or preparation for hemodialysis can be instituted. Once a firm diagnosis of renal failure is established, the institution of each hemodialysis appears to result in a higher percentage of return of renal function.

It has been recommended by some that any urine volume below 30 ml/hr signals danger of impending renal failure. It is thought that a particularly useful test of impending tubular necrosis is a measurement of the urine-to-plasma ratio with regard to urea nitrogen. When the ratio is 10 or below, it is indicative of renal failure; however, when the ratio is 30 or above the patient is most likely suffering from dehydration alone. In the range between 10 and 30 the situation is considered to be impending or possibly incipient but still potentially reversible tubular necrosis.

With most individuals once the diagnosis of renal tubular damage has been ascertained, every effort should be made to restrict the intake of water, sodium chloride, and particularly potassium. Since patients subjected to open-heart surgery will not have a prolonged period of intestinal ileus, they will be taking oral fluids relatively soon, and excessive loading with fluids and potassium is possible. In renal failure any tendency for the serum sodium level to fall is usually indicative of excessive fluid intake.

## POSTOPERATIVE FEVER AND INFECTION

Preoperative precautions such as antibacterial showers, clean linen, pulmonary prophylaxis, and preoperative antibiotic administration as well as intensive protective measures in the postoperative period have made major problems with infection relatively rare in the cardiac surgical patient.

### ■ What are common causes for temperature elevations seen during the postoperative period?

Fevers occurring in the first 24 to 48 hours postoperatively are usually associated with varying degrees of atelectasis and retained pulmonary secretions, as in most postoperative surgical patients. These temperatures are usually under 102° F orally and respond most often to continuation of the antibiotics, vigorous suctioning, deep breathing, coughing and other pulmonary modalities, and the simple administration of rectal acetaminophen (Tylenol) or salicylates. When the rectal temperatures persist at 101° to 102° F, simple cooling measures or use of a cooling blanket are helpful. Some of the temperature elevations immediately following use of the pump are also probably associated with increased red blood cell destruction, fluid shifts, etc.

Total refractoriness of fever to all therapeutic modes suggests CNS involvement, possibly from poor cerebral perfusion or embolic phenomenon.

High fevers occurring between the third and fifth days may indicate pulmonary infection as a result of nonresolved atelectasis, or possible urinary infection or septicemia. Any fevers that develop late or are refractory to active therapeutic regimens are evaluated with cultures of the wounds, sputum, blood, and urine. If the temperature elevations persist, antibiotics are withheld for 12 to 24 hours while blood cultures are reobtained, preferably during periods of temperature spikes.

Fevers that occur between the seventh and tenth days are more indicative of fluid accumulations or cavity infections, and careful scrutiny of all wound areas will not infrequently reveal serum or infected accumulations. Another cause, although rare, is pulmonary embolic phenomenon and is usually associated with dyspnea, slight tachycardia, mild hypertension, and pleural or pericardial friction rubs.

High fever on the seventh to tenth postoperative days can also indicate endocarditis and/or infection of a prosthetic graft or valve. When this is suspected, both venous and arterial blood samples are submitted for culture and sensitivity. Occasionally arterial blood samples have been responsible for establishing the diagnosis of mycotic infections of prosthetic valves.

It is relatively common to have low-grade temperature elevations persist despite antibiotics and appropriate hydration and in the face of normal white blood cell counts and sedimentation rates. On the recommendation of the cardiologist or epidemiologist all antibiotics and most nonessential drugs are often withheld, with frequent return of the temperature to normal.

Fever during the second postoperative week associated with pleuritic pain, pericardial friction rub, ECG evidence of pericarditis, and occasionally high lymphocyte and eosinophil counts may constitute a form of postcardiotomy syndrome that is treated initially with salicylates and/or acetaminophen (Tylenol) and occasionally with steroid medication (10 mg of prednisone four times a day for a period of 3 days), frequently with dramatic response.

The fever of bacterial endocarditis is often associated with chills and moderate to marked elevation of the white blood cell count and sedimentation rate. The signs and symptoms usually occur anywhere from the first week to multiple months after the surgical procedure. (More delayed onset of signs and symptoms is not uncommon in fungal endocarditis.) Dyspnea, peripheral embolic phenomenon (with peripheral petechiae or Quincke's pulse), splenomegaly, and/or the development of new murmurs are all significant signs in bacterial endocarditis.

Again, it is emphasized that the incidence of incisional, pulmonary, and sternal infections has been almost nil with diligent preoperative, postoperative, and operative precautions and with the use of antibiotics in *all* these phases.

## GASTROINTESTINAL COMPLICATIONS

Complications of the gastrointestinal tract are usually quite rare and are kept to a minimum because of certain basic standards of care.

### ■ How are gastrointestinal complications prevented?

Whenever there is evidence by physical examination or on the postoperative chest x-ray films of gastric distention, nasogastric tubes are placed for decompression of the stomach.

Liquids and ice chips are withheld until gastrointestinal activity is evident. Since sucking of ice chips is accompanied by moderate amounts of swallowed air for such a small fluid yield, I believe it is imperative that the patient be given nothing orally for a maximum of 24 and often 36 hours in the immediate postoperative period.

Individuals who have experienced problems with gastric hypersecretion, duodenal ulcer, peptic esophagitis, or acid indigestion will agree that coffee, tea, apple juice, and salty bouillons create epigastric distress and appear to produce moderate hyperacidity and distress. Therefore once bowel sounds are heard and abdominal distention is not present, a bland palatable diet is instituted. Once this is tolerated for 12 to 24 hours, the patient is allowed a more select or therapeutic diet (diabetic, low salt, etc.). In no case in the immediate postoperative period is coffee, hot spicy soup, or bouillon allowed because of gastric acid secretion and fear of bronchial aspiration.

Gastrointestinal bleeding, particularly in patients with peptic esophagitis and duodenal ulcer, is not uncommon and is diagnosed in a manner similar to a routine workup.

## INVOLVEMENT OF THE CENTRAL NERVOUS SYSTEM

Postoperative minor or major psychotic reactions, focal neurologic deficit, or total flaccid paralysis and coma can all occur during the postoperative phase.

### ■ What frequent abnormalities of the CNS are manifested postoperatively and what is the cause and treatment?

Major and minor personality disorders are not infrequently seen in postoperative patients. Occasionally specific causes are evident, such as a history of chronic alcoholic intake or preoperative personality problems treated with tranquilizing medications. However, frequently there is no history or specific etiology to explain postoperative signs and symptoms of paranoia, agitation, intermittent lack of coherence, disorientation, memory lapses, hallucinatory episodes, or bizarre motor actions during rest. The combination of the stress of the surgery, some degree of atherosclerotic cerebrovascular insufficiency, constant deprivation of sleep, or possibly embolization of small amounts of air or other minute particulate matter during the pump run are all possible contributing factors.

These conditions usually require a magnitude of reassurance for the patient, relatives, and practitioners. Ignoring or antagonizing the irrational, confused patient usually only intensifies the problem. Appropriate sedation and establishment of sleep for the patient appears to be the single most important therapy, and this is frequently accomplished by withholding all activities if possible from midnight until 5:00 or 6:00 A.M. (with a respectively quiet unit during those hours) and utilization of a mild tranquilizing medication such as diazepam (Valium). In uncontrollable patients or those with a history of chronic ethanolism, chlorpromazine (Thorazine), chlordiazepoxide (Librium), or in dire necessities, IV alcohol is used. The majority of the confusion and bizarre activity episodes usually subside within 72 to 96 hours, but this period seems like weeks and months to the family and professional staff. With recovery, the patient can usually recall the episode in a very hazy postnightmarish manner, and this recall is often present for months or years.

■ **What are the less common but more serious CNS abnormalities that can occur?**

Total lack of consciousness without response to pain or other stimuli can occur in the immediate postoperative period from cerebral edema, continual embolization of air during the pump run, massive intracerebral embolization of clot or debris, or even intracerebral hemorrhage.

Generalized stupor and lack of response with focal signs are more often associated with small embolic phenomenon but nevertheless can be associated with postoperative sequelae or even death.

Progressive lightening of the coma with improvement is an encouraging sign, and when it occurs within the first 24 to 48 hours, carries a prognosis of minimum residual sequelae.

If no major response is obtained in the first 3 to 4 hours and there is no evidence to support analgesic dosage, then neurologic consultation is obtained and a postoperative EEG is immediately secured and compared with the preoperative study. Caloric tests of the eardrums and evaluation for doll's eyes are performed by the neurologist or neurosurgeon. If there is any question of brain damage, methods to decrease cerebral edema are instituted. Corticosteroids given three or four times a day are administered over a 3- to 4-day period, the head and torso are maintained at approximately 30 degrees of elevation to decrease cerebral edema, overhydration is avoided with administration of adequately balanced salt solutions, and the judicial use of diuretics is instituted. Osmotic diuretics, such as mannitol and urea compounds (Urevert) are used less frequently today because of the associated rebound edema phenomena that can complicate recovery.

During this phase of CNS insult it is imperative that appropriate ventilation with normal or high concentrations of oxygen be maintained with normal or minimally elevated partial pressures of carbon dioxide.

Additional treatment includes hypothermia to decrease the metabolic needs of the CNS, diphenylhydantoin, (Dilantin) or diazepam (Valium) to control seizures or convulsions, and when the suspected etiology is embolizing clot, utilization of heparin anticoagulation, when safe.

In cases where the specific etiology of the strokelike symptoms is not established, selective carotid arteriograms may be required. However, most symptomatic carotid artery stenosis or ulcerations have been discovered and evaluated preoperatively by auscultation and/or arteriography and surgically corrected before any cardiac surgical procedure is performed.

Occasionally patients will demonstrate delayed effects from analgesics and/or muscle relaxants used during surgery. These patients will frequently appear alert enough to be extubated, giving the surgeon a false sense of security. Then, as the patient is ready to leave the hospital, he will develop shallow respirations, become hypercapnic, and require emergency assisted ventilation and reintubation.

## OTHER COMPLICATIONS

■ **What other complications can occur in the postoperative cardiac surgical patient?**

Fluid and electrolyte imbalances not infrequently occur; however, the administration of and reasons for appropriate electrolyte therapy have previously been described (Chapter 12).

Myocardial ischemia, infarction, or congestive failure can occur in these coronary occlusion–prone patients, but the management of these conditions is similar to that of any patient with these diagnoses. It is essential that these complications be recognized promptly so that the patient does not leave the unit or hospital with an existing infarction, impending arrhythmia, or congestive heart failure.

Psychologic dependency occurs in a fair number of cardiac surgical patients as a result of their having been in an atmosphere offering continuous expert attention. When transferred after 3 or 4 days to telemetry on the ward, it is important that the patient be assured that this transfer is an indication of excellent postoperative recovery.

## BIBLIOGRAPHY FOR CHAPTERS 10-13


Alexander, J. W.: Nosocomial infections, Curr. Probl. Surg., Aug., 1973.

Aspinall, M. J.: Nursing the open heart surgery patient, New York, 1973, McGraw-Hill Book Co.

Austen, W. B., and Mundth, E. D.: Postoperative intensive care in the cardiac surgical patient, Prog. Cardiovasc. Dis. **11**:229, 1968.

Bachmann, F.: Disseminated intravascular coagulation, Disease-A-Month, Dec., 1969.

Bachmann, F., and Pichairut, O.: Surgical bleeding, Med. Clin. North Am. **56**:207, 1972.

Bartlett, R. H., Gazzaniga, A. B., and Geraghty, T. R.: The yawn maneuver: prevention and treatment of postoperative pulmonary complications, Surg. Forum **22**:196, 1971.

Bartlett, R. H., Gazzaniga, A. B., and Geraghty, T. R.: Respiratory maneuvers to prevent pulmonary complications: a critical review, J.A. M.A. **244**:1017, 1973.

Bartlett, R. H., Gazzaniga, A. B., Brennan, M., and Hanson, E. L.: Studies in pathogenesis and prevention of postoperative pulmonary complications, Surg. Gynecol. Obstet. **137**:925-933, 1973.

Beall, A. C., Jr., Fred, H. L., and Cooley, D. A.: Pulmonary embolism, Curr. Probl. Surg., Feb., 1964.

Behrendt, D. M., and Austen, G. W.: Patient care in cardiac surgery, Boston, 1972, Little, Brown & Co.

Brandenberg, R. O.: Medical problems of aortic valve replacement, Prog. Cardiovasc. Dis. **7**: 531, 1965.

Buchbinder, N. A., and Roberts, W. C.: Left-sided valvular acute infective endocarditis, Am. J. Med. **53**:20-35, 1972.

Burman, S. O.: Intra-aortic balloon pumping for low cardiac output syndromes, Surg. Clin. North Am. **55**:101-105, 1975.

Bushnell, S. S.: Respiratory intensive care nursing, Boston, 1973, Little, Brown & Co.

Calvin, J. W., Stemmer, E. A., Steedman, R. A., and Connolly, J. E.: Clinical application of parasternal mediastinotomy, Arch. Surg. **102**: 322-325, 1971.

Clowes, G. H. A., Jr.: Surgery of the lung, esophagus and mediastinum. In Kinney, J. M., et al., editors: Manual of preoperative and postoperative care, Philadelphia, 1967, W. B. Saunders Co.

Cohn, H. E., and Capelli, J. P.: The diagnosis and management of oliguria in the postoperative period, Surg. Clin. North Am. **47**:1187, 1967.

Connolly, J. E., Wakabayashi, A., German, J. C., Stemmer, E. A., and Serres, E. J.: Clinical experience with pulsatile left heart bypass without anti-coagulation for thoracic aneurysms, J. Thorac. Cardiovasc. Surg. **62**:568-576, 1971

Constant, J.: Bedside cardiology, Boston, 1969, Little, Brown & Co.

Cooley, D. A., and Hallman, G. L.: Surgical treatment of congenital heart disease, Philadelphia, 1966, Lea & Febiger.

Damman, J. F., Jr., Thumg, N., Christlieb, I. I., Littlefield, J. B., and Muller W., Jr.: The management of the severely ill patient after open-heart surgery, J. Thorac. Cardivasc. Surg. **45**:80, 1963.

Danielson, G. K., and Ellis, F. H., Jr.: Low cardiac output and cardiac arrhythmias after open heart surgery. In Hardy, J. D.: Critical surgical illness, Philadelphia, 1971, W. B. Saunders Co.

Dismukes, W. E., et al.: Prosthetic valve endocarditis, Circulation **48**:365-377, 1973.

Ellis, F. H., Jr.: Surgery for acquired mitral valve disease, Philadelphia, 1967, W. B. Saunders Co.

Engleman, R. W., et al.: Cardiac tamponade following open-heart surgery, Circulation **41** (suppl. 11):165-171, 1970.

Finland, M.: Current problems in infective endocarditis, Mod. Concepts Cardiovasc. Dis. **41**: 53-58, 1972.

Fraser, R. S., Rossall, R. E., and Dvorkin, J.: Bacterial endocarditis occurring after open heart surgery, Can. Med. Assoc. J. **96**:1551-1558, 1967.

Friedman, B.: Cardiac surgery: dependency and apprehension complicate nursing care. Cardiac surgery: skilled nursing during the critical postoperative period, Nursing '74 **4**:33-40, 1974.

Goldin, M. D.: Intensive care of the surgical patient, Chicago, 1971, Year Book Medical Publishers, Inc.

Gott, V. L., Brawley, R. K., Donahoo, J. S., and Griffith, L. S. C.: Current surgical approach to ischemic heart disease, Curr. Probl. Surg., May, 1973.

Guntheroth, W. G., Morgan, B. C., and Mullins, B. S.: Effect of respiration and venous return and stroke volume in cardiac tamponade. Mechanism of pulsus paradoxus, Circ. Res. **20:** 381, 1967.

Harrison, D. C., Kerber, R. E., and Alderman, E. L.: Pharmacodynamics and clinical use of cardiovascular drugs after cardiac surgery, Am. J. Cardiol. **26:**385-392, 1970.

Hegeman, C. O., Rappaport, I., and Berger, W. J.: Superficial temporal artery cannulation, Arch. Surg. **99:**619-623, 1969.

Holzer, J., et al.: Effectiveness of dopamine in patients with cardiogenic shock, Am. J. Cardiol. **32:**79-83, 1973.

Hudak, C. M., Gallo, B. M., and Cohn, T.: Critical care nursing, Philadelphia, 1973, J. B. Lippincott Co.

Javid, H., et al.: Neurological abnormalities following open-heart surgery, J. Thorac. Cardiovasc. Surg. **58:**502-509, 1969.

Juler, G. L., Stemmer, E. A., and Connolly, J. E.: Complications of prophylactic digitalization in thoracic surgery patients, J. Thorac. Cardiovasc. Surg. **58:**352-360, 1969.

Kantrowitz, A. R., Phillips, S. J., Butner, A., Tjønneland, S., and Haller, J. D.: Technique of femoral artery cannulation for phase-shift balloon pumping, J. Thorac. Cardiovasc. Surg. **56:**219, 1968.

Karliner, J. S.: Dopamine for cardiogenic shock, J.A.M.A. **226:**1217, 1973.

Kinney, J. M.: The recovery room and intensive care patient. In Kinney, J. M., et al., editors: Manual of preoperative and postoperative care, Philadelphia, 1967, W. B. Saunders Co.

Kirklin, J. W.: Advances in cardiovascular surgery, New York, 1973, Grune & Stratton, Inc.

Kirklin, J. W., and Nunn, S. L.: The cardiovascular system in care of the surgical patient. In Kinney, J. M., et al., editors: Manual of preoperative and postoperative care, Philadelphia, 1967, W. B. Saunders Co.

Kloster, F. L., Bristow, J. D., and Griswold, H. E.: Medical problems in mitral and multiple valve replacement, Prog. Cardiovasc. Dis. **7:**504, 1965.

Laufman, H.: Hematologic crises in surgery. In Hardy, J. D.: Critical surgical illness, Philadelphia, 1971, W. B. Saunders Co.

Levitsky, S.: New insights in cardiac trauma, Surg. Clin. North Am. **55:**43-54, 1975.

McGoon, D. W.: Techniques of open-heart surgery for congenital heart disease, Curr. Probl. Surg., Apr., 1968.

Meltzer, L. E., Pinneo, R., and Kitchell, J. R.: Intensive coronary care, Philadelphia, 1970, The Charles Press, Publisher.

Moffitt, E. A., Sessler, A. D., and Kirklin, J. W.: Postoperative care in open-heart surgery, J.A.M.A. **199:**129, 1967.

Nelson, R. M., Jenson, C. B., and Smoot, W. M., III: Pericardial tamponade following open-heart surgery, J. Thorac. Cardiovasc. Surg. **58:** 510-516, 1969.

Netter, F. H.: Heart, Ciba Collection of Medical Illustrations, Summit, N. J., 1969, Ciba Publications.

Neville, W. E.: Cardiopulmonary bypass for open-heart surgery. In Cooper, P.: The craft of surgery, Boston, 1964, Little, Brown & Co.

Neville, W. E.: Extracorporeal circulaion, Curr. Probl. Surg., July, 1967.

Neville, W. E.: Care of the surgical cardiopulmonary patient, Chicago, 1971, Year Book Medical Publishers, Inc.

New, H. C.: Antimicrobial agents—mechanisms of action and clinical usage, Curr. Probl. Surg., June, 1973.

Oaks, W. W., and Moyer, J. H.: Pre- and postoperative management of the cardiopulmonary patient, New York, 1970, Grune & Stratton, Inc.

Parmley, L. F., Manion, W. L., and Mattingly, T. W.: Nonpenetrating traumatic injury of the heart, Circulation **18:**371, 1958.

Payne, D. D., De Weese, J. A., Mahoney, E. B., and Murphy, G. W.: Surgical treatment of traumatic rupture of the normal aortic valve, Ann. Thorac. Surg. **17:**223, 1974.

Quick, A. J.: Bleeding problems in clinical medicine, Philadelphia, 1970, W. B. Saunders Co.

Randall, H. T.: Fluid and electrolyte therapy. In Kinney, J. M., et al., editors: Manual of preoperative and postoperative care, Philadelphia, 1967, W. B. Saunders Co.

Roberts, W. C., Buchbinder, N. A.: Right-sided infective endocarditis, Am. J. Med. **53:**7-19, 1972.

Secor, J. S.: Coronary care—a nursing specialty, New York, 1971, Appleton-Century-Crofts.

Shaw-Mirany, J.: Technical advances in resection and graft replacement of thoracic, abdominal and peripheral aneurysms, Surg. Clin. North Am. **55:**57-77, 1975.

Soroff, H. S., Birtwell, W. C., and Giron, F.: Assisted circulation. In Norman, J. C., editor: Cardiac surgery, New York, 1972, Appleton-Century-Crofts.

Spodick, D. H.: Acute cardiac tamponade, pathology, physiology, diagnosis and management, Prog. Cardiovasc. Dis. **10:**64, 1967.

Standards for cardiopulmonary resuscitation (CPR) and emergency cardiac care (ECC), J.A.M.A. **227**(suppl.):834-865, 1974.

Stock, J. P. P.: Diagnosis and treatment of cardiac arrhythmias, New York, 1969, Appleton-Century-Crofts.

Tector, A. J., Reuben, C. F., Hoffman, J. F.,

Gelford, E. T., Healon, W., and Morman, L.: Coronary artery wounds treated with saphenous vein bypass grafts, J.A.M.A. **225**:282, 1973.

Van Meter, M.: Chest tubes—basic techniques for better care, Nursing '74 **4**:48-55, 1974.

Von Hippel, A.: Chest tubes and chest bottles, Springfield, Ill., 1970, Charles C Thomas, Publisher.

Wakabayashi, A., Connolly, J. E., Stemmer, E. A., and Nakamura, Y.: Clinical experience with heparinless, veno-arterial bypass without oxygenation for the treatment of acute cardiogenic shock, J. Thorac. Cardiovasc. Surg. **68**:687-695, 1974.

Walter, C. W.: Blood donors, blood transfusions. In Kinney, J. M., et al., editors: Manual of preoperative and postoperative care, Philadelphia, 1967, W. B. Saunders Co.

Wheat, M. W., et al.: Acute dissecting aneurysms of the aorta, J. Thorac. Cardiovasc. Surg. **58**: 344, 1969.

Wilson, J. W.: The pulmonary cellular and subcellular alteration of extracorporeal circulation, Surg. Clin. North Am. **54**:1203-1220, 1974.

Yang, S. S., Bentivoglia, L. G., Maranhao, V., and Goldberg, H.: From cardiac catheterization data to hemodynamic parameters, Philadelphia, 1972, F. A. Davis Co.

*chapter 14*

# Management of endocrine and metabolic disturbances

BERNHARD G. ANDERSON

The endocrine system consists of glands that secrete hormones directly into the bloodstream. As customarily defined, the endocrine glands include the pituitary, thyroid, parathyroid, and adrenal glands, the ovaries, the testes, and the islet cells of the pancreas. The hypothalamus, part of the brain, secretes "releasing" factors, or hormones that release or inhibit the secretion of the hormones of the anterior pituitary gland. In pregnancy the placenta has important endocrine functions.

A wide variety of other organs and cells secrete hormones directly into the blood but are not usually classified as endocrine glands. The kidney secretes erythropoietin, which stimulates red blood cell production, and renin, which raises the blood pressure and affects aldosterone secretion by the adrenal cortex. Gastrointestinal hormones include secretin and gastrin. Prostaglandins, kinins, and serotonin are chemical compounds found in blood that are of diverse or uncertain origin and have important physiologic effects. They are sometimes classified as hormones, although not customarily included as part of the endocrine system. The endocrine status of the pineal gland and the thymus is uncertain.

Metabolism refers to a complex variety of biochemical processes occurring in organs, tissues, and cells of the body and concerned with the utilization of oxygen and food for energy and growth. Metabolic disorders are usually considered in relation to specific metabolic processes: diabetes mellitus and carbohydrate metabolism, diabetes insipidus and water metabolism, parathyroid disease and calcium metabolism, etc. Hormones serve as regulators of many metabolic processes, and it is therefore appropriate to consider endocrine and metabolic disorders together.

The endocrine glands and the hormones they secrete have important interrelationships and influences on many body functions both in health and in disease. This chapter is concerned with the major endocrine problems in the management of critically ill patients.

The following topics are discussed:

- Adrenocortical hormones
- Adrenocortical insufficiency
- Pheochromocytoma
- Calcium disorders
- Thyroid disorders
- Diabetic ketoacidosis
- Hyperglycemic nonketotic coma
- Lactic acidosis
- Hypoglycemia
- Diabetes insipidus
- Inappropriate antidiuretic hormone (ADH) syndrome

## Adrenocortical hormones

### ■ What are the adrenocortical hormones?

The adrenal cortex secretes a variety of steroids, the most important being cortisol and aldosterone. Androgens, estrogens, and progestins are also secreted but are physiologically less important. Cortisol, the major glucocorticoid, contributes to the maintenance of the blood glucose level mainly by promoting glyconeogenesis from amino acids; thus it is a protein catabolic. Cortisol increases the glomerular filtration rate and thus enhances water diuresis. Glucocorticoids also have lympholytic and eosinopenic effects and tend to increase the number of erythrocytes present. Various other glucocorticoid effects include stimulation of the CNS, increased gastric acidity, and fat mobilization. Of great importance are the anti-inflammatory and immunosuppressive actions of glucocorticoids. These actions are the basis for the therapeutic use of cortisol and related glucocorticoids in a wide variety of diseases. Aldosterone, the major mineralocorticoid, promotes the retention of sodium and the excretion of potassium by the kidneys. Cortisol, although primarily a glucocorticoid, has mineralocorticoid effects in large amounts.

Corticotropin (ACTH), secreted by the anterior pituitary gland, stimulates the adrenal cortex to produce cortisol. Diurnal variation in the release of corticotropin normally occurs so that it is released in the greatest amounts about 4 A.M. to 6 A.M. and in the least amounts about 12 hours later. The secretion of cortisol closely follows the release of corticotropin. A servoregulatory mechanism operates to stimulate the release of corticotropin when the plasma cortisol level falls and to suppress corticotropin when the plasma cortisol level rises. Stress—including trauma, infections, psychic factors, and a wide variety of illnesses—stimulates the release of corticotropin and consequently the secretion of cortisol. Stressful stimuli apparently induce the hypothalamus to secrete corticotropin-releasing factor.

Aldosterone is not under direct corticotropin control but is regulated mainly by the renin-angiotensin system. Aldosterone secretion increases in response to a reduction in intravascular volume, such as occurs with sodium depletion and acute hemorrhage.

Synthetic adrenocortical steroids have been produced that have potent glucocorticoid effects with little or no mineralocorticoid effects. These agents include prednisone, prednisolone, triamcinolone, and dexamethasone. They are widely used for their anti-inflammatory effects, and they have all the other glucocorticoid properties of cortisol except producing sodium retention.

## Adrenocortical insufficiency

### ■ What is adrenocortical insufficiency, and what treatment is recommended?

Acute adrenocortical insufficiency may be caused by bilateral adrenal hemorrhage or infarction and is precipitated by stress in patients with chronic adrenocortical insufficiency, anterior pituitary insufficiency, and adrenocortical suppression from glucocorticoid therapy. The usual clinical manifestations include weakness, hypotension, shock, fever, and reduced consciousness. Hyperpigmentation of the skin and mucous membranes is seen in patients with chronic primary adrenocortical insufficiency. The serum sodium level is usually low and the potassium level high in primary adrenocortical failure, but not in cases secondary to pituitary insufficiency or suppression by previous corticosteroid treatment. The blood glucose level tends to be low and the blood urea nitrogen elevated. The diagnosis is confirmed by finding a low value for plasma cortisol or 17-hydroxycorticosteroids, but treatment must be started immediately on reasonable suspicion without awaiting laboratory confirmation.

TREATMENT. The treatment includes the following:

1. Hydrocortisone, 100 mg given by IV route, should be given stat. A soluble preparation of hydrocortisone such as the hemisuccinate or phosphate form is used. Additional hydrocortisone in 5% dextrose and normal saline solution is given by IV infusion at a rate of 10 mg of hydrocortisone/hr for 24 hours; alternatively, 50 mg of hydrocortisone can be given by IM route every 6 hours.

2. A 1000 ml IV infusion of 5% dextrose in normal saline solution should be started immediately. The total fluid replacement in the first 24 hours is about 3000 ml. Thereafter 1000 ml of 5% dextrose in normal saline solution given daily is usually adequate, with 5% to 10% dextrose in water making up the remainder of the fluid requirement.

3. No potassium is given in the first 24 to 48 hours because the serum potassium level is already elevated. Later maintenance

amounts of potassium will be needed, usually 40 to 60 mEq daily given as potassium chloride.

4. Vasopressors such as norepinephrine or metaraminol may be needed if the hypotension does not respond to hydrocortisone and fluid and sodium replacement.

5. The hydrocortisone dose is reduced to 25 mg every 6 hours on the second or third day and progressively reduced to reach maintenance amounts of 20 to 30 mg daily in divided doses within 1 week. This can usually be given orally after the acute crisis has subsided.

6. A mineralocorticoid is usually needed to promote sodium retention when the hydrocortisone dose is less than 60 mg/day. Fludrocortisone is given orally; the average dose is 0.1 mg daily.

7. Fluids can be given orally as soon as tolerated, followed by a regular diet that usually obviates the need for sodium and potassium supplements.

8. Precipitating causes and concurrent diseases should be identified and treated appropriately.

*Secondary adrenocortical insufficiency* is treated as outlined with certain modifications. Cortisol is deficient, but aldosterone secretion is not greatly decreased. Therefore sodium depletion is uncommon, and mineralocorticoids are seldom needed.

*Management of stress* in patients with adrenocortical insufficiency is concerned with providing optimum support for patients with chronic adrenal insufficiency, hypopituitarism, or recent adrenal corticosteroid therapy (within 6 months) who have major acute illnesses, trauma, or are undergoing surgery. Similar management is appropriate for patients undergoing elective bilateral adrenalectomy. Hydrocortisone is given by IV route at a rate of 10 mg/hr beginning 30 minutes to 1 hour before the induction of anesthesia. Alternatively, hydrocortisone can be given by IM route in doses of 50 mg every 6 hours. Some practitioners prefer to give cortisone acetate by IM route in doses of 50 to 100 mg beginning 12 hours before surgery. The other details of management are similar to those described previously.

## Pheochromocytoma

■ **What is pheochromocytoma, and what management modalities should be considered?**

Paroxysmal or sustained hypertension occurs in patients with pheochromocytoma, a tumor of the adrenal medulla or sympathetic nerve endings. These tumors secrete norepinephrine and epinephrine, are uncommon, and are curable by surgery. Labile hypertension associated with palpitation, headache, and excessive sweating are characteristic manifestations. The diagnosis is established by finding an excessive urinary excretion of catecholamines or their metabolites. Hypertensive crises may occur. Preoperative and postoperative care requires special pharmacologic management.

### *Specific drugs*

Phentolamine (Regitine) and phenoxybenzamine (Dibenzyline) are useful in controlling blood pressure. Both are $\alpha$-adrenergic blocking agents; they inhibit the effects of catecholamines but do not alter their synthesis or degradation. Phentolamine is a short-acting preparation; repeated IV doses of 1 to 5 mg may be needed to control paroxysmal hypertension. Phenoxybenzamine is longer acting; oral doses of 40 to 100 mg every 12 hours are given for more sustained control of the hypertension. Propranolol (Inderal), a $\beta$-adrenergic blocker, is useful in controlling catecholamine-induced arrhythmias, tachycardia, angina, and sweating. Doses of 40 mg or more every 4 to 6 hours may be needed.

Drugs to be avoided because they release catecholamines include metaraminol (Aramine), $\alpha$-methyldopa, guanethidine, and the tricyclic antidepressants. Organic iodine dyes used in arteriography are potent releasers of catecholamines; therefore arteriography should not be performed until blockage is adequately established with phenoxybenzamine.

### *Surgical management*

In preparation for the surgical removal of a pheochromocytoma patients are usually treated with phenoxybenzamine for 2 weeks or longer to stabilize the blood pressure.

Opinions differ concerning the advisability of continuing administration of the drug up to the time of surgery or suspending it 2 to 3 days before surgery. Hypotension may follow the removal of a pheochromocytoma. IV norepinephrine is given under careful monitoring to raise the blood pressure. Blood volume restoration is important to control postoperative hypotension; these patients tend to have decreased plasma volume.

## Calcium disorders

■ **What causes calcium disorders in critically ill patients, and what therapeutic measures may be taken?**

Calcium is important in various membrane transport systems, which accounts for its effects on nerve, muscle, and heart function. About one half of the calcium in the blood plasma is bound to plasma proteins or complexed with other ions; the other half is ionized and physiologically available. Although the *total* calcium concentration in the serum is usually measured, the *ionized* calcium is the important fraction that determines its physiologic activity. Thus the total calcium concentration may be low in patients with low plasma protein levels but the ionized calcium fraction may be normal. Alkalosis decreases and acidosis increases the ionized fraction of calcium. Hypercalcemia depresses neuromuscular excitability and causes bradycardia, cardiac arrhythmias, and impaired renal function. Hypocalcemia increases neuromuscular excitability and causes tetany.

Calcium metabolism is regulated by parathyroid hormone, thyrocalcitonin, and vitamin D. A deficiency of parathyroid hormone leads to hypocalcemia, whereas an excess of parathyroid hormone produces hypercalcemia. This hormone has two major effects: (1) it maintains the plasma concentration of calcium at its normal level, 9 to 11 mg/100 ml, and (2) it promotes the renal excretion of phosphate. Thyrocalcitonin, which is secreted by the thyroid gland, lowers the plasma calcium concentration. Vitamin D promotes calcium absorption from the gut, contributes to the maintenance of a normal plasma calcium concentration, induces the calcification of new bone, and increases the renal excretion of calcium.

### *Hypercalcemia*

Hypercalcemia may be caused by tumors metastatic to bone and less commonly by neoplasms that secrete a parathyroid hormone–like substance. Hyperparathyroidism is a classic cause of hypercalcemia. Less common causes of hypercalcemia include hypervitaminosis D, the milk-alkali syndrome, multiple myeloma, sarcoidosis, Paget's disease with immobilization, thiazide diuretics, hyperthyroidism, and adrenal insufficiency.

TREATMENT. The urgency and vigor with which treatment must be pursued depends on the severity of the hypercalcemia. A patient with a serum calcium concentration in excess of 15 mg/100 ml is usually in critical condition and requires intensive care. It is important to monitor the fluid intake and output, body weight, serum electrolyte levels, ECG, and central venous pressure. Fluid overload must be prevented. Adverse changes in the serum concentrations of sodium, potassium, calcium, and magnesium may occur. Agents that lower the serum calcium include the following: (1) drugs that increase the urinary excretion of calcium, such as saline and furosemide; (2) drugs that increase calcium precipitation or retard bone dissolution, such as phosphates and mithramycin; and (3) measures that decrease the gastrointestinal absorption of calcium. Thyrocalcitonin might be effective but is not generally available.

The specific treatment recommended is as follows:

1. Hydration is induced with isotonic sodium chloride solution, 3 to 5 L given over 24 hours.

2. Furosemide is administered in doses of 80 to 120 mg to induce sodium and calcium excretion.

3. Phosphates are given, provided renal function is adequate and the patient is not hyperphosphatemic. Preparations containing monobasic and dibasic sodium and potassium phosphate may be given orally; the equivalent of 2 to 3 g of phosphorus is given daily in divided doses. Neutra-Phos-K contains 1

g of phosphorus/300 ml. Phospho-Soda contains 1 g of phosphorus/8 ml; 4 ml diluted in 200 ml of water can be given three or four times daily. Preparations of neutral phosphate can be given by IV infusion slowly, 50 mM over 6 to 8 hours, but the use of these preparations is hazardous.

4. Mithramycin may be effective in patients with hyperphosphatemia or impaired renal function. A single dose of 25 $\mu$g/kg in normal saline solution given over 3 to 4 hours may be adequate to lower the serum calcium concentration to normal within 48 to 72 hours.

5. Prednisone, 60 to 80 mg daily, may be helpful, but its effects are too slow (several days) in an acute situation, and it is usually ineffective in patients with hyperparathyroidism.

### *Hypocalcemia*

Acute hypocalcemia develops within a few hours postoperatively if the parathyroid glands have been damaged or inadvertently removed in patients undergoing thyroidectomy. Increased neuromuscular irritability with tetany occurs. (Tetany is also seen with alkalosis, but the serum calcium is normal.) Chronic hypocalcemia occurs in hypoparathyroidism, rickets, and osteomalacia and may be a manifestation of magnesium deficiency. The Chvostek sign (twitching of the side of the face in response to tapping on the facial nerve in front of the ear) is usually positive.

TREATMENT. Treatment consists of the administration of calcium, vitamin D, and possibly parathyroid hormone, as follows:

1. In an emergency IV calcium infusion is promptly effective. Calcium gluconate, 10 ml of a 10% solution, should be given slowly. Great caution is mandatory if the patient is receiving digitalis or its glycosides because of the synergistic effects of calcium and digitalis on the heart. In less acute situations calcium salts can be given orally; 10 to 25 g of calcium lactate or calcium gluconate may be needed daily. Dietary calcium should be increased but dietary phosphates decreased. Milk products should be avoided because they are rich in phosphates as well as calcium. Sedation may be helpful.

2. Hypocalcemia after thyroid or parathyroid surgery may be temporary, lasting only a few days or weeks. If the condition appears to be permanent or cannot be controlled by calcium orally, vitamin D is prescribed. Calciferol in doses of 200,000 units daily is given, with reduction of the doses as the serum calcium concentration is restored to normal. Dihydrotachysterol may be preferred because of its quicker onset and shorter duration of action. The dosage range is 1.0 to 1.5 mg/day. The serum calcium concentration should be monitored frequently (initially every week, then less often) to maintain the serum calcium level at about 9 to 10 mg/100 ml. Hypercalcemia from overtreatment must be avoided.

3. Parathyroid hormone would be logical therapy, but suitable preparations are unavailable for clinical use.

## Thyroid disorders

■ **On what basis are the diagnoses of thyroid storm and myxedema coma made, and what plans of care should be considered?**

Thyroid function is not altered acutely during the course of nonthyroidal illness, but two thyroid disorders are encountered that do require intensive care—thyroid storm and myxedema coma.

### *Thyroid storm*

Thyroid storm (thyrotoxic crisis) is an acute severe exacerbation of hyperthyroidism. Although rare, it is fatal if untreated and has a significant mortality even with prompt treatment. The "storm" may be precipitated by trauma, surgery, or intercurrent diseases in patients with hyperthyroidism. Extreme tachycardia, atrial fibrillation, fever, and profound weakness occur together with the usual manifestations of hyperthyroidism, including warm, moist skin, tremor, and muscle weakness with or without goiter and ophthalmopathy. The diagnosis of thyroid storm in a patient with hyperthyroidism is arbitrary; the customary criteria include fever in excess of 100° F orally (without other cause) and a heart rate in excess of 140 beats/min. Laboratory data to confirm the diagnosis include elevated values for free and total thyroxine in the serum, and usually an abnormally high level of thyroid uptake of radioactive iodine. The urgency is such that treatment must be started before laboratory confirmation of the diagnosis can be obtained.

TREATMENT. Specific treatment is directed at inhibiting the secretion of excess thyroid hormone and counteracting its effects. The treatment should be delivered as follows:

1. Antithyroid drugs are given in large doses—propylthiouracil, 200 mg, or methimazole (Tapazole), 20 mg, every 6 hours orally or by gastric intubation (no parenteral forms of these drugs are available). These block the synthesis of new thyroid hormone.
2. Iodine in the form of sodium or potassium iodide, 0.5 to 1.0 g, is given orally or by IV route every 12 to 24 hours, but not until the patient has received a blocking dose of propylthiouracil or methimazole. Iodides inhibit the synthesis and release of thyroxine from the thyroid.
3. Adrenergic blocking agents are helpful because some of the effects of excess thyroxine are mediated by increased sensitivity to the effects of catecholamines. Oral guanethidine and IM reserpine have been used. The most effective drug currently available is propranolol in doses of 40 mg or more every 4 to 6 hours.

Supportive treatment includes the following measures:

1. Fluids are given to correct dehydration and replace losses of sodium and potassium.
2. Dextrose with large amounts of vitamin B complex vitamins are administered. The hypermetabolism associated with hyperthyroidism requires increased amounts of vitamin B.
3. Hydrocortisone, 200 to 300 mg daily, is often recommended (although adrenal insufficiency is ordinarily not present).
4. Hypothermia may be needed if cool wet packs or ice packs are ineffective.
5. Digoxin or shorter acting glycosides may be needed, as well as quinidine or other antiarrhythmic agents. The dose of digoxin may be larger than usual because of the accelerated metabolism.
6. Diuretics may be needed if congestive heart failure or pulmonary edema occurs.
7. Sedation with phenobarbital or diazepam may be helpful.
8. Appropriate treatment of precipitating or concurrent diseases should be initiated.

Improvement should occur within 24 to 48 hours, with recovery from the acute storm within a few days. Appropriate treatment of the hyperthyroidism is then continued until definitive therapy can be implemented.

### *Myxedema coma*

Myxedema coma is a severe state of hypothyroidism. It occurs in patients with untreated hypothyroidism of long duration. Although uncommon, it is extremely important to recognize the disorder and treat it effectively because it is fatal if untreated and has a high mortality rate even with treatment. The characteristic signs of myxedema (severe hypothyroidism) are usually present: typical facies, nonpitting edema, cold dry skin, myoedema and delayed relaxation of tendon reflexes (unless the patient is areflexic), bradycardia, and usually hypotension. Mental obtundation is severe. Hypothermia is common, several degrees below normal, but may not be apparent using the usual clinical thermometer.

Precipitating factors include infection, trauma, cerebral vascular thrombosis, and drugs that depress the CNS. Carbon dioxide retention may occur in association with alveolar hypoventilation. Hyponatremia may occur in association with the inappropriate secretion of antidiuretic hormone.

Laboratory data specifically include abnormally low values for total thyroxine concentration in the serum. The cerebrospinal fluid protein level may be elevated.

The ECG usually shows sinus bradycardia, low voltage of the QRS complexes, and low or flat T waves.

TREATMENT. Treatment may need to be started on the basis of reasonable suspicion without waiting for the results of confirmatory laboratory tests despite the hazard in patients with heart disease.

Treatment with thyroid hormone is specific. IV levothyroxine sodium is given, usually in a dose of 0.5 mg. Some practitioners prefer to give 0.25 mg initially and 0.25 mg again in 24 hours. As an alternative, liothyronine (triiodothyronine) may be given in doses of 25 $\mu$g every 6 to 12 hours. This is given orally because parenteral preparations are not usually available. As the patient improves, maintenance therapy with oral levothyroxine can be started. The usual dose varies from 0.1 to 0.3 mg daily.

Supportive measures are instituted as follows:

1. Ventilation, even assisted ventilation, if necessary, and the judicious use of oxygen are important.
2. Prevention of further heat loss is important, and gentle external warming may be used cautiously.
3. Fluid replacement should be accomplished slowly; excess sodium should be avoided. Dilutional hyponatremia may be encountered, requiring water restriction.
4. Hydrocortisone, 200 mg daily in divided doses, is recommended because of the possibility of adrenocortical insufficiency.
5. Digitalis may be needed in the treatment of congestive heart failure. The dose may be lower than usual because of the hypometabolism.
6. Appropriate treatment for precipitating and concurrent diseases should be initiated.

## Diabetic ketoacidosis

### ■ What is diabetic ketoacidosis, and how is it treated?

This metabolic emergency is caused by a deficiency of insulin or resistance to its action. The failure to metabolize glucose leads to overproduction of glucose by the liver and hyperglycemia. The metabolism of fat is accelerated but is incomplete; this produces an accumulation of ketones, acetoacetic acid, and $\beta$-hydroxybutyric acid. A severe degree of metabolic acidosis results together with excessive amounts of acetone and ketones in the blood and urine. The osmotic diuresis produced by the hyperglycemia results in severe dehydration with depletion of sodium and potassium.

The clinical manifestations include weakness, dehydration with polyuria and polydipsia, hyperpnea, and coma in severe cases. Ketoacidosis is precipitated in patients with diabetes mellitus by intercurrent diseases, chiefly infections, trauma, or failure to take insulin. Ketoacidosis sometimes occurs as the presenting problem in patients with previously unrecognized diabetes mellitus.

Laboratory data include the following: blood glucose level elevated, usually in the range of 400 to 800 mg/100 ml; serum pH low (a pH of 7.1 indicates a doubling of the hydrogen ion concentration); serum bicarbonate level low, less than 10 mEq/L in severe cases; strongly positive tests for acetone and glucose in the serum and urine; and leukocytosis. The serum sodium concentration may be low, normal, or high, depending on the severity of dehydration and degree of sodium depletion. The serum potassium level is often normal despite a severe potassium deficit, because the acidosis causes an intracellular-to-extracellular shift of potassium. The severity of the patient's condition is more closely related to the degree of acidosis than to the degree of hyperglycemia.

TREATMENT. The following treatment should be instituted promptly:

1. Short-acting (or "regular") IV insulin should be given in a dose of 50 to 100 units, with 50 to 100 units given subcutaneously. Doses of insulin are repeated at hourly intervals, 50 to 100 units subcutaneously, until the blood glucose level has fallen to half its initial value, or below 300 mg/100 ml. Thereafter smaller doses of insulin are given at less frequent intervals as control of the hyperglycemia and ketoacidosis is achieved. If the response is inadequate within a few hours, indicating an unusually severe degree of insulin resistance, the dose of insulin is doubled every 2 hours and IV hydrocortisone, 100 to 200 mg, is given. Rarely several

thousand units of insulin will be required, but usually several hundred units of insulin is adequate. (Recently the administration of small amounts of insulin by slow IV infusion has been advocated as an alternative to conventional methods.)

2. IV fluids are given to correct dehydration; several liters are usually needed in the first 24 hours. Normal or half-normal saline solution is recommended. Sodium bicarbonate, 50 to 150 mEq, can also be given initially, particularly if the acidosis is severe.

3. Dextrose is not given initially because it is hypertonic and cannot be utilized. After the insulin effect is established and the blood glucose level falls below 300 mg/100 ml, 5% dextrose in water is given to prevent hypoglycemia, furnish energy, and inhibit ketoacidosis.

4. Potassium replacement is not usually started immediately because of the acidosis and possible hyperkalemia. But as soon as the insulin becomes effective, potassium will be needed, usually 3 to 4 hours after insulin administration is begun. IV potassium chloride or phosphate is given at a rate of 20 mEq/hr; 100 to 200 mEq may be needed in the first 12 hours.

5. Precipitating factors and diseases should be sought and treated appropriately.

After the acute situation is controlled, usually within 24 hours, intermediate or long-acting (lente or NPH) insulin is used. When tolerated, an appropriate diet is provided. Less intensive therapy is indicated for milder cases of diabetic ketoacidosis.

### *Monitoring procedures*

Monitoring procedures are essential in the management of these patients. Frequent determinations of the blood glucose, pH, and electrolyte levels are extremely useful. Hourly tests of the urine for glucose and ketones are desirable during the early phase. The ECG may provide evidence of hypokalemia. Accurate records of fluid intake and output are indispensable. A "flow sheet" that shows the essential data in readily comprehensible form is most helpful.

### *Surgical procedures*

Surgical procedures require special management in diabetic patients. For patients taking insulin, one half of the usual daily dose of lente or NPH insulin is given on the morning of surgery, together with a slow infusion of 5% dextrose in water. This may be supplemented with additional short-acting insulin, depending on the blood glucose levels. Usually the urine is tested for glucose and acetone every 2 to 4 hours postoperatively, and insulin is given, depending on the urine glucose concentration and the response to previous doses of insulin. As the patient improves and is able to tolerate food, a return to the previously established insulin regimen can be accomplished. Hypoglycemia must be carefully watched for and promptly treated.

## Hyperglycemic nonketotic coma

■ **How is the diagnosis made and what is the treatment for hyperglycemic nonketotic coma?**

This syndrome occurs in patients with maturity-onset diabetes mellitus, although it can occur at any age and in insulin-dependent diabetic patients. The characteristic features of this disorder are severe dehydration and hyperglycemia without ketoacidosis, hence the term "hyperglycemic nonketotic hyperosmolar coma." The syndrome is precipitated by concurrent disease, often infections. Relative insulin deficiency leads to hyperglycemia and osmotic diuresis. In the absence of adequate fluid replacement, extremely severe dehydration occurs. Mental obtundation is profound, with or without coma. The condition is fatal if untreated.

TREATMENT. Treatment consists of the administration of fluids and insulin. Hypotonic saline solution, a 0.45% solution of sodium chloride, is given initially. Dextrose solutions are contraindicated until the blood glucose concentration has decreased significantly; then dextrose solutions are given to provide water without excess sodium. Water deficits of 8 to 10 L or more are common. Potassium replacement will almost always be needed, and larger amounts will usually be required earlier than in patients with diabetic ketoacidosis.

Insulin should be given promptly. There is some evidence that the insulin requirements in hyperglycemic nonketotic coma are less than in diabetic ketoacidosis. However, excessive insulin resistance as well as insulin sensitivity does occur in this syndrome, and the insulin requirements usually approximate those in diabetic ketoacidosis. Regular insulin, 50 units/hr, is recommended, with modification of the dose and frequency of administration depending on the response.

Lactic acidosis occasionally occurs as a complication and requires bicarbonate therapy.

Concurrent diseases must be sought and treated appropriately.

## Lactic acidosis

■ **When may lactic acidosis be anticipated, and what immediate steps should be taken to correct this condition?**

This disorder is relatively uncommon but can be extremely serious. It occurs in a wide variety of diseases and is usually precipitated by anoxia. Diabetic as well as nondiabetic patients may be affected. The serum lactate is elevated and the lactate:pyruvate ratio usually exceeds 10:1. Sodium bicarbonate is given to correct the acidosis, fluid deficits should be corrected, and insulin may be needed in diabetic patients.

## Hypoglycemia

■ **What is hypoglycemia, and how is it treated?**

The brain is dependent almost entirely on glucose for its metabolism. Therefore it is extremely important that hypoglycemia be recognized and treated promptly. Among the critically ill, hypoglycemia is probably most commonly encountered in diabetic patients receiving insulin. Other causes include impaired liver function with inadequate food intake, adrenal insufficiency, insulinomas and other insulin-producing tumors, and a variety of drugs, but mainly the sulfonylureas and phenformin (oral antidiabetic agents). Neuromuscular irritability, tremor, excess sweating, and tachycardia occur in response to epinephrine release by the adrenal medulla. With more severe degrees of hypoglycemia convulsions or coma may occur. The blood glucose concentration is usually less than 50 mg/100 ml. Treatment should be started on reasonable suspicion without awaiting the results of the blood glucose determination.

TREATMENT. Treatment with glucose is specific. IV dextrose should be given in severe situations; 10 to 25 g is usually adequate, but more may be needed. Because of its high viscosity, 50% dextrose solution is difficult to inject, and 20% solutions are easier. Alternatively, glucagon can be given subcutaneously, intramuscularly, or intravenously in doses of 1 to 5 mg; it is effective in patients with excess insulin, but not in patients with impaired liver function.

For the milder hypoglycemic reactions to insulin in diabetic patients orally administered orange juice in amounts of 120 to 180 ml may be sufficient. Frequent feedings, especially bedtime feedings, are helpful to prevent hypoglycemia in patients treated with long-acting insulin.

For severe cases of hypoglycemia in patients with insulin-producing tumors diazoxide may be helpful, as well as cortisone acetate or other glucocorticoids.

## Diabetes insipidus

■ **On what is the diagnosis of diabetes insipidus based, and which treatment modalities should be considered?**

The antidiuretic hormone (ADH) vasopressin controls the reabsorption of water by the kidneys. ADH is secreted by specialized cells in the hypothalamus and stored in the posterior lobe of the pituitary gland. The secretion of ADH is regulated by osmoreceptors located in the anterior hypothalamus. These receptors are sensitive to changes in the osmolality of the plasma. The plasma osmolality increases with a rise in solutes (or loss of water) and decreases with a loss of solutes (or gain of water) in the plasma. An increase in plasma osmolality stimulates the secretion of ADH, which promotes the renal tubular reabsorption of water. A decrease in plasma osmolality inhibits the secretion of ADH and thus promotes the renal excretion of water.

Diabetes insipidus is characterized by severe polyuria and polydipsia caused by inadequate ADH activity. The cause of the disorder is a lesion of the hypothalamic nuclei that secrete ADH or of the posterior lobe of the pituitary. Brain tumors or trauma are common causes, but some cases are without known cause. These patients excrete large amounts of dilute urine, 4 to 10 L/day. This is accompanied by intense thirst so that the patients consume large amounts of water. Provided the patient has free access to water, osmotic equilibrium can be maintained; however, unconscious patients and those who for any reason cannot drink freely are subject to severe dehydration, which can be fatal. The diagnosis is suggested in patients with head trauma or recent pituitary surgery who pass excessive amounts of urine with low specific gravity (less than 1.010). This must be distinguished from impaired renal concentrating ability, a response from diuretic agents, or fluid overload.

TREATMENT. Treatment with vasopressin is effective. For acute or temporary situations aqueous pitressin is used because of its short duration of action. The usual dose is 5 to 10 units given subcutaneously every 4 to 6 hours. (Because of its vasoconstrictive effects, it should be used with caution in patients with coronary artery disease.) For more sustained effect pitressin tannate in oil is used. Each ampule contains 5 units/ml. The IM dosage range is 0.2 to 1.0 ml, and the duration of action varies from 24 to 72 hours. The dose and frequency of administration should be adjusted to the individual patient's need, so as to maintain a urine volume of 1 to 3 L/24 hours. The ampule should be warmed to body temperature and shaken thoroughly to ensure that the active drug is suspended evenly in the oil. Fluid intake and output should be carefully monitored. The patient's daily weight and determination of urinary specific gravity or osmolality are helpful guides.

#### *Nephrogenic diabetes insipidus*

Nephrogenic diabetes insipidus is a renal tubular defect characterized by an inability of the kidneys to respond to ADH. There is no deficiency of ADH in this condition; therefore the administration of pitressin or vasopressin is not effective treatment. Restriction of fluids and the administration of thiazide diuretics may be helpful. The mechanism of action of these drugs is incompletely understood; probably they are effective by inducing a sodium deficit.

### Inappropriate ADH syndrome

■ **What is the significance of inappropriate ADH syndrome?**

This disorder is characterized by the ability to secrete a dilute urine in the presence of decreased plasma osmolality and normal renal function. The physiologic events resemble those that occur following the administration of excessive amounts of ADH: the plasma osmolality and serum sodium concentration are low, whereas the urine contains sodium and is relatively concentrated. Edema is not usually present. Excessive ADH activity has been detected in some of these patients.

This syndrome has been described in a variety of clinical situations, including CNS disorders, anesthesia or surgical stress, chronic lung disorders, myxedema, and various malignant neoplasms.

TREATMENT. Treatment is simple; strict limitation of fluid intake will usually correct the hyponatremia. The condition is resistant to the administration of sodium, particularly isotonic saline solution.

## SUMMARY

Endocrine and metabolic disturbances occur in a variety of conditions in critically ill patients. Stress initiates an adrenal response, mediated by the hypothalamus and anterior pituitary gland, that provides increased amounts of adrenocortical hormones, which are important in many metabolic processes. Although adrenal insufficiency is uncommon, adrenocortical steroids are frequently used in pharmacologic doses for their anti-inflammatory and supportive effects. Diabetes mellitus is relatively common and diabetic ketoacidosis is often precipitated by acute illness. Hyperglycemic nonketotic coma has been recognized in recent years as a serious complication of acute diseases associated with dehydration in mildly diabetic patients. Hypercalcemia occurs in a variety of disorders that disturb calcium homeostasis. Thyroid function is not ordinarily disturbed in patients with nonthyroidal diseases, but hyperthyroid crisis and myxedema coma, although rare, require prompt intensive treatment. Derangements of water and electrolyte metabolism are common in critically ill patients and closely related to various endocrine functions.

Specific plans for treatment are presented for the major endocrine and metabolic disorders that occur in critically ill patients.

## BIBLIOGRAPHY

Bondy, P. K., and Rosenberg, L. E., editors: Duncan's diseases of metabolism, ed. 7, Philadelphia, 1974, W. B. Saunders Co.

Foster, D. W.: Insulin deficiency and hyperosmolar coma. In Stollerman, G. H., editor: Advances in internal medicine, vol. 19, Chicago, 1974, Year Book Medical Publishers, Inc.

Rosenfeld, M. G., editor: Manual of medical therapeutics, ed. 20, Boston, 1971, Little, Brown & Co.

Sawin, C. T.: The hormones. Endocrine physiology, Boston, 1969, Little, Brown & Co.

Williams, R. H., editor: Textbook of endocrinology, ed. 5, Philadelphia, 1974, W. B. Saunders Co.

*chapter 15*

# Management of renal failure

D. E. GENTILE

## ■ What is the functional role of the kidneys?

In man, kidneys are paired organs, each weighing about 140 g, located retroperitoneally in the dorsal part of the abdomen, partially above and below the twelfth ribs. Although small in size, they receive approximately 20% to 25% of the cardiac output each minute. Microscopically each kidney contains 1 to 1.25 million functional units, the nephrons, one of which is illustrated in Fig. 15-1. Filtration of the plasma takes place at the glomerulus, and the filtrate thus formed is altered in its course through the nephron by tubular reabsorption and secretion until an appropriate (for the body's needs) quantity and quality of urine is produced at the terminal portion of the nephron. The calyces, pelves, ureters, and bladder are simply conduits and do not further alter the composition of the urine.

Renal function is complex and not limited to the elimination of urea and other waste products of metabolism from the body via the urine. Normally functioning kidneys allow man a considerable amount of freedom in the type and amount of food and liquid ingested and the environmental conditions that are endurable. By producing urine that is hypertonic (concentrated) or hypotonic (dilute), relative to the "tonicity" of plasma water, and by varying the excretion of electrolytes, the kidneys contribute greatly to the maintenance of the normal composition of body fluids, a state necessary for the proper function of all body cells and organs. Because the urinary excretion of acids or alkali can be altered to help maintain body fluid pH within narrow limits, the kidneys together with the lungs and the body buffer system protect man from major swings in pH that may result from the ingestion of excessive acids or alkali, from the production of acid from neutral dietary precursors, or from clinical conditions leading to excessive losses of acids or alkali from the body, as may be seen in severe vomiting or diarrhea.

Apart from these "regulatory" functions, the kidneys play a role as endocrine organs by producing hormones that affect red blood cell formation (erythropoietin), blood pressure control (renin and prostaglandins), and

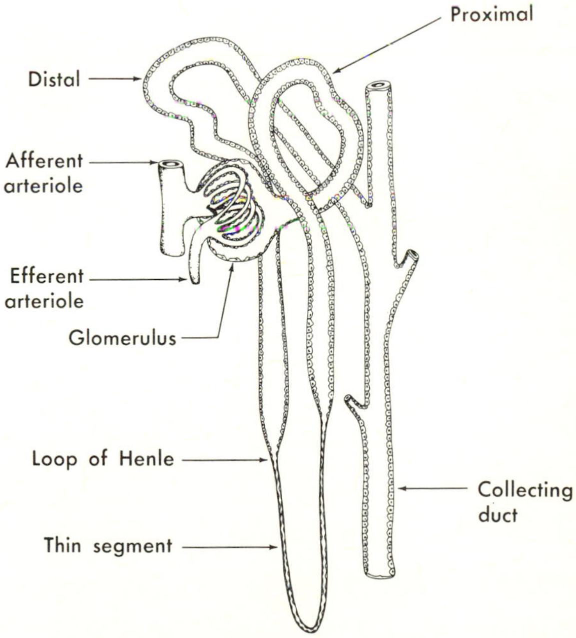


**Fig. 15-1.** Diagram of nephron.

the secretion of aldosterone by the adrenal glands (renin-angiotensin system). An additional aspect of kidney function includes metabolic processes, for example, the conversion of vitamin D to an active metabolic form and the degradation of insulin, parathormone, and gastrin.

Since the kidneys are involved in numerous and fundamental processes, it is easy to see why there are far-reaching, complex, and serious manifestations of renal functional impairment. Fortunately the large number of nephrons present in each kidney comprise a "reserve force," so that although subtle biochemical changes may be present with mild to moderate degrees of kidney disease, relatively normal homeostasis may be maintained, and the patient may feel quite well until 70% to 80% of the nephron mass has been destroyed.

### ■ How does examination of the urine help in the evaluation of kidney function? What are the components of routine urinalysis?

Simple *observation* of the urine can provide evidence of disease of the urinary tract or kidneys. For instance, if the urine is cloudy, the presence of pyuria (pus cells in the urine) and thus urinary tract infection may be suspected. Red urine will usually indicate the presence of blood but may be caused by hemoglobin or myoglobin in the urine and may be seen in certain types of porphyria or in some persons after the ingestion of beets. Other colors may be seen after the ingestion of certain dyes (methylene blue plus medications containing various dyes).

Milky urine may be seen when pus, phosphate crystals, and, in rare cases, lymphatic fluid are present in the urine. Foamy, sticky urine is characteristic of marked proteinuria.

The *specific gravity* is a measurement of the density of the urine and is affected by the number as well as the molecular weight of the solids present. Specific gravity should always be interpreted in the context of the patient's state of hydration. Normal kidneys can vary urinary specific gravity over a wide range (1.001 to 1.040), producing high specific gravity (concentrated) urine when the patient has been without fluids for some time and is relatively dehydrated. Low specific gravity (dilute) urine is present normally when the patient has taken in (or has been administered) more fluids than are absolutely required. The specific gravity can be misleading when large amounts of glucose are present, giving falsely high readings. The specific gravity may be inappropriately high in clinical states where a positive water balance exists, such as congestive heart failure and hypoalbuminemia. In these situations, although intrinsic renal damage is not present, diminished renal blood flow leads to inappropriate urinary concentration.

Although not performed as part of the routine urinalysis, measurement of the urine *osmolality* gives more precise information than specific gravity about urinary concentration and dilution and is often used in cases where such information is needed.

Measurement of the urinary *pH* may provide information relating to the patient's acid-base balance and will also indicate abnormal renal responses to an existing acid-base problem. Inherited or acquired defects in the acidification process of the urine (renal tubular acidosis) are frequently associated with alkaline urine in the presence of metabolic acidosis. A clue to the diagnosis is the inappropriate pH of the urine in a situation where normal kidneys would be elaborating maximally acidified urine. Inappropriate acidification of the urine can be seen in cases where marked body potassium depletion exists, as in prolonged vomiting caused by duodenal ulcer with obstruction.

Urine is routinely tested for the presence or absence of *glucose*. A positive test is usually caused by the presence of an elevated serum glucose level. In normal situations glucose is filtered at the glomerulus and completely reabsorbed by the proximal tubules when serum glucose concentration is normal or slightly elevated. In abnormalities of glucose reabsorption (renal glycosuria) glucose is present in the urine despite a normal serum concentration.

Qualitative tests for *protein* are part of the routine urinalysis. A commonly used test is the addition of sulfosalicylic acid to the clear supernatant of centrifuged urine with observation of the degree of precipitation present. This gives semiquantitative information on the amount of protein present. When abnormal amounts of protein are present qualitatively, quantitative tests are performed on timed (12- or 24-hour) collections. Up to 150 mg of protein may be present normally in 24 hours. In a variety of kidney diseases abnormal amounts of protein are present, and qualitative tests will be positive for protein. In general the largest amounts of protein are seen in patients with primary glomerular diseases, especially those producing the nephrotic syndrome.

*Microscopic examination* of the centrifuged urinary sediment is a critical test. Whenever possible, it should be performed carefully on the first morning specimen (usually the most concentrated). The sediment is, in a sense, a biopsy without surgery or needle aspiration of the kidney and can provide specific information when performed by an experienced observer. The presence of an excessive number of casts and the type of cells or crystals contained in them may give positive identification of the disease process present. The presence of red blood cells in casts, for instance, strongly suggests glomerulonephritis; white blood cell casts indicate pyuria as originating from one or both kidneys. Other formed elements such as *oval fat bodies* (lipid-laden tubular epithelium), *doubly refractile fat bodies* (cholesterol esters), and *crystal casts* give specific information indicating the disease state producing renal functional impairment.

## ■ What is the significance of serum creatinine, creatinine clearance, and blood urea nitrogen?

The most common quantitative estimate of kidney function used clinically is *creatinine clearance. Creatinine* is an inert substance that is formed from the dehydration of creatine in muscle, is not metabolized further (significantly), and is excreted, for practical purposes, simply by the process of filtration at the renal glomerulus. Its production (and thus excretion) is a function of the muscle mass of the individual. Males have greater creatinine production and excretion than females, the difference between the two being proportional to muscle mass. Despite the facts that (1) measurement of the serum creatinine is not exact because of the presence of an interfering noncreatinine chromogen in the serum and (2) small amounts of creatinine are added to the urine by tubular secretion, as well as glomerular filtration in man, for clinical purposes the creatinine clearance is equivalent to the *glomerular filtration rate* (GFR), as shown in the following formula:

$$\text{GFR} = \frac{U_{cr} \times V}{P_{cr}}$$

where $U_{cr}$ = urinary creatinine concentration, V = urinary flow rate (usually milliliters per minute), and $P_{cr}$ = plasma creatinine concentration. Average GFR values for normal young men is 125 ± 15 ml/min/1.73 $m^2$ of body surface area. For normal young women the average is 110 ± 15 ml/min/1.73 $m^2$ of body surface area.

Since urine flow rate is used in the calculation of GFR, accurately timed collections of urine are necessary for valid results. The serum creatinine level is inversely proportional to the creatinine clearance, but because normal serum creatinine concentrations can vary according to the size and muscle mass of the patient, a single serum creatinine determination may not provide precise information regarding the absolute level of renal function. For example, a serum creatinine concentration of 3.0 mg/100 ml in a 90-pound woman may indicate renal functional impairment comparable to that seen in a 200-pound muscular man whose serum creatinine concentration is considerably higher.

*Blood urea nitrogen* (BUN) is a measure of the major end product of protein metabolism in man (urea). The BUN is normally below 20 mg/100 ml and rises when renal functional impairment is present. Since urea is reabsorbed by the tubules, its clearance may be affected by the urine flow rate. The level of BUN is affected not only by changes in glomerular filtration and urine flow rate but also by the rate of urea production. BUN may be elevated in the presence of stable renal function following the ingestion of large protein loads and also in situations where rapid protein breakdown is taking place, such as in patients who have suffered extensive trauma, those who have infection, and in others following major surgery. These factors must be considered before drawing conclusions about renal functional status simply from the level of BUN. For example, in a patient who has extensive gastrointestinal bleeding (protein load) or is extremely catabolic the BUN may rise significantly with only a small increment in the serum creatinine level. This situation is called *prerenal azotemia* and means that nonrenal factors are accountable for a demonstrated rise in BUN.

Many of the routinely measured electrolytes and blood chemistries are affected by renal abnormalities and will be discussed, where pertinent, subsequently. X-ray and isotope studies provide much information about the structure and function of the urinary tract. These tests provide data of diagnostic and therapeutic significance but are not, in the strictest sense, studies of renal function.

■ **Of what use is renal biopsy in the diagnosis and management of kidney disease?**

Evaluation of kidney tissue by routine microscopy, by special immunofluorescent techniques, and by electron microscopy has provided help in the diagnosis of specific renal and systemic disorders and serves as a guide to the therapy and prognosis in many renal (especially glomerular) disorders. Whereas renal biopsy may be performed as an open surgical procedure, the technique of percutaneous renal biopsy is most commonly used.

■ **What precautions are taken before performing renal biopsy?**

The following checks should be made:

1. The presence and location of two kidneys should be demonstrated.
2. Coagulation studies should be normal.
3. Urinary tract infection should be ruled out.
4. The patient should be cooperative and understand the reason for the biopsy as well as the potential benefits and risks involved.

■ **What are some potential complications of renal biopsy?**

Bleeding may take place. This may occur into the renal collecting system, producing gross hematuria, sometimes with clot formation and renal colic, or it may be perinephric (retroperitoneal); in addition, significant bleeding can be hidden and only become evident when a blood pressure or hematocrit drop is noted.

Bleeding of a minimum amount is routine. On rare occasions (less than 1%) bleeding is sufficient to require transfusion. Bleeding massive enough to require nephrectomy is even less common.

The close monitoring of vital signs and the observation of the urine after biopsy is required to detect early signs of significant bleeding. Grossly bloody urine is not uncommon and is more likely to occur in severely uremic patients or patients with uncontrolled hypertension. Bright red urine may be present when relatively small amounts of blood are present, and it is useful to quantitate the amount of bleeding by centrifugation of the urine in a hematocrit centrifuge.

Injury, or sampling of other structures, although uncommon, may occur. Infection is also rare. The exact frequency of the occurrence of atrioventricular fistula is unknown, but rarely is it of clinical significance.

## ACUTE RENAL FAILURE

■ **What is acute renal failure?**

Acute renal failure is the sudden onset of diminished renal function usually, but not always, accompanied by oliguria. (Oliguria is customarily defined as a urine output of less than 400 ml/24 hr.) There are occasional cases of true acute renal failure wherein normal or large amounts of urine are formed. In these instances the condition is called *nonoliguric acute renal failure.* Sudden failure of kidney function may occur in patients with previously normal kidneys or in those who have preexisting kidney disease. The designation of acute signifies not only the nature of onset but also suggests the possibility of reversible renal failure.

### ■ How can acute renal failure be distinguished from chronic renal failure?

Chronic renal failure is the result of a parenchymal disease process of both kidneys that has been present for months or years with gradual, irreversible deterioration of renal function. Urine output is often normal until the latest stages of the disease. In rare situations chronic renal failure may have an "acute" course, as in certain cases of *rapidly progressive glomerulonephritis, bilateral renal cortical necrosis,* and *multiple myeloma.* At times it is difficult to distinguish acute from chronic renal failure or to quantitate the effects of an acute insult on renal function in a patient with underlying kidney disease. It is critical to make the distinction, since specific treatment for remediable causes of acute deterioration of renal function will have a favorable impact on the patient's long-term course.

In the evaluation of any patient with renal failure it is important to review completely the patient's medical history for information concerning previous kidney disease or hypertension. A review of past medical records, if available, will provide useful information whether there is positive evidence of renal involvement or not.

Evaluation of kidney size and the absence or presence and severity of anemia may also provide differential information. With chronic parenchymal renal disease and renal failure of a severe degree there is usually a reduction in the size of the kidneys. Evaluation of renal size can be accomplished by kidney-ureter-bladder (KUB testing), tomography, or infusion intravenous pyelogram (IVP) with tomography.

Although visualization of the kidneys using contrast material and x-ray films may not be ideal, sufficient information can be obtained by utilizing large doses of contrast material. This rule of diminished renal size in chronic disease is not absolute, however, since there are certain chronic disease processes that may be associated with normal or large kidneys even though significant renal failure is present. Examples of these include *polycystic kidney disease, diabetic glomerulosclerosis,* and *renal amyloidosis.*

Anemia of chronic renal failure will be discussed later in greater detail, but in general chronic renal failure is accompanied by anemia that becomes more severe as the level of renal function diminishes. The presence of normal or near-normal hemoglobin concentration and hematocrit level in a patient with significant renal functional impairment who is not dehydrated suggests the presence of a relatively recent deterioration of renal function.

### ■ What are the causes of acute renal failure?

#### *Renal ischemia*

Renal ischemia may result from hypotension following traumatic, surgical, or obstetric hemorrhage; *disseminated intravascular coagulation;* severe dehydration from gastrointestinal or other fluid losses, for example, exposure to excessive environmental heat; "third spacing," as may be seen following extensive third-degree burns or following bowel surgery; and after vascular surgery, especially of the aorta and/or renal arteries.

#### *Toxins*

Certain drugs and chemicals exert specific nephrotoxicity. A partial list of these includes the following:

*Agents that may cause acute renal failure*
- Antibiotics: gentamicin, kanamycin, colistin, neomycin, amphotericin, sulfonamides
- Metals: mercury, lead, arsenic
- Carbon tetrachloride
- Ethylene glycol
- Radiographic contrast materials
- Anesthetic agents: methoxyflurane, halothane
- DDT and other insecticides

*Agents that may cause interstitial nephritis*
Analgesics: phenacetin
Methicillin

*Agents that may cause nephrotic syndrome*
Penicillamine
Trimethadione, paramethadione
Gold

With both "ischemic" and "toxic" acute renal failure the pathologic lesion often seen is necrosis of the renal tubules. Thus a common synonym for acute renal failure associated with these causes is *acute tubular necrosis.* It is of interest, however, that tubular necrosis may not be seen on renal biopsy or at autopsy in a significant number of cases of acute oliguric renal failure following an ischemic episode. The renal histology may appear normal, suggesting that a purely functional abnormality may be present, perhaps related to the abnormal distribution of renal blood flow.

### *Parenchymal renal disease*

Severe acute glomerulonephritis of any type may lead to acute oliguric renal failure. Diffuse interstitial nephritis of acute onset and unknown origin as well as interstitial nephritis related to drugs and infection has been noted to produce acute renal failure. In patients with underlying vascular disorders, such as diabetes mellitus, *necrotizing papillitis* may result from infarction of the renal papillae caused by a combination of medullary interstitial infection and vascular insufficiency. Papillary necrosis may also occur as the result of prolonged, excessive ingestion of phenacetin and perhaps other analgesics, but leads to gradual chronic renal functional impairment rather than this acute renal failure.

### *Nephron obstruction*

Intrarenal (nephron) obstruction may occur as the result of deposition of a number of materials, including uric acid crystals, oxalate crystals, the precipitation of sulfonamides, and the precipitation of abnormal globulins such as those found in the urine of patients with multiple myeloma. In each of these cases the presence of large amounts of a relatively insoluble substance and dehydration of the patient combine to produce precipitation of the substance in nephrons.

## ■ What is prerenal failure?

Normal renal blood flow is approximately 1200 ml/min and comprises approximately 20% of the cardiac output. In situations where vascular volume depletion exists, defense mechanisms to maintain circulation to other vital organs result in decreased blood flow to the kidneys. As a result, renal function tests may be abnormal and urine flow rate may diminish, although parenchymal renal damage has not occurred. When this happens, it is important to detect the problem early and take measures to correct it rapidly before full-blown true acute renal failure develops. Close clinical surveillance alone may give sufficient clues to establish the presence of volume depletion. If the patient develops oliguria while under clinical observation, a review of the recent trend in body weight may demonstrate inordinate weight loss over several days, suggesting negative water balance. Measurements of the central venous pressure or the pulmonary wedge pressure, if low, provide evidence for volume depletion. If the patient is not absolutely confined to bed, the simple observation of a postural (standing) drop in blood pressure may give added weight to the possibility that volume depletion exists.

A trial of IV fluids, including normal saline solution, mannitol, or a solution containing albumin may lead to correction of vascular volume deficit, increased rates of urine formation, and restoration of the BUN and serum creatinine concentration toward normal. The amount of the solutions given and the rates at which they are given depend on the degree of volume depletion that is suspected clinically, the age and cardiovascular status of the patient, and the response of arterial pressure and central venous pressure or pulmonary wedge pressure to the fluid administration. An important point to keep in mind is the fact that concentrated albumin solutions increase vascular volume to a greater degree than would be expected from the volume of solution administered, since the colloid osmotic pressure of protein infused leads to a shift of water from "compartments" outside of the blood vessels to the vascular compartment. When these diagnostic or therapeutic fluid administration maneuvers are made, the most serious potential complication is circulatory overload with congestive heart failure and pulmonary edema. This danger is increased when acute renal failure is present.

At times when the circulatory state and the state of hydration of the patient are equivocal or the patient has known or suspected borderline cardiac function, it is safer to attempt to stimulate renal perfusion and urine formation by the administration of potent diuretics such as furosemide or ethacrynic acid. It is frequently necessary to give relatively large IV doses of these agents in order to determine if a response will take place. Doses in the range of 200 to 600 mg of furosemide are generally safe but should not be given rapidly or directly into a central venous pressure catheter. In the latter instance the potential for causing cardiac arrhythmias exists. Larger doses of these drugs have been reported to produce transient or permanent deafness on rare occasions. Care should be taken not to administer large doses to patients who are receiving potentially ototoxic antibiotics such as aminoglycosides (for example, gentamicin), since the combined effects of the diuretic and antibiotic are more likely, although not proved, to cause eighth nerve damage.

### ■ What measures should be taken to exclude urinary obstruction as a cause for acute oliguria?

Obstruction to the flow of urine must always be considered when evaluating a patient with acute oliguria. Obstruction of the ureters, bilaterally, is unusual but can occur.

When the clinical situation strongly suggests obstruction, bilateral retrograde catheterization of the ureters may be performed in an effort to rule out obstruction. This should not be done without considerable forethought in light of the potential hazards of the procedure in a critically ill patient. Isotope scanning techniques may safely help to rule out obstruction.

### ■ What are the causes of bilateral ureteral obstruction?

The causes of bilateral ureteral obstruction are as follows:

1. Pelvic tumor with local invasion
2. Retroperitoneal lymphadenopathy, as seen with lymphomas and leukemia
3. Idiopathic retroperitoneal fibrosis
4. Deposition of urate crystals in the ureters (This may be seen in patients with extreme hyperuricemia following treatment of neoplasms with cytotoxic agents or following the injection of radiologic contrast materials in hyperuricemic, dehydrated patients.)
5. Accidental ligation of both ureters during pelvic surgery
6. Bilateral ureteral calculi (rare)

### ■ What specific problems are seen in patients with acute renal failure?

The specific problems seen in these patients may be summarized as:

1. Nutritional complications
2. Water balance difficulties
3. Electrolyte disturbances
4. Uremic manifestations
5. Infection
6. Gastrointestinal bleeding

This list may oversimplify the problems encountered in the management of patients with acute renal failure. More commonly than not the patient is desperately ill as a result of recent severe trauma or burns or extensive surgery, with or without infection. Thus the problems caused by the patient's underlying disease state are compounded by a second, critical clinical problem. Treatment with drugs is made more complicated and recovery from the primary problem that led to the development of acute renal failure is made more tenuous.

### ■ What are the nutritional requirements of patients with acute renal failure?

Patients who have acute renal failure following trauma, burns, or surgery are extremely catabolic, breaking down their own tissue stores to meet their massively increased energy requirements. Over a relatively short time period severe nutritional deficits can occur and, perhaps more important, excessive breakdown of protein stores leads to a rapid rise in BUN. This in turn leads to the early development of uremia. For many years it has been recognized that the provision of nonprotein calories may decrease the rate of protein breakdown, and the usual treatment was the administration of hypertonic glucose solutions or, if the patient could take food orally, carbohydrate and fat calories were given. Quantitative limits were placed on this form of treatment because fluid intake was limited by the presence of oliguria and because of difficulties encountered in administering IV hypertonic solutions. In addition, the necessary level of conservation of protein breakdown could not be effectively accomplished. Similar problems were encountered in attempting to achieve oral nutritional replacement therapy because patients were frequently anorexic and had nausea and vomiting. In the case of a patient who does not require hemodialysis therapy, supportive dietary measures can be utilized but usually at the expense of nutritional needs. If the patient is not ill enough to need dialysis, a temporary state of malnutrition may be tolerated until recovery occurs.

It has been shown that *total parenteral nutrition* utilizing a mixture of essential amino acids and hypertonic glucose solutions administred via a caval catheter may be used to satisfy the nutritional needs of some patients, especially those who are not oliguric. This form of therapy is based on the observation that the administration of essential amino acids may produce better utilization of protein nitrogen.

The absolute caloric needs vary according to the underlying disease states. Severely burned or posttraumatic patients may initially have a caloric requirement of 4000 to 5000 calories/day.

Patients who require dialysis (the majority of patients with acute renal failure) can have more effective alimentation and/or caloric intake than those treated conservatively, since frequent dialysis allows restoration of fluid balance and removal of potentially toxic protein metabolites, as well as the maintenance of normal serum electrolyte concentrations. Special aspects of nutrition in dialysis patients will be discussed in Chapter 17.

Anabolic steroids have been used to minimize negative nitrogen balance in acute renal failure, but their effects have not been dramatic.

### ■ How is rational fluid therapy achieved in the conservative management of acute renal failure?

Since oliguria is present in most patients with acute renal failure, overhydration and circulatory overload are a constant threat. It is virtually impossible to give a patient no fluid because of the need for medications and calories. The general goals in management are to produce negative water balance when the patient is overhydrated at the onset, or to maintain a zero water balance if the patient is normally hydrated. (In the situation where the patient is underhydrated to begin with, trials at restoration of normal hydration in an effort to reestablish urine flow will, ideally, have led to a state of normal hydration.) Estimation of the state of hydration must be made from day to day by physical examination, looking for the presence or absence of edema, hypertension, postural hypotension, abnormal skin turgor, and pulmonary congestion.

*Accurate daily weight* of the patient is of critical importance in assessing water balance, since sharp swings in body weight over short time periods are attributable to changes in water balance rather than to changes in dry body mass. Since a gradual fall in dry mass can be expected to occur because of the catabolic state of the patient and inadequate nutrition, a fall in body weight of about ½ pound/day is expected if water balance is achieved.

A number of formulas have been devised for calculating fluid requirements, for example, an intake of 500 ml plus the measured output for 24 hours. These formulas are useful for initiating therapy but must be altered according to the patient's specific needs as determined by weight changes and physical findings. Patients who are febrile or exposed to high ambient environmental temperatures will require more fluid administration than those who are not, since insensible water loss and perspiration will be greater at higher temperatures.

### ■ What are the manifestations of hyperkalemia and what measures are taken to prevent them?

The clinical environment in which acute renal failure develops sets the stage for dramatic increases in the level of serum potassium. Trauma, surgery, and infection all lead to cellular breakdown with the release of intracellular potassium to the circulation. When coupled with the inability to excrete potassium, concomitant extracellular acidosis secondary to renal failure, and tissue ischemia secondary to hypotension and poor perfusion, rapid rises in serum potassium levels can take place. Although flaccid paralysis and anxiety may occur as a result of hyperkalemia, the most serious adverse effects are on cardiac conduction. Characteristic changes are seen in the ECG, generally when the serum potassium concentration reaches and exceeds 6.5 mEq/L (Fig. 15-2). As the serum potassium levels increase in the toxic range, there is progressive evidence of cardiac depression, and death can occur from cardiac standstill or ventricular fibrillation in a matter of minutes. Unfortunately

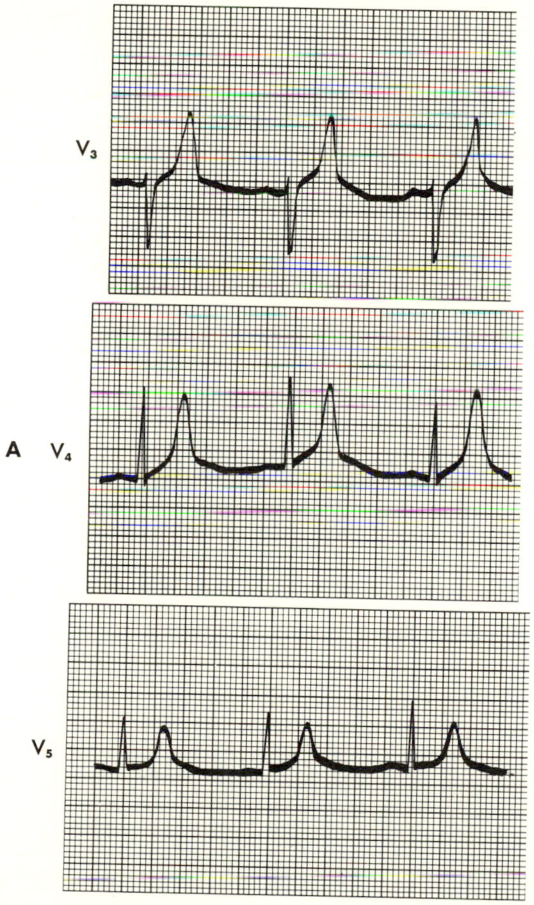


**Fig. 15-2. A,** Peaked T wave with narrow base from a patient with a serum potassium concentration of 6.6 mEq/L.

*Continued.*

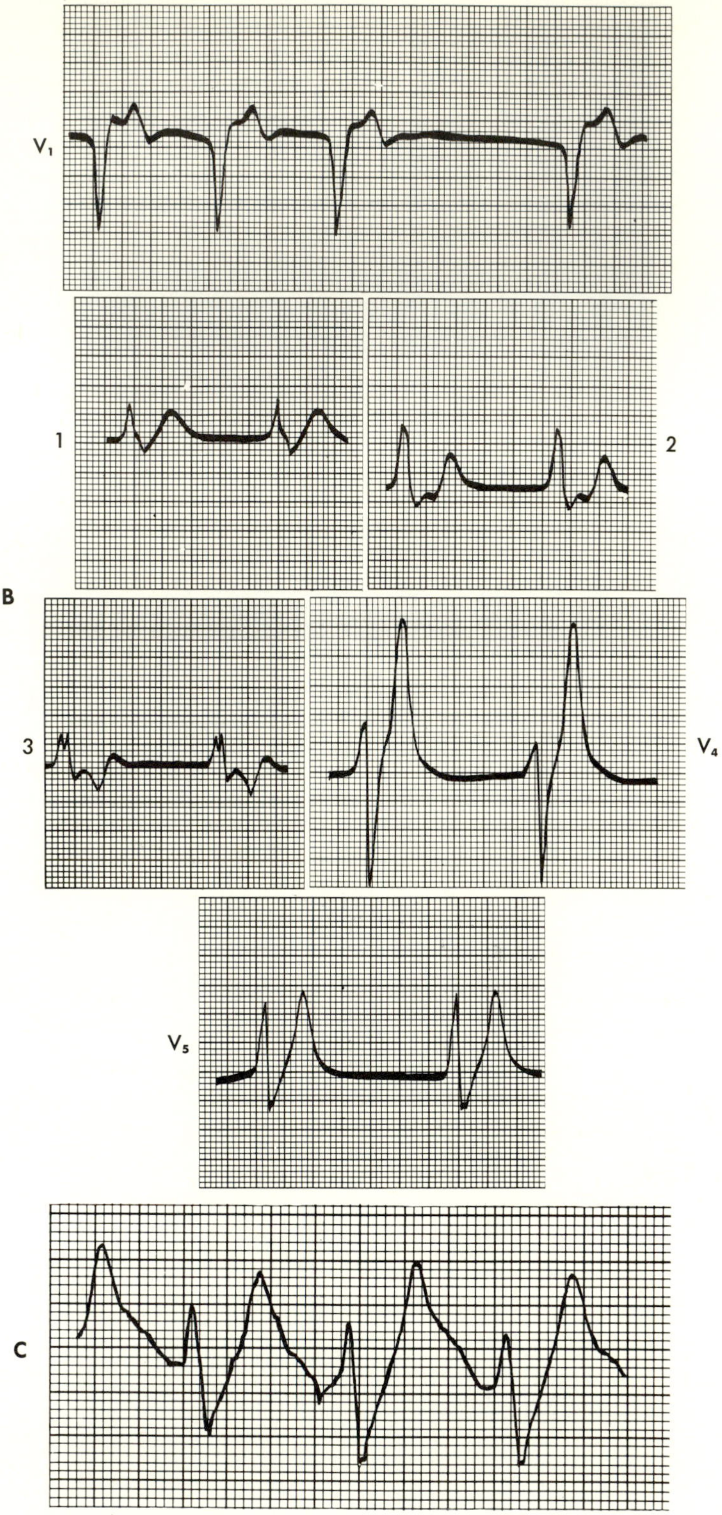


**Fig. 15-2, cont'd. B,** Wide QRS complex with loss of P waves and peaked T waves from a patient with a serum potassium concentration of 7.5 mEq/L. **C,** Very wide QRS complex, AV dissociation, and "sine" wave pattern from a patient with a serum potassium concentration of 8.3 mEq/L.

there is no direct correlation between the absolute serum level of potassium and the changes seen in the ECG; cardiac monitoring and serial ECG's are necessary for observation of the effects of potassium toxicity. This lack of correlation exists because the ratio of the extracellular to intracellular concentrations of potassium, rather than the serum level per se, is responsible for the deleterious electrical effects.

A rising serum potassium concentration in the toxic range comprises a *medical emergency that requires immediate measures for control.* Removal of potassium from the body is specifically desired and is most effectively achieved by dialysis (most efficiently by hemodialysis). Fatal levels of hyperkalemia may develop before the preparation for dialysis can be made, and one or all of the following measures may be used definitively or as interim therapy:

1. *Infusion of sodium bicarbonate.* Sodium ion antagonizes the effect of potassium on the myocardial cell membrane, and the rise in extracellular pH caused by the bicarbonate leads to a movement of potassium into the cells.

2. *Calcium solutions* (calcium gluconate or calcium chloride). Calcium ion antagonizes the effect of potassium at the myocardial cell membrane.

3. *Glucose and insulin infusion.* This combination causes the movement of potassium into the cells temporarily. One unit of regular insulin is given for every 3 to 4 g of glucose. Thus 50 ml of 50% dextrose in water can be given with 8 units of regular IV insulin.

4. *Cation-exchange resins* (specifically sodium polystyrene sulfonate [Kayexalate]). These selectively exchange sodium (to the patient) for potassium (from the patient) and can be given either orally or by retention enema. When given orally or by enema with 70% sorbitol or 20% dextrose in water, the resultant loss of water via the gastrointestinal tract may enhance the removal of potassium. When given by retention enema, it is imperative that the enema be retained for a period of 30 to 60 minutes in order to allow efficient exchange to take place. A theoretical exchange of 3 mEq of potassium/g of resin used is predicted but somewhat less occurs in clinical use.

These measures may be sufficient treatment in themselves but more often than not peritoneal dialysis or hemodialysis must be instituted to maintain safer serum potassium levels. Control of potassium intake is mandatory in the subsequent management of the patient.

### ■ What consideration must be given to other ions in the management of acute renal failure?

In oliguric acute renal failure sodium restriction is necessary to avoid hypertension and congestive heart failure. In the nondialyzed oliguric patient absolute avoidance of sodium is necessary. Low concentrations of serum sodium may sometimes be observed but are more often caused by dilution of the extracellular fluid by excessive water administration prior to the recognition of oliguria rather than to true sodium depletion. In nonoliguric patients measurement of the sodium excretion will be necessary to arrive at a rational prescription for appropriate sodium intake.

Low serum levels of calcium may be observed in some patients and are related to phosphate retention. No clinical symptoms are usually observed unless the rapid correction of acidosis is achieved by the administration of alkali. Frank tetany may develop under these circumstances and will require the administration of calcium. Antacid therapy is usually given to minimize the occurrence of gastrointestinal ulceration. Aluminum hydroxide gels should be used for this purpose, since other antacids contain magnesium that may be absorbed in sufficient quantities by the gastrointestinal tract, further increasing the level of serum magnesium, which is already elevated by the presence of renal failure. Specific therapy for acidosis is not usually given, but protein restriction instituted to minimize azotemia will diminish acid production from metabolism. In modern medical practice calcium, phosphate, magnesium, and acid-base metabolism are more effectively managed with dialysis therapy.

**■ What factors affect survival in acute renal failure?**

As already pointed out, acute renal failure does not usually occur as an isolated condition but as a complication of serious medical problems. Thus the nature and severity of the underlying problem are the ultimate factors in survival. A patient with third-degree burns over 90% of the body surface, for example, has a poor prognosis whether or not renal failure develops. Dialysis therapy has resulted in an improvement in the mortality statistics for posttraumatic acute renal failure from a World War II death rate of greater than 90% to one of approximately 67% among Korean War casualties.

Although the survival rate did not improve during the Vietnam war, the *incidence* of acute renal failure in severely traumatized military men was decreased by two thirds. Refinement of surgical, cardiovascular, and fluid and electrolyte resuscitative techniques very likely have played a major role in this reduced morbidity. Most of the worldwide experience shows little improvement in survival during recent years, owing in part to the fact that patients in older age groups and those undergoing bold modern surgical procedures present more serious and complicated medical problems than were seen before.

The chief cause of death among patients with acute renal failure is infection. This is especially true in patients who have had abdominal injuries and/or abdominal surgical procedures. Whether the presence of renal failure makes these patients more susceptible to infection or longer survival allows infectious complications to develop is not definite, but both factors are probably significant.

The presence of an indwelling urethral catheter is a potential source of urinary tract infection and sepsis. This form of instrumentation is unnecessary in most patients with acute renal failure and should be avoided.

Another relatively common complication in some reports is gastrointestinal bleeding. The combination of stress and the effects of uremia in producing defects in coagulation plays a role in producing this complication.

**■ Does renal function return to normal following recovery from acute renal failure?**

In cases of acute renal failure associated with renal hypoperfusion or tubular necrosis virtually complete recovery of renal function can be expected. Measurements of glomerular filtration rate usually approach normal after several weeks or months. Occasionally abnormalities in concentrating ability and other discrete tubular functions have been seen for a number of months after recovery. There is no known increased susceptibility to the development of a second episode of acute renal failure. If acute renal failure is associated with glomerulonephritis, interstitial nephritis, papillary necrosis, or bilateral cortical necrosis, residual renal functional impairment and hypertension are more likely to develop.

## CHRONIC RENAL FAILURE

Diffuse parenchymal renal disease, regardless of etiology, ultimately leads to the development of *end-stage renal failure* with the symptom complex of uremia. Although specific diseases may impart particular characteristics to the clinical picture, patients who have far-advanced kidney failure can effectively be considered as a single group. The specific cause of the uremic syndrome is unknown, but its development is related to the retention of toxic products of protein metabolism, as well as to general derangement of the body's content and concentration of normal constituents such as sodium, potassium, bicarbonate, hydrogen ions, calcium, phosphorus, and magnesium. The following discussion will consider the manifestations or consequences of chronic renal failure and the general principles involved in conservative management.

**■ What diseases cause chronic renal failure?**

There is considerable overlapping in any classification of renal disease. The partial list given here serves to indicate the variety of disease processes that lead to renal failure:

1. Glomerular disease (*acute* and *chronic glomerulonephritis* of diverse etiologies). *Systemic lupus erythematosus* and other col-

lagen vascular diseases can be included in this category even though they produce significant vascular and interstitial lesions.

2. Primary interstitial lesions. This includes *chronic pyelonephritis* and *nephritis of analgesic abuse.*

3. Congenital renal anomalies. *Polycystic kidney disease, medullary cystic disease,* and *hypoplastic kidneys* are the most common causative agents in this category.

4. Obstructive uropathy. Obstruction may occur at any point in the urinary tract and may be intrinsic or extrinsic. Thus obstruction may be caused by urethral stricture or posterior urethral valves with vesicoureteral reflux, or there may be obstruction of the ureters, either congenital or caused by involvement by neoplasm or urinary stones.

5. Other. Other categories of renal disease include metabolic disorders such as gout and nephrocalcinosis secondary to hyperparathyroidism, vascular disease such as nephrosclerosis related to hypertension, and tubular disorders such as the Fanconi syndrome.

### ■ Is there a difference between chronic renal failure and uremia?

In the strictest sense there is a difference. As renal function deteriorates, abnormalities in the blood and body chemistries are present and will become more abnormal as the destruction of the nephron population takes place. Anemia and hypertension may be present as well, but the patient may continue daily activities with no awareness of the chronic illness present. At some point in time a variety of symptoms will develop, including fatigability, somnolence, nausea and vomiting, pruritus, muscle cramps, paresthesias, easy bruisability, and symptoms of circulatory overload. These symptoms, some or all of which may be present in a single patient, signify the presence of symptomatic uremia.

### ■ What hematologic abnormalities are present in uremia, and how are they managed?

Normocytic normochromic anemia is a common concomitant of renal failure. The more severe the renal failure, the more severe is the anemia. Both decreased red blood cell production and shortened survival of red blood cells contribute to the anemia. Decreased production of erythropoietic factor from diseased kidneys (the chief source of this substance in the body) is the major cause of decreased red blood cell production, whereas unknown factors in uremic serum and changes in small blood vessels as a result of hypertension lead to a shortened life span of red blood cells. Other factors contributing to anemia are the propensity of uremic patients to bleed from the gastrointestinal tract and possibly diminished iron absorption from the intestines.

The treatment of anemia is generally not effective unless uremic factors are removed. Occasionally transfusions are necessary because of symptoms directly attributable to anemia, especially in patients with significant coronary vascular disease. Because of hypertension and chronic circulatory overload, packed red blood cells should be used. If the patient is a candidate for renal transplantation, transfusion should be given only when absolutely necessary, and frozen deglycerinated (washed) red blood cells should be used whenever possible. This will minimize the chances of the patient developing hepatitis and the formation of cytotoxic antibodies, which can lead to an increased incidence of transplant rejection. Treatment with vitamins and iron does not lead to an improvement in anemia in patients not receiving maintenance hemodialysis.

Bleeding, especially from the gastrointestinal tract and mucous membranes of the nose and mouth, is a common consequence of uremia. While the primary cause of bleeding may be disturbances in these tissues themselves, a qualitative defect in platelet function plays an important contributing role. This abnormality can be corrected by dialysis.

Decreased leukocyte counts are seen in uremic patients and may be associated with increased susceptibility to infections. Multiple factors in a general debilitating illness, however, probably contribute to this decreased resistance to infection.

### ■ Is hypertension inevitable in uremia?

Most patients with advanced renal failure have hypertension. However, those that do not have hypertension exhibit relatively large urinary volumes and rates of sodium excretion. These patients are likely to have primary interstitial rather than glomerular disease and frequently have a background of obstructive uropathy.

Hypertension, when present, is related to salt and water excess and/or the effect of increased renin production by diseased kidneys. The principles of treatment include the achievement of optimum salt and water balance by diet manipulation and the use of diuretics and various antihypertensive agents suited to the specific needs of the patient. As with other causes of hypertension, optimum control of blood pressure is required to decrease the likelihood of coronary and cerebrovascular complications and also to prevent additional damage to already severely compromised kidneys. Drugs commonly used in the treatment of hypertension include diuretics (thiazides, furosemide, and ethacrynic acid), methyldopa, hydralazine, propranolol, guanethidine, and diazoxide.

### ■ Pericarditis is a common manifestation of uremia. How is it recognized and treated?

Prior to the availability of hemodialysis and transplantation, pericarditis was usually present shortly before the death of a patient with uremia. More recently it has been recognized that pericarditis may occur prior to the terminal phase of renal disease and may occur in patients whose uremia is relatively well controlled by hemodialysis. Pericardial inflammation may be present with or without chest pain and can be detected by careful frequent examination of the heart, listening closely for a pericardial friction rub.

In uremia there is a tendency for the formation of hemorrhagic pericardial fluid that may rapidly increase in quantity and produce *cardiac tamponade,* that is, interference with blood return to the heart and thus decreased cardiac output as a result of "constriction" of the heart by fluid under considerable pressure in the pericardial cavity. When tamponade is developing, the pericardial friction rub may disappear, but there are increasing signs of elevated jugular venous pressure. Arterial blood pressure will fall, a narrow pulse pressure will be noted, and paradoxical pulse (systolic pressure decreased more than 10 mm Hg in inspiration as compared to expiration) will be present.

The patient who is at risk for developing uremic pericarditis must be closely monitored with regard to these clinical signs. Emergency measures will be required to reverse the serious hemodynamic complications of cardiac tamponade. Pericardiocentesis setup should be immediately available and used when clinically indicated. The removal of fluid from the pericardial sac by needle aspiration may result in dramatic improvement, but this may be only temporary, because rapid reaccumulation of fluid can occur and because the pericardial fluid may be "loculated" and thus not adequately removed by one or two needle aspirations. In these cases open (surgical) pericardiotomy may be required with the creation of a pericardial "window" to allow continuous drainage of newly formed pericardial fluid into the mediastinum. At times it is necessary to excise the visceral pericardial membrane in order to reduce the surface producing the inflammatory fluid, to allow free drainage of the mediastinum, and to prevent development of adherent, constrictive pericarditis. The infusion of steroids into the pericardial cavity has been used following either pericardiocentesis or open pericardiotomy with apparent reduction in the inflammatory response that produces pericardial effusion.

### ■ What are the gastrointestinal manifestations of uremia?

Anorexia, nausea and vomiting, and gastrointestinal bleeding caused by "uremic enterocolitis" are commonly seen. These add to the discomfort and disability of the patient and require supportive therapy. The bleeding that occurs, while usually not massive, may lead to sufficient blood loss to make transfusion necessary. Conservative treatment with diet, as discussed subsequently, in addition to antiemetic drugs will lead to relief of some of these symptoms if sufficient residual renal function is present.

**■ What are the neurologic manifestations of uremia?**

The most marked neurologic symptoms are as follows:

1. Somnolence and lethargy, loss of deductive ability, delusions, hallucinations, progressive obtundation, and finally coma when an advanced degree of azotemia is present
2. Peripheral neuropathy, both sensory (paresthesias and loss of vibratory position and sense) and motor, with variable degrees of weakness
3. Possibly seizures (frequently associated with hypertension)
4. Neuromuscular irritability with cramping, muscle twitching, shooting pains, gross myoclonic jerks, and asterixis (flapping tremor similar to that seen in severe liver disease and with respiratory acidosis)

**■ Why does bone disease occur in association with uremia?**

Marked disorders of calcium and phosphorus metabolism occur in renal failure. These are caused by several metabolic abnormalities, including the following:

1. *Disordered vitamin D metabolism.* This leads to reduced responsiveness to the administration of normal or very large doses of vitamin D. The liver and the kidneys are responsible for the conversion of vitamin D to its (presently known) most active form, 1,25-dihydroxycholecalciferol. A deficiency of this metabolite leads to the decreased absorption of ingested calcium from the intestine. Over a period of time this contributes to diminished mineralization of bone. In children growth is affected and ricketslike lesions develop. In adults bone pain and pathologic fractures may occur. Vitamin D affects bone metabolism directly, but the significance of this action is presently not well understood.

2. *Secondary hyperparathyroidism.* This occurs as a result of retention of phosphate with consequent lowering of serum calcium levels as renal failure progresses. Again, there is demineralization of bone and the characteristic bone lesion of hyperparathyroidism, that is, *osteitis fibrosa cystica,* develops. Mobilization of calcium from bone in the presence of high serum phosphate levels may lead to deposition of calcium phosphate in many tissues of the body *(metastatic calcification).* When deposition is in critical areas, significant symptomatology may occur, such as heart block from deposition in the cardiac conduction system and painful arthritis from deposition in the synovium and bursa of joints. Pruritus is associated with increased calcium deposition in the skin, and "uremic red eyes" occur with conjunctival deposits.

3. *Chronic metabolic acidosis.* This probably contributes to bone demineralization but is not the major factor in producing this complication.

**■ Are measures taken to prevent or minimize skeletal complications?**

Efforts are made to maintain normal concentrations of calcium and phosphorus in the serum, although this by no means guarantees the desired result. Therapeutic efforts include the following:

1. The provision of adequate dietary calcium, in the range of 1.2 g/24 hr for adults, should be undertaken.

2. The reduction and maintenance of serum phosphate at normal levels should be accomplished with the use of aluminum hydroxide gels. (Magnesium-containing gels are contraindicated because magnesium absorption may take place and contribute further to the already increased levels of serum magnesium seen in renal failure.) *Aluminum hydroxide should be given immediately following a meal.*

3. Vitamin D may be given, but large doses are required. Because of abnormal rates of metabolism, there is the distinct possibility of "overshooting" the desired effect,

with the result being that increased metastatic calcification may take place. The recent discovery and isolation of 1,25-dihydroxycholecalciferol may help to make treatment safer and more effective.

4. Correction of metabolic acidosis, when severe, should be achieved.

5. Partial or complete parathyroidectomy may be necessary, depending on the long-range therapeutic plans for the patient and the severity of the disorder.

Additional measures are taken in patients whose renal functions have deteriorated sufficiently to require maintenance hemodialysis.

## ■ What is uremic pneumonitis?

X-ray and pathologic findings similar to those seen in pulmonary edema are found in patients with uremia. Since hypertension and circulatory overload are commonly present, it is difficult to separate purely cardiovascular factors from metabolic factors that may be causing these findings. It is entirely possible that exudate formed from uremic capillary abnormalities is the cause for the x-ray appearance of the "uremic lung," but the evidence is not conclusive. This finding usually accompanies far-advanced uremia, and control is achieved by eliminating uremia by conservative means or by dialysis and also by relieving circulatory congestion.

Another finding related to the lungs in uremia is pleuritis with friction rub and pleural effusion. Again, this is usually seen with advanced renal failure.

## ■ What are the dermatologic manifestations of uremia?

Pruritis is a common and sometimes persistent complaint of uremic patients. The cause for this is not known but has been related to calcium deposition in the skin.

Uremic patients have a distinctive yellowish pallor that may be related to the retention of "urochrome" pigment plus the effects of anemia.

Purpura and ecchymosis are commonly seen and are related to abnormal platelet function, perhaps increased capillary fragility, and other unknown factors.

Rashes are commonly seen. The fact that uremic patients receive multiple medications probably contributes to this manifestation.

## ■ What is the role of diet in the treatment of uremia?

Although a specific uremic "toxin" has not been identified, it is clear that the end products of protein metabolism play a major part in producing uremic symptoms. The symptoms are usually not evident until marked impairment of renal function exists, and restriction of protein intake is not necessary until symptomatic uremia is present. Diets high in essential amino acids (high biologic value protein) have been found to have a greater effect on reducing azotemia (and also uremic symptomatology) than diets low in protein but not high in essential amino acids. When protein-restricted diets containing high biologic value protein are given with sufficient carbohydrate and fat calories (approximately 30 calories/kg), reduction in BUN and improvement in symptoms occur in patients with marked renal functional impairment, that is, creatinine clearance less than 5 ml/min. As a result, dialysis therapy may be deferred for several months. Adequate nutritional and social (and emotional) requirements of the patient rarely allow reduction of protein intake below 0.5 to 0.7 g of protein/kg of body weight. Lack of patient acceptance of the diet is the main obstacle to "successful" dietary management.

Sufficient intake of vitamins is necessary. Other factors in dietary management include the close supervision of calcium, sodium, potassium, and water balance of uremic patients. Considerable individualization of diet is required for each patient, depending on the peculiarities of mineral balance observed.

## ■ What renal and extrarenal factors can be controlled to produce optimum renal function in patients with advanced renal failure?

The appropriate measures to take include the following:

1. Ideal control of hypertension
2. Elimination of urinary infection
3. Control of congestive heart failure
4. Prevention of volume depletion (dehydration)
5. Removal of urinary obstruction
6. Elimination of protein loads that may be produced by gastrointestinal bleeding or by tissue catabolism secondary to infection or to the use of drugs that lead to protein breakdown, such as adrenocorticosteroids and tetracyclines
7. Correction of electrolyte imbalances, especially sodium depletion

## ■ What problems related to drug therapy exist in patients with renal failure?

The metabolism of many drugs requires excretion by the kidney or conversion to inactive forms by the kidney. It is evident that the dosage of many drugs must be altered in patients with renal failure in order to avoid dangerous side effects and complications. The following list shows several drugs commonly used in uremic patients, the dose of which may be unchanged in some cases or reduced in others as renal functional impairment progresses:

*Drugs that should be avoided in renal failure*

Antibiotics: tetracycline, chlortetracycline, demethylchlortetracycline, cephaloridine, nitrofurantoin, nalidixic acid, neomycin

Other agents: triamterene, spironolactone, azathioprine, chlorpropamide, phenformin, gold

*Drugs that should be significantly reduced in dose in renal failure*

Antibiotics: gentamicin, kanamycin, streptomycin, amphotericin, polymyxin B, colistin, vancomycin, pentamidine (?)

Other agents: phenobarbital, procainamide, quinidine, allopurinol, digoxin, tolbutamide (?)

*Drugs that require little or no change in dose in renal failure*

Antibiotics: cephalothin, chloramphenicol (decreased dose with associated hepatic disease), erythromycin, clindamycin, ampicillin, carbenicillin, cloxacillin, methicillin, penicillin G, doxycycline

Other agents: acetylsalicylic acid, secobarbital, codeine, diazepam, glutethimide, morphine, lidocaine, atropine, propranolol, diazoxide, hydralazine, methyldopa, furosemide, diphenylhydantoin

## BIBLIOGRAPHY

Bennett, W. M., Singer, I., and Coggins, C.: A practical guide to drug usage in adult patients with impaired renal function, J.A.M.A. **214:**1468-1475, 1970.

Bennett, W. M., Singer, I., and Coggins, C.: A practical guide to drug usage in adult patients with impaired renal function—a supplement, J.A.M.A. **223:**991-997, 1973.

Lewis, E. J., and Magill, J. W., editors: Proceedings of the Conference on Nutritional Aspects of Uremia, Oct. 23, 1967, Am. J. Clin. Nutr. **21:**349-643, 1968.

Papper, S.: Clinical nephrology, Boston, 1971, Little, Brown & Co.

Pitts, R. F.: Physiology of the kidney and body fluids, Chicago, 1974, Year Book Medical Publishers, Inc.

Strauss, M. B., and Welt, L. G., editors: Diseases of the kidney, Boston, 1971, Little, Brown & Co.

*chapter 16*

# Principles of hemodialysis

STANLEY M. ROSEN

The kidney is particularly susceptible to damage in those situations responsible for admission to intensive care units. Hypotension, dehydration, surgery, anesthesia, and sepsis all make the patient susceptible to prerenal and intrinsic renal failure. Processes involved in the management of the primary illness may also contribute to renal damage. Inadequate care of urinary catheters or decreased resistance to bacteria may result in urinary tract infection and gram-negative septicemia. The emergence of gram-negative and resistant organisms during the progress of the disease often requires the use of potentially nephrotoxic antibiotic and chemotherapeutic agents.

Renal failure in this situation is frequently multifactorial but fortunately is usually reversible over a period of time extending from a few days to several months. Ninety-five percent of patients recover from the renal failure within 21 days, providing they receive suitable supportive therapy, which may include hemodialysis.

This chapter is intended to be an introduction to hemodialysis for personnel who work in an intensive care unit and who might be asked to assist a specialized hemodialysis team in the management of such patients.

Although most patients receive hemodialysis for renal failure, the procedure is also used in some circumstances associated with drug overdose.

## BASIC CONSIDERATIONS

### ■ What is hemodialysis?

Dialysis is the diffusion of dissolved particles from one fluid compartment to another across a semipermeable membrane. The fluid compartments in hemodialysis consist of blood and dialysis fluid, respectively. The semipermeable membrane consists of cellophane.

### ■ Can all dissolved particles pass across the semipermeable membrane?

Particles must be below a certain size to pass across the semipermeable membrane. The precise size of the particle depends on the specific membrane. Semipermeable membranes may be considered to act as filters containing holes. The holes cannot be visualized even with the most powerful microscope, but particles smaller than the size of the holes pass across the membrane, whereas particles larger than the size of the holes are unable to do so. Membranes for hemodialysis have been chosen so that particles of molecular weight greater than 40,000 cannot pass across the membrane. Thus serum proteins and blood cells cannot pass across the membrane, nor can bacteria or other infective organisms commonly found in tap water.

Particles below molecular weight 40,000 will pass through the "theoretical holes" with varying ease according to the size and shape of the particle. The smaller the particle, the more easily it passes. The more the particle approximates a sphere, the more easily it will pass across the membrane. Thus ions, for example, sodium, potassium, calcium, citrate, and chloride, pass through the membrane with the greatest ease, whereas certain vitamins, for example, vitamin $B_{12}$ (molecular weight approximately 1000) pass through with more difficulty.

### ■ Can particles move in both directions across the membrane?

Yes. The particles will move from the fluid compartment containing the higher concentration to that containing the lower concentration. Thus if potassium is in higher concentration in blood, it will move from the blood to the dialysis fluid compartment. If bicarbonate is in higher concentration in the dialysis fluid compartment, it will move into the blood compartment.

The speed at which the movement takes place is determined not only by the size and shape of the particle but also in accordance with the difference in concentration of that substance between the two compartments, that is, the concentration gradient.

### ■ What criteria determine the composition of the dialysis fluid?

The composition of the dialysis fluid is chosen so that at the end of dialysis the concentration of substances in the blood reaches a desired level.

Since one of the purposes of dialysis in renal failure is to remove the waste products of protein breakdown, for example, urea and creatine, the concentration of these substances in dialysis fluid is zero. The concentration is kept to a minimum by continuously replacing the dialysis fluid coming into contact with the membrane.

Other retained substances such as potassium are more easily dialyzable and could produce serious deleterious effects on cardiac function if not removed from blood.

Plasma bicarbonate is usually decreased in renal failure. To correct this disturbance, the movement of bicarbonate should be from the dialysis fluid to blood. Bicarbonate should therefore be at a higher concentration in the dialysis fluid than in blood. The pH of dialysis fluid should approximate that of blood (pH 7.4). Unfortunately at this pH bicarbonate is unstable and decomposes to carbon dioxide and water. For this reason acetate replaces bicarbonate in the fluid. This substitution is possible because acetate is rapidly metabolized to bicarbonate in the patient's liver.

Calcium and magnesium ions easily pass across the dialysis membrane. Serum calcium would fall unless calcium ions were added to the dialysis fluid in an amount equivalent to that in blood. This equals approximately half the total serum calcium.

A basic composition used for dialysis fluid is as follows:

| | |
|---|---|
| $Na^+$ | 135 mEq/L |
| $K^+$ | 1 mEq/L |
| $Cl^-$ | 102 mEq/L |
| Acetate | 38 mEq/L |
| $Ca^{++}$ | 3 mEq/L |
| $Mg^{++}$ | 1 mEq/L |

### ■ When are modifications of the basic composition made?

When the patient has a serum sodium concentration differing by more than 10% of normal, that is, by more than 14 mEq from normal, modifications are indicated. If the serum sodium concentration is very low and it is suddenly corrected completely, pulmonary edema may develop.

If severe hyperkalemia is present, a sudden decrease to normal concentration could precipitate cardiac arrhythmias. This effect is facilitated if the patient has been treated with digitalis preparations. Under these circumstances the serum potassium concentration is reduced more slowly by decreasing the gradient for potassium across the membrane, that is, by increasing the potassium concentration in the dialysis fluid. This can be done by adding a known amount of potassium chloride to the dialysis fluid.

For example, if the serum potassium concentration is 8.5 mEq/L, it is necessary to decrease it to a level below the toxic range (approximately 7.0 mEq/L). To avoid doing this too quickly, the dialysis fluid concentration should be increased to 4.0 mEq/L.

### ■ Is sterile water required to manufacture dialysis fluid?

No. Infective agents will not pass across the membrane.

### ■ Can the dialysis fluid solutes be dissolved in tap water?

It depends on the ionic content of the tap water. In hard water areas calcium concentration might be high enough to cause deleterious effects such as nausea and vomiting. A water softener could be used to counteract this problem.

■ **How can water be removed from blood across the semipermeable membrane?**

Water molecules will only pass across the membrane if they are propelled by a pressure. There are three ways of creating this pressure gradient from blood to dialysis fluid: (1) increase the pressure in the blood compartment, (positive pressure), (2) decrease the pressure in the dialysis fluid compartment (negative pressure), or (3) use dialysis fluid of higher osmotic pressure than blood.

■ **What is osmotic pressure?**

A solution consists of a solvent, for example, water, and a solute, for example, glucose. If two glucose solutions of different concentration are placed on either side of a membrane, then water will move from the solution of low glucose concentration to that of high concentration, because the concentration of water molecules in the high glucose concentration will be less and water molecules will move along the concentration gradient. The pressure generated by the movement of water is called the osmotic pressure.

■ **What is the technical term used to denote (1) the difference of pressure across the membrane and (2) the movement of fluid from blood to dialysis fluid?**

The difference in pressure is called the pressure gradient. The movement of fluid is called ultrafiltration.

■ **Are the fluids in the blood and dialysis compartments static during hemodialysis?**

No. Both compartments are moving at flow rates determined by the required rate of transfer of solutes. In general the greater the flow rate of blood and dialysis fluid, the more solute would be transferred. However, the practical gain achieved by increasing blood flow rate above 300 ml/min and dialysis fluid above 500 ml/min is not significant.

■ **Can the efficiency of a dialysis system be measured?**

Yes. It can be calculated in the manner that renal clearance is calculated, that is, the amount of blood completely cleansed of waste products expressed in milliliters per minute.

■ **What determines the efficiency of a dialyzer?**

Two major points must be considered:

1. The effective surface area of the membrane with which the blood and dialysis fluid are in contact.
2. The physical characteristics of the membrane. In general thinner membranes will be more efficient, but there is a practical limit because the membrane tears more easily as it becomes thinner. Strength can be imparted to the membrane by impregnating it with copper to produce Cuprophan. Under these conditions, it can be used in as thin a sheet as 0.0005 inch.

■ **What are the relationships of the blood and dialysis fluid compartments to the membrane in the dialyzers?**

The three arrangements most commonly used are the flat layer, the coil, and the hollow fiber.

The flat layer dialyzer consists of two sheets of membrane sandwiched between rigid support boards. Blood flows between the two membranes and dialysis fluid flows between the membranes and the outer supporting boards.

The coil kidney consists of a cellophane tube or tubes supported by a backup screen wound around a central core. The coil is placed in a canister. Blood flows through the cellophane tube(s), and dialysis fluid is pumped through the base of the canister between the layers of the coil.

The hollow fiber kidney consists of thousands of hollow fibers composed of regenerated cellulose with lumina of 200 $\mu$ enclosed in a rigid transparent plastic case. Blood flows through the lumen of the fibers and dialysis fluid flows through the plastic case on the outside of the fibers.

## VASCULAR ACCESS

■ **How is blood supplied from the patient to the artificial kidney?**

The technique used for vascular access may vary according to the number of times dialysis may be required.

■ **What is the commonest method for vascular access in intensive care units?**

The arteriovenous (A-V) shunt, or Quinton Scribner shunt, is most commonly used. Teflon cannulas are tied into an artery and a corresponding vein. The commonest sites for use are the radial and posterior tibial arteries. The cannulas are attached to polymeric silicone (Silastic) tubes subcutaneously. The Silastic tube is then brought through the skin and the end connected to the artificial kidney when required. Otherwise the ends of the arterial and venous Silastic tubes are connected to each other to maintain a continuing flow through the cannulas to minimize blood clotting (Fig. 16-1).

The A-V shunt can be constructed within

A

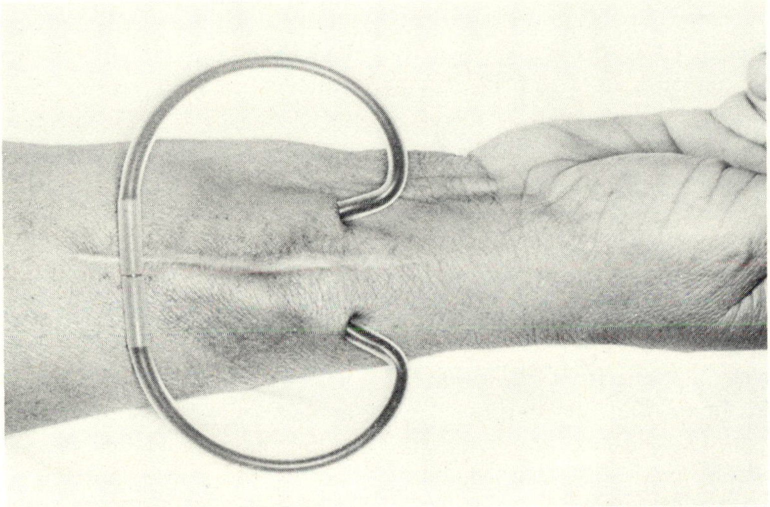

B

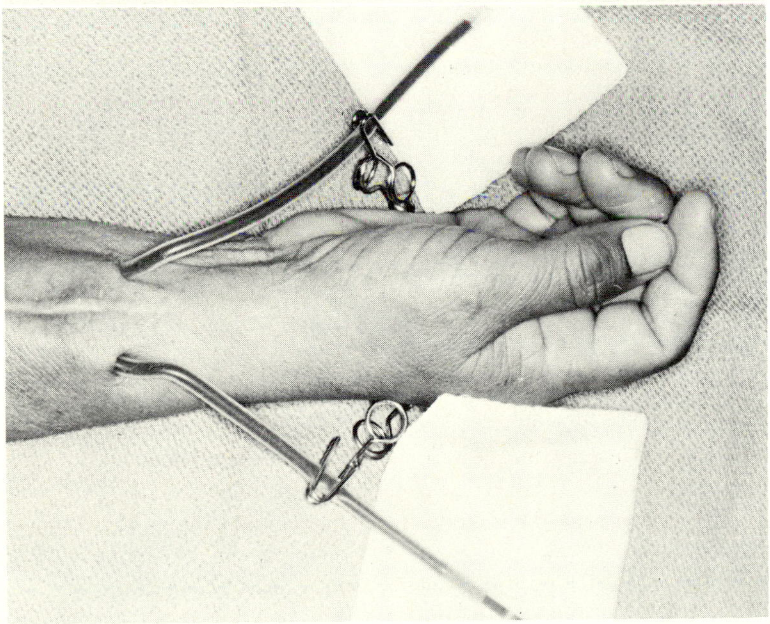

**Fig. 16-1. A,** A-V shunt connected together with Teflon adapter. **B,** Shunt shown with arterial and venous sides disconnected. Note bulldog clamps on each side of shunt.

an hour. It can be used immediately, although electively a waiting period of 24 hours to allow complete blood stasis is desirable. The shunt should be constructed whenever possible in the operating room, but under emergency conditions it can be inserted in an intensive care unit.

### ■ What is the major complication of the A-V shunt?

Clotting of blood in the shunt is the major difficulty encountered. A variety of causes may contribute to this complication.

Restriction of blood flow in the limb will slow return through the veins and facilitate clotting. Blood pressure and other cuffs should not be used on these limbs. Patients are also instructed not to rest with their body pressing on the limb.

Infection is a very serious complication. It can result in clotting of the shunt or destruction of the vessel walls, with the potential for serious and fatal hemorrhage. The chances of infection are minimized by meticulous cleansing of the skin in the neighborhood of the shunt. The infecting organism is usually *Staphylococcus,* and until a sensitivity result is available, the infection should be treated with sodium methicillin (Staphcillin). Infection with other organisms, for example, *Pseudomonas,* has been sporadically reported.

Hypotension also facilitates clotting. This may occur as the result of dehydration, shock, septicemia, blood loss, or reduced cardiac output.

The blood of some patients is hypercoagulable.

### ■ Are there any signs to indicate that a shunt is clotting?

Blood flowing through an external shunt is at body temperature and causes the Silastic to feel warm to the touch. There is also usually a thrill felt and a bruit heard over the shunt.

As blood flow slows through the shunt, the Silastic feels cooler, the thrill and bruit disappear, and the color of the blood column becomes darker. Eventually clots can be seen through the wall of the tubing.

### ■ Can clots be removed from the shunt?

Yes. If the underlying cause has been reversed and the clot has not been left for too long, it may be removed. This process ("declotting") should be performed as soon as possible and becomes extremely difficult after 6 hours.

### ■ What is the procedure for declotting a shunt?

The shunt area must be exposed under sterile conditions. The equipment required includes (1) two 18-inch lengths of polyethylene tubing (outside diameter of 0.05 inch) that can be connected to 2 × 2 ml syringes, (2) drapes and dressing, (3) two cannula clamps, (4) heparin, (5) saline solution (warm), (6) cup for heparin, (7) small jug for discarded fluid, (8) gloves, and (9) tapes.

The Teflon connector is removed from the shunt. If blood flows back through the Silastic, a cannula clamp should be applied immediately. Declotting of the arterial cannula is performed first. Visible clots are removed by gentle traction with a sterile sponge. Then a 20 ml syringe containing heparin solution (40 mg in 1 L) is connected and aspiration performed. Aspiration is repeated after a small amount of heparin solution has been injected. Declotting of the arterial cannula is complete only when the blood pushes back the barrel of the syringe. If declotting is incomplete, the polyethylene catheter is inserted into the Silastic tube, which is irrigated with warm heparinized saline solution. If this is unsuccessful, use of a Fogarty catheter may be necessary, and visualization of the cannula and artery using x-ray techniques and radiopaque media may be advantageous.

After completing the procedure on the arterial side the cannula should be filled with 10 ml warm heparinized saline solution and the Silastic tube clamped. Declotting should then be attempted on the venous side using a similar procedure.

If one side cannot be declotted, the other cannula should be kept patent by infusing heparinized saline solution with a constant infusion pump until the clotted cannula can be replaced.

### ■ Are there other techniques for vascular access?

If only one dialysis is anticipated, a long Teflon catheter can be introduced percutaneously through the femoral veins on either side into the inferior vena cava. The catheter with the tip higher in the cava is used for the "venous" return from the kidney and the lower catheter is used to aspirate blood via a pump to the kidney.

Subcutaneous fistulas between an artery and vein can also be created for vascular access, but generally these are only constructed for maintenance dialysis in terminal renal failure. Various techniques are used for this procedure. One technique for creating the fistula is to create a side-to-side anastomosis of the radial artery and a nearby vein. Blood will then flow directly from the artery into the superficial venous system, which will dilate. The dilated veins can be punctured by two needles on repeated occa-

A

B

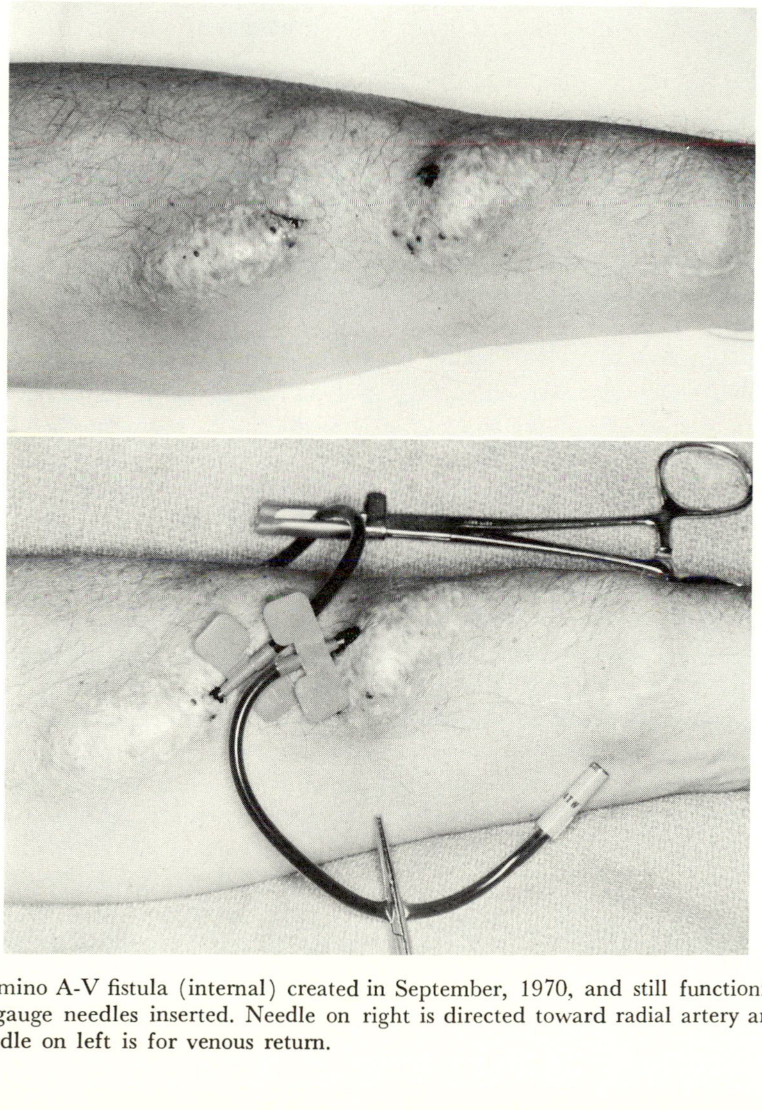

**Fig. 16-2. A,** Cimino A-V fistula (internal) created in September, 1970, and still functioning. **B,** Cimino fistula with 14-gauge needles inserted. Needle on right is directed toward radial artery and uses arterial blood flow. Needle on left is for venous return.

sions. The needle nearer the anastomosis is used to pump blood to the artificial kidney and the other needle is used for return of blood to the patient (Fig. 16-2).

Another variant of this technique is to use a bovine vascular graft interspersed at either the radial or femoral artery.

## ANTICOAGULATION

### ■ How is the blood passing through the artificial kidney prevented from clotting?

Heparin is infused into the blood as it leaves the patient at the rate of 100 mg/hr for an adult. This maintains the clotting time of the blood in the artificial kidney at more than 30 minutes, but also prolongs the clotting time of the blood in the patient's own circulation. This technique is therefore called *systemic heparinization.*

### ■ Is it possible to prolong clotting time in the artificial kidney without a corresponding increase in the patient's circulation?

This of course is necessary in those circumstances where the patient is already bleeding or has an additional predisposition to bleeding, such as may occur in postoperative conditions.

Protamine sulfate neutralizes the effect of heparin and can be added to the blood as it returns from the artificial kidney to the patient. Approximately 1 mg of protamine sulfate neutralizes 1.5 mg of heparin. However, the potency of both drugs varies from batch to batch, and clotting times of the patient's blood and extracorporeal blood should be checked at 30- to 60-minute intervals. Rates of infusion should be adjusted until the patient's clotting time is less than 15 minutes with liberal regional heparinization or less than 10 minutes with rigid regional heparinization. The clotting time of artificial kidney blood should be more than 30 minutes.

### ■ How are clotting time tests performed at bedside?

These are performed by a modification of the Lee-White test. In this procedure 1 ml of blood is apirated from the respective blood line using a 2 ml disposable plastic syringe with a 20-gauge needle. The time is noted on a chart. The needle is removed from the syringe and the blood gently transferred to a carefully cleaned and dried glass test tube, which is placed in a rack without agitating the blood. The sample is checked at 10-minute intervals by gently tilting the tube to a 45-degree angle. The time is recorded when the blood becomes thick enough so that it is immobile when the test tube is completely inverted.

Accurate clotting times can only be obtained if each aspect of the test is performed in minute detail.

## MONITORING

### ■ What parameters are monitored during hemodialysis?

With regard to the patient, the weight, vital signs, blood pressure, and any symptoms are checked.

The patient's weight is always measured at the beginning and end of dialysis, the difference in weight being equivalent to the amount of fluid lost or retained. The frequency of weighing during dialysis depends on the stability of the patient's circulation. Patients who are acutely or seriously ill should be dialyzed on a weighing bed so that weight can be monitored at 30-minute intervals or more frequent intervals when required.

The same comments apply to vital signs, blood pressure, and symptomatology.

Observation of the equipment should detect blood leak, flow on "arterial" line, pressure on "venous" line, air bubble on "venous" line, temperature of dialysis fluid, conductivity of dialysis fluid, and electrical mains failure.

A blood leak detector is fitted to the line carrying dialysis fluid away from the artificial kidney. By this means a small leak in the artificial kidney can be detected. Equipment monitors are linked to a central console box that will emit a visual and auditory signal when that monitor registers the limit of tolerance for a particular parameter. The monitor may be linked into a feedback mechanism to minimize the danger from an unplanned situation.

The blood leak detector has a negative feedback mechanism to the pump aspirating blood from the patient, so that when a blood leak develops, the flow of blood from the patient stops. A similar feedback mechanism switches off the blood pump if the conductivity meter monitoring the composition of dialysis fluid is not within specified limits.

An arterial pump monitor indicates when the blood flow from the patient reaches a critically low level. This warns the dialysis supervisor that the patient's circulation may be failing, or there is a block of outflow of blood from the patient.

The return line from the kidney to the patient has a bubble trap because gases may diffuse from the dialysis fluid to the blood. The bubbles that form in the blood are caught in the bubble trap chamber. On the bubble trap is a detector to indicate if the level of air in the bubble trap is too low. This protects the patient from an air embolus. Attached to the bubble trap is a side arm on which the pressure in the venous side of the kidney is measured.

Ultrafiltration is determined to a major extent by the pressure in the kidney, which can be increased as required by tightening a clamp on the venous line. Limits of tolerance for venous pressure are set by the dialysis supervisor according to the desired ultrafiltration required. If the alarm is triggered because the pressure is too low, the supervisor tightens the clamp. The pressure might rise too high because of increased blood flow through the kidney or might be a warning of obstruction in the venous line or cannula. This monitor may also have a feedback mechanism to switch off the blood pump in order to avoid rupture of the kidney membrane.

## COMPLICATIONS

■ **What action should be taken if there is a separation of connection at any point in the dialysis circuit?**

The blood pump should be stopped immediately and a clamp placed on both sides of the break. The connection at that point should be inspected for malfunction and replaced as necessary. This complication results from poor technique.

■ **What causes a blood leak through the membrane and how can it be corrected?**

Warning of a blood leak may be given by a monitor that detects particles in the outflow of the dialysis fluid. Occasionally false alarms are provided by air bubbles. If the leak is so small that the fluid is not discolored, blood may be detected by the use of Hemastix or by centrifuging the fluid for red blood cells (a red button would be seen at the bottom of the tube).

Large leaks tend to occur early in dialysis and are usually caused by faulty construction, storage, or "priming" of the kidney.

■ **What is "priming" of the kidney?**

The term "priming" refers to the technique whereby the artificial kidney is rinsed with heparinized saline solution before dialysis commences. This wets the surface of the membrane to enable resultant physical changes to occur and impregnate it with heparin. At the start of dialysis the circuit is left filled with heparinized saline solution unless the patient is critically ill and has an unstable hemodynamic system. Under these latter circumstances heparinized blood from the blood bank is used.

If the circuit is primed too quickly, a high pressure might be generated and perforation of the membrane ensue.

■ **What action should be taken with a large blood leak that grossly discolors the dialysis fluid?**

Dialysis should be stopped immediately.

■ **What should be done if the leak is small and the fluid is only faintly tinged?**

The leak may seal itself, but it would be hazardous to use high transmembrane pressure for the remainder of the dialysis. Recurrent small leaks are an indication to discontinue dialysis because a large leak could ultimately ensue.

## ■ What are the causes of hypotension?

The basic causes of hypotension include the following:

1. Excess ultrafiltration is the commonest cause and can be verified by comparing the patient's weight with that at the start of dialysis if the patient is on a weighing bed. Otherwise the degree of ultrafiltration will have to be estimated from the venous and dialysis fluid pressures and other causes of hypotension ruled out.
2. Blood loss may occur from the circuit or a bleeding site in the patient such as gastric or intestinal mucosal erosions and sites of trauma. Critically ill patients are most likely to bleed, and matched blood should be available for them before dialysis is started.
3. Excess blood may accumulate in a coil kidney that is distensible to some degree. This is equivalent to bleeding the patient.
4. The action of hypotensive medication might be accentuated during minimum ultrafiltration.
5. Endotoxin shock and pyrogen reactions may precipitate hypotension.

## ■ How should these causes of hypotension be managed?

Blood flow should be decreased, and the patient should be kept horizontal and saline solution administered if the cause is solely excessive ultrafiltration. Otherwise blood or other volume expanders, for example, plasma, may be necessary. The patient's condition should be meticulously monitored until blood pressure is restored to normal.

## ■ Are there any other causes of hypotension to be considered?

Pulmonary and air embolus might be considered and cardiac ischemia is always a possibility in a seriously ill and elderly patient. Uremic bleeding into the pericardial sac may restrict filling of the heart and reduce cardiac output.

## ■ Why might pyrogenic reactions occur?

Fever and chills during dialysis may be caused by contamination of the circuit with endotoxins from organisms destroyed during sterilization of the circuit. Blood transfusions may also be responsible, as may drug reactions. Septicemia from an infected blood access site is another possible factor.

## ■ Sometimes the patient's symptoms worsen during dialysis instead of improving. Why does this happen?

This may be the result of the dialysis disequilibrium syndrome. During dialysis urea and other solutes may be removed from blood at a rate faster than they move from tissue into blood. This creates a higher gradient for these solutes between tissue and blood. Consequently, an osmotic gradient is created, with fluid moving into cells from the bloodstream. Tissue edema ensues, and severe and fatal symptoms may result from cerebral edema.

The earliest symptom of dialysis disequilibruim syndrome is increasing apathy followed by confusion and disorientation. Increased twitching and convulsions ultimately occur. There may also be a rise in pulse, blood pressure, and respiratory rate. Death may result from cardiac arrest or pulmonary edema.

Dialysis disequilibrium syndrome can be avoided by dialyzing at a slower rate for short periods of time until extreme changes of biochemistry have been corrected.

## ■ Nausea and vomiting are common symptoms in any complications of dialysis. What are the most frequent causes?

The most commonly occurring factors in producing nausea and vomiting during dialysis are as follows:

1. Hypotension
2. Hypertension from fluid overload or dialysis disequilibrium syndrome
3. Gastric erosions
4. Dialysis disequilibrium syndrome
5. Anxiety
6. Medications
7. Hard water syndrome (In some areas local tap water contains a high concentration of calcium. Unless the water is treated with a softener or deionizer, the patient develops hypercalcemia and vomiting.)

**■ Headache can also be troublesome. What can be done to minimize it?**

Avoidance of dialysis disequilibrium syndrome, tension situations, and control of hypertension minimize headache.

**■ Cardiac arrhythmias are not uncommon in the intensive care situation. What facilitates them during dialysis?**

During dialysis cardiac arrhythmias may result from the following situations:

1. Hypoxia secondary to hypotension stresses a diseased myocardium.
2. Volume overload results in pulmonary edema, hypoxia, and cardiac arrhythmia.
3. Rapid reduction in serum potassium, especially in a digitalized patient, predisposes to cardiac arrhythmias.
4. A hematocrit that is inappropriately low for renal failure may indicate cardiac arrhythmias.

**■ How can chest pain be interpreted?**

Chest pain may be caused by any of the following:

1. It may result from cardiac ischemia, precipitated hypotension, or pulmonary edema.
2. Embolism of air or clot may produce a pleuritic pain and shock.
3. Pericarditis is a common complication of renal failure and is manifested by a scratchy or sharp substernal pain aggravated by respiration. The great dangers of pericarditis during dialysis are hemopericardium and cardiac tamponade.

**■ What is one of the most dramatic complications of dialysis?**

Convulsions may dramatically complicate dialysis. Causes include dialysis disequilibrium syndrome, hypertension, hypotension, cerebrovascular disease, or severe sudden changes in water and electrolyte composition. The latter may result from faulty composition of the dialysis fluid. Routine measures for managing convulsions should be instituted, anticonvulsants administered, and dialysis discontinued until the situation can be assessed by a physician. A sample of dialysis fluid should be taken for analysis.

**■ What other complications may constitute a life-threatening situation?**

Breathlessness as a result of fluid overload, congestive heart failure, pulmonary embolus, or dialysis disequilibrium are considered serious and even life-threatening conditions. Of course breathlessness may be the simple hyperventilation of anxiety.

**■ What may be a very annoying complication but not of serious consequence?**

Muscle cramp may be caused by rapid changes in water and sodium composition and can be offset by the infusion of saline solution.

**■ Is hemodialysis used to treat any other problem apart from renal failure?**

Yes. It can be used to treat overdose of certain drugs. The ease with which a drug is dialyzed depends on the blood concentration and the percentage of drug bound to serum proteins. Because proteins are not dialyzable, the more the drug is bound to serum protein, the less it is dialyzable.

The drugs for which dialysis is most commonly used are salicylates and the long-acting barbiturates.

If a drug is excreted through the renal route, dialysis would be essential for removal of that drug if renal failure exists.

**■ Are therapeutic drugs and essential body constituents removed by dialysis?**

Yes. Blood levels of some drugs, for example, diphenylhydantoin (Dilantin), are diminished by as much as 75% during a routine dialysis treatment and have to be replaced.

Water-soluble vitamins are removed in significant amounts, and replacement therapy is also essential for these substances.

**BIBLIOGRAPHY**

Pendras, J. P., and Stinson, G. W., editors: The hemodialysis manual, Seattle, 1970, Edmark Corporation.

Rosen, S. M.: Renal failure during and after shock, Int. Anesthesiol. Clin. **4**:861-881, 1969.

*chapter 17*

# Insight into short- and long-term hemodialysis treatments

N. DABIR VAZIRI
MARY ROBERTA McMAHON

In the predialysis era potentially reversible acute renal failure was associated with a high mortality rate. Return to the normal state for surviving groups involved prolonged periods of convalescence and disability. Management of such patients at that time consisted of rigid dietary restriction of fluids, proteins, sodium, and potassium. The consequence of this dietary restriction was a catabolic state with loss of muscle mass and other tissues that prolonged the recovery time and delayed the assumption of normal activities following the improvement of renal function.

Because of their uremic environment, malnutrition, and underlying disorders, patients were decidedly prone to develop systemic infections. Sepsis was the most common cause of death in patients with acute renal failure. Among those who survived, additional catabolic effects of systemic infection further prolonged the convalescent period. Uremic pericarditis with its serious consequences, that is, pericardial tamponade and constrictive pericarditis, was very common. Uremic neuropathy was frequently seen. Sensory and motor neuropathies were quite disabling and could last for many months after recovery from acute renal failure.

Anemia was invariably present and often very profound. Severe fluid overload and resultant congestive heart failure and pulmonary edema were extremely prevalent. These could occur even in the face of the most severe restriction of sodium and fluid intake with total body weight loss. It was the endogenous water from tissue breakdown that overloaded patients' damaged hearts, not the ingested or parenterally infused fluids.

End-stage chronic renal failure was a hopeless and terminal condition. With the advent of dialysis techniques and their proper use the high mortality and morbidity associated with acute renal failure has improved significantly, and patients with acute renal failure are allowed adequate dietary protein intake and are dialyzed early before uremic symptoms and complications supervene. Therefore positive nitrogen balance is maintained and wasting and uremic complications are prevented while the acute renal failure follows a course toward complete recovery. When the kidney function improves, the patient is in a good physical and mental condition and is able to resume normal life.

End-stage renal failure is no longer synonymous with death. Patients with nonfunctioning kidneys can be maintained on long-term dialysis for many years with relative comfort and productivity. It should be mentioned, however, that even though the development and perfection of dialysis technology has been one of the greatest breakthroughs in the field of medicine, it is far from being a perfect substitute for a normal kidney.

The kidney can be envisioned as a gland with both endocrine and exocrine functions. The result of its exocrine function is the formation of urine, which is the end product of glomerular filtration, tubular secretion, and tubular reabsorption. The kidney is responsible for elimination of metabolic waste products, excretion of exogenous toxins, maintenance of acid-base balance, and fluid and electrolyte homeostasis. Excretory function of the kidney is a smooth, sensitive, and continuous process and responds to physiologic needs of the body so properly that the composition and volume of body fluids are kept within normal limits despite wide variability of dietary content and fluid intake.

In addition to their excretory role, kidneys serve the following important endocrine functions:

1. Kidneys are responsible for the production of *erythropoietin,* a polypeptide hormone that regulates erythrocyte formation in the bone marrow. Lack of erythropoietin in patients with end-stage renal failure is one of the causes of the anemia that is always associated with renal failure.

2. Conversion of *vitamin D* to its active metabolite (1,25-dihydroxycholecalciferol) occurs in the kidney. In the absence of a functional kidney, dietary vitamin D or its endogenous counterpart remains inactive. Therefore a state of vitamin D resistance supervenes, resulting in the development of rickets or osteomalacic bone disease.

3. Kidneys secrete *renin,* which, by generating angiotensin II, regulates extracellular fluid volume and arterial blood pressure. Angiotensin II is one of the most potent vasoactive agents and causes severe vasoconstriction and raises the blood pressure. It is also capable of stimulating the secretion of aldosterone, which is a sodium-conserving hormone. By virtue of its sodium-conserving properties, aldosterone can expand extracellular volume.

4. A variety of prostaglandins is produced by the kidneys.

5. Kidneys are target organs for parathyroid hormone, aldosterone, and antidiuretic hormone (ADH).

6. Kidneys are responsible for the degradation of 20% of the insulin secreted by the pancreas.

From the preceding discussion it becomes obvious that the kidney is an important member of the endocrine system. It directly secretes hormones, regulates secretion of some hormones by other glands, responds as target organ to hormones produced elsewhere in the body, and participates in the deactivation of some hormones. Needless to say, dialysis does not replace the endocrine function of the kidneys. It is not even an adequate substitute for their excretory function, since it lacks the smoothness and continuity of normal renal operation.

Dialysis treatments are given intermittently, which results in rapid changes in the composition and volume of the internal milieu. They permit the accumulation of waste products, hydrogen ion, sodium, potassium, other substances, and frequently excess water during the interdialysis intervals. Therefore dialysis patients undergo recurrent fluctuation of the composition and volume of body fluids, which is contrary to the normal physiologic state and has adverse short- and long-term consequences.

By expressing these negative views, I do not intend to be pessimistic, but rather to present a realistic view. In fact, during the past 10 to 15 years with the development and evolution of dialysis technology, a great deal of progress has been made in the management of end-stage renal failure.

## ■ What are the basic elements in hemodialysis?

The basic elements involved in the process of hemodialysis are patient, dialyzing membrane (artificial kidney), and dialysis machine, the source of dialysis fluid. Accessory devices, that is, connecting tubes and various pumps, etc., are obviously necessary to bring these elements together and make the process mechanically feasible.

### *Patient*

The patient serves as the source of the blood; therefore it is necessary to have access to the bloodstream. Various means of providing access to the bloodstream exist and have been discussed elsewhere. These include the Scribner arteriovenous shunt, the Allen-Brown shunt, the arteriovenous fistula, the saphenous vein, and the bovine carotid artery grafts. In emergency situations blood access can be provided by the transcutaneous insertion of special catheters in femoral veins.

*Dialyzer*

Dialyzers consist of permeable membranes across which exchange processes between blood and dialysis fluid take place. They are usually made of cellophane or Cuprophan, which are cellulose derivatives. The basic difference between various dialyzers is in their physical arrangement. Several sizes of each kind are usually available. In the following paragraphs we will try briefly to describe the basic structure of the various commercially available dialyzers.

*Coil hemodialyzers.* In coil hemodialyzers the dialyzing membrane is made into a tubelike structure that is wound around a central core and supported by woven screens or unwoven lattices. Dialysate reaches the membranes through the perforations in the

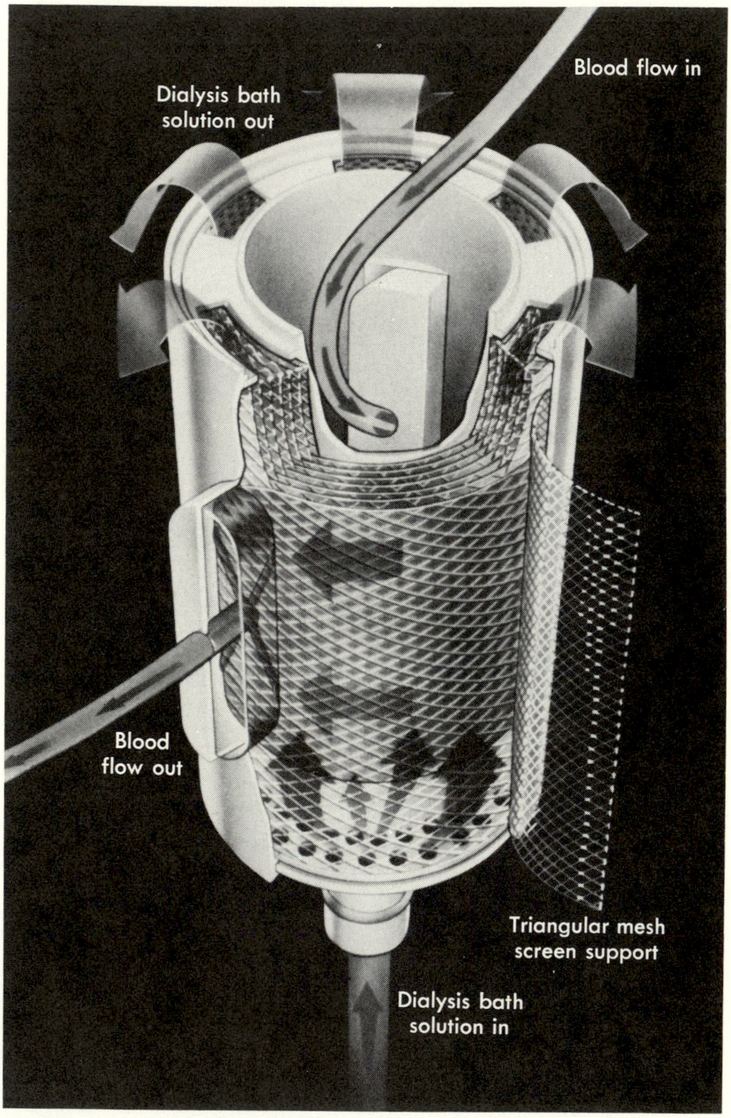


**Fig. 17-1.** Ultra-Flow II Coil Hemodialyzer. (Courtesy Travenol Laboratories, Inc., Morton Grove, Ill.)

supporting structure, while the blood is continuously pumped into the tubelike membrane (Fig. 17-1). Depending on the number of coils (1, 2, or 4), total surface area (0.7 to 2.5 $m^2$), kind of cellulose used (cellophane, Cuprophan), width of the blood channels, and supportive structure, a multitude of coil hemodialyzers have been manufactured.

***Parallel flow hemodialyzers (Kiil).*** The parallel flow dialyzers consist of two dialyzing membranes placed between two supportive surfaces in parallel fashion. Blood flows between the two membranes and dialysate flows on the outside (Fig. 17-2). These dialyzers are characterized by small priming volumes and low internal resistance.

***Hollow fiber or capillary dialyzers (Dow).*** The hollow fiber hemodialyzers consist of a large number of microtubules made of deacetylated cellulose acetate. The capillaries are jacketed in a plastic cylinder and sealed on each end into a tube sheet (Fig. 17-3). Blood passes through the capillaries continuously, while dialysate flows in and out of the plastic case, bathing blood-containing microcapillaries. Capillary dialyzers are characterized by their small size, easy storage, and very small priming volumes; however, because of thrombogenicity these require larger doses of heparin.

### *Dialysis machine (dialysate source)*

The dialysis machine is responsible for the production and delivery of dialysate. Many brands of dialysis machines are available. Depending on the mechanics of dialysate production, these machines can be categorized into four groups.

***Central delivery system.*** In the central delivery system large volumes of dialysate are made by mixing appropriate amounts of concentrated solution to treated water. Dialysate is then delivered through pipelines to each individual patient treated in the dialysis unit. This system has several advantages: the size of the individual machines is quite small, the risk of mistakes in making individual baths is nonexistent, the problem of malfunction of the proportioning system is avoided, and the patient care area remains clean.

There are some disadvantages: the large size of initial investment and the inability to make adjustments according to individual patient needs.

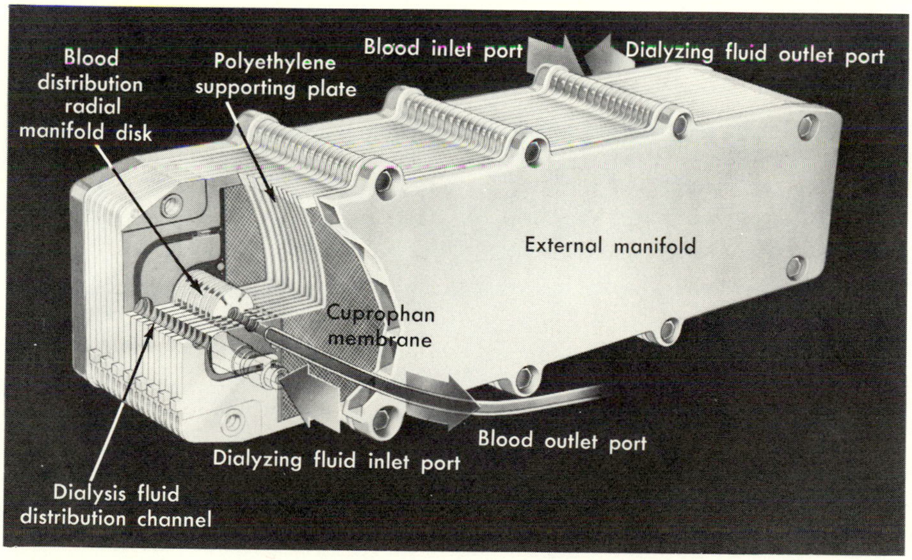


**Fig. 17-2.** Parallel Plate Dialyzer. (Courtesy Travenol Laboratories, Inc., Morton Grove, Ill.)

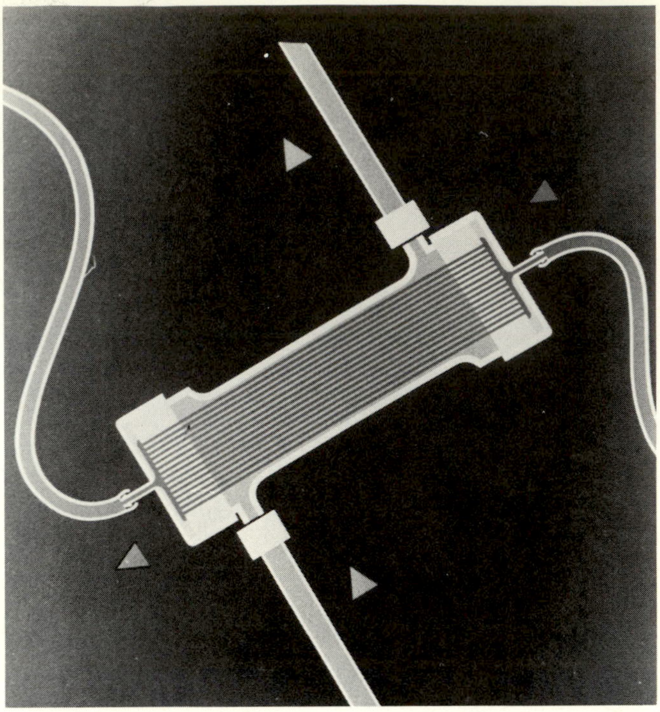

**Fig. 17-3.** Hollow Fiber Artificial Kidney. (Courtesy Cordis-Dow Corporation, Miami, Fla.)

***Batch system.*** In a batch system each machine has its own tank with an average capacity of 120 L of dialysate. The tank is filled with treated water, and the proper amount of concentrate is then added to provide ideal concentration. The advantage of this system is the possibility of making individual adjustments in dialysate composition depending on biochemical abnormalities. The disadvantages include the large size of each machine, the spillage of water and dialysate on the floor during mixing and draining processes, and the possibility of making mistakes by adding too much, too little, or no dialysate to the tank with its serious consequences.

***Proportionating machines.*** In the proportionating system treated water enters the machine from a central reservoir and is mixed with the concentrated solution on a continuing basis. Fresh dialysate is produced in this manner and delivered to the dialyzer. The advantage of these machines is their small size. Their disadvantage is the risk of malfunction of the proportionating pump, which can have serious consequences.

***Dialysate regenerating system.*** The dialysate regenerating machines have recently been introduced on the market and have practically eliminated the need for large volumes of dialysate. Only 1 to 2 L of dialysate is needed for the operation of these machines. In contrast to all the other systems, the dialysis fluid is not discarded after passage through the dialyzer; instead it is passed through two cartridges containing various adsorbents. The adsorbents remove various metabolic waste products as well as potassium ion, phosphorus, calcium, magnesium, etc., and refresh the dialysate, which can be recirculated. To avoid hypocalcemia, calcium is constantly infused into the venous line.

As a result, portable dialysis machines no bigger than a suitcase have become a reality. A stable, well-trained dialysis patient will no longer be imprisoned by the giant kidney machine in the future and will be able to travel with more freedom.

### ■ What are the indications for short-term hemodialysis?

The indications for short-term hemodialysis can be divided into two major categories: renal and nonrenal. The renal indications include acute renal failure and reversible deterioration of stable chronic renal disease. The nonrenal indications to be considered are intoxication with dialyzable drugs; severe fluid overload refractory to other modalities of treatment; metabolic acid-base balance disturbances, for example, lactic acidosis or severe metabolic alkalosis; severe electrolyte abnormalities, for example, hyperkalemia, hypercalcemia, hypermagnesemia, or hyponatremia; and marked hyperuremia.

### ■ When is the right time to start hemodialysis treatment in acute renal failure?

With the increasing availability and improvement of dialysis techniques, the approach to the management of acute renal failure has changed considerably. Dietary protein restriction as a means of uremia control is no longer justifiable. Dialysis treatment should be started early rather than late. Most nephrologists believe that dialysis should be started before the patient becomes symptomatic. The following findings call for the initiation of dialysis without delay:

1. Hypercatabolic states as suggested by the rapid rise of creatinine and urea such as is seen in patients with systemic infection and crushing injuries
2. Marked azotemia (BUN more than 100 mg)
3. Hyperkalemia
4. Marked metabolic acidosis
5. Any of the following uremic symptoms: Gastrointestinal manifestations—anorexia, nausea, or vomiting; CNS symptoms—reversal of sleep patterns, changes of mental status, asterixis, or convulsions; cardiovascular manifestations—pericarditis, congestive heart failure, or pulmonary congestion; or hematopoietic system symptoms—bleeding diathesis (platelet dysfunction resulting from uremia) or anemia

### ■ Are there any contraindications to the use of hemodialysis?

There are no absolute contraindications to the use of hemodialysis; however, under the following conditions hemodialysis may be difficult or somewhat dangerous:

1. Hemodialysis is not recommended when systemic heparinization is contraindicated, for example, in the presence of actively bleeding peptic ulcers, fresh intracranial hemorrhage or head trauma, or hypersensitivity to heparin preparations. Under most circumstances the use of regional heparinization or miniheparinization (administration of very small amounts of heparin) allows hemodialysis to be used with a minimum of difficulty. If major problems are anticipated, peritoneal dialysis should be considered. In the presence of pericarditis regional or miniheparinization should be used to avoid hemopericardium and tamponade.
2. Patients with severe cardiovascular disease and instability may present problems in hemodialysis. These patients may not tolerate the relatively rapid changes of internal milieu and intravascular volumes imposed by hemodialysis. They should undergo peritoneal dialysis.
3. Young children and elderly patients in whom the creation and maintenance of functioning vascular access is difficult should not undergo dialysis. These patients may be better treated with peritoneal dialysis.
4. Patients suffering overdoses of drugs that have high tissue- and protein-binding action respond to peritoneal dialysis better than hemodialysis, for example, those patients with diphenylhydantoin (Dilantin) and glutethimide poisoning.

### ■ What are the criteria for starting maintenance dialysis in patients with chronic renal failure?

Patients with chronic renal failure should be monitored closely. It is often possible to predict the course of the disease with some certainty when the patient has been studied for some time. It is ideal to create an arteriovenous fistula or one of the other means of internal vascular access a few months prior to the expected date when dialysis will be needed. The availability of a reliable vascular access for use when it is needed gives a sense of security to both patient and physician. In general when creatinine clearance falls below 10 ml/min or when the first symptoms of uremia develop, dialysis should be started; patients who start later respond less favorably to dialysis. The indications for the immediate initiation of dialysis in patients with chronic renal failure are the same as those for patients with acute renal failure.

### ■ What are the requirements for admission to a long-term dialysis program?

With the wide availability of federal funds for the care of patients with end-stage renal failure, the acceptance standards for a long-term dialysis program set by dialysis committees have become quite liberal. Factors such as age and underlying systemic disorder are no longer used as reasons for denying a patient the right to live in most centers. In other words, the patient is the main decision-maker; patients with terminal metastatic cancer who do not wish to continue the agony are not treated with dialysis. The acceptance of patients with profound psychiatric disorders is frequently a difficult decision. These patients can cause severe disturbances in the dialysis units, terminate their lives by opening the vascular access, project their paranoid ideas on dialysis personnel, and become a source of threat to the others. Nevertheless, in the opinion of some practitioners psychiatric disorder does not justify denial of a person's right to live.

### ■ What are the objectives of home dialysis programs, and what criteria are required?

Because of the tremendous financial impact of in-center maintenance dialysis, home dialysis programs have been strongly supported and encouraged by the federal government and private agencies. The average cost of dialysis was estimated as $6300 for home and $23,000 for in-center dialysis in 1972 in California. In addition to its much lower cost, home dialysis provides a more complete and natural rehabilitation.

The following lists some of the criteria required for a home hemodialysis program:

1. Physical structure of the patient's residence should be suitable for installation of water deionizer, reservoir, plumbing system, dialysis machine, and drainage system.
2. Patient should be eager to participate and assume the major role in self-dialysis with minimum assistance at home.
3. Patient should be trainable and reliable.
4. Availability of a willing and interested related dialysis assistant, for example, spouse, parent, or child, is an absolute requirement, since even when the patient is perfectly self-sufficient, there are emergency situations where the aid of a second person is vitally important. However, since severe psychologic problems such as role reversal, emotional blackmailing, sense of dependency for life on the other person, and severe guilt feelings in cases of real or potential mistakes can be and have been encountered, the tendency is to assign the patient the major role in self-dialysis and use the assistant for minor tasks and emergency situations.

### ■ Should dialysis patients be given any special diet?

Restriction of dietary sodium, potassium, and fluid intake is frequently necessary in dialysis patients. A day-to-day weight change in dialysis patients reflects the balance of their fluid intake and output rather than a real alteration of lean body mass. Patients with good urine output may be allowed more or less liberal fluid intake. In general a weight gain of 0.5 kg/day is permitted between dialyses. A "no-added" salt (4 g/day), low potassium, and liberal protein diet is usually prescribed.

These statements hold true both in acute and chronic renal failure patients treated with hemodialysis. It is worthwhile to mention that salt substitutes contain large amounts of potassium and should not be used in patients with renal failure.

### What drugs are routinely prescribed for dialysis patients, and what is the reason behind their use?

Since intermittent dialysis does not completely remove all the dietary phosphorus, the plasma phosphorus concentration is frequently elevated. Prolonged elevation of serum phosphorus levels results in soft tissue and vascular calcifications and progressive bone damage. For this reason hyperphosphatemia should be controlled. This is achieved by the use of phosphate-binding antacids (aluminum hydroxide) that bind dietary phosphate and prevent its absorption from the intestines. The dose of aluminum hydroxide should be adjusted by careful monitoring of the plasma phosphorus level. In order to achieve its maximum phosphate-lowering effect, aluminum hydroxide should be given with or after each meal. Because of its abundance in various foods, a low phosphate diet is not practical.

Since water-soluble vitamins are lost with dialysis, supplementation with therapeutic multivitamins is necessary. Folic acid loss is particularly significant and if not replaced results in severe anemia. The daily use of 1 to 2 mg of folic acid is mandatory to prevent folate deficiency anemia.

A small amount of iron is lost with each dialysis, and iron absorption is frequently impaired in patients with renal failure. As a result, some of these patients are iron deficient. When iron deposits in the patient's bone marrow are reduced or lacking, the administration of oral or parenteral iron will be helpful.

Patients who have excess iron stores because of repeated transfusions should not be given additional iron, since it can cause hemosiderosis and organ damage.

Patients with chronic renal failure are frequently in a negative calcium balance. Their fecal calcium content is often more than their dietary intake. A variety of therapeutic approaches have been taken to overcome this problem, including the use of high calcium dialysates (3.5 mEq/L), therapeutic doses of vitamin D, and oral administration of calcium carbonate. Variable results have been reported with each of these modalities. It is mandatory that hyperphosphatemia be controlled before attempts are made to improve calcium balance. If the serum calcium level is raised by any of the means just mentioned while the serum phosphorus level is elevated, calcium phosphate will precipitate in vascular walls and soft tissues, causing vascular and tissue damage.

### What are the major criteria by which adequacy of dialysis is judged?

Several parameters are used to judge adequacy of dialysis treatment:

1. Patient's general condition and sense of well-being
2. Degree of anemia and its progression or improvement
3. Nerve conduction velocity (NCV) and electromyographic (EMG) abnormalities (NVC and EMG studies are most commonly used to assess the adequacy of dialysis. These studies can be done serially twice a year.)
4. Degree of azotemia as judged by average plasma urea and creatinine levels
5. Fluid balance, blood pressure control, and cardiac status
6. Muscle mass and dry body weight
7. Presence or absence of uremic symptoms

The deterioration of these parameters calls for more intensive dialysis treatment.

### What is the minimum dialysis requirement per week?

No single figure suits all dialysis patients. Depending on the patient's residual renal function, size, and dietary and metabolic load, the dialysis requirements vary. In other words, a special dialysis program in terms of length and frequency should be tailored for each individual patient. However, the average patient requires a minimum of 18 hr/m$^2$ of dialysis per week.

*The hour–square meter concept* refers to the product of dialysis time in hours multiplied by the surface area of the dialyzing membrane. For instance, when a patient is dialyzed three times a week, 6 hours each time with a dialyzer with a 1 $m^2$ surface, the weekly dialysis will be 18 hr/$m^2$, as calculated below:

$$3.0 \times 6.0 = 18 \text{ hr/week}$$
$$T \times S = 18.0 \times 1.0 = 18 \text{ hr/m}^2$$

in which T = time on dialysis in hours per week and S = surface area of dialysis membrane in square meters.

According to this concept, the dialysis time can be shortened if the dialysis surface is increased. By utilizing large surface area dialyzers or two dialyzers in parallel or in series, a significant reduction of dialysis time has become possible.

Although the clearance of small molecules, for example, urea and creatinine, with the large surface area, fast dialysis technique is satisfactory, its efficiency in removing mid-sized molecules, which are thought to be responsible for uremic neuropathy, may be suboptimal. The technique is still quite new, and more experience is required to answer this and many other questions that may be raised in the future.

## ■ What is the extent of rehabilitation?

The degree of rehabilitation is quite variable. Approximately 28% of these patients are capable of doing all usual activities, 34% are unable to perform strenuous work, 24% are unable to do ordinary activities, and 14% need assistance for primary self-care.

## ■ What is the long-term survival rate of patients on maintenance hemodialysis treatment, and how does it compare with the figures for renal transplantation survival?

The mortality rate in the long-term dialysis population is approximately 10% per year. According to some statistics, home dialysis is slightly superior with respect to survival to in-center dialysis. This has not been a consistent finding, however, and it may reflect a greater physical and psychologic stability among home dialysis patients as compared to the in-center dialysis group. Table 17-1 shows the 1- and 2-year survival statistics obtained from three different sources.

**Table 17-1.** Survival statistics of patients on maintenance hemodialysis*

| *Source* | *Type of program* | *1-year survival (%)* | *2-year survival (%)* |
|---|---|---|---|
| European Dialysis and Transplantation Association | In-center | 84 | 72 |
| | Home | 92 | 85 |
| Peter Bent Brigham Hospital | In-center | 93 | 86 |
| | Home | 88 | 78 |
| 1972 National Dialysis Registry | | 90 | 80 |

*In comparison with renal transplantation, dialysis is superior to cadaver and inferior to live related renal transplantation as far as mortality rates are concerned.

## ■ What is the significance of the dialyzability of various drugs?

It is quite important to know if a drug is dialyzable or not, and if it is, to what extent. Dialysis can be used to enhance the elimination of dialyzable drugs from the body in cases of drug overdose. Patients with renal failure frequently have multiorgan disorders requiring multiple drug therapy. Furthermore, because of their increased susceptibility, the incidence of infections requiring antibiotic therapy is quite high in these patients. Sufficient blood levels of antibiotics or other drugs are quite vital to obtain the pharmacologic effects. If the drug is dialyzable, its plasma concentration may fall below therapeutic levels following dialysis. As a result, the underlying disorders will cease to be under control. By proper adjustment of the dose and administration of dialyzable drugs at the end of dialysis, this problem can be avoided. Table 17-2 provides information as to the dialyzability of some of the more commonly used drugs.

**Table 17-2.** Dialyzable drugs

| *Drug* | *Significant dialysis of drug* |
|---|---|
| *Antimicrobial agents* | |
| Aminosalicylic acid | Yes (H)* |
| Amphotericin B | No (H) |
| Cefazolin | No (H, P) |
| Cephalosporins | |
| Cephalexin | Yes (H, P) |
| Cephalothin | Yes (H, P) |
| Chloramphenicol | No (H, P) |
| Chloroquine | ? |
| Clindamycin | No (H, P) |
| Colistimethate | Yes (P)<br>No (H) |
| Erythromycin | ? |
| Ethambutol | Yes (H, P) |
| Flucytosine | Yes (H, P) |
| Gentamicin | Yes (H)<br>No (P) |
| Isoniazid | Yes (H, P) |
| Kanamycin | Yes (H, P) |
| Lincomycin | No (H, P) |
| Methenamine mandelate | ? |
| Nalidixic acid | ? |
| Neomycin | Yes (H)<br>No (P) |
| Nitrofurantoin | Yes (H) |
| Penicillins | |
| Amoxicillin | Yes (H) |
| Ampicillin | Yes (H)<br>No (P) |
| Carbenicillin | Yes (H)<br>No (P) |
| Cloxacillin | No (H) |
| Dicloxacillin | No (H) |
| Methicillin | No (H, P) |
| Nafcillin | No (H) |
| Oxacillin | No (H, P) |
| Penicillin G | No (H, P) |
| Pentamidine | ? |
| Pyrimethamine | ? |
| Quinine | Yes (H)<br>No (P) |
| Rifampin | ? |
| Streptomycin | Yes (H, P) |
| Sulfamethoxazole trimethoprim | Yes (H) |
| Sulfisoxazole | Yes (H, P) |
| Tetracyclines | |
| Doxycycline | No (H, P) |
| Minocycline | ? |
| Tetracycline | No (H, P) |
| Vancomycin | No (H, P) |
| *Analgesics, antihistamines, narcotics, and narcotic antagonists* | |
| Analgesics (nonnarcotic) | |
| Acetaminophen (Tylenol) | Yes (H)<br>No (P) |
| Acetylsalicylic acid (aspirin) | Yes (H, P) |
| Phenazopyridine (Pyridium) | ? |
| Antihistamines | |
| Chlorpheniramine maleate (Chlor-Trimeton) | ? |
| Diphenhydramine (Benadryl) | ? Yes (H) |
| Narcotics and narcotic antagonists | |
| Codeine | ? |
| Meperidine (Demerol) | ? |
| Methadone | ? |
| Morphine | ? |
| Naloxone (Narcan) | ? |
| Pentazocine (Talwin) | ? |
| Propoxyphene (Darvon) | No (H, P) |
| *Sedatives, hynotics, and tranquilizers* | |
| Barbiturates | |
| Amobarbital (Amytal) | No (H, P) |
| Phenobarbital | Yes (H, P) |
| Secobarbital (Seconal) | No (H, P) |
| Benzodiazepines | |
| Chlordiazepoxide (Librium) | No (H) |
| Diazepam (Valium) | No (H) |
| Ethchlorvynol (Placidyl) | Yes (H, P) |
| Glutethimide (Doriden) | No (H, P) |
| Lithium carbonate | Yes (H, P) |
| Meprobomate (Miltown, Equanil) | Yes (H, P) |
| Methaqualone (Quaalude, Mandrax) | Yes (H) |
| Phenothiazines | No (H, P) |
| Tricyclic antidepressants | |
| Amitriptyline (Elavil) | ? Yes (P)<br>No (H) |
| Desipramine (Norpramin) | ? |
| Imipramine (Tofranil) | ? Yes (P)<br>No (H) |
| Nortriptyline (Aventyl) | ? Yes (P)<br>No (H) |
| *Cardiovascular, antihypertensive, and diuretic agents* | |
| Antiarrhythmic agents | |
| Lidocaine | ? |

*H = hemodialysis; P = peritoneal dialysis.

*Continued.*

**Table 17-2.** Dialyzable drugs—cont'd

| *Drug* | *Significant dialysis of drug* |
|---|---|
| *Cardiovascular, antihypertensive, and diuretic agents—cont'd* | |
| Antiarrhythmic agents—cont'd | |
| Procainamide (Pronestyl) | Yes (H) |
| Propranolol (Inderal) | No (H) |
| Quinidine | Yes (H, P) |
| Antihypertensive agents | |
| Diazoxide | Yes (H, P) |
| Guanethidine | ? |
| Hydralazine (Apresoline) | No (H, P) |
| Methyldopa (Aldomet) | Yes (H, P) |
| Minoxidil | ? |
| Reserpine | No (H, P) |
| Cardiac glycosides | |
| Digitoxin | No (H, P) |
| Digoxin | No (H, P) |
| Ouabain | No (H, P) |
| Diuretics | |
| Acetazolamide | ? |
| Ethacrynic acid | ? |
| Furosemide | ? |
| Mercurials | ? |
| Metolazone | No (H) |
| Spironolactone | ? |
| Thiazides | ? |
| Triamterene | ? |
| *Miscellaneous agents* | |
| Anticoagulants | |
| Heparin | No (H) |
| Warfarin | ? |
| Antineoplastic and immunosuppressive agents | |
| Alkylating agents | ? |
| Azathioprine (Imuran) | Yes (H) |
| Cyclophosphamide (Cytoxan) | Yes (H) |
| Methotrexate | Yes (H) |
| *Miscellaneous agents—cont'd* | |
| Corticosteroids | |
| Cortisone | No (H) |
| Dexamethasone | ? |
| Hydrocortisone | ? |
| Methylprednisolone | No (H) |
| Prednisolone | ? |
| Prednisone | ? |
| Drugs for treatment of arthritis and allied conditions | |
| Allopurinol | ? |
| Colchicine | ? |
| Gold sodium thiomalate | ? |
| Indomethacin | ? |
| Phenylbutazone | ? |
| Probenecid | ? |
| Drugs used in neurologic disorders | |
| Diphenylhydantoin (Dilantin) | Yes (H) |
| Levodopa | ? |
| Neostigmine | ? |
| Primidone (Mysoline) | Yes (H) |
| Trihexyphenidyl (Artane) | ? |
| Trimethadione (Tridione) | ? |
| Hypoglycemic agents | |
| Acetohexamide | ? |
| Chlorpropamide | No (P) |
| Insulin, regular (crystalline) | ? |
| Phenformin | ? |
| Tolbutamide | No (H) |
| Other drugs | |
| Atropine | ? |
| Clofibrate | ? |
| Penicillamine | ? |
| Propylthiouracil | ? |
| Theophylline (aminophylline) | ? |
| Tubocurarine | ? |

## BIBLIOGRAPHY


Arthur, G., et al.: Clinical maintenance hemodialysis with a sorbent-based low-volume dialysate regeneration system, Trans. Am. Soc. Artif. Intern. Organs **17**:253-256, 1971.

Bailey, G. L., editor: Hemodialysis principles and practice, New York, 1972, Academic Press, Inc.

Bennett, W. M., Singer, I., and Coggins, C. J.: A guide to drug therapy in renal failure, J.A.M.A. **230**:1544-1553, 1974.

Knepshield, J. H., et al.: Dialysis of poisons and drugs—annual review, Trans. Am. Soc. Artif. Intern. Organs **19**:599, 1973.

Pendras, J. P., and Stinson, G. W., editors: The hemodialysis manual, Seattle, 1970, Edmark Corporation.

Shaldon, S.: Haemodialysis in chronic renal failure, Postgrad. Med. J. suppl., p. 3, Nov., 1966.

Shimizu, A., et al.: Straight arteriovenous shunt for long-term hemodialysis, J.A.M.A. **216**:645-647, 1971.

*chapter 18*

# Complications of hemodialysis and their management

N. DABIR VAZIRI

End-stage renal disease, once a terminal event, is now being converted by dialysis technology to a chronic debilitating condition. Life itself may be prolonged for many years, but its quality is widely variable because of medical and nonmedical problems. Long-term dialysis patients, in addition to being susceptible to the diseases contracted by other persons, are prime targets for many other disorders that are more or less peculiar to them. This chapter is intended to briefly review these complications and discuss their prevention and management.

These complications may be related to vascular access difficulties, defective dialysis apparatus, improper fluid composition, anticoagulation, dialysis of essential nutrients, infections, consequences of shunt declotting procedure, rapid alterations of extracellular fluid volume and composition, failure to adhere to the dietary and drug regimen, socioeconomic and psychologic problems, hyperlipidemia and accelerated atherosclerosis, chronic anemia, renal osteodystrophy, secondary hyperparathyroidism, hypertension, dialysis-associated pericarditis, or other cardiac complications.

## ■ What are the complications caused by the rapid changes of extracellular fluid volume and composition imposed by dialysis?

### *Hypotension*

Hypotension is discussed in detail in Chapter 16.

### *Transient dyspnea at end of dialysis*

Occasionally patients develop a transient tachypnea and mild shortness of breath immediately after completion of dialysis. This seems to be related to a mild but sudden increase of intravascular volume resulting from the rapid return of blood content from the artificial kidney and tubing system to the patient. In a short period of time the excess fluid is sequestered throughout the extracellular compartment and symptoms improve.

### *Disequilibrium syndrome*

Disequilibrium syndrome is a clinical disorder that occurs during or immediately after dialysis. It may be mild, manifesting with headaches, nausea, vomiting, and drowsiness. When severe, it presents with involuntary jerking movements, disorientation, psychosis, convulsions, and coma. It is accompanied by EEG changes that point to the CNS origin of these clinical manifestations. The EEG changes consist of diffuse slowing of the basal rhythm and occasional paroxysms of high voltage spikes. Pathologically swelling of nerve cells and cerebral edema characterize this syndrome. The syndrome is most likely to occur with the first few dialyses in the following situations:

1. In severely azotemic patients
2. When prolonged and overly efficient dialysis is given
3. In the presence of preexisting neurologic disorder

The disorder occurs paradoxically while biochemical abnormalities of the patient's extracellular fluid are being corrected.

The pathogenesis of the syndrome is not well understood. However, it seems to be caused by a disequilibrium between intracellular and extracellular fluids. This results from slowness of the exchange processes across the cell membrane. The following factors have been incriminated in the pathogenesis of disequilibrium syndrome:

1. Reduction of extracellular fluid osmolality resulting from the removal of urea by dialysis and, more importantly, a drop in its sodium concentration.* Lower extracellular fluid osmolality relative to intracellular fluid causes a shift of water into the cell and resultant cell swelling.

2. Increased intracellular and cerebrospinal fluid acidosis. Dialysis can rapidly correct the extracellular fluid acidosis by increasing its bicarbonate concentration. With correction of renal acidosis, pulmonary compensation will disappear. As a result, the partial pressure of carbon dioxide ($P_{CO_2}$) rises. In contrast to bicarbonate ions, $CO_2$ equilibrates across the cell membrane quite rapidly. Therefore $P_{CO_2}$ inside the cell rises while bicarbonate is still low; as a result intracellular pH falls. The same mechanism is operative across the blood-brain barrier, causing cerebrospinal fluid acidosis.

3. Reduction of oxygen delivery to the tissues. This relates to the effect of blood pH on the oxygen-hemoglobin dissociation curve. In the presence of acidosis the affinity of hemoglobin for oxygen is reduced. As a result, a more complete unloading of oxygen is expected at the tissue level. Rapid correction of acidosis with dialysis reverses this effect and may transiently impair tissue oxygen delivery in these anemic patients.

TREATMENT AND PREVENTION. Several modalities of treatment and prevention have been used with variable results. By slow IV infusion of mannitol or hypertonic sodium chloride solutions during dialysis, the symptoms may be minimized or eliminated. This is accomplished through maintaining extracellular fluid osmolality. The administration of diphenylhydantoin (Dilantin) prior to dialysis can reduce the symptoms.

In my experience the best way of preventing disequilibrium syndrome is to reduce the duration and flow rates of the first few dialysis treatments and increase their frequency. This results in the gradual rather than sudden correction of extracellular fluid abnormalities, allowing parallel correction of intracellular fluid with time.

### *Postdialysis syndrome*

Postdialysis syndrome is a very common problem among the long-term dialysis population. It manifests as weakness, fatigue, and dizziness, and occasionally with headaches, nausea, and muscle cramps. Symptoms start after dialysis and last 12 to 24 hours. The problem reappears with each dialysis and is very annoying. I believe this syndrome is a mild recurrent form of disequilibrium syndrome.

### *Paradoxical hypertension*

Severe hypertension can occur when the patient undergoes drastic ultrafiltration. This is called paradoxical because the usual response is hypotension rather than hypertension. It is caused by the increased release of vasoactive agents, that is, renin-angiotensin and catecholamines, in response to volume depletion. Treatment consists of the IV infusion of saline solution to replete intravascular volume and relieve vascular hyperreactivity.

## ■ What complications can arise from the dysfunction of dialysis apparatus and inappropriate dialysate formulation?

### *Mechanical blood loss*

Blood losses caused by rupture of the dialysis membrane or disconnection of the tubing system are discussed elsewhere.

*The sodium concentration in all conventional dialysates is around 130 mEq/L. It is about 155 mEq/L in the water fraction of plasma and extracellular fluid. Therefore most dialysates are hypotonic with respect to sodium and are capable of reducing the extracellular fluid sodium concentration.

### *Clotting of artificial kidney*

Clotting occurs when the patient is not adequately heparinized and/or the blood flow through the dialyzer is slow. In microcapillary kidneys many of the microfibers may be occluded by blood clots without being noticed. This can markedly reduce the efficiency of dialysis. With coil dialyzers clotting is readily suspected by a rapid increase of the venous resistance and visual detection of the clot in the tubing system. Because of their relatively large priming volume, clotting in coil dialyzers is associated with significant blood loss.

Adequate anticoagulation with careful monitoring of clotting time and provision of good blood flow are essential for the prevention of this problem.

### *Hemolysis*

Hemolysis is occasionally seen in dialysis patients under the following circumstances:

1. Dialysis against hypotonic bath. This is occasionally encountered when the person who is responsible for dialysis forgets or fails to add adequate amounts of concentrate to the tank before dialysis is started. Malfunction of the proportionating machines can also create a similar problem. Exposure to hypotonic medium results in the swelling and rupture of red blood cells as they pass through the dialyzer.

Patients often complain of shortness of breath, chills, back pain, feeling badly, nausea, and vomiting. Because of the release of hemoglobin into plasma, blood content of the venous line appears glossy and simulates cherry syrup. Dialysis should be discontinued immediately. Serial hematocrit and electrolyte determinations should be performed. The patient's blood should be typed and cross matched and transfusion started if a significant drop in hematocrit is observed or if the patient becomes symptomatic from the acute exacerbation of anemia. Because of the release of intracellular potassium, serum potassium levels may rise to dangerous concentrations and should be carefully watched. In order to avoid this serious complication, the routine measurement of dialysate conductivity before starting dialysis should be mandatory.

2. Tight occlusion of the blood pump. This results in traumatic breakdown of the red blood cells as they pass through the pump. Finding many red blood cell fragments (schistocytes) on a smear taken from the blood leaving the pump suggests the diagnosis and calls for correction of the problem.

3. Copper-induced acute hemolysis. A few cases of acute hemolysis resulting from dialysis with copper-contaminated dialysates have been reported in the literature. Contamination was caused by the release of copper from copper tubing in dialysate-making machines. In all cases water deionizer was exhausted, allowing delivery of acid water capable of dissolving copper, to the dialysate-making machine. Greenish discoloration of the dialysate should indicate the possibility of copper contamination.

4. High dialysate temperature. Excess heating of dialysis fluid is another cause of hemolysis during the dialysis procedure.

### *Air embolism*

Air embolism is one of the most serious complications of hemodialysis. The following conditions can predispose to the development of air embolism:

1. Use of a blood pump
2. High negative pressure that sucks the air from around the needle and releases the dissolved gas as free bubbles in the blood
3. Empty bottles connected to the blood line
4. Defective and broken lines, providing an entrance for air into the blood line

I have seen fatal cases of air embolism subsequent to starting the machine with an *unprimed* kidney and tubing system! The severity of the disorder depends on the volume and rapidity of air entering the circulation, as well as on the patient's position at the time of the incident. A small amount of air slowly infused into the circulation is dissolved in the plasma and usually causes no significant problems. When a sizable bolus of air rapidly enters the venous circulation, it finds its way along the bloodstream toward the right atrium and ventricle. Subsequent contractions of the heart against the air-blood mixture create tremendous amounts of foam, filling the right ventricle and pulmonary vascular bed and impeding blood return to the left ventricle and systemic circulation. Some air bubbles find their way through the naturally occurring central pulmonary arteriovenous shunts or cardiac septal defects to various organs, including brain and retinal vessels.

Clinical findings consist of sudden onset of dyspnea, cough, cyanosis, respiratory arrest, and loss of consciousness. Churning of the foam may be audible on auscultation of the heart, and air bubbles may be seen in retinal vessels on careful funduscopic examination. Examination of the tubing system frequently reveals the presence of residual air in the tubing system, helping to establish the diagnosis.

The best treatment for air embolism, similar to every other disorder, is its prevention. This is achieved by avoiding high negative pressures, checking for defective and leaky tubing systems, using collapsible plastic instead of rigid glass IV fluid containers, and clamping the IV line before the container is completely empty. Electronic air-detecting devices are also helpful.

In the case of suspected air embolism, *dialysis should be stopped* and the source of air eliminated immediately. The patient should be placed *on the left side* with the feet higher than the head, trying to trap the air bolus in the right atrium and allow enough time for its resolution in the blood. Oxygen should be administered in high concentration. In the case of respiratory arrest or severe distress, *assisted respiration is necessary.* A *needle aspiration* of the right side of the heart to remove the trapped air and foam may be necessary to make resuscitative measures successful.

If available, the patient should be placed in a hyperbaric chamber. Under high barometric pressures the solubility of nitrogen in the plasma increases; air bubbles disappear and clinical improvement ensues. Decompression of the chamber should be performed very slowly, since sudden decompression results in the appearance of air bubbles in the blood and diffuse fatal air embolization.

### *Leukopenia*

The number of circulating white blood cells drops significantly during the first 30 minutes of dialysis. It returns toward normal in about 1 hour. Margination of the white blood cells along the tubing system, dialysis membranes, and vessel walls seems to be responsible for the phenomenon. I should mention that this phenomenon occurs invariably with each dialysis in all patients and has no known adverse effects.

### *Hypernatremia*

Hypernatremia is another complication caused by the inappropriate formulation of dialysate. Severe hypernatremia with a hyperosmolar state has occurred as a consequence of ion-exchange water softener malfunction, allowing delivery of water with a high sodium concentration to the dialysate-making machine. Headaches, excess thirst, blurry vision, and disorientation characterize this syndrome.

### *Water intoxication*

Water intoxication is also caused by the inappropriate formulation of dialysis fluid when its sodium concentration is below 120 mEq/L. It presents with signs of increased intracranial pressure, that is, headaches, nausea, vomiting, confusion, convulsion, and coma.

### *Hypokalemia*

Most dialysis patients are dialyzed against zero or very low potassium baths. Although this is often necessary for the removal of excess potassium, at times a profound hypokalemia is encountered. Clinically hypokalemia presents with muscular weakness, ileus, and cardiac arrhythmias that could be life threatening in digitalized patients. Therefore serum potassium concentrations should be checked periodically to avoid this complication.

### *Hard water syndrome*

The calcium content of tap water can be quite high. Ion-exchange water softeners are used to remove the calcium content of tap water. Malfunction of the water softener can release excess calcium into the water. When this water is mixed with ordinary concentrate, the resultant dialysate will have a very high calcium concentration. Dialysis against such dialysate will result in the influx of calcium from the bath to the patient and cause hypercalcemia. Clinical symptoms include weakness, lethargy, anorexia, vomiting, hypertension, and burning of the skin. The diagnosis is confirmed by measurement of the calcium content of the bath and the patient's plasma.

Treatment and prevention are obvious, that is, correction of the malfunctioning apparatus and calcium concentration of dialysate.

### *Fluoride excess*

The fluoride content of dialysates is quite high in cities where water supplies are artificially fluorinated or areas where the content of fluoride in the water is naturally high. Fluoride can cause osteosclerosis and some other bony and dental changes, but it has generally been thought to be harmless. Recently, however, the possibility of its role in the pathogenesis of progressive renal osteodystrophy has been raised. Therefore the safety of high fluoride dialysate is quite uncertain at the present time.

### *Hyper- and hypoglycemia*

At the present time most conventional hemodialysis fluids are either glucose free or contain no more than 200 mg of glucose. Therefore hyperglycemia and reactive hypoglycemia secondary to hemodialysis are no longer observed. However, in the past when baths containing high concentrations of glucose were used for ultrafiltration purposes, these complications were commonly seen. With peritoneal dialysis, in which the dialysates have a high glucose content, hyper- and hypoglycemia remain among the consequences of this procedure. For further information, refer to Chapters 19 and 20.

## ■ What are the complications caused by failure to adhere to the dietary and drug regimen?

Despite the wide variability of dietary intake, the volume and composition of the body fluids remain relatively unchanged. Kidneys play a major role in maintaining the homeostasis of the internal milieu, which is vital to the proper function of all the cells and organ systems.

Dialysis patients who are functionally or anatomically without kidneys lack these regulatory mechanisms. Therefore the volume and composition of their body fluids alter every time they eat or drink.

Although dialysis treatment is intended to replace the excretory function of the kidney, because of its intermittent nature, it does not simulate the function of normal kidneys, which have the minute-to-minute control of homeostasis of the internal milieu. The purpose of dietary and drug regimens prescribed for these patients is to minimize these fluctuations, which have immediate and long-term adverse effects on various organs. The dietary and drug regimens recommended for dialysis patients were discussed earlier in detail. Here I will discuss various problems that can result from failure to adhere to these recommendations.

### *Fluid overload*

The ingestion of excess fluid by these patients results in expansion of their body fluids, including the intravascular and interstitial compartments. This in turn elevates the blood pressure and increases the load on the heart, resulting in congestive heart failure and pulmonary edema.

In catabolic patients endogenously produced water from the breakdown of tissues can produce congestive heart failure and pulmonary edema in the absence of excess exogenous fluid intake and weight gain.

The ingestion of excess salt can cause expansion of the extracellular fluid by shifting water from the intracellular to the extracellular compartment. Therefore fluid and sodium ion intakes should be restricted to prevent these catastrophic events. When they happen, emergency dialysis with ultrafiltration should be performed. If this is not possible, phlebotomy with plasmaphoresis and the return of packed red blood cells should be considered.

### *Hyperkalemia*

Renal failure patients cannot handle large loads of potassium. The ingestion of potassium-rich foods, for example, fruits and milk, results in a rapid rise of their serum potassium. Severe hyperkalemia causes muscle weakness and even paralysis of various muscle groups, including the respiratory muscles. It has serious cardiac toxicity. As plasma potassium increases above 6 to 7 mEq/L, the T waves become tall and peaked, the P-R interval is prolonged, P waves disappear, QRS complexes are prolonged, and idioventricular rhythm and cardiac arrest follow sequentially with gradual increments of plasma potassium.

Emergency treatment is necessary if fatal cardiac complications are to be avoided. Potassium ion can be driven into the cells by IV infusion of sodium bicarbonate or insulin and glucose mixtures. IV calcium gluconate counteracts the cardiac effects of hyperkalemia, but it is dangerous in digitalized patients.

A sodium-polystyrene sulfonate (Kayexalate)–sorbitol mixture (ion-exchange resin) given orally or by enema can lower plasma potassium ion by removing it through the gastrointestinal tract. Emergency dialysis against zero or, if not available, a low potassium ion bath is the most direct answer.

It should be noted that hyperkalemia may occur in postsurgical catabolic patients (sepsis or crush syndrome), or patients with hemolysis or gastrointestinal bleeding in the absence of exogenous potassium ion intake. This is caused by the release of potassium ion secondary to the breakdown of tissues or red blood cells. Frequent dialysis treatments and administration of Kayexalate are helpful in bringing this hyperkalemia under control.

### *Hyperphosphatemia*

Intermittent dialysis is not adequate to remove all the phosphorus that enters the body fluids from dietary sources and bone resorption. Hyperphosphatemia is therefore a common finding in dialysis patients. Aluminum hydroxide administered with meals binds dietary phosphate and prevents its absorption. It is routinely prescribed for dialysis patients to control hyperphosphatemia. Failure to administer aluminum hydroxide results in lowering of the serum calcium level, increased vascular and soft tissue calcification, and progression of renal osteodystrophy. To adjust the dose of aluminum hydroxide and determine the reliability of the patient in taking the drug, the serum phosphorus level should be checked at regular intervals.

### *Hypermagnesemia*

The kidney is the main route of magnesium ion ($Mg^{++}$) excretion. Use of $Mg^{++}$-containing antacids or laxatives by renal failure patients can result in marked elevation of plasma $Mg^{++}$. Hypermagnesemia results in development of the following:

1. Depression of neuromuscular conductivity and thereby weakness of skeletal muscles, hypo- and areflexia, and paralysis of respiratory muscles
2. Suppression of the CNS, resulting in confusion, lethargy, and coma
3. Cardiac conduction and contractility defects, resulting in various blocks and cardiac arrest

To prevent these complications, the use of $Mg^{++}$-containing antacids and laxatives should be prohibited in renal failure patients. Treatment includes dialysis using a low $Mg^{++}$ bath.

### *Megaloblastic anemia*

Failure to take folic acid supplements results in the deterioration of preexisting anemia in these patients. This is discussed in some detail with respect to the drug regimen (Chapter 17).

## ■ What problems can arise in association with the vascular access?

A multitude of local and systemic complications can arise from vascular access, whether it is one of the internal or external arteriovenous shunts.

### *Clotting*

Thrombosis is the most common complication of arteriovenous shunts. Disappearance of the thrill and bruit and, in the case of external shunts, visual detection of clot in the cannulas confirm the diagnosis. Predisposing factors include the following:

1. Reduced blood flow through the shunt caused by hypotension, pericardial tamponade, tight bandage, or sleeping on the extremity bearing the shunt may contribute to the development of thrombosis.
2. There is a high incidence of clotting of the blood access following major surgical procedures, regardless of their nature. This has been attributed to the so-called hypercoagulable state secondary to surgically induced tissue damage (release of tissue thromboplastin, etc.).
3. Local trauma and multiple punctures can induce thrombosis by damaging the endothelium.
4. Local infections predispose to thrombosis.

External shunts can be declotted, as discussed elsewhere. In the case of internal shunts, surgical thrombectomy has been tried with variable success.

Heparin infusion through a T tube intermittently every 4 hours or continuously by a Harvard pump can be given on a short-term basis to prevent recurrent clotting. Small doses of coumadin, dipyridamole (Persantine), or aspirin have been used successfully on a long-term basis.

### *Embolization*

The injection of heparinized saline solution into the arterial cannula during the declotting procedure can dislodge the clot and push it upward against the blood flow. The clot can then be carried to various organs by the bloodstream. When the injected volume is high enough to move the clot to the aortic arch, cerebral embolization can occur. With lower volumes embolization and ischemic necrosis of the extremity may develop.

Pulmonary embolism following declotting of the venous cannulas has also been reported. Arterial embolization can be prevented by avoiding the injection of more than 1 to 2 ml of declotting solution into the arterial line. Treatment consists of emergency embolectomy whenever possible following angiography.

### *Infection*

Blood access infections can be local or become systemic. In general infections are more common but easier to control in external arteriovenous shunts. They are less common but more difficult to eradicate in internal shunts. Local infections consist of cellulitis, abscess formation, or infection around the cannula. These infections have at times caused separation of the cannula and life-threatening blood loss. They are usually caused by *Staphylococcus aureus,* but other organisms such as *Streptococcus* and *Pseudomonas* are also seen. Meticulous shunt care and systemic antibiotics may eradicate the infection; however, at times removal of the cannula or closure of the internal shunt is necessary.

Systemic infections include septicemia, septic pulmonary embolism with resultant lung abscess, and endocarditis. One of the problems that is occasionally encountered is persistent fever in a patient with internal or external shunt who has no evidence of local infection. The question that arises is whether the shunt should be dismantled or not. In my experience infection without local manifestation is quite uncommon. Nevertheless, endovasculitis of arteriovenous fistula can present with minimum local signs and yet behave as endocarditis. Endovasculitis should be treated just as endocarditis, with 4 weeks of treatment using appropriate antibiotics. If antibiotics fail to improve the symptoms of infection, the shunt should be dismantled.

Vancomycin, which is effective against *Staphylococcus,* is a favorite antibiotic in the treatment of blood access infections. Because of its long half-life in patients without kidney function, injection of 1000 mg of vancomycin every 10 days provides adequate coverage.

### *Pseudoaneurysm*

Pseudoaneurysm is an uncommon complication of external arteriovenous shunts. It is usually seen in shunts that have survived an episode of local infection and presents as a pulsatile mass.

### *Phlebitis*

Phlebitis can be seen with both external and internal shunts. It presents with severe pain, since blood with arterial pressure flows through the inflamed vein. A cord may be palpable along the vein. It usually results in clotting of the shunt. Anticoagulation therapy with elevation and heat application are used to treat this condition.

### *Skin erosion*

Skin erosion consists of ulceration of the skin overlying the subcutaneous segment of cannula. The development of erosion is often followed by local infection and subsequent clotting of the shunt. Prevention includes leaving some subcutaneous soft tissue between the cannula and overlying skin at the time of shunt placement. Padding with sterile cotton at pressure points is helpful after the shunt is inserted.

### *Dermatitis*

Dermatitis is a common complication. It is usually caused by hypersensitivity to adhesive tapes, antibiotic ointments, or pHisoHex. It responds to the discontinuation of the allergen and the use of corticosteroid-containing ointments.

### *Joint separation*

Joint separation results from separation of the external ends of the arterial and venous cannulas. When occurring at night or remaining unnoticed, this can result in life-threatening blood loss. This is more likely to happen when the shunt is old and the external ends are worn out. For this reason old shunts should be trimmed for a tight connector fit.

### *Cannula avulsion*

The most common cause of cannula avulsion is local shunt infection resulting in weakening or necrosis of the vessel wall. Suicidal or accidental pulling of the shunt has also been reported. Cannula avulsion is associated with significant blood loss.

### *High output cardiac failure*

External arteriovenous shunts usually do not cause high output cardiac failure, since their flow rate is about 200 to 350 ml/min, which is only a small fraction of the cardiac output. However, arteriovenous fistulas, saphenous vein grafts, and bovine grafts that have very high blood flows can impose a significant load on the heart and cause cardiac enlargement and failure. Measurement of cardiac output before and after temporary obstruction of the arteriovenous shunt demonstrates its hemodynamic significance. Determination of pulse rate before and after temporary manual occlusion of the shunt is a simple bedside examination to demonstrate significant arteriovenous shunting. If the pulse rate drops by 10 or more counts per minute or cardiac output increases significantly following temporary occlusion of the shunt, the patient's cardiac failure is likely to improve by surgical correction of the shunt directed toward reducing its flow.

### *Steal syndrome*

In the presence of an external or internal arteriovenous shunt, which is a low resistance circuit, more blood preferentially flows through the arteriovenous shunt. If the patient also has peripheral vascular disease, shunting of the blood away from the extremity will cause ischemia. Ischemia may present as intermittent claudication, pain on elevation of the involved extremity, cooler temperature compared to the contralateral side, decreased arterial pulses, and prolonged blanching time. At times ischemic gangrene results. Treatment consists of reduction of the blood flow through the shunt or its surgical removal.

## ■ What are the complications of anticoagulation in dialysis patients?

Anticoagulation is necessary to prevent clotting of the blood during its extracorporeal circulation. Systemic or regional heparinization is used for this purpose. *Bleeding* from various sources, for example, intracranial, gastrointestinal, wound, or intrapericardial, can occur subsequent to heparinization. Uremic patients, because of their underlying platelet dysfunction, are even more prone to serious bleeding disorders following heparinization than are other patients. Patients in whom systemic anticoagulation is contraindicated may be dialyzed with *regional heparinization.* This involves the continuous infusion of heparin into the arterial line of the dialyzer to prevent clotting outside the body. Equivalent amounts of protamine sulfate are simultaneously infused into the venous line to neutralize the effect of heparin when the blood returns to the circulation. Accordingly, by this pharmacologic maneuver adequate anticoagulation is achieved in the extracorporeal circuit without affecting the systemic coagulation profile.

One of the problems frequently encountered following regional heparinization is *heparin rebound.* This presents as depression of the coagulation parameters and occasionally bleeding a couple of hours after termination of the procedure. It is caused by faster metabolism of protamine sulfate as compared to heparin, which results in the appearance of heparin effect after the protamine sulfate is completely metabolized. Administration of additional protamine sulfate at this time reverses the rebound phenomenon.

The development of *allergic reaction* to the animal protein content of heparin occasionally creates a major problem. Heparin allergy usually presents as severe pruritus following the administration of heparin. The solution to this problem is to switch from pork mucosa heparin to beef lung heparin.

## ■ What are the infectious complications of hemodialysis?

It is a well-known fact that uremia lowers the resistance to infection. The repeated transfusions required by some hemodialysis patients expose them to blood-borne infections. Furthermore, the use of external shunts or repeated cannulations of internal fistulas with each dialysis provide a convenient port of entry for various organisms. The infections that are more commonly seen in this population include blood access infections, viral hepatitis, cytomegalovirus infections, and pyrogenic reaction.

### *Blood access infections*

Local and systemic infections originating from the blood access were discussed earlier.

### *Viral hepatitis*

Viral hepatitis is one of the most serious problems associated with chronic dialysis. Dialysis patients and staff are frequently exposed to blood and its derivatives. Many outbreaks of hepatitis among the patients and staff have occurred in dialysis units, resulting in tremendous morbidity and significant mortality.

Two major forms of viral hepatitis exist: hepatitis B (long-incubation, $Au_1$-positive, HAA-positive, or serum hepatitis) and hepatitis A (short-incubation, $Au_1$-negative, or HAA-negative hepatitis). In contrast with the old concept, hepatitis A can be transmitted not only by the oral route but also through parenteral means. Similarly, hepatitis B can be transmitted not only parenterally, but also through oral, respiratory, sexual, and personal contact.

Although the use of blood and its derivatives is the major cause of hepatitis, HAA-positive hepatitis may occur in untransfused persons. This probably results from the transmission of the virus from one patient to the other by contaminated dialysis equipment, personnel, toilet facilities, dining utensils, personal contacts, etc. The incidence of anicteric asymptomatic disease with chronic antigenemia is quite high among dialysis patients. It is frequently severe and symptomatic among the dialysis personnel with transient antigenemia. Because of the prevalence of asymptomatic disease in patients, it is necessary to perform monthly screening tests, liver function tests, and HAA antigen determinations. There are no false positive results for HAA, but depending on the sensitivity of the testing method and the time of sampling in relation to the time of exposure, there is a 20% to 50% chance of registering a false negative result. Therefore a negative HAA test does not rule out hepatitis B.

Abnormal liver function does not always indicate viral hepatitis. The differential diagnosis list is long and includes infectious and noninfectious causes.

*Noninfectious causes of hepatitis*

Drugs: methyldopa (Aldomet), methyltestosterone chlorpromazine, diphenylhydantoin (Dilantin), indomethacin (Indocin), griseofulvin, synthetic estrogens and progestins, etc.

Toxins: alcohol, plasticizers used in manufacturing dialysis tubing, inorganic phosphorus, carbon tetrachloride, etc.

Anesthetics: halothane and methoxyflurane

Postsurgical: probably caused by morphine, produces benign and self-limited hepatic dysfunction

*Infections*

Cytomegalovirus, miliary tuberculosis, leptospirosis, tularemia, brucellosis, amebiasis, mononucleosis, hepatitis associated with pneumonia and sepsis, etc.

*Miscellaneous*

Hemosiderosis secondary to repeated transfusions and parenteral iron, cirrhosis, neoplasm, biliary obstruction, etc.

Since hepatitis A and B are both transmitted by oral and parenteral routes, the prevention and control methods are the same and are aimed at two fronts:

1. Prevent the introduction of the virus to the unit.
   a. Restrict transfusions and use frozen packed red blood cells when necessary. Hepatitis viruses are destroyed as a result of the procedures necessary to prepare frozen packed red blood cells; therefore the use of this preparation minimizes the risk of hepatitis.
   b. Screen dialysis candidates and prospective personnel for liver function and the presence of HAA.
2. Take measures to prevent the spreading of the disease when hepatitis has occurred.
   a. Exercise meticulous nursing techniques of aseptic and contagion precautions.
   b. Screen patients and personnel monthly for liver function and the presence of HAA.
   c. Personnel contracting hepatitis should be excused from work until such time when the HAA test is negative.
   d. Limit blood transfusions to very symptomatic patients or in preparation for surgery. The advantage of using frozen packed red blood cells over the use of other products was discussed earlier.
   e. Serve meals with disposable utensils and prohibit eating and smoking by the personnel in the unit.
   f. Separate the patients' toilet facilities from those of the personnel. Install knee-operated faucets and pedal-operated soap dispensers.
   g. Enforce personal hygiene.
   h. Vigorously cleanse the dialysis machine following rupture of the coil.
   i. Avoid spilling blood and other fluids on the floor.

This list of precautionary measures is by no means complete, and the reader is referred to specific sources for additional information.

### *Cytomegalovirus infection*

Cytomegalovirus infection is seen in immunosuppressed hosts. It can cause hepatitis, pericarditis, nephritis, enteritis, pneumonitis, and mononucleosis-like syndromes.

### *Pyrogenic reaction*

Pyrogenic reaction results from the passage of some bacterial endotoxins from the bath into the circulation. It presents with fever and shaking chills during or shortly after dialysis. It is caused by bacterial growth in the tap water used for making dialysate. Pyrogenic reaction is not a true infection, since the bacteria do not enter the body.

## ■ What complications can arise from chronic renal failure in dialysis patients?

With the advent of the dialysis technique the natural course of end-stage renal failure has changed. With partial substitution of the excretory function of the kidney by long-term dialysis, patients can live for many years despite a lack of functioning kidneys. As a result, many metabolic defects that would not have become manifest fully had the patient died of uremia will do so with prolongation of life. These include renal osteodystrophy, peripheral neuropathy, nerve deafness, anemia, pericarditis, accelerated atherosclerosis and hyperlipidemia, and sexual problems.

### *Renal osteodystrophy*

Renal osteodystrophy consists of one or a combination of several of the following disorders:

1. Renal dwarfism, which refers to growth retardation caused by the onset of renal failure early in life.

2. Ricketts or osteomalacic bone disease, which is caused by the impaired metabolic activation of vitamin D by the kidney. Vitamin D in its original form is biologically inert and needs metabolic activation in the liver and kidney in order to become biologically active. In the absence of a functioning kidney vitamin D remains inactive, resulting in the development of osteomalacic bone disease and the impairment of calcium absorption from the intestines.

3. Bone disease related to increased parathormone secretion. The impairment of phosphate excretion in chronic renal failure results in the elevation of plasma phosphate. Since the product of calcium and phosphate is constant ($CA \times PO_4 = K$), an elevation of serum phosphate results in a lowering of serum calcium. Furthermore, as discussed earlier, the impairment of vitamin D metabolism in renal failure interferes with calcium absorption from the intestines and bones and further depresses the plasma calcium level. A reduction of the plasma calcium level stimulates the parathyroid gland to secrete large amounts of parathyroid hormone. Parathyroid hormone causes bone resorption to normalize serum calcium level. Prolonged elevation of parathyroid hormone results in development of osteitis fibrosa cystica. Bone pain, fragility, x-ray abnormalities, and severe pruritus are among the clinical findings of secondary hyperparathyroidism.

4. Soft tissue and vascular calcifications. This is caused by high phosphate levels enhancing the precipitation of calcium phosphate in soft tissues and vessel walls. Vascular calcifications probably contribute to these patients' ischemic heart disease and peripheral vascular insufficiency.

5. Osteosclerosis. Osteosclerosis is apparent on x-ray films as a relative increase in radiopacity of some areas of the skeleton. This increased density does not mean stronger bony structure; rather, it has been shown to be abnormal and fragile. Osteosclerosis is caused either by the abnormal deposition of calcium and phosphate in immature matrix and/or is a reflexion of fluoride toxicity, as discussed earlier.

A variety of therapeutic modalities have been advocated for the treatment and prevention of renal osteodystrophy. These include control of hyperphosphatemia by dialysis and phosphate-binding agents, such as aluminum hydroxide, by far the most important and effective therapy; dialysis against high calcium baths, that is, 3.5 to 4 mEq/L, to suppress parathyroid hormone and improve negative calcium balance; administration of oral calcium carbonate; use of therapeutic doses of vitamin D; or performance of subtotal parathyroidectomy, which frequently alleviates pruritus and improves bone disease.

Dialysis against high calcium baths and the administration of oral calcium carbonate or therapeutic doses of vitamin D can be quite dangerous if carried out without controlling hyperphosphatemia, since by elevating the level of plasma calcium while the serum phosphate level is high, soft tissue and vascular deposition of calcium can be enhanced, which is quite damaging.

### *Peripheral neuropathy*

Peripheral neuropathy is one of the known complications of uremia. Dialysis treatment can slowly improve the patient's peripheral neuropathy. However, nerve conduction studies and electromyography frequently show residual abnormalities. There is indirect evidence to suggest that the accumulation of some as yet unidentified middle molecules normally cleared by the kidney is responsible for the development of peripheral neuropathy. The clearance of these molecules by dialysis is reduced when the dialysis time is short and flow rates of blood and dialysate are high. Such inadequate dialysis treatments can result in the development of progressive disabling neuropathy, although the patient's urea and creatinine levels are adequately reduced.

### *Nerve deafness*

Nerve deafness of varying severity is very common among long-term dialysis patients.

The pathogenesis of this deafness is not clearly understood. It may be part of the uremic neuropathy, but the possibility of exposure to ototoxic drugs cannot be ruled out. Recently preparations used for the sterilization and preservation of dialysis membranes and tubing systems have been incriminated.

### *Anemia*

Anemia is an almost universal finding among the dialysis population. It is disabling and very difficult to control. Multiple factors are involved in the pathogenesis of this anemia:

1. Lack of *erythropoietin,* a polypeptide hormone secreted by the kidneys that is responsible for the formation of red blood cells by the bone marrow.

2. Defective iron utilization by erythroid precursors. The amount of iron stored in the reticuloendothelial cells of these patients is usually increased, but it cannot be utilized for hemoglobin synthesis. This abnormality is commonly seen in most of the chronic diseases.

3. Blood loss. Because of uremic platelet dysfunction, gastrointestinal and other sources of occult blood loss are common in these patients. Furthermore, with each dialysis, some, although a small amount of blood, is lost.

4. Short red blood cell life span. The uremic environment has adverse effects on erythrocytes and results in the premature destruction of red blood cells. When red blood cells from normal persons are transfused into a uremic patient, the life span of these cells shortens. Transfusion of a uremic patient's red blood cells to a normal person normalizes the cells' life span. These data indicate that the early destruction of red blood cells in uremic patients is caused by the abnormal environment, not an intrinsic defect in the red blood cells.

5. Decreased iron absorption from the gastrointestinal tract has been demonstrated.

6. Folic acid, which is essential for red blood cell production, is washed out of the circulation during dialysis.

7. Bone marrow depression, caused by the uremic environment, deficiency of erythropoietin, and the lack of various essential nutrients, plays a major role in the pathogenesis of anemia in dialysis patients.

8. Drug-induced anemia, for example, by methyldopa (Aldomet), should always be suspected.

The treatment of the anemia of chronic renal failure presents an extremely difficult problem. *Folic acid* in doses of 1 to 2 mg/day should be given to all dialysis patients to make up for losses with dialysis. Oral or parenteral *iron* should be given only to those patients in whom the saturation of iron-binding proteins is low and the bone marrow iron stores are depleted.

*Testosterone derivatives* stimulate erythrogenesis in the bone marrow in the presence of some erythropoietin. They are used orally as methyltestosterone on a daily basis or in IM injectable depot forms given every 1 to 4 weeks. These derivatives are almost always effective in raising the patient's hematocrit by a few points. Their drawbacks, however, include androgenic effects on female patients (increased hair growth and voice changes), possible atherogenic effect, and cholestatic jaundice caused by methyl derivatives.

*Cobalt compounds* can raise the hematocrit through stimulating an impairment of oxygen utilization by the cells, which signals the bone marrow to produce more red blood cells. Improvement of tissue oxygenation, which is the goal in the treatment of anemia, is not achieved by the use of cobalt compounds.

*Blood transfusions,* although resulting in the dramatic improvement of anemic symptoms and providing a sense of strength and well-being, produce only transient effects and are associated with great risks. The adverse consequences of repeated transfusions are as follows:

1. High risk of viral hepatitis and transmission of other infectious agents such as cytomegalovirus and various bacteria that contaminate blood during its preparation.

2. Suppression of the patient's own erythrogenic mechanism because of the availability of exogenous red blood cells.

3. Hemosiderosis. With each transfusion a

significant amount of iron enters the body and must be stored in reticuloendothelial cells following the destruction of red blood cells. The accumulation of enormous amounts of iron in the liver, pancreas, heart, skin, and other tissues damages these organs.

4. The development of antibodies against white blood cell and platelet antigens results in febrile reactions during future transfusions.

5. The formation of antibodies against various minor blood group antigens with multiple transfusions makes it difficult to find compatible blood for emergency or elective purposes in the future.

Therefore it is recommended that transfusions be restricted for the treatment of highly symptomatic patients or in preparation for surgery.

### *Pericarditis*

Two distinct forms of pericarditis can be recognized in these patients:

1. Uremic pericarditis. This is a fibrinous and hemorrhagic pericarditis that is found in untreated or underdialyzed patients. It improves and gradually clears with adequate dialysis treatments.

2. Dialysis-associated pericarditis. This occurs in the face of adequate dialysis treatment. It is also fibrinous and hemorrhagic and presents with fever, leukocytosis, chest pain, pericardial friction rub, and effusion. It usually does not respond to more adequate dialysis treatment. Its etiology is as yet obscure. Viral, bacterial, and fungal cultures and serologic tests have been unrevealing. Improvement may follow the use of indomethacin (Indocin) or corticosteroids.

At times pericardial effusion increases and pericardial tamponade results. This requires emergency pericardiocentesis and decompression of the heart chambers to improve the cardiac output and reduce venous pressure. Occasionally surgical pericardiectomy or creation of a pericardial window should be performed.

Patients with pericarditis should be closely monitored for the development of cardiac tamponade. Rapid distention of the jugular veins, arterial hypotension, marked paradoxical pulse pressure (more than 10 mm Hg), dyspnea, hepatomegaly, and hepatojugular reflux suggest significant pericardial effusion and cardiac tamponade.

These patients should undergo dialysis with regional or miniheparinizations to avoid hemopericardium.

### *Accelerated atherosclerosis and hyperlipidemia*

Coronary artery disease is the most common cause of death among long-term dialysis patients. The incidence of myocardial infarction in these patients is several times higher than that of patients with type II hyperlipidemia. It takes only a few years to develop a severe atherosclerosis that would have otherwise taken many decades. Although the pathogenesis of accelerated atherosclerosis in dialysis patients is not clearly understood, several factors seem to be responsible:

1. Hypertension. The majority of dialysis patients are hypertensive. This hypertension is usually but not always volume dependent. It drops following dialysis with ultrafiltration and gradually rises again with reexpansion of the extracellular volume between dialyses. It is often difficult to use antihypertensive drugs to control this hypertension. With the use of these drugs the patient's blood pressure drops to subnormal levels during and after dialysis, which interferes with the dialysis procedure and with the patient's activity afterward.

2. Fluctuations of intravascular volume impose an excess load on the heart and cause cardiomegaly and recurrent episodes of cardiac failure.

3. Anemia and the presence of arteriovenous shunts produce a high output state that further increases the load on the heart.

4. Vascular calcification, discussed with renal osteodystrophy, enhances the development of coronary artery disease.

5. Type IV hyperlipidemia with marked elevation of plasma triglyceride levels is extremely prevalent among dialysis patients. The pathogenesis of this hyperlipidemia is not well understood yet. Whatever the causes

of hyperlipidemia, it contributes to accelerated atherosclerosis.

6. The level of uric acid in these patients is frequently above normal.

7. A diabetic glucose tolerance curve is usually exhibited. Abnormal carbohydrate metabolism is a well-known phenomenon in these patients.

8. Testosterone preparations commonly used for the treatment of anemia are known atherogenic substances.

All these factors and perhaps other as yet unrecognized conditions predispose these patients to accelerated atherosclerosis and death from ischemic heart disease and cerebrovascular accidents. There is no definite treatment or prevention for this complication. Nevertheless, at the present state of knowledge the following steps appear to be advisable in reducing the risk and severity of the disorder:

1. Low carbohydrate and saturated fat diet
2. Adequate hypertension control
3. Use of lipid-lowering drugs when necessary
4. Avoidance of androgenic steroids when possible
5. Control of hyperphosphatemia and hyperparathyroidism

### *Sexual problems*

Impotency, sterility, and amenorrhea are extremely common among dialysis patients. Androgenic steroids sometimes improve impotence in male patients, but the effect is transient. Psychotherapy may be helpful.

## ■ What are the socioeconomic and psychologic impacts of long-term dialysis?

Maintenance dialysis is a very expensive treatment. It can easily drain all the financial resources of an average family in a short period of time. Although the various governmental agencies will cover the expenses involved in the care of end-stage renal disease, this usually does not begin until all the family resources are exhausted. Poor state of health and disruption of the patient's time schedule caused by the time spent for dialysis itself and the traveling to and from the dialysis center frequently interfere with the patient's work and productivity.

Depending on dialysis for living, fear of sudden death from disruption of vascular access, hyperkalemia or pulmonary edema, severe dietary restrictions, impaired sexual activity, changes of self- and body images because of disfiguring external and internal shunts and multiple surgical scars, sense of being rejected from society, and many other social, personal, financial, and psychologic problems are faced by these patients every day. Each patient's reaction to the stress is somewhat different. Depression and denial are commonly encountered, whereas suicide by opening the shunt or ingestion of large quantities of potassium-containing foods and other self-destructive means are rarely seen.

Psychotherapy, especially the help and support of social workers and dialysis personnel, is extremely important in improving the patient's psychologic attitude.

## BIBLIOGRAPHY

Abram, H. S., Moore, G. L., and Westervelt, F. B.: Suicidal behavior in chronic dialysis patients, paper presented at the one hundred twenty-third annual meeting of the American Psychology Association, May, 1970.

Bailey, G. L., editor: Hemodialysis principles and practice, New York, 1972, Academic Press, Inc.

Bennett, W. M., Singer, I., and Coggins, C. J.: A guide to drug therapy in renal failure, J.A.M.A. **230**:1544-1553, 1974.

Bussell, J. A., Abbott, J. A., and Lim, R. C.: A radial steal syndrome with arteriovenous fistula for hemodialysis, Ann. Intern. Med. **75**: 387, 1971.

Editorial: Air embolism, Dialysis & Transplantation J., pp. 13-17, April/May, 1972.

Arthur, G., et al.: Clinical maintenance hemodialysis with a sorbent-based low-volume dialysate regeneration system, Trans. Am. Soc. Artif. Intern. Organs **17**:253-256, 1971.

Halper, I. S.: Psychiatric observations in chronic dialysis program, Med. Clin. North Am. **55**: 177, 1971.

Kaegi, A., et al.: Arteriovenous-shunt thrombosis, N. Engl. J. Med. **290**:304-306, 1974.

Kennedy, A. C., et al.: The pathogenesis and prevention of cerebral dysfunction during dialysis, Lancet **1**:790-793, 1964.

Kjellstrand, C. M., et al.: Considerations of the middle molecule hypothesis 11—neuropathy in nephrectomized patients, Trans. Am. Soc. Artif. Intern. Organs **19**:325, 1973.

Knight, A. H., et al.: Hepatitis-associated antigen and antibody in haemodialysis patients and staff, Br. Med. J. **3**:603-606, 1970.

Manzler, A. D., and Schreiner, A. W.: Copper-induced acute hemolytic anemia, Ann. Intern. Med. **73**:409-412, 1970.

Port, F. K., Johnson, W. J., and Klass, D. W.: Prevention of dialysis disequilibrium syndrome by use of high sodium concentration in the dialysate, Kidney Int. **3**:327-333, 1973.

Siddiqui, J. Y., et al.: Causes of death in patients receiving long-term hemodialysis, J.A.M.A. **212**: 1350-1354, 1970.

Thomas, P. K., et al.: The polyneuropathy of chronic renal failure, Brain **94**:761-780, 1971.

Tyler, H. R.: Neurologic disorders in renal failure, Am. J. Med. **44**:734-748, 1968.

*chapter 19*

# Principles of peritoneal dialysis

N. DABIR VAZIRI

The term "dialysis" refers to the diffusion of water and solutes across a permeable membrane separating two fluid compartments. Factors governing this process are the permeability characteristics of the membrane, the osmotic and hydrostatic pressures on each side, and the differential concentration of individual solutes in each compartment. *Water* molecules move freely across the membrane. Although this movement is bidirectional, the net transport of water occurs from the hypotonic to the hypertonic compartment. The rate and the direction of *solute* transport depends on the size of the molecules, the differential concentrations in each compartment, and the mass flow. The smaller the molecule, the higher is its permeability. However, if a highly diffusible substance binds with high molecular weight substances, such as proteins, the molecule will lose its diffusibility.

Hydrostatic forces are also important in the mass transport of water and solutes. The direction of movement is from the high pressure to the low pressure compartment. The result of these various interactions is the achievement of a state of *equilibrium* in which the algebraic sum of osmotic and hydrostatic forces becomes equal on both sides of the membrane. Therefore no *net* water and solute transport can occur, since the rate of transport in one direction is equal to the other. Diffusion and mass transport processes are quite rapid in the beginning but slow down in time as pressure and concentration gradients gradually dissipate. These principles form the basis for the use of *dialysis treatment* in clinical medicine. This treatment is aimed at the elimination of endogenous or exogenous toxins, the correction of electrolyte and acid-base abnormalities, and/or the removal of excess fluids. This requires a mechanism that brings the patient's circulating blood in contact with a physiologic solution through a permeable membrane. In such a system undesirable compounds present in patient's blood can be washed out by diffusion into the dialysate. Furthermore, equilibration of the patient's plasma with dialysate that has desirable electrolyte concentrations helps to normalize the patient's electrolyte and acid-base abnormalities.

Dialysis involves three major elements:

1. Blood
2. Dialyzing membrane
3. Dialysis fluid (dialysate)

Accessory devices are obviously necessary to bring these elements together and to make the process mechanically feasible. In peritoneal dialysis, the mesenteric and peritoneal capillary circulation provides the blood supply. The peritoneal membrane, consisting of the capillary wall, a thin layer of connective tissue, and the mesothelial lining, makes up the dialyzing membrane.

With this brief introduction the basic concepts and techniques involved in peritoneal dialysis will be presented and an attempt made to answer some of the questions that are important in understanding these concepts and in managing patients undergoing peritoneal dialysis.

## ■ How is the peritoneal catheter inserted?

It should be ascertained that the bladder is empty and there are no masses in the way before attempting to insert the catheter. This is done by careful examination of the abdomen and straight catheterization of the bladder when necessary. Failure to do so may result in catastrophic entry to a distended bladder, an abdominal aortic aneurysm, a tumor mass, or a polycystic kidney instead of the peritoneal cavity.

To reduce the patient's anxiety, premedication may be given with diazepam (Valium) or other preferred medications. The patient should be in the supine or semisupine position. The skin under the umbilicus is shaved properly, cleansed with iodine or other preferred solutions, and draped as for a laparotomy. The skin and underlying tissue are deeply infiltrated with a local anesthetic agent, for example, 1% procaine. An extremely small midline incision is made about one third of the way from the umbilicus to the pubic bone. The scalpel blade is inserted into the anterior wall of the abdomen until it is felt to grate on the linea alba. A small incision is extended in the linea alba. The reason for selecting the midline for introducing the catheter is its relative avascularity, which reduces the risk of significant bleeding. Through this incision the catheter with the stylet in place is inserted. With a short thrust the peritoneum is penetrated. The patient may experience some pain as the parietal peritoneum is stretched and should be made aware ahead of time that this pain will occur in order to prevent uncontrolled movements that may interfere with proper catheter placement.

It may be advisable to ask the patient to contract the abdominal wall muscles while the catheter is being pushed through the incision. As soon as the peritoneum is pierced, the stylet should be removed and the catheter advanced. It should be aimed posteriorly and inferiorly toward the small pelvis through right or left paravertebral gutter. Usually about 50 cm of the catheter enters the abdomen. Some of the older catheter sets include a trocar through which the peritoneal catheter is advanced, and the trocar is re-

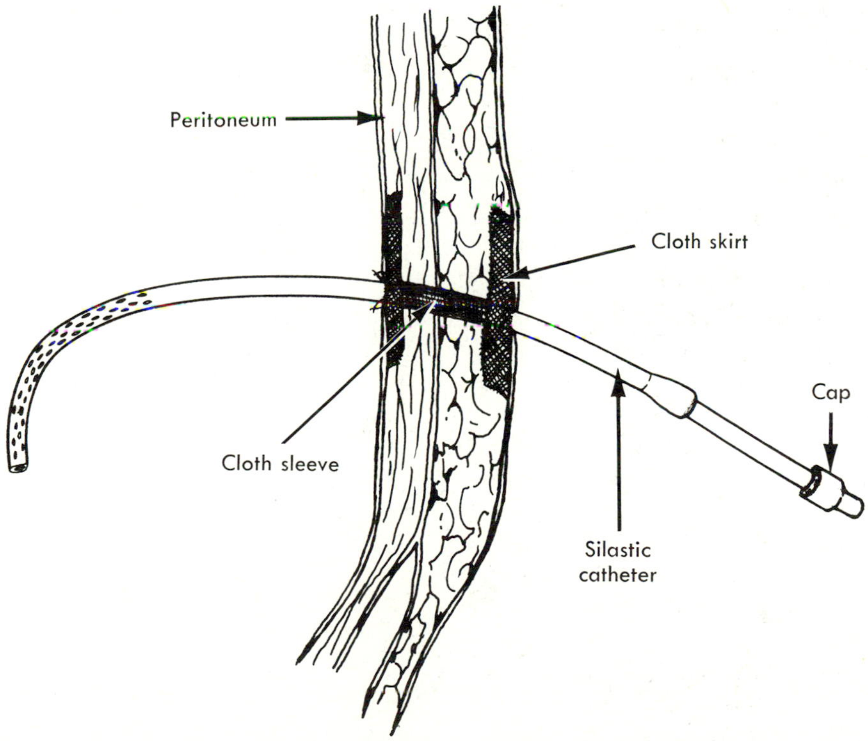


**Fig. 19-1.** Schematic of Tenckhoff's catheter in place.

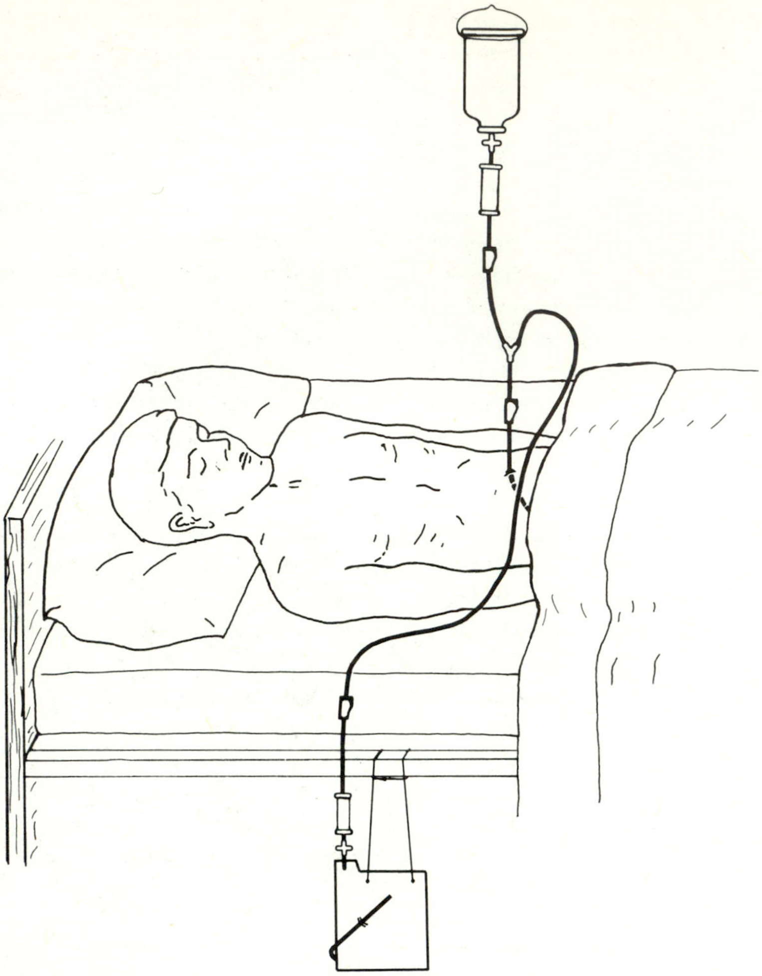

**Fig. 19-2.** Peritoneal dialysis.

moved after the catheter is properly placed. The position of the catheter is important in ensuring an adequate flow of irrigation fluid. The catheter is usually advanced with ease. Difficulty in passing the catheter is usually caused by the presence of the omentum in the way and rarely by its extra- or retroperitoneal localization. The difficulty is usually overcome by manipulating the catheter or infusing 1 or 2 L of dialysis fluid through the catheter and subsequently readjusting and advancing it.

Needless to say, the team performing the procedure should wear masks, gloves, hats, and sterile gowns and should exercise extreme aseptic measures. To prevent the inadvertant displacement of the catheter, a couple of stitches are placed along the incision and the catheter is tied to the skin. The catheter is then connected to the inflow system (Figs. 19-1 and 19-2).

## ■ What is the dwell time?

Dwell time refers to the period of time between the end of inflow and the beginning of drainage.

## ■ What about the volume, duration, and number of passages?

It is important to remember that the *dialysis fluid should be warmed to body temperature* before it is used. Introduction to the peritoneal cavity of the fluid at a subnormal temperature not only causes discomfort to the patient, but also reduces the efficacy of dialysis by constricting the peritoneal vascular bed and reducing its blood flow. With regard to volume, up to 2 L of fluid is allowed to flow into the peritoneal cavity by gravity as rapidly as possible with each passage. This should take no longer than 5 to 10 minutes. If the flow is slow, the catheter should be repositioned, since its tip may be buried in the omentum. The volume of administered fluid on each run should be tailored according to the patient's size, age, and pulmonary status. The introduction of large amounts of fluid into the abdomen of a patient with respiratory failure may adversely affect pulmonary ventilation by restricting the diaphragmatic excursion, particularly in the supine position. This is mostly a hypothetical consideration, however, and with proper positioning of the patient and slight adjustment of fluid volumes such problems are readily avoided.

Fluid is allowed to remain in the peritoneal cavity for 15 to 30 minutes. During this time the necessary exchanges between fluid and circulating blood in the peritoneal capillaries take place. The abdomen is drained by a siphon effect through the closed system. When the system is patent, the gravity drainage should occur quite rapidly and should take no longer than 10 minutes. When the flow slows down, manual compression of the abdomen toward the catheter may result in a temporary increase of flow into the drainage container. This procedure is repeated continuously for 12 to 48 hours and occasionally for 72 hours, depending on the clinical response and the nature of the disease for which peritoneal dialysis is being used. It should be kept in mind that the *longer the duration of the procedure the higher is the risk of peritoneal infection. Specimens of drainage fluid should be sent for bacterial culture and sensitivity tests periodically.* Careful records should be kept of the exact time of starting and ending each exchange, the drugs added, the vital signs, and the fluid balance. When dialysis is completed, the catheter is removed and the wound closed with additional stitches or clamps and covered with sterile gauze.

## ■ What are the clearance and the role of dwell time?

The effectiveness of dialysis is indicated by the peritoneal clearance. Clearance can be simply defined as the volume of plasma that is completely cleared of the substance under consideration in 1 minute by peritoneal dialysis. It is calculated using Van Slyke's formula:

$$C = \frac{U \times V}{P}$$

in which C = clearance in milliliters per minute, U = concentration in outflow fluid, P = concentration in blood or plasma, and V = rate of dialysate flow in milliliters per minute.

Clinical and experimental investigations have shown that urea and potassium have the highest peritoneal clearances. The clearances of creatinine, uric acid, phosphate, and sulfate are almost equal, at a level lower than urea and potassium and higher than calcium and magnesium.

Serial measurements of urea concentration in dialysate fluid have shown that the concentration rises quite rapidly during the first 20 to 30 minutes. Thereafter urea enters the peritoneal fluid at a much slower rate. This is caused by a reduction of the concentration gradient with time; in fact, in 2 hours a state of equilibrium is achieved. Urea and other clearance studies have been done using various dialysate flow rates. Urea clearance improves as the dialyzing rate is increased. A maximum clearance of 28.5 ml/min is achieved with a dialyzed volume of 3.5 L/hr. Further increases in dialyzed volume result in a reduction of urea clearance. Therefore *a dialysis volume of 2.5 to 3.5 L/hr provides the most efficient and economical condition.*

## ■ What is meant by continuous as opposed to intermittent flow?

Two basic ways of irrigating the peritoneum exist—continuous flow and intermittent flow.

In the continous method two catheters are placed. Dialysate enters through one and drains through the other on a continuing basis.

The popular method is intermittent flow, in which a predetermined volume of dialysate is rapidly infused into the peritoneal cavity. Some time is allowed for equilibration and the exchange processes between fluid and blood, following which the old fluid is drained and fresh fluid introduced.

The risk of infection, leakage, and traumatic complications is highest using the continuous method, for obvious reasons, and the urea clearance is lower as a result of the short cut taken between the inflow and outflow channels, shorter equilibration time, and lower concentration gradients.

## ■ What is the ideal composition of irrigating fluid?

There is no single ideal dialysis fluid. The ideal fluid for one patient with a particular problem may be unsuitable for another person with a different problem. In general the dialysis fluid should have the following properties:

1. It must permit the maximum diffusion of metabolic waste products or exogenous toxins.
2. It must be capable of correcting the patient's volume abnormalities, for example, volume overload.
3. It should be able to normalize the patient's electrolyte abnormalities.

When the purpose of dialysis is merely the elimination of uremic toxins or dialyzable exogenous poisons, dialysis fluid should contain physiologic concentrations of electrolytes and 1.5% glucose. When hyperkalemia is present, a potassium-free dialysate should be used to enhance the elimination of excess potassium. In cases of hypercalcemia or hypermagnesemia, calcium and magnesium ions should be reduced or preferably removed from the dialysate, respectively.

When fluid overload is the major problem, a hypertonic solution containing 4% to 5% glucose should be used. Frequently multiple problems coexist, requiring complex considerations. In fact, as the patient's clinical and biochemical status changes during and or as a result of dialysis, the composition of fluid may need to be changed and proper adjustments made to meet new physiologic requirements; therefore close follow-up and the frequent clinical and laboratory evaluation of patients undergoing short-term peritoneal dialysis is quite important. Many of the necessary alterations can be made by using different commercially available dialysates of various composition and by the addition of necessary substances to them. However, there have been occasions when a homemade peritoneal dialysate specifically designed for certain patients has been necessary. For instance, almost all the commercial preparations contain lactate and a few of them acetate as the base substance. These organic anions are readily converted to bicarbonate under ordinary circumstances. However, patients with lactic acidosis are not capable of converting lactate. Therefore the use of lactate-base dialysates not only fails to correct the patient's acid-base disturbance, but will even exaggerate it. In such situations I have ordered bicarbonate base dialysate to be made. Because of the pharmacologic incompatibility of calcium ion and magnesium ion with bicarbonate (precipitation of calcium and magnesium bicarbonate), the solution must be free of calcium and magnesium ions. Use of this dialysate has been very successful in improving the patient's acid-base balance, and by careful monitoring of the patient's serum calcium and magnesium levels and the IV infusion as needed of calcium ion compounds, the development of significant hypocalcemia or hypomagnesemia in these patients has been prevented.

Fructose and sorbitol have been used in place of glucose to generate osmotic forces for the removal of excess fluids. Peritoneal dialysis with solutions containing sorbitol has occasionally caused reversible alterations of mental status, mild liver function test abnormalities, nausea, and vomiting. For this reason the Food and Drug Administration has recently removed these products from U.S. markets; however, 1.4 to 1.8 g sorbitol solutions are still used in other countries. Table 19-1 provides the list and composition of most of commercially available peritoneal dialysis fluids.

**Table 19-1.** Commercially available peritoneal dialysis solutions

| *Manufacturer* | *Product* | *Available sizes (ml)* | *pH* | *Components (mEq/L)* | | | | | | |
|---|---|---|---|---|---|---|---|---|---|---|
| | | | | $Na^+$ | $K^+$ | $Ca^{++}$ | $Mg^{++}$ | $Cl^-$ | *Lactate* | *Acetate* |
| Abbott Laboratories | Inpersol D-1.5-W | 1000, 2000 | 5.2 | 140.5 | 0 | 3.5 | 1.5 | 101 | 44.5 | 0 |
| | Inpersol D-4.25-W | 200 | | 140.5 | 0 | 3.5 | 1.5 | 101 | 44.5 | 0 |
| Cutter Laboratories, Inc. | Peridial 1.5D | 1000, 2000 | 5.4 | 132 | 0 | 3.5 | 1.5 | 102 | 35 | 0 |
| | Peridial 4.25D | 2000 | 5.4 | 132 | 0 | 3.5 | 1.5 | 102 | 35 | 0 |
| McGaw Laboratories | Peritoneal dialysis solution with 1.5% dextrose | 1000, 2000 | | 140 | 0 | 4.0 | 1.5 | 100.5 | 0 | 45 |
| | Peritoneal dialysis solution with 1.5% dextrose and low sodium | 1000, 2000 | | 132 | 0 | 3.5 | 1.5 | 102 | 35 | 0 |
| | Peritoneal dialysis solution with 4.25% dextrose | 2000 | | 140 | 0 | 4.0 | 1.5 | 100.5 | 0 | 45 |
| | Peritoneal dialysis solution with 4.25% dextrose and low sodium | 2000 | | 132 | 0 | 3.5 | 1.5 | 102 | 35 | 0 |
| Travenol Laboratories | Dianeal with 1.5% dextrose | 1000, 2000 | 5.5 | 141 | 0 | 3.5 | 1.5 | 101 | 45 | 0 |
| | Dianeal K with 1.5% dextrose | 1000 | 5.5 | 141 | 4 | 3.5 | 1.5 | 101 | 45 | 0 |
| | Dianeal 137 with 1.5% dextrose | 2000 | 5.5 | 132 | 0 | 3.5 | 1.5 | 102 | 35 | 0 |
| | Dianeal K-141 with 1.5% dextrose | 2000 | 5.5 | 132 | 4 | 3.5 | 1.5 | 106 | 35 | 0 |
| | Dianeal with 4.25% dextrose | 2000 | 5.0 | 141 | 0 | 3.5 | 1.5 | 101 | 45 | 0 |
| | Dianeal 137 with 4.25% dextrose | 2000 | 5.5 | 132 | 0 | 3.5 | 1.5 | 102 | 35 | 0 |
| | Dianeal K-141 with 4.25% dextrose | 2000 | 5.5 | 132 | 4 | 3.5 | 1.5 | 106 | 35 | 0 |

### ■ What drugs, if any, are added to dialysis fluid?

To prevent clotting of the catheter it is customary to add 500 to 1000 units of *sodium lipoheparin* to each 2 L of dialysis fluid for the first two to four runs. If the drainage fluid remains or turns clear, no more heparin is used in subsequent passages. However, if the return is blood tinged, heparin use should be continued until the drainage fluid clears.

When the patient has peritonitis or contamination has occurred during the procedure, antibiotics can be mixed with the fluid. Highly effective local and systemic levels of antibiotics are usually achieved by the addition of antibiotics to peritoneal dialysis fluid (Table 19-2).

Most of the peritoneal dialysates are potassium free. To avoid hypokalemia the patient's plasma potassium levels should be carefully monitored. When the plasma potassium level is normal or subnormal, 2 to 4 mEq of potassium chloride can be added to each liter of dialysate to maintain a normal potassium balance.

Isoproterenol (Isuprel) can be added to the dialysis fluid to improve the efficiency of dialysis. This improvement is the result of increased peritoneal blood flow and vasodilatation.

Albumin has been added to dialysates in order to enhance the removal of protein-bound substances such as salicylates. This is quite costly and should be used only in cases of severe intoxication.

Dialysis with cotten seed oil has been used in the treatment of patients with intoxication with glutethimide and other lipid-soluble agents. This procedure carries with it the risk of fat embolism and is quite messy.

**Table 19-2.** Intraperitoneal antibiotics

| *Antibiotic* | *Dose (mg/L)* | *Safe blood level (μg/ml)* | *Half-life* |
|---|---|---|---|
| Ampicillin | 50 | 50-100 | Short |
| Keflin | 50 | 50-100 | Short |
| Carbenicillin | 200 | 200 | Short |
| Methicillin | 100 | 100-200 | Short |
| Gentamicin | 10 | 10-12 | Long |
| Kanamycin | 10 | 10-15 | Long |
| Vancomycin | 15 | 15-25 | Long |
| Amphotericin | 2.5 | 2.5 | Long |

Peritoneal dialysis with fluids containing tromethamine (THAM) has been used in the treatment of patients with barbiturate overdose. THAM is an organic base that can bind weak acids and their salts. Therefore its addition to peritoneal dialysis fluids enhances the elimination of barbiturates from the circulation. Because of its affinity for weak acids, it can lower the $P_{CO_2}$ in the blood, which is transient and clinically unimportant. Its absorption from the peritoneum is quite slow, which is a point in favor of its use.

### ■ What are the causes of poor drainage and dialysis fluid retention, and what can be done?

A mild to moderate positive balance is commonly seen with the first few runs of peritoneal dialysis. This is caused by pooling of small amounts of fluid in parts of the peritoneal cavity that are not readily drained by the catheter when the catheter tip is not located in the most dependent part of the small pelvis. This should not cause any undue anxiety, since with subsequent passes the balance becomes progressively negative. However, if the drainage stops or slows down while significant amounts of fluid are still in the abdomen, this may indicate that the catheter tip is buried in the omentum. By applying mild pressure to the lower abdomen on both sides, elevating the head of the bed, rotating the patient or carefully repositioning the catheter, the drainage can usually be improved and the retention eliminated. If all these measures fail, the catheter should be removed and examined for clots in the lumen. Sometimes catheter malfunction is caused by peritonitis, ileus, or constipation. The other cause of drainage problems is malplacement of the catheter outside the peritoneum, that is, within the adipose tissue of the abdominal wall or retroperitoneal space. This is occasionally encountered when the procedure is performed by an inexperienced person on an obese patient and calls for the removal of the catheter and its proper replacement.

## ■ Does the body absorb the glucose content of the peritoneal dialysate?

The concentration of glucose in peritoneal dialysis fluids is much higher than in plasma. This concentration gradient results in the diffusion of glucose from the peritoneal cavity to circulating blood. At a dialyzed volume of 2.5 L/hr a total of 300 to 750 g of glucose may be absorbed per day, which provides a large quantity of calories. In nondiabetic patients the blood sugar level can rise to as high as 330 mg/100 ml. Although this may not create any major problems in nondiabetic patients, it can produce significant difficulties in diabetic patients. Therefore blood sugar levels should be carefully monitored and the insulin dose adjusted in diabetic patients.

## ■ Is ultrafiltration possible using peritoneal dialysis, and if so, how?

In contrast to hemodialysis, the control of hydrostatic forces for the purpose of ultrafiltration is not possible in peritoneal dialysis. However, *osmotic forces can be used very effectively*. By adding high concentrations of glucose, fructose, or sorbitol to the dialysate, it can be made hypertonic (2.5% to 4% glucose or 1.5% to 1.8% sorbitol). This hypertonicity results in the movement of water from intravascular to peritoneal spaces and in the removal of large quantities of water. For the purpose of effective ultrafiltration *shorter transit times* (10 to 20 minutes) are desirable. With prolonged dwell times increasing amounts of osmotic agent are absorbed into the circulation, which not only limits the effective ultrafiltration but can also create serious complications.

## ■ What are the indications for short-term peritoneal dialysis?

Under most circumstances peritoneal and hemodialysis can be utilized interchangeably. The choice between the two is usually made on medical grounds. However, simplicity of the technique, possibility of rapid initiation, independence from the surgical team to provide vascular access, complicated space-occupying machinery, and lack of the need for specially trained personnel tend to favor the choice of peritoneal dialysis over hemodialysis.

In some patients peritoneal dialysis is superior to hemodialysis. Patients who need only one or two dialyses may better be managed by peritoneal dialysis. For example, when dialysis is needed to treat severe intractable congestive heart failure, significant amounts of fluid can be removed by peritoneal dialysis over 1 to 2 days. Furthermore, acute hemodynamic changes that may occur with hemodialysis and can cause cardiovascular complications are avoided.

Intoxication with drugs that have low circulating levels and high tissue- and protein-binding capacities will respond to peritoneal dialysis, which is a slow and prolonged process, more readily than to hemodialysis. Drugs such as diphenylhydantoin (Dilantin) and glutethimide fall into this category.

In situations where anticoagulation is contraindicated, for instance, in patients with internal bleeding, cerebral trauma, or hemorrhage and following neurosurgical procedures or hemorrhagic pericarditis, peritoneal dialysis is safer than hemodialysis.

In very young children, elderly patients, and those with severe cardiovascular diseases or shock, peritoneal dialysis is preferable.

Because of its lower risk of intermittent bacteremia, hypotension, and bleeding caused by heparinization, peritoneal dialysis is probably superior to hemodialysis following open-heart surgery, particularly prosthetic valve replacement.

Patients with acute renal failure after various major abdominal or transabdominal retroperitoneal surgeries have undergone peritoneal dialysis with satisfactory results. Therefore recent abdominal surgery does not seem to be a contraindication to peritoneal dialysis. However, in the presence of fresh wounds and multiple drains it may be quite a messy procedure. It should be noted that many postoperative patients have ileus, which renders catheter insertion somewhat difficult, and also atelectasis, which predisposes to pulmonary infections. These patients should be treated with intermittent positive pressure breathing (IPPB) and pulmonary toilet. In addition, the volume of their peritoneal dialysis exchanges should be reduced to avoid further compression and atelectasis of the lung tissue. The general indications for short-term peritoneal dialysis are as follows:

1. Acute renal failure
2. Reversible deterioration of chronic renal failure
3. Various intoxications
4. Severe fluid overload refractory to other therapeutic means
5. Acid-base disturbances
6. Major electrolyte and some metabolic disturbances
7. In awaiting the maturation of arteriovenous fistula and the initiation of chronic hemodialysis
8. In treatment of peritonitis by adding antibiotics to dialysis fluids

Beneficial results have been reported with peritoneal dialysis in acute hemorrhagic pancreatitis. The improvement has been attributed to the removal of vasoactive substances released from necrotic pancreatic and other tissues.

## ■ Are there any contraindications to the use of peritoneal dialysis?

There are no absolute contraindications to peritoneal dialysis, especially if the risk of hemodialysis is higher than that associated with peritoneal dialysis. The following list enumerates those conditions in which peritoneal dialysis may be associated with a high incidence of various complications:

1. In the presence of diffuse skin infection or cellulitis of the abdominal wall the catheter can transport the pathogenic organisms to the peritoneal cavity and cause peritonitis.

2. Diffuse intra-abdominal malignancy and previous peritonitis are associated with a higher risk of viscus perforation. This is also true in cases involving small children and cachectic individuals. Under these circumstances prior infusion of some dialysate into the peritoneal cavity through a 15-gauge, 10 cm long needle to distend the abdomen followed by aspiration of fluid from the projected site of catheter insertion ensures free access to the peritoneal cavity and reduces the risk. Surgical insertion of the catheter under direct vision is the other alternative.

3. With severe bleeding diathesis, the correction of the hemostatic abnormality, if possible, prior to catheter placement is ideal. If not possible, surgical placement of the catheter under direct vision may be the procedure of choice.

4. Peritoneal catheter insertion in patients with ileus is associated with an increased risk of viscus perforation, drainage difficulty, and poor clearance. Furthermore, severe bowel distention may preclude the use of adequate exchange volumes.

5. The presence of abdominal drains may result in a leakage of the fluids and peritoneal infection.

6. In the presence of diaphragmatic gaps the dialysate may find its way up to the thoracic cavity and embarrass pulmonary function. By placing the patient in a sitting or semisitting position, the difficulty may be eliminated.

7. Preexisting asymptomatic hernias may enlarge or become symptomatic as a result of peritoneal dialysis. This is caused by the increased intraperitoneal tension generated by large volumes of fluid. It can be prevented by avoiding abdominal overdistention and by the use of local supportive devices.

8. The inability to maintain adequate dietary intake is a definite contraindication to long-term peritoneal dialysis. This is because of the significant obligatory protein loss with peritoneal dialysis that results in a depletion syndrome if the dietary intake is insufficient.

## ■ Can peritoneal dialysis be performed in the presence of acute peritonitis?

The answer is definitely yes. In fact, by combining the systemic and local antibiotic therapy, faster and more complete recovery of peritonitis can be accomplished. It is important to mention that the degree of protein loss with peritoneal dialysis is much greater in patients with peritonitis than those without peritonitis. It could be as much as 60 g or more daily.

### ■ How does peritoneal dialysis compare with hemodialysis and what are the major differences, advantages, and disadvantages?

1. The surface area of the artificial kidney is variable, depending on the choice of dialyzer. The surface area of the adult peritoneum is fixed at about 1.8 $m^2$ (almost equal to skin surface).

2. The permeability characteristics of the membranes are different. The peritoneal membrane is much more permeable, allowing the passage of larger molecules, in contrast to artificial kidney membranes that have limited permeabilities.

3. Blood flow, hydrostatic pressure, and dialysate flow rate can be easily regulated in hemodialysis by means of the various pumps and clamps, whereas only dialysate flow can be altered in peritoneal dialysis.

4. Hemodialysis baths are always isosmolar, and ultrafiltration is achieved by manipulation of the hydrostatic forces. In the case of peritoneal dialysis, hydrostatic forces are almost constant, but osmotic forces are variable.

5. With hemodialysis the clearance of small molecules is several times higher than in peritoneal dialysis. This results in a rapid correction of extracellular fluid biochemical abnormalities, which may cause disequilibrium syndrome. Because of the slowness of biochemical changes in peritoneal dialysis, disequilibrium syndrome is practically nonexistent.

6. In hemodialysis abrupt changes of blood volume caused by extracorporeal circulation may result in hypotension at the onset of the treatment or during ultrafiltration, and mild congestive heart failure at the end on return of the blood, which suddenly increases the load on a borderline compensated heart.

7. With peritoneal dialysis it is easy to change the composition of dialysate as the patient's laboratory findings and state of hydration change. This is more difficult in the case of hemodialysis because of the rapidity of the patient's biochemical changes and the large volume of dialysis fluids.

8. Because of its relatively low clearance rates, peritoneal dialysis may not be an adequate treatment for hypercatabolic patients in whom tremendous amounts of waste products are generated. Under these circumstances the use of long and frequent hemodialysis treatments with or without peritoneal dialysis is advisable.

9. Hemodialysis is more efficient in the rapid correction of severe fluid overload and pulmonary edema. The same is true in the case of severe hyperkalemia and other electrolyte abnormalities.

10. Peritoneal dialysis is associated with a loss of 20 to 80 g of protein daily.

11. The longer duration of peritoneal dialysis and the maintenance of the same position in bed is frequently tiresome.

12. The consequences of the absorption of large amounts of glucose with peritoneal dialysis has been discussed.

13. Peritoneal dialysate should be sterile. This is not a requirement for hemodialysis fluids, since bacteria cannot pass through hemodialysis membranes.

14. There is no need for systemic or regional heparinization during peritoneal dialysis. This is an absolute necessity in the case of hemodialysis; therefore peritoneal dialysis may be the procedure of choice in patients who should not be treated with anticoagulants.

15. There is no need for a vascular access in peritoneal dialysis and no risk of air embolism, clotting, rupture of the dialyzer, or many other complications that are associated with hemodialysis.

## BIBLIOGRAPHY

Andersson, G., et al.: Glucose absorption from the dialysis fluid during peritoneal dialysis, Scand. J. Urol. Nephrol. **5**:77-79, 1971.

Baran, H., et al.: Kinetics of protein loss during peritoneal dialyses, Pol. Med. J. **11**:277-280, 1972.

Boen, S. T.: Kinetics of peritoneal dialysis, Medicine **40**:243, 1961.

Brewer, T. E., et al.: Indwelling peritoneal (Tenckhoff) dialysis catheter. Experience with 24 patients, J.A.M.A. **219**:1011-1015, 1972.

Deger, G. E., and Wagoner, R. D.: Peritoneal dialysis in acute uric acid nephropathy, Mayo Clin. Proc. **47**:189-192, 1972.

De Santo, N. G., et al.: Haematoma of rectus abdominis associated with dialysis, Br. Med. J. **3**:281-282, 1972.

Edwards, D. H., Gardner, R. D., and Williams, D. G.: Rupture of a hernial sac: a complication of peritoneal dialysis, J. Urol. **108**:255-256, 1972.

Gault, M. H.: Peritoneal solutions, Can. Med. Assoc. J. **108**:325-327, 1973.

Greenblatt, D. J.: Fatal hypoglycaemia occurring after peritoneal dialysis, Br. Med. J. **2**:270-271, 1972.

Henderson, L. W.: Peritoneal ultrafiltration dialysis: enhances urea transfer using hypertonic peritoneal dialysis fluid, J. Clin. Invest. **45**: 950-955, 1966.

Holm, J., Lied En, B., and Lindqvist, B.: Unilateral pleural effusion—a rare complication of peritoneal dialysis, Scand. J. Urol. Nephrol. **5**:84-85, 1971.

Kahn, S. I., Garella, S., and Chazan, J. A.: Nonsurgical treatment of intestinal perforation due to peritoneal dialysis, Surg. Gynecol. Obstet. **136**:40-42, 1973.

Kessler, J.: Peritoneal dialysis and dialysate volumes, N. Engl. J. Med. **286**:110, 1972.

Mattocks, A. M., and El-Bassiouni, E. A.: Peritoneal dialysis: a review, J. Pharm. Sci. **60**: 1767-1782, 1971.

Maxwell, M. H., et al.: Peritoneal dialysis. I. Technique and applications, J. Am. Med. Assoc. **170**:916, 1959.

Pirpasopoulos, M., et al.: A cost-effectiveness study of dwell times in peritoneal dialysis, Lancet **2**:1135-1136, 1972.

Rae, A., and Pendray, M.: The advantages of peritoneal dialysis in chronic renal failure, J.A.M.A. **225**:937-941, 1973.

Raja, R. M., et al.: Hyperosmotic coma complicating peritoneal dialysis with sorbitol dialysate, Ann. Intern. Med. **73**:993-994, 1970.

Rosato, E. E., et al.: Peritoneal lavage treatment of experimental pancreatitis, J. Surg. Res. **12**: 138-140, 1972.

Scurrell, A. M.: Peritoneal dialysis—a five-year evaluation, Nurs. Times **69**:929-931, 1973.

Sharma, B. K., et al.: Peritoneal dialysis in resistant congestive heart failure and pulmonary oedema, J. Indian Med. Assoc. **58**:159-162, 1972.

Sheppard, J. M., et al.: Lactic acidosis: Recovery associated with use of peritoneal dialysis, Aust. N.Z. J. Med. **2**:389-393, 1972.

Stoltz, M. L., Nolph, K. D., and Maher, J. F.: Factors affecting calcium removal with calcium-free peritoneal dialysis, J. Lab. Clin. Med. **78**: 389-398, 1971.

Vidt, D. G.: Recommendations on choice of peritoneal dialysis solutions, Ann. Intern. Med. **78**:144-146, 1973.

Wardle, E. N.: Simple method for detection of infection of peritoneum during dialysis, Br. Med. J. **2**:518-520, 1973.

*chapter 20*

# Long-term peritoneal dialysis

**N. DABIR VAZIRI**

Long-term peritoneal dialysis can provide a valuable adjunct in the management of patients with end-stage renal failure. The high risk of peritonitis, the need for repeated painful insertions of peritoneal catheters, and the high cost of dialysis fluids were among the factors limiting the utilization of peritoneal dialysis on a long-term basis in the past.

With the advent of implantable peritoneal catheters, automated dialysis machines, and improved aseptic techniques, home and in-center long-term peritoneal dialysis procedures are gaining increased popularity among physicians and patients. The implanted catheter provides a long-term access to the peritoneal cavity, thereby eliminating the need for the painful reinsertion of the catheter with each dialysis and reducing the risk of infection.

The catheters (Tenckhoff catheters) are made of Silastic, which is soft, pliable, quite compatible with peritoneal membrane, and therefore nonirritating. The part of the catheter that lies in the wall of the abdomen is equipped with one or two Teflon cuffs. Fibroblasts grow into the Teflon cuffs and provide satisfactory fixation of the catheter to the abdominal wall.

Automated machines provide unlimited amounts of sterile pyrogen-free dialysate by mixing a sugar-electrolyte concentrate with water. Pure pyrogen-free sterile water is produced in the machine from tap water by several processes, including reverse osmosis, heating, and filtration through several membranes and cartridges. Therefore the problem of handling large volumes of expensive premade dialysates and its tremendous financial impact has been resolved.

A predetermined volume of dialysate is delivered and drainage disposed of intermittently through a closed system. The dialysate temperature, inflow, outflow, and dwell times are automatically regulated.

In contrast to hemodialysis, peritoneal dialysis is a slow and smooth process, and sudden hemodynamic changes requiring close attention and immediate action are not expected.

The procedure can be started by an unattended, trained patient at home, proceed during sleep and be terminated in the morning. As a result, daytime activity will not be compromised, since all the required 30 to 40 hours of dialysis per week can be done at night.

At the present time the number of institutions providing in-center and home dialysis programs is limited and the cost of operation is higher than that of hemodialysis. In the near future, however, we will undoubtedly witness the universal expansion of this technique with a lower cost of operation.

## ■ What are the causes of failure of the indwelling catheter to drain properly?

*Diagnosis and management*

Failure of the indwelling catheter to drain properly may be caused by one of the following problems:

1. Malposition of the catheter. This usually results from omental entanglement during implantation of the catheter. It should be suspected when the catheter malfunction occurs during the early postimplantation period. Upper or midabdominal pains are frequently observed when suctioning is applied. The pain is caused by traction of the omentum with suctioning. The diagnosis is confirmed by abdominal x-ray studies following injection of

3 to 5 ml of contrast medium (Renografin). It is corrected by repositioning of the catheter.

2. Internal obstruction. This is usually caused by tissues sucked into the catheter lumen through its side perforations. It is more commonly seen in children and is more likely to occur when the side perforations are large. The diagnosis is confirmed by injection of radiopaque dye into the catheter under an image intensifier. An attempt should be made to remove the incarcerated tissue fragments and reposition the catheter. If this fails to solve the problem, a new catheter should be placed.

3. Obstruction caused by peritoneal infections. This is usually associated with asymptomatic or mild or recurrent infections and may be a sequela of a healed infection. The development of pain with rapid infusion of dialysate suggests the diagnosis. Anatomic confirmation can be achieved by x-ray study of the abdomen following injection of 10 to 20 ml of radiopaque dye into the catheter. The study will show poor diffusion of the dye throughout the abdomen and perhaps encasement of the catheter by surrounding tissues. Catheter replacement followed by 3 to 4 weeks of intraperitoneal and systemic antibiotic therapy will solve the problem.

4. Constipation. Constipation is one of the causes of functional and reversible catheter obstruction. A history of constipation, negative x-ray studies, and improvement following the use of purgatives suggest the diagnosis. Measures that improve bowel function will correct catheter malfunction.

## ■ What are the primary indications for long-term peritoneal dialysis?

There are certain groups of patients who do not tolerate hemodialysis treatment well and may be better treated with long-term peritoneal dialysis. These include the following:

1. Young children. Although providing vascular access and performing hemodialysis is possible even in infants, the procedure is difficult and hard to maintain. Furthermore, hemodialysis is psychologically much more traumatic than painless peritoneal irrigation through an implanted catheter during sleeping hours at home, which allows full-time school attendance and liberal activities. Early renal transplantation is the other alternative. However, because of the accompanying long-term steroid therapy, children undergoing transplantation usually grow and mature very poorly. For this reason it is advisable to defer transplantation to a later time when reasonable growth and maturation have occurred. This classic concept has been recently challenged. In the interim these patients should be maintained on long-term dialysis and a high protein calorie diet.

2. Elderly patients. The elderly, particularly those persons over 60 years of age with major cardiovascular disorders, are good candidates for long-term peritoneal dialysis. Providing and maintaining functional vascular access is frequently difficult in these patients because of prevalent atherosclerotic peripheral vascular disease. In addition, these patients are frequently sensitive to the sudden hemodynamic changes and rapid alterations of the biochemical composition of internal milieu imposed by hemodialysis. For these reasons they react more favorably to long-term peritoneal dialysis.

3. Patients with severe cardiovascular disease and instability. These persons are better candidates for peritoneal dialysis regardless of age.

4. Patients with contraindications to systemic or regional heparinization. These patients may have to use peritoneal dialysis. Recurrent bleeding peptic ulcer disease, dissecting aneurysms, or hypersensitivity to various heparin preparations are a few examples of the disorders affecting these persons.

5. Patients who lack reliable vascular access routes for hemodialysis. The number of suitable vessels for creation of vascular access and the survival of each vascular access route are limited. Consequently, with passage of time hemodialysis patients, particularly *diabetic* patients, run out of reliable vascular access routes. This has always been a frustrating experience for those practitioners who deal with patients on long-term hemodialysis. However, with the advent and perfection of

the long-term peritoneal dialysis technique, lack of vascular access is no longer a hopeless situation.

6. Patients who require home dialysis but who live alone. For reasons of safety and simplicity unattended persons are quite capable of performing peritoneal dialysis with automated machines. This is not true with hemodialysis, in which life-threatening complications can occur at any minute.

7. Patients who exhibit an inability to learn hemodialysis techniques. Self-hemodialysis techniques are more complicated than peritoneal dialysis techniques. In addition, the cannulation of arteriovenous fistulas and various grafts is quite painful. Home dialysis candidates who cannot or refuse to learn hemodialysis techniques should be considered for a long-term home peritoneal dialysis program.

8. Patients who refuse transfusions because of ethnic beliefs. These persons should not undergo hemodialysis, since major blood loss or hemolysis necessitating transfusion is among the more common complications of hemodialysis. Peritoneal dialysis is the proper choice in these patients.

9. Hemodialysis and transplant candidates awaiting fistula maturation or transplantation surgery. These patients can be treated with peritoneal dialysis in the interim period.

## ■ How are fluid retention and hypertension controlled in patients on long-term peritoneal dialysis?

Fluid and sodium intakes should be restricted in these patients. In addition, the osmolality of the dialysate should be adjusted by changing the dialysate glucose concentration so that fluids retained between dialyses can be removed. A 1.5% glucose dialysate usually does not remove any fluids; 2% to 2.5% solutions are suitable for most patients.

Hypertension frequently remains a problem despite control of extracellular fluid volume, requiring antihypertensive drugs or even bilateral nephrectomy.

## ■ What are the complications of peritoneal dialysis?

The complications of peritoneal dialysis can be divided into several categories:

1. Related to insertion of catheter
2. Caused by infection
3. Metabolic complications
4. Miscellaneous complications

### *Complications directly related to insertion of catheter*

***Intestinal perforation.*** Intestinal perforation is likely to occur when too much force is exerted to penetrate the peritoneum. Patients with ileus, diffuse intra-abdominal carcinomas, adhesions, previous peritonitis, and large uteruses are more prone to this complication. Surgical intervention may be necessary in such circumstances. However, according to a recent report, several patients with intestinal perforation subsequent to peritoneal catheter insertion have been treated conservatively with antibiotics and supportive measures with good results.

***Bladder perforation.*** Perforation of the bladder has been reported in patients with urinary retention and distended bladder. For this reason it is mandatory to empty the bladder before attempting to insert the peritoneal catheter.

***Intraperitoneal bleeding.*** Rupture of small abdominal wall vessels is not an uncommon complication. It presents with bloody fluid return that should clear readily. The addition of 5 mg heparin to each liter of dialysate is helpful to prevent obstruction of the catheter by blood clots. Heparin can be discontinued after the fluid turns clear. Large vessel injury is very unlikely; however, rapid development of shock and heavy bloody return should suggest this possibility or, alternatively, rupture of one of the solid organs. A mild bloody return may be indicative of peritoneal infection or neoplasm. It is occasionally seen during the first few days of the menstrual period even in the absence of endometriosis.

*Hematoma* of the abdominal rectus muscle and retroperitoneal penetrations are occasionally encountered.

### *Complications caused by infections*

***Peritonitis.*** Peritonitis is one of the major complications of peritoneal dialysis. Although it is frequently caused by infection, aseptic peritonitis is encountered with some frequency.

STERILE PERITONITIS. Sterile peritonitis is an aseptic inflammation caused by low dialysate pH, its marked hypertonicity and chemical impurities, and the presence of blood or pyrogens in the fluid. It is associated with symptoms of peritoneal irritation and an increased number of white cells in the drainage fluid. White cell counts in the fluid may be as high as 50 cells/mm$^3$ or more, and this makes the fluid turbid. Sterile peritonitis can result in adhesion formation and peritoneal fibrosis.

INFECTIOUS PERITONITIS. Although some investigators have speculated that the infectious organisms originate from the bowels as a result of catheterization-induced lacerations, the most likely possibility is that the organisms are carried through the skin to the peritoneum by the catheter. It is important to realize that symptoms of peritonitis in these patients are frequently very mild or nonexisting. A high index of suspicion is necessary to make the diagnosis in early stages.

Late obstruction of the catheter that fails to correct with the irrigation may be the first sign of peritonitis. A low-grade fever, reduced appetite, weakness, or malaise are sometimes present. Mild abdominal discomfort and slight rebound tenderness or a blood-tinged fluid return may be the presenting signs.

*Infected catheter exit* or *subcutaneous catheter tract* should raise suspicion. With gram-negative infections a full-blown sepsis may develop. *By far the most common finding is turbidity of the drainage fluid. White blood cell count in the fluid frequently exceeds 300 to 500 cells/mm$^3$.*

The gram stain may confirm the presence of bacteria in the peritoneal fluid. Cultures and sensitivity tests should be done and treatment started immediately. The choice of antibiotic is dependent on the findings of a gram-stained smear. Appropriate changes can be made later when the results of the culture and sensitivity testing become available, or if peritonitis fails to respond in 24 to 48 hours.

*Treatment includes the addition of appropriate antibiotics and heparin to the irrigation fluid, which provides effective local and systemic antibiotic concentrations and prevents obstruction of the catheter by fibrin clots.* Unless the patient is markedly septic, there is no need for the administration of antibiotics through other routes. Small exchange volumes are used to reduce discomfort, and irrigation is carried on continuously for 3 to 4 days, by which time the infection should have cleared. Every-other-day dialysis with heparin and antibiotic-containing fluid is then carried on for 3 weeks more. If the biologic half-life of the antibiotic used is short (for example, cephalosporins), oral or parenteral administration will be indicated to maintain optimum plasma and tissue levels on the days off of dialysis. Failure to respond to therapy or recurrence of infection may call for removal of the old catheter and placement of a new one in a different site.

*Daily fluid culture and sensitivity tests are mandatory during treatment,* since resistant organisms may emerge and new organisms superimpose, requiring a change in strategy. Delayed or inadequate treatment of peritonitis results in adhesion formation and peritoneal fibrosis that will complicate future catheterizations and markedly reduce the peritoneal dialysis clearances to the extent that peritoneal dialysis may have to be abandoned. Furthermore, protein losses with peritoneal dialysis increase tremendously in the presence of peritonitis, reaching levels as high as 60 to 80 g/day. Recommended intraperitoneal antibiotics and their doses are given in Table 19-2 (p. 356).

Since *Staphylococcus aureus* is one of the major causes of peritonitis in these patients, cephalothin may be a good starting drug while awaiting the results of the culture and sensitivity tests.

Loading doses of gentamicin, vancomycin, and kanamycin should be given parenterally prior to the initiation of their peritoneal administration. Since chloramphenicol requires metabolic activation for its antimicrobial effect, its direct peritoneal use is ineffective.

### *Metabolic complications*

***Protein amino acid and vitamin losses.*** As discussed earlier, protein loss with dialysis fluid is a problem in long-term peritoneal dialysis patients. Under ordinary circumstances it is 10 to 20 g/dialysis, which amounts to 30 to 60 g/week. When peritonitis is present, losses can increase five to ten times. Although amino acid and vitamin losses have not been investigated thoroughly yet, their losses should be similarly significant. Even calorie malnutrition may occur despite the absorption of large quantities of glucose from the bath. To avoid protein and vitamin depletion a high protein diet with multiple vitamins and 2 to 4 mg/day of folic acid should be prescribed. If the patient is catabolic, parenteral hyperalimentation may be necessary. Patients who cannot maintain a good protein intake should not be treated with peritoneal dialysis; hemodialysis may be a better choice.

***Consequences of glucose absorption.*** For obvious reasons a high glucose concentration in the peritoneal dialysate results in the absorption of large quantities of glucose into the circulation. This may be beneficial to patients with calorie malnutrition. In other patients it can cause obesity, hyperlipidemia (type IV), and hyperglycemia that may even require small doses of regular insulin (blood sugar levels more than 400 mg/L) for its control. In diabetic patients the insulin requirement may change, and the insulin dose should be adjusted before their discharge to a home dialysis program.

*Hyperosmolar coma* caused by the preferential movement of water across the peritoneal membrane against a high osmotic gradient was discussed earlier. It is not uncommon with acute peritoneal dialysis, but because of the stability of the patients and the interrupted nature of the treatment (every other day), hyperosmolar coma is very rare in patients on long-term peritoneal dialysis, since the resultant mild hyperosmolar states are corrected by ingestion of free water and endogenous water production.

***Electrolyte disturbances***

HYPOKALEMIA. Patients dialyzed against zero or very low potassium dialysates may develop hypokalemia, which can cause weakness, ileus, and cardiac arrhythmias. This could be quite dangerous in patients receiving digitalis preparations.

HYPOCALCEMIA. Hypocalcemia may develop when a low calcium ion bath is used.

HYPERNATREMIA. Because of the excess loss of free water, hypernatremia may occur. This was discussed earlier.

***Hypoglycemia.*** A hypoglycemia attack can occur following the termination of peritoneal dialysis. This is frequently seen when dialysates with high glucose concentrations are used. The pathogenesis of this hypoglycemia is as follows: Because of its high concentration in dialysis fluid, glucose is absorbed in large quantities during dialysis. This raises the levels of plasma glucose, which, in turn, stimulates insulin secretion by the pancreas. With the termination of dialysis, the influx of glucose to the circulation ceases immediately, but because of its long half-life, the insulin level remains elevated for several hours. During this period of time recurrent endogenous insulin reactions can occur. This reaction is self-limited and is treated with IV infusion of glucose and oral carbohydrates, just as reactions caused by exogenous insulin are treated. The development of palpitation, diaphoresis, agitation, confusion, coma, convulsion, etc. after peritoneal dialysis should suggest the diagnosis, and prompt treatment of hypoglycemia should be started. Failure to treat hypoglycemia may result in permanent brain damage.

### *Miscellaneous complications*

***Ascites formation.*** Some patients develop progressive and recurrent ascites during the interdialysis intervals, following the discontinuation of peritoneal dialysis, after renal transplantation, or when switching to hemodialysis programs. The reason for this phenomenon is not clear. However, it seems to be related to the prolonged use of low pH and hypertonic dialysates, which is believed to cause aseptic inflammation of the peritoneal membranes. The fluid is quite rich in protein and relatively cell free. At times the rate of its accumulation is such that unless it is regularly drained, it can cause respiratory embarrassment. In these cases, if the catheter is not infected, it should be left in place for some time to drain the fluid, hoping that it will clear spontaneously.

***Pleural effusion.*** Pleural effusion in patients with chronic renal failure may be caused by fluid retention and congestive heart failure. Acute massive effusion following peritoneal dialysis, however, is probably caused by a shift of the intra-abdominal fluid to the thoracic cage through a preexisting or evolving diphragmatic defect.

***Abdominal pain.*** Peritoneal dialysis through the indwelling Silastic catheter should be painless. The presence of pain may be caused by one or a combination of the following conditions:

1. Peritonitis (as previously discussed)
2. Adhesions around catheter
3. Low dialysate pH (less than 5.5)
4. Free air within the peritoneal cavity as a result of inadequate deaeration of fluid by the machine or inadvertent infusion of air into the peritoneal cavity and characterized by pain in the shoulders and interscapular area following assumption of an upright position; can be corrected by assuming Trendelenburg or knee-chest position to let the air out through the catheter
5. Unrelated disorders such as appendicitis, peptic ulcer disease, and gaseous distention of intestines

## BIBLIOGRAPHY

Baillod, R. A., et al.: Home dialysis in children and adolescents, Proc. Eur. Dialysis Transplant. Assoc. **9:**335-342, 1972.

Berlyne, G. M., et al.: Amino acid loss in peritoneal dialysis, Lancet **1:**1339-1341, 1967.

Boen, S. T.: Kinetics of peritoneal dialysis, Medicine **40:**243, 1961.

Boyer, J., et al.: Hyperglycemia and hyperosmolality complicating peritoneal dialysis, Ann. Intern. Med. **67:**568-572, 1967.

Crossley, K., et al.: Intraperitoneal insulin for control of blood sugar in diabetic patients during peritoneal dialysis, Br. Med. J. **1:**269-270, 1971.

Edwards, S. R., and Unger, A. M.: Acute hydrothorax, a new complication of peritoneal dialysis, J.A.M.A. **199:**853-855, 1967.

Henderson, L. W.: Peritoneal ultrafiltration dialysis: enhances urea transfer using hypertonic peritoneal dialysis fluid, J. Clin. Invest. **45:** 950-955, 1966.

Johnson, P. J.: Bidirectional permeability of human peritoneum to substances of widely varying molecular weight, Master's thesis, University of Washington, 1973.

Lindner, A., and Tenckhoff, H.: Nitrogen balance in patients on peritoneal dialysis, Trans. Am. Soc. Artif. Intern. Organs **16:**255-259, 1970.

Mallette, W. G., et al.: A chemically successful subcutaneous peritoneal access button for repeated peritoneal dialysis, Trans. Am. Soc. Artif. Intern. Organs **10:**396-398, 1964.

Maxwell, M. H., et al.: Peritoneal dialysis. I. Technique and applications, J.A.M.A. **170:**916-924, 1959.

Rae, A., and Pendray, M.: The advantages of peritoneal dialysis in chronic renal failure, J.A.M.A. **225:**937-941, 1973.

Simmons, J. M., et al.: Relation of calorie deficiency to growth failure in children on hemodialysis and growth response to calorie supplementation, N. Engl. J. Med. **285:**653-656, 1971.

Stauch, M., et al.: Factors influencing protein loss during peritoneal dialysis, Trans. Am. Soc. Artif. Intern. Organs **13:**172-175, 1967.

Tenckhoff, H.: Peritoneal dialysis today: a new look, Nephron **12:**420-436, 1974.

Tenckhoff, H., et al.: One year's experience with home peritoneal dialysis, Trans. Am. Soc. Artif. Intern. Organs **11:**11-14, 1965.

*chapter 21*

# Management of the burn patient

**PATRICIA ALLYN**
**ROBERT BARTLETT**

The skin is a remarkable organ, protecting the body from the environment and keeping fluids in and infection out. Burn damage to the skin of any magnitude is a serious injury. Nowhere in medicine is the coordination of a team of doctors, nurses, therapists, technicians, and laboratory and operating room personnel so important. The seriously burned patient is the ultimate challenge in critical care because of the complexity of medical and nursing management. Even though the magnitude of injury may be massive and prolonged, survival and rehabilitation can be expected as soon as the burn surface is covered with healthy skin.

## ■ What is the pathophysiology of burns?

Thermal injury to the skin causes cellular necrosis, capillary damage, capillary thrombosis, and denaturation of collagen and other proteins in the skin and subcutaneous layers. The depth of the burn is proportional to the amount of heat and length of time it is applied (Table 21-1).

A first-degree burn causes erythema of the skin and only slight damage to the uppermost layers, occasionally causing blistering. Second-degree burn encompasses all the range between this and the extreme of third-degree burn but by definition implies that some of the layer of epithelial cells that generates new skin is intact. Second-degree burns can therefore be expected to heal by the generation of new skin and reepithelialization. A third-degree burn is that in which the skin and all its appendages (sweat glands, hair follicles, and sebaceous glands) are completely destroyed by the injury, so that the patient has a thick layer of coagulated necrotic skin (eschar) on top of viable subcutaneous fat. Third-degree burns will always require skin grafting or some other method of closure for healing to be complete. Fourth-degree burns extend into muscle and bone.

Immediately after the injury, it is often difficult to judge the depth of the burn, but some general characteristics can usually be recognized. The capillary injury of second- and third-degree burns results in leakage of plasma from blood into the interstitial space of the subcutaneous fat and damaged skin. In addition, large amounts of water are lost from the surface of the burn by evaporation. This is most obvious in second-degree burns where the surface is moist and oozing plasma, but the charred eschar of third-degree burns is also very permeable to water vapor. The evaporation of water from the surface causes cooling of the patient. The loss of plasma into the burned area and loss of water from the burned area to the atmosphere results in a rapid diminution of blood volume, specifically plasma volume, causing a concentration of red blood cells or a rise in hematocrit. As the blood volume falls and the hematocrit rises, viscosity increases, making it harder for the heart to pump the small amount of blood remaining. Cardiac output falls, perfusion of other vital organs falls, and unless the fluid is replaced, the patient with a major burn will die very promptly from plasma loss. Consequently, most of the effort in the first 2 days after an extensive burn is directed at replacing plasma that has been lost into the tissues and dealing with the later resorption of this plasma back into the vascular space.

**Table 21-1.** Characteristics of various depths of burns

| *Depth of burn* | *Cause* | *Surface* | *Color* | *Pain sensation* |
|---|---|---|---|---|
| First degree | Sun or minor flash | Dry, no blisters | Erythematous | Painful, hyperesthetic |
| Second degree | Flash or hot liquids | Blisters, moist | Mottled red | Painful, hyperesthetic |
| Third degree | Flame | Dry | Pearly white or charred | Little pain, anesthetic |
| Fourth degree | Sustained flame or electrical | Charred, cracked | Charred, black | Little |

## INSTRUCTIONS FOR COMPLETING THIS FORM

**1 COLOR IN THE BURN**

Shade or color in the body diagrams to represent as closely as possible how the burn looks to you when viewing the patient from directly anterior and/or directly posterior direction. Ignore the dashed lines on the diagrams while doing this.

**2 CIRCLE AGE FACTOR**

Since body proportions change from infancy to adulthood and since these changes mainly affect relative head and lower extremity proportions, this table allows you to choose the most appropriate body proportions for the age of the patient. Ages 0, 1, 5, 10, and 15 years and adult are given. Choose the age closest to that of the patient and use the H (head), T (thigh), and L (leg) percentage factors in the colunm below the age selected. To avoid mistakes, circle these numbers.

**3 CALCULATE EXTENT OF BURN**

Each body part listed in the calculation table is indicated on the anterior and posterior body diagrams by dashed lines. The percentage of total body surface area for each body part is printed either on the diagram or in the age factor table (step 2). If the shaded or colored area in the body diagram covers an entire body part, the whole percentage figure for that part is entered into the calculation table. If the shaded area covers only a fraction of a body part, then that fraction of the percentage figure is entered. For example, if an anterior chest burn covered about one third of the trunk, then one third of 13, or 4%, would be entered in the space for "trunk" in the anterior column. When all body parts have been considered, subtotals are made for anterior and posterior burned areas. The grand total then represents an estimate of the percent of total body area burned. This number is most frequently referred to as the "size of the burn."

Plasma loss begins immediately after the burn and continues at a high rate for 12 to 15 hours, after which it gradually diminishes; the edema phase is generally finished within 48 hours.

All of these phenomena become more severe with increasing depth and extent of the burn. The extent is expressed as the percentage of body surface involved with second-, third-, and fourth-degree burn. This is estimated by mapping the burn on a chart and calculating the percent of body involved (Fig. 21-1).

The second largest problem confronting the patient with major burns is infection. Once the edema phase has been passed and the patient is taking nourishment orally and normal hemodynamics have been reestablished, a large amount of necrotic skin exposed to the atmosphere on one side and covered by subcutaneous fat on the other side is left. This necrotic skin is an excellent culture medium and becomes colonized with bacteria quite rapidly. The principal effort of burn care between the fourth day and the

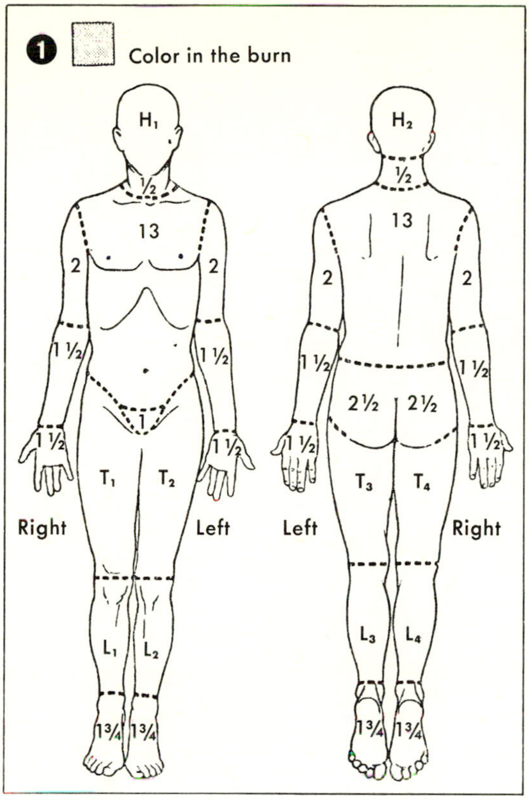


❸ Calculate extent of burn

| | Anterior | Posterior |
|---|---|---|
| Head | $H_1$ | $H_2$ |
| Neck | | |
| Right arm | | |
| Right forearm | | |
| Right hand | | |
| Left arm | | |
| Left forearm | | |
| Left hand | | |
| Trunk | | |
| Buttock | | |
| Perineum | | |
| Right thigh | $T_1$ | $T_4$ |
| Right leg | $L_1$ | $L_4$ |
| Right foot | | |
| Left thigh | $T_2$ | $T_3$ |
| Left leg | $L_2$ | $L_3$ |
| Left foot | | |
| Subtotal | | |
| % Total area burned | | % |

❷ Circle age factor

Percent of areas affected by growth

| | Age 0 | 1 | 5 | 10 | 15 | Adult |
|---|---|---|---|---|---|---|
| $H_{(1 \text{ or } 2)}$ = ½ of the head | 9½ | 8½ | 6½ | 5½ | 4½ | 3½ |
| $T_{(1,2,3 \text{ or } 4)}$ = ½ of a thigh | 2¾ | 3¼ | 4 | 4¼ | 4½ | 4¾ |
| $L_{(1,2,3 \text{ or } 4)}$ = ½ of a leg | 2½ | 2½ | 2¾ | 3 | 3¼ | 3½ |

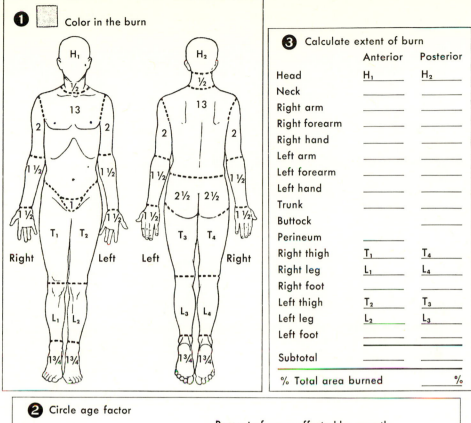

**Fig. 21-1.** Estimation of size of burn by percent.

fourth week is devoted to preventing infection in this necrotic skin while waiting until the surface is healed or ready for grafting.

The subcutaneous fat will generally not accept a skin graft until it has formed a significant layer of granulation tissue with its rich capillary bed that will vascularize and maintain a split-thickness skin graft in a viable condition. Granulation tissue begins to form at the interface between healthy and damaged tissue within days of the burn, but the complete formation of granulation tissue requires 3 to 6 weeks. The time from burn to grafting can be shortened by debriding eschar and assuring good nutrition.

Preventing infection in the eschar is accomplished with topical surface antibiotic agents that keep the eschar free of invasive infection with bacteria. Associated with this, daily cleansing and antiseptic washing of the surface with removal of dead tissue decreases the exposure of the surface to bacteria and minimizes the chance for infection. Most of the drugs used to destroy bacteria on the surface of the eschar also inhibit granulation tissue and epithelialization and therefore prolong the time for healing somewhat.

Other organs besides the heart and skin are vulnerable in the burn patient. Pulmonary complications are the most common cause of death after burn injury. This may be because of smoke inhalation, fluid overload, pulmonary capillary damage, or a combination of these. Renal failure may occur, particularly in fourth-degree burns associated with myoglobin or hemoglobin urea. Paralytic ileus is common if septicemia occurs. Stress ulcers with upper gastrointestinal bleeding are also associated with sepsis. CNS symptoms are common and reversible, ranging from confusion or depression to seizures and coma.

During the weeks before surface healing or grafting, careful attention must be paid to joints, muscles, and ligaments under the area of the burn. Immobilization may result in contractures and loss of function very rapidly, so that exercise of the full range of motion of all joints in the area of the burn and night splinting to prevent deformity are essential parts of burn management. Proper nutrition is also essential, as grossly excessive amounts of calories are required to run the metabolic machinery after a severe burn. After discharge these patients should be observed for several months to assist with their complete rehabilitation and return to normal life.

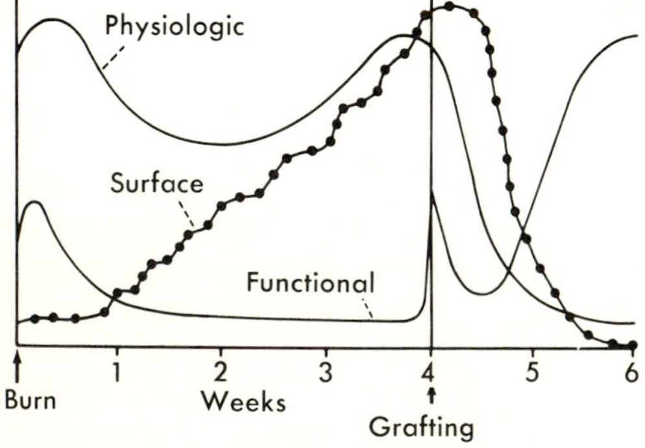


**Fig. 21-2.** Emphasis in burn management.

## ■ How is the determination made as to the degree of emphasis to be placed on the physiologic, surface, and functional management of the burn patient?

The physiologic, surface, and functional management processes involved in treating the burn patient are equally important in assuring good results but require different emphasis at different times. This changing emphasis is diagrammed in Fig. 21-2. Physiologic management is of primary importance during the resuscitation phase and remains important until the time the surface is covered. Direct surface management is of minimum importance for the first few days following the burn injury but becomes progressively more important until the time of grafting, when surface management is paramount. Functional management must be stressed within the first 24 hours of burn injury to prevent tissue damage that may lead to irreversible structural loss. This is particularly true in severe burns of the hands and the eyes. As long as joint motion is maintained during emergency management, little attention need be paid to functional management until the time the surface is covered with skin. Beyond that time, functional management becomes the most important aspect of care and continues to be of major importance for 6 to 12 months.

Although the individual aspects of care can be described in this fashion, the team approach to the patient requires that each individual who approaches the burn patient must be well versed in all aspects of management and their interrelationships. This is particularly important with regard to psychologic management and rehabilitation. All burn patients should be treated as any other ill patient in the hospital. Cosmetic appearance and function should be discussed freely but minimized in the acute phase and throughout the patient's course. If the patient leaves the hospital with a healthy mental status, social adjustment will be much easier.

## ■ What survival rates are anticipated in the care of burn patients?

Survival is expected for patients less than 60 years of age with uncomplicated burns covering up to 60% of the body surface. Death in these patients is usually related to smoke inhalation or other concomitant injury. Among young patients with burns over 60% to 80% of the body surface 50% survive, but survivors with burns of over 80% are rare. Death is usually caused by pulmonary insufficiency. At Orange County Medical Center 93% of the patients who survived major disfiguring or deforming burns underwent successful rehabilitation and resumed normal life.

This chapter outlines a plan for the critical care of the burn patient. Although there are several alternative methods of physiologic and surface care, these methods have produced the best results in burn care today based on survival, hospital stay, and rehabilitation. Other management approaches will be mentioned where appropriate. The interested reader is referred to the bibliography for further details.

## PHYSIOLOGIC MANAGEMENT

Major emphasis is placed on physiologic management from the time of admission until the time that the surface is ready for skin grafting. During this time all major organ systems are vulnerable to failure in the burn patient, and organ function must be carefully monitored and failure prevented or vigorously treated when it occurs. Specific areas of concentration in physiologic management are outlined in Fig. 21-3.

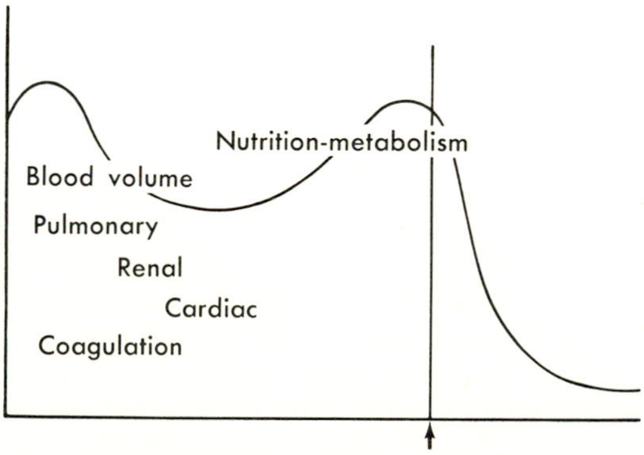


**Fig. 21-3.** Physiologic management.

### ■ What initial measures should be considered in the care of the critically burned patient?

All patients with second- or third-degree burns over greater than 20% of the body surface area should be admitted. All children and infants with second- or third-degree burns over 15% or more of the body surface area should be admitted. The full management protocol outlined here should be instituted for all patients who are admitted to the hospital and then modified according to physiologic response.

#### *Emergency care*

Rapid cooling of a thermal injury will minimize the depth of tissue damage and is the only appropriate first aid that should be carried out at the scene. If the patient is seen during or immediately after the burn or if the surface is no longer warm, topical cooling is not necessary; in fact, it may be detrimental. Beyond that time the surface should be simply covered with a sheet or towel (which need not be sterile) and the patient should be prepared for transfer to a burn center. A third- or fourth-degree burn will not be painful, and although the patient will be apprehensive and worried, medication for pain will not be required. Second-degree burns are quite painful on exposure to air. This pain may be alleviated by wet dressings applied to the surface. Tepid water on a towel or sheet will suffice during transfer. No other topical agents should be applied; no débridement should be done. A large IV line should be attached and colloid infusion begun if 30 minutes or more will elapse before the patient arrives in the burn unit.

#### *Emergency room care*

All clothing should be completely removed to facilitate examination, and the patient should be covered with a clean sheet. Vital signs should be measured and blood drawn to evaluate complete blood count (CBC), blood urea nitrogen (BUN), blood sugar, type and cross match, and carboxyhemoglobin. If the patient is hypotensive or appears to have any signs of respiratory distress or facial burns, arterial blood gases should be measured. Simultaneously, one large plastic catheter should be inserted into a peripheral vein for fluid administration and a central venous catheter of the largest possible diameter should be inserted by direct puncture or cutdown. Venipuncture and cutdown procedures may be performed through burned tissue with impunity. The position of the central venous catheter must be verified by chest x-ray film, usually taken in the emergency room. Fluid infusion may be begun in the peripheral venous catheter and dextrose and water infusion in the central venous catheter. A bladder catheter should be placed to measure urine output and a nasogastric tube should be passed. Chest x-ray films should be taken, and the patient readied for transfer to the critical care area. Diazepam (Valium) may be given by IV route for sedation. Rarely narcotics may be required for pain. All of this should be accomplished in 15 minutes or less.

If the patient has obvious respiratory distress, severe deep burns around the head and neck, or burn injury extending into the palate or pharynx on direct examination, tracheal intubation will be necessary. A nasotracheal tube should be passed when feasible, but prolonged and repeated attempts at intubation may exacerbate the edema; this job should be performed by the most experienced member of the team. If intubation is impossible, tracheostomy may be done, but only on extremely rare occasions.

Concomitant injuries may be cared for after an adequate airway is established. If the patient has a condition requiring immediate operation (compound fractures, intracranial bleeding, intra-abdominal bleeding), he should be taken to the operating room and treatment for the burn surface becomes of low priority. Closed fractures are splinted. Skeletal traction, if necessary, may be carried out through burned tissue without concern.

### *Burn unit admission*

If the patient is significantly hypotensive, is suffering severe respiratory insufficiency, or has an initial blood pH below 7.30, he should be taken directly from the emergency room to the burn unit. If these findings are not present, the patient should be taken to a hydrotherapy room, preferably adjacent to the burn unit, where he should be weighed and bathed in a large tub with warm water, sodium hypochlorite, and Betadine solution. All loose tissue should be debrided at this time without anesthesia. Blisters should be opened and debrided, and all hair-bearing areas near or in the burn area shaved. If foreign material such as dirt and tar is present, more extensive cleaning may be required. Pain medication may be given by IV route for the first time during this phase of management. It is not necessary to shave the entire head in burns of the face or scalp. If the patient's condition is unstable, débridement, washing, and dressing should be carried out as quickly as possible in bed in the burn unit while more intensive monitoring and therapy is taking place.

After the initial cleaning of the surface, topical antibiotic dressings should be quickly applied and the patient placed in bed in the burn unit in a semisitting position. Hands and feet should be elevated if burned. ECG monitoring is initiated at this time, along with hourly measurement of blood pressure, pulse, central venous pressure, urinary output, respiratory rate, tidal volume, and fluid intake. Temperature should be monitored continuously; an over-the-bed radiant heater may be added to prevent hypothermia (Fig. 21-4).

This phase of management should take no longer than 1 hour. Consideration should then be given to placement of an intra-arterial catheter, a pulmonary artery catheter, and Kirschner wire pins in fingers for severely burned hands; escharotomies should be performed on any area that appears to be constricting. Arterial catheters should be placed for any patient with severe smoke inhalation injury, any patient who requires

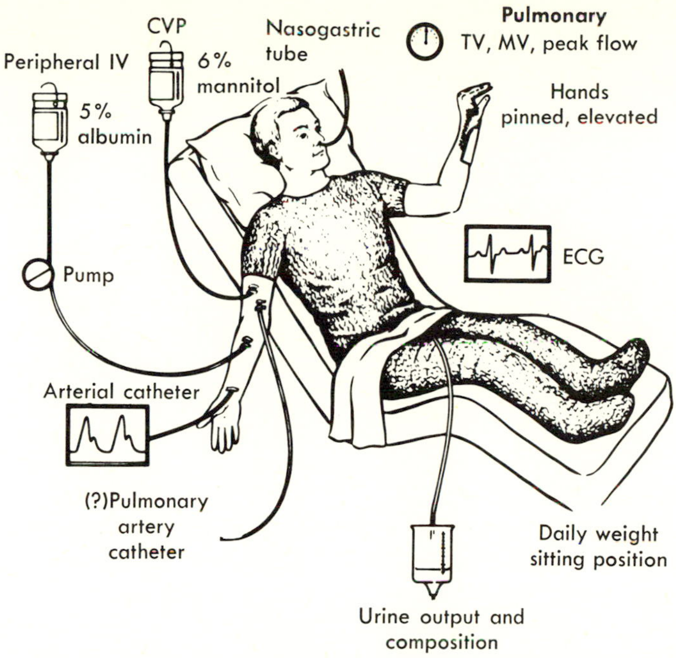


**Fig. 21-4.** Initial management and monitors.

intubation, or any patient with unstable blood pressure. Pulmonary artery catheters should be floated into patients with preexisting myocardial disease, massive burns, or preexisting pulmonary disease. Metal pins should be placed to maintain the proximal interphalangeal joints in full extension for patients with third-degree burns of the hands. Hand management is discussed extensively later. The hands should be placed in anticlaw splints and elevated.

Escharotomies should be carried out early in the course of management for all patients who have extensive circumferential burns of extremities, neck, or chest. When in doubt, the escharotomy should not be done, and the blood supply or chest expansion carefully monitored at hourly intervals, escharotomy being performed within the first 6 to 12 hours if significant constriction occurs. Escharotomy usually can be done without anesthesia using a knife blade or cautery, and bleeding from the skin edges is minimal. If bleeding does occur, it must be controlled with electrocautery. If the patient requires escharotomy, an extensive procedure should be done, extending down to and including fingers, on both sides of the wrist or ankle, and proximal to normal tissue, which may include the chest wall. Escharotomies over the chest wall to facilitate chest expansion should be done in grid fashion, including both vertical and horizontal incisions. IV morphine or similar narcotics should be used for pain. IV diazepam (Valium) or similar drugs should be used to calm agitated patients. Ketamine anesthesia is useful when pin placement is required, but this should not be used to anesthetize the patient simply because of agitation.

Once the initial management is instituted as outlined in Fig. 21-4, attention should be turned to hemodynamic and fluid resuscitation.

## ■ What should be known about hemodynamics and blood volume in the care of the burn patient?

Fluid management is the most important part of the early care of the burn patient. The goals of successful fluid management are to maintain adequate perfusion and supply metabolic demands while maintaining pace with the rate of plasma loss into and water evaporation through the burned surface; this should not result in an overload of the extracellular space in the lungs with large amounts of salt and water. Studies by Moore[1] showed that a large burn can sequester approximately 10% of the body weight in the extracellular space, and the fluid that is sequestered is essentially plasma. This fluid is reabsorbed after 48 hours and excreted over the ensuing 7- to 10-day period. These studies are incorporated into the "Brigham Burn Budget," which we follow.

Although a 5% albumin colloid solution is preferred for further resuscitation, many centers achieve good results by infusing crystalloid solutions such as lactated Ringer's solution only. Studies by Monafo and coworkers[2] and Moylan and associates[3] suggest that the total amount of sodium ion is the critical factor in successful burn resuscitation. This has led some investigators to infuse hypertonic saline solution or lactated Ringer's solution to provide the required amount of sodium ion with less fluid volume. Several formulas have been devised to calculate the fluid requirements of the burn patient. The Baxter formula dictates the use of 4 ml of Ringer's lactate solution per kilogram per percent burn. We recommend that crystalloid solutions be avoided during resuscitation because they may preferentially collect in the interstitial space in the lung, leading to pulmonary complications hours or days later. Burn formulas for fluid management are loose approximations to provide a general idea of the amount of fluid to have on hand during the acute management stage.

The fluid plan followed in the University of California Irvine Medical Center burn unit is outlined in Fig. 21-5. Simply stated, a plasma substitute is infused at a rate sufficient to maintain adequate arterial perfusion. This will require approximately 10% of the body weight in colloid solution during the first 48 hours, half of that during the first 12 hours. Blood pressure, central venous pressure, urine output, and hematocrit are measured every hour initially, and every 2 to 4 hours thereafter until the patient's condition becomes stable. Urinary output should remain between 20 and 50 ml/hr in adults, and mean arterial pressure should remain above 80 mm Hg. If the mean arterial pressure is below 80 mm Hg or if the urine output is less than 20 ml/m²/hr, the infusion rate is increased until these parameters are improved, or until the central venous pressure is 10 cm $H_2O$ or the pulmonary artery diastolic pressure is 20 cm $H_2O$. The hematocrit is a valuable index of plasma loss in the burn patient. The hemato-

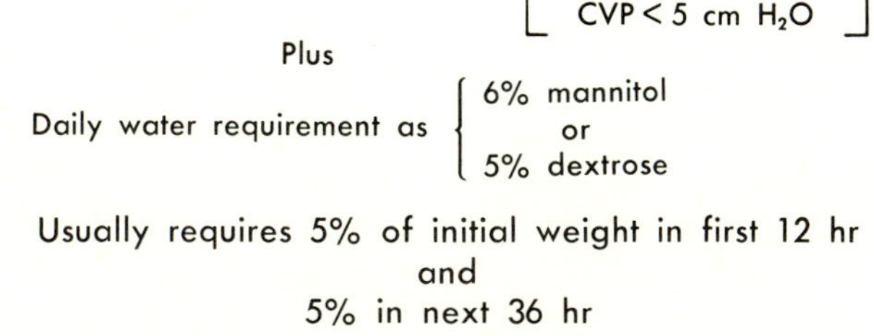

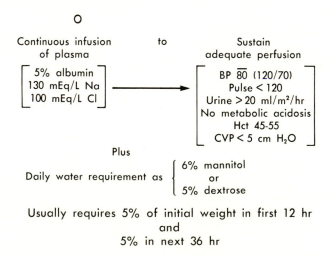


**Fig. 21-5.** University of California Irvine Medical Center burn "formula."

crit should be carefully followed and maintained between 40% and 50% with plasma infusion. A rapidly dropping hematocrit during resuscitation is usually a sign of excessive plasma infusion and is treated by slowing the infusion, not by transfusion of blood. Some red blood cells are lost in the presence of burn injury but generally not enough to require a transfusion.

The relationship between the blood volume and cardiac function is monitored by estimating perfusion by the criteria just mentioned and measuring central venous or right atrial pressure. The patient should be in normal acid-base status without metabolic acidosis. Usually the severely burned patient will have a moderate respiratory alkalosis. If metabolic acidosis exists, it should be treated with sodium bicarbonate or tromethamine (THAM) buffer, followed promptly by a more rapid infusion of plasma substitute.

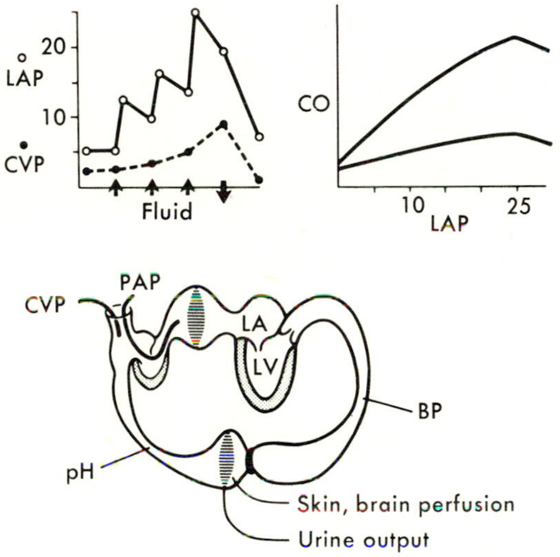


**Fig. 21-6.** Central venous and pulmonary artery pressure monitoring.

Pulmonary artery pressure monitoring[5] provides a much more sensitive index of blood volume and cardiac function relationships than central venous pressure monitoring. Pulmonary artery pressure monitoring should be instituted in any patient who remains hypotensive or acidotic while on an appropriate fluid replacement regimen or in any patient who has signs of myocardial depression with central venous pressure above 10 cm $H_2O$. The relationships between pulmonary artery and central venous pressure monitoring are shown in Fig. 21-6, and interpretation of the pulmonary artery pulse contour as a guide to fluid management is shown in Fig. 21-7. It is suggested that correct fluid resuscitation is usually associated with a central venous pressure of 0 to 5 cm $H_2O$; central venous pressure over 10 cm $H_2O$ is usually associated with left ventricular failure and pulmonary edema accumulation.

Water with 5% dextrose in solution should be infused to replace insensible water losses, which will usually be excessive if the burn surface is wet and exudative. Occlusive

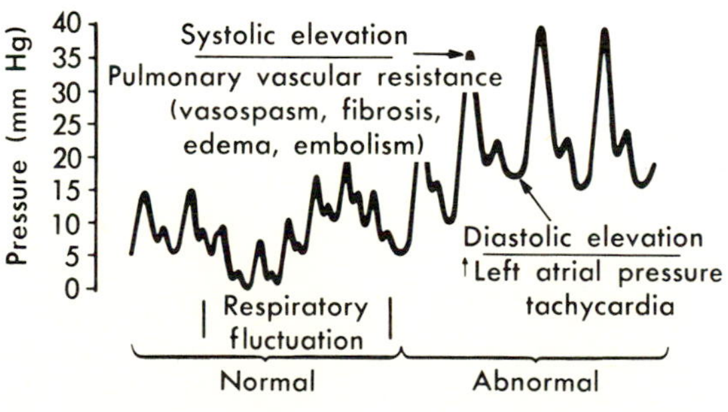


**Fig. 21-7.** Pulmonary artery pressure interpretation. (From German, J. C., Allyn, P. A., and Bartlett, R. H.: Arch. Surg. **106:**788, 1973.)

dressings minimize surface evaporation to some extent. The water requirement for an adult will be approximately 2000 ml/day. The water requirement for a child or infant can be calculated as 1000 ml/$m^2$ of body surface area or as three fourths of the estimated blood volume. Electrolytes should be infused if electrolyte solution is lost through vomiting, diarrhea, or nasogastric tube suction. Initially there may be hemoglobin or myoglobin in the plasma from hemolysis and muscle destruction. In this case, infusion of a diuretic drug is instituted to attempt to prevent acute renal failure secondary to pigment casts. In general the insensible water loss is replaced with 5% mannitol solution during the first 24 hours if pigment is present in the serum or urine. Mannitol, ethacrynic acid, or furosemide may also be used. There is no need for additional diuretic drugs. The urine output is such a valuable monitor of fluid replacement and perfusion that artificially changing the volume or composition of the urine with potent diuretics is not a wise practice. Fluid management continues with the previously mentioned parameters in mind until capillary integrity is reestablished and spontaneous diuresis occurs, usually 48 to 72 hours after the burn. If the fluid is reabsorbed from the burn area, renal function must be excellent to prevent hypervolemia.

## ■ How is renal damage in the burn patient detected and managed?

Although cardiac output may fall early after burn injury, properly managed fluid resuscitation will avoid classic acute tubular necrosis in virtually every case. If fluid resuscitation is inadequate for any reason and acute tubular necrosis does occur, it may present as anuric or polyuric renal failure. In either case, renal damage is best detected by abnormalities of urinary electrolytes, so that all urine is saved in 24-hour intervals for the first 3 days after the burn has occurred. In this way urinary electrolytes and urea can be present with the stress of the burn. Urinary sodium levels will be less than 10 mEq/L and urinary potassium levels higher than 60 mEq/L. Urine urea levels should be 10 to 20 times the blood urea. If the urinary sodium concentration is over 50 mEq/L, and the potassium concentration is under 20 mEq/L, renal tubular damage is present.

When renal failure does occur following burn injury, it is usually associated with hemolysis or muscle destruction. When fourth-degree burns are suspected, induced diuresis with mannitol or furosemide should be instituted.

When renal failure occurs in burn patients secondary to pigment load, acute tubular necrosis, or relative renal insufficiency with normal urine volume, renal function should be replaced or augmented with dialysis. Peritoneal dialysis can be carried out, but hemodialysis is preferred. As soon as the diagnosis of renal failure is made, an arteriovenous shunt should be placed, preferably through nonburned tissue to permit securing of the shunt. Daily dialysis may be instituted and carried out for 6 to 8 hours prior to tubbing and debriding daily. The use of vigorous hemodialysis in the five massively burned patients at Orange County Medical Center prolonged life in three patients to the point where grafting was possible. Only 22 cases of dialysis treatment of renal failure in burned patients have been reported in the literature (including the five cases just cited) with four survivors.[6]

### *Technical considerations in dialysis*

Aggressive hemodialysis in the massively burned patient requires the assemblage and coordination of a team of medical, nursing, and allied critical care personnel. Hemodialysis is definitely preferable to peritoneal dialysis, except in small children. A standard silicone rubber shunt may be placed in any available extremity, usually in an area of burn eschar. Because of the quality of the tissue, great care must be taken to avoid dislodging the shunt during dialysis, hydrotherapy, and dressing changes. Burn patients exhibit definitely hypercoagulable signs during the second and third week following the burn injury, and clotting of the venous limb of the shunt is a common complication, resulting in many revisions. The shunt is commonly used to infuse hypertonic glucose solutions during hyperalimentation. Infection around the shunt or septicemia from the shunt has not been a problem. The treatment protocol may include daily tubbing in a Hubbard tank containing water and chlorine bleach and cleaning the burn surfaces with Betadine solution. The surface should be dressed with antibiotics (mafenide acetate [Sulfamylon Cream] or silver sulfadiazine). The shunt area should be thoroughly washed and redressed daily, along with the rest of the burn area.

On the few occasions where arteriovenous hemodialysis has resulted in sustained hypotension in a patient with precarious hemodynamic status, venovenous dialysis has been achieved by the passage of a large catheter into the inferior vena cava for outflow with a peripheral vein used as a return route. It is easy to achieve flows of 200 to 300 ml/min with this technique and hypotension does not result, but the large caval catheter cannot be left in position and must be replaced with each dialysis.

Hemodialysis flows of 200 to 300 ml/min may be used, usually with ultrafiltration and regional heparinization. The patient should be weighed daily after dialysis, with all dressings off, and prior to hydrotherapy. Weight loss during dialysis should be monitored by the use of a bed scale. It is easiest to begin dialysis early in the morning and continue until 1 or 2 P.M. The patient is usually mentally and physiologically most stable immediately after dialysis, at which time all dressings should be removed and the patient tubbed, debrided, redressed, and returned to bed. Bleeding with dressing and débridement has been less following dialysis than when dialysis is done after débridement. As in any high mortality group of patients, one of the most important aspects of patient care is the maintenance of enthusiasm and optimism among the treatment team.

## ■ What pulmonary complications may be anticipated in the burn patient?

Pulmonary complications are the most common cause of death in burn patients. For example, in a series of 100 patients reviewed in the Orange County Medical Center burn unit in 1971 and 1972, 22 had pulmonary complications, and 19 of these patients died. This 20% incidence and 86% mortality associated with pulmonary complications is typical of results from other units. The factors in the pathogenesis of pulmonary complications are outlined in Fig. 21-8. Exogenous factors (primarily smoke inhalation) and endogenous factors (circulating myocardial depressants and other humoral factors) combine to produce alveolar collapse and increased interstitial water in the lung. This results in hypoxemia and decreased functional residual capacity and further complicates peripheral perfusion. The edematous lung is susceptible to infection, and bacterial pneumonitis is a common fatal complication.

Lung damage from smoke inhalation is caused by the toxic effects of volatile vapors from completely burned materials on the respiratory epithelium and alveoli. These vapors, which include formaldehyde and other aldehydes and ketones, are formed when wood, upholstery, paint, etc. burn. Lung damage occurs when the fumes are inhaled over a prolonged period of time. Consequently, pulmonary damage from smoke inhalation occurs in patients who have been in fires in enclosed spaces. The best indicator of smoke inhalation is the presence of soot in the sputum, and this may persist for several days. Carboxyhemoglobin may indicate the severity of smoke inhalation if measured soon after the injury.

Smoke inhalation alone carries a high mortality from brain death secondary to hypoxia or overwhelming pulmonary insufficiency in the first few hours. The patient who survives a smoke inhalation injury more than 12 hours has a good prognosis. Smoke inhalation in association with any surface burn creates more serious pulmonary problems than smoke inhalation or burn alone.

Endogenous pulmonary damage from inadvertent fluid overload may be minimized

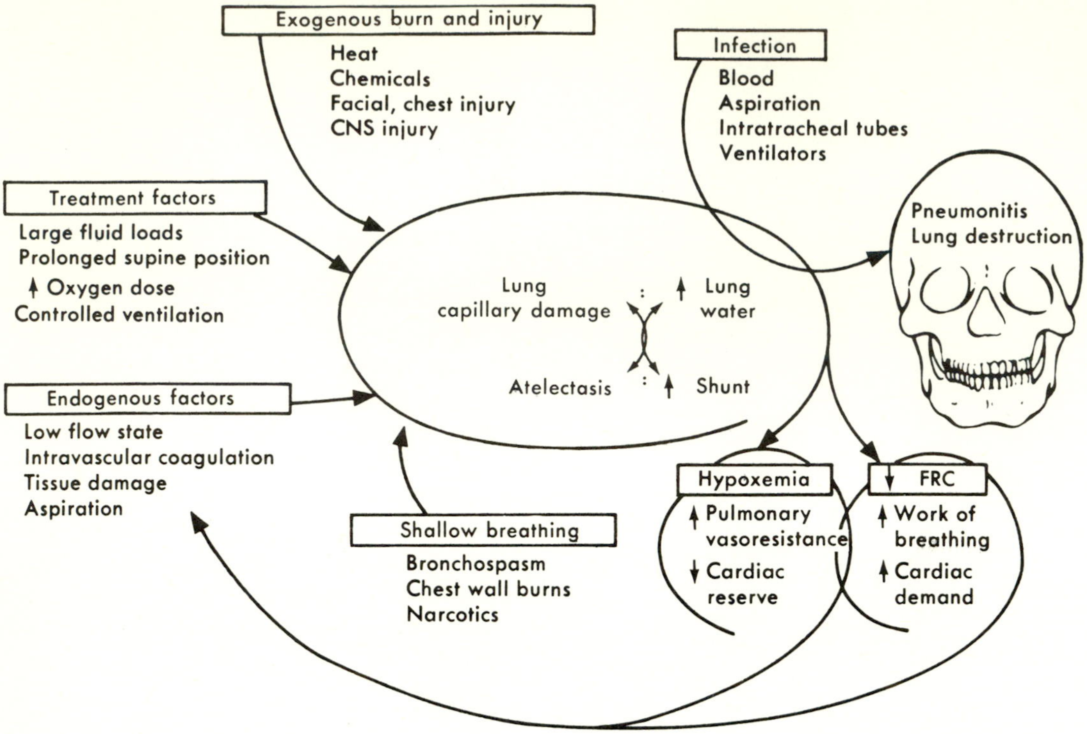


**Fig. 21-8.** Pathogenesis of pulmonary insufficiency. (Modified from Achauer, B. M., et al.: Ann. Surg. **177**:311, 1973.)

by using colloid solution for resuscitation and by using pulmonary artery pressure as a guide to fluid replacement as previously outlined. Avoiding endotoxin in the bloodstream by debriding eschar and keeping the surface clean and avoiding low-flow states with potential intravascular coagulation and lysosomal enzyme release are also important in preventing pulmonary capillary damage and myocardial depression. Circulating myocardial depressants have been identified in burned skin, and this may add to interstitial pulmonary edema.

Pulmonary complications secondary to upper airway obstruction from burn edema itself are managed by intubation of the trachea through the nose or the mouth for the 4 or 5 days during the edematous phase. Tracheostomy is usually not necessary to relieve upper airway obstruction. Management with a mechanical ventilator is also unnecessary for the patient with upper airway obstruction.

The best guide to pulmonary parenchymal damage is arterial $P_{O_2}$ at a known concentration of oxygen in inspired air ($F_{I_{O_2}}$). Hypoxemia during air breathing may be the only sign of impending pulmonary damage early after the burn. Chest x-ray films are usually normal during the first 24 hours. Progressive hypoxemia is one of the indications for mechanical ventilation with lung parenchymal damage. An indwelling arterial catheter should be placed in all patients whose history or blood gas concentrations suggest impending pulmonary complications, and intubation with mechanical ventilation is instituted when indicated. The use of intentional dehydration with diuretics and positive end-expiratory pressure is helpful in smoke inhalation syndrome. Large doses of corticosteroids may be given to the smoke inhalation patient to minimize edema and humoral damage to lung capillaries, although the value of this medication has not been definitely proved.

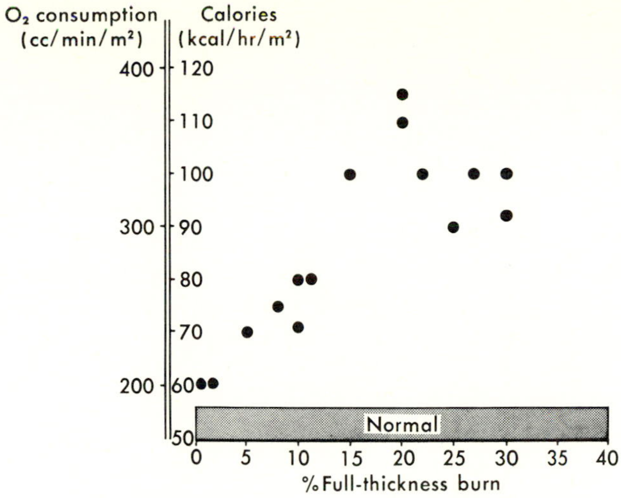


**Fig. 21-9.** Caloric expenditure vs full thickness burn.

Using the principles of recognition, prevention, and management, the incidence of pulmonary complications in the University of California Irvine Medical Center burn unit has decreased to 15%, with an overall mortality of 50%.

## ■ What nutritional and metabolic management modalities should be considered?

Burn injury imposes a hypermetabolic catabolic state with increased caloric expenditure and rapid wasting of fat and lean body mass. The patient with a moderate burn can lose 10% of body weight in a period of 2 to 3 weeks. Patients who rapidly lose 15% to 20% of body weight reach a state of energy crisis characterized by hypothermia, bradycardia, coma, and hyponatremia that has a high mortality rate if not promptly treated with calories. The hypermetabolic state has been related to heat loss as a result of water evaporation from the surface.[9] Water loss through burn or eschar reaches a level two to three times the amount of water loss through intact skin. This is minimized by the occlusive dressings that are used in our unit. The complications of desiccation evaporation (hypernatremia, rising hematocrit, and intense thirst) are not seen in our patients. Studies by Zawacki[10] and other investigators have shown that when water loss is totally eliminated by occlusive plastic dressings, the hypermetabolic state persists. The hypermetabolic state seems to be related to the extent and the depth of the burn and is associated with high catecholamine levels and high steroid levels. In patients who are not septic this hypermetabolism reaches an extreme two times the baseline level.

Although some have considered that the hypermetabolic state always occurred and was attended with lean tissue loss, this is not necessarily the case. In a recent study measuring caloric expenditure by indirect calorimetry, it was found that weight loss could be prevented and could, in fact, be promoted during the healing phase of burn injury by meeting the caloric expenditure on a day-to-day basis. Normal caloric expenditure is 40 to 55 calories/m$^2$/hr. In burn patients a caloric intake of at least 100 calories/m$^2$/hr should be assured by oral intake, tube feeding, or occasionally by IV nutrition. This should be accompanied with careful measurement of body weight daily. If the patient loses weight on this regimen, indirect calorimetry should be carried out and actual caloric expenditure calculated.

Higher metabolic rates are associated with a larger percentage of burn and with the amount of third-degree burn. Caloric intake is calculated daily, and if the intake falls behind caloric expenditure on oral intake, a nasogastric feeding tube should be passed and tube feedings added. The tube feeding may be formulated by a hospital dietary department and should have a milk and meat base. The caloric strength can be varied from ¾ to 1½ calories/ml. If caloric requirements cannot be met by oral intake and gastric tube feeding, IV nutrition may be instituted using 10% Intralipid by a peripheral vein or 25% glucose by a central venous catheter. Both of these IV caloric substrates should be supplemented with 5% amino acid solution as a nitrogen source. The average caloric expenditure between the first and third weeks of burn management from this study is illustrated in Fig. 21-9. These charts can be used to estimate caloric expenditure based on total body surface burn or, better, on percent of full-thickness burn.

Maintaining good nutrition, particularly positive caloric and nitrogen balance, is essential in achieving survival and satisfactory healing in all extensively burned patients. Appetite is poor in burn patients, and almost every patient with burn covering 50% or more of total body surface will require tube feedings.

## ■ What changes in coagulation and platelet mechanisms may be anticipated in the burn patient?

Extensive changes in coagulation and platelet mechanisms occur in burn patients. These changes were not widely recognized and were incompletely studied until recently. In a recent report[12] detailed studies of coagulation, platelet count and function, and fibrinolysis were made in 11 extensively burned patients.

Hemostasis is normally accomplished by a series of enzyme reactions involving the soluble protein clotting factors and ending in the formation of fibrin, as well as the adhesion and aggregation of platelets, forming a platelet plug. Fibrin clots contain plasminogen, which becomes activated to plasmin, a fibrinolytic enzyme, and destroys fibrin, resulting in fibrin degradation products (FDP). Partial thromboplastin time, prothrombin time, and thrombin time are screening tests that cover clotting factors I to XII. The changes that occur in clotting factors after burn injury with colloid resuscitation include a drop in clotting factor level (manifested as a rise in screening test time) occurring during the first 24 to 48 hours following burn injury. This is primarily caused by dilution with the fluid used for resuscitation. Factor VIII is manufactured by the liver in response to stress, and its level rises during this period. The clotting factors gradually increase thereafter, reaching normal or supernormal levels associated with shorter screening test times, so that the burn patient exhibits hypercoagulable signs between the second and fourth weeks following burn. The drop in clotting factors does not reach clinically significant levels in these patients. Fibrinolysin (plasminogen-plasmin) activity is not elevated in burn patients, and FDP levels remain normal (essentially absent) throughout the course of burn injury.

The most significant changes occur in platelet count and function, as shown in Fig. 21-10. Platelet count drops following burn injury, partly as a result of dilution and partly from other mechanisms that remain to be determined. The platelet count reaches the lowest level on the second or third day following burn and is associated with platelet malfunction (thrombocytopathia) at the same time. Any surgical procedure carried out during this time may encounter severe bleeding typical of thrombocytopenia and thrombocytopathia, that is, gradual continued oozing that stops with cautery or direct pressure and starts again within an hour and is unresponsive to further mechanical efforts at control. This type of bleeding can cause exsanguinating hemorrhage but is misleading because of the slow continuous oozing nature of the bleeding. When this type of bleeding occurs, it must be treated with platelet concentrates or fresh blood with active platelets. Platelet count returns to normal by the end of the first week and is above normal from the second to the fifth week following burn injury.

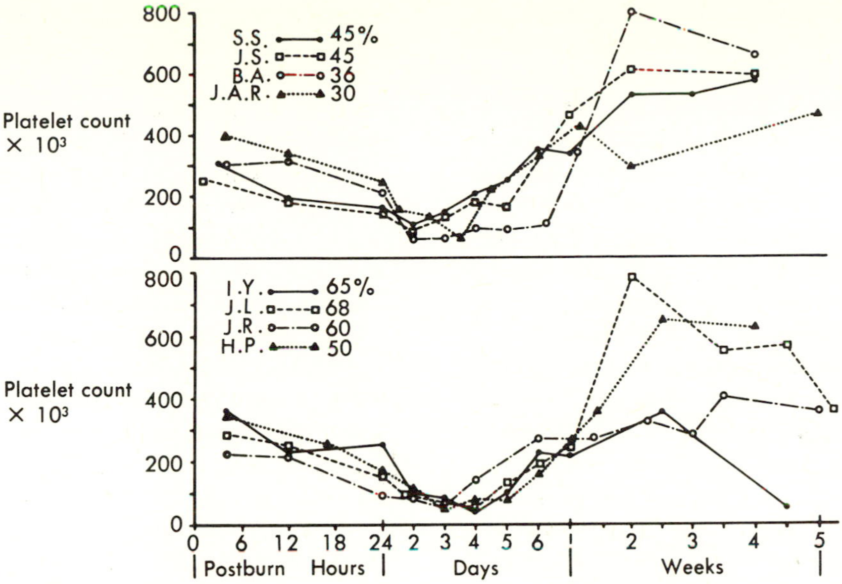


**Fig. 21-10.** Platelet concentration in burned patients.

Hence if surgical procedures are required early in the course of mangement, they should be done within the first 24 hours, if possible, or delayed until the platelet count has begun to rise. Rising platelet count is associated with a return of normal platelet function. The use of fresh-frozen plasma, vitamin K, or other efforts aimed at supporting clotting factors are unnecessary maneuvers. Since there is no evidence of consumption coagulopathy as such, heparin therapy is contraindicated. During the late healing phase and at the time of grafting the patient's blood is truly hypercoagulable; granulating beds that are debrided are commonly seen to clot very promptly. Thromboembolic phenomena, however, are exceedingly rare in burn patients. The mechanism of thrombocytopenia and the role of platelet-active durgs in the prevention of thrombocytopenia are under investigation. If gram-negative septicemia occurs in a burn patient, thrombocytopenia will result, and this is a good guide to sepsis. One patient in the series mentioned previously developed thrombocytopenia associated with *Klebsiella* septicemia from a septic thrombophlebitis. This is also the only patient (I. Y.) who showed a delayed drop in platelet count in Fig. 21-10.

Thrombocytopenia per se should not be treated unless associated with significant bleeding. The prophylactic administration of platelets simply because the count is low is not indicated and is in fact contraindicated, as platelet antibodies may develop.

Blood transfusion is required frequently in the management of burn patients, particularly when active surface eschar excision is carried out. The average requirement of a patient burned over 50% of the body is 10 to 20 units of blood during hospitalization.

## ■ What should be known about immunology and reticuloendothelial function in the burn patient?

Host defense mechanisms against bacteria, fungus, or viral infection must be maintained in the burn patient. Reticuloendothelial function, including phagocytosis, bacterial clearance, and bacterial killing by circulating white cells and tissue histiocytes, has been extensively studied in burn patients. Severe leukocytosis in the range of 20,000 to 50,000/mm³ (primarily with polymorphonuclear leukocytes and monocytes) is common in extensively burned patients.

Serum immunologic factors follow patterns similar to serum clotting factors, with initial depression followed by return to normal and maintenance of normal or slightly elevated levels throughout the course of treatment. This includes the study of immunoglobulins, complement, and antibody responses. Cellular immunologic responses in the form of lymphocyte physiology have been studied by Munster and associates[14] and others. They show a predominance of $\beta$-lymphocytes following burn injury with significant alteration in cellular immunity.

The supplementation of immune responses by bacterial vaccines or passive immunization with hyperimmune serum has been extensively investigated in burn patients, particularly with regard to *Pseudomonas aeruginosa.* This line of investigation has not been pursued in the Orange County Medical Center burn unit, as septicemia is exceedingly rare (three to four instances per year) and is usually associated with diverse organisms among which no particular endemic strain predominates. In fact, studies related to sepsis in general, rare new opportunistic organisms, methods of surface bacterial counting, wound biopsy, and control of surface sepsis with biologic dressings have all been unnecessary, because surface infection and systemic infection simply do not occur. This is primarily the result of maintaining adequate nutrition, as mentioned previously, and maintaining a clean burn surface, as mentioned subsequently.

### ■ What gastrointestinal management modalities should be considered?

Patients with extensive burns develop ileus for the first day or two following burn injury, and a nasogastric tube should be utilized with all burn patients for gastric suction during this time. One or two hourly instillations of antacid may be carried out during the acute period, followed by the placement of antacid or food in the stomach at least every hour during the remainder of the course of extensively burned patients. As soon as peristalsis returns, as evidenced by active bowel sounds and passage of stool or flatus, feeding is begun, preferably directly by mouth or by nasogastric tube if the patient cannot eat. Occasionally ileus may complicate later phases of burn management, and this is managed by nasogastric suction. Rarely bleeding may occur from the gastric mucosa, which is evidenced by occult blood–positive gastric aspirate. Extensive bleeding should be unusual, and gastric bleeding requiring transfusion or operation is rare. In many adult burn units stress ulcer with burn injury (Curling's ulcer) is a common occurrence.[16] Lack of Curling's ulcer in some burn units may be associated with the frequent instillation of antacid or food into the stomach and the lack of sepsis. The best treatment for massively bleeding stress ulcers in other patients may be extensive subtotal or total gastrectomy.

Pancreatitis has complicated burn management in four patients at the Orange County Medical Center, all of whom were extensively burned patients with very deep burns. Pancreatitis has occurred late in the course of management and has been associated with deep muscle necrosis, ileus, and peritonitis. This complication was lethal in two of the four patients involved. The etiology is unknown. Pancreatitis should be considered in patients with extensive burn injury, ileus, and peritoneal findings.

### ■ What CNS and neuropsychiatric management modalities should be considered?

"Burn encephalopathy" has been described and is usually associated with sepsis, hypoxia, smoke inhalation, shock, or hyponatremia. A toxin in burned skin has been described that may alter brain capillary permeability.[17] Abnormal CNS function is common in major burn patients and ranges from confusion and disorientation to stupor, seizures, and coma. This encephalopathy is usually not associated with septicemia and the exact cause is unknown. This metabolic encephalopathy is totally reversible and essentially never leaves organic sequelae.

Reversible peripheral neuropathies have been reported following burn injury, and muscle weakness is a common complaint. Weakness usually occurs in directly burned and grafted areas; the exact cause is difficult to delineate.

Psychiatric and psychologic management plays a major part in burn patient care. Many burn patients have psychologic disorders before burn injury, in fact, causing burn injury. These include senility, chronic brain syndrome, alcoholism and its sequelae, drug abuse and its sequelae, and a variety of personality disorders. If the patient was not psychologically disturbed before burn injury, he may become so, particularly if the burn will be disabling or severely disfiguring. Every effort should be made to treat the burn patient as capable of total rehabilitation. Burn scars should be freely discussed but minimized, and the patient should be assured that reconstructive procedures will make the appearance acceptable. At the same time every patient should be cautioned that every burned area will result in scarring; his adjustment to this fact must begin early in the course of management. All the staff involved with the care of burn patients should be encouraged to participate in the psychologic care from the time of admission, primarily by this type of prophylaxis. The help of a psychiatrist is rarely necessary but extremely valuable on occasion.

## SURFACE MANAGEMENT

■ **What surface management is recommended?**

During the first week of hospitalization the wound itself is of secondary importance to physiologic considerations. However, the essence of burn care revolves around burn wound management. An interest in topical antibiotics and the use of total exposure treatment in the last two decades has diverted attention from aggressive mechanical care of the burn wound. It is recommended that appropriate burn unit protocol include the following: vigorous daily cleaning of the burn surface in a hydrotherapy tank, direct débridement, and tangential excision of eschar at frequent intervals followed by semiocclusive dressings. Use of this type of surface management virtually eliminates burn wound sepsis so that patient isolation, precautionary procedures, and efforts at quantitating surface flora are unnecessary. As long as the surface is kept clean, the type of surface antibiotic used is relatively unimportant. The vehicle and ease of application become the major considerations. This type of surface management is continued until the entire burn surface is covered with healthy granulation tissue, at which time split-thickness skin grafting is done. This usually occurs 20 to 25 days after burn injury. Grafting may be done with a combination of postage stamp, mesh graft, and sheet graft techniques, and a 95% to 100% take may be expected with every grafting procedure.

The only satisfactory alternative method of surface care is immediate or early (first 5 days) excision of eschar down to viable tissue or fascia and immediate surface coverage either with autograft or skin substitute followed by autograft.[18] This approach has been evaluated from time to time, and it has been found to be a favorable one for only small burns (15% of body surface or less). Inadequate graft take (40% to 60%) in most early excisions merely results in a fresh wound that requires formation of granulation tissue before regrafting can be done. This results in no ultimate saving of time and the possible risks associated with a major operative procedure early in the patient's course. Satisfactory temporary skin coverage would make this surface management technique preferable to current methods. This method of surface care will become preferable when satisfactory skin substitutes are developed. Silicone membrane, homograft, and pigskin in this connection have all been found to be lacking.[19, 20] The use of true skin transplantation (homograft associated with pharmacologic immune suppression) after early excision has been satisfactorily carried out by Burke[21] in a few massively burned pediatric patients. Further evaluation of this radical procedure and continued evaluation of skin substitutes will eventually lead to early excision and coverage as a method of choice. Specific details in surface management protocol are outlined in Fig. 21-11.

Recommended protocol involves open

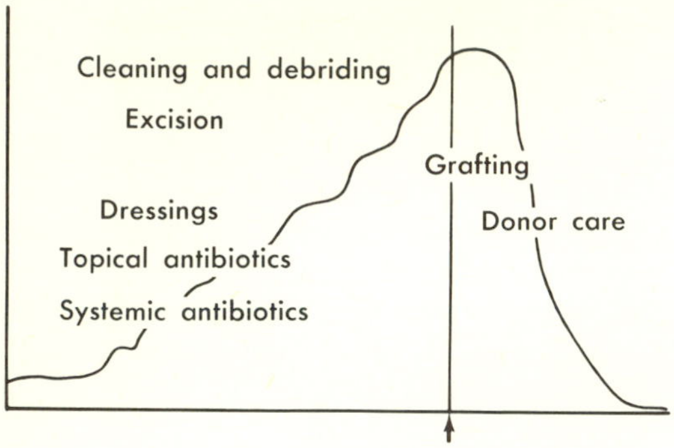


**Fig. 21-11.** Surface management.

wards without isolation precautions, cleaning and tubbing in water and hypochlorite solution carried out every day and pursued to the point of documented sterility after tubbing each day, excison of eschar beginning as soon as the platelet count is adequate and continued until a satisfactory granulating wound is obtained, and closed wounds with occlusive dressing using topical antibiotic cream, permitting the total mobility of patients.

### *Open wards*

The philosophy of open wards is possible because of adequate surface management and is very important in the physiologic and psychologic care of the patient. The only precautions are covering of street clothes with a gown when entering the burn unit and washing of hands between caring for each patient when the patients or bedside accoutrements are handled.

### *Cleaning*

Cleaning of the surface must be carried out at 24-hour intervals to be effective. Bacteria multiply in a logarithmic fashion and may reach levels capable of invasive infection if the surface is allowed to go more than 24 hours without vigorous cleaning and antiseptics. The burn surface is cleaned by immersion in water containing sodium hypochlorite solution (Clorox, in a ratio of 1:300 units of water). This amount of hypochlorite corresponds to 1 gallon per Hubbard tank, ½ gallon per small tank, or one glass per bathtub or large bucket. The hypochlorite destroys the bacteria it contacts and also coagulates proteins on the surface to facilitate cleaning and removal. After immersion in the warm hypochlorite tub for 10 to 20 minutes the surface should be actively cleaned by scrubbing with a soft cloth using Betadine solution. The surface should be cleaned until all protein exudate has been removed from the surface, and eschar, debrided deep dermal or fat tissue, or granulation tissue is exposed. This is commonly associated with a small amount of bleeding. Loose necrotic tissue, if present, should be removed by sharp débridement; this may be done without anesthesia but does require heavy narcotic dosage on a daily basis. Every patient should be cleaned in this fashion every day, regardless of the extent of the burn. Rarely, a massively burned patient or smoke inhalation patient with unstable pulmonary or hemodynamic status may be cleaned in bed, but this is difficult. Patients should be submerged in the hypochlorite tub with central venous catheters, fresh incisions, all manner of open wounds, fractures, chest tubes, arterial catheters, tracheostomy wounds, etc. It is interesting that osteomyelitis associated with the presence of skeletal pins and wound infection in fresh operative sites are virtually absent with this surface cleaning protocol.

### *Excision of eschar*

The excision of eschar should be begun as soon as adequate platelet count and function is assured (beginning on the fifth or sixth day following the burn) and carried out every 3 to 4 days until a satisfactory granulation surface is present. Excision may be carried out tangentially using hand-held dermatomes of the Weck, Goulian, or Campbell grafting knife variety. The first excision may be done without anesthesia and carried to the point of pain or bleeding. This is partly therapeutic but primarily diagnostic to identify areas of second- and third-degree burn. Major débridement is associated with bleeding and is never begun until a solid IV line is in place and blood is available.

Following this initial débridement, sub-

A

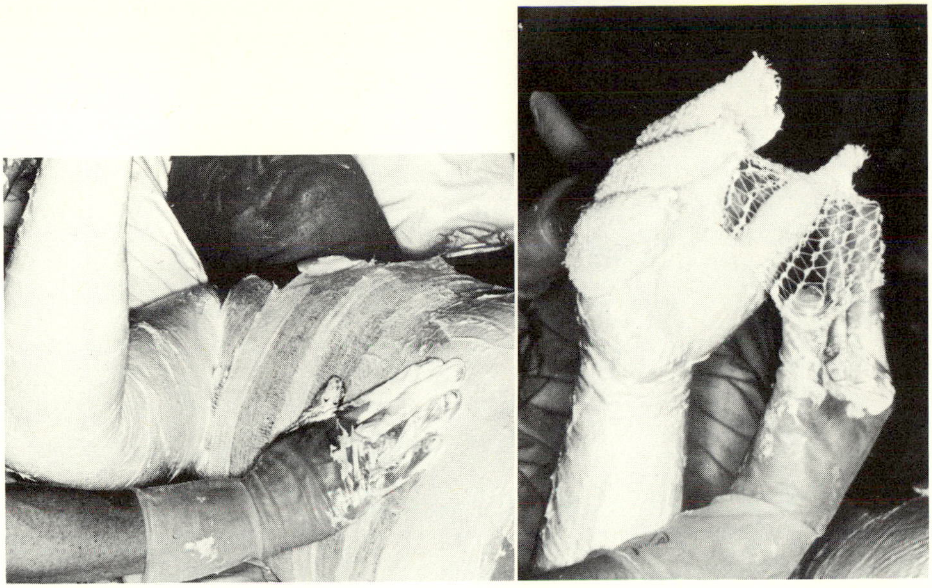

B

**Fig. 21-12.** Dressing technique.

sequent excisions may be carried out utilizing IM ketamine anesthesia in a dose of 3 to 4 mg/kg. *Ketamine* has greatly facilitated burn management and is used extensively. Gag and cough reflexes are preserved with ketamine anesthesia, the patient is semiresponsive, excessive muscle tone and posturing result, maintaining normal body temperature, and the drug can be administered to patients in the tub in any position. Over 1000 doses of ketamine anesthetic have been administered in this fashion to burn patients at University of California Irvine Medical Center with no significant physiologic complications. Psychologic complications in the form of "bad trips" or frightening nightmares occurred in 16% of patients initially. This has decreased to approximately 5% with the extensive use of diazepam (Valium) during induction and during emergence from ketamine anesthesia.

The tangential excision may be carried out in vigorous fashion down to fat or fascia where necessary, limited by the appearance of viability and bleeding. Major bleeding may be controlled with electrocautery carried out simultaneously with the débridement. Total hemostasis with cautery must be achieved before surface dressings are applied. The only significant complications that have followed this type of management have been those related to the underestimation of bleeding, causing hypovolemia with shock requiring fluid and blood transfusion for resuscitation.

### *Closed wounds*

Closed wounds may be achieved by the application of topical antibiotic cream dressings after tubbing. Dressing may be carried out by burn unit critical care staff. Antibiotic cream impregnated into fine-mesh gauze rolls should be applied to the surface. Supplemental antibiotic cream may be added to the surface lightly and the entire dressing held in place with an elastic netting (Surgifix) dressing. Care must be taken to avoid circumferential wrapping, particularly in the early phase, when edema is present. These techniques are illustrated in Fig. 21-12.

After dressings are applied patients should be encouraged to be up and around. Any patient who is satisfactorily ambulatory may be discharged home to return at 24-hour intervals for cleaning, tubbing, débridement, and re-dressing until the time of grafting. Burns covering up to 40% of the body may be primarily managed on an outpatient basis unless significant pulmonary, nutritional, metabolic, or social complications do not permit this management.

The type of topical antibiotic is not particularly important from a bacteriologic point of view as long as the surface is vigorously cleaned daily. Consequently, the material that has the best application characteristics without pain and is the most economical is the favored material. At present this is *silver sulfadiazine* (Silvadene), a hydrophilic cream containing 1% silver sulfadiazine that has good bactericidal properties and is not painful on application. Mafenide acetate (Sulfamylon Cream) has equal bactericidal properties and ease of applicability, but it is associated with a burning pain on application and may cause mild metabolic acidosis by carbonic anhydrase inhibition. The 1% *sodium sulfadiazine* solution may be prepared in the pharmacy and has good working characteristics and an adequate bactericidal activity, although it is not as good as silver sulfadiazine in this regard. Consequently, sodium sulfadiazine is recommended for use in small burns, on an outpatient basis, or in the treatment of major burns with open areas after grafting. Silver sulfadiazine and sodium sulfadiazine are virtually free of complications. Although skin sensitivity and rash have been reported, this has been observed in only three cases. *Candida albicans* and *Staphylococcus aureus* are commonly cultured from the surface in small amounts in patients treated with silver sulfadiazine. Gram-negative organisms are also found in patients treated with sodium sulfadiazine. This topical colonizing flora is insignificant, does not cause invasive infection, and is not specifically treated until the time of grafting.

*Betadine* ointment has good bactericidal properties and causes mild burning on application but is in a gel base that is difficult to manage. It becomes liquid at body temperature and runs freely from the surface, staining linen and personnel. *Neosporin* has caused deafness in some patients and should not be used for topical burn care. *Furacin* is readily available, painless on application, and moderately inexpensive. It is associated with a 10% to 30% skin sensitivity and is not recommended for use for that reason. The use of *0.5% silver nitrate solution,* reapplied frequently to gauze dressings, has been practiced in many institutions. This is an excellent bactericidal agent but forms a black silver chloride precipitate on virtually all surfaces with which it comes in contact. Consequently, it is unpopular as a topical agent. Use of this material may be associated with marked electrolyte abnormalities. A comparison of various antibiotic preparations is shown in Table 21-2.

**Table 21-2.** Topical antibiotic preparations

| *Preparation* | *Cost/ 100 g* | *Cost/day (adult, 50% burn)** |
|---|---|---|
| Mafenide (Sulfamylon Cream) in 454 g jar | $1.49 | $14.90 (2.2 pounds) |
| Silver sulfadiazine (Silvadene) in 400 g jar | $2.60 | $26.00 (2.2 pounds) |
| Betadine ointment in 454 g jar | $2.40 | $54.40 (5 pounds) |
| Furacin ointment in 2270 g jar | $0.95 | $9.50 (2.2 pounds) |
| Neosporin in 15 g tube† | $6.34 | |

*1975 prices.
†Not used for large burns.

## ■ How is a granulating wound managed?

After eschar is removed granulation tissue begins to form on the surface. Commonly a period of several days exists wherein healthy granulation tissue is present, associated with remnants of eschar, coagulated dermis, exposed muscle, bone, tendon, or fat. During this time the granulation tissue may be managed with a topical antibiotic dressing along with the rest of the surface, as described previously. This keeps the granulation area clean and free from invasive infection. The surface will remain healthy if nutrition is good. Skin grafting may be carried out when the entire surface is ready. The use of human homograft skin,[22] banked frozen homograft skin,[23] fresh xenograft (pig) skin, and frozen radiated banked xenograft skin[24] is advocated in many other centers. All these techniques of management of the granulating wound have been evaluated and found to be equal or inferior to the dressings previously outlined. Skin prostheses such as silicone rubber membrane and collagen membrane have been extensively evaluated and are not significantly better than gauze dressings alone. Eventually a skin prosthesis will be available that has good adherence and bactericidal properties. At that time this material will be the preferred management for granulating wounds.

The granulation tissue can be managed in this fashion for as long as 3 or 4 weeks if necessary. This is required only when a burn cannot be completely covered at the time of the initial grafting (burns greater than 40% of body surface area). Granulation tissue dressed in conventional fashion for longer than 1 month becomes progressively fibrotic associated with poor blood supply, a pale firm appearance, and a fascia-like appearance when scraped and debrided. This "hypermature" granulation tissue can be avoided by periodic débridement of the granulation tissue by mechanical means or the use of topical 1% silver nitrate.

After skin grafting the areas of granulation tissue are commonly left between postage stamp grafts or interstices in mesh grafts. These areas may be managed by the techniques just outlined with daily vigorous removal of protein transudate from the surface.

## ■ What factors should be considered when grafting is required?

The philosophy of grafting techniques should be to achieve total autogenous skin coverage at the earliest possible time. This should be done in the interest of patient survival and may sometimes be done at the expense of late cosmetic results but never at the expense of functional result. For example, in a patient with third-degree burns of hands, face, and all of both legs, the legs would be grafted first to achieve surface coverage and survival, with hands and face taking second priority. With surface management as outlined above, grafting would usually be carried out between 20 and 25 days after the burn, permitting grafting of hands and face 1 to 2 weeks later. This policy does not result in severe disfigurement or disability problems. The postage stamp method used for most grafting results in a checkerboard appearance. In general, however, the cosmetic late results of stamp grafting compare favorably with sheet or mesh grafting and the advantages of the technique as outlined subsequently warrant its use.

After considering the priority of surface to be covered, the next consideration is to achieve the surface coverage rapidly. It is recommended that no more than 2 hours be spent in the operating room performing a grafting procedure (except for the hands or face, which may require longer). Approximately 30% to 40% of the body surface area may be covered with graft at a single sitting in 2 hours with an expectation that 95% to 100% will take in every patient.

## ■ How should donor sites be managed?

It is recommended that split-thickness skin graft ranging from 0.008 inch in small children to 0.012 inch in adults be used. These thin grafts promote good surface takes. Over hands and face thicker grafts may be used (up to 0.014). After skin is taken from the donor site the surface should be allowed to clot by exposure to air. Material to be applied to the donor site should be saturated with blood to allow fibrin to mesh into its surface. Clots should be gently wiped off and the donor site material (thin silicone membrane at present) applied to the surface. This may be held in place with tape if extensive turning is required. Donor site covers should be rolled where necessary to eliminate transudate. They should be left in place until the donor site heals and the material falls off spontaneously. If donor site coverages are rubbed off in the process of extensive turning and grafting, silicone membrane may be replaced or dressing with silver sulfadiazine instituted. Donor sites provide excellent models of partial skin damage and are commonly used for studies of topical agents or skin substitutes. Although infection in donor sites is extremely unusual, these sites should be treated with topical cleaning when it does occur. Donor sites heal well in 7 to 10 days regardless of the method of management. The major consideration in selecting a dressing for donor sites is to leave the patient mobile and free of pain. Silicone membrane has the best characteristics in this regard.

### ■ What operating room policies should be considered?

Every patient undergoing skin grafting should be tubbed in hypochlorite solution prior to going to the operating room. All hair-bearing skin in areas of potential donor sites should be shaved in the tub at the same time. The burns should be topically washed with Betadine and wrapped in moist towels.

In the operating room the following equipment is necessary for all burn grafting: heating blanket on the bed, temperature sensor in the patient, at least one good IV line for major grafting, and ECG monitoring. Ketamine anesthesia associated with diazepam (Valium) is recommended, and narcotics and nitrous oxide may be given at the discretion of the anesthesiologist. Endotracheal intubation is never necessary despite extensive turning and revision of position. Temperature must be followed carefully. Blood loss should be followed primarily by pulse rate or blood pressure where appropriate, although in many patients the blood pressure cannot be measured because of the lack of an available site. Often the task of an extensive grafting appears to be so massive that the novice surgeon is frozen into immobility. All members of the grafting team must be exhorted to continue to participate rapidly in the various procedures in order to achieve a short time for the patient to be under anesthesia.

After grafting is completed and the grafts are held in place with nylon netting or sutures, the patient may be returned directly to the burn unit. Grafts and/or donor sites on extremities should have topical pressure applied by firm Kerlix gauze wrapping immediately after grafting; this should be left in place overnight and carefully removed the next day. Wrapping should never be placed over unprotected graft or over hands or face, and wrapping is not practical on the trunk.

Extra donor skin that is removed in the operating room and not required for grafting should be placed in saline solution with antibiotics and refrigerated for possible future use. This skin may be used up to 1 week following grafting for application to granulating areas. In general the preservative solution is prepared with 1 g of cephalothin (Keflin)/L of saline solution.

### ■ How is late surface care managed?

After grafting, the mesh and sheet grafts should be cared for by frequent (every 4 hours) pressure with cotton-tipped applicators to eliminate any transudate or exudate. Grafts should be left exposed to the air during this period. Collections under grafts should be aspirated or removed through small incisions. Sheet grafts and mesh grafts should be left exposed at all times except on those rare occasions when stents are used, in which case the grafts should be left exposed beginning 48 hours after grafting. Rolling and cleaning of the surface by the critical care unit staff should be carried out until the grafts are firmly adherent (3 to 5 days). On the third or fourth day the patient may be gently dipped in the hypochlorite tub without vigorous cleaning. On the fifth day all netting and rubber covers may be gently removed. On the sixth or seventh day the use of closed dressings with silver or sodium sulfadiazine may be reinstituted if there are any open areas on the surface.

As soon as the surface is completely covered with skin, light gauze and elastic wraps may be applied to all grafts on extremities and mobility encouraged. When total surface coverage has been achieved, the patient should be measured for elastic pressure garments over grafted or healed second-degree burn areas. Elastic wraps should be continued until that time to maintain pressure on the burns, to mold collagen into a flat pattern, and to protect the delicate new epithelium.

The healed second-degree or grafted third-degree surface always itches and has varying degrees of pain. Itching may be treated with antihistamines (diphenhydramine [Benadryl] or hydroxyzine [Atarax]), and pain may usually be adequately treated by topical pressure. The healed surface always proceeds through a period of hypertrophy of scar with rapidly proliferating collagen and fibroblasts below the epithelium, resulting in a raised, erythematous, itchy, and hyperesthetic surface. This process continues for 4 to 6 months following the burn, then gradually regresses over the ensuing year as fibrosis eliminates the capillary bed in hypertrophic scar. Hypertrophic scarring can be minimized by topical application of pressure as outlined subsequently. All patients should be cautioned that hypertrophic scarring will inevitably occur. Resurfacing or reconstructive procedures are contraindicated until prompted by joint deformity or psychologic disability. The surface becomes dry very easily, and the patient should be advised to use lanolin ointment on the surface to maintain lubrication.

## FUNCTIONAL MANAGEMENT

### ■ What functional management modalities should be considered?

Cases in which the patient survives a major burn but becomes a physical or social cripple should not occur. Proper functional management, as outlined in Fig. 21-13, will prevent this situation. Functional management in the acute phase is as essential a part of critical care as physiologic monitoring or surface cleaning.

### *Prophylaxis*

***Joint function.*** The prevention of contracture deformity requires meticulous attention to detail. Characteristically the burn patient

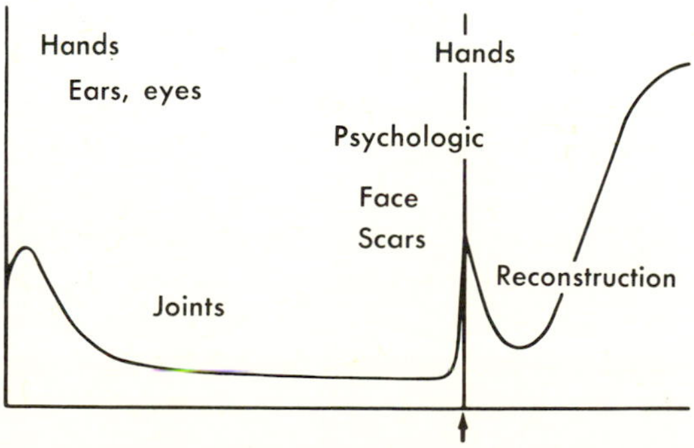


**Fig. 21-13.** Functional management.

attempts to maintain a fetal-like position, one of flexion and adduction. This position must be assiduously avoided, as it leads to contracture. The major concern is with those patients who have burns that cross the flexor surface of the joint or that are lateral to this surface. Efforts toward preventing disabling contractures should begin on admission to the burn unit with proper positioning and splinting.

***Hand.*** Splints should be fabricated and applied, even if the patient's fingers have been pinned.

***Elbows.*** Elbows should be placed in full extension and supination. If this position is difficult to maintain, extension splints may be necessary.

***Neck.*** Deformities of the neck are severely disabling and great care should be taken to prevent such contractures. The neck should be positioned in hyperextension. *No pillows should be used!* A crib mattress placed on top of a regular mattress with the head over the edge of the crib mattress is a good method for positioning. An isoprene neck conformer may be fabricated and applied as soon as the edema decreases. This device should be worn essentially 24 hours each day.

***Axilla.*** The patient should be positioned with the arms in 90 degrees of abduction. If this position is difficult to maintain, elbow splints will assist.

***Hips.*** The lower extremities should be placed in full extension with the legs abducted approximately 15 degrees to prevent dislocation at the hip and flexion contractures. The prone position is excellent if the patient can tolerate it.

***Feet.*** The feet should be held in 90 degrees of flexion to prevent heel cord shortening. This position may be maintained by using a footboard or posterior splints.

### ■ How often should exercise of the range of motion be employed?

Maintaining joint range of motion in the burn patient is a prime concern, as any limitation will affect the patient's ultimate functional level. Each joint should be taken though the complete range of motion at least once daily. If the patient is responsive, he should be taught self-ranging. If any loss of range is observed, the occupational therapist should be notified so that corrective measures can be taken before the contracture becomes established. The hand is an exception to this procedure. If the burn is second-degree or less, full range of motion is encouraged. If the patient has third-degree burns crossing the dorsum of the hand, extreme flexion may damage the extensor hood mechanisms and should be used with caution.

On healing of second-degree burns the patient should be encouraged to move as much as possible. Early attention to self-care needs such as feeding and hygiene should be encouraged. Splinting devices should be applied mainly at night to maintain the proper functional position, and the patient should be involved in active exercise during the day.

## ■ How are grafting and skeletal traction managed?

If pins are used in the wrist for positioning after grafting, wrist flexion should be avoided, as this results in mechanical hyperextension of the metacarpophalangeal joints and flexion of the proximal interphalangeal joints. The patient (while in traction) should be taught isotonic exercises to prevent loss of muscle bulk and weakness.

## ■ What techniques may be employed in postgrafting functional management?

The goal of the entire burn team should be to assist the patient in reaching the highest possible functional level.

### *Pressure and collagen molding*

Collagen molding in the healing burn by the application of continuous pressure can improve the ultimate appearance of healed or grafted burns. Two weeks after healing or grafting, the occupational therapist should measure the patient for pressure garments to cover all major burn areas. Once fitted, the patient should be instructed to wear the garment 24 hours each day. If additional pressure is indicated for specific areas of scarring, individually fitted isoprene inserts may be fabricated for placement under the garment. The patient should be encouraged to wear the pressure garments until the grafts have matured, approximately 1 year after the burn.

### *Prophylactic splints*

Prophylactic splints may be used primarily as a precaution against contracture or to prevent recurrence of a contracture. These splints are usually worn at night for a length of time determined by the practitioner or therapist.

### *Active splints*

***Progressive splinting.*** Progressive splinting is a useful tool for improving range of motion when established contractures occur. The splints may be fabricated from isoprene and applied directly to the flexor surface of the extremity. The progressive splinting process calls for continuous wearing of the splint from one therapy session to the next. The range of the splint is gradually increased on a daily basis until full range of motion is achieved.

***Dynamic splints.*** Dynamic splints are splints that allow the patient to perform active motion. These splints are particularly helpful in reducing edema in the newly (after 5 days or more) grafted hand.

***Exercise.*** After healing of second-degree burns or grafting of third-degree burns, a vigorous exercise program should be initiated. The patient should be treated at least once daily with passive stretching and active and resistive exercise. Passive exercise must begin early after healing or grafting if functional use of the extremity is to be accomplished. Active exercise should be stressed, particularly in the activities of daily living. Resistive exercise should be given to prevent imbalance of muscle power and generalized weakness and as an assist for overcoming contractures. The patient should be encouraged to take an active role in the rehabilitative process. Each patient should be instructed in a home program and given written directions for exercise and splinting. By the time the patient is discharged from occupational therapy, he should be wearing the pressure garment as prescribed and should be reliably doing passive stretching and exercise as outlined by the therapist.

### ■ What vocational rehabilitation assistance is available?

Vocational rehabilitation should be available for those patients having difficulty returning to their former employment. The patient may be referred directly to the state department of vocational rehabilitation or may be referred to the occupational therapy department, who will contact a vocational counselor.

### ■ What protocol for hand management should be employed?

Prompt and early management of burned hands is required for a satisfactory functional result. As soon as the immediate physiologic needs have been met and stabilized, a hand management plan should be initiated. Usually the hand burn victim has an extensive total body burn. The dorsum of the hand is almost always involved, and this thin skin is easily destroyed, exposing and damaging extensor tendons and the dorsal hood. Palmar burns are unusual, and deformity from palmar burns is rare. Because of edema and extensive tendon exposure, the patient tends to keep the hands in metacarpophalangeal hyperextension, proximal interphalangeal flexion, and distal interphalangeal flexion. This position is most comfortable and is naturally assumed. It will lead to severe disability associated with extensor tendon rupture and boutonnière deformity if not quickly managed.

Principles of management require *proximal interphalangeal and distal interphalangeal joint fixation in extension* to prevent extensor tendon rupture with *metacarpophalangeal joint motion,* including a full 90 degrees of flexion to stretch the metacarpophalangeal collateral ligaments. This is usually accomplished by simple elevation, active and passive motion, and anticlaw splints. The patient with obvious third-degree burns of the hand and arm is treated according to the protocol outlined by Achauer et al.[25]

## SUMMARY

The physiologic management principles in the acute burn patient are the same principles that apply to any generalized or localized capillary leak syndrome (pancreatitis, peritonitis, anaphylaxis, portal vein thrombosis, etc.). Careful cardiac and pulmonary monitoring and therapy are essential. Equally important are surface management and functional management. These modalities are often not considered part of critical care or the duty of the burn practitioner. These *are* responsibilities of the critical care physicians, nurses, and allied team members and are of the most critical nature and must not be neglected.

## REFERENCES


1. Moore, F. D.: The body weight burn budget—basic fluid therapy for the early burn, Surg. Clin. North Am. **50:**1249-1265, 1970.
2. Monafo, W. W., Chuntrasakul, C., and Ayvazian, V. H.: Hypertonic sodium solutions in the treatment of burn shock, Am. J. Surg. **126:**778, 1973.
3. Moylan, J. A., Jr., Reckler, J. M., and Mason, A. D., Jr.: Hypertonic lactate saline resuscitation in thermal injury, Surg. Forum **22:**49-51, 1971.
4. Baxter, C. R.: Fluid therapy of burns, sixth national burn seminar, J. Trauma **7:**69-73, 1967.
5. German, J. C., Allyn, P. A., and Bartlett, R. H.: Pulmonary artery pressure monitoring in acute burn management, Arch. Surg. **106:**788, 1973.
6. Bartlett, R. H., Gentle, D. E., Allyn, P. A., Nitta, D. E., and Quasha, A.: Hemodialysis in the management of massive burns, Trans. Am. Soc. Artif. Intern. Organs **19:**269-276, 1973.
7. Achauer, B. M., et al.: Pulmonary complications of burns: the major threat to the burn patient, Ann. Surg. **177:**311, 1973.
8. Zikria, B. A., Ferrer, J. M., and Floch, H. F.: The chemical factors contributing to pulmonary damage in smoke poisoning, Surgery **71:**704, 1972.
9. Gump, F., and Kinney, J. M.: Caloric and fluid losses through the burn wound, Surg. Clin. North Am. **50:**1235-1248, 1970.
10. Zawacki, B. E.: The microcirculation of skin after burning: its relation to tissue edema and viability, sixth annual meeting of the

American Burn Association, Cincinnati, Ohio, 1974.
11. Bartlett, R. H., Allyn, P. A., Geraghty, T., and Wetmore, N.: Nutritional management based on oxygen consumption and caloric balance measurements, sixth annual meeting of the American Burn Association, Cincinnati, Ohio, 1974.
12. Bartlett, R. H., Fong, S. W., Woldanski, C. A., Williams, G., Hardeman, J., and Anderson, W.: Changes in coagulation and platelet function following burn injury, sixth annual meeting of the American Burn Association, Cincinnati, Ohio, 1974.
13. Bartlett, R. H., and Allyn, P. A.: Pulmonary management of the burned patient, Heart & Lung **2**:714-719, 1973.
14. Munster, A., et al.: Cell-mediated immunity after thermal injury, Ann. Surg. **177**:139-143, 1973.
15. Alexander, J. W., et al.: Prevention of invasive Pseudomonas infection in burns with a new vaccine, Arch. Surg. **99**:249-256, 1969.
16. Artz, C. P.: Curling ulcer, annual report, Ft. Sam Houston, Texas, 1954, Brooke Army Medical Center, Surgical Research Unit.
17. Allgower, M., Burri, C., Cueni, L., Engley, F., Fleisch, H., Gruber, U. F., Harder, F., and Russell, R. G. G.: Study of burn toxins, Ann. N.Y. Acad. Sci. **150**:807-815, 1968.
18. Haynes, B. W., Jr.: Early excision and grafting in third degree burns, Ann. Surg. **169**:736-747, 1969.
19. German, J. C., Wooley, T. E., Achauer, B., Furnas, D. W., and Bartlett, R. H.: Porcine xenograft burn dressings—a critical reappraisal, Arch. Surg. **104**:806-808, 1972.
20. Tavis, M., Harney, J., Thornton, J., Woodruff, A., and Bartlett, R. H.: Modified collagen membrane as a skin substitute: preliminary studies, sixth annual meeting of the American Burn Association, Cincinnati, Ohio, 1974.
21. Burke, J. F.: The use of skin transplantation and immunosuppression in the treatment of extensive full thickness thermal burns, fifth annual meeting of the American Burn Association, Dallas, Texas, 1973.
22. Shuck, J. M., Pruitt, B. A., Jr., and Moncrief, J. A.: Homograft skin for wound coverage, Arch. Surg. **98**:472, 1969.
23. Berggren, R. B., and Lehr, H. B.: Viability of frozen human skin, Mod. Med. **34**:134, 1966.
24. Rappaport, I., Pepino, A. T., and Dietrick, W.: Early use of xenografts as a biological dressing in burn trauma, Am. J. Surg. **120**:144-148, 1970.
25. Achauer, B. B., Bartlett, R. H., Furnas, D. W., Allyn, P. A., and Wingerson, E.: Internal fixation in the management of the burned hand, Arch. Surg. **108**:814-820, 1974.

## BIBLIOGRAPHY

Artz, C. P., and Moncrief, J. A.: The treatment of burns, ed. 2, Philadelphia, 1969, W. B. Saunders Co.

Boswick, J. A., editor: The surgery of burns, Surg. Clin. North Am. **50**:entire issue, 1970.

Feller, I.: International bibliography on burns, Ann Arbor, Mich., 1969, American Burn Research Corporation.

Feller, I., and Archambeault, C.: Nursing the burned patient, Ann Arbor, Mich., 1973, Institute for Burn Medicine.

Furnas, D. W.: A bedside outline for the treatment of burns, Springfield, Ill., 1969, Charles C Thomas, Publisher.

Lynch, J. B., and Lewis, S. R.: Symposium on the treatment of burns, vol. 5, St. Louis, 1973, The C. V. Mosby Co.

Monafo, W. W.: The treatment of burns, St. Louis, 1971, Warren H. Green, Inc.

Moyer, C. A., and Butcher, H. R., Jr.: Burns, shock, and plasma volume regulation, St. Louis, 1967, The C. V. Mosby Co.

Polk, H. C., Jr., and Stone, H. H.: Contemporary burn management, Boston, 1971, Little, Brown & Co.

*chapter 22*

# Care of the neurologic patient

HARRY FRIEDMAN

The majority of neurologic syndromes encountered in day-to-day clinic or office practice do not reach the level of critical care requirements such that minute-to-minute observation is mandatory. Although many of these conditions progress inexorably to death, such as progressive degenerative processes, these disorders require little more than good custodial care. It is primarily in the areas of trauma to the brain, spinal cord, and contiguous structures, neoplasia, certain infectious-inflammatory processes, toxic states, and vascular disease that emergency situations arise that require decisive and aggressive approaches at all echelons of management. The purpose of this chapter is to point out those entities in neurologic-neurosurgical practice that may be encountered in the foregoing categories wherein the application of high standards of diagnostic skill and management, as well as quality critical care, must be exercised. Although rare or extremely unusual complications will not be discussed, the usual and some unusual complications will be mentioned. Diagnostic studies, including biochemical, neurophysiologic, and neuroradiologic studies, will be considered. The limitations as well as the usefulness of the lumbar puncture will be stressed. Diagnostic and therapeutic neuropharmacology will be mentioned.

Recognizing the importance of critical care, there will be sections dealing with general treatment measures as well as bedside critical care management in specific or unusual situations.

In enumerating those neurologic or neurosurgical conditions that could be classified as "true emergencies," the list would include acute bacterial meningitis, cerebral hemorrhage in its various forms, acute cerebral vascular occlusion, decompensation of the CNS in the presence of neoplasms, pituitary apoplexy, some forms of cerebral trauma such as depressed skull fractures, cerebral contusion, the various traumatic cerebral hemorrhages, spinal cord injury, status epilepticus, and certain intoxications. The cardinal signs of deterioration and usual means of management will be discussed.

## TRAUMA

### ■ What are the general principles of treating the severely head-injured patient?

The focus of primary care should be on prevention of secondary CNS damage, since complications that follow such trauma can be more detrimental than the initial injury itself.

A thorough history and complete physical examination are of vital importance in predicting the patient's subsequent course. For example, different kinds of automobile accidents can produce different injuries depending on the direction of impact to the head. Motorcycle and bicycle accidents may produce depressed skull fractures, whereas falls and diving accidents and those associated with a moving vehicle often result in spinal injuries.

Gunshot and stab wounds of the head produce deep injuries with retained foreign bodies that often lead to serious complications and severe infections; in addition, air and cerebrospinal fluid leaks are commonly seen in such patients.

Preexisting medical problems such as those seen in diabetes, cardiac disturbances, hys-

**Table 22-1.** Signs associated with head injury and observations or treatment

| *Sign* | *Observation/treatment* |
|---|---|
| Oculomotor or third cranial nerve paralysis resulting from direct injury; compression of nerve between the temporal lobe uncus and tentorium caused by hematoma or edema or kinking around posterior cerebral artery; most significant cranial nerve in indication of rising intracranial pressure | Observe briskness of reaction of pupil to light by checking each pupil individually with flashlight to measure direct, not consensual, reaction; darken room; approach laterally; check every 15 min at first. Observe changes in speed of reaction. Observe difference in size of pupils (ipsilateral dilation with third nerve compression). Report change in equality *immediately;* dilation with fixation is a late sign with a poor prognosis.<br>Observe for other eye signs. While checking eyes, look for foreign bodies, including contact lenses, and remove, if possible. |
| Increased systolic pressure and/or widened pulse pressure and slow pulse caused by increased systole from attempt to transport sufficient oxygen in face of rising intracranial pressure, pulse eventually slowing reflexly as blood pressure rises | Check blood pressure and pulse every 15 min at first. Look for other injuries if blood pressure falls and pulse increases.<br>Be sure airway is adequate for oxygenation, especially in presence of facial, neck, and chest injuries. |
| Decreased movement, strength, and sensation in extremities resulting from lesion and/or increased pressure in cerebral hemisphere or brain stem, compression of motor fibers from midbrain to spinal cord against the tentorium, or spinal cord injury | Check every 15 min for spontaneous equal movement of all extremities. If an extremity does not move spontaneously, record type of stimuli, if any, that causes movement. Check for purposefulness of movements. Check strength and equality of handgrips; check for drift of outstretched arms.<br>Observe for decorticate and decerebrate posture. (Decorticate posture involves abducted and rigidly flexed arms. Decerebrate posture characterized by rigidly extended extremities, arched back, and toes turned inward.) |
| Seizures resulting from direct trauma to cerebral tissues, cerebral edema, foreign bodies in brain, or hypoxia | Note beginning point, progression, and duration.<br>Suction excessive saliva; stay with patient; protect the airway.<br>Try to differentiate drowsiness and confusion of postictal state from progressive irritability and lethargy associated with increasing intracranial pressure. |
| Vomiting caused by increased intracranial pressure or swallowing blood, especially if food or alcohol was ingested just prior to accident | Observe vomiting, which may be projectile.<br>Suction promptly; remove suction catheter from tubing and put tubing directly in mouth to remove large, undigested food particles that obstruct catheter.<br>Turn patient to side to prevent aspiration; keep entire spine in straight alignment when turning.<br>Pass nasogastric tube as ordered.<br>Remove foreign bodies from mouth, including dentures. Look for sources of bleeding in mouth. |
| Restlessness resulting from rising intracranial pressure, pain, hypoxia, or urinary retention | Elevate head of bed 30 degrees unless contraindicated by shock; never put in Trendelenburg position. Avoid having bright lights on face continuously.<br>Maintain a relatively quiet environment with few distractions.<br>Make instructions to patient simple and understandable; avoid speaking in loud tones even if patient is loud and abusive. |

**Table 22-1.** Signs associated with head injury and observations or treatment—cont'd

| *Sign* | *Observation/treatment* |
|---|---|
| | Check for distended bladder and catheterize, especially if abdominal trauma is suspected.<br>Restrain as needed; patient may require leather restraints. Improperly applied or excessive restraint can increase restlessness further. Only protective covering to keep patient from removing tubes and dressings may be needed and can be made by placing a folded washcloth in the palm of hand with finger surfaces separated and then wrapping a 3-inch elastic bandage around entire hand and up the arm about 6 inches. Tape securely; remove at least every 8 hours to check circulation to hands. |
| Cerebrospinal fluid leakage usually caused by disruption of mucous membranes in basilar skull fracture, primarily risking infection | Observe for clear drainage from nose and ears; bloody drainage that produces a relatively colorless halo around a spot of blood usually indicates the presence of cerebrospinal fluid leak (bull's eye sign).<br>If drainage is excessive, use only a loose, dry sterile dressing.<br>Use good hand washing technique.<br>Do not suction nasally in presence of this drainage.<br>Discourage nose blowing or sneezing. Cerebrospinal fluid produces a positive reaction on dextrose testing. |

teria, and epilepsy as well as alcoholic or drug ingestion frequently precipitate a fall, leading to serious head injuries. The seriousness of these injuries may be compounded by the chronic use of drugs such as anticoagulants. In these instances treatment of the preexisting problem should be undertaken simultaneously with the CNS injury evaluation.

The level of consciousness can be altered by other factors also, such as concurrent abdominal injury (ruptured spleen, contused kidney, lacerated liver, or perforated urinary bladder), causing a rapid or insidious blood loss that can seriously compromise the body's total circulating blood volume and the large amount of oxygenated blood required by the brain. *Head injury alone does not cause shock.* Hypovolemia may cause hypoxia of the neuronal and support cells, further edema of the cerebral tissue, and loss of consciousness. Hypovolemia and hypoxia from chest injuries (pneumothorax, hemothorax, or flail chest) can result in the same problem. In addition to causing a reduced level of consciousness, hypoxia causes restlessness that can contribute to a rise in intracranial pressure.

Head injuries are commonly accompanied by neck injuries, which should always be suspected until proved to be absent. High cervical cord laryngeal or tracheal damage may alter the level of consciousness. Since consciousness, or the patient's awareness of self and surroundings, is a result of total body function, the practitioner must always suspect and observe for associated conditions that may alter the patient's consciousness. It is important to assess the patient's orientation to time, place, and person. The head-injured patient should be aroused during normal sleeping hours and questioned regarding these three aspects as part of routine patient care and observation.

The neurologic signs listed in Table 22-1 are usually associated with changes in the patient's sensorium, and appropriate intervention is recommended. The usual pharma-

**Table 22-2.** Common drugs, dosages, and routes of administration used in the care of the head-injured patient

| *Drug* | *Dose* | *Route* | *Comments* |
|---|---|---|---|
| Methylprednisolone (Solu-Medrol) | 20-40 mg every 6 hr | IV, then IM | Dose tapered gradually as discontinued, or depot injection given day before termination of steroid if given for more than 3 days; antacid given with each dose to prevent GI bleeding from stress or steroid; steroid used to decrease cerebral edema |
| Mannitol, 20% | 30-50 ml/hr | IV | Diuretic to reduce extracellular fluid volume and decrease cerebral edema if hematoma is absent |
| Phenobarbital | 30-60 mg every 4 hr | IV, IM, or PO | Anticonvulsant; more rapid acting than diphenylhydantoin |
| Diazepam (Valium) | 5-10 mg initially, then repeated every 30 min as needed | IV | Anticonvulsant for persistent unrelieved seizures; may be necessary initially until diphenylhydantoin level effective; patient observed for respiratory depression and depression of level of consciousness |
| Propoxyphene (Darvon) | 32-65 mg every 3-4 hr as needed | PO | Analgesic |
| Acetaminophen (Tylenol) | 325-650 mg every 3-4 hr as needed | PO or PR | Analgesic, antipyretic |
| Acetylsalicylic acid (aspirin) | 300-600 mg every 3-4 hr as needed | PO or PR | Analgesic, antipyretic |
| Codeine | 30 mg every 3-4 hr as needed | IM or PO | Narcotic analgesic |
| Tetanus toxoid | 0.5 ml | IM | For active immunity |
| Human tetanus immune globulin (Hyper-Tet) | 250-500 units | IM | For passive immunity |

cologic preparations and dosages used in the care of the head-injured patient are outlined in Table 22-2.

Whether surgery is needed or not, several treatment modalities can be followed. The patient should be on the side or back with nasogastric drainage to prevent aspiration. The head of the bed should be elevated 30 degrees to enhance venous drainage. Oxygenation with mask or binasal cannula at 5 to 6 L/min should be given. IV fluids should be kept below 2 L/24 hr. Steroid solutions using either methylprednisolone (Solu-Medrol) or dexamethasone (Decadron) should be given every 6 hours together with antacids either by nasogastric tube or in the form of IM injection of anticholinergic medication, for example, glycopyrrolate (Robinul). Because of the danger of adrenal suppression, tapering dosages of corticosteroids should be given, starting on the fourth or fifth day. Caution should be exercised in giving antiedemic agents until the presence of an intracranial clot is ascertained, since decompression pharmacologically may precipitate further bleeding.

The following factors related to bedside clinical management should be considered: frequent turning and use of sheepskin, footboards, antiembolic stockings, and cardiac monitoring. In addition, periodic observation of electrolyte concentrations, arterial blood gas levels, glucose concentration, and blood urea nitrogen (BUN) should be performed. Indwelling bladder catheters should be avoided, if possible. Since fever is often present in head injuries, this should be treated with appropriate antipyretics; the indiscriminate

**Table 22-3.** Classification of various types of acute head injuries and treatment

| *Anatomic location* | *Type of injury* | *Usual CNS signs or symptoms* | *Treatment* |
|---|---|---|---|
| Skull | Linear fracture | Those of underlying brain injury | Observation if uncomplicated |
| | Depressed fracture | Same as linear fracture | Surgical decompression with brain débridement or hemorrhage evacuation as indicated |
| | Frontal basilar fracture | Cerebrospinal fluid rhinorrhea, periorbital ecchymoses, pneumocephalus | Elevation of head, antibiotics, surgical closure if rhinorrhea persists for more than 1 week or if recurrent episodes of meningitis occur |
| | Petrobasilar fracture | May be associated with CN VII and CN VIII dysfunction, otorhinorrhea, Battle's sign | Observation, possibly antibiotics |
| Meninges and their spaces | Epidural hemorrhage | "Lucid interval," progressive deterioration, ipsilateral dilated pupil, skull fractures crossing meningeal artery groove | Urgent decompression |
| | Dural laceration | Those of underlying brain injury, venous oozing (if compound injury) from lacerated dural sinus | Elevation of head and packing of wound, surgical débridement and closure |
| | Subdural hemorrhage | Those of underlying brain injury, progressive deterioration, may be acute or chronic | Evacuation of hemorrhage |
| | Subarachnoid hemorrhage | May be mild or severe depending on brain injury and presence or absence of associated arterial spasm | Observation if uncomplicated by collection of blood or other surgical CNS lesion |
| Brain | Concussion | Mild headache, nausea, vomiting, dizziness; no focal signs or unconsciousness | Observation |
| | Contusion | History of unconsciousness, transient focal signs, prolonged elevated intracranial pressure, possibly signs of severe focal damage with cerebral edema | Observation if mild or transient; steroids, hyperventilation, intracranial pressure monitoring, internal decompression if severe |
| | Laceration | As with contusion | Exploration and débridement if suspected; often an incidental finding during decompression |
| | Intracerebral hemorrhage | Usually associated with deepened consciousness and focal signs of damage | Evacuation of clot; if in frontal, occipital, or temporal lobe, subtotal lobectomy |

use of antibiotics should be discouraged and should be reserved for use when clear indications of infection are present or imminent. The bowel regimen, including use of stool softeners and periodic enemas, should be instituted early. Early and frequent mobilization of joints and extremities will help prevent pressure sores, contractures, calcium loss, and negative nitrogen balance. In addition, this will help promote venous drainage and maintain muscle tone.

The onset of shock in the head-injured patient demands that a search be made in other body cavities for its cause, since head injuries do not cause shock, as emphasized previously.

Table 22-3 summarizes the various head injuries and indicates appropriate treatment.

■ **What ancillary diagnostic tests may be performed in the workup of the head-injured patient?**

Skull x-ray films, including anteroposterior, Towne, and stereoscopic horizontal beam brow-up lateral views, should be obtained. The horizontal beam brow-up lateral view should be obtained rather than the often performed vertical beam lateral view with the patient's head rotated in the supine position, since a cervical spine fracture may be present associated with the head injury. Also, pneumocephalus is easier to observe if the head is in the brow-up position. Stereoscopic films help delineate the location and extent of fracture and/or foreign bodies.

Cervical spine x-ray films to show C7-T1 should be routinely performed in the head-injured patient for the reasons alluded to previously.

Echoencephalography is often performed. The results of this study should not preclude more definitive evaluation, particularly of the severely injured patient.

Arteriography should be performed in the patient who has demonstrated focal signs but whose condition is stable. Both sides of the head should be studied, either with bilateral injections of contrast material or by the cross-compression technique utilizing a single site of injection. The patient who has not shown focal signs, who has not had asymmetric pupils (in the absence of orbital injury), and who is reasonably alert can usually be safely observed without having arteriography. The patient suffering a head injury who has asymmetric pupils should undergo exploratory surgery immediately without expending valuable time to perform diagnostic studies. The coexistence of orbital trauma should not deter immediate exploration, since severe intracranial trauma capable of producing a dilated pupil may be present.

Computerized axial tomography is a radiologic technique that can very accurately locate lesions and may give a clue as to the nature of the lesion.

Caloric irrigation of the external ear canals coupled with determination of doll's eye responses (oculocephalic reflex) may be helpful in determining the extent of brain stem injury.

■ **What is the general plan for treating the comatose patient in the emergency room when no history is available?**

1. Rapidly examine pupils, response to pain, and presence of focal neurologic signs, and determine vital signs and external signs of trauma.
2. Draw blood for electrolyte, glucose, BUN, toxicology screening, and arterial blood gas tests.
3. Give by IV route 50 ml of a 50% glucose solution.
4. Provide airway and oxygen; endotracheal tube is preferred.
5. Obtain ECG.
6. Obtain x-ray films, including arteriograms.
7. Perform lumbar puncture after ascertaining that no mass effect is present on arteriography.
8. Insert nasogastric tube.

■ **What conditions may cause increased intracranial pressure?**

1. Cellular and/or vascular disease or injury, producing cerebral edema or bleeding
2. Space-occupying lesions
3. Obstruction of ventricular and cerebrospinal fluid pathways
4. Interference with venous drainage from intracranial cavity
5. Meningitis
6. Hypoxia, acute or chronic

■ **What are the signs and symptoms of increased intracranial pressure?**

1. Increasing headache with or without vomiting
2. Restlessness
3. Diminishing alertness and noticeable changes in the level of consciousness
4. Irregular pupils that may be dilated on the side of a hemorrhage
5. Decreased pulse rate
6. Decreased respirations (Periods of apnea may eventually occur.)
7. Possibly a gradual increase in blood pressure

8. Possible weakness or paralysis on one side of the body
9. Convulsions
10. Increased cerebrospinal fluid pressure

The critical care practitioner caring for the neurosurgical patient must make continuous, astute, intelligent observations and must also have the ability to interpret and record his or her observations in order that life-saving measures may be instituted at the appropriate moment. Organ swelling (the result of fluid or mass) elsewhere in the body presents only modest implications; however, brain edema, hematoma formation, and progressive hydrocephalus threaten life itself. Irreversible damage may occur when nerve cells are rendered hypoxic, as when increased pressure is developing and impairing CNS circulation, since nerve cells cease functioning under such conditions.

Experience has shown that, despite all the space-age monitoring devices now available for use in critical care, close observation by the bedside practitioner of specific *body functions* serves as the best guide for assessing intracranial pressure. Some important areas of observation to be considered in the care of the seriously ill neurologic patient are consciousness, blood pressure and pulse, pulmonary signs, vomiting, weakness or paralysis, temperature, respiration, pain, and convulsion. As techniques for constant monitoring of intracranial pressure directly are perfected, earlier detection of pressure increases will be enhanced.

### *Consciousness*

The practitioner should be aware that actual *squeezing of the brain* may occur as pressure builds up in the cranial cavity, especially if caused by a space-occupying lesion. As the intracranial pressure begins to increase, the patient may appear asymptomatic.

Diffuse compression may affect numerous brain regions, including the reticular formation. The result is that confusion, disorientation, and delerium are often observed during the early stages of increased intracranial pressure. Deep coma and other complications may follow unless early corrective measures are taken to decrease the pressure.

### *Blood pressure and pulse*

One of the most reliable indications of rising intracranial pressure is pulse slowing, which reflexly occurs as extracranial carotid circulation encounters an abnormally elevated head of pressure in the intracranial circulation as a result of alterations in autoregulatory mechanisms. Blood pressure may rise, but this is usually a terminal event as autoregulation fails and the full head of pressure is transmitted into the arterial circulation.

### *Ocular signs*

Normally the pupils are equal in size and react on exposure to light. Neurologically injured patients should be observed closely for changes in the pupils' size, equality, and reaction to light. Should an intracranial hemorrhage occur, a dilated, fixed pupil may be observed on the affected side, that is, it will not react on exposure to a light directed on the pupil. A fixed dilated pupil demands emergency action.

Funduscopic examination may reveal the presence of subhyaloid or splinter hemorrhages, the former suggesting intracranial hemorrhage and the latter suggesting increasing intracranial pressure. Papilledema is rarely seen before 18 to 24 hours. If present, vision is usually unaffected.

Medial deviation of an eye may result from increased intracranial pressure causing traction on the sixth cranial nerve with resultant paresis of the lateral rectus muscle.

Skew deviation of the eyes may be the result of cerebellar or brain stem compression.

### *Vomiting*

Vomiting, sometimes projectile, is a common symptom of increased intracranial pressure; the characteristics and frequency of all vomiting should be reported to the principal practitioner.

Since vomiting or strain of any kind, for example, while using the bedpan, should be avoided in order to avoid further increase in the pressure, the bedside practitioner should do everything possible to control vomiting, strain in defecation, or undue patient activity.

### *Weakness or paralysis*

Progressive hemiparesis, spasms, and hypertonicity may be the result of compression of a hemisphere or of the brain stem. The first indication that progressive hemiparesis is impending may be a positive Babinski response (a fanning and dorsiflexion of the toes when the sole of the foot is stroked). This should be reported immediately to the principal practitioner.

### *Temperature*

A hyperthermic condition will increase the patient's metabolic needs; therefore it is important that every measure be employed to avoid an increase in body temperature.

### *Respiration*

The most important task that the bedside practitioner must carry out religiously is to maintain a clear airway. Increased intracranial pressure and hypoxia in the respiratory center of the medulla will result in respiratory changes. The hypoxia itself increases cerebral edema. The early signs of respiratory failure are irritability, anxiety, and restlessness. The respiratory rate begins to rise and becomes shallow, the nares flare in and out, there is a decrease in the tidal volume and vital capacity (the use of bedside spirometric measurements is helpful), the pulse rate and blood pressure rise, sweating and cyanosis occur, and consciousness is lost. Again, the body's compensatory mechanisms come into play, and the accessory muscles of respiration work at an early stage; then the chest wall and abdomen cease to move. Snoring and stertorus respirations may be noted initially, followed by Cheyne-Stokes type respiration as progress toward death occurs. Altered respiratory states are extremely serious in the neurologic patient and immediate corrective action must be initiated if possible.

The patient may require mouth-to-mouth respiration or intubation and mechanical ventilatory support until the increased intracranial pressure has been brought under control.

### *Pain*

Since headache is a significant symptom of increasing intracranial pressure, it is important to record its location, duration, and severity.

### *Convulsion*

Accurate observation and recording may provide vital information that will be useful in the treatment of the patient, since the type of seizures may indicate the area of the brain being focally irritated. The bedside practitioner should protect the patient (use of padded tongue blades, plastic airways, and *firm* padding of some kind to prevent the patient from self-harm as a result of falling against bed rails, etc.) and observe the seizure, noting kind; movements (clonic or tonic); duration; level of consciousness *preceding, during,* and *after* the seizure; and when the seizure began to progress.

## ■ How is the patient with spinal injury handled?

Although opinion varies as to the definitive treatment of spinal fractures as far as timing and type of surgery, certain points need to be stressed regarding early care. The patient should be immobilized in a supine position on a sheepskin or alternating pressure mattress. Stabilization of the head (with sandbags and a towel roll placed under the neck) should be instituted until definitive treatment is performed. The two-mattress bed technique or Circ-O-Lectric bed should be used for the patient with cervical spine injury in traction. The Circ-O-Lectric bed can also be used for patients with thoracic or lumbar spine fractures. Early tracheostomy may be necessary.

Patients with residual function in extremities can be managed on a regular bed with a trapeze bar attached. Constant catheterization should be avoided to minimize infection and to enhance bladder training; instead, intermittent catheterization should be performed. Vital signs should be observed, especially in high spinal injuries because of vasomotor instability. In addition, initially temperature-regulating mechanisms may be disturbed, resulting especially in the preservation of heat, for example, the lightest bedclothes may produce high rises in temperature. A bowel regimen should be instituted early, consisting of the administration of stool softeners, laxatives, and enemas to prevent impaction.

### ■ How are patients with malingering or hysterical brain or spinal cord injury detected?

All patients, regardless of the initial impression or the patient's past history, should be treated as if certain injury exists. In two areas, however, suspicion may be aroused; these are the apparently unconscious patient and the apparently paralyzed patient.

False unconsciousness may be suspected in an individual suffering an injury too minor to have produced unconsciousness and exhibiting fluttering or opening and closing of the eyelids. Catatonic posturing may be possible, for example, an extremity may maintain itself in a raised position. The patient may resist verbal commands or application of painful stimuli, but may awaken quickly when ammonia is applied to the nostrils.

The state of hysterical spinal injury may be suspected when a nonanatomic sensory pattern is present, and no lesion may be localized on x-ray films. Caution must be used here, since a myelopathy may be produced in the absence of fracture. The application of painful stimuli will aid in exposing the hysterical or malingering state.

### ■ How is status epilepticus handled?

Diphenylhydantoin in the usual dosages for acute seizures is generally ineffective because of its slow metabolism in the liver. Currently IV or IM phenobarbital, diazepam, or IV sodium amobarbital may be given according to the following schedule:

Phenobarbital: adult, 30 to 60 mg given by IM route every 4 to 6 hours, with 20 to 30 mg given by IV route slowly for the initial therapy

Sodium amobarbital: adult, 250 to 500 mg given by IV route every 4 hours, with drip of 1 g in 1 L of fluids to run 24 hours, then stop to allow patient to awaken; constant monitoring of vital signs is imperative

Diazepam: adult, 5 to 10 mg given by IV route slowly or 5 to 10 mg given by IM route every 6 hours

Diphenylhydantoin: adult, 100 mg given by IM or IV route to institute chronic treatment

## CEREBROVASCULAR ACCIDENTS

### ■ How is the diagnosis of stroke made?

Stroke, or cerebrovascular accident (CVA), is manifest by the sudden appearance of symptoms referable to a particular vascular distribution after other cerebral catastrophes such as trauma, tumor, or abscess have been eliminated as possibilities. The latter is important, since mass lesions may be silent until they suddenly deteriorate; this is unusual, however, since a careful history will usually reveal that subtle symptoms have been present over a period of time. The cardinal sign of CVA is its suddenness in onset in the absence of prior deterioration. It may be manifest by either interruption of blood flow to an area by thrombosis or embolization or by hemorrhage, either intracerebral or subarachnoid.

Occlusion of the common carotid artery may produce a picture of total contralateral hemiparesis or hemiplegia; dysphasia or aphasia, if involving the dominant hemisphere; and contralateral visual field involvement. Cortical and deep sensory involvement may be present. A lesion in the area of the anterior cerebral artery may produce contralateral leg weakness and may include the contralateral face by involving the artery of Heubner proceeding to the face area of the internal capsule. Middle cerebral artery occlusion produces contralateral hemiparesis or hemiplegia involving mainly face and arm, speech difficulty if in the dominant hemisphere, and right-side field deficits.

### ■ How is the patient with uncomplicated subarachnoid hemorrhage treated?

Early arteriography and lumbar puncture should verify the diagnosis of subarachnoid hemorrhage (SAH) and the location of the aneurysm, as well as the hemodynamic characteristics of the cerebral circulation around the aneurysm. For the patient who is to have a direct surgical approach to the aneurysm, it is best to delay surgery until 10 to 14 days after the bleeding episode to allow spasm to subside. Meanwhile the patient is to maintain strict bed rest and quiet environment, lying flat in bed with nothing given rectally, although stool softeners and antihypertensive medication of the nonrauwolfia type may be given if the systemic blood pressure rises to a high level.

For an aneurysm of the internal carotid artery that is to be treated by common carotid artery gradual ligation, surgery can be carried out early by the same principles of care just outlined, which will continue to apply until complete occlusion is accomplished.

## ■ What are the usual causes of embolization to cerebral arteries?

Cerebral embolization arises from cardiac causes such as chronic atrial fibrillation, cardioversion-initiated or spontaneous fragmentation of mural thrombi (as from old myocardial infarction), fragmentation of valvular vegetations, paradoxical embolization through patent foramen ovale, and as a complication of cardiac surgery.

## ■ What is the medical treatment of stroke?

Adequate nutrition, oxygenation, and early rehabilitation of such patients are indicated. In acute stroke an adequate airway must be provided, and aspiration should be prevented. Nasal oxygenation to maintain a high $P_{O_2}$ to the marginal areas of ischemia (too high a $P_{O_2}$ may produce cerebral vasoconstriction) should be provided. A mixture of oxygen and carbon dioxide at about 6 L/min will provide the high $P_{O_2}$ required plus a measure of vasodilatation to enhance flow. If the patient cannot swallow, IV nutrition may be given, but nasogastric feedings are more desirable, since the tube serves as a means of emptying the stomach between feedings, if necessary, to reduce the possibility of aspiration while providing a route of nutritional support not possible with conventional means of IV feeding. Anticoagulation should be considered for the patient with transient ischemic attacks, especially if an ulcerative plaque is observed on arteriogram. Also, the patient with brain stem ischemia should be considered for anticoagulation. Aqueous heparin in a dose of 4000 to 5000 units given by IV administration every 6 hours should be adequate. It should not be used if blood pressure is very high.

## ■ When is surgery indicated for stroke?

This depends on the manifestation of the stroke. There are three general areas for surgical intervention: carotid artery stenosis or occlusion, intracerebral hematoma, and cerebral aneurysm. These are discussed here in general terms. Acute occlusion of the extracranial portion of the carotid artery, if discovered within the first 6 to 8 hours, should be considered a possible indication for exploration. Waiting too long may predispose the patient to developing a hemorrhagic infarct in the area of ischemia. Also, the patient with transient ischemic attacks referable to a specific carotid stenosis should be considered for endarterectomy.

The patient who has suffered an intracerebral hematoma, especially of the nondominant hemisphere or of the cerebellum, should be considered for early surgical removal of the clot. The same is true for the patient suffering an intracerebral hematoma from rupture of an intracranial aneurysm. Otherwise the SAH patient should have a period of waiting before definitive surgery on the aneurysm should be considered, as noted previously.

## ■ How is cerebellar hemorrhage best managed?

This is best handled by early surgical decompression. The diagnosis is made in a patient usually with a hypertensive history who develops sudden, severe headache with vomiting, unsteady gait, and other specific signs of cerebellar dysfunction. Ventriculography, arteriography, or computerized axial tomography may support the diagnosis, but little time should be lost in performing decompression, since progression to the comatose and decerebrate state can occur quite rapidly. With a history and physical examination suggesting this picture, it is justifiable to operate without performing contrast studies, since the course may be rapid and irreversible and valuable time may be lost.

### ■ What are some of the neurologic complications of cardiovascular surgery?

The embolization of cholesterol plaques is the usual cause of neurologic dysfunction. Air and fibrin clot embolization from valves can occur. Also, a hypercoagulable state may occur. There is recent evidence that fat embolization can occur after median sternotomy. Focal neurologic deficits may occur after carotid artery surgery because of the embolization of fibrin clots, incomplete plaque removal, improper shunt positioning, and intimal dissection with arterial occlusion. Paraplegia caused by intercostal artery interruption, especially of the great radicular artery of Adamkiewicz, may occur after aortic surgery.

### ■ What are the potential complications of common carotid artery ligation?

There are three potential sources of complications: ischemia, embolization, and carotid artery erosion. Ischemic symptoms, that is, focal deficits, may arise during the turning down of the clamp. This is treated by reopening the clamp. Embolization may occur near the completion of occlusion when a bruit appears, signaling turbulence at the clamp site, or if the clamp has been placed too far from the carotid bifurcation. If embolization is suspected, immediate arteriotomy with evacuation of the clot is necessary.

Rarely a clamp erodes the artery. This may be signaled by slow swelling at the surgical site or a slow ooze of blood from the incision, or it may be catastrophic with a large gush of blood and rapid swelling. Direct pressure should be applied until the artery can be exposed and repaired.

## CNS INFECTIONS

### ■ What are the most common meningeal infecting agents in descending order of frequency, and what is the most effective antibiotic treatment for these?

1. Viral agents (enterovirus, mumps). Treatment is supportive in most cases, although cytosine arabinoside may be given in papovavirus infections.
2. *Neisseria meningitidis.* Penicillin G (adult, 20 million units/day), ampicillin (400 mg/kg/day given by IV route in children 2 months of age or older), or a sulfonamide may be given.
3. *Haemophilus influenzae* (in children 7 years of age or younger). Ampicillin (100 to 200 mg/kg/day) or chloramphenicol (50 to 100 mg/kg/day) is recommended.
4. *Diplococcus pneumoniae.* Penicillin G (20 million units/day) or erythromycin (1 to 4 g/day) may be administered.
5. *Streptococcus pyogenes* (groups A and B). Penicillin G or erythromycin is recommended.
6. *Escherichia coli* (or other gram-negative bacilli, especially in neonates and after neurosurgical procedures). A combination of ampicillin with gentamicin (6 mg/kg/day) or kanamycin may be given. Cephalosporins are also useful. Gram-negative ventriculitis may be treated by a combination of intraventricular gentamicin and carbenicillin.
7. *Coagulase-positive Staphylococcus* (brain abscess, surgical infection). Penicillin G, ampicillin, or methicillin (100 to 300 mg/kg/day) may be used.
8. *Mycobacterium tuberculosis.* Isoniazid (adult, 30 mg/kg/day), ethambutol (15 mg/kg/day), or streptomycin (adult, 1 g/day, children, 20 mg/kg/day) is effective. Pyridoxine should be given to patients taking isoniazid.
9. *Cryptococcus neoformans* and other fungi. Amphotericin B (adult, 1 to 2 g/day) is recommended.
10. *Listeria monocytogenes.* Penicillin G or ampicillin may be given.
11. *Enterococcus* (in neonates). Penicillin G or ampicillin may be given.

12. *Treponema pallidum.* Penicillin G or tetracycline (20 mg/kg/day) is useful.
13. *Leptospira.* Penicillin G or a tetracycline is the preferred treatment.

### ■ What are the usual causes of brain abscess?

Retained foreign bodies introduced by trauma such as depressed bone fragments, hair, clothing, and dirt form one group causing brain abscess. Another, although less likely, is abscess complicating meningitis associated with frontobasilar or petrobasilar skull fractures. Chronic purulent otitis media is associated with brain abscess. Metastatic abscess from another source of infection such as the pulmonary or cardiac system accounts for some brain abscesses.

Cerebral aneurysms may result from mycotic cardiac emboli and may lodge in the walls of cerebral arteries. They usually cause episodes of SAH. Characteristically they are multiple and located in areas considered unusual for congenital aneurysms, that is, they are along the smaller, more distal branches of the major cerebral circulations. Frequently SAH is the first clinical manifestation of subacute bacterial endocarditis. Furthermore, the patient who demonstrates low-grade fever with the appearance of a diastolic murmur, or splinter, or petechial hemorrhage with neurologic deterioration may have either cerebral abscess or cerebral mycotic aneurysm.

### ■ How may the patient who presents with focal neurologic deficits and purulent discharge from the ear be best managed?

A rapid but careful neurologic history and examination should be performed to determine the duration of the suspected cerebral lesion and whether it is located in cerebellum or temporal lobe, the two most likely locations of focal cerebritis or abscess resulting from chronic purulent otitis. Temporal lobe abscess usually produces contralateral hemiparesis, dysphasia if in the dominant hemisphere, and occasionally visual field impairment along with papilledema. Cerebellar abscess usually produces ipsilateral dystaxia, dysmetria, and nystagmus on the side of the lesion. One must be careful not to confuse unsteadiness with hemiparesis.

Following this procedure, drainage material is sampled for culture and sensitivity, and the patient is given large doses of antibiotics, following which cerebral arteriography is performed to help delineate the location of the lesion. The otolaryngologist then will perform a mastoidectomy to institute drainage. Immediately after this the neurosurgeon should carry out the appropriate procedure, either excision of the abscess or aspiration and drainage. If it is determined that the cerebral lesion is focal cerebritis rather than abscess, the administration of large doses of IV antibiotics is the treatment of choice until the cerebritis resolves or an abscess finally walls off. If the latter occurs, the appropriate neurosurgical procedure should be instituted.

Early drainage of the otitis is required to prevent sepsis and to enhance recovery from the subsequent craniotomy, particularly if only a drainage procedure is performed, since continuing bacterial contamination will probably produce continuing infection. Furthermore, sudden rapid neurologic deterioration can occur as a result of cerebral edema, increased intracranial pressure, or subdural or intraventricular rupture of the abscess.

### ■ What are some of the acute and chronic complications of meningitis?

Focal or generalized convulsive seizures are commonly seen and may actually be the presenting symptoms. Generalized sepsis may occur, and particularly in meningococcal meningitis, the Waterhouse-Friderichsen syndrome (WFS) with adrenal and circulatory collapse can occur. WFS may actually be a manifestation of disseminated intravascular coagulopathy with the adrenal dysfunction being actually a secondary, not a primary, phenomenon. It is thought that the adrenal gland may suffer ischemic changes as a result of platelet aggregations and thus, in part at least, produce the systemic deterioration characteristic of WFS.

Chronic complications include cerebral or

subdural abscess, usually from late or incomplete therapy. Normal pressure hydrocephalus is occasionally seen as a late effect caused either by blockage of the cerebrospinal fluid outflow at the aqueduct or absorption over the cerebral convexity at the pacchionian granulations.

### ■ What should be known about infectious polyneuritis?

Infectious polyneuritis is best known as the Guillain-Barré syndrome and is often considered to be a true medical emergency.

If the course of the disease indicates a rapidly ascending paralysis, mechanical ventilation may be indicated, and preparation for a possible tracheostomy should be carried out. Special bedside care may be required in order to observe and record the patient's progress properly. Bulbar signs such as hoarseness, choking, or respiration by accessory muscles indicate that mechanical ventilation may be imminently necessary.

The unique symptom is a bilateral facial palsy. Other symptoms besides paralysis include painful tactile and thermal hyperesthesia, usually aural in distribution, or hypoesthesia and tenderness of muscles. Extraocular muscle function may be impaired. Cerebrospinal fluid shows an elevated protein content without a corresponding increase in cells. A recent history of possible viral exposure may strengthen the suspicion that this disease is present.

## CNS TUMORS

### ■ Why might patients with a cerebral tumor undergo sudden deterioration?

The two primary causes of sudden change are hemorrhage and edema. Hemorrhage within the tumor produces an intracerebral hematoma with sudden increase in intracranial pressure. Edema in the area of the brain around a tumor may increase as the tumor size increases. During hypoxic or ischemic episodes or during sudden pH changes or other as yet unknown occurrences, cerebral compensation fails, with subsequent sudden increase in cerebral edema and thus increased intracranial pressure.

In general the more malignant types of tumor hemorrhage, probably because they may have abnormal vessels within the tumor or may erode normal cerebral vessels. Glioblastoma multiforme, metastatic malignant melanoma, and other malignant metastatic tumors produce hemorrhage.

Sudden deterioration caused by edema or hemorrhage requires immediate oxygenation, ventilatory support, large IV and IM doses of steroids, and immediate surgical decompression. Mannitol or urea may be given but should be reserved for the period immediately preceding and during craniotomy.

### ■ When should a spinal cord tumor be handled as an emergency?

Whether the patient has a history of previous malignancy or not, if progressive signs and symptoms referable to a particular level of the spinal cord are present and especially if these findings are less than 1 week in duration, early surgical decompression should be accomplished. If there are no roentgenographic findings coincident with the level of neurologic deficit, a myelogram to confirm the level should be performed prior to surgery and a marker placed over the spine at the proper level. The time spent waiting for surgery should be kept to a minimum, since recovery of lost neurologic function or prevention of further deterioration is enhanced by early decompression.

## COMPLICATIONS THAT MAY FOLLOW DIAGNOSTIC NEUROLOGIC PROCEDURES

### ■ What is the usefulness of the lumbar puncture?

In clinical practice the lumbar puncture (LP) is most helpful in determining the presence or absence of SAH and the presence or absence of an infection or inflammatory process. Regarding the former, uniform color in three tubes indicates the presence of SAH, and a yellow supernatant indicates that it is at least 12 hours old. A traumatic LP may be indicated by variations in the amount of blood in the collecting tube and a clear, colorless supernatant, especially if the clinical history suggests a course lasting more than 12 hours. The presence of clear, colorless cerebrospinal fluid with a lymphocytic response is usually suggestive of aseptic (viral) meningitis or tuberculous or fungal meningitis. The clinical picture and appropriate smears will help differentiate between these. A cloudy cerebrospinal fluid is usually present with acute bacterial meningitis.

### ■ What are the contraindications to LP?

The presence of papilledema until the mass effect in the head is excluded, a pineal shift on the Towne projection of skull x-ray films, and focal neurologic signs before a mass effect is excluded (usually by arteriography) usually contraindicate LP. There is rarely a need to perform LP in a case of head injury or suspected tumor, since other studies will be more definitive, and LP may produce a rapid deterioration.

### ■ What are some complications of neuroradiologic procedures and their treatment?

Carotid arteriography may be associated with the production or aggravation of focal neurologic signs by means of intra-arterial thrombosis or occlusion requiring exploration for the reestablishment of flow, sheath injections, accidental air injection, or embolization from the needle or adjacent atheromatous plaques. Hemorrhage into adjacent tissues can cause pain, swelling, and tracheal compression. This may require endotracheal intubation or tracheotomy. Allergic reactions to the contrast material may occur and are treated as any allergic reaction.

**Table 22-4.** Endocrine-metabolic states associated with CNS disease

| *Metabolic disturbance* | *Associated neurologic state* | *Clinical diagnosis* | *Laboratory diagnosis* | *Treatment* |
|---|---|---|---|---|
| Panhypopituitarism | Pituitary adenoma; may be sudden as in pituitary apoplexy | Headaches, visual field deficit, endocrine disturbance | Low thyroid-stimulating hormone levels, low 17-hydroxycorticoid and 17-ketogenic steroid levels, low gonadotropin levels | Removal of tumor, hormonal replacement |
| Inappropriate secretion of antidiuretic hormone | Several, including SAH, subdural hematoma, tumor | Hyponatremia | Low serum sodium level, high urine sodium level; low serum osmolality, high urine osmolality; high urine specific gravity; normal renal and adrenal function | Treatment of underlying CNS condition; restriction of fluids; administration of concentrated saline solution (for example, 300 ml of 3% sodium chloride) if total body sodium depletion is suspected |
| Hyperosmolar nonketotic acidosis | Head injury, usually | Stupor, hyperglycemia | High serum glucose, acidosis, no acetone in serum | IV insulin |
| Diabetes insipidus | Pituitary tumor; usually postoperative complication of pituitary surgery; blunt head trauma | Marked diuresis of a dilute urine (several hundred milliliters per hour) | Low urine specific gravity | Aqueous pitressin for first 3 days; pitressin tannate in oil after first 3-4 days; fluids to match urine output plus approximately 500 ml/24 hr; electrolyte levels monitored |

Retrograde brachial arteriography may cause catheter embolization (if one is used), arterial spasm, or embolization distally with varying degrees of ischemia to the forearm and hand. Spasm may be treated with local injections of lidocaine or simple warm packs. Occlusion by embolus requires immediate arteriotomy and evacuation of thrombus. The median nerve may be injured by too medial a needle passage. Dissecting hematoma in the neurovascular compartment may cause compression of the median and ulnar nerves and of the brachial artery. This requires instant fasciotomy and hematoma evacuation.

Pneumoencephalography may be associated with severe headache, nausea, and vomiting. These are best treated by placing the patient in a flat position and administering appropriate medication. Seizures or a sudden increase in intracranial pressure may occur, especially if an irritating lesion is already present. Anticonvulsant medication, antiedema agents, and definitive treatment of the offending lesion will usually handle these complications. One must always observe for temporal lobe or cerebellar herniation in the presence of mass lesions.

Ventriculography may be attended by the same complications, except that herniation is less likely to occur.

Myelography is sometimes accompanied by headache, unsteadiness, nausea, and vomiting. An additional hazard is the production of increased neurologic deficits when the needle is placed below the level of the block. Early decompression of the lesion causing the block is necessary to avoid this occurrence.

### ■ How do various drugs affect pupillary size (acute intoxication)?

Morphine, heroin, and nerve gases produce meiosis.

Dilated pupils may be produced by the following (pupillary response is spared): glutethimide, atropine, cocaine, amphetamines, ganglionic blockers, botulism, alcohol (may produce unequal pupils), and LSD-type drugs.

### ■ What conditions and/or drugs may bring about papilledema (not caused by intracranial mass lesions)?

The conditions and/or drugs producing papilledema are as follows:

| | |
|---|---|
| Hyperthyroidism | Lead poisoning |
| Hypervitaminosis A | Chronic steroid administration |
| Hypoparathyroidism | Steroid withdrawal |
| Addison's disease | Birth control pills |
| Systemic lupus erythematosus | Nalidixic acid |
| Diabetes mellitus | Tetracycline |
| Guillain-Barré syndrome or other conditions causing an increase in cerebrospinal fluid protein | Tuberculous meningitis |
| Hypertension | Sarcoidosis |
| Rocky Mountain spotted fever | Polycythemia vera |
| Bilateral ischemic optic neuropathy (giant cell arteritis) | Sickle cell anemia |
| | Upper cervical spine masses |
| | Leukemia |
| | Thrombotic thrombocytopenic purpura |
| | Hurler's syndrome |

Table 22-4 identifies several endocrine and/or metabolic states associated with CNS disease and indicates the appropriate treatment for each.

## BIBLIOGRAPHY

Aaron, H., editor: Handbook of antimicrobial therapy, New Rochelle, N.Y., 1974, Medical Letter, Inc.

Advisory Council for the National Institute of Neurological Disease and Blindness: A classification and outline of cerebrovascular disease, Neurology **8:**1-34, 1958.

Bartter, F. C., and Schwartz, W. B.: The syndrome of inappropriate secretion of antidiuretic hormone, Am. J. Med. **42:**790-806, 1967.

Bruce, D. A., Langfitt, T. W., Miller, J. D., Schultz, H., Vapalahti, M. P., Stancek, A., and Goldberg, H. D.: Regional cerebral blood flow, intracranial pressure and brain metabolism in comatose patients, J. Neurosurg. **38:** 131-144, 1973.

Caveness, W. F., and Walker, A. E.: Head injury, Philadelphia, 1966, J. B. Lippincott Co.

Coates, J. B., and Meirowsky, R. M.: The Neurosurgery of trauma, Office of the Surgeon General, Washington, D. C., 1965, United States Army.

DeBakey, M. E., Crawford, E. S., Cooley, D. A., Morris, G. C., Garrett, H. E. and Fields, W. S.: Cerebral arterial insufficiency: one to eleven year results following arterial reconstructive operation, Am. Surg. **161**:921-945, 1965.

Dennis, L. H., Cohen, R. J., Schachner, S. H., and Conrad M. E.: Consumptive coagulopathy in fulminant meningococcemia, J.A.M.A. **205**: 183-185, 1968.

Fisher, C. M., Picard, E. H., Polack, A., Dalal, P., and Ojemann, R. G.: Acute hypertensive cerebellar hemorrhage: symptoms and surgical treatment, J. Nerv. Ment. Dis. **140**:38-57, 1965.

Friedman, H., and Odom, G. C.: Expanding intracranial lesions in geriatric patients, Geriatrics **27**:105-115, 1972.

Lundberg, N., Troupp, H., and Loren, H.: Continuous recording of the ventricular fluid pressure in patients with severe, acute traumatic brain injury, J. Neurosurg. **22**:581-590, 1965.

Merritt, H. H.: A textbook of neurology, ed. 5, Philadelphia, 1973, Lea & Febiger.

Murphy, F., and Maccubbin, D. A.: Carotid endarterectomy: a long term follow-up study, J. Neurosurg. **23**:156-168, 1965.

Odom, G. L., Tindall, G. T., Cupp, H. B., and Woodhall, B.: Neurosurgical approach to intracerebral hemorrhage in cerebrovascular disease, J. Nerv. Ment. Dis. **41**:145-168, 1966.

Plum, F., and Posner, J. B.: The diagnosis of stupor and coma, ed. 2, contemporary neurology series, Philadelphia, 1972, F. A. Davis Co.

Salmon, J. H.: Ventriculitis complicating meningitis, Am. J. Dis. Child. **124**:35-40, 1972.

Toole, J. F., and Patel, A. N.: Cerebrovascular disorders, New York, 1967, McGraw-Hill Book Co.

Whisnant, J. P., Matsumoto, N., and Eleveback, L. R.: The effect of anticoagulant therapy on prognosis of patients with transient cerebral ischemic attack in a community, Mayo Clin. Proc. **48**:844-848, 1973.

Youmans, J. R.: Neurological surgery, New York, 1973, W. B. Saunders Co.

*chapter 23*

# Clinical management of the obstetric patient

**IRENE MATOUSEK**
**CHESTER B. MARTIN**

There are sound reasons for the different management of women who are critically ill at any point in pregnancy from conception until the physiologic puerperal recovery approximately 6 weeks after delivery. First, there are alterations in maternal physiology and anatomy that may change or obscure physical findings or responses to stressful circumstances or medications. Second, there is the presence of the fetus, dependent for life support on a relatively intact maternal physiology.

In very early pregnancy the embryo is undergoing rapid proliferation of cells and differentiation of body systems. At this time pharmacologic insults from the administration of drugs are likely to occur. Hazards from radiation are also well documented, and there is serious cause to believe that an unfavorable maternal environment with altered body chemistry and a deficient supply of oxygen may have equally grave consequences.

### ■ When does pregnancy become a concern in the management of a critical care patient?

Pregnancy should be a concern from conception onward. It may be worthwhile to consider every woman during the reproductive years, from approximately age 12 to age 50, as a likely candidate for pregnancy unless proved otherwise. A rapid pregnancy screening test of urine and/or serum may be helpful in verifying an early pregnancy when history or clinical examination findings are equivocal.

When the patient is known to be pregnant, the inclusion of pregnancy on the patient's problem list ensures consideration of pregnancy in selecting clinical diagnostic techniques, therapeutic plans, and management. A critical illness of almost any sort may cause the pregnancy to terminate spontaneously. The termination of pregnancy in a critically ill woman may often result in the birth of a compromised infant.

It may be well to consider the advantages to the fetus of transportation, in utero, to a site where *both* mother and infant may have intensive care immediately available.

## PHYSIOLOGIC CHANGES IN PREGNANCY

### ■ What are some of the important changes in maternal physiology during pregnancy?

The pregnant patient has an increase in blood volume, heart rate, and cardiac output (the amount of blood pumped each minute by the heart). Her blood pressure tends to be lower than in the nonpregnant state, especially during the middle period of pregnancy. The energy cost and increased cardiac work required by exercise is greater during pregnancy than at other times. This is of particular significance in the pregnant woman with cardiac or pulmonary disease and may reduce the tolerance for exercise or stress in such patients.

Kidney blood flow and urine filtration are

normally increased by 30% to 50% during pregnancy. In addition, there is normally a dilatation of the ureters and slowing of urine flow during pregnancy. These changes predispose the pregnant patient to urinary tract infections, which, if severe, can be a threat to both maternal and fetal health.

### ■ What is the role of nutrition in pregnancy?

Although good nutrition is important at any time, it is especially so during pregnancy. Inadequate nutrition may contribute to many of the complications of pregnancy, including impaired fetal growth and preeclampsia-eclampsia. (See subsequent discussions.)

### ■ What are the important changes produced by the enlarging uterus?

As it grows, the uterus progressively displaces the other abdominal contents of the abdomen. In most normal women, the displacement produces no symptoms or at most contributes slightly to unpleasant symptoms such as heartburn and epigastric fullness after meals. In women with deformities of the thoracic spine and rib cage, however, the upward displacement of abdominal contents may displace the diaphragm and restrict its movements sufficiently to produce respiratory embarrassment.

The displacement of many abdominal organs from their normal position, and the forward displacement of the abdominal wall by the enlarging uterus may alter the physical signs accompanying many acute intra-abdominal diseases and trauma. For example, in appendicitis the abdominal tenderness and localized signs of peritoneal irritation may appear much later in the course of the disease during pregnancy than in the nonpregnant state, and the tenderness when it appears may be located at or above the level of the umbilicus rather than in the usual right lower quadrant position. Similarly, with intra-abdominal bleeding or gastrointestinal perforation, signs of peritoneal irritation may appear only quite late in the course of the disease, and the early absence of these signs may lead to an initial misdiagnosis and mismanagement.

In the last third of pregnancy the weight of the uterus and its contents is carried anterior to the normal axis of weight bearing. This plus the hormone-induced softening of the connective tissue supports of joints predisposes the pregnant patient to postural back pain and, indeed, acute back injury.

Also during the last third of pregnancy the enlarging uterus compresses the pelvic veins and inferior vena cava. This in turn leads to slowing of the blood circulation in the pelvic and leg veins and predisposes the pregnant patient to the development of thrombophlebitis and thromboembolism, especially if she is immobilized because of illness or injury. Even ambulatory women have an increased risk of developing venous thrombosis, especially if there is any preexisting venous disease. Such measures as elastic support stockings, avoidance of long standing, and elevation of the legs when at rest are thus indicated in pregnant women with a history of thrombophlebitis or with existing varicose veins; leg elevation, elastic stockings, and regular examination for evidence of thrombophlebitis are indicated whenever a pregnant patient is immobilized or confined to bed because of illness or injury. It is important that the stockings be removed at least every 4 hours and reapplied to prevent constriction and impairment of blood flow. At the time of removal passive movement of the lower extremities may assist blood flow.

### ■ What are the goals for fetal management during critical care of the obstetric patient?

The primary goal is to provide the best possible maternal environment for the growing fetus. The developing fetus is dependent on its mother for an uninterrupted supply of oxygen. This in turn requires an intact supply of maternal red blood cells, adequate maternal blood pressure to ensure perfusion of the placenta, and sufficient arterial oxygen tension to promote diffusion across the placenta. Accordingly, transfusion should be considered for correction of severe anemia. Hypotension should be corrected by the restoration of effective blood volume (avoiding vasoconstrictive drugs, if possible, since these may impede uterine blood flow). Oxygen should be administered when there is maternal hypoxemia, hypotension, or severe anemia.

The fetus must be protected from pharmacologic and biochemical insults. The fetus very rapidly reflects altered maternal biochemical states. Almost all drugs cross the placenta, and many affect the fetus or newborn adversely.

The fetus is dependent on the mother for an adequate heat-losing mechanism. The high metabolic rate of the fetus creates heat, which must be transported to the mother for dissipation. This mechanism is essential to avoid stressing the fetal organism, both through the increased consumption of oxygen during hyperthermia and exhaustion of the cardiovascular system, which increases heart rate and cardiac output in an attempt to lose heat. The safe heat tolerance level for the human fetus is unknown, but it may be lower than that of the child or adult. Serious consideration should be given to treating the sustained elevation of temperature in critically ill pregnant women directly through the use of evaporation, cold packs, or other means.

The fetus is also dependent on the mother for nutrition. The essential substrates appear to be glucose and amino acids. Although the fetus apparently can tolerate short periods of deprivation, there is evidence that its neurologic development may be impaired by maternal ketoacidosis. For this reason the critically ill pregnant woman should receive sufficient calories to prevent the development of starvation, ketosis, and acidosis.

## OBSTETRIC PROBLEMS IN THE FIRST HALF OF PREGNANCY

The most commonly encountered pregnancy-related problems requiring critical care during the first half of pregnancy are abortion, ectopic pregnancy, and pernicious vomiting.

### Abortion

Abortion legally denotes the termination of pregnancy prior to the stage of fetal viability, that is, prior to 20 weeks after the last menstrual period (LMP), in most jurisdictions in the United States. Abortions may be spontaneous or induced; induced abortions further may be either therapeutic (performed through legitimate medical care channels) or illegal (criminal).

#### ■ What are the symptoms and findings in spontaneous abortion?

The first clinical signs of spontaneous abortion are usually the appearance of vaginal bleeding accompanied by lower abdominal cramping pain. The bleeding results from separation of the placenta, whereas the cramps represent intense uterine contractions. The stage of abortion marked only by uterine bleeding with or without accompanying cramps but before dilatation of the cervix has begun is called "threatened abortion."

With further evolution of the abortion process the cervix begins to efface and dilate as a result of the uterine contractions. When the cervical dilatation and effacement can be detected on clinical examination, the abortion is said to be "inevitable." Considerable placental separation has usually occurred by this stage, and the bleeding may become quite heavy.

Dilatation of the cervix is usually followed shortly by expulsion of the products of conception (embryo or fetus, fetal membranes, and placenta). The expulsion phase is frequently accompanied by a further increase in the amount of vaginal bleeding. An incomplete abortion is one in which the conceptus has been partially expelled, but additional fragments of the placenta and fetal membranes remain within the uterus. A complete abortion is one in which all of the products of conception have been expelled. The stage of complete abortion is usually followed by a reduction in the severity of the cramps and in the amount of vaginal bleeding. During the latter half of the first trimester and in the first half of the second trimester the expulsion of the products of conception may occur piecemeal over several hours, and it is not unusual for fragments of placenta and fetal membranes to remain within the uterus following expulsion of the major portion of the products of conception. Retention of these placental fragments in utero may cause continued bleeding, and the degenerating placental material provides a rich growth medium for bacteria, which enter the uterine cavity through the dilated cervix. For this reason and in order to minimize the duration of pain and the amount of blood loss, incomplete abortion is usually terminated by curettage, and curettage is frequently performed even though the abortion may seem to have proceeded spontaneously to completion.

## ■ What are the chief critical care problems in spontaneous abortion?

The major problems of spontaneous abortion relate to blood loss, infection, and operative injury during completion of the abortion.

Any patient undergoing abortion is at risk for a major hemorrhage. Assessment of the amount of blood loss already sustained, establishment of a route for the rapid IV administration of fluids or blood, and arranging for the availability of cross-matched blood for replacement should be done very early in the care of these patients. These steps should be performed even if the patient is only experiencing minor bleeding when she is first seen, because the amount of hemorrhage may increase dramatically at any time.

When the patient is seen with threatened abortion signaled only by mild cramps and scanty vaginal bleeding, adequate treatment may consist of starting an IV infusion, restricting oral intake (in case later operative intervention is required), and observing her while at bed rest for a time. In a large proportion of these early cases the symptoms will subside, and the pregnancy will continue uneventfully. In other patients the pain and bleeding will increase and require evacuation of the uterus by curettage. When the patient is initially seen at the stage of inevitable or incomplete abortion, preparations should be set in motion for early curettage in order to minimize the amount of pain, the amount of blood lost, and the likelihood of ascending uterine infection. The oral administration of liquids, food, or medication should be avoided in anticipation of the use of anesthesia.

Serious intrauterine infection is not frequent in patients with spontaneous abortion unless the patient has delayed for a considerable time before seeking medical care. All patients should be examined for evidence of infection, however, because of the potential gravity of this complication. Suggestive findings include fever, uterine tenderness, and foul-smelling vaginal discharge or placental fragments. Hypotension and tachycardia disproportionate to the estimated amount of blood lost are potentially very serious clinical signs. Infected abortion can become a life-threatening complication because of the possibility of septicemia, septic shock, and invasive pelvic infections with virulent strains of *Streptococcus, Escherichia coli,* or *Clostridium,* which may inhabit the vagina and cervix.

In order to minimize the likelihood of introducing additional pathogenic organisms into the vaginal tract of patients undergoing abortion, pelvic examination should be carried out only following antiseptic cleansing of the vulva, and only sterile gloves and instruments should be employed. The number of pelvic examinations should be kept to the minimum required for diagnosis and treatment.

Operative injury to the uterus, cervix, and, in rare instances, even the bowel or pelvic supporting tissues may occur during the course of curettage and completion of an abortion despite the exercise of careful judgment and the employment of skillful technique. Simple uterine perforation usually requires only observation to exclude intra-abdominal bleeding from the perforation site. More serious injuries may require active intervention. Since an injury may go unrecognized at the time by even an experienced surgeon, all patients should be observed carefully for evidence of blood loss or peritoneal irritation for several hours following curettage.

## ■ What critical complications may occur with therapeutic abortion?

The complications of the therapeutic termination of pregnancy depend on the means employed to empty the uterus. In the first trimester this is usually evacuation of the products of conception by means of a suction curette. The chief hazards of this route are laceration of the cervix during dilatation and perforation of the uterus during curettage. Either of these accidents may be followed by serious hemorrhage. In addition, perforation of the uterus may result in inadvertent injury to the bowel, with resulting peritonitis. Uterine infection may occur, even though the dilatation and curettage were carried out under surgical asepsis. The infection may become apparent early during the postoperative period or may appear several days later (especially if a few placental fragments have been left in the uterus). Patients should be observed for several hours under recovery room conditions following suction curettage in order to detect hemorrhage or peritonitis from unrecognized injuries. The patient should also be instructed on discharge to be alert for symptoms and signs of delayed postoperative infection and to return immediately should symptoms appear.

## ■ What are the problems associated with therapeutic abortion during the second trimester?

In the second trimester the uterus is larger, its contents are bulkier and more substantial, and the techniques for terminating pregnancy are less satisfactory than in the first trimester. The most widely used technique for therapeutic abortion in the second trimester has been the intra-amniotic injection of hypertonic solutions, especially sodium chloride. These hypertonic solutions kill the fetus and damage the placenta and decidua, resulting in labor and expulsion of uterine contents. The hazards associated with the use of hypertonic solutions include the following:

1. Rapid movement of fluid into the amniotic space, causing hypotension
2. Inadvertent IV injection, resulting in shock
3. Accidental injection into the myometrium, causing uterine necrosis and peritonitis
4. Release of clot-promoting substances from the degenerating placenta and decidua into the circulation, producing disseminated intravascular coagulation with consumption of clotting factors and a secondary bleeding disorder
5. In patients with cardiac and renal disease, retention of the excessive sodium within the vascular system and vessel walls, resulting in edema, hypertension, and even cardiac failure
6. With hypertonic glucose solutions, serious intrauterine infection

Although these complications are relatively infrequent, their occasional occurrence makes it advisable that patients undergoing midtrimester abortion be observed carefully for evidence of one or another of these problems for several hours following the intra-amniotic installation of the hypertonic solution. Many authorities believe that these patients should be kept in the hospital until abortion has been completed.

The use of hypertonic injections into the amniotic cavity has been combined with the IV administration of oxytocin in order to shorten the injection-delivery time. This combination has also been found to result in an increased incidence of some of the complications mentioned previously. The addition of uterine stimulation with oxytocin to that resulting from the hypertonic solutions may also result in uterine rupture.

Another technique that has been employed for second trimester abortion is the use of laminaria (dried seaweed that swells on absorption of water) or a bougie (such as a Foley catheter with a large volume bag) to effect a gradual dilatation of the cervix, followed by the administration of oxytocin to produce labor and evacuation of the uterus. The occasional hazards of this technique include infection resulting from instrumentation of the cervix and uterine rupture resulting from overstimulation with oxytocin. These techniques should be applied only in the hospital setting and only with close observation to detect complications at their earliest occurrence.

Recently prostaglandins have become available for use in second trimester abortion. These are naturally occurring substances that have among their actions stimulation of myometrial contractility. The prostaglandins of the $E_2$ and $F_{2\alpha}$ types have been administered by a variety of routes, but the most popular one at present is the intra-amniotic injection of the prostaglandin. The most serious complication associated with these agents has been the occasional occurrence of uterine rupture, especially rupture of the posterior portion of the lower uterine segment or upper cervix. Less threatening side effects include nausea, abdominal cramps, diarrhea, and fever. Some patients also develop an acute elevation in blood pressure following the administration of prostaglandins. The potential complications and side effects demand that these agents be used only in the hospital setting, where facilities for close observation and immediate treatment of complications are available.

#### ■ What are the serious complications that may occur following illegal abortion?

The most frequent complications following illegal abortion are the same ones that occur after spontaneous or therapeutically induced abortion: hemorrhage, infection, and trauma. The frequency of these complications is probably increased, because the criminal abortionist is likely to be relatively uneducated, unskilled, and in some cases flagrantly careless and dirty. In addition, the patient is likely to delay seeking medical care, in the hope that her problem will go away and that she may remain undetected. When these patients do seek medical attention, they are likely to be suffering from severe and protracted hemorrhage or advanced pelvic or systemic infection. There may be intraperitoneal bleeding or peritonitis as a result of uterine perforation, and occasionally foreign bodies such as catheters and other objects are found within the abdominal cavity as a testimony to the abortionist's lack of skill. The patient known or suspected to have had a criminal abortion should have abdominal x-ray films taken to detect intraperitoneal air resulting from uterine perforation, intra-abdominal foreign bodies, and evidence of infection with gas-forming organisms in the pelvis. Many criminal abortion patients are critically ill when they are brought to the hospital and may require immediate, vigorous therapy of hypovolemic shock and advanced sepsis.

In some cases criminal abortion has been attempted by the injection of necrotizing solutions or pastes into the uterus. In these patients there may be extensive necrosis of pelvic tissue and advanced infection. Tetanus or gas gangrene infections may be present. Some of these substances may be nephrotoxic, moreover, adding the problems of renal shutdown to those of shock and sepsis.

### Ectopic pregnancy

#### ■ What is ectopic pregnancy?

Ectopic pregnancy refers to the implantation of the conceptus outside the main portion of the uterine cavity. This ectopic implantation most frequently occurs in the fallopian tube, but may also occur on the pelvic peritoneum and surface of other intra-abdominal organs (abdominal pregnancy), on the ovary (ovarian pregnancy), in the intramyometrial portion of the uterine tube (cornual pregnancy), or in the cervical canal (cervical pregnancy). Ectopic pregnancies rarely survive beyond the first trimester. Rupture of the implantation site (tube or uterine cornu) or placental separation are the usual events that terminate the pregnancy, and either can cause profuse intra-abdominal hemorrhage. Some abdominal pregnancies survive into the second or third trimester; however, the incidence of placental insufficiency and maternal complications (for example, bowel obstruction) is high and delivery of a live, mature fetus is unusual.

#### ■ What are the symptoms of ectopic pregnancy?

The most frequent symptom of ectopic pregnancy, especially tubal pregnancy, is abdominal pain. Other very common symptoms include vaginal bleeding and a history of delayed or missed menstrual period. Symptoms of shock may also be present.

Important physical findings suggesting ectopic tubal pregnancy include a pelvic mass —usually unilateral or posterior to the uterus—and the aspiration of nonclotting blood on culdocentesis. The uterus may be normal in size or enlarged one and one-half to two times. Hypotension, tachycardia, and pallor may be present if the intraperitoneal bleeding is severe.

■ **What are the initial critical steps in the management of ectopic pregnancy?**

The initial management steps in cases of suspected ruptured or bleeding ectopic pregnancy consist of establishing a large caliber IV line, assessing adequacy of circulation, and sending a blood sample for type and cross match. The patient should be observed carefully and frequently for evidence of actual or impending shock during the time when diagnostic procedures and preparations for definitive therapy are being carried out.

### Pernicious vomiting

■ **What is pernicious vomiting (hyperemesis gravidarum)?**

Many pregnant patients experience some nausea and vomiting during the first trimester. These symptoms probably result from hormonal stimulation of the "vomiting center" in the brain stem. Usually the nausea and vomiting are mild and disappear toward the end of the first trimester. In a small minority of women, however, the nausea and vomiting are severe and protracted and may result in dehydration and ketoacidosis. Repeated episodes of nausea and vomiting can interfere markedly with maternal nutrition.

■ **What is the danger of pernicious vomiting to the pregnancy?**

In one large study of women with hyperemesis gravidarum there was a high incidence of abortion in patients suffering repeated episodes of severe nausea and vomiting. In addition, more recent studies have shown that there is an increased incidence of neurologic abnormalities in the infants of women who experienced ketonemia and ketonuria from any cause during their pregnancies.

■ **Which patients with nausea and vomiting of pregnancy require urgent care?**

The pregnant woman who presents with clinically apparent dehydration clearly needs hospitalization for correction of her fluid and electrolyte abnormalities. In addition, the urine of any pregnant woman with a history of more than occasional vomiting should be tested for the presence of acetone. Any pregnant woman exhibiting acetonuria is a candidate for hospitalization and IV fluid therapy. In many patients with hyperemesis gravidarum, the nausea and vomiting will subside when the patient is admitted to the hospital and her fluid and electrolyte abnormalities are corrected. Other patients will require antinauseant medications for relief of the nausea and vomiting. These medications should be selected carefully, especially during the first trimester, because some of them have been suspected of causing congenital anomalies.

## OBSTETRIC PROBLEMS IN THE SECOND HALF OF PREGNANCY

■ **What are the obstetric and other pregnancy-related problems requiring critical care during the second half of pregnancy?**

The most important disorders—from the standpoint of severity or frequency—requiring critical care during the second half of pregnancy include bleeding complications (such as placenta previa and abruptio placentae), hypertensive disorders, premature rupture of the fetal membranes, and premature labor. Urinary tract infections may occur at any time during pregnancy, but these can become life-threatening complications, especially for the fetus, during the latter months.

All pregnant patients become critical care patients during labor, delivery, and the early postpartum hours. Although most women go through the peripartum time without incident, the potential for damaging or life-threatening complications for both fetus and mother is at its greatest during this time.

Although many intercurrent medical diseases may complicate the management of pregnancy, certain maternal diseases such as diabetes, heart disease (especially obstructive valvular disease), chronic renal disease, and acute febrile illnesses are particularly noteworthy because of their relative frequency and because of the urgent maternal or fetal complications sometimes associated with them.

### ■ What are the important bleeding complications during the second half of pregnancy?

The most important obstetric complications associated with vaginal bleeding during late pregnancy are placenta previa and premature separation of the placenta (abruptio placentae). Trauma to the vagina and cervix and lesions such as cervical erosions and cervical cancers may also cause bleeding during pregnancy, as at other times. Bleeding during the early or late postpartum period may result from lacerations of the uterus, cervix, or vagina; failure of the uterine muscle to contract following separation of the placenta; or the presence of fetal membranes within the uterus.

### ■ What is the clinical situation characteristic of placenta previa?

Placenta previa refers to implantation of the placenta in the lower portion of the uterine cavity, adjacent to or even covering the cervical opening. Bleeding occurs when a portion of the placenta separates as a result of the normal thinning of the lower uterine segment and dilatation of the upper cervix, which takes place prior to labor in late pregnancy. Placental separation and consequent bleeding may also occur as a result of mechanical disturbance of the upper cervix or lower uterine segment that may occur during intercourse or vaginal examination.

The bleeding in placenta previa is typically painless and unassociated with regular uterine contractions. The uterus is soft and not tender. Because the placenta occupies the lower portion of the uterus, the fetal presenting part (breech or vertex) is usually displaced upward and may be palpated as "floating" relatively high above the pelvic inlet. In many cases the long body axis of the fetus may be oriented transversely or obliquely (transverse or oblique lie) instead of the usual position parallel to the maternal body axis. The fetal heart tones are usually normal and without the irregularity suggesting fetal distress, unless the amount of maternal blood lost has been great enough to produce (maternal) hemorrhagic shock.

Episodes of bleeding from placenta previa usually subside spontaneously unless interference causes additional placental separation or progressive labor has begun. Since even gentle manipulation of the cervix may dislodge additional portions of the placenta and produce further bleeding, it is of utmost importance to avoid this possibility. For this reason vaginal examination should not be performed on any patient suspected of having placenta previa unless the patient is in the operating room, prepared for surgery, and with anesthesia and surgical personnel in attendance (a "double set-up" examination, so-called because one is prepared to carry out a cesarean section or induction of labor in vaginal delivery, depending on the findings). The double set-up examination is reserved for patients with vaginal bleeding after 36 or 37 weeks of pregnancy, at which time the fetus is considered to be mature enough to withstand delivery. Earlier than this time, patients known or suspected to have placenta previa are managed expectantly with bed rest under close medical observation in order to permit the pregnancy to continue to the stage of fetal maturity.

### ■ What are the clinical characteristics of premature separation of the placenta?

The symptoms and findings resulting from premature separation of the normally implanted placenta vary according to the degree of placental separation and, to a lesser extent, according to the mechanism responsible for the separation. The degree of premature separation can range from detachment of all or a major part of the placenta (abruptio placentae) to separation of only a small portion of the placental edge. The mechanism involved in the major placental separations appears to be most often disruption of the wall of one or more of the arteries supplying maternal blood to the placenta, permitting the escape of maternal blood under high pressure into the decidua (endometrium of pregnancy). The extravasated blood may dissect extensively in the decidual layer, leading to the separation of increasing amounts of the placental area. The most frequent cause of these arterial ruptures is thought to be focal degeneration and necrosis in the arterial wall. Such lesions occur with increased frequency in pregnancies complicated by chronic hypertensive disease, and abruptio placentae occurs more often in hypertensive than in normotensive pregnant women.

Less extensive and less dramatic placental separations result from local disruption of the placental attachments, especially at the placental margin. Such local separations may result from stresses imposed by unequal growth of the placenta and uterine wall and perhaps also tensions on the placental attachments occurring during uterine contractions. The maternal blood escaping into the decidua in these local separations is not under high arterial pressure, and the separation is less likely to extend.

Although only a small proportion of placental separations result from external trauma, trauma can indeed produce either local or extensive placental separation. Placental separation is more likely to occur in cases of abdominal trauma; however, severe accelerations or decelerations, as during automobile accidents, may stress the placental attachment to the point of separation even though there is no direct injury to the abdomen. The possibility of premature separation of the placenta should thus be kept in mind in the assessment of women who experience trauma during pregnancy.

The pregnant woman who has experienced a major degree of placental separation presents a fairly characteristic clinical picture. Vaginal bleeding is usually present, and this can be copious. In a small portion of cases the bleeding from placental separation is retained behind the placenta (concealed abruptions), and in these patients vaginal bleeding will be absent. Continuous abdominal and/or low back pain is likely to be present, and this may be severe. The uterus is frequently tender to palpation, especially if the area of abruption involves the anterior uterine wall.

Uterine contractions are usually present, and in some patients with severe abruptions very frequent uterine contractions combined with an increase in the resting tension (hypertonus) gives the impression of a continuous uterine contraction that does not relax. The fetal heart tones may be absent, or a slow or irregular fetal heart rate may give evidence of fetal distress. Major degrees of placental separation may be recognized easily from the history and physical findings.

The smaller degrees of premature separation of the placenta are more difficult to diagnose with certainty from the clinical findings alone. In particular it may be difficult to distinguish between a marginal separation of the placenta and bleeding from placenta previa without the aid of specialized techniques such as ultrasound or radioisotope scanning to demonstrate the placental location. Uterine pain, tenderness, and contractions may be minimal or absent with small placental separations. One important clue may often be obtained on abdominal examination, that is, the finding that the fetal presenting part (vertex or breech) is dipping deeply into the pelvis, and this suggests that a major degree of placenta previa is unlikely to be present. On the other hand, this finding does not exclude a marginal or low-lying placenta; thus digital vaginal examination should only be performed under the double set-up conditions unless placental localization studies have excluded placenta previa.

### ■ What are the management principles in premature separation of the placenta?

When the clinical symptoms and findings indicate a major degree of placental separation, prompt termination of the pregnancy by induction of labor or cesarean section is indicated. The fetal heart rate should be monitored continuously and the fetus delivered by cesarean section if distress occurs. Induction of labor with fetal monitoring is usually also indicated for lesser degrees of premature placental separation when the complication occurs during the last 3 or 4 weeks of pregnancy, after the fetus has reached adequate maturity. Earlier than this time, the pregnancy may be managed expectantly under close observation if the bleeding subsides and there is no evidence of fetal distress.

## ■ What other major maternal complications may occur with abruptio placentae?

Hemorrhagic shock is a frequent complication of major placental abruptions because of the extensive maternal blood loss that may occur. In many patients, however, the blood pressure is maintained at normal or even elevated levels for a time even though major hemorrhage has occurred. If this possibility is not recognized, one may be lulled into a false sense of security in managing patients with placental abruption, only to be rudely surprised when circulatory collapse occurs abruptly. The patient with severe abruptio placentae, that is, the patient with abdominal pain and a tense, tender uterus, has probably lost 1000 to 1500 ml of circulating blood volume within a relatively short time after the onset of the abruption. In these patients it is a good practice to begin replacement with electrolyte solutions immediately after the complication is diagnosed. The urine output is usually a good indicator of the adequacy of the blood volume, and a low or falling output (below 50 to 75 ml/hr) suggests inadequate replacement. If the urine volume does not begin to increase following infusion of 1000 to 1500 ml of fluid, however, one should be wary of the possibility that acute renal failure has occurred. A central venous pressure catheter should be inserted at this point, if this has not already been done, and used as a guide to further fluid therapy in order to avoid volume overload and pulmonary edema.

Another major complication that may accompany abruptio placentae is the occurrence of a coagulation disorder. The most frequent coagulopathy encountered with abruptio placentae is disseminated intravascular coagulation with consumption of multiple clotting factors. In a very much smaller proportion of patients a fibrinolytic state may dominate. A blood sample for observation of clot formation and possible lysis should be drawn periodically throughout the management of patients with abruptio placentae. Even when a coagulopathy develops, however, specific replacement of fibrinogen and other clotting factors is usually necessary only if cesarean section delivery is required.

The third major complication that may accompany abruptio placentae is acute renal failure. This occurs primarily because of renal ischemia resulting from severe blood loss. In patients with disseminated intravascular coagulation, fibrin thrombi in the renal glomerular capillaries may add to the impairment of kidney function.

## ■ What other problems cause vaginal bleeding in late pregnancy?

Lacerations of the vagina or cervix may produce copious bleeding because of the increased vascularity of these tissues during pregnancy. These lacerations may result from sexual activity or attempts to terminate the pregnancy. Caustic chemicals such as potassium permanganate are occasionally used for douching, and these may cause vaginal or cervical ulcerations with heavy bleeding. Cervical cancers may also be responsible for heavy bleeding during pregnancy. Vaginitis, cervicitis, or cervical erosions tend to produce only scanty bleeding, spotting, or blood-tinged discharge. Bloody mucous may be expelled at the onset of labor ("bloody shows"). Any vaginal bleeding during late pregnancy must be assessed with caution, however, for the initial bleeding from placenta previa or premature placental separation may be very scanty in amount.

Rarely an abnormal insertion of the umbilical cord into the placenta or an atypical path of umbilical vessel branches will bring these fetal vessels close to the internal cervical opening, where they may be torn during cervical dilatation or vaginal examinations in labor. Fetal hemorrhage from these vessels can rapidly bring about fetal distress. For this reason the fetal heart rate should always be monitored for evidence of fetal distress when vaginal bleeding occurs in late pregnancy, even when there is no evidence of abruptio placentae or placenta previa.

### ■ What are the initial measures in the management of the patient with vaginal bleeding in late pregnancy?

Patients with vaginal bleeding in late pregnancy should immediately have the following procedures done:

1. A rapid assessment of the amount of blood lost
2. Provision made for blood replacement
3. An IV line placed for fluid therapy
4. Other indicated physiologic support such as oxygen administration

The first step is a rapid assessment of the amount of bleeding that has occurred or is occurring. When the patient describes bleeding greater than the peak of menstrual flow, or if there is blood on the legs or clothing, it is wise to proceed as if a major bleeding complication is present. When abdominal pain and uterine tenderness are present, the possibility of abruptio placentae with concealed hemorrhage should be considered, even though external bleeding is minimal or absent. A large caliber IV line should be established immediately and kept open with a balanced electrolyte or normal saline solution. Tachycardia, hypotension, and pallor usually indicate that a major degree of blood loss has already occurred, and fluids should be administered rapidly. In any case blood should be tested for type and cross match.

After these steps have been accomplished, additional history may be obtained and physical examination carried out in order to determine further the cause of the bleeding. A gentle, careful speculum examination may be carried out in order to inspect the vagina and cervix for local lesions; however, pelvic examination may easily provoke an immediate massive hemorrhage. Therefore digital palpation of the upper vagina and cervix *should not* be performed except in the operating room under double set-up conditions, and even then only if the decision has been made to terminate the pregnancy. The fetal heart tones should be checked as part of the initial assessment, and continuous monitoring of the fetal heart rate (using external techniques) should be begun if the presumptive diagnosis is abruptio placentae or placenta previa or if the mother appears to be hypovolemic. When fetal distress is present, the administration of oxygen to the mother by means of a face mask may benefit the fetus while preparations are being made for definitive treatment.

The data base should be completed as soon as the patient's condition permits. This will include a well-defined history either from the patient or her family, a review of available records, completion of the physical examination, and steps to obtain information from other pertinent sources such as the physician's office, clinic, or hospital.

### ■ What are abnormally elevated levels of blood pressure during pregnancy?

The expected blood pressure in young women during the childbearing years tends to be lower than the "normal" 120/80 mm Hg. The blood pressure tends to fall slightly during pregnancy in normal women, averaging about 5 mm Hg below nonpregnant levels during the latter part of the first trimester, the second trimester, and the early part of the third trimester. The midpregnancy fall in blood pressure may be exaggerated in patients with chronic hypertension. For this reason blood pressures greater than about 125/80 mm Hg should be regarded with suspicion during pregnancy.

### ■ What are the hypertensive disorders that may complicate pregnancy?

Blood pressures greater than 140 mm Hg systolic and 90 mm Hg diastolic are definitely abnormal during pregnancy. Lower readings are abnormal when they represent a rise of 30 mm Hg systolic or 15 mm Hg diastolic over nonpregnant or early pregnancy blood pressure.

The group of hypertensive diseases that may complicate pregnancy includes the following four categories:

1. *Preeclampsia-eclampsia.* This is a syndrome of unknown cause that occurs only during pregnancy or the early postpartum period. Preeclampsia is characterized by hypertension, generalized edema, and proteinuria. In eclampsia convulsions and/or coma are also present.

2. *Chronic hypertension* This category includes women known or suspected to have chronic hypertensive disease. The elevated blood pressure may be the result of essential vascular hypertension, or it may be secondary to other maternal disease such as chronic renal disease or collagen vascular disease.

3. *Chronic hypertension with superimposed preeclampsia-eclampsia.* This category includes patients with chronic hypertension who develop a further increase in their blood pressure accompanied by proteinuria and/or edema during the latter half of pregnancy. Approximately one fourth of patients with chronic hypertension develop superimposed preeclampsia during pregnancy.

4. *Late or transient hypertension.* In this category are patients who develop an elevation in blood pressure during the third trimester of pregnancy or within the first 24 hours after delivery but whose blood pressure returns to normal within 10 days after delivery. These patients are distinguished from those with preeclampsia by the absence of generalized edema or proteinuria.

## ■ What are the consequences of hypertensive disease for the pregnant patient?

Patients with chronic hypertension have a 25% chance of developing a further increase in blood pressure, together with evidence of impairment of renal function, during pregnancy. In addition, chronic hypertension is often accompanied by changes in the arteries supplying the maternal blood to the placenta, resulting in impaired placental and fetal growth and an increase in the incidence of premature delivery and low birth weight infants. There is also a two- to threefold increase in the frequency of abruptio placentae in patients with chronic hypertension.

Women who develop severe preeclampsia, eclampsia, or preeclampsia superimposed on chronic hypertension are at increased risk for the occurrence of stroke or other vascular accident or cardiac failure. Other serious complications of preeclampsia-eclampsia include impaired kidney and liver function and blood coagulation defects. The maternal blood supply to the uterus is also impaired in preeclampsia-eclampsia, and fetal growth retardation, asphyxia, and even death may occur. Preeclampsia-eclampsia may develop and progress very rapidly, and patients with this complication of pregnancy require close observation and often intensive medical care.

## ■ What are the critical observations in pregnancies complicated by hypertension?

The pregnant woman with elevated blood pressure should be checked immediately for the presence of hand or face edema and proteinuria. The occurrence of either of these findings suggests that preeclampsia, alone or superimposed on hypertensive disease, is present. Dependent leg edema alone is not a pathologic finding, since this may occur in a large proportion of pregnant women. The pregnant patient with generalized edema and/or proteinuria should receive prompt assessment by a specialist in obstetrics.

The hypertensive pregnant patient should also be questioned about the occurrence of severe headaches, visual disturbances, paresthesias or weaknesses, and epigastric pain. She should be examined for hyperactivity of the deep tendon reflexes (especially the knee jerks). The presence of any of these findings suggests that an eclamptic convulsion may be imminent, and immediate obstetric consultations should be obtained. In addition, the patient should be kept in quiet surroundings and stimulated as little as possible. Seizure precautions should be taken.

A number of regimens have been employed for the prevention of control of eclamptic seizures. Parenteral magnesium sulfate therapy has been proved to be effective and is widely used. An initial loading dose of 2 to 4 mg of 10% magnesium sulfate may be given slowly by IV route to achieve rapid serum levels. This may be followed by the continuous administration of 1 to 1.5 g/hr using a constant infusion pump, or by IM administration of 10 g of 50% magnesium sulfate initially, followed at 4-hour intervals by repeat IM doses of 5 g. The patient receiving magnesium sulfate therapy should be monitored carefully for evidence of magnesium-induced depression of the CNS or myocardium. The most frequent sign of magnesium excess is absence of the knee jerks. Signs of greater toxicity include slowing of the respiration below 12 breaths/min or the heart rate below 60 beats/min. The findings of absent knee jerks requires only that the infusion be stopped or that the next scheduled dose of IM magnesium sulfate be delayed. CNS or cardiac depression should be reversed immediately using IV calcium gluconate. Magnesium is excreted by the kidney, and the maintenance doses of magnesium sulfate should be reduced or withheld if the urine output falls below 50 ml/hr. On the other hand, the continued presence of hyperactive deep tendon reflexes demonstrates that inadequate magnesium levels are present and indicates that an increase in the dose of magnesium sulfate is needed.

Patients with severe preeclampsia or eclampsia, alone or superimposed on chronic disease, require intensive nursing observation with careful attention to airway, intake and output, and vital signs. An obstetrician-gynecologist experienced in the management of complicated pregnancy should supervise management and be available for immediate consultation.

Although delivery "cures" preeclampsia-eclampsia, the need for intensive observation and care extends 24 to 48 hours into the postpartum period, because approximately one fourth of eclamptic seizures and other serious complications may occur during this time.

### ■ What is the relationship between urinary tract infection and pregnancy?

It is questionable whether pregnancy actually increases the incidence of bacterial infection of the urinary tract. The incidence of significant asymptomatic bacteriuria in pregnant women has been reported to be between 4% and 7% by many investigators, and a similar incidence has been observed in nonpregnant women. On the other hand, pregnancy does appear to increase the likelihood that a woman with a low grade asymptomatic urinary tract infection may develop acute pyelonephritis, and this may be a severe complication for both mother and fetus.

### ■ What special problems accompany acute pyelonephritis during pregnancy?

The special problems of acute pyelonephritis during pregnancy relate to the effect of maternal fever on fetal well-being and to the possible occurrence of premature labor during the acute episode. The likelihood of fetal distress resulting from hyperthermia, relative hypoxia, and cardiovascular stress increases as the maternal temperature rises above 101° F. Thus measures to reduce maternal temperature such as physical cooling and administration of antipyretics may be part of the initial therapy of acute pyelonephritis during pregnancy. Dehydration and electrolyte imbalance should also be corrected promptly. Uterine contractions that may develop into progressive, premature labor may not be reported by the acutely ill patient and may not be noticed by medical attendants concentrating on other phases of the illness; pregnant patients with acute pyelonephritis should be observed frequently and specifically for the presence or absence of uterine contractions. Although in most patients the excessive uterine activity subsides with bed rest, hydration, and lowering of maternal fever, a few patients require specific therapy (for example, IV ethanol) to suppress the uterine activity. Consultation with an obstetric specialist should be obtained if regular uterine contractions develop during the course of acute pyelonephritis.

## ■ What other medical or surgical illnesses cause problems during pregnancy?

Almost any medical or surgical disease may occur coincident with pregnancy. In the management of these intercurrent illnesses one must consider both the effect of pregnancy on the disease and the effect of the disease on pregnancy. Drugs that are known or suspected to have adverse effects on the embryo or fetus should be avoided whenever possible. Diagnostic x-ray examination, especially of the abdomen, should be performed only if necessary for the differential diagnosis or management of the patient. Maternal hypotension, blood volume deficits, and electrolyte abnormalities must be corrected promptly in order to minimize the effect of acute illness on the fetus. Administration of oxygen to the mother during episodes of maternal circulatory or respiratory embarrassment or during periods of high fever may prevent or correct fetal distress from hypoxia. In other instances these measures can sustain the fetus while preparations are being made for emergency delivery. With survival rates and long-term prognosis for premature infants improving steadily, consideration may be given to the termination of pregnancy for fetal indications at any time from 27 or 28 weeks after the LMP onward, when the abnormality producing the fetal distress cannot be corrected and the maternal condition permits.

Some of the more important medical diseases that are affected by pregnancy or that alter the management of pregnancy include diabetes, heart disease, chronic renal disease, and acute febrile illnesses.

## ■ What are the major problems in diabetic pregnancy?

Pregnancy may make latent diabetes manifest and may complicate the management of known diabetes. Nausea and vomiting in the first trimester may interfere with food intake and thus may increase the incidence of symptomatic hypoglycemia in insulin-requiring diabetic patients. Although the embryo and fetus appear to be relatively tolerant to hypoglycemia, these episodes should be recognized promptly and treated appropriately. The possibility of hypoglycemia should be kept in mind in the differential diagnosis of disturbances of consciousness and "anxiety" symptoms in early pregnancy.

Most diabetic pregnant women experience an increase in insulin requirement during the latter half of pregnancy. These patients may develop ketoacidosis when these requirements are not met or as a result of stress during an acute, intercurrent illness. Because ketoacidosis may result in death or impaired neurologic development of the fetus, the diabetic pregnant patient should be observed carefully for evidence of ketoacidosis, especially when an infection or other acute stress is present.

The incidence of intrauterine fetal death in late pregnancy is increased in diabetic patients. Measures such as fetal heart rate monitoring and estriol determinations make it possible to recognize the endangered fetus in time to prevent a fatal outcome. An obstetric consultant should thus be involved in the management of any diabetic pregnant patient.

## ■ How does pregnancy complicate the management of patients with heart disease?

The increased blood volume, heart rate, and cardiac work during pregnancy make the cardiac patient more likely to develop congestive heart failure. In general patients with class I and II cardiac disease tolerate pregnancy well, but heart failure may occur even in some of these patients during pregnancy. The pregnant cardiac patient is most likely to develop congestive failure at 28 to 32 weeks of gestation (near the end of the phase of rapid blood volume expansion), during labor and delivery, and during the first 2 days of the puerperium. Acute pulmonary edema may develop particularly rapidly during labor or immediately following delivery. Acute congestive failure may also occur at other times during pregnancy, especially if the stress of major illness or trauma is added. The management of congestive heart failure and acute pulmonary edema is the same during pregnancy as at other times.

**■ What problems does pregnancy introduce for the management of chronic renal disease?**

The patient with chronic renal disease who has minimum or absent proteinuria, no elevation of the blood urea nitrogen or creatinine levels, and no hypertension can usually tolerate pregnancy successfully. Patients with more severe renal disease are at increased risk to develop progressive deterioration in renal function during pregnancy. Normotensive patients may become hypertensive, and hypertensive patients may experience a further increase in blood pressure during pregnancy. The increasing renal impairment and hypertension may occur as a result of progression of the primary renal disease or as manifestations of a suprimposed preeclampsia-eclampsia. These patients may become candidates for intensive care because of renal failure or because of a hypertensive crisis. The occurrence of either of these latter complications is usually an indication for termination of pregnancy, even if the fetus has not reached the stage of viability.

**■ What complications does pregnancy introduce into the management of acute intra-abdominal disease?**

Especially during the latter half of pregnancy, the presence of the gravid uterus may alter the clinical signs of acute intra-abdominal disease (for example, the location and characteristics of pain and tenderness) and make the presence or absence of these signs less reliable in differential diagnosis. Uterine contractions may occur either as part of the primary illness or following abdominal surgery, thus adding the problems of management of impending or actual premature labor to those of the primary disease process. Fetal distress may occur when shock or high fever is part of the maternal disease process. The patient with acute abdominal disease during pregnancy thus requires extra observation directed at the early detection of increased uterine activity or fetal distress.

The bedside clinician must be aware that labor and delivery are not only possible but likely to occur. Vigilance for the first evidence of labor is needed for the critically ill pregnant patient who is likely to go into labor and deliver before term. This is true whether the illness is directly related to her pregnancy or not. The woman whose condition is not improving is at the greatest risk of labor. When disease or its treatment impairs the sensorium, the woman herself may be unable to communicate the sensations of labor contractions.

**■ What are the warning signs of labor in the critically ill patient with an altered sensorium?**

During labor uterine contractions lasting from 30 to 60 seconds usually occur at regular intervals. The following physiologic and behavioral changes may accompany uterine contractions and be observed in cyclic intervals: increased respiration rate, change in pulse rate, increase in systolic and diastolic blood pressure, restlessness, and moaning. Additional physical evidence suggesting labor and/or impending delivery are bloody vaginal discharge, rupture of the bag of waters, grunting or expulsive efforts, and bulging of the perineum.

### *Vaginal discharge*

A clear, sticky mucous secretion is normally present in pregnancy. This may not be externally apparent until the last trimester. At times this vaginal discharge may be slightly milky colored or pale yellow. The quantity of normal vaginal discharge should not require use of a sanitary napkin. A sudden increase in the quantity of normal mucous secretion warrants further investigation. Particularly in women with first pregnancies, an increased vaginal discharge that is tinged with either brown or pinkish blood streaks may be evidence that the cervix is softening and beginning to dilate. When these signs are present, the patient should be examined for the presence of regular uterine contractions signifying labor. Bleeding from the vagina, whether old or fresh, may signify either labor or a complication and warrants immediate medical attention.

*Rupture of membranes*

A gush of fluid usually signifies the rupture of the fetal membranes. The fetal heart rate should be observed immediately on discovery of ruptured membranes to detect slowing or irregularity, which might signify umbilical cord prolapse and compression. When abnormal fetal heart tones are found, the mother should be placed in knee-chest or deep Trendelenburg position in an attempt to relieve cord compression. Should the maternal positioning be impossible, an attempt to displace the fetal presenting part manually should be made. In any case, oxygen should be administered to the mother and medical help obtained immediately.

When rupture of the membranes is suspected, immediate assessment should be made to determine whether labor is present, since it is possible for the membranes to rupture only a brief period of time before the delivery of the infant. The fluid has a characteristic fleshy odor and normally is a clear, watery color with specks of white vernix. However, a yellow color or a heavy "grass" green color usually indicates the presence of meconium and requires immediate medical attention.

Incontinent urination should not be confused with leakage of amniotic fluid. The distinctions may be made by several tests, the simplest of which is recognition of the characteristic odor of urine, very unlike the odor of amniotic fluid.

When the fluid has been collected in a container that is clean and free of soap or other foreign materials, the pH of amniotic fluid is alkaline, whereas usually the pH of urine is acid. However, it is well to remember that both protein and blood in the urine may change the pH to an alkaline reaction.

***Premature rupture of membranes.*** The fetal membranes may rupture prior to the onset of labor. This provides a route of entrance for pathogenic organisms into the immediate environment of the fetus, which normally is sterile. The immediate recognition of leakage of amniotic fluid is important to the welfare of the fetus. There is risk of sepsis to the fetus once the sterile environment is destroyed. In many instances the fetus, even though of small size, has a better chance for survival outside of the mother rather than remaining in the uterus. The risk of infection increases with time. For this reason delivery before 24 hours has elapsed is often desirable. It may be necessary to perform a sterile speculum examination to confirm leakage of amniotic fluid. Preferably such assessment should be made prior to any sterile vaginal examination. The only equipment required is a sterile vaginal speculum, sterile ring forceps or other forceps of sufficient length to reach the cervical end of the vaginal canal, a sterile glass slide, and nitrazine or other paper suitable for testing pH. Unless pooling fluid is seen in the posterior fornix it may be necessary to collect a specimen from the vaginal pool for both pH testing and examination for ferning when the fluid dries on a glass slide; pH testing is invalid in the presence of infection or blood.

## ■ What is the significance of vena caval syndrome?

In the last trimester of pregnancy the uterus is a large, heavy organ and lies over the inferior vena cava. This anatomic relationship may favor a diminished blood flow from the venous system into the right atrium. The diminished blood flow in turn mimics the clinical symptoms of shock caused by a serious decrease in cardiac output. The patient may exhibit a rapid thready pulse, pallor, and perspiration. A feeling of light-headedness or faintness accompanies lowered blood pressure.

When these symptoms are present without a significant blood loss or a causal relationship, the vena caval syndrome of pregnancy should be suspected. Treatment is simple and relief of all the symptoms exceedingly prompt. The patient should be turned to the left lateral position, thus allowing the shift of gravity to take the weight of the uterus off the inferior vena cava. If there are reasons why the patient cannot be turned to the side, manual deviation of the uterus to the left side of the patient may also bring about relief from these symptoms.

This syndrome is more likely to occur

when the abdominal wall is well developed and in good tone, aiding in compression of the intra-abdominal organs.

## SUPPORT AND COMFORT MEASURES

### ■ How can the patient's anxiety be relieved?

The presence of a calm clinician who relates to the patient in a warm, human manner does much to allay patient anxiety and fear. Although the critical care unit is completely familiar to the practitioner, the visual impact of complex equipment combined with strange noises makes this an alien and frightening environment for the patient. A simple explanation of the purpose of the equipment and orientation to the procedures should be offered to all patients. For pregnant patients additional equipment for fetal monitoring must be explained.

### ■ What can be done to alleviate the mother's fears caused by her separation from the infant?

Following delivery, the mother's physical condition prevents her from making visits to the infant. Polaroid pictures of the infant are easily made and offer the mother visual evidence of the infant's condition. Often the infant will be shown in an incubator, possibly wired to monitors. It may be well to inform the mother about such devices and their benign nature before pictures are shown. When the neonate is very ill, personal contact from the neonatal intensive care staff may be beneficial.

### ■ What is the appropriate manner of dealing with the infant's death?

The death of an infant is difficult at any time. The family who bears this loss together with concern for a critically ill mother requires understanding and sympathy from the practitioners. This can be expressed by allowing them to talk about their loss and grief. The desire to talk about the infant's death is normal and a necessary part of the grieving process. Families may wish to see and hold the infant after death. Arrangements for privacy and for family members to mourn with the mother can be facilitated by the nursing personnel. The practitioner should ask the family if they wish to meet with the chaplain or have a pastor visit to provide the solace of spiritual support.

## MONITORS FOR PREGNANT PATIENTS

There may be times when the intensive care unit is the most suitable location for a patient during labor. Initial provisions should include plans for the place of delivery. Under these circumstances a variety of techniques requiring special equipment may be used that are unique to pregnancy and labor. It may be advantageous to have a listing in the intensive care unit of such equipment and its location together with a description of the procedures. Suggested equipment is discussed subsequently.

The first phase of fetal monitornig is preparation. All necessary equipment and supplies must be at hand and in working condition.

The patient needs instruction and explanation of what will be done and why monitoring is valuable to her. The procedure for application may be explained as very similar to a vaginal examination. The mother might like to know that the record of the infant's heartbeat provides the best possible information about his condition. The audible heartbeat may be played at times so the mother may hear the infant. After the monitor has been functioning for a while, the alert patient may appreciate being shown a strip and given a brief explanation of the tracing.

Data collection and interpretation require skill. The practitioner must look at the strip every few minutes and recognize all deviations from normal fetal heart rate patterns.

### ■ What are the techniques for monitoring during labor?

The fetal heart may be heard by stethoscopic auscultation. Uterine contractions may be perceived objectively by palpation through the maternal abdominal wall. Direct observation by trained personnel has been the historical approach to obstetric patients. These clinical measures require constant attendance, are subject to the usual human limitations, and at best provide a minuscule sample of data. In the main there are two general approaches using external or direct monitoring systems. External systems do not require penetration of the maternal or fetal body. Therefore the cervix may be closed, and labor is not a prerequisite. Fetal signals are picked up through the maternal abdomen, and rupture of the amniotic sac is not required. These advantages permit the collection of data from periods as early as the eleventh week of gestation.

### ■ What techniques of monitoring uterine activity are employed?

Various types of tokodynamometers that record uterine activity are available. They provide continuous records of data obtained externally from equipment that encircles the woman's abdomen. Data about the frequency of uterine contractions and the intensity of the contractions is suggested.

Direct monitoring of uterine activity is accomplished by placing an intrauterine catheter and recording pressure changes. Intrauterine techniques measure both resting tone and the amplitude of uterine contractions. The intrauterine technique has the disadvantage that the membranes must be ruptured. Direct techniques permit more precise data collection and allow the elimination of interfering signals. In addition, the degree of uterine activity can be deduced from the frequency, intensity, and duration of uterine contractions. Less than a minute between successive uterine contractions may indicate an excessive degree of uterine activity, and the principal practitioner should be notified immediately. If the patient is receiving oxytocin and the physician is not immediately at hand, the oxytocin should be discontinued pending the arrival of the physician. Turning the patient on her side may relieve too frequent uterine contractions occurring in the absence of uterine stimulant medication.

## FETAL MONITORING

### ■ How is the fetal heart rate monitored?

#### *Ultrasound*

Ultrasound instruments, which use the Doppler principle, send a sound impulse from a transducer that also reads the echoes resulting from movement. Cardiac action can be heard fairly easily. The swishing sound of blood flowing through a large vessel such as the umbilical cord may be detected as well. A special transducer that can be connected to a fetal monitor may provide both an auditory and visual record of fetal cardiac action. It is necessary to have conducting jelly as well as the recording instrument and the transducer.

The sounds of fetal cardiac action may be detected as early as 10 or 11 weeks of intrauterine life when ordinary auscultation is not productive. Compact portable units are available. They have the advantage of external use and do not require the rupture of membranes.

#### *Phonocardiography*

Fetal phonocardiography employs a microphone held in contact with the maternal abdomen. Both a visual record and audible sounds may be obtained. Like other external techniques, it may be used prior to as well as during labor and does not require either dilatation of the cervix or ruptured membranes.

#### *Fetal electrocardiogram (Fig. 23-1)*

An electrode is attached directly to the fetal presenting part that transmits fetal heart patterns to a recorder. Direct fetal monitoring provides the advantages of continuous data as opposed to intermittent data from auscultation, a record of variations in beat-to-beat rates that reflect fetal adaptive mechanisms, and responses of fetal heart rate to uterine activity. The fetal QRS complex is detected by means of a spiral electrode attached to the fetal scalp; a catheter is placed within the uterus attached to a strain gauge so that not only the timing and duration but also the intensity of uterine contractions can be measured. This continuous monitoring

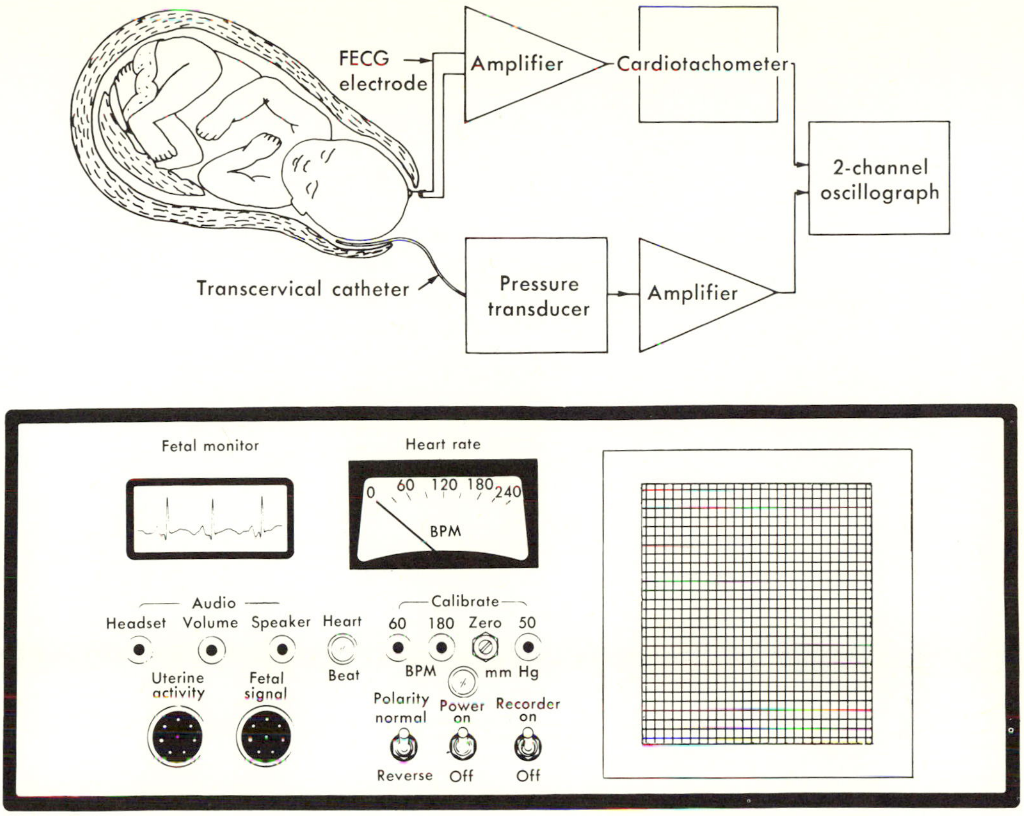


**Fig. 23-1. A,** Technique for fetal intensive care. Specially designed electrode is attached to presenting part of fetus to obtain FECG, which is then fed to an amplifier and signal conditioning circuit. Instantaneous cardiotachometer measures interval between successive FECG's and plots continuous graph. Output of cardiotachometer is displayed on one channel of two-channel oscillograph. Intrauterine pressure is obtained from intrauterine catheter inserted transcervically into uterus just beyond biparietal diameter of fetal head. Catheter is attached to pressure transducer, whose output is amplified and displayed beneath fetal heart rate record on other channel of oscillograph. **B,** Panel of fetal monitor, incorporating in single package components of block diagram in **A.** It can be used to obtain either indirect or direct fetal heart rate and uterine contraction monitoring techniques. (From Hon, E. H.: An introduction to fetal heart rate monitoring, New Haven, Conn., 1971, Harty Press, Inc.)

of the fetal heart together with uterine contractions provides information about fetal conditions and early indication of fetal distress. The fetal heart rate is observed in the period between uterine contractions to determine the *baseline fetal heart rate.* The normal fetal heart rate pattern consists of a baseline heart rate usually between 120 and 160 beats/min. Baseline variability and fluctuations of 5 to 20 beats/min are normal. A decrease in baseline variability may be caused by certain drugs such as atropine, tranquilizers, or magnesium sulfate, as well as barbiturates and narcotics. In the absence of drugs the baseline fetal heart rate and its variability can be considered to give information about the status of the fetus, particularly the activity of the CNS. A decrease in the baseline variability in the absence of drugs indicates depression of the CNS activity and often reflects fetal hypoxia and acidosis.

■ **What fetal heart rate patterns can be expected in association with uterine contractions?**

The fetal heart rate is observed during uterine contractions (Fig. 23-2). The normal

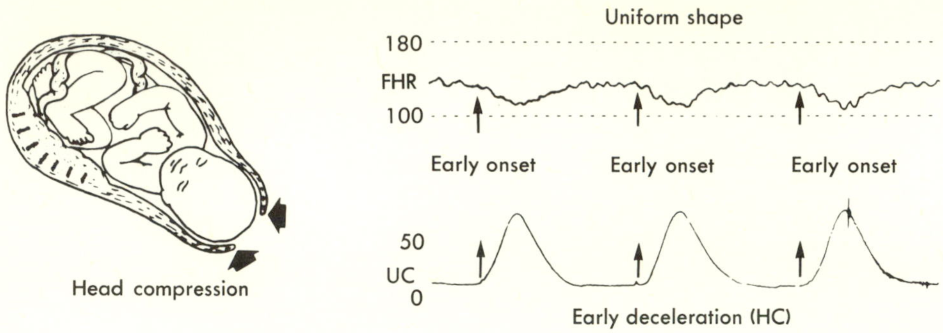


**Fig. 23-2.** This fetal heart rate deceleration pattern is thought to be caused by fetal head compression. It is of *uniform shape,* reflects shape of associated intrauterine pressure curve, and has its onset *early* in contracting phase of uterus. Hence it has been labeled "early deceleration." HC = head compression, UC = uterine contraction. (From Hon, E. H.: An introduction to fetal heart rate monitoring, New Haven, Conn., 1971, Harty Press, Inc.)

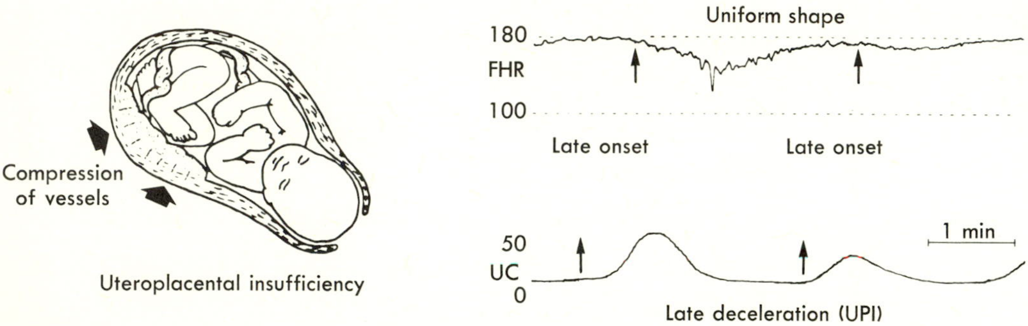


**Fig. 23-3.** This fetal heart rate deceleration pattern is thought to be caused by acute uteroplacental insufficiency resulting from decreased intervillous space blood flow during uterine contractions. It is also of *uniform shape* and also reflects shape of associated intrauterine pressure curve. In this case, however, in contradistinction to the early deceleration pattern of Fig. 23-2, its onset occurs *late* in contracting phase of uterus. Hence it has been labeled "late deceleration." This fetal heart rate deceleration pattern is considered indicative of uteroplacental insufficiency. UPI = uteroplacental insufficiency. (From Hon, E. H.: An introduction to fetal heart rate monitoring, New Haven, Conn., 1971, Harty Press, Inc.)

fetus may show no change in heart rate in response to uterine contractions. Periodic changes in the fetal heart rate in association with uterine contractions may in some cases be a normal feature of labor and in others indicate the occurrence of fetal stress as a result of uterine contractions. Three major types of deceleration patterns have been described by Hon[1] and others.

In the early deceleration pattern the heart rate rarely falls below 100 to 110 beats/min at the low point of the deceleration. This pattern is not associated with fetal hypoxia or depressed infants in the absence of other problems.

A second deceleration pattern is a late deceleration pattern thought to represent fetal hypoxia resulting from insufficient uteroplacental exchange (Fig. 23-3). This pattern, similar to the early deceleration pattern, tends to be uniform and U shaped. The late deceleration pattern begins relatively late, that is, 20 to 30 seconds after the onset of the uterine contraction, and the low point of the deceleration occurs near the end of the uterine contraction or even as the uterine

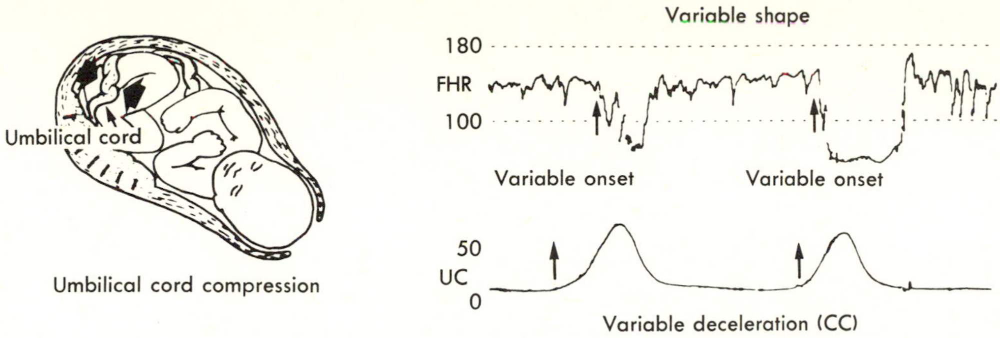


**Fig. 23-4.** This fetal heart rate pattern is thought to be caused by umbilical cord occlusion. It is of *variable shape,* does not reflect shape of associated intrauterine pressure curve, and its onset occurs at a variable time during contracting phase of uterus. CC = cord compression. (From Hon, E. H.: An introduction to fetal heart rate monitoring, New Haven, Conn., 1971, Harty Press, Inc.)

pressure is returning to baseline levels. This pattern always indicates fetal hypoxia, and when it is associated with a flat baseline fetal heart rate, it indicates that significant fetal distress is present. When late deceleration cannot be corrected, immediate delivery is indicated.

The most common fetal heart rate pattern is variable deceleration, believed to be caused by umbilical cord compression (Fig. 23-4). This is an irregular deceleration pattern that may occur at almost any time during the contraction. The degree of deceleration frequently does not reflect the intensity of contraction. For example, several contractions of equivalent magnitude may be accompanied by variable decelerations of quite different degrees. The healthy fetus can tolerate brief episodes of cord compression lasting up to 30 or 45 seconds without distress. Longer periods of cord compression, particularly those in which the fetal heart rate falls below 60 to 70 beats/min and in which the duration of the deceleration exceeds 45 to 60 seconds, may be associated with the occurrence of progressive fetal hypoxia and acidosis. In these instances the deterioration in fetal condition will often be reflected as well in a progressive decrease in baseline variability and increase in baseline fetal heart rate.

In summary, prolonged severe variable decelerations, that is, those lasting longer than 45 to 60 seconds and with the heart rate falling to 60 to 70 beats/min or below, or late decelerations of any magnitude indicate fetal distress. When these patterns are associated with a flat baseline fetal heart rate, the situation is likely to be grave, with significant hypoxia and acidosis already present.

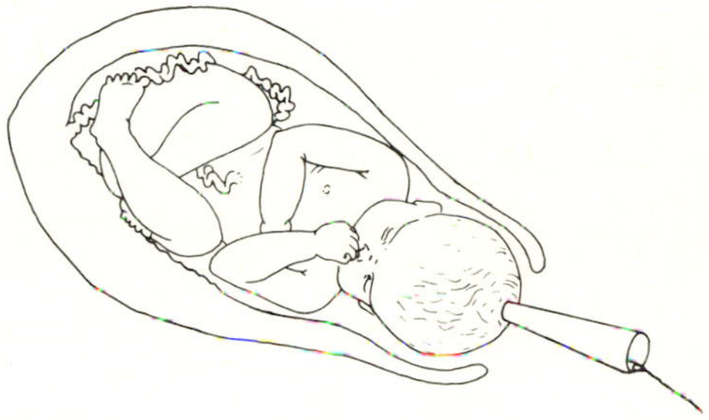

**Fig. 23-5.** Fetal scalp blood sampling. Endoscope is inserted transvaginally for direct visualization of fetal scalp, and light is attached to light source. (From Della Pietra, E. R.: Intrapartum maternal and fetal monitoring, Los Angeles, 1974, Postgraduate Division, School of Medicine, University of Southern California.)

Periodic fetal heart rate accelerations also occur in association with uterine contractions and with fetal movement between contractions. Such fetal heart rate accelerations usually have no pathologic significance and in fact usually reflect a healthy fetus.

## ■ Of what use is fetal scalp blood sampling?

Another means of assessment of fetal condition during labor is fetal scalp blood sampling (Fig. 23-5). In this technique a small sam-

## FETAL MONITORING

### PREPARATION

It may be desirable to continue maternal care in an intensive care unit during labor. In these circumstances the obstetrician requires the following supplies for fetal monitoring:

1. A functioning fetal monitoring system such as Corometrics (Fig. 23-1)
   a. A sterile unit containing a fetal scalp electrode
   b. An introducer and uterine catheter
2. A light source
3. A 30 ml container of sterile distilled water for flushing the intrauterine catheter
4. Two 5 ml syringes

### IMMEDIATE ASSISTANCE IN THE EVENT OF DELIVERY

Even with diligent observation, it is still possible for labor to be undetected. Measures to ensure an immediately clear airway and provision for gas exchange, rapid drying, and prevention of chilling may mean the difference between survival of an intact infant and serious jeopardy or loss of life.

### DELIVERY SUPPLIES

Preparations may be made to have a warmed incubator and a sterile pack containing two pairs of scissors, two cord clamps, a number of towels, a blanket for the infant, and a sterile bulb aspirator at hand. When possible, equipment for newborn resuscitation should be readily available.

### NEWBORN RESUSCITATION

1. Laryngoscope with premature blade
2. Sterile Kole tracheal tubes, sizes 1.5, 2.0, 2.5, 3.0, and 3.5
3. DeLee aspirator
4. Infant bag for ventilation, 0.5 L with a T assembly adapter

Where umbilical cord catheterization might be used, the following drugs may be kept at hand:

1. 50% glucose for IV use
2. Calcium gluconate solution
3. $H_2CO_3$ ampules
4. Epinephrine, 1:10,000 concentration
5. Sterile equipment for umbilical cord catheterization

### FETAL SCALP SAMPLING EQUIPMENT

1. Container of ice
2. Long, heparinized capillary tubes
3. Magnet
4. Sterile supplies or disposable kit
   a. Blade holder and blade
   b. Cone-type endoscope
   c. Ring forceps
   d. Gauze pledgets
   e. Antibacterial cleansing agent
   f. Sterile towels

ple of blood is obtained from a lancet puncture in the fetal scalp and is analyzed especially for the pH, but also for carbon dioxide and oxygen tensions. Particularly in the critical care patient it may be necessary to obtain a simultaneous maternal arterial or venous blood sample in order to interpret the fetal pH, since the presence of a maternal acidosis, either metabolic or respiratory, may alter the interpretation of the fetal data. The chief role of fetal scalp blood sampling would appear to be in the interpretation of equivocal fetal heart rate patterns, although in a few centers fetal scalp blood sampling is used as the major means of assessment of fetal condition during labor. A list of the equipment necessary for fetal scalp blood sampling is found in the boxed material on p. 430.

Nursing care, associated with fetal monitoring, includes frequent observation of the tracing for the presence of periodic deceleration in the fetal heart rate or the presence of a flat baseline. Anything suspicious should be called to the physician's attention immediately. Immediate intervention is indicated when abnormal fetal heart rate patterns are recognized. For example, when variable decelerations are present the patient should be turned on her side in an attempt to eliminate deceleration. Repeated changes in position may be necessary in order to relieve cord compression. The Trendelenburg position may be necessary to eliminate deceleration patterns unaffected by turning the patient from side to side. When other decelerations are present, the patient should be turned on her side in order to remove any element of vena caval compression with supine hypotension. In either case oxygen can be administered to the mother by face mask.

## REFERENCE

1. Hon, E. H.: An introduction to fetal heart rate monitoring, New Haven, Conn., 1971, Harty Press, Inc.

## BIBLIOGRAPHY

Della Pietra, E. R.: Intrapartum maternal and fetal monitoring, Los Angeles, 1974, Postgraduate Division, School of Medicine, University of Southern California.

Hellman, L. M., and Pritchard, J. A.: Williams obstetrics, ed. 14, New York, 1971, Appleton-Century-Crofts.

Martin, C. B., Jr., Ulene, A., and Guzinski, J. M.: Module, care of the pregnant patient: submodule, problems in pregnancy, Raritan, N. J., 1974, Ortho Pharmaceutical Corporation.

Matousek, I.: Fetal nursing during labor, Nurs. Clin. North Am. 1972.

Woolley, A. S.: Excellence in nursing in the coronary-care unit, Heart & Lung, **1**:785, 1972.

*chapter 24*

# Critical care of the neonate

ROBERT F. HUXTABLE
EARLENE SCHARPING

In the past many inappropriate and sometimes misleading terms have been used to describe the neonate. These have included "premature," "postmature," "small for dates," "dysmature," "intrauterine growth retardation," and "low birth weight." For many years all infants weighing less than 2500 g at birth were classified as "premature." Actually a very significant proportion of these were small for gestational age and more mature than weight alone would suggest. These loosely applied terms, although partially accurate, fail to direct attention to the problems the infant will likely encounter. The infant of low birth weight caused by inadequate gestation is likely to have respiratory distress syndrome, whereas the one small for gestational age may suffer the effects of hypoglycemia.

It is much more valuable to assign the newborn infant to one of the following nine categories that provide mortality statistics and help in the anticipation of likely problems. Classification is based on weight and gestational age. Infants *above the ninetieth, between the tenth and ninetieth,* and *below the tenth per weight percentile* are called *large* (LGA), *appropriate* (AGA), and *small* (SGA) *for gestational age,* respectively. Those of *less than 38 weeks, 38 to 42 weeks,* and *greater than 42 weeks* of gestation are called *preterm* (PrT), *term* (T), and *postterm* (PoT), respectively. It is useful to classify every infant in this manner and display the classification in clear view on the bassinet or incubator as follows:

| | PrT | T | PoT |
|---|---|---|---|
| LGA | | | |
| AGA | | | |
| SGA | | | |

## THERMAL REGULATION

■ **Why is thermal regulation of such critical importance in the neonatal period?**

There are two basic reasons for thermal regulation during the neonatal period:

1. The newborn loses heat more rapidly and has different mechanisms for heat production than the older child.
2. A body temperature change on either side of a point known as the "thermoneutral point" results in increased oxygen consumption and increased consumption of substrates for the generation of heat.

The four mechanisms of heat transfer must be considered. Heat transfer by *conduction* occurs when the skin is in contact with a surface of different temperature, such as a cold scale platform or table. Heat loss by conduction is reduced by interposing a material that conducts heat poorly, such as fabric. Heat loss by *convection* occurs as a result of the transfer of heat into the molecules of a moving gas of lower than body temperature; thus heat loss can be considerably greater in drafty rooms. Even though the air temperature is appropriate and no convection currents are present in an incubator, the infant may have significant heat loss by *radiation*. Radiant heat energy is exchanged between two solid surfaces of different temperature. Therefore if an incubator canopy is near a cold window, its heat radiates to the window, reducing its temperature below that of the infant. The infant then radiates heat to the incubator canopy of lower than body temperature. The fourth mechanism of heat loss is by *evaporation*. This is a very efficient and rapid mechanism of cooling because of the large number of calories consumed in converting a unit weight of water from the liquid to the gas phase. It is probably the most important mechanism of thermal stress in the delivery room.

■ **What is the significance of brown fat?**

When under thermal stress, an older child or adult generates heat by increased physical activity or by shivering. The newborn infant does not possess this capability but has a unique mechanism for nonshivering thermogenesis consisting of the metabolism of stores of high energy brown fat. This unique adipose tissue is found in most newborn mammals and has been described as brown because of its rich vascular supply. In utero malnutrition results in depletion of white fat, whereas brown fat is preserved. Conversely, autopsy studies have shown that newborn infants who are well nourished at birth and are subjected to cold stress deplete brown fat whereas white fat is preserved. Brown fat stores normally gradually disappear during the first year of life, the time corresponding to the development of the shivering thermogenesis mechanism.

■ **Why is thermal regulation a greater problem for preterm than term infants?**

The preterm infant has smaller fat stores for metabolism and heat production. The ratio of surface area to body weight is greater than that of the term infant, resulting in relatively greater consequences of heat loss by any of the four mechanisms. Because of nervous system immaturity, the preterm baby is hypotonic and unable to assume the flexed posture that preserves heat by reducing exposed surface area.

■ **At what temperature should the skin of preterm and term infants be maintained?**

When monitoring skin temperature with a thermistor, usually placed over the upper abdominal skin, the term infant's temperature should be maintained at 36.1° C. Infants weighing less than 1500 g should be maintained at 36.6° C.

■ **What environmental temperature is recommended for neonates in various weight groups?**

Suggested starting points are 34.9° C for a 1000 g infant, 33.5° C for a 2000 g infant, and 30° C for larger term infants. These are only rough guides and should be modified accordingly by taking the infant's temperature at least once each hour until it is stable and every 3 hours thereafter.

■ **What is the effect of administering cold oxygen to the face of a newborn infant by mask?**

The thermal receptors in the skin of the face are much more sensitive to cold than other areas of the skin of the newborn infant. Exposure of the face to cold reflexly initiates production of norepinephrine, resulting in an abrupt increase of metabolism and oxygen consumption. This may occur in the presence of normal environmental and body core temperatures. It is therefore important to warm and humidify oxygen before it is delivered by face mask.

■ **Why is thermal regulation of greater importance to a preterm infant with respiratory distress syndrome than to a well term infant?**

Anaerobic metabolism occurring during hypoxia and resulting in acidemia occurs at an even greater rate when metabolic demands are increased and further exaggerate the acidemia. Hypoxia alone results in increased pulmonary vascular resistance caused by blood vessel constriction. This effect is made more pronounced by acidemia.

■ **Other than radiant heat warmers and incubators, how can supplementary heat be administered to the infant under urgent circumstances?**

An ordinary gooseneck lamp, chemical heat packs, or rubber gloves filled with warm water can be quickly and conveniently used. Care must be exercised to avoid burns of the skin. This can be achieved usually by wrapping warm packs in diapers. The temperature of the water should not exceed 45° C.

## INFECTION

■ **Why are the fetus and neonate uniquely susceptible to infection?**

Two principal reasons may be given: opportunity for exposure to infection and peculiarities of immunity. It is convenient to classify infections as transplacental or acquired during or after birth. Transplacental infections are acquired by the fetus as a result of an infection in the mother at any time during pregnancy. These infections tend to be nonbacterial and include *cytomegalovirus infection, rubella, syphilis,* and *toxoplasmosis.* It is possible for a transplacental infection to occur while the infection is asymptomatic in the mother, as is common with cytomegalovirus infection. Rubella, on the other hand, tends to produce symptoms in the mother, although these might be quite mild.

A *herpes virus infection* might be acquired by a newborn during the process of birth as a result of contacting genital herpetic lesions in the mother.

Infections acquired during or after birth are caused mainly by *bacteria.* The risk of infection of the infant is probably increased by prolonged ruptured membranes (greater than 24 hours). When there is no evidence of infection of the mother at the time of birth and when there has not been prolonged rupture of the membranes, bacterial neonatal infection does not tend to occur until after 48 hours of age.

The immune system in the neonate with respect to immune globulin production is also unique. Of the immunoglobulins IgG, IgM, and IgA, the only one that passes freely from the mother to the fetus is IgG. During fetal life IgA and IgM remain at very low levels. The fetus can, however, produce IgM as a result of transplacental infection, and IgM determination in the neonate is used as a screening test for transplacental infection. Values above 20 mg/100 ml have diagnostic value; however, lower values are not conclusive evidence against transplacental infection. The fetus develops the ability to produce IgM in response to infection at about 20 weeks of gestation.

■ **What bacterial organisms are newborn infants most susceptible to?**

Neonatal infections are most commonly caused by gram-negative rods, *Escherichia coli* being the most common. Other gram-negative rods causing infection include *Klebsiella, Proteus,* and *Pseudomonas.* Remaining bacterial infections are caused mainly by gram-positive cocci, including *Staphylococcus* and *Streptococcus.* At the present time group B *Streptococcus* is assuming increasing importance.

■ **What are the most common modes of transmission for nursery-acquired infections?**

Infecting organisms are most commonly transferred to patients via the epithelial scales from the hands of personnel attending patients. Thus the most important method of preventing the spread of infection in nurseries is hand washing. The second major source of infection is contaminated equipment.

■ **What infections most clearly justify removal of the infant from the nursery?**

Gastroenteritis caused by specific bacterial organisms (especially enterpathogenic *E. coli*) and staphylococcal disease clinically manifested by abscess formation clearly justify removal from the nursery. Other infections can generally be handled in the nursery by "unit isolation," in which case the infant is kept in an incubator and has contact with a minimum number of personnel.

■ **What hand washing program would be appropriate for a newborn nursery?**

A 3-minute scrub of the hands and forearms to the elbows on entering the nursery for the day is appropriate. This should be done either with an iodophor- or hexachlorophene-containing preparation. Following the initial 3-minute scrub, there should be a 30-second scrub between handling patients.

■ **What are the clinical signs of sepsis?**

It is important to remember that the clinical manifestations of sepsis in the newborn are subtle and often referred to as "SSS," or the soft signs of sepsis. Often the practitioner feels subjectively that the infant is just "not doing well." Signs include poor feeding, gastric residuals, abdominal distention, increasing frequency of apnea and bradycardia, color change, poor muscle tone, temperature instability, and jaundice.

■ **What action should be taken when sepsis is suspected?**

The following plan of action should be instituted in the case of suspected sepsis:

1. When there have been prolonged ruptured membranes but mother and infant are both well, culture the throat and the periumbilical skin and observe.
2. When there have been prolonged ruptured membranes and mother has signs of infection such as fever and foul-smelling amniotic fluid, culture as for a septic workup and start treatment as in subsequent step.
3. When there are clinical signs of sepsis, promptly perform a septic workup. Include cultures of the throat, periumbilical skin, urine, blood, and spinal fluid. Also determine spinal fluid total and differential cell count, glucose and protein concentrations, and bacterial content by gram stain.

Antibiotic treatment usually consists of a combination of penicillin and amnioglycoside. The most frequently used combination at present is penicillin or ampicillin and kanamycin. When the infection is thought to be hospital acquired, gentamicin is usually substituted for kanamycin.

When there is evidence of staphylococcal disease suggested by pustules or pyropneumothorax, nafcillin is appropriately substituted for penicillin.

If after 5 days all cultures are negative and the infant is doing well, antibiotics may be discontinued. If the blood cultures are positive and cerebral spinal fluid culture negative, treatment for 7 to 10 days is usually sufficient. Treatment for meningitis as proved by positive spinal fluid culture should be more prolonged in order to prevent relapse, usually in the range of 3 weeks. Meningitis caused by *Pseudomonas* is also treated by the intrathecal administration of antibiotics. Newborn infants tend to metabolize and excrete antibiotic drugs more slowly than older children; therefore infections are treated with smaller and less frequent doses of drugs.

■ **Is there any value in performing routine throat cultures of nursery personnel?**

No. Many of the staff members are colonized with coagulation-positive *Staphylococcus* and impose no increased risk to patients. Cultures of personnel should be performed only in connection with specific infection problems in the nursery.

## SHOCK, ACID-BASE, AND FLUID PROBLEMS

■ **What factors lead to shock in the neonate?**

Any factors leading to a significant disturbance in cardiopulmonary function can produce the clinical syndrome of shock. These include inadequate oxygenation (as seen in respiratory distress syndrome, pulmonary infections, CNS drug depression, and obstructed airway disease), hypovolemia (from hemorrhage or excessive water loss), and septicemia.

■ **What are the clinical manifestations of shock?**

The intense peripheral vascular constriction, a compensatory mechanism, results in extreme pallor and cyanosis around the mouth and in the nail beds. Heart rate and respiratory rate are increased. Blood pressure is decreased. In contrast to the adult, whose blood pressure falls early in shock, the compensatory mechanisms in the newborn infant tend to sustain the blood pressure for a longer period of time. The normal mean arterial pressure of the neonate is 35 to 45 mm Hg and should be measured under conditions predisposing to shock when a central arterial catheter is in place. Indirect methods of blood pressure measurement are less reliable, but the recently available Doppler or ultrasound methods have increased the reliability of this approach.

### ■ What are the first steps in the treatment of shock?

Although the underlying cause must ultimately be corrected, immediate treatment is directed at relief of the compromised cardiopulmonary system and includes the following points: (1) Proper thermal regulation is necessary. It should be remembered that oxygen consumption is increased on either side of the thermoneutral point. (2) Oxygen requirements must be supplied by whatever means is appropriate to the situation. (See discussion of respiratory problems.) (3) Correction of the acid-base balance must be achieved. Very frequently the patient is acidemic and often has a combination of respiratory and metabolic acidosis. (4) Blood volume expansion is necessary in hypovolemic states. (5) A proper fluid and electrolyte balance must be maintained. It should be recognized that electrolyte concentration alone does not determine the presence of total body deficit. For example, some infants with severe water loss through diarrhea have higher than normal sodium concentrations even though there is a total body sodium depletion.

### ■ What is the most common form of acid-base disturbance seen in the neonate?

The imbalance most commonly seen is that of acidemia caused by respiratory insufficiency. This is manifested by arterial pH less than 7.35, $P_{O_2}$ less than 50 mm Hg, and $P_{CO_2}$ greater than 43 mm Hg. The sum of the effects of carbon dioxide retention resulting from hypoventilation and lactic acid production caused by anaerobic metabolism determines the degree of acidemia. Correction therefore must include both improved ventilation and improved oxygenation. These goals may be achieved by the proper combination of increased respiratory rate, tidal volume, ambient oxygen concentration, cardiac output, alveolar capillary diffusion rate, oxygen-carrying capacity of the blood, and blood volume in hypovolemic states.

### ■ How does the fluid and electrolyte economy in a neonate differ from that in an older child or adult?

Infants are much more susceptible to disorders of hydration than older persons for several reasons. Early in the neonatal period renal function is immature, and compensatory excretion and reabsorption mechanisms are not yet functioning efficiently. The rate of turnover of fluid per unit of body weight in an infant is about three times that of an adult, and their body water stores can therefore be depleted much faster. An infant with diarrhea may lose more than 50 ml of fluid/kg of body weight in a single day. The percent of total body water in the infant is approximately 75% to 80% of the body mass as compared to 55% for the adult female. The normal newborn has a physiologic loss of 5% to 10% of body fluid during the first few days of life.

### ■ What are the signs of dehydration in an infant?

Dry mucous membranes, depressed anterior fontanelle, poor skin turgor, decreased urine output, and increased blood urea nitrogen characterize dehydration.

### ■ Under normal circumstances what are the fluid requirements for a term infant?

Approximately 100 ml/kg/day is the normal requirement. Low birth weight infants weighing less than 1500 g require 100 to 125 ml/kg/day. An infant with respiratory problems or one exposed to increased radiant energy (under a radiant warmer or bilirubin lights) may have increased insensible losses and require more than 150 ml/kg/day. The best guides are serial weight determinations and serial determinations of urine specific gravity, with an attempt made to maintain it between 1.005 and 1.015.

■ **What are the normal values and daily maintenance requirements for electrolytes in the neonatal period?**

The values are as follows: sodium, 138 to 145 mEq/L; potassium, 3.5 to 5.5 mEq/L; and chloride, 95 to 110 mEq/L. The daily requirements for sodium are 3 to 5 mEq/kg and for potassium, 2 mEq/kg.

■ **How can the degree of fluid deficit be estimated?**

Losses of 5%, 10%, and 15% of body weight result in mild, moderate, or severe dehydration, respectively. A 5% loss results in dry skin and mucous membranes, decreased amount of urine, and slight fontanelle depression. A 10% loss results in circulatory disturbances manifested by mottled skin, tachycardia, severely reduced urine output, significantly depressed fontanelle, sunken eyes, and loss of elasticity of the skin. A 15% loss results in a moribund condition and demands immediate attention for the survival of the patient.

## HEMATOLOGIC PROBLEMS

■ **What are the more common types of hemolytic disease of the newborn (erythroblastosis fetalis)?**

The expression "erythroblastosis fetalis" has generally been replaced by "hemolytic disease of the newborn." The more severe type is caused by Rh sensitization of the mother. The mother who has no Rh antigen on the red blood cells and is therefore capable of forming Rh antibodies does so as a result of receiving the transmission of very small amounts of fetal blood through the placenta. This happens during labor; therefore these cells can be destroyed by giving anti-Rh antibody to the mother shortly after the infant's birth. The more severe form of hemolytic disease occurs in the infant of a mother who has been sensitized by a previous pregnancy and received no Rh antibody. AO and BO incompatibilities are the other more common types. Neither tends to be as severe as Rh incompatibility; however, BO tends to produce more severe disease than AO incompatibility. These latter types are frequently successfully treated by placing the infant under light.

■ **What risks to the infant result from such a hemolytic process?**

The antibodies produced by the mother against fetal blood cross the placenta, enter the fetal circulation, and attach to the red blood cells of the fetus, which carry the Rh antigen. This results in hemolysis, or breakdown, of the red blood cell walls and production of free hemoglobin in the circulation. There are two consequences of this. The infant becomes anemic and has reduced oxygen-carrying capacity in the blood. When severe enough, this can lead to heart failure. In addition, the large amount of hemoglobin released is converted to bilirubin and high concentrations of bilirubin can produce brain damage.

■ **How is hyperbilirubinemia clinically manifested in the neonate?**

Increased bilirubin concentration in the blood and tissue is clinically observed as jaundice, or a yellow color in the skin and conjunctivae. Jaundice is not seen until bilirubin exceeds 5 to 7 mg/100 ml. Normal variations in color vision lead to difficulty in estimating bilirubin by inspection. After a neonate has been placed under a light, the estimate of bilirubin from skin color tends to be low.

■ **Is jaundice normal in the newborn?**

There is a normal rate of red blood cell breakdown leading to bilirubin production during fetal life. It is eliminated by way of the mother's circulation; therefore the normal newborn is not jaundiced. After delivery the mother's circulation is no longer available to effect the elimination of bilirubin, and some infants become jaundiced during early neonatal life. This *physiologic jaundice,* or *icterus neonatorum,* typically begins after 24 hours, peaks at 3 to 4 days, and falls to the normal value within 7 to 14 days. In contrast to this course, jaundice occurring during the first 24 hours or after a week of age suggests a pathologic cause that should be investigated.

■ **What types of bilirubin are found circulating in the blood?**

Bilirubin is found in the conjugated and unconjugated form. In the conjugated form bilirubin has chemically interacted with glucuronic acid. This chemical reaction takes place in the liver. This conjugated form is nontoxic. The free or unconjugated form of bilirubin is lipid soluble and is toxic to the CNS. The unconjugated form can be bound by albumin in the circulation, reducing the concentration of unconjugated bilirubin and the probability of toxicity. The premature infant has a less mature conjugating system in the liver and is therefore more likely to become jaundiced even when the rate of red blood cell destruction is not increased.

■ **What situations increase the likelihood of bilirubin toxicity?**

The preterm infant appears to be more subject to CNS bilirubin poisoning than the term infant. Exchange transfusion in the term infant is considered mandatory when the indirect or unconjugated bilirubin concentration reaches 20 mg/100 ml. The preterm infant who is not ill is considered a possible candidate for exchange transfusion when the unconjugated bilirubin concentration is in the range of 15 to 20 mg/100 ml. Certain problems in ill preterm infants increase bilirubin toxicity and lead to the consideration of exchange transfusion when unconjugated bilirubin concentration is less than 15 mg/100 ml. When the serum albumin is low, less free bilirubin is bound and a higher concentration of the toxic form is found. The degree of binding to albumin is affected by the blood pH. When there is a high concentration of circulating hydrogen ion, the albumin binding of bilirubin is reduced. Hypoglycemia results in increased circulating nonesterified fatty acids, which also displace bilirubin from albumin. Some drugs, such as sulfisoxazole, compete with bilirubin for albumin binding.

■ **How is hyperbilirubinemia treated?**

There are various modes of therapy recommended. These include no treatment, light treatment, and exchange transfusion.

*No treatment*

Physiologic jaundice found after the first 24 hours of age and peaking on the third to fourth day usually does not exceed 12 mg of total bilirubin/100 ml and requires no treatment.

*Light treatment*

Less severe and more slowly progressing jaundice is commonly found in preterm infants and in association with ABO incompatibility and can very often successfully be treated by placing the infant under light. The light usually used is emitted by fluorescent bulbs. Although the light appears white, the effective portion of the radiant energy acting on bilirubin is in the wavelength range of blue light. During the time the infant is under light the eyes are covered to avoid any possible damage to the retina. The recommended intensity of light is between 200 and 400 footcandles. This is commonly referred to as *phototherapy* and has been shown to reduce bilirubin concentration by an average of 1.5 to 2 mg/ml over a 12- to 24-hour period.

*Exchange transfusion*

More severe and rapidly progressive forms of jaundice, as well as jaundice in ill preterm infants, is treated by exchange transfusion. This is done by placing a plastic catheter in either the umbilical artery or umbilical vein and alternately withdrawing infant blood and infusing donor blood. The total volume used is usually twice that of the infant's blood volume. This will replace approximately 85% of the infant's blood with donor blood. Although phototherapy is not appropriate for the treatment of the ill infant with one of the more severe forms of hyperbilirubinemia, it can reduce the need for repeated exchange transfusions.

■ **Other than blood incompatibilities, what is the single most important cause of jaundice in the newborn infant?**

The most important cause of jaundice exclusive of blood incompatibilities is infection.

■ **Other than Rh and ABO hemolytic disease, what are the causes of anemia in the newborn?**

Blood loss from any cause results in anemia. This may occur before, during, or after the process of birth. It may result from birth trauma, placental injury, or twin-to-twin transfusion. Anemia results from late clamping of the cord when the infant is held above the level of the placenta. Hemolytic disease other than that described with relation to Rh and ABO incompatibility may result from a deficiency of certain red blood cell enzymes, making the cells more subject to hemolysis. One of the more common of these is glucose-6-phosphate dehydrogenase deficiency.

■ **What are normal levels of hemoglobin and hematocrit in the newborn infant?**

The term infant of normal birth weight has a mean hemoglobin concentration of 17 g/100 ml of blood during the first day of life. The mean hematocrit during this time is 51%.

■ **Are there any problems associated with excessive circulating red blood cells?**

A high hematocrit may result from delayed clamping of the cord while the infant is held below the placental level and less frequently may result from twin-to-twin transfusion. Hematocrit value is considered excessive and may lead to clinical problems if over 70%. Concentrations above this produce excessive viscosity of the blood and reduced flow. This can lead to CNS and cardiopulmonary symptoms.

■ **Is any treatment ever required for high hematocrit?**

It is probably wise when the hematocrit is excessively high to reduce it to approximately 60 by a partial exchange transfusion with albumin or plasma. This reduces blood viscosity and peak bilirubin level resulting from the breakdown of the excessive number of red blood cells.

■ **What is meant by the term "DIC?"**

These initials refer to *disseminated intravascular coagulation.* This entity is found in extremely ill infants, especially those in shock and those with severe bacterial infections. There is spontaneous disseminated coagulation in the small blood vessels, resulting in the consumption of blood factors normally involved in the coagulation process. Thus it is sometimes referred to as *consumption coagulopathy.* This situation results in a tendency to bleed into the skin, mucous membranes, urinary tract, or intestines. Platelet counts and coagulation factor concentrations are low. Since fibrin is formed in the coagulation process and is subsequently split by enzyme action, the presence of excessive fibrin split products in the circulating blood is also supportive of the diagnosis. In some instances heparin is administered to control the coagulation process.

## RESPIRATORY SYSTEM DISORDERS

■ **What is the most common reason for admission of a newborn infant to an intensive care unit?**

A primary respiratory problem is the most common reason for admission. Approximately one half of all newborns admitted to the intensive care unit are admitted because of respiratory difficulty.

■ **What is the most common type of respiratory disorder leading to admission of the newborn?**

This disease is called *idiopathic respiratory distress syndrome, or hyaline membrane disease,* and typically occurs in preterm newborn infants. These two terms, both misnomers, are by common usage employed to describe a symptom complex that centers on low lung compliance caused by insufficient surfactant production. This may result from immaturity, insufficient surfactant production as a result of hypoxia, chemical or thermal injury to the surfactant-producing cells, increased surfactant utilization, or a combination of these. Surfactant is a phospholipid compound that makes it possible for alveoli to expand more easily. That is to say, less mechanical force is required to bring air into the alveoli of the lungs when surfactant is in the alveolar lining fluid. In the absence of the surfactant the alveoli tend to remain collapsed. The blood passing collapsed alveoli picks up little or no oxygen. Arterial blood therefore contains less than the normal amount of oxygen, and the tissues become hypoxic. The metabolism of tissues continues, however, and in the absence of sufficient oxygen this metabolism produces lactic acid. Both hypoxia and acidemia act on the small blood vessels in the lung, causing them to constrict. This constriction increases the resistance to blood flow through the lungs, causing large amounts of blood to be shunted through the ductus arteriosus and the foramen ovale, thus bypassing the lung and leading to even greater hypoxia and acidemia. The pathophysiologic process therefore tends to be self-perpetuating.

■ **From the answer to the previous question, what would be logical approaches to the prevention or treatment of respiratory distress syndrome?**

The prevention of preterm birth will probably ultimately become the most important method of preventing the disease. Currently the prevention of fetal hypoxia during labor and of cold distress of the newborn after delivery is helpful. A surfactant production system operating at a marginal level can be so damaged by hypoxic and thermal stress as to function subnormally and lead to respiratory distress syndrome (RDS).

It is beneficial to increase the oxygen tension and content of circulating blood. This effort is first made by increasing oxygen concentration in the gas surrounding the infant's head. If arterial blood oxygen tension does not exceed 50 ml Hg while the infant is breathing 60% oxygen, continuous positive air pressure (CPAP), as described subsequently, should be employed.

When oxygen enrichment of the atmosphere alone does not result in sufficient oxygenation, measures should be taken to expand the collapsed alveoli. If the infant is breathing spontaneously, this is achieved by applying CPAP. This is usually done by intubating the infant with a 2½ to 4 mm diameter endotracheal tube, the size depending on the infant's size, and attaching the tube to a system that does not allow the airway pressure at the end of the expiration to fall to atmospheric pressure. With this system the infant is not allowed to exhale as much gas as previously and consequently does not empty the alveoli. This establishes a functional residual capacity (FRC). Pressures applied are usually initially 4 to 6 cm $H_2O$ and are increased or decreased, depending on the infant's response. The infant who is not breathing spontaneously is put on positive end-expiratory pressure (PEEP). This expression is generally accepted as describing respiratory assistance employing a respiratory assistance device such as a Bennett, Bird, or Bourns respirator with positive end tidal pressure.

Control of the acidosis is achieved by administering a buffer solution. Sodium bicarbonate is most commonly used; less frequently tromethamine (THAM) is used. Sodium bicarbonate should be infused slowly; usual doses for half correction of base deficit require at least 5 minutes for infusion.

■ **What are two important complications of respirator therapy?**

1. Infection from contaminated equipment may occur. Respirator tubing and nebulizers must be changed at frequent intervals.
2. Pneumothorax may develop. Equipment for the emergency management of pneumothorax should be immediately at hand for any patient who is on a respirator or receiving PEEP.

**■ What happens when at term the fetus in the uterus becomes hypoxic as a result of occlusion of the umbilical cord?**

The fetus passes meconium into the amniotic fluid and develops gasping respirations. Depending on the severity of hypoxia, meconium aspiration resulting from this process may be minimal to severe. When severe, it is referred to as the *massive meconium aspiration syndrome*. If the fetus has not been monitored during labor, the first clue may be meconium staining of the amniotic fluid after the membranes rupture. Amniotic fluid stained with meconium is sterile and produces chemical irritation in the small airways. They become partially obstructed, producing air trapping. The volume of the chest is increased, and the anteroposterior diameter may be unusually large.

**■ How should meconium aspiration be managed?**

When it is obvious in the delivery room that the neonate has aspirated meconium, the airway should be suctioned repeatedly through a laryngoscope until as much meconium as possible has been removed. This is enhanced by saline gavage, which probably reduces the severity of the disease.

**■ A term infant develops respiratory distress and poor color immediately after birth. Amniotic fluid is normal, and fetal monitoring has been normal. On inspection the abdomen appears smaller than normal. What is the infant's problem?**

Reduced size of the abdomen in a newborn with respiratory distress suggests *diaphragmatic hernia,* in which a large proportion of the abdominal viscera has herniated through the diaphragm, occupying space that would normally be occupied by lung. In respiratory assistance, bag and mask should not be used because this would only force more air into the intestine and further compress the lung. Respiratory assistance should be given by endotracheal intubation. When this diagnosis is made, arrangements should be made for direct admission into the operating room, and the infant should be immediately placed under the supervision of the anesthesiologist and surgeon.

**■ A term infant, appearing to be normal at birth, regurgitates and becomes blue at the first feeding. What is the most likely problem?**

Esophageal atresia and tracheoesophageal fistula should be suspected. There is a variety of combinations of these lesions, but by far the most common type is esophageal atresia with a fistula between the trachea and distal esophageal pouch. Continuous suction in the upper pouch and gastrostomy to prevent the aspiration of gastric content make it possible to delay surgical repair until optimum conditions can be met.

**■ Why is it important to administer oxygen therapy to infants under very carefully monitored conditions?**

Injury to the retina is produced by high arterial oxygen tension. Infants younger than 36 weeks of gestation are especially subject to this damage. The maximum tolerable arterial oxygen tension is not known with certainty, and small preterm infants have been known to develop retinopathy of the preterm infant (retrolental fibroplasia) even when there has been no oxygen enrichment. At present the goal of oxygen therapy is to sustain an arterial oxygen tension somewhere in the range of 50 to 70 mm Hg or a capillary oxygen tension around 35 to 45 mm Hg. The retina responds to high oxygen tension by constriction and overgrowth of the capillary blood vessels. This is followed by hemorrhage and scar formation, causing contraction and retinal detachment.

Toxicity to the lung may result. Microscopically detectable damage to lung cells can be caused by breathing only moderately increased oxygen concentrations for short periods of time. Clinically important oxygen lung damage is usually associated with breathing more than 70% oxygen for more than 4 days. Oxygen damage to the lung leads to oxygen dependency that may last for weeks to months. However, after many months the lung function and chest x-ray films may completely return to normal.

■ **What are some important aspects of resuscitation of the newborn infant in the delivery room?**

As soon as the infant is delivered, the nostrils and the oropharynx should be suctioned with a bulb syringe. The cord is cut and clamped, and the infant is dried immediately to prevent heat loss by evaporation. The infant is placed under a radiant heat warmer and the Apgar score is assessed at age 1 minute. An Apgar score of 3 or below is that of a severely depressed infant who requires immediate resuscitation. After suctioning the pharynx clear of mucous the airway should be intubated under direct vision with a laryngoscope. Blood, mucous, and aspirated meconium should be cleared from the airway by suction and positive pressure ventilation with oxygen should be instituted. At this point oxygenation is much more important than the administration of alkali. A 1-minute Apgar score of 4 to 7 is that of a moderately depressed infant who will often respond to simple stimulation of the skin or inflation of the airway by mask and bag. An Apgar score above 7 is found in nondepressed infants. Vigorous and possibly traumatic efforts to stimulate a depressed infant, such as hot and cold applications and rectal dilation, are not recommended. These maneuvers consume time that is best applied to clearing the airway and achieving proper oxygenation. The Apgar score is then evaluated at age 5 minutes. The 5-minute Apgar score is more closely predictive of the long-term effects of birth anoxia.

The newborn infant does have some anatomic peculiarities that are important in resuscitation. The tongue is relatively large. The nares are narrow and the glottis is high. The cricoid ring is narrow and the mandible is short. The airway is placed in proper alignment for intubation by placing the head in the "sniffing position" with the shoulders only slightly raised and the chin protruding. This is in marked contrast to the appropriate position for the adult (hyperextension). It is important for the operator to have adequate assistance. The vocal cords can often be brought into clearer view by a slight depression of the anterior neck over the laryngeal area.

If no heartbeat is heard, external cardiac massage should be initiated. This is accomplished by applying pressure using the index and middle fingers over the lower sternal area at a rate of 120 compressions/min. This should be in a ratio of 3:1 in relation to assisted respirations, which are given at a rate of 40 respirations/min. Care should be exercised to avoid injury to the sterum, liver, and spleen.

## CARDIOVASCULAR SYSTEM ABNORMALITIES

■ **What types of congenital heart disease are most likely to be seen in a neonatal intensive care unit?**

Transposition of the great vessels and hypoplastic left heart syndrome most frequently present problems, and during the early part of the course may be difficult to distinguish from primary lung disease.

■ **What observations might be helpful in distinguishing between heart and lung disease?**

Extreme desaturation of arterial blood caused by congenital heart disease results from large fixed right-left shunts. That is to say, the fraction of blood not flowing through the lungs is large. In this case, allowing the infant to breath high concentration oxygen would have a minimum effect on arterial oxygen tension. It is therefore sometimes helpful to apply the test of breathing 100% oxygen. If the oxygen tension rises appreciably, it is more likely that the infant has primary lung disease than primary congenital heart disease. There are some infants, however, with severe respiratory distress syndrome who cannot be distinguished from those with congenital heart disease by this test. In this situation the diagnostic assessment must be based on history and physical and radiographic findings to make the best judgment possible. When it is of extreme importance to identify heart disease for therapeutic reasons, it may be necessary to perform cardiac catheterization. Distinguishing heart and lung disease may be so difficult, even for very experienced staff, that infrequently an infant with respiratory distress syndrome undergoes catheterization.

■ **What type of supportive care should infants acutely ill with congenital heart disease be given?**

Optimum oxygenation, proper thermal regulation, and meeting nutritional needs are important. The infant should also be observed closely for signs of heart failure.

■ **How is heart failure in the newborn infant diagnosed?**

The most useful signs of heart failure are tachypnea, tachycardia, heart enlargement, and liver enlargement. It is not necessary that a murmur be present, and some of the more severe forms of congenital heart disease are not accompanied by heart murmur. In contrast to the adult, the newborn in congestive heart failure does not typically have pulmonary rales and peripheral edema. Fluid retention is best identified by the close observation of weight.

■ **What is the treatment for congestive heart failure in the neonate?**

The following treatment regimen should be employed:

1. Digitalization. (See Table 24-6 for digoxin dosage.)
2. Supplementary oxygen. Care is taken to avoid overoxygenation because of the possibility of eye and lung toxicity.
3. Control of acid-base balance.
4. Temperature regulation at the thermoneutral point. (Oxygen consumption is increased by either hypo- or hyperthermia.)
5. Oral feedings should be withheld if the respiratory rate is high enough to produce the danger of aspiration.
6. Correction of anemia by blood transfusion.
7. Diuretics. Furosemide is usually used if rapid diuresis is required, and a mercurial diuretic is used if a more prolonged, smoother effect is desired.

■ **How should a neonate be monitored for digitalis toxicity?**

An ECG rhythm strip should be run prior to each dose of digoxin. The effect of digitalis is assessed by its effect on conduction as manifested by prolongation of the P-R interval and reduction of heart rate. The next dose should generally be withheld if the rate is less than 100 beats/min.

■ **What heart rate should be considered bradycardia in a newborn?**

Below 90 beats/min should be considered bradycardia.

■ **Would a heart murmur in a newborn infant ever be considered normal?**

Heart murmurs are very common in normal newborn infants as well as older children. The sound heard as a result of turbulent blood flow. The murmurs are often transient and rapidly changing during the neonatal period. Frequently a changing murmur is related to changing flow through the ductus arteriosus as it is closing. In the absence of associated symptoms and signs suggestive of heart disease it is best to avoid ascribing major significance to murmurs heard in early infancy and to follow the course over a longer period of time before alerting the parents.

■ **When does the ductus arteriosus usually close?**

In the healthy infant it usually closes functionally within the first 24 hours. However, anatomically it may remain open for a longer period of time, requiring, in some infants, several months for closure. The small preterm infant with respiratory distress tends to have more frequent difficulty with prolonged patent ductus arteriosus. It is not unusual for an infant of this type to require surgical ligation of the ductus arteriosus because of intractable heart failure and persistent need for high oxygen concentration and respiratory support.

■ **What normally causes the ductus arteriosus to close?**

Increased oxygen tension in the blood is usually responsible. During fetal life the oxygen tension experienced by the ductus is in the range of 25 to 30 mm Hg. At the time of birth the oxygen tension rises abruptly. The ductus is quite sensitive to this increase and responds by constricting. Disorders resulting in protracted hypoxemia delay closure of the ductus.

## NEUROLOGIC DISORDERS

■ **Does the immaturity of the CNS in the preterm infant result in CNS abnormalities found in long-term follow-up?**

Early studies revealing that "very low birth weight infants" (1000 to 1500 g) had a high incidence (greater than 50%) of CNS damage suggested that the immaturity alone may have been responsible for a significant proportion of the long-term CNS deficits. With the improved care provided by modern neonatal critical care units the long-range prognosis appears to be improving so much that this formerly held concept is probably inaccurate; thus we are led to believe that the main causes of long-lasting CNS damage are hypoxia, CNS hemorrhage, hypoglycemia, hyperbilirubinemia, and CNS infections occurring before or after birth.

■ **What clinical manifestations of neurologic disturbance are present in the newborn?**

Early in the course of the neurologic disturbance the muscle tone tends to be diminished and the reflexes small or absent. Seizure activity associated with hypoxia, hypoglycemia, or hypocalcemia may be so subtle as to be easily overlooked and may be seen only as increased muscle tone of an extremity, repetitive eye blinking, drooling, chewing movements, and sometimes only as apnea. More conspicuous seizure activity may be localized or may consist of generalized convulsive movements.

■ **What are the causes of seizures in the newborn infant?**

Hypoxia, hypoglycemia, hypocalcemia, infection, disorders of amino acid metabolism, alkalosis (as from hyperventilation), hypomagnesemia, hyperbilirubinemia, pyridoxine deficiency, hypo- or hypernatremia, drug withdrawal in the infant of an addicted mother, and CNS hemorrhage may cause seizures.

■ **What would be an appropriate initial workup for a neonate with seizures?**

Evaluation of blood sugar and serum calcium concentrations and septic workup, including spinal fluid analysis, are appropriate. If these are not informative, a more detailed workup may include investigations for transplacental infections, screening for metabolic disorders, and administration of pyridoxine during an EEG.

## ENDOCRINE-METABOLIC DISORDERS

The endocrine and metabolic problems associated with newborns, the clinical and laboratory diagnostic signs by which the disorder is identified, and appropriate immediate management are summarized in Table 24-1. All the conditions listed can lead to severe illness in the newborn infant.

## DIGESTIVE SYSTEM

■ **What is the significance of the delayed passage of meconium?**

Over the first 24 hours 98% of infants pass meconium. The delayed passage of meconium, particularly if there is associated abdominal distention or vomiting, should lead to suspicion of obstruction somewhere in the lower intestine. Possible causes of obstruction include meconium plug syndrome, Hirschsprung's disease, imperforate anus, atresia of the colon, and meconium peritonitis associated with cystic fibrosis.

■ **Is it possible to determine whether the blood vomited or passed rectally by the neonate is of maternal origin?**

Yes. The distinction can usually be made by an Apt test. There is a difference between the susceptibility of fetal and adult hemo-

**Table 24-1.** Endocrine-metabolic problems

| *Disorder* | *Diagnostic clues* | *Management* |
|---|---|---|
| Myasthenia gravis | Infant with respiratory insufficiency soon after birth; mother with myasthenia gravis; course self-limited, usually resolving in a few weeks | Respiratory support with bag or respirator; edrophonium (Tensilon) test and treatment with pyridostigmine (Mestinon); drug tapered as symptoms diminish |
| Galactosemia | Jaundice, sepsis, copper reducing substance in the urine; specific test on red blood cells for uridine diphosphoglucose transferase positive | Control of infection; reduction of bilirubin by light; exchange transfusion if necessary; lactose-free diet; genetic counseling |
| Hypoglycemia | Apnea, poor color, convulsions in infant of a diabetic mother; infant small for gestational age; high hematocrit; hemolytic disease | Early feeding; IV glucose; adrenocortical steroids if glucose alone not effective |
| Hypocalcemia | Low birth weight; traumatic delivery; jittery infant; seizures; laryngospasm; Low serum calcium levels (below 7 mg/100 ml) | Administration of calcium gluconate, preferably by oral route (when urgency requires IV administration, great care taken to avoid extravasation); tissue necrosis resulting from IV calcium administration common |
| Disorders of amino acid metabolism such as maple syrup urine disease or methylmalonic aciduria | Acidemia, difficult to control and unexplained by respiratory status; ketonemia; elevation of amino acid concentrations on specific chromatographic tests; seizures | Buffers to modify acidemia and anticonvulsant therapy until specific dietary or vitamin therapy can be administered; genetic counseling |
| Late metabolic acidosis of the preterm infant | Preterm infant doing well first few days, but after 1 or 2 weeks taking feedings poorly, failing to gain weight; low blood pH (below 7.25) | Small doses of sodium bicarbonate added to formula to bring prompt improvement of symptoms |
| Virilizing adrenal hyperplasia (adrenogenital syndrome or congenital adrenal hyperplasia) | Virilized genitalia, more conspicuous in female; vomiting followed by shock; serum potassium levels high (cardiac arrhythmias) and sodium levels low; elevated blood pregnanetriol levels | IV sodium chloride, deoxycorticosterone for emergency treatment; adrenocortical steroids for prolonged treatment; genetic counseling |

globin to the effects of alkali. This effect is observed as a simple color change.

■ **A 3-week-old male infant develops projectile vomiting of nonbile-stained material, weight loss, dehydration, and scanty stools. This age, sex, and symptom complex is characteristic of what problem?**

Hypotrophic pyloric stenosis should be suspected. In addition to the symptoms, physical findings include impaired nutrition and hydration, gastric waves proceeding from the left to the right over the left upper and central abdomen, and a palpable mass often described as an "olive" at the position of the pylorus.

■ **A 3-week-old infant suddenly develops vomiting of bile-stained material, abdominal distention, and signs of shock. Why is it important that the correct diagnosis be made quickly?**

This clinical complex is characteristic of malrotation of the intestine and midgut volvulus. It is important to make the correct diagnosis quickly because delay can result in the loss of a large amount of bowel resulting from circulatory impairment produced by the volvulus. This entity is a major contributor to the severe instances of short bowel syndrome.

■ **A preterm infant who has had respiratory distress syndrome appears to be recovering from a respiratory problem. At 10 days of age he develops rapid onset of abdominal distention, gastric residuals, temperature instability, and shocklike state. What is the most probable diagnosis and what is the pathogenesis of this disease?**

Necrotizing enterocolitis (NEC) should be suspected. When this clinical complex is seen, the diagnosis is supported by findings on x-ray examination of thickened bowel wall, gas in the bowel wall, free gas in the peritoneal cavity, and gas in the portal circulation. This gas is hydrogen that is generated by anaerobic bacteria in the intestines and will often disappear after feedings have been stopped. Discontinuing feedings early in the course of the disease and treating the shock are probably the most important features of successful management.

The etiology of this disease is as yet unclear. NEC has been described only in recent years. Therefore it is probably a result of one of the newer forms of management of low birth weight infants or is occurring in infants who would not formerly have survived long enough to develop the disorder. It tends to develop within 5 to 21 days of age. At the present time the most logical causes seem to include a prior period of hypoxia or infection or a combination of both of these. It has been demonstrated that aortic blood flow may be very significantly decreased by the placement of aortic catheters via the umbilical artery. This could result in reduced mesenteric artery flow, and the tips of such catheters should probably be placed no higher than the aortic bifurcation.

■ **What are the limitations on feeding a preterm infant with respiratory distress syndrome?**

Early feeding is considered important in preterm infants. Early feeding decreases the likelihood of hypoglycemia and the peak bilirubin level. It is wise, however, to delay feedings when the respiratory rate is excessively high. Distention of the stomach can reduce movement of the diaphragm, and the possibility of regurgitation and aspiration is greater. It is usually best to delay oral feedings by nipple or gavage until the respiratory rate is below 60 respirations/min.

## NORMAL VALUES

Tables 24-2 to 24-6 and the boxed material on p. 447 list various normal values used in the care of the neonate.

**Table 24-2.** Temperature equivalents

| *Centigrade* | *Fahrenheit* | *Centigrade* | *Fahrenheit* |
|---|---|---|---|
| 34.0 | 93.2 | 38.6 | 101.4 |
| 34.2 | 93.6 | 38.8 | 101.8 |
| 34.4 | 93.9 | 39.0 | 102.2 |
| 34.6 | 94.3 | 39.2 | 102.5 |
| 34.8 | 94.6 | 39.4 | 102.9 |
| 35.0 | 95.0 | 39.6 | 103.2 |
| 35.2 | 95.4 | 39.8 | 103.6 |
| 35.4 | 95.7 | 40.0 | 104.0 |
| 35.6 | 96.1 | 40.2 | 104.3 |
| 35.8 | 96.4 | 40.4 | 104.7 |
| 36.0 | 96.8 | 40.6 | 105.1 |
| 36.2 | 97.1 | 40.8 | 105.4 |
| 36.4 | 97.5 | 41.0 | 105.8 |
| 36.6 | 97.8 | 41.2 | 106.1 |
| 36.8 | 98.2 | 41.4 | 106.5 |
| 37.0 | 98.6 | 41.6 | 106.8 |
| 37.2 | 98.9 | 41.8 | 107.2 |
| 37.4 | 99.3 | 42.0 | 107.6 |
| 37.6 | 99.6 | 42.2 | 108.0 |
| 37.8 | 100.0 | 42.4 | 108.3 |
| 38.0 | 100.4 | 42.6 | 108.7 |
| 38.2 | 100.7 | 42.8 | 109.0 |
| 38.4 | 101.1 | 43.0 | 109.4 |

To convert centigrade to Fahrenheit:

$$(9/5 \times \text{Temperature}) + 32$$

For example: To convert 40° C to Fahrenheit
$9/5 \times 40 = 72 + 32 = 104°$ F

To convert Fahrenheit to centigrade:

$$(\text{Temperature} - 32) \times 5/9$$

For example: To convert 98.6° F to centigrade
$98.6 - 32 = 66.6 \times 5/9 = 37°$ C

## NORMAL VALUES AND INFORMATION FOR NEWBORN INFANTS

**BILIRUBIN**

12 mg/100 ml or less

**BUN**

20 mg/100 ml or less

**ELECTROLYTES**

| | |
|---|---|
| Chloride | 95-110 mEq/L |
| Potassium | 3.5-5.5 mEq/L |
| Sodium | 138-145 mEq/L |

**GLUCOSE**

30+ mg/100 ml — Hypoglycemia in term infants <30 mg/100 ml, Hypoglycemia in preterm infants <20 mg/100 ml } during first 24 hr. Give IV glucose, 10% solution or stronger.

**HEMATOCRIT**

45%-65% — If above 65%, consider partial exchange of 10% blood volume for same volume of plasma.

**CALCIUM**

8-10.5 mg/100 ml — Treat if below 7 mg/100 ml or if symptomatic between 7-8 mg/100 ml.

**PHOSPHORUS**

3.5-8 mg/100 ml — This may be as high as 10 if calcium is low because of a transient hypoparathyroidism.

**MISCELLANEOUS**

| | |
|---|---|
| Respiratory rate | 35 respirations/min (range 20-60 respirations/min) |
| Heart rate | 140 beats/min (range 120-160 beats/min) |
| Length | 50 cm |
| Head circumference | 35 cm |
| Weight (mean at term) | |
| Male | 3350 g |
| Female | 3250 g |
| Neonatal mortality rate | 17.8/1000 (United States, 1972) |
| Normal blood gas values (first week) | |
| pH | 7.30-7.40 |
| $P_{CO_2}$ | 35 mm Hg |
| $P_{aO_2}$ (arterial) | 60-90 mm Hg |

Retrolental fibroplasia related to $P_{aO_2}$, not $F_{IO_2}$ (fraction of inspired oxygen).

Any infant on any additional oxygen must be monitored with frequent blood gas determinations (this includes infants on oxygen concentration below 40%).

Most common antibiotic combination in neonatal sepsis

Ampicillin (100-200 mg/kg/24 hr every 12 hr IV) or penicillin (50,000-100,000 units/kg/24 hr every 12 hr IV) may be used with kanamycin (15 mg/kg/24 hr) or gentamicin (5-6 mg/kg/24 hr, usually given IM, but may be given IV).

**Composition by percentages**

| | *Protein* | *Fat* | *Carbohydrate* | *Minerals* |
|---|---|---|---|---|
| Cow's milk | 3.3 | 3.7 | 4.8 | 0.7 |
| Breast milk | 1.2 | 3.5 | 7.0 | 0.2 |

**Table 24-3.** Gram equivalents of pounds and ounces

| | *Pounds* | | | | | | | |
|---|---|---|---|---|---|---|---|---|
| *Ounces* | *1* | *2* | *3* | *4* | *5* | *6* | *7* | *8* |
| 0 | 454 | 907 | 1361 | 1814 | 2268 | 2722 | 3175 | 3629 |
| 1 | 482 | 936 | 1389 | 1843 | 2296 | 2750 | 3204 | 3657 |
| 2 | 510 | 964 | 1418 | 1871 | 2325 | 2778 | 3232 | 3686 |
| 3 | 539 | 992 | 1446 | 1899 | 2353 | 2807 | 3260 | 3714 |
| 4 | 567 | 1021 | 1474 | 1928 | 2381 | 2835 | 3289 | 3742 |
| 5 | 595 | 1049 | 1503 | 1956 | 2410 | 2863 | 3317 | 3771 |
| 6 | 624 | 1077 | 1531 | 1985 | 2438 | 2892 | 3345 | 3799 |
| 7 | 652 | 1106 | 1559 | 2013 | 2466 | 2920 | 3374 | 3827 |
| 8 | 680 | 1134 | 1588 | 2041 | 2495 | 2948 | 3402 | 3856 |
| 9 | 709 | 1162 | 1616 | 2070 | 2523 | 2977 | 3430 | 3884 |
| 10 | 737 | 1191 | 1644 | 2098 | 2552 | 3005 | 3459 | 3912 |
| 11 | 765 | 1219 | 1673 | 2126 | 2580 | 3033 | 3487 | 3941 |
| 12 | 794 | 1247 | 1701 | 2155 | 2608 | 3062 | 3515 | 3969 |
| 13 | 822 | 1276 | 1729 | 2183 | 2637 | 3090 | 3544 | 3997 |
| 14 | 851 | 1304 | 1758 | 2211 | 2665 | 3119 | 3572 | 4026 |
| 15 | 879 | 1332 | 1786 | 2240 | 2693 | 3147 | 3600 | 4054 |

**Table 24-4.** Conversion of inches to centimeters

| *Inches* | *cm* | *Inches* | *cm* | *Inches* | *cm* |
|---|---|---|---|---|---|
| 10 | 25.40 | 15 | 38.10 | 20 | 50.80 |
| 10½ | 26.67 | 15½ | 39.37 | 20½ | 52.07 |
| 11 | 27.94 | 16 | 40.64 | 21 | 53.34 |
| 11½ | 29.21 | 16½ | 41.91 | 21½ | 54.61 |
| 12 | 30.48 | 17 | 43.18 | 22 | 55.88 |
| 12½ | 31.75 | 17½ | 44.45 | 22½ | 57.15 |
| 13 | 33.02 | 18 | 45.72 | 23 | 58.42 |
| 13½ | 34.29 | 18½ | 46.99 | 23½ | 56.69 |
| 14 | 35.56 | 19 | 48.26 | 24 | 60.96 |
| 14½ | 36.83 | 19½ | 49.53 | | |

**Table 24-5.** Neonatal fluid and electrolyte needs

| | |
|---|---|
| *Water requirements* | |
| Full-term infant | 100 ml/kg/day |
| Healthy infant under 1500 g | 100-125 ml/kg/day |
| Infant with respiratory distress syndrome under 1500 g | 125-150 ml/kg/day |
| First day of life | 80-100 ml/kg/day |
| *Electrolytes* | |
| Sodium | 3-4 mEq/kg/day (maintenance) |
| Potassium | 2 mEq/kg/day (maintenance) |
| Calcium | 200 mg calcium gluconate/kg/day (maintenance) 400-800 mg calcium gluconate/kg/day (treatment) |
| *Caloric requirement* | 120-150 calories/day for growth |
| *Colloid* | |
| Packed red blood cells | 2 ml/kg for each gram hemoglobin is to be raised |
| Whole blood | 6 ml/kg for each gram hemoglobin is to be raised |
| Plasma or plasmanate | 10 ml/kg |

**Table 24-6.** Common drug dosages for the neonate

| | |
|---|---|
| *Antibiotics* | |
| Ampicillin | 100-200 mg/kg/24 hr |
| Gentamicin | 5-6 mg/kg/24 hr |
| Kanamycin | 15 mg/kg/24 hr |
| Nafcillin | 20-30 mg/kg/24 hr |
| Polymixin B | 1.5-2.5 mg/kg/24 hr |
| Polymixin E | 3-5 mg/kg/24 hr |
| Penicillin G | 50,000-100,000 units/kg/24 hr |
| *Cardiovascular medications* | |
| Atropine | 0.01 mg/kg/dose |
| Digoxin | 0.05 mg/kg total digitalizing dose (Give ½ total dose stat and remainder in two divided doses at 4-6 hr.) |
| Epinephrine | 1:1000 dilution 0.01 ml/kg/dose |
| *Metabolic correction agents* | |
| Calcium gluconate, 10% | 200-400 mg/kg/24 hr |
| Glucagon | 300 mg/kg/24 hr |
| Neo-Calglucon | 500 mg/kg/24 hr |
| *Sedatives* | |
| Chlorpromazine (Thorazine) | 1.0 mg/kg/24 hr |
| Phenobarbital | 5-8 mg/kg/24 hr |

## SUMMARY

In this chapter on critical care of the neonate we have covered thermal regulation, infection, shock, acid-base, and fluid problems and have developed a body system–oriented approach to the problem, including consideration of the hematologic, respiratory, cardiovascular, neurologic, endocrine, and gastrointestinal systems.

Although problems have often been discussed individually, actual neonatal critical care often becomes very complex as a result of interwoven problems. The infant born preterm, following premature rupture of the membranes, is at increased risk for *infection, thermal stress, respiratory distress, cardiovascular problems* (patent ductus arteriosus), *eye damage* (retrolental fibroplasia), *lung damage* (bronchopulmonary dysplasia), *malnutrition, necrotizing enterocolitis, metabolic problems* (hypoglycemia, hypocalcemia), *hyperbilirubinemia,* and *anemia.* Successful management of such a complex group of problems requires carefully coordinated efforts of a dedicated, well-equipped, disciplined team as well as a large financial commitment.

## BIBLIOGRAPHY

Aladjem, S., and Brown, A. K., editors: Clinical perinatology, St. Louis, 1974, The C. V. Mosby Co.

Avery, M. E., and Fletcher, B. D.: The lung and its disorders in the newborn infant, Philadelphia, 1974, W. B. Saunders Co.

Gluck, L.: Modern perinatal medicine, Chicago, 1974, Year Book Medical Publishers, Inc.

Harper, R. G., and Yoon, J. J.: Handbook of neonatology, Chicago, 1974, Year Book Medical Publishers, Inc.

Klaus, M. H., and Fanaroff, A. A.: Care of the high-risk neonate, Philadelphia, 1973, W. B. Saunders Co.

Korones, S. B.: High-risk newborn infants, St. Louis, 1972, The C. V. Mosby Co.

*chapter 25*

# Critical care of infants and children after the neonatal period

STANLEY M. KEGEL
MELVILLE I. SINGER

## ■ Why is there a need for a separate section of discussion of critical care in infants and children?

Children are not little adults. There are major differences in the metabolic processes in adults and children. Diseases are frequently different, as are responses and toxicity with relation to medications. Drugs commonly used in adults are frequently inadequately tested for use in children, and there may be major differences in the absorption and activity of these medications between the tablet and liquid forms. Although neoplastic and degenerative diseases form a major part of adult medicine, infections, accidents, and congenital anomalies are more common in children. A knowledge of the diseases prevalent in childhood and the metabolic responses of children are essential to proper treatment.

### Unexpected toxicity

A few examples will help clarify the differences between children and adults with respect to drugs. Oxygen has widely been used in the treatment of respiratory failure. High oxygen concentrations were used for many years in the treatment of premature infants with respiratory distress, resulting in the blinding of many children from retrolental fibroplasia caused by damage to the eye from oxygen. The use of chloramphenicol in small infants resulted in a shocklike state, the so-called gray babies, with many deaths until the inability of the neonate to metabolize chloramphenicol was demonstrated. Although adults may tolerate a wide range of fluid therapy without serious results, small errors in fluid therapy in children can result in circulatory overload, dehydration, or major electrolyte disturbances. A knowledge of the immaturity of the kidney and liver in infants and children is essential in determining the dosage and frequency of drugs detoxified or excreted by these organs.

## ■ How should drug doses for children be calculated?

Drug action, absorption, detoxification, and excretion are related to the metabolic rate of the child rather than body weight or age. Metabolic rate is most closely related to surface area.

Older rules for drug dosage such as Young's rule:

$$\frac{\text{Age (yr)} \times \text{Adult dose}}{\text{Age (yr)} + 12}$$

Fried's rule for infants:

$$\frac{\text{Age (mo)} \times \text{Adult dose}}{150}$$

or Clark's rule:

$$\frac{\text{Weight (lb)} \times \text{Adult dose}}{150}$$

are very inaccurate and usually result in infants and small children receiving ineffective doses of medication.

For most drugs the formula:

$$\frac{\text{Body surface area}}{1.72} \times \text{Adult dose}$$

will give a safe and effective dosage for children. In infants under 1 month of age the calculated dose should be reduced by 50%.

The nomogram derived from West's surface area nomogram can be used to calculate the portion of an adult dose a child should receive (Fig. 25-1). If the nomogram for surface areas is not used, the surface area (SA) can be calculated by the formula:

$$\text{SA (m}^2\text{)} = \frac{4 \text{ Weight (kg)} + 7}{\text{Weight (kg)} + 90}$$

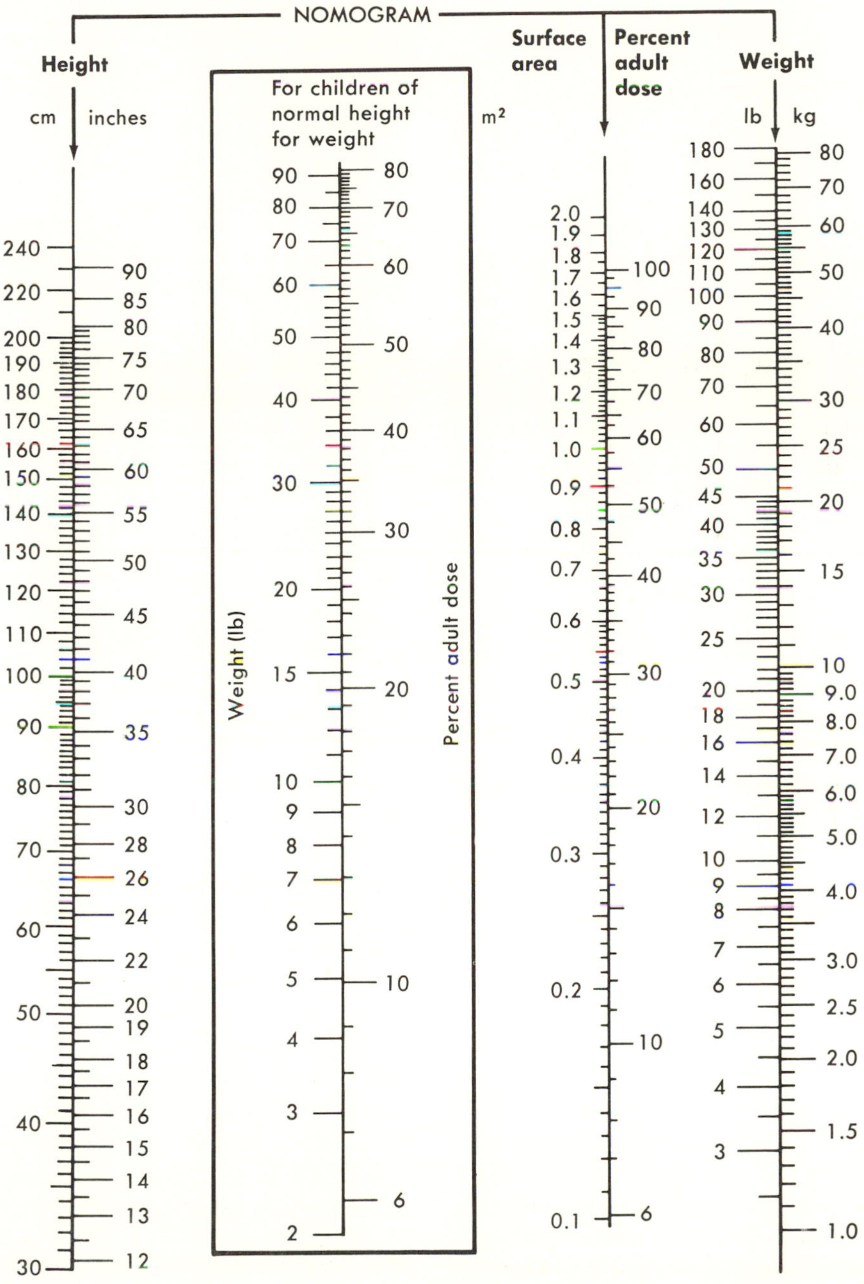


**Fig. 25-1.** Modified West surface area nomogram for estimating drug dosage in children. (Modified from Nelson, W. E.: Textbook of pediatrics, ed. 8, Philadelphia, 1964, W. B. Saunders Co.)

**Table 25-1.** Calculation of children's drug dosages

| *Age* | *Approximate weight (pounds)* | *Portion of adult dose* |
|---|---|---|
| 2 mo | 11 | 1/6 |
| 5 mo | 14 | 1/5 |
| 9 mo | 19 | 1/4 |
| 15 mo | 25 | 3/10 |
| 2 yr | 28 | 1/3 |
| 4 yr | 38 | 2/5 |
| 7 yr | 50 | 1/2 |
| 9 yr | 65 | 3/5 |
| 11 yr | 75 | 2/3 |

**Table 25-2.** Simple guide to body surface area from weight in pounds*

| *Weight (pounds)* | *Body surface area ($m^2$)* |
|---|---|
| 6 | 0.2 |
| 12 | 0.3 |
| 18 | 0.4 |
| 24 | 0.5 |
| 35 | 0.6 |
| 42 | 0.7 |
| 49 | 0.8 |
| 56 | 0.9 |
| 63 | 1.0 |
| 70 | 1.1 |

*Up to 24 pounds, multiples of 6 + 1; over 24 pounds, multiples of 7 + 1.

For children of average height and weight the approximations in Tables 25-1 and 25-2 are helpful if it is impossible to calculate the surface area.

■ **In the immediate treatment of acute poisoning, what are the indications and contraindications for emptying the stomach, and what means of accomplishing this should be used?**

Syrup of ipecac is the safest and most effective agent to use because it removes both the toxic agent and the emetic. The dose is 15 ml in a 1- to 5-year-old child and 30 ml in an older child, followed by a glass of water, and may be repeated in 30 minutes if vomiting has not occurred. Parenteral emetics are more dangerous and should rarely be used. Gastric lavage is less effective and is indicated primarily in the comatose child with an endotracheal tube to protect the airway or when emetics have been unsuccessful.

The induction of emesis is contraindicated if the patient is comatose or convulsing, if petroleum distillates or corrosives have been ingested, or if hematemesis has occurred. There is good evidence that the major toxicity of hydrocarbons such as cleaning fluids, gasoline and kerosene, lighter fluid, furniture polishes, and mineral sealing oils is induced by inhalation rather than ingestion. The emesis or lavage fluid should be saved for future laboratory analysis.

■ **What other measures are indicated in the acute treatment of a poisoning victim?**

Following induction of emesis or gastric lavage, activated charcoal is effective in promoting the absorption of many drugs. Activated charcoal given 30 minutes after the ingestion of aspirin, as an example, will result in a 50% reduction of maximum serum salicylate level. Charcoal is effective in the removal of most analgesics (salicylates, propoxyphene, acetaminophen); alkaloids (digitoxin, ergotamine); sedatives (barbiturates, glutethimide, ethchlorvynol); and antidepressants (chlorpromazine, imipramine, nortriptyline), as well as a variety of other commonly prescribed drugs (amphetamine, quinidine and quinine, diphenylhydantoin, primaquine, chloroquine, isoniazid).

While most effective if given within 30 minutes of ingestion, charcoal is still effective in binding poisons that have already passed through the pylorus. Charcoal is most effective against drugs that are slowly absorbed from the gastrointestinal tract.

Universal antidote, a combination of activated charcoal with magnesium oxide and tannic acid, is less effective than activated charcoal alone. Other absorbents such as evaporated milk and attapulgite are also less effective than powdered charcoal.

■ **If the poison is unknown, what signs and symptoms are helpful in making a correct diagnosis?**

1. Phenothiazines frequently present with a picture of "pseudotetanus" with ataxia, oculogyric crisis, and the jaws locked in an open position.
2. Tricyclic antidepressants such as imipramine will frequently present with cardiac arrhythmias in association with convulsions or coma.
3. Agitation, hallucinations, dilated pupils, fever, and flushed dry skin usually indicate the presence of an atropine-like agent or LSD.
4. Vomiting, hyperpnea, fever, and an odor of acetone on the breath frequently indicate salicylate intoxication.
5. Increased salivation and tearing, urination and defecation, and constricted pupils suggest organic phosphate or mushroom poisoning.
6. Constricted pupils associated with respiratory or neurologic depression should be considered indicative of narcotic poisoning until proved otherwise.

### ■ What are the manifestations of salicylate intoxication?

Salicylates remain the most frequent cause of poisoning in preschool children. Over half of the cases of salicylism that require hospitalization are the result of chronic therapeutic ingestion rather than acute poisoning. Salicylate toxicity is caused by the direct effect on the gastrointestinal tract, the results of increased metabolism, the derangement of carbohydrate metabolism, the stimulation of the medullary respiratory center, and interference with blood coagulation processes.

Local gastrointestinal irritation results in vomiting, abdominal pain, and gastrointestinal bleeding. Bleeding occasionally may be severe enough to cause anemia and shock.

Salicylates stimulate the respiratory center of the CNS located in the medulla. This effect results in increased ventilation, decreased $P_{CO_2}$ and a respiratory alkalosis. In response to the respiratory alkalosis the renal excretion of sodium, potassium, and bicarbonate is increased, reducing the body's ability to compensate for the developing metabolic acidosis.

Salicylates also increase the metabolic rate, probably by uncoupling oxidative phosphorylation. This increases oxygen consumption, carbon dioxide formation, and heat production. Respiratory and cardiac rate and cardiac output are increased because of the increased metabolic demands. The increased heat production results in increased water loss by sweating, aggravating the water loss caused by the hyperventilation. If the aspirin was given for a febrile illness, severe hyperpyrexia may occur.

Salicylates also interfere with carbohydrate metabolism. Either hyperglycemia or hypoglycemia may occur. Hyperglycemia is in part a result of the release of epinephrine by stimulation of the hypothalamic sympathetic centers. However, salicylates also decrease aerobic metabolism and increase glucose-6-phosphatase activity, which increases the blood glucose level. Hypoglycemia may be caused by increased peripheral utilization of glucose and interference with glyconeogenesis. The brain glucose concentration may be reduced despite normal or elevated serum glucose levels by interfering with oxidative phosphorylation in the brain. Salicylates interfere with the Krebs cycle, resulting in increased fat mobilization and utilization and formation of organic acids (especially lactic, pyruvic, and acetoacetic acids), ketosis, and ketonuria.

Hyperventilation, sweating, vomiting, and diarrhea all lead to increased water and electrolyte loss. Initially urine loss is also increased as a response to the respiratory alkalosis, and further diuresis occurs as a response to the ketosis, hyperglycosuria, and metabolic acidosis. Because of the decreased extracellular water volume, effective sweating no longer occurs, increasing the hyperpyrexia and accentuating the dehydration. Intracellular shifts of potassium as well as vomiting and kaliuresis may result in severe hypokalemia that must be corrected when treating the acidosis. Shock and renal failure may occur.

Finally salicylates have prolonged effects on the coagulating mechanisms, resulting in increased capillary fragility, thrombocytopenia with impaired platelet aggregation, and decreased prothrombin and factor VII levels. Derangement of clotting may last for several weeks after a single dose of salicylates.

## ■ How should salicylism be treated?

First, further salicylate absorption must be prevented. The induction of emesis by administering syrup of ipecac should be immediately instituted if the patient is awake. If confused or comatose, gastric lavage with normal saline solution is preferable. Lavage or emetics should be followed by the use of activated charcoal. These measures should be attempted up to 10 hours after salicylate ingestion. They are much less effective in the treatment of chronic toxicity.

If the patient is in shock, immediate expansion of the circulating blood volume is indicated. From 350 to 500 ml of a plasma expander/$m^2$ should be given in a 45- to 60-minute period. Plasmanate is most effective, but sodium bicarbonate, lactated Ringer's solution, or isotonic saline solution may be used. Dextran is contraindicated, as it may aggravate the derangement of the clotting mechanisms.

In the absence of an adequate clinical response such as improved blood pressure, pulses, and capillary filling time and increased urine production, fluids can be continued at this rate for another hour.

Once shock has been corrected and the patient regains the ability to urinate, the fluid deficit should be treated. This may require 2500 to 5000 ml/$m^2$ in the first 24 hours. A hypotonic electrolyte solution containing 5% glucose, 20 to 40 mEq of sodium, and 20 to 40 mEq of potassium/L is optimal.

Hyperpyrexia should be treated by sponging with tepid water; ice water sponging may cause cutaneous vasconstriction, interfering with heat loss, or may cause shivering, increasing heat production, and should not be used.

Fluids should contain sufficient sodium bicarbonate to alkalinize the urine. A urine pH greater than 7.5 will increase the amount of salicylates in urine fivefold. The use of 3.5 to 5 mEq of 7.5% sodium bicarbonate/kg over a 4-hour period is usually sufficient to alkalinize the urine. Bicarbonate should be used cautiously until blood pH is obtained to ensure that the child is not in respiratory alkalosis. Acetazolamide, a carbonic anhydrase inhibitor, can be used in place of sodium bicarbonate to achieve an alkaline urine or as an adjunct to it. A single dose of 5 mg/kg is usually effective.

As the dehydration and acidosis are treated, frequent determinations of blood gas, electrolyte, and glucose levels are necessary to prevent severe hypoglycemia or hypokalemia. In the presence of hypoglycemia 10% glucose solutions are preferable. Oral potassium supplementation should be started when the patient is able to tolerate oral feedings.

Exchange transfusion, peritoneal dialysis, and hemodialysis are effective but should be reserved for patients with severe salicylism, coma, renal failure, or failure to respond to other means of therapy. Although hemodialysis is the most effective of these techniques, peritoneal dialysis is more generally available in the critical care unit.

Vitamin K has been widely employed to treat the coagulation disorders, although its efficacy has been questioned.

## ■ What are the symptoms of organic phosphate pesticide poisoning?

Organophosphorus drugs such as malathion and parathion are rapidly replacing DDT and other chlorinated hydrocarbons for pesticide control. These drugs act by inactivating acetylcholinesterase, the enzyme that hydrolyzes acetylcholine. This results in prolonged autonomic and peripheral nervous system stimulation. These drugs are not physiologically active. Toxicity depends on the relative rate of metabolic conversion to an active agent and the rate of detoxification and excretion. Drugs such as barbiturates, narcotics, phenothiazines, and theophyllines potentiate conversion and thus increase toxicity. Children appear to be especially susceptible to these drugs.

With moderate exposure to organophosphorus compounds, constriction of pupils, tearing, nasal congestion, headache, and increased salivation will occur. More severe exposure results in excessive salivation, fasciculation of skeletal muscles, abdominal cramps, diarrhea and vomiting, bronchospasm, bradypnea, respiratory paralysis, stupor, and finally shock, coma, and death. With a large dose death may occur within minutes. Most deaths occur during the first 24 hours, and patients surviving for 48 hours usually recover completely.

### ■ How should organic phosphate poisoning be treated?

Emesis should be induced using syrup of ipecac, and the exposed skin and eyes should be thoroughly washed. Contaminated clothing must be removed. If the patient has severe respiratory symptoms, an airway should be established with an endotracheal tube to prevent aspiration of vomitus. If the patient is stuporous or comatose, gastric lavage with saline solution should be done immediately.

Atropine blocks the action of acetylcholine. A dose of 1 to 2 mg in small children to 5 mg in adults should be given by the IV or IM route at 10- to 20-minute intervals until flushed skin, dilated pupils, and tachycardia occur. There is evidence that metaraminol (Aramine) reduces the side effects of atropine while enhancing its effect against acetylcholine. It should be given at double the dose given of atropine.

Pralidoxime (Protopam) should be given in an IV dosage of 50 mg/kg every 12 hours. A maximum of 2 g total dosage should not be exceeded. This drug acts by breaking the covalent bond between acetylcholinesterase and the alkylphosphate, reactivating the acetylcholinesterase.

As atropine has little effect on the skeletal muscle sites, pralidoxime is most effective in relieving paralysis of the respiratory muscles. It is also effective in controlling parasympathetic symptoms but is very slow acting when compared to atropine.

If respiratory failure or bronchospasm exists, an airway and mechanical ventilation may be necessary.

Although recovery usually occurs within 48 hours, the patient will be more susceptible to these drugs for as long as 6 months. Further exposure must be prevented.

## Drowning

### ■ What physiologic changes occur in drowning?

Ten percent of the accidental deaths in the United States are caused by drowning. Of these, 40% involve children under 5 years of age.

The physiologic changes are caused not only by the direct effects of hypoxia, but also result from the differences between the aspirated fluid and plasma. Thus the physiopathology of saltwater as compared to freshwater drowning is quite different.

The primary disturbance is acute ventilatory insufficiency with arterial hypoxia and metabolic acidosis. The presence of fluid irregularly distributed in alveoli causes a large shunting of unoxygenated blood to the pulmonary venous system. This is aggravated by pulmonary edema caused by increased capillary permeability and pulmonary hemorrhage and by decreased lung compliance.

In freshwater drowning fluid rapidly enters the circulation, resulting in hemodilution, hemolysis of red blood cells, hemoglobinemia, and hyperkalemia. The increased circulatory blood volume leads to circulatory overload, congestive heart failure, and pulmonary edema, aggravating the perfusion-diffusion defect. The pulmonary edema and decreased compliance are increased in freshwater drowning by the washing out of surfactants. Protein, sodium, and chloride are drawn into the alveolar spaces, increasing the hemodilution. The combination of asphyxia with hypoxia and hyperkalemia predispose to ventricular fibrillation.

In saltwater drowning there is an increased concentration of electrolytes. Fluids leave the intravascular spaces, resulting in hemoconcentration and hyperelectrolytemia. The increased electrolyte concentrations act as a chemical irritant, resulting in inflammation and pulmonary edema with patchy areas of atelectasis and emphysema developing. Decreased pulmonary compliance is less severe in saltwater drowning because of the lack of damage to surfactants. The marked shift of fluids into the pulmonary spaces leads to hemoconcentration, decreased circulating blood volume and shock. A significant drop in blood pressure is an ominous sign in saltwater drowning and is frequently preceded by a drop in central venous pressure. Serious cardiac arrhythmias are less frequent in saltwater drownings.

Hypoxia, hypercapnia, and acidosis are the major physiologic effects. The metabolic acidosis with the rise in organic acids progresses until adequate oxygen therapy is given. Bronchospasm is common. Abdominal distention is usually caused by swallowing large amounts of fluids that may be vomited later and aspirated. A tachycardia is usually present, and extrasystoles or a gallop rhythm may signify developing cardiac failure with increasing pulmonary and cardiac insufficiency. Hypoxemia and hypercapnia increase, resulting in increasing neurologic depression, seizures, and coma. Decerebrate rigidity, persistent seizures, and EEG changes frequently indicate irreversible brain injury and death follows. Persistent severe hypoxia in a patient being administered oxygen should be considered ominous.

## ■ How should a drowning patient be treated?

The primary treatment consists of maintenance of adequate ventilation and oxygenation. Oxygen should be given in adequate concentrations to achieve normal arterial oxygen levels. A patent airway must be maintained. Frequent suction may be necessary. An endotracheal tube or tracheostomy is frequently necessary to maintain the airway. Intermittent or continuous positive pressure breathing may be required to decrease pulmonary edema, to maintain an adequate oxygen diffusion, and to expand atelectatic portions of the lungs. The aspiration of gastric contents is indicated to reduce the possibility of vomiting. IV sodium bicarbonate should be used to treat the metabolic acidosis. Blood gases and electrolytes must be carefully monitored to determine the amount of ventilatory support, oxygen, and bicarbonate needed. Diuretics such as furosemide should be used to treat the marked hemodilution or cardiac failure. Digitalization is indicated in the presence of congestive failure. Isoproterenol and steroids may be given by aerosol and parenterally to reduce bronchospasm. Parenteral steroids are also beneficial in preventing or reducing the cerebral edema secondary to hypoxia. Antibiotics should be given to prevent aspiration pneumonitis. In saltwater drowning a rapid infusion of plasma should be given to treat shock and restore the intracellular volume. Freshwater drowning patients may require packed cell transfusions to restore the reduced oxygen-carrying capacity caused by hemolysis and hemodilution. In the presence of severe cardiac decompensation and pulmonary edema a partial exchange transfusion using whole blood or packed cells may be necessary to prevent further overloading of the circulation. Succinylcholine (Anectine) or curare-like drugs should be used if necessary to synchronize the patient with the respirator. Diazepam or other anticonvulsants should be given as required to control seizures. It is advisable to keep the patient normothermic in order to reduce oxygen requirements. If severe cerebral edema is suspected, hypothermia may be advisable, but shivering should be controlled by the use of parenteral chlorpromazine (Thorazine). After shock has been controlled the patient should be maintained at 1200 to 1500 ml of fluids/$m^2$ daily using a multiple electrolyte solution. Serum electrolytes including calcium and magnesium should be carefully monitored.

Controlled studies are now being done in several centers throughout the country to treat severely affected drowning patients who are not expected to survive with long-term cardiopulmonary bypass procedures using membrane oxygenators. Although this technique appears to be promising, it should be considered experimental at this time.

Patients who respond within 24 hours usually make complete recoveries. Patients who have been in a coma for prolonged periods occasionally completely recover but usually have extensive brain damage.

## Croup and related disorders

### ■ What is the cause of infectious croup?

The croup syndrome is caused by inflammation or obstruction of the epiglottis, larynx, or trachea. It is manifested by inspiratory stridor, usually with hoarseness and a barking cough. It is most often caused by *Haemophilus influenzae* type B, *Corynebacterium diphtheriae,* or viruses.

### ■ How should viral croup be treated?

Viral croup (or laryngotracheobronchitis) usually begins with hoarseness and a barking cough that is worse at night. Mild fever and anorexia may be present. With increased swelling of the vocal cords or subglottic tissues, hoarseness becomes more severe and breathing becomes labored with inspiratory stridor. If the child becomes restless because of air hunger, becomes cyanotic or appears to be exhausted, tracheostomy or intubation may be necessary; however, these procedures are much less often necessary than in epiglottitis. The use of racemic epinephrine by nebulization has been very effective in some centers in decreasing respiratory distress and reducing the necessity of tracheostomy. A mucopurulent exudate is frequently present in croup. The use of tracheostomy or endotracheal tubes is helpful not only in relieving obstruction but also to remove these secretions. Mist and oxygen are the primary initial treatment. Steroids, although never proved to be beneficial in controlled studies, are routinely used by some physicians.

### ■ What are other causes of croup and how should they be managed?

Spasmodic croup is most likely allergic and is characterized by minimum findings of inflammation, daytime remissions, and frequently a history of previous attacks. High humidity is usually sufficient to give relief.

Foreign bodies, angioneurotic edema of the larynx or epiglottis, and retropharyngeal abscesses may also present a crouplike syndrome.

Although many physicians use corticosteroids as anti-inflammatory agents in the croup syndrome, their efficacy has been convincingly demonstrated only in allergic states such as angioneurotic edema and spasmodic croup. Antibiotics are indicated for *Haemophilus influenzae* and *Corynebacterium diphtheriae* infections but are also used for the treatment of infections in patients with foreign bodies.

### ■ How should acute epiglottitis be treated?

Acute epiglottitis usually presents as a severe crouplike syndrome of sudden onset. It occurs most frequently in children 3 to 7 years of age and is almost always caused by *Haemophilus influenzae* type B. *Staphylococcus aureus* and $\beta$-hemolytic *Streptococcus* type A are occasionally the offending organisms. Epiglottitis is characterized by the sudden onset of respiratory distress, barking cough, sore throat, and fever that may rapidly progress to severe respiratory obstruction. Marked drooling caused by the inability to swallow is characteristic. The cherry red swollen epiglottis can be seen on examination of the posterior pharynx. A safer means of demonstrating the swollen epiglottis is by lateral x-ray films of the neck. The difficulty in breathing is characterized by inspiratory stridor, a barking cough, and use of the accessory muscles of respiration. With increasing obstruction marked anxiety, air hunger, restlessness, increasing retractions, and cyanosis develop. Increasing cyanosis and impending exhaustion indicate death may occur unless an adequate airway is assured. In the early treatment of epiglottitis the use of high humidity and mist to decrease swelling is indicated. Oxygen should also be given. *Haemophilus influenzae* is usually responsive to ampicillin, although strains resistant to this antibiotic have appeared recently in the United States. Chloramphenicol is the alternate drug for the treatment of *Haemophilus influenzae* infections and should be considered if ampicillin-resistant strains are prevalent in the community.

In some centers routine tracheostomy is recommended for the treatment of acute epiglottitis. In other centers this procedure is delayed, providing personnel and equipment are available for an emergency trache-

**Table 25-3.** Oratracheal tube specifications in pediatrics

| *Age* | *French size* | *Length (cm)* |
|---|---|---|
| Newborn | 11-14 | 3 |
| 1-6 mo | 15-16 | 4 |
| 6-12 mo | 17-18 | 4 |
| 12-18 mo | 19-20 | 5 |
| 18-36 mo | 21-22 | 5 |
| 3-4 yr | 23-24 | 6 |
| 5-7 yr | 25-26 | 6-7 |
| 8-9 yr | 27-28 | 7 |
| 10-11 yr | 29-30 | 8 |
| 12-14 yr | 32-34 | 8 |

ostomy at the bedside. Tracheostomy should not be delayed if there is increasing air hunger or restlessness, cyanosis while receiving oxygen, or a rise in arterial $P_{CO_2}$ or if signs of exhaustion or mental confusion develop. It is preferable that a tracheostomy be done in the operating room following endotracheal intubation. However, in an emergency immediate tracheostomy should be carried out in the critical care unit. Recent studies have demonstrated that endotracheal intubation is as effective as tracheostomy in the treatment of epiglottitis. This must be done by an experienced intubator so that the obstruction is not acutely aggravated by trauma. Typical tube sizes and lengths are found in Table 25-3. The advantages of intubation include a decreased risk of the procedure and a decreased duration of the artificial airway and of the hospitalization. Intubation should be continued for 48 hours.

### ■ How should laryngeal diphtheria be treated?

Laryngotracheal diphtheria, although rare today, must be considered in inadequately immunized children. The presence of a membranous tonsillopharyngitis, marked cervical adenopathy, or severe toxicity suggests the presence of diphtheria. Increasing obstruction with progressive cyanosis, coma, exhaustion, and death may occur or sudden severe hypoxia may occur from detachment and aspiration of a piece of membrane. An adequate dose of diphtheria antitoxin must be given promptly. Antibiotics are less effective but should also be used. Tracheostomy may be necessary.

## Other respiratory problems

### ■ How can pertussis be differentiated from croup and how is it managed?

Pertussis (whooping cough) may be confused with croup because of the marked inspiratory stridor. Pertussis is manifested by sudden paroxysms of short rapid coughs that terminate in a prolonged inspiration with a typical high-pitched whoop. A series of coughing paroxysms and whoops may occur until a mucous plug is dislodged. Vomiting frequently follows the attack. The typical paroxysm usually does not occur until the third week of the illness. The early phase presents as an upper respiratory infection frequently with a night cough. Petechiae, subconjunctival hemorrhages, epistaxis, and subarachnoid hemorrhages are common in the paroxysmal stage and are caused by the marked increase in venous pressure. Seizures resulting from severe hypoxia may occur during paroxysms.

There is usually an elevation of the white count with the increase entirely caused by lymphocytes. At times the lymphocyte count may be as high as 100,000 and leukemia considered. The higher the white count, the worse is the prognosis.

Management includes bed rest with oxygen, humidity, and sedation. Pertussis hyperimmune globulin should be given to infants and severely ill patients. Antibiotics are less effective in decreasing morbidity and mortality but should be used to control contagiousness. To terminate a severe attack, suction of the posterior pharynx will frequently dislodge a thick mucous plug.

### ■ What pulmonary problems are associated with prolonged respiratory care for hyaline membrane disease?

Bronchopulmonary dysplasia is a pulmonary disorder seen primarily in small premature infants requiring prolonged mechanical assistance and oxygen therapy usually exceeding 10 days. Infants with bronchopulmonary dysplasia after recovering from hyaline membrane disease continue to have chronic respiratory symptoms or symptoms develop after a relatively well period. X-ray films reveal diffuse, coarse, fibrotic, and inflammatory changes with air bronchograms. Bronchopulmonary dysplasia is believed to be caused by oxygen toxicity. Similar changes are seen in animals and adults receiving oxygen concentrations greater than 60% via respirators. Superimposed pneumonia, primarily caused by gram-negative organisms, is believed to be an additional factor resulting in severe inflammation and destruction of the lung tissues. The disease slowly regresses over several years. There is no known treatment. The incidence of this illness can probably be reduced by limiting the duration of respiratory therapy, giving minimum concentrations of oxygen, closely monitoring arterial $P_{aO_2}$, and intensively treating secondary infections.

## ■ What other pulmonary problems are unique to premature infants?

The Wilson-Mikity syndrome occurs in premature infants who either had no evidence of hyaline membrane disease or who had a short illness not requiring ventilatory assistance. These infants develop progressive hyperpnea, cyanosis, cough, and retractions. The illness progresses for 2 to 6 weeks and then reaches a plateau lasting several weeks. Rales appear at this time. If the infant survives the acute stage, symptoms slowly regress and complete recovery as evidenced by clinical and roentgenographic examination occurs in 3 to 24 months. X-ray films reveal nonspecific interstitial thickening with patchy areas of atelectasis and multiple cystlike areas of emphysema. The cause is unknown, and there is no treatment except for supportive care using humidity and low concentrations of oxygen. Steroids and antibiotics have not been demonstrated to be helpful and are indicated only for documented complicating pneumonia.

## ■ How can lobar emphysema be recognized in children?

Congenital lobar emphysema may be noted shortly after birth but more commonly presents as respiratory distress usually associated with a respiratory infection at 1 to 2 months of age. Emphysema of a single lobe is commonly caused by a deficiency in the bronchial cartilage but may result from partial obstruction of a bronchus internally by a plug or externally by tumors or cardiovascular structures. Wheezing is usually present, and in severe cases cyanosis and retractions are prominent. Physical examination reveals evidence of overexpansion and decreased breath sounds on the affected side as well as shift of the heart and mediastinal structures to the opposite side. X-ray films confirm the radiolucent lobe, frequently with herniation of the lung to the opposite side and atelectasis of the remaining lung on that side. It can be differentiated from pneumothorax by the presence of lung markings throughout the affected lung. Early bronchoscopy is indicated. If a plug or foreign body cannot be found, surgical removal of the involved lung may be necessary.

## ■ What congenital anomalies cause obstructive respiratory disease after the newborn period?

Tracheomalacia is a disorder consisting of tracheal rings that are too pliable and collapse easily with respiration. Although symptoms may be present from birth, they become more severe during early infancy and are frequently aggravated by respiratory infections. Clinically infants exhibit inspiratory stridor, expiratory wheezes, tachypnea, and cough. Complicating lower respiratory infections with cyanosis and distress are common. Symptoms increase during crying or feeding but are present at rest. Many infants assume an opisthotonic position that maximally opens the respiratory passageways. Bronchoscopy is indicated to rule out a laryngeal web or other surgically correctable lesion. A barium swallow esophagogram should be obtained to rule out the presence of a vascular ring. Treatment is nonspecific and consists of control of secretions by humidity and expectorants and treatment of complicating infections with antibiotics. These children usually show definite improvement by 6 months of age with complete recovery by 1 to 2 years of age.

Vascular rings present a picture of progressive stridor and wheezing usually associated with dysphagia when solid feeding is started. The presence of aberrant vessels forming a complete ring around the esophagus and trachea is demonstrable by esophagograms and confirmed by angiography. The most common aberrant vessel, an anomalous right subclavian artery, does not produce symptoms. The most severe cases are usually associated with a double aortic arch. The rare anomalous left pulmonary artery does not produce dysphagia and is the only lesion producing an anterior constriction of the trachea. Treatment of vascular rings is surgical after clearing of secondary pulmonary infections. Symptoms frequently persist after surgery because of associated tracheomalacia.

## ■ What type of tracheoesophageal fistulas may not be symptomatic during the newborn period?

Tracheoesophageal fistulas without esophageal atresia (H-type tracheoesophageal fistula) usually are not diagnosed in the neonatal period. The diagnosis should be suspected in any infant with recurrent pneumonia without apparent cause or in infants who develop spells of choking, coughing, cyanosis, or respiratory distress following the ingestion of formula. Physical examination reveals evidence of pulmonary infection and usually a distended abdomen caused by air in the stomach. Infants develop repeat episodes of pneumonia, especially in the right lower lobe. Diagnosis is by esophagography via pressure injection of contrast media or by esophagoscopy or bronchoscopy. Treatment is surgical following treatment of the respiratory infection, and complete recovery can be expected.

## ■ What is *Pneumocystis* pneumonia and how should it be managed?

Primarily affecting premature and debilitated infants, interstitial plasma cell pneumonia is an illness caused by a protozoan, *Pneumocystis carinii*. It is also common in children with immunologic disorders such as agammaglobulinemia and thymic dysplasia and in children with leukemia or lymphomas who have received steroid or immunosuppressive therapy.

It occurs primarily between 6 and 16 weeks of age, although it is not uncommon under 1 year of age. Hospitalized children appear to be most susceptible to *Pneumocystis* pneumonia.

The onset is insidious with poor feeding, irritability, and failure to thrive preceding tachypnea, cyanosis, and respiratory distress. Fever is unusual. Auscultation of the chest may be normal or reveal scattered rales and rhonchi. X-ray films reveal a characteristic infiltration radiating bilaterally from each hilus with sparing of peripheral lung fields.

The diagnosis usually requires lung biopsy either by needle aspiration or open thoracotomy. The organism may occasionally be demonstrable in sputum or bronchial washing. Special silver stains are usually necessary to demonstrate the organism.

Treatment consists of the use of ultrasonic nebulization and oxygen therapy. Steroids, antibiotics, and gamma globulin are ineffective. Pentamidine isothionate is the only available drug beneficial in the treatment of *Pneumocystis* infections. The dose for children is 100 to 150 mg/m$^2$ daily. Hypoglycemia, azotemia, and liver toxicity are common in patients treated with this drug. Gavage feedings and IV fluid therapy are usually necessary. IV alimentation may be necessary in some children. The mortality rate associated with *Pneumocystis* pneumonia is 30% to 50%.

## ■ What is the pathophysiology of bronchiolitis?

Bronchiolitis is a severe respiratory illness affecting primarily infants, usually under 6 months of age. Most cases are caused by respiratory syncytial virus, although parainfluenza and adenovirus can produce a similar illness. Approximately 10% of infants requiring hospitalization for bronchiolitis later develop asthma. It is not known whether a predisposing tendency to asthma results in a more severe illness or whether damage to the bronchioles predisposes the patient to asthma later.

The primary lesion in bronchiolitis is bronchiolar obstruction by edema, lymphocytic infiltration, and plugs of mucus and cellular debris. As resistance to airflow in a tube is inversely proportional to the fourth power of the radius, thickening of the bronchioles in infants will cause a markedly greater increase in resistance than in the larger airways of older children and adults. Thus older children will usually have a milder respiratory illness without significant obstruction to airflow.

The bronchiolar thickening results in disturbances in air exchange. Some degree of hypoxemia is usually present even though the infant is not visibly cyanotic. Hypercapnia develops much later in the illness and is a sign of severe disease with respiratory failure.

Bronchiolitis usually starts as a mild upper respiratory infection followed in several days by a paroxysmal cough, wheeze, and difficulty in feeding. The temperature is usually normal and tachypnea and tachycardia are present. Because of obstruction to airflow, respiratory efforts increase and retractions are noted. However, retractions are less prominent than is seen in upper airway obstruction such as croup. The chest becomes overinflated, and the liver and spleen become palpable.

This combination of respiratory distress, tachycardia, and hepatomegaly is frequently misdiagnosed as congestive heart failure. Auscultation of the lungs usually reveals poor air exchange. Rales and a mild wheeze are usually present. Mild dehydration is frequently present because of the inability to feed.

Chest x-ray films reveal overexpansion with patchy areas of atelectasis that are easily misdiagnosed as pneumonia. Secondary pneumonia should be suspected when there is a fever and leukocytosis. Pneumothorax and mediastinal emphysema may occur but are rare.

■ **How should bronchiolitis be managed?**

Because hypoxemia is usually present, oxygen therapy is indicated. Concentrations above 40% are rarely necessary. Arterial $P_{O_2}$ can be monitored by percutaneous arterial punctures. Although there is little evidence that high humidity decreases the bronchiolar edema, it should be used. Ultrasonic nebulizers produce much smaller droplets and are more likely to be helpful in bronchiolitis than the usual mist tent. Because of the difficulty in feeding and mild dehydration, the severely affected infant with this illness should receive IV maintenance fluids. Antibiotics should not be used unless there is evidence of secondary bacterial infection. Controlled studies have shown no beneficial effect of antibiotics as prophylaxis against bacterial complications. Steroids, although extensively used, are not beneficial except in the occasional child believed to be allergic. As these infants rarely are in congestive failure, digitalization is not usually indicated. Tracheostomy and endotracheal intubation will not relieve the obstruction. Endotracheal intubation is indicated only in the infant with severe respiratory failure requiring mechanical ventilation.

Bronchodilators such as aminophylline and isoproterenol may be helpful in some cases. A trial of 5 mg/kg of IV aminophylline is worthwhile in the infant in severe respiratory distress or if cyanosis is present during oxygen administration.

Bronchiolitis is usually self-limited. The mortality is less than 1% except in debilitated children. Complete recovery without sequelae can be expected.

## Cystic fibrosis and its complications

■ **What is the earliest manifestation of cystic fibrosis?**

Meconium ileus is present in 10% to 15% of all patients with cystic fibrosis. This is a form of intestinal obstruction caused by the accumulation of abnormal puttylike meconium resulting from a lack of pancreatic enzymes. Meconium ileus may be complicated by associated intestinal atresia or stenosis, volvulus, or perforation with intestinal obstruction.

In a minority of cases the obstruction can

be relieved by the use of meglumine diatrizoate (Gastrografin) enemas under careful observation by a radiologist-surgeon team. Surgery is usually required. Atretic, gangrenous, and markedly dilated areas must be resected. A Mikulicz resection with a double-barrel ileostomy or an ileostomy with a single-barrel end-to-side anastomosis is most commonly required. Pancreatic enzymes or 5% *N*-acetylcysteine are commonly used to irrigate the distal bowel in order to free the inspissated meconium. Total parenteral alimentation is frequently necessary in these children. Pancreatic enzymes are employed as soon as feeding can be instituted either orally or by gastrostomy. Vigorous treatment of respiratory infections and careful attention to protein, electrolyte, caloric, and blood requirements are essential during the postoperative period.

■ **What problems are associated with the sweat disturbance in patients with cystic fibrosis?**

All patients with cystic fibrosis lose excessive amounts of both sodium and chloride in their sweat. This is the basis of the pilocarpine iontophoresis sweat test for the diagnosis of cystic fibrosis. Patients with this disease have sweat chloride concentrations above 60 mEq/L and sodium concentrations above 70 mEq/L. Under conditions of increased sweating, severe hyponatremic hypochloremic dehydration may occur, and the patient may present with "heat stroke," circulatory collapse, or coma. Dehydration should be suspected with fevers, during hot weather, following periods of strenuous physical activity, or while in unventilated mist tents. The hypochloremia and hyponatremia may be aggravated by the use of ultrasonic nebulization with water, as large quantities of water may be absorbed into the circulation as well as electrolytes lost into the pulmonary alveoli. When present, the electrolyte disturbance should be treated by parenteral replacement. It can usually be prevented by adding salt to the dietary intake during periods of fever or when sweating is increased. This may be incorporated in the preparation and seasoning of food and need not be given separately. Infants in the first year of life require 1 g of salt (¼ teaspoon) daily. In the second and third years ½ teaspoon should be given. Older children will require ¾ to 1 teaspoon supplemental salt in the diet.

■ **What is the management of the respiratory disease in the child with cystic fibrosis?**

Treatment is directed toward relieving respiratory obstruction and controlling secretions, management of the accompanying infections, and therapy for respiratory failure and other complications.

Therapy aimed at the bronchial obstruction is directed toward decreasing the viscosity of pulmonary secretions and improving the pulmonary hygiene. A water-saturated atmosphere enables the patient to mobilize secretions. Compressed air is used unless hypoxia exists. If oxygen is required, it should be given at the lowest concentration effective in relieving symptoms. Many of these patients have chronic respiratory failure with hypercapnia. In these patients the respiratory center in the medulla may be insensitive to carbon dioxide levels and driven by the hypoxia. Sudden correction of the hypoxia in these patients may result in respiratory arrest. In addition, high concentrations of oxygen may impair ciliary activity, irritate the bronchial mucosa and alveoli, and cause vasomotor changes.

The ultrasonic nebulizer is more effective than the compressed air nebulizer in increasing the deposition of water in the tracheobronchial tree. Ultrasonic nebulization can provide particles of 1 to 5 $\mu$ in size, which will reach the small bronchioles. If water is used for nebulization, large quantities of water may enter the circulation, resulting in hemodilution, hyponatremia, and hypochloremia. Circulatory overload and congestive failure may occur. Dilute saline (0.25 to 0.5 normal) solutions should be used to prevent this complication. A 10% propylene glycol solution can be used in air compressor nebulization to stabilize particle size. Acetylcysteine has been used by nebulization to thin secretions but must be used very cautiously because it is irritating and will frequently result in a marked increase in pulmonary secretions. The cautious use of this drug, especially for the treatment for localized disease under direct vision during bronchoscopy, can be very effective in selected patients with increasing respiratory failure despite intensive conservative management.

Chest physical therapy and postural bronchial drainage are important adjuncts in the treatment of pulmonary disease. These procedures should be done before meals or at least 1 to 2 hours after eating. They are especially effective at bedtime to help clear the airways and reduce nocturnal coughing. Two to four treatments per day are optimal. Procedures that help loosen secretions and facilitate bronchial drainage include clapping, deep breathing, assisted coughing, thoracic squeezing, and vibration. With localized lung disease the drainage of the affected bronchi should precede that of uninvolved areas. With generalized disease the lower lobes are drained first, followed by the middle lobe, the lingula, and the upper lobes. The order should be reversed in infants and postoperative patients.

Intermittent positive pressure breathing may be effective in relieving obstruction and in administering antibiotics and other medications. However, this procedure is not without risk and must be used with caution, as it may spread pulmonary infection or cause air trapping or pneumothorax. Short periods of therapy are advisable and pulmonary function studies should be monitored. Saline solution, bronchodilator drugs, antibiotics, and enzymes can be given by this means. The use of $\beta$-2-adrenergic agents such as isoetharine (Bronkosol) are preferable to isoproterenol or epinephrine because of their reduced cardiac effects. The simultaneous aerosol and systemic administration of antibiotics may be especially effective in *Pseudomonas* and staphylococcal infections. Local irritation, toxicity, and allergic reactions can result from the aerosol administration of antibiotics.

Penicillin (100,000 to 200,000 units), methicillin (250 to 500 mg), neomycin (100 to 200 mg), kanamycin (50 to 100 mg), polymyxin (4 mg), colistin (10 to 20 mg), gentamicin (10 to 20 mg), and carbenicillin (250 to 500 mg) can be administered daily by aerosol therapy. Mucolytic agents such as acetylcysteine may be of value in selected patients but more frequently result in an increased production of secretions and prolonged morbidity and duration of the hospitalization. In patients with progressive respiratory disease and pulmonary failure the use of endotracheal tubes, tracheostomy, or bronchoscopy may be necessary to remove secretions and provide ventilatory support.

### ■ How should pulmonary infection be treated in cystic fibrosis?

Patients with cystic fibrosis must be assumed to have mixed infections caused by resistant organisms. *Staphylococcus aureus* and gram-negative rods, especially *Pseudomonas aeruginosa* and *Klebsiella pneumoniae,* remain the most common pulmonary pathogens. The current trend is to use antibiotics intermittently for the treatment of exacerbations rather than to use continuous antibiotic therapy. Adequate cultures and sensitivity studies are imperative prior to instituting antimicrobial therapy. Until these studies are reported, a combination of antibiotics should be chosen, based on the sensitivity patterns of pathogens in the local community. Usually initial treatment will consist of a penicillinase-resistant penicillin such as oxacillin with a drug effective against gram-negative organisms such as colistin or carbenicillin. Maximum therapeutic dosages are necessary and in the acutely ill patient should be given parenterally.

Typical dosages that can be given are found in Table 25-4 on p. 464.

### ■ What is cor pulmonale and how can it be recognized in cystic fibrosis?

Continuous or intermittent obstruction of the airways causes pulmonary vasoconstriction as a result of hypoxia and acidosis. The occurrence of airway obstruction from early infancy may retard maturation of the pul-

**Table 25-4.** Dosages of antibiotics used for cystic fibrosis patients

| *Drug* | *Route* | *Dose/day* | *Maximum dose/day* |
|---|---|---|---|
| Penicillin | Oral, IV, IM | 50,000 U/kg | 20,000,000 U |
| Methicillin | IV, IM | 100-200 mg/kg | 4-6 g |
| Ampicillin | Oral, IM | 100-200 mg/kg | 3-4 g |
| Oxacillin | Oral, IV | 100-200 mg/kg | 4-6 g |
| Carbenicillin | Oral, IV | 300-400 mg/kg | 20-25 g |
| Cephalothin | IM, IV | 50-100 mg/kg | 4-12 g |
| Chloramphenicol | Oral, IV | 50-100 mg/kg | 2-4 g |
| Erythromycin | Oral | 50-100 mg/kg | 2-4 g |
| Kanamycin | IM | 15 mg/kg | 1-1.5 g |
| Lincomycin | IM, IV | 20-30 mg/kg | 1.5-2 g |
| Streptomycin | IM | 20-40 mg/kg | 1-2 g |
| Colistin | IM | 4-7 mg/kg | 200-300 mg |
| Gentamicin | IM | 4-7 mg/kg | 200-300 mg |
| Tetracycline | Oral, IV | 50-100 mg/kg | 2-4 g |

monary arterioles, with retention of thick, reactive arteriolar musculature. The acute development of more severe obstruction may then result in severe vasoconstriction. If the right ventricle cannot eject the required cardiac output against the increased afterload, right ventricular dilatation and acute right heart failure ensue. With chronic respiratory failure, intimal changes occur, resulting in obstructive pulmonary hypertension, right ventricular hypertrophy, and eventually chronic right heart failure. Small thrombi or emboli may aggravate these changes. The airway obstruction may be in the upper or lower respiratory tract. Children with cystic fibrosis may have upper respiratory obstruction as a result of nasal polyps or enlarged adenoids and tonsils severe enough to cause hypoxia and pulmonary vasoconstriction.

Heart failure may be difficult to distinguish in cystic fibrosis patients with chronic respiratory disease. The emphysema may displace the liver inferiorly, suggesting hepatomegaly. Visible neck vein distention may be present. Rales, dyspnea, and tachycardia are seen with acute respiratory disease. Poor nutrition or absorption may result in significant hypoproteinemia with resulting ascites and peripheral edema. An acute fluid overload from oral or parenteral intake or absorption of fluids from aerosol therapy may result in circulatory overload and heart failure in the absence of cor pulmonale.

The ECG is frequently of value in the diagnosis of cor pulmonale. In the emphysematous patient without cor pulmonale deep S waves in the right precordial lead are typical. This is frequently misdiagnosed as left ventricular hypertrophy. With acute right heart failure, a significant shift of the frontal QRS complex of at least 60 degrees is typical. With chronic right heart failure, the typical right ventricular hypertrophy and peaked P waves suggesting right atrial enlargement are found. Chest x-ray films usually reveal cardiac enlargement with dilatation of the large central pulmonary arteries tapering to small pulmonary arteries peripherally. In active infection pulmonary vascular disease may not be readily distinguishable. Echocardiography will reveal right ventricular dilatation, paradoxic motion of the ventricular septum, and increased thickness of the right ventricle wall. Satisfactory echos are frequently difficult to obtain in the presence of emphysema. Hypoxia and acidosis are present. In cor pulmonale the pH and $P_{aO_2}$ are reduced, and the $P_{aCO_2}$ is elevated. The pH is frequently reduced greater than the elevation of $P_{aCO_2}$ because of associated metabolic acidosis. Normal respiratory values for children may be found in Table 25-5. With chronic cor pulmonale, polycythemia and clubbing are typical.

## ■ What is the treatment for cor pulmonale?

Since the basis of cor pulmonale is obstructive disease of the airways with hypoxemia and acidosis, the primary treatment is the im-

**Table 25-5.** Normal respiratory values in children

| | *Newborn* | *Infants* | *Children* |
|---|---|---|---|
| Respiratory frequency | 40-60 | 20-30 | 20-30 to 6 yr, 15-20 over 6 yr |
| pH | 7.30-7.40 | 7.30-7.40 | 7.35-7.45 |
| $P_{aCO_2}$ | 30-35 | 30-35 | 35-45 |
| $P_{aO_2}$ | 60-90 | 80-100 | 80-100 |
| Tidal volume (cc/kg) | 5-6 | 7-8 | 7-8 |
| Dead space (cc/kg) | 2 | 2 | 2 |

provement of ventilation. If there is upper airway obstruction, removal of enlarged nasal polyps, adenoids, and tonsils may result in significant improvement in cardiac function. Steroids have been used to shrink nasal polyps or prevent their recurrence. Vigorous management of the lower respiratory disease and impaired ventilation is necessary. Oxygen therapy should be initiated to improve the hypoxemia. It must be remembered that in children with chronic respiratory failure and chronic hypercapnia, the central respiratory center may be insensitive to the $P_{CO_2}$ elevation, and the hypoxemia may provide the only stimulus to maintain respiration. The administration of oxygen to these children may decrease respirations, resulting in increased carbon dioxide narcosis and respiratory arrest. Assisted ventilation will be necessary in these children and should not be delayed, being performed if necessary with endotracheal intubation or tracheostomy.

As acidosis also increases pulmonary vasoconstriction, this should be corrected with the use of sodium bicarbonate or tromethamine (THAM). While many authors recommend THAM in these patients because plasma bicarbonate is already high, it offers no advantage over bicarbonate and is more apt to result in respiratory arrest.

Some studies have suggested that tolazoline (Priscoline) may be of value in lowering the pulmonary vascular resistance. It is more apt to be of value in acute hyperactive cor pulmonale than in the more chronic obstructive form. Further studies of this and other pulmonary vasodilators are necessary.

Digitalis glycosides, by their positive inotropic effect on the heart, improve the efficiency of the heart in patients with cor pulmonale. Digoxin (Lanoxin) is most commonly used in children because of its rapid action and short duration of toxicity. Since a therapeutic response to digitalis may be difficult to distinguish because of the pulmonary disease, serum digoxin determinations may be necessary to determine the adequacy of digitalization and the presence of toxicity.

Salt restriction and diuretics are also useful in improving cardiac function but must be used cautiously because of increased salt losses in the sweat in these patients. Because of the increased vascular and extracellular fluid volume in heart failure and the tendency to hyponatremia and hypochloremia in cystic fibrosis, water restriction is important in these children. It must be remembered that a low serum sodium level is not indicative of low total body sodium. Furosemide has replaced mercurial diuretics as the drug of choice in heart failure in children. Salt restriction should be moderate. Potassium replacement is necessary when diuretics are used unless spironolactone (Aldactone) is used as a second diuretic. Replacement of chloride by oral ammonium chloride may be necessary with the frequent use of diuretics but should be used cautiously because it will increase the acidosis. Hypokalemia and hypochloremia may be avoided by using diuretics every other day rather than daily.

Anemia aggravates the congestive heart failure by decreasing the oxygen-carrying capacity, thus increasing the necessary cardiac output to meet the metabolic requirements. The cyanotic patient in chronic respiratory failure should be polycythemic. A "normal" hematocrit or hemoglobin in these patients indicates a significant anemia and should be treated. Small transfusions of packed red blood cells should be considered. If large transfusions are necessary, a partial exchange transfusion with packed cells may prevent severe cardiac decompensation. Salt-free albumin transfusions may be necessary if significant hypoproteinemia is present.

The correction of the pulmonary insufficiency remains the most important goal in the treatment of right heart failure caused by cor pulmonale, the other measures being only supportive.

## ■ What is the pathogenesis of disseminated intravascular coagulation?

Disseminated intravascular coagulation (DIC) is a disease process caused by the consumption of plasma clotting factors and platelets, resulting in thrombi in small vessels followed by a hemorrhagic diathesis.

DIC commonly occurs in infections by bacteria that form endotoxins. It occurs most frequently in meningococcal infections and sepsis caused by gram-negative rods but may be seen in other infections, including streptococcal and staphylococcal disease, varicella, rickettsial infections, and generalized vaccinia. DIC may also be seen in patients with cyanotic congenital heart disease, especially during surgery using the pump oxygenator; severe burns or trauma; malignancies; snake bites; drug intoxications; anaphylactic reactions; and giant cavernous hemangiomas.

The process in infections caused by endotoxin-producing bacteria is believed to be direct damage to the vascular endothelium and activation of Hageman factor. In burns or trauma tissue thromboplastin is formed. In patients with giant hemangiomas platelets aggregate and release platelet thromboplastin. Each of these defects initiates a series of reactions resulting in the conversion of prothrombin to thrombin, which activates fibrinogen into fibrin, the formation of intravascular thrombi, and the depletion of platelets and plasma clotting factors. Factors depleted during the process include antihemophilic factor, proaccelerin, prothrombin, and fibrinogen. As fibrin is deposited, fibrinolysins are activated and split fibrin into products that act as anticoagulants until they are removed by the reticuloendothelial system.

These processes result in thrombi and emboli that produce tissue ischemia and necrosis, depletion of clotting factors, and the effects of fibrin products, which lead to widespread hemolysis, hemolytic anemia caused by red blood cell fragmentation by fibrin strands in peripheral vessels and, if severe, shock and death.

The diagnosis is made by the demonstration of abnormalities of coagulation, including low platelet count, prothrombin time, and partial thromboplastin time, and by the presence of fibrinolysins and fibrin split products. The euglobulin lysis time and cryofibrinogen tests are valuable in determining the presence of these latter two groups. Specific determination of multiple factors may be necessary for differentiation of DIC from other hemorrhagic diatheses.

## ■ What is the treatment of DIC?

Heparin is the drug of choice in DIC. It is given by IV route in doses of 1 to 1.5 mg (100 to 150 units)/kg every 4 to 6 hours. This is continued until coagulation factors return to normal. In severe cases the replacement of depleted factors by transfusion of platelet concentrates and fresh-frozen plasma should also be used. Antifibrinolytic agents such as ε-aminocaproic acid (Amicar) should not be used in the treatment of DIC.

Survival depends on the correction of causative factors and shock and on the extent of damage to major organs. Specific antibiotics for the bacterial infection are necessary. Shock must be vigorously treated with fluids and colloids. Large dosages of steroids are indicated in endotoxic shock. The correction of anemia, dehydration, acidosis, and other metabolic disturbances may be required, as may the use of peritoneal dialysis or hemodialysis if renal failure develops.

The mortality remains high despite heparinization and adequate correction of the coagulopathy.

## VOMITING

■ **What is the most common cause of severe vomiting in infants and how should it be managed?**

Congenital hypertrophic pyloric stenosis is the most common cause of upper gastrointestinal obstruction in children. It is eight times more frequent in males than females, is frequently familial, and most often occurs in the firstborn child. It is characterized by vomiting, usually beginning in the second or third week of life and becoming progressively more frequent and projectile in nature. Weight loss and dehydration ensue, and death may occur if treatment is delayed. The obstruction is caused by thickened pyloric musculature. The vomiting is of gastric fluids containing hydrochloric acid and potassium, resulting in a metabolic alkalosis. The thickened muscle is usually palpable as an "olive" in the right upper quadrant, and visible gastric peristaltic waves are usually seen. Laboratory studies reveal an elevation of pH and plasma carbon dioxide content and decreased serum chloride and potassium. Hemoconcentration is frequently present.

The initial treatment is directed toward correction of the dehydration and alkalosis. The IV administration of saline solutions with supplemental potassium chloride (20 to 40 mEq/L) should be used rather than prepared multiple electrolyte solutions such as Isolyte P or M, as these solutions are constituted for the treatment of acidosis. Gastric replacement solution or other acidifying solutions such as ammonium chloride are rarely necessary. When the dehydration and electrolyte derangement are corrected, surgery is indicated. The Fredet-Ramstedt procedure consists of splitting the thickened pyloric muscles. Recovery is rapid, and oral feedings are usually initiated as soon as the infant awakens from the anesthesia. Glucose water is usually given for the first few feedings, followed by increasing amounts of formula.

## REYE SYNDROME

■ **What is Reye syndrome?**

Reye syndrome (pronounced "rye," as in the grain) is a virus-associated encephalopathy first described by Dr. R. D. J. Reye. The clinical diagnosis is made when the following criteria are fulfilled:

1. Prodromal viral illness
2. Protracted vomiting within a week after the onset of the viral illness
3. Delirium and stupor beginning soon after the onset of vomiting
4. Absence of focal neurologic signs
5. Abnormalities of liver function as demonstrated by elevated enzyme (particularly SGOT) levels, increased blood ammonia, and abnormal prothrombin time
6. No (or slight) jaundice
7. Normal cerebrospinal fluid protein and cell count
8. Fatty infiltration of the liver (usually found at autopsy)

■ **What is the clinical picture of Reye syndrome?**

Lovejoy et al. in 1974[1] proposed a system of clinical staging that would allow interpretation of the therapeutic effectiveness of different modes of therapy. They described stage 1 as being associated with vomiting, lethargy, liver dysfunction, and a mildly abnormal EEG. Stage 2 is associated with delirium, combativeness, hyperventilation, hyperactive reflexes, liver dysfunction, and a somewhat more severely abnormal EEG. The third stage is associated with obtundation or coma, evidence of decortication, liver dysfunction, and also a moderately severe abnormal EEG. Stage 4 represents a deepening coma, decerebration, a cephalocaudal progression of brainstem dysfunction, and often improvement in liver dysfunction associated with a severely abnormal EEG. The final stage 5 is associated with seizures, loss of reflexes, respiratory arrest, correction of liver dysfunction, and an isoelectric EEG. Lovejoy et al. believed that stages 1 through 3 were compatible with full recovery, but a poor outcome was predicted when there was rapid passage through the first three stages, the presence of seizures in stage 2, a presenting blood ammonia concentration of greater than 300 $\mu$g/100 ml, increased spinal fluid pressure in stage 3, a markedly increased prothrombin time in stage 3, or a severely abnormal EEG.

### ■ Which viral infections lead to Reye syndrome?

In 1974 about 350 cases were reported to the Center for Disease Control in Atlanta. Of these, 55 followed type B influenza, 25 were apparently secondary to chickenpox, another 20 succeeded non-upper respiratory infection, and the remainder followed various upper respiratory illnesses. The two largest groups, those associated with influenza B and upper respiratory infections, shared another characteristic. The median age of incidence was 11 years for both, with peak rates clustered in children aged 12 to 15 years. In contrast, in the 25 patients whose encephalopathy followed chickenpox the median age was 6 years.

The mechanism by which viral infections are linked to Reye syndrome is unknown. The viral infection may be related to direct damage to the liver, CNS or secondary toxic damage, or a postviral immunologic reaction.

### ■ What is the treatment of Reye syndrome?

There are many unanswered questions with regard to Reye syndrome relative to etiology, optimum therapeutic management, and subsequent capabilty to prevent this disorder. A prospective study is being carried out with regard to therapy so that we may know what is the best approach for these patients. Until further information is available, the correct therapeutic approach is not known. It does appear from recent information that corticosteroid therapy to reduce brain edema may be an important facet to therapy. In addition, most investigators still prefer to use exchange transfusions in the treatment of these children. Measures such as the infusion of insulin and glucose to reduce fatty acid accumulation may also be useful and can be utilized at the same time. Other therapeutic approaches include the use of peritoneal dialysis and the administration of the amino acid L-citrulline to reduce serum ammonia levels.

## HEMOLYTIC UREMIC SYNDROME

### ■ What is the hemolytic uremic syndrome and what causes it?

The hemolytic uremic syndrome is the most common cause of acute renal failure in infants. The sexes are affected equally. There is usually a seasonal incidence, with the peak occurring in late summer or early fall. Involvement of more than one member of the family has been reported on several occasions. Definite evidence for infection as a cause of this condition has largely been negative, although several viruses have been isolated in individual cases.

### ■ What are the clinical features of the syndrome?

The disease attacks infants who previously were well; more rarely it occurs in older children. There is a prodromal stage that lasts from a few hours to several days. The most common symptoms in this stage are gastrointestinal disorders, diarrhea is quite characteristic, and there may be abdominal pain, vomiting, and occasionally hematemesis. Fever occurs in about half the cases; temperature is usually moderate (38° to 39° C). There may be enlargement of the lymph nodes or rash. The syndrome may also develop without any prodromal symptoms. The principal signs of the disease in the acute phase are the simultaneous appearance of hemolytic anemia, hematuria or anuria, and thrombocytopenia.

### ■ Is the hemolytic anemia severe?

The hemolytic anemia is rapid in the onset and very severe and may worsen in subsequent exacerbations. The red blood cell count may fall to 2 million/$mm^3$ in 24 hours. The hemolytic nature of this anemia is demonstrated by a high level of reticulocytes in circulating blood and an increase in erythroblastosis in the bone marrow with the passage of normoblasts in the peripheral blood. Generally the serum bilirubin level is only slightly elevated. The red blood cells are very deformed, and there are numerous schistocytes. Although the deformities are not specific, they are a constant feature of this syndrome.

### ■ Are there disturbances of coagulation?

Coagulation disorders are almost a constant feature, often appearing at the onset of the disease, and are manifested by purpura, cutaneous ecchymosis, and gastrointestinal bleeding. Cerebral hemorrhage is rare but has been seen. The bleeding time is frequently prolonged, and in nearly every case there is considerable thrombocytopenia with a platelet count below 100,000. The half-life of the platelets is diminished. The thrombocytopenia rarely persists for more than 8 days. There is a variability in the coagulation factors from patient to patient and from day to day. However, these factors suggest that localized intravascular coagulation does play a part in the pathophysiology of the syndrome.

### ■ What are the renal manifestations?

The renal manifestations appear at the same time as the anemia and are manifested either by signs of acute glomerulonephritis with or without a decrease in urine output or by total anuria. When the urine output is maintained, there is nearly always hematuria (often macroscopic) and proteinuria that may be sufficient to produce the nephrotic syndrome with edema. The blood urea nitrogen is nearly always elevated on the first examination. Anuria at the onset is very common in infants. The few milliliters of urine that are passed contain a very large number of red blood cells, and there is a special risk of hyperkalemia in these infants because of hemolysis.

### ■ How are the cardiovascular system and CNS affected?

Blood pressure is elevated in more than half of the cases. The hypertension may appear in the initial stages. It is generally moderate with systolic blood pressures of 140 mm Hg but rarely may be more severe and can lead to cardiac failure. Neurologic signs are particularly common in infants. Convulsions may occur at the onset of the disease. The cerebrospinal fluid is generally normal.

### ■ What is the prognosis of this condition?

The majority of children under the age of 2 years recover without ill effects. In children more than 2 years of age the prognosis is not as good. Two thirds of these cases proceed to progressive renal failure with malignant hypertension. There has never been demonstrated a relapse of the hemolytic uremic syndrome after recovery or a deterioration in renal function in patients clinically cured after the acute episode. However, hypertension and later neurologic complications have been reported.

### ■ How is the syndrome treated?

In the absence of precise etiology the specific treatment is based on the hypothesis that there is a process of intravascular coagulation in the hemolytic syndrome. The logical treatment is to use heparin to prevent the formation of new fibrin deposits or to accelerate the process of fibrinolysis by plasminogen activators. Heparin therapy has been used for some years. It is impossible to be certain that the treatment is effective in view of the unpredictable course of the untreated disease and the absence of any controlled trials. Despite this, heparin is widely used. The daily dose of heparin in infants is 8 to 10 mg/kg/24 hours injected continuously into a vein by means of an infusion pump. The therapy is controlled by measuring the clotting time twice a day using micromethods. Treatment is generally continued for 10 to 15 days. If there is a risk of hemorrhage from a therapeutic maneuver such as peritoneal dialysis, the action of heparin should be neutralized by protamine immediately before the particular procedure and the heparin therapy resumed immediately afterward. Therapy by fibrinolysis activators such as streptokinase and urokinase has been used, but there is no real proof of effectiveness.

Anemia is cautiously corrected by transfusion. Hypotensive drugs are used to control blood pressure. Steroid therapy is ineffective.

### ■ How is renal failure treated?

Early and intensive treatment of the acute renal failure has considerably improved the prognosis of the hemolytic uremic syndrome of infants. This includes the control of hyperkalemia by oral or rectal administration of exchange resins and/or varied and successive IV infusions, limitation of fluid administration, and peritoneal dialysis.

■ **How is peritoneal dialysis performed?**

There are many techniques of peritoneal dialysis that have been utilized. The following is a brief outline of one method of management that can be utilized in the critical care unit.

Patients may be premedicated, depending on their state of awareness. Skin, subcutaneous tissues, and peritoneum are anesthetized with 1% procaine or lidocaine at a site lateral to the rectus muscle. If the liver is enlarged, the right upper quadrant is avoided; otherwise upper and lower quadrants on either side are suitable. A No. 18 lumbar puncture needle is inserted into the peritoneal cavity and connected to the dialysis administration set. Approximately one third of the calculated volume of dialysis fluid, warmed to body temperature, is administered and the lumbar puncture needle is removed. A 0.5 cm incision is then made in the skin, and an adult-size disposable catheter with a self-contained trocar is advanced until the peritoneal cavity is entered. This is indicated by a sudden decrease in resistance. The trocar is then removed, and the catheter is advanced toward the pelvis. The correct position of the catheter is confirmed by the influx of the previously infused fluid. No sutures are required, and the catheter is kept in place with adhesive tape.

■ **Why inject fluid before placing the catheter?**

The intraperitoneal administration of dialysis fluid prior to insertion of the catheter facilitates the flow by allowing the catheter to lie free within the peritoneal cavity.

■ **What kind of and how much dialysis fluid is used?**

The dialysis fluid utilized will vary with the requirements, and it may be necessary to add heparin in a dose of 5 mg/L. The fluid is administered over 10 to 15 minutes. Prophylactic antibiotics are not required. The fluid is allowed to equilibrate over 30 minutes and then is drained in 10 to 15 minutes. In children 6 to 14 years of age 1 L fluid exchanges are performed. In younger children and infants 50 to 100 ml/kg exchange is recommended. The length of dialysis and the total amount of fluid exchanged depends on the requirements of the patient.

■ **What causes hyperkalemia?**

Increased serum potassium occurs as a result of inadequate renal excretion (acute renal failure) or the accidental administration of potassium.

■ **How is hyperkalemia controlled?**

In the presence of renal failure a slow rise in serum potassium can usually be controlled with ion-exchange resins. In an emergency a level of 8 to 9 mEq/L may be corrected as indicated subsequently. A serum potassium level of 7 mEq/L not responding to conservative management is an indication for dialysis. The emergency treatment of elevated serum potassium includes the following measures:

1. Slow IV infusion of sodium bicarbonate (3 ml/kg) up to a total of 50 ml
2. Administration of 25% to 50% glucose to provide a dose of 0.5 g of glucose/kg/hr by slow IV drip with 1 unit of regular insulin added to each 2 g of glucose

For the slow increase in serum potassium caused by renal failure sodium polystyrene sulfonate (Kayexalate) resin may be given orally in a dose of 1 g/kg up to 20 g mixed with 50 to 75 ml of water or a dose of 2 g/kg up to 40 g mixed with 100 ml of water as a retention enema. Repeat doses of Kayexalate resin should be based on determinations of the serum potassium level.

The T wave of the ECG provides a means of observing changes in cellular potassium without serum determinations. As the potassium concentration increases, the T wave increases in height and becomes sharply spiked.

■ **What are hypoxic spells?**

One of the complications of cyanotic congenital heart disease is the so-called hypoxic spells, also known as blue spells, anoxic spells, paroxysmal dyspnea, syncopal attacks, and paroxysmal hyperpnea. These spells are characterized by an increasing rate and depth of respiration with increasing cyanosis often associated with crying, progressing to limpness and syncope, and occasionally ending in convulsions, cerebrovascular accidents, and/or death. These episodes occur in the tetralogy of Fallot, pulmonary atresia, tricuspid atresia, and similar cyanotic congenital defects, but are rarely if ever found in transposition of the great arteries.

■ **What causes hypoxic spells?**

The precise etiology of these episodes is not clear. Several theories have been proposed to explain them, and indeed the true etiology may be a combination of all these theories. Hyperpnea or an increase in the depth and rate of respiration appears to be crucial to the beginning of the spell. In normal individuals hyperpnea will increase arterial oxygen saturation. However, in patients with right-to-left shunts hyperpnea causes a decrease in arterial oxygen saturation. Similarly, in the normal individual hyperpnea leads to increased cardiac output of both right and left ventricles, whereas in patients with a fixed resistance to the flow of blood into the lungs, there is an increase in systemic blood flow without a similar increase in pulmonary flow. This leads to a decrease in arterial $P_{O_2}$ and pH and an increase in $P_{CO_2}$. These changes tend to stimulate respiration and a vicious cycle is begun.

Another theory of the etiology of these spells suggests that they are caused by obstructive spasm of the right ventricular infundibulum, which may occur as a result of the release of catecholamines. This increase in infundibular obstruction thus decreases pulmonary blood flow and leads to similar changes that result in an increase in respiratory activity. Other explanations of the spells are related to a sudden decrease in systemic vascular resistance or in the development of metabolic acidosis secondary to hypoxia.

■ **When do these spells occur?**

The onset of the symptoms may be as early as the first month of life but may occur as late as 12 years of age or older. The peak incidence is between 2 and 3 months of age. In the more severely cyanotic infants the attacks may occur at any time of the day, but in patients with only occasional episodes the attacks commonly occur in the morning after a full night of sleep. Crying, defecation, and feeding are frequent precipitating events. Curiously the attacks are not restricted to patients with severe cyanosis. They have been observed in patients with normal arterial saturations at rest, and some patients with severe desaturation do not develop spells. However, the arterial oxygen saturation during a spell is always low.

■ **How is the spell treated?**

The treatment of a hypoxic spell requires placement of the child in the knee-chest position, administration of oxygen, and IM administration of morphine sulfate in a dose of 0.1 to 0.2 mg/kg of body weight. Occasionally the IV administration of sodium bicarbonate in a dose of 1 to 3 mg/kg will combat metabolic acidosis.

Some patients with relative anemia will require the transfusion of packed red blood cells or the administration of iron to increase the oxygen-carrying capacity of the blood. Propranolol in a dose of 1 mg/kg/day given every 6 hours night and day has been reported to prevent hypoxic episodes, and IV propranolol may be used in treating an infant where other measures are not successful. Usually one hypoxic episode is an absolute indication for some type of surgery to improve pulmonary blood flow.

## CONGESTIVE HEART FAILURE

■ **What is heart failure?**

Heart failure is defined as the state in which the heart fails to maintain an adequate circulation for the needs of the body despite a satisfactory venous filling pressure.

The heart compensates for the increased demands of the body by changing the strength of cardiac contraction and varying the heart rate. The strength of cardiac contraction for short-term needs is increased by adrenaline, sympathetic tone, and increased diastolic filling of the ventricles. For long-term needs increased cardiac contraction is maintained by cardiac hypertrophy. Drugs such as digitalis also increase the strength of cardiac contraction. (The effect on the strength of cardiac contraction by a drug is known as an inotropic effect.) An increase in heart rate increases cardiac output until a critical rate is reached (about 180 beats/min). Above the critical rate cardiac output falls because the decrease in diastolic time prevents adequate filling of the ventricles. At this point coronary flow becomes inadequate, and the mechanical efficiency of the heart falls. Cardiac failure occurs when the previously mentioned mechanisms fail and the ventricles become overdistended in diastole. Cardiac failure may occur with high cardiac output such as in thyrotoxicosis, anemia, and arteriovenous fistula, but it is more commonly seen with low cardiac output. The increased diastolic pressure of the failing ventricle raises left atrial and pulmonary venous pressure, reducing lung volume. The increased right atrial and peripheral venous pressure rises, distending the liver and peripheral veins. Cerebral and coronary circulation are maintained at almost normal levels initially, but renal blood flow is reduced, leading to oliguria, salt and water retention, and edema. Cardiac failure may occur as a result of increased pressure work of the heart, such as with valvular stenosis; increased volume work of the heart, such as with left-to-right shunts; or damaged ventricular muscle, such as in myocarditis or cardiomyopathy. In the postoperative period cardiac failure may occur from an overloaded vascular system, as with overtransfusion of blood or other fluids, sudden onset of arrhythmias, or anoxemia.

**■ What are the signs and symptoms of heart failure?**

The manifestations of heart failure are related to impaired myocardial performance and systemic and pulmonary venous congestion.

**■ What are the signs of an impaired myocardium?**

Cardiac enlargement on chest x-ray films is a most consistent sign of decreased cardiac function and is produced by ventricular dilatation. Tachycardia above 160 beats/min in infants and above 120 beats/min in older children is commonly seen with heart failure. Rates above 220 beats/min should raise the question of paroxysmal supraventricular tachycardia, which may be the cause of congestive heart failure rather than its result. A gallop rhythm is frequently heard in infants and children with congestive heart failure. Cold extremities with weakly palpable peripheral pulses and lowered blood pressure are commonly seen. Bounding arterial pulses in the presence of congestive heart failure are suggestive of a high output state such as patent ductus arteriosus or systemic arteriovenous fistula.

**■ How is systemic venous congestion manifested?**

The signs of systemic venous congestion include enlargement of the liver, which is usually tender with a rounded edge, and neck vein distention, which can be readily seen in the older child. In the infant this is difficult to assess because of the short neck. Peripheral edema is a rare finding in cardiac failure in infants and young children. Facial edema is more common in a child. Ascites and anasarca are rare except in older children with restrictive pericardial disease or severely compromised myocardial function.

**■ How is pulmonary venous congestion manifested?**

Tachypnea is a common sign of pulmonary congestion, and respiratory rates greater than 60 respirations/min are not uncommon in infants. Wheezing is a frequent sign of left ventricular failure in infants and may be confused with bronchiolitis. Rales are usually not heard in infants and young children with congestive heart failure. Sweating, growth failure, and chest deformity are frequently seen in patients with long-standing chronic congestive heart failure.

### ■ How is heart failure treated?

The treatment of congestive heart failure is directed toward improving myocardial performance and reversing the deranged function of other organ systems. Frequent clinical reappraisal is necessary during treatment to reach the optimum degree of improvement in myocardial performance.

Digitalis is the drug of choice for the management of congestive heart failure. Digoxin is the most widely used digitalis glycoside for infants and children and is available in oral and parenteral preparations. One must be aware of the varying response of patients to this drug and prepared to adjust the dose depending on the reaction of the individual. This is particularly true in patients with inflammatory disease of the myocardium where there is an increased sensitivity to digitalis glycosides. Orders for the use of digitalis must be explicitly written to include the type of glycoside, the route of administration, the dose in milligrams or micrograms, and the number of milliliters containing this dose. It is important to realize that the oral preparation of digoxin (Lanoxin) contains 0.05 mg/ml, whereas the parenteral form contains 0.25 mg/ml, and the pediatric parenteral form contains 0.1 mg/ml. Recent reports have indicated a variation in the effectiveness of differing digoxin preparations, and it is recommended that only the Burroughs Wellcome brand of digoxin, Lanoxin, be used in infants and children.

### ■ How is digoxin administered?

The total digitalizing dose for a given patient is calculated on the basis of body weight and age; the following list may serve as a guide:

| | |
|---|---|
| Birth to 2 mo | 0.05 mg/kg |
| 2 mo to 2 yr | 0.075 mg/kg |
| 2 yr to 5 yr | 0.06 mg/kg |
| Over 5 yr | 0.05 mg/kg |

One half of the digitalizing dose is given immediately and the remainder in two equal doses at 4- to 6-hour intervals. In extremely urgent situations or if perfusion is severely impaired, the initial dose may be given by the IV route, but more commonly digitalization is accomplished by the IM route. The patient must be watched for evidence of digitalis toxicity, and evaluation of the heart rate and rhythm are particularly necessary prior to the administration of the last one fourth of the digitalizing dose. Adequacy of the total digitalization should be evaluated 4 to 6 hours following the administration of the calculated total digitalizing dose, and if digitalization is complete without evidence of toxicity, orders should then be written for maintenance digitalis, which may be given orally or parenterally. The daily maintenance digoxin dose is one fourth of the total digitalizing dose and is given in two equal doses at 12-hour intervals. Orders should always be written indicating that a dose should be withheld and the patient reevalulated if the heart rate falls below 100 to 120 beats/min for infants and 60 to 80 beats/min in older children or if irregularity is noted. Digitalis toxicity should be treated by immediate cessation of administration, followed by frequent ECG monitoring. With mild intoxication the signs of toxicity will usually disappear in 2 to 3 days. With evidence of severe toxicity or in the presence of hypokalemia the administration of potassium by slow IV infusion at a dose not to exceed 0.5 mEq/kg/24 hr in a patient who has voided is most effective. Procainamide (2.5 mg/kg) or propranolol (0.1 mg/kg) may be given slowly by IV route for severe ventricular arrhythmias caused by digitalis.

### ■ Why and how are diuretics used?

Since abnormal salt and water retention are major manifestations of congestive heart failure, and since the overloaded circulation further hinders myocardial performance, diuretic therapy occupies an important place in the management of congestive heart failure. Furosemide (Lasix) is the most effective diuretic agent available and can be administered by either IV or IM route in a dose of 1 to 2 mg/kg. Meralluride (Mercuhydrin) is a somewhat less potent mercurial diuretic that can be given by IM route in a dose from 0.25 ml for infants to 1.5 ml for older children and adolescents.

Common oral diuretics used in infants and children include chlorothiazide (Diuril), which is given in a dose of 25 mg/kg/day to a maximum of 250 mg/day in two divided doses, and spironolactone (Aldactone), which is given in a dose of 0.7 mg/kg/day in two divided doses.

Other therapeutic measures useful in the treatment of acute congestive failure include elevation of the head and shoulders to an angle of 45 degrees, bed rest, reduction in feedings, decreased intake of sodium, administration of oxygen in up to 50% concentrations with increased humidity up to 80%, and administration of antibiotics if infection is suspected. In acute pulmonary edema, sedation with morphine sulfate (0.1 mg/kg) and tourniquets on three extremities rotated every 10 to 15 minutes may be helpful. If pulmonary edema has been precipitated by rapid infusion of fluids or blood, removal of blood by venipuncture may be of value.

## ARRHYTHMIAS

Abnormal cardiac rhythm in the pediatric patient is of importance when it affects the cardiac output, and in a postoperative patient it can lead to ineffective cardiac pumping. Anoxia, drugs, uremia, or surgical trauma to the conducting system must be considered as possible causes of arrhythmias. The diagnosis of arrhythmia must be made by interpretation of the ECG and may be classified into ectopic beats, tachycardias, and heart block.

### ■ What is the significance of ectopic beats?

Single ectopic beats may originate in the atrium, junctional or nodal area, or ventricle. They may occur singly or in a repetitive fashion associated with normal beats such as in a bigeminy or trigeminy. Those ectopic beats arising in the atrial or nodal areas usually do not require treatment. Ventricular premature beats, if they are frequent or if they occur from more than one focus, may be a prelude to more severe ventricular arrhythmias. Digitalis toxicity often leads to ventricular arrhythmias. Treatment is most often effective with lidocaine, procainamide, quinidine, and propranolol.

Frequent unifocal ventricular ectopic beats including bigeminy may occur in children with no heart disease. Treatment is usually not necessary.

### ■ What are tachycardias and how are they treated?

Tachycardias include sinus tachycardia, paroxysmal supraventricular tachycardia, and ventricular tachycardia. Sinus tachycardia is usually present at rates between 150 and 200 beats/min. The rate will usually vary slightly in the ECG, and each ventricular complex is preceded by P waves. Treatment should be directed to the cause of sinus tachycardia, such as fever or congestive heart failure. Paroxysmal supraventricular tachycardia is very common in infants but can occur at any age. Heart rates are usually in excess of 160 beats/min and frequently above 220 beats/min. There may be a history in an older patient of recurrences of tachycardia. The ECG demonstrates the tachycardia occurring at an extremely regular rate without variation. P waves are frequently not visible, but in the rare instance when they are present, there is usually a prolonged P-R interval. The physiologic effect of the tachycardia is to shorten diastole, leading to inadequate cardiac filling and the development of congestive heart failure. The treatment of choice in children is the administration of digitalis, which will cause a reversal of the tachycardia. In a patient in extremis cardioversion has been effective to restore normal heart rate. Ventricular tachycardia, which is recognized by the widened abnormal ventricular beats, is of major significance because of the inadequate ventricular filling produced, the resultant diminished cardiac output, and the tendency for ventricular tachycardia to proceed to ventricular fibrillation. Immediate treatment is indicated and the IV administration of lidocaine first as a bolus and then as a drip is usually the first modality utilized. Procainamide and propranolol can be used by IV route. Cardioversion may be necessary to restore normal rhythm. Should the tachycardia proceed to ventricular fibrillation, cardiopulmonary resuscitation and electrical defibrillation are needed.

Atrial fibrillation or flutter, which is occasionally seen in the pediatric age group, is usually associated with a rapid ventricular rate. Initial treatment usually consists of the administration of digitalis to slow the ventricular response and the subsequent administration of quinidine to correct the fibrillation "flutter" to sinus rhythm.

### ■ What is heart block?

Heart block occurs in three degrees. First-degree heart block, which is manifested by prolongation of the P-R interval on the ECG, indicates a delay in the transmission of electrical impulse from the sinus pacemaker through the internodal area. It may be present in rheumatic fever as well as toxic states and is sometimes found in congenital cardiac abnormalities, including endocardial cushion defects or corrected transposition. It occurs after digitalis administration but does not indicate toxicity.

Second-degree heart block is manifested by the failure of an occasional sinus beat to be followed by a ventricular response. This may occur on a regular basis or may be demonstrated by an increasing P-R interval with final failure of the ventricular response (Wenckebach phenomenon).

Third-degree heart block describes a condition where there is no relationship between the atrial and ventricular beats. It may be congenital in origin, secondary to surgical interruption of the bundle of His, or induced by drugs such as digitalis or quinidine. The ventricular rate usually ranges from 30 to 45 beats/min and can produce symptoms related to insufficient cardiac output. Emergency treatment of complete heart block may require the administration of isoproterenol (Isuprel), temporary cardiac pacing, or a permanent pacemaker.

### ■ How does the treatment of cardiac arrest differ in infants and children?

Cardiac arrest is in a sense a severe form of cardiac arrhythmia in which there is failure of the heartbeat. It requires immediate cardiopulmonary resuscitation, including establishment of an airway, ventilation of the patient, and closed chest cardiac massage. It is important to remember in the establishment of an airway in a child that overextension of the head can compress the trachea and close it. Ventilation is most effectively provided by mouth-to-mouth resuscitation, but in a critical care unit intubation and bag ventilation can be effectively performed. Closed chest resuscitation in a newborn or small infant requires the use of two-finger pressure over the midsternum, gradually increasing to one-hand pressure on the lower portion of the sternum in an older child. The sternum should be massaged at a rate of 80 to 100 times/min, with one respiration for about every five chest movements. Sodium bicarbonate should be administered as soon as possible, since acidosis develops rapidly. An ECG should be obtained to determine whether ventricular fibrillation is present, and electrical defibrillation should be administered. Other drugs useful in stimulating the arrested heart include isoproterenol, epinephrine, and calcium chloride.

It should be pointed out that resuscitation of a child with cyanotic congenital heart disease is very difficult and seldom successful because of the inability to oxygenate the patient's blood caused by the right-to-left shunt and/or obstruction of the flow of blood to the lungs as a result of the cardiac defect.

Table 25-6, on p. 476, indicates drug dosages used in children for the treatment of arrhythmias and congestive heart failure.

## SHOCK

### ■ What is shock?

Shock is a term used to describe a syndrome in which the patient exhibits a number of characteristic signs. These include ashen skin; oral mucous membranes that are pale and dry; cold, clammy extremities; decrease in temperature; a fast, thready pulse;

**Table 25-6.** Drug dosages and therapeutic measures not given in the text

| *Agent* | *Dosage* |
|---|---|
| *Antiarrhythmic drugs* | |
| Lidocaine | |
| Bolus | 1 mg/kg by IV every 3-5 min |
| Drip | 50 ml 2% in 200 ml 5% glucose in water to make 4 mg/ml |
| Procainamide | |
| IV | 2.5 mg/kg by slow IV push |
| Oral | 7 mg/pound |
| Quinidine | 30 mg/kg/day |
| Propranolol | 0.1 mg/kg by slow IV push |
| *Cardiotonic drugs* | |
| Epinephrine | 0.5 μg/kg/min IV drip |
| In cardiac arrest | 1-4 ml of 1:10,000 dilution |
| Isoproterenol (Isuprel) | 1 mg in 250 ml 5% glucose in water to make 4 μ/ml given as IV drip and titrated to heart rate |
| Calcium chloride | 1-4 ml 10% by slow IV push |
| *Diuretics* | |
| Mannitol | 1 g/kg by slow IV drip |
| Furosemide (Lasix) | 1-2 mg/kg by IV push |
| Chlorothiazide | 5-15 mg/pound/day orally in 2 doses |
| Spironolactone | 1.5 mg/pound/day |
| Meralluride (Mercuhydrin) | 0.1 ml/10 pounds by IM every 1-2 days |
| *Antihypertensive drugs for acute glomerulonephritis* | |
| Hydralazine hydrochloride (Apresoline) | 0.15 mg/kg by IM every 12 hr |
| Reserpine | 0.07 mg/kg by IM every 12 hr |
| *Cardiopulmonary resuscitation drugs* | |
| Sodium bicarbonate | 2-5 mEq/kg by IM, repeated at 5-10 min intervals |
| Cardioversion (electrical defibrillation) | 5 watt-seconds/kg (if > 50 kg, 400 watt-seconds) |

low blood pressure; CNS depression or restlessness; thirst; and decreased or absent urinary flow. These signs are either caused by the decreased blood flow that is a major part of shock or are the result of compensatory sympathetic activity. Shock is not a single entity but may be caused by a variety of factors and mechanisms. The common denominator is a reduction in blood flow and resulting abnormalities of tissue metabolism. Shock may be produced by a loss of blood volume (hypovolemia), such as in acute blood loss with hemorrhagic or traumatic shock; a loss of plasma, such as in burn shock or dehydration; secondary to a disturbance in cardiac filling, such as pericardial tamponade, or cardiac emptying, such as in myocardial disease or inflammation; abnormalities of the blood vessels, such as in neurogenic shock, which is a mild form of shock that may be caused by certain humeral influences on blood vessels; and bacteria, which is known as endotoxic shock or septic shock. Shock can also be produced by respiratory failure secondary to hyaline membrane disease. It can also be caused by the positive pressure of ventilation used to treat this condition, if used to excess, which can interfere with the filling of the heart. It can also occur secondary to a ruptured omphalocele or to hemorrhage caused by DIC.

When the insult causing shock is not severe, various compensatory mechanisms can serve to maintain the cardiovascular system. If the shock is severe and of prolonged duration, the circulation deteriorates and the shock condition is said to be decompensated. Continuation of the shock condition leads to irreversible shock and death.

### ■ What is the pathophysiology of shock?

The pathophysiology of shock is best illustrated by blood loss. Following reduction of blood volume, compensation occurs by a decrease in venous capacity and an increase in cardiac emptying. There is vasoconstriction of the blood vessels in the limbs, splanchnic organs, and kidneys, so that there is preferential blood circulation to the heart and brain. Initially the sympathetic nervous system helps to maintain the arterial blood pressure. The vasoconstriction of the splanchnic and renal vessels leads to metabolic acidosis, and the acidosis results in the decreased ability of the cardiovascular system to respond to catecholamines, the mediating agent of the sympathetic nervous system. As acidosis increases, capillary sphincter tone decreases, and this leads to an increase of blood flow into the capillary beds, which results in an engorgement of capillaries and transudation of fluid into the extracellular space. In general when the blood volume is reduced to 60% to 70% of normal, signs of shock are clearly evident. If these volume deficiencies remain uncorrected, the reductions of volume, pressure, and flow, instead of being minimized by compensatory mechanisms, may become progressively more severe.

### ■ What parameters should be monitored in shock?

In the management of the patient with shock it is important to monitor central venous pressure, blood pressure, cardiac output if possible, blood gas concentrations, urinary output, body weight, hematocrit and white blood cell count, sodium, potassium, chloride, blood urea nitrogen, and creatinine concentrations, and in the newborn, glucose levels.

### ■ How is shock treated?

Treatment of the condition involves first treating the primary causes, if known. Respiratory assistance with tracheostomy or an endotracheal tube may be necessary. In shock associated with increased central venous pressure myocardial failure must be considered, and treatment utilizing digitalis and diuretics would be indicated. Abnormal heart rhythm or rates must be controlled. Acidosis must be corrected. In the patient with shock and low venous pressure the replacement of blood or electrolytes is mandatory. In patients with a mild decrease in urinary output the use of mannitol is sometimes helpful. Isoproterenol (Isuprel) in a dose of 0.25 $\mu$g/kg/min given by IV drip is sometimes helpful in improving myocardial function and peripheral perfusion. Antibiotics are indicated if there is evidence of infection. The use of steroids is open to question.

## FLUID AND ELECTROLYTE THERAPY

### ■ Why is fluid balance so important in infants and children?

Even in health the amounts of water, electrolytes, and calories are relatively greater in children than in adults. Water constitutes a greater proportion of the body of a child and the daily turnover of fluid is greater. Infections that bring about increased losses of water are more common in childhood, and the body's responses to them are more violent. Fever, vomiting, and diarrhea are more frequent and relatively more severe. Therefore in children and infants the maintenance or restoration of normal fluid and electrolyte balance often overshadows specific therapy in importance. This applies to the greatest extent in diarrheal disease, but the fluid management of other conditions associated with fever or vomiting, severe burns, and many surgical conditions is a necessary part of any plan of therapy.

### ■ What are the clinical features of dehydration?

The clinical assessment of dehydration is of great importance. It should be remembered that the usual electrolyte studies give information as to the concentration of electrolytes, and only by inference based on clinical observation and history can one judge abnormalities in the total amounts of electrolytes and fluid. In the infant signs of dehydration are sunken fontanelle, sunken eyes, and skin that has lost its elasticity. The last is most easily demonstrated on the skin of the abdomen, which, when picked up, remains in sharp folds. In cases in which water loss has been predominant and the retention of electrolytes has occurred, a doughy thick consistency of the skin may be noted. In older children the severity of dehydration may be difficult to evaluate clinically. In severe cases in which there is poor peripheral circulation the skin is often gray and the extremities are cold and blue. In the child where the loss of water is greater than the loss of electrolytes, there will be elevated levels of sodium and chloride in the serum. As dehydration progresses, renal function diminishes and the dehydration produces high fever, further augmenting the water loss. In severe cases signs of CNS dysfunction are frequent, with convulsions that do not respond to calcium or measures taken to reduce the fever. This type of dehydration is known as hypernatremic dehydration.

### ■ What types of fluid are available for parenteral therapy?

Solutions available for parenteral fluid and electrolyte therapy include glucose and water, which is usually given in concentrations of 5% or 10%; sodium chloride, most commonly used as physiologic saline solution (0.85% sodium chloride); Ringer-type solutions, which are essentially sodium chloride with trace minerals added; and polyionic solutions such as Darrow's, Butler's, and lactated Ringer's or Hartman's solution. Potassium chloride is available to be added to infusions, and alkalinizing solutions such as sodium bicarbonate and sodium lactate are available for the correction of acidosis.

### ■ How are parenteral fluids administered?

Fluids are most efficiently administered by the IV route. This can be by means of a scalp vein needle or a butterfly needle, which is a short segment of straight needle of varying sizes from 18 to 25 gauge connected to a piece of plastic tubing through which the IV solution can be administered. The advantage of these scalp vein needles is that they can be immobilized readily and maintained in a vein. The most frequent sites for administration are in the scalp veins or veins in the hand, wrist, ankle, or foot. IV fluids can also be administered by direct cannulation of larger veins with a metal or plastic needle; they can be given via a cutdown, most commonly in the ankle; and recently in children over 15 pounds, we have been introducing a large plastic catheter into the femoral vein by percutaneous Seldinger technique and advancing this into the inferior vena cava for both the administration of fluid and electrolytes and the measurement of central venous pressure.

### ■ How are the electrolyte and water requirements estimated?

Calculation of the fluid used to treat dehydration and electrolyte imbalance consists of two parts: maintenance, which is the intake required by a well infant or child of the same age and size, and replacement, which is the amount required to replace abnormal fluid or electrolyte losses that have occurred and may still be going on.

### ■ How are the maintenance requirements calculated?

Maintenance requirements in an infant or child are most accurately calculated on the basis of the rate of metabolic turnover and are based on the metabolism of 100 calories. Water and electrolyte needs can be determined from caloric turnover. The basic formula for water maintenance by caloric needs is 100 ml/kg for the first 10 kg, 50 ml/kg for the next 10 kg, and 25 ml/kg for each kilogram more than 20 kg. Corrections must then be utilized for changes in body temperature and activity. Less exact but clinically effective calculations can be obtained from formulas using surface area or body weight. For all infants from age 1 week to adult life the normal requirements per square meter are as follows: water, 1500 to

2000 ml; sodium, 35 to 50 mEq; and potassium, 30 to 40 mEq. These requirements can also be estimated on the basis of body weight. For infants under 1 year of age 150 ml/kg of body weight is the maintenance water requirement. From ages 1 to 2 years the requirement is 125 ml/kg, and from 2 to 4 years of age 100 ml/kg is needed. After the age of 4 years the amount gradually decreases to 70 ml/kg at 10 years of age. The requirements for sodium of an infant 1 to 6 months of age are 15 mEq/day, for 6 months to 2 years of age they are 22 to 30 mEq/day, and for older children 30 to 60 mEq/day is required. Requirements for potassium of infants weighing up to 10 kg are 3 mEq/kg/day; for children weighing 10 to 20 kg the requirements are 1 to 2 mEq/kg/day; and for children weighing 20 to 70 kg 1 mEq/kg/day is required.

**■ How is replacement therapy calculated?**

Replacement therapy is estimated on the basis of the patient's body weight. The amount of fluid lost is estimated from the following considerations: loss of 5% of the body weight in fluid is the smallest amount clinically detectable, and loss of 20% is about the maximum compatible with life. Children moribund from dehydration are therefore estimated to have lost 20% of their body weight. Moderately dehydrated children are estimated to have lost about 10% of body weight. In mild dehydration the weight loss is assumed to be 5% of body weight. Fluid used for replacement therapy is essentially saline solution modified to include potassium if there is potassium deficiency and bicarbonate or lactate if there is acidosis. In a patient in a moribund state and in circulatory collapse the initial fluid should be isotonic saline solution, plasma, albumin solution, or blood. The primary object in this case is to restore circulating blood volume. In this instance 20 to 30 ml/kg or 350 ml/m$^2$ is injected over the first hour. At the end of this time the rate of administration is changed to permit normal replacement. Essentially calculations are made for the total needs of the infant based on maintenance plus replacement therapy. This is given over a 24-hour period, depending on the infant's condition. The initial therapy may be given more rapidly if there is circulatory embarrassment. In a patient with hypernatremia it is essential to correct electrolyte and fluid imbalance slowly so as not to produce cerebral edema or changes in brain volume.

## PATENT DUCTUS ARTERIOSUS

**■ Why is patent ductus arteriosus common in premature infants?**

In the fetus the ductus arteriosus provides a channel allowing 50% to 60% of the cardiac output to be ejected into the descending aorta without first passing through the lung vessels. At birth there is a sudden rise in systemic vascular resistance caused by the closure of the placental circulation and a drop in pulmonary vascular resistance caused by expansion of the lungs with dilatation of the pulmonary vessels. Thus almost immediately after birth the systemic and pulmonary resistances are approximately equal, and there is little or no flow through the ductus arteriosus in either direction. The ductus arteriosus in the term infant is exquisitely sensitive to the rise in oxygen concentration, resulting in constriction of the ductus followed by structural closure in the first few days of life.

It has been long recognized that the ductus arteriosus frequently remains patent in premature infants and may not close spontaneously for many months. Animal studies have demonstrated that the response of the ductus musculature to oxygen concentration depends on the gestational age of the fetus. It has been estimated that two thirds of all infants with birth weights less than 1750 g have delayed closure of the ductus arteriosus and that the ductus is patent in virtually all infants with birth weights under 1000 g. Suggested causes have included the high threshold of ductus tissue to oxygen, lower pulmonary capillary $P_{O_2}$ as a result of inadequate ventilation because of weak respiratory musculature or pathologic processes such as hyaline membrane disease, and immature development of the ductus musculature. The latter cause is unlikely, as the ductus can be demonstrated to constrict quite readily with the infusion of acetylcholine and other drugs. The higher incidence of patent ductus arteriosus (PDA) in both term and premature infants born at high altitudes certainly results from the lower $P_{O_2}$ at high altitudes.

## ■ How does PDA present in the premature infant?

The pattern of presentation is closely related to the size of the infant. In infants weighing over 1750 g PDA presents in a pattern similar to term infants. Usually no murmur or other abnormal findings are noted until 4 to 6 weeks of age. At that time a soft systolic ejection-type murmur is usually heard along the left sternal border. Over the next several weeks to months the murmur becomes louder, the pulses become bounding, and the maximum location of the murmur moves higher to the area of the second intercostal space at the left midclavicular line. In early infancy the findings frequently suggest an interventricular septal defect. The typical machinery murmur extending into diastole may not be present until 6 months to 1 year of age. Some of these infants with large ductus and low pulmonary vascular resistance develop evidence of congestive heart failure, gain weight slowly, or develop recurrent lower respiratory tract infections. Most remain asymptomatic except for the physical findings indicating PDA.

In infants weighing between 1500 and 1750 g the findings usually occur earlier. These infants typically have little if any respiratory distress and appear to be doing well until 1 to 2 weeks of age, when a systolic murmur is heard at the upper left sternal border. Over the next several days the murmur becomes louder and more prolonged, frequently extending into diastole, and the pulses are noted to be brisk to bounding. The precordium may be hyperactive, and a third sound is frequently noted at the apex. Many of the infants will develop mild respiratory distress at this time. In most infants after 2 to 3 weeks the murmur becomes shorter and softer, pulses diminish, and by 6 weeks of age there is no further evidence of PDA. However, some infants develop evidence of congestive heart failure, and occasionally apneic spells occur. The earlier findings in premature infants appear to be caused by a more rapid fall in pulmonary vascular resistance than occurs in term infants.

Infants with birth weights between 1000 and 1500 g usually have moderate to severe respiratory distress from birth. The infant usually begins to improve after several days and may no longer require oxygen or respiratory assistance. Typically 5 to 8 days after birth a systolic murmur will be heard over the pulmonic area in these infants and may be heard only intermittently for the first few days. The murmur becomes louder and longer, frequently extending into diastole, and pulses become bounding. There is usually an increase in respiratory effort with sternal retractions, indicating the development of congestive heart failure. Increased oxygen is required to prevent hypoxia, and the infant usually requires continuous positive air pressure (CPAP) to maintain adequate pulmonary functions. Increasing end-expiratory pressures become necessary, and frequently the infant will have apneic spells requiring stimulation or the frequent use of respiratory assistance. The heart may be larger than on previous x-ray examinations, but pulmonary vascularity is difficult to differentiate from pulmonary disease.

Infants weighing less than 1000 g almost always have respiratory distress from birth and may require a respirator to assist in breathing. Findings of PDA usually develop at 3 to 5 days of age. If the infant is breathing spontaneously, the development of apneic spells, increasing retractions, and an increase in the required end-expiratory pressure usually indicate the presence of a significant PDA. If the infant is on a respirator, increasing pressures will usually be required for the maintenance of adequate ventilation to prevent a rising $P_{CO_2}$. Occasionally a murmur is present. However, murmurs usually cannot be heard if the infant is on a respirator or receiving CPAP therapy. Pulses usually become stronger, and if an arterial catheter is in place, a wide pulse pressure is noted.

### ■ How can congestive heart failure caused by PDA be distinguished from progressive pulmonary disease in the premature infant?

The diagnosis of congestive heart failure is usually not difficult in the term or premature infant without respiratory distress. However, there is little in the physical examination that can readily distinguish whether the symptoms are caused by the cardiac or pulmonary disease. The bounding pulses and murmurs present only confirm that the ductus is patent. Rales are frequently present in either condition, and the liver is usually not markedly enlarged even in the presence of congestive heart failure. X-ray films usually reveal evidence of hyaline membrane disease with a vascularity that is not distinguishable. The heart may be mildly to moderately enlarged.

If an arterial catheter is in place in the upper to midthoracic descending aorta, a single film aortogram can be obtained by rapidly hand-injecting 2 ml of half-strength sodium diatrizoate (Renografin-76) and obtaining a posteroanterior chest film at the end of the injection. If the infant is in congestive heart failure with a large left-to-right shunt, marked filling of the pulmonary arteries will usually be seen. Centers experienced in obtaining echocardiograms on infants have been impressed with the use of measures of left atrial size by this technique to determine the significance of PDA. Normally in infants weighing less than 1300 g the left atrial dimension is 4 to 5 mm, those weighing between 1300 and 2000 g, 5 to 9 mm, and those weighing over 2000 g, 9 to 12 mm. If the left atrial diameter is over 9 mm in premature infants weighing less than 1300 g, over 14 mm in infants weighing from 1300 to 2000 g, or over 17 mm in infants weighing over 2000 g, significant left-to-right shunt with congestive heart failure can be assumed. The ratio of the left atrium to aortic size can also be used. In normal term or premature infants the left atrial:aortic ratio is $0.71 \pm 0.13$. In infants in congestive failure the left atrial: aortic ratio will be $1.19 \pm 0.18$ or greater.

Several precautions are necessary in using echocardiograms in infants. It is important that a transducer of the proper size be used. The transducer should measure 5 MHz or greater with a diameter of no more than ⅜ inch. Infants who are undergoing retractions or who have chest deformities will usually have a pancaked left atrium. The usually obtained echocardiogram transecting the pulmonary outflow tract, aortic valve, and left atrium will reveal a normal-sized left atrium and normal left atrial:aortic ratios even in the presence of severe congestive heart failure. To obtain accurate measurements in these infants, the transducer must be placed in the suprasternal notch and directed down and slightly to the left. In this position the beam will transect the right pulmonary artery, arch of the aorta, left atrium, and mitral valve and will give accurate measurements of aortic and left atrial size. Evidence of the accuracy of this method of determining heart failure in these infants can be demonstrated by the rapid fall in left atrial size and left atrial:aortic ratio measurements in those infants who respond to digitalization, the rapid fall to normal of these measurements after surgery in infants with clinical improvement, and the lack of improvement with surgery in those infants undergoing surgery who had normal left atrial measurements.

### ■ How should the older infant with PDA be managed?

The asymptomatic infant at 2 weeks to 6 months of age with findings typical of PDA needs no treatment. Surgery can be done electively at 1 year of age if the ductus does not close spontaneously.

The infant with evidence of congestive heart failure should be digitalized. Term infants over 1 month of age usually require 60 to 75 mg/kg of digoxin (Lanoxin) as a digitalizing dose. Premature infants are more sensitive to digitalis glucosides than larger infants. A dose of 40 $\mu$g of digoxin/kg of body weight is usually adequate for digitalization in these infants. Maintenance requirements are usually 10 to 15 μg/kg given in two divided doses. In acute heart failure salt restriction and diuretics are also helpful. SMA S:26 and Similac PM 60:40 (not regular Similac) have the lowest sodium content of the readily available formulas. Lonolac, a formula very low in sodium, should not be used because of failure to gain weight. Infants on solid feedings should have foods strained in a blender rather than canned baby food, which has a very high sodium content. In the hospitalized infant with congestive heart failure furosemide (Lasix), 1 mg/kg, should be given parenterally. Less ill infants can be given chlorothiazide oral suspension (Diuril), 15 mg/pound/day. The infant with severe congestive heart failure may be improved significantly by a course of catecholamines administered by a constant infusion pump. Epinephrine, 0.2 to 0.4 mg/kg/min, or isoproterenol, 0.1 to 0.25 mg/kg/min, can be given for several hours to prepare the child for cardiac catheterization or surgery. These drugs have a positive inotropic effect, improve cardiac function, and may be life saving in the critically ill infant. The older child with congestive heart failure should have surgery as soon as failure and infections are controlled. Cardiac catheterization is probably indicated only in those infants in whom the diagnosis is in doubt or a second lesion is suspected.

### ■ How should the premature infant with early evidence of PDA be managed?

The larger premature infant who develops evidence of PDA at 7 to 14 days of age without symptoms requires no treatment. If the infant is anemic, small transfusions should be given until the hematocrit is 40% to 45%. Raising the hematocrit is frequently associated with closure of the ductus within 1 or 2 days. If congestive failure develops, this should be treated and the infant should be taken to surgery as soon as the condition stabilizes. The infant with apneic spells should also have surgical closure of the PDA if a significant left-to-right shunt can be demonstrated by echocardiography, cardiac catheterization, or aortography.

The management is more difficult in the younger infant with respiratory distress, as it is difficult to distinguish the part played by the ductus from that of the respiratory disease. Transfusions, digitalization, diuretics, and oxygen are indicated, and respiratory assistance may be necessary. Indications for surgery differ in centers throughout the country. There is no doubt that many of these infants with large left-to-right shunts caused by PDA will survive without surgery. However, these infants will frequently require long periods of respiratory support and high oxygen concentrations and are likely to develop bronchopulmonary dysplasia. It is in this group of infants that the use of echocardiography using the suprasternal notch approach is of most value.

Those infants in which the left atrial size fails to decrease following digitalization or those having a significant increase in left atrial size following a good response to conservative management should have surgical closure of the ductus performed as soon as possible. Surgery is not indicated in those infants without left atrial enlargement, as their symptoms are probably caused by the pulmonary disease.

Cardiac catheterization prior to surgery is indicated only if there is a question of a more complex cardiac lesion or if adequate echocardiographic studies are not available. Cardiac catheterization carries a significant risk in an ill premature infant requiring respiratory assistance, and if necessary, a rapid study sufficient to make a diagnosis is preferable to a complete physiologic study. Prevention of hypothermia and acidosis during catheterization is important. Minimum amounts of contrast media should be used, as these drugs are very hypertonic and will draw large amounts of fluid into the circulation, resulting in severe overloading of the circulation and an increase in congestive heart failure and pulmonary edema. There is usually a rapid improvement in premature infants with large left-to-right shunts caused by PDA following surgery, and respiratory assistance and oxygen therapy can usually be gradually discontinued over a short period of time.

## HYPERVISCOSITY

### ■ What is the hyperviscosity syndrome?

Neonates may be severely polycythemic because of excessive placental-fetal transfusion at birth or maternal-fetal or twin-to-twin transfusions. Severe polycythemia is also seen in dysmaturity and small-for-date infants believed to be the result of chronic hypoxia in utero. It has been well recognized that these polycythemic infants have a high incidence of hypoglycemia and hypocalcemia with seizures, lethargy, vomiting, and feeding problems. It is less well recognized that these infants frequently present with a course suggesting transposition of the great vessels or other forms of severe cyanotic heart disease, and the syndrome is frequently not recognized until after a normal cardiac catheterization and angiocardiographic study. The infant is plethoric and cyanotic with the cyanosis in the legs frequently appearing greater than that in the arms and face. Respiratory distress may be present. A loud single second sound is heard at the upper left sternal border. A systolic murmur may be present at the lower left sternal border. The liver may be enlarged. The syndrome is seen only in infants with hematocrits above 70%, and the average hematocrit in symptomatic infants is 77%. Polycythemic blood has high viscosity. This results in a decrease in the rate of blood flow and by physical factors alone increases pulmonary vascular resistance to a greater extent than systemic resistance. This results in pulmonary hypertension and a reversal of flow through the ductus arteriosus. The resulting hypoxemia further increases pulmonary vascular resistance by vasoconstriction and prevents closure of the ductus. The high pulmonary pressure is transmitted to the right ventricle, which must act against an increased afterload to eject its contents. Right ventricular end-diastolic pressure increases and with it there is an increase in right atrial pressure that becomes higher than left atrial pressure. This causes the foramen ovale to open and a right-to-left shunt occurs at this level as well. Thus there is a persistence of the fetal circulation in these children. Blood gas determinations reveal a very low $P_{O_2}$ and oxygen saturation. It must be remembered that sampling from a catheter in the low thoracic or abdominal aorta includes blood that has been shunted right to left through the ductus.

Treatment is by erythropheresis, that is, phlebotomy with replacement of the same quantity of plasma. Enough blood should be removed to reduce the hematocrit to 65%. Symptoms caused by the pulmonary hypertension and persistent fetal circulation will usually be rapidly improved. Lethargy and other evidences of CNS depression are also frequently improved unless resulting from hypocalcemia or hypoglycemia. Serum glucose and calcium levels should be monitored and glucose or calcium given if low. Recognition of this syndrome can prevent unnecessary cardiac catheterization in these ill infants as well as rapidly curing their illness.

## REFERENCE

1. Lovejoy, F. H., Jr., Smith, A. L., Bresnan, M. J., Wood, J. N., Victor, D. I., and Adams, P. C.: Clinical staging in Reye's syndrome, Am. J. Dis. Child. **128**:36, 1974.

## BIBLIOGRAPHY

Avery, M. E.: The lung and its disorders in the newborn infant, ed. 2, Philadelphia, 1968, W. B. Saunders Co.

Coleman, A. B., and Alpert, J. J.: Poisoning in children, Pediatr. Clin. North Am. **17**:471-753, 1970.

Cooke, R. E.: Biologic basis of pediatric practice, New York, 1968, McGraw-Hill Book Co.

Guide to diagnosis and management of cystic fibrosis, Atlanta, 1971, Cystic Fibrosis Foundation.

Kendig, E. L., Jr.: Pulmonary disorders. In Kendig, E. L., Jr., editor: Disorders of the respiratory tract in children, vol. 1, ed. 2, Philadelphia, 1972, W. B. Saunders Co.

Rowe, R. D., and Mehrizi, A.: The neonate with congenital heart disease, Philadelphia, 1968, W. B. Saunders Co.

Royer, P., Habib, R., Mathiew, H., and Broyer, M.: Pediatric nephrology, Philadelphia, 1974, W. B. Saunders Co.

Rudolph, A. M.: Congenital diseases of the heart, Chicago, 1974, Year Book Medical Publishers, Inc.

Shirkey, H. C.: Pediatric dosage handbook, ed. 2, Washington, D.C., 1973, American Pharmaceutical Corporation.

*chapter 26*

# Pathophysiology and treatment of circulatory shock

CLAYTON H. SHATNEY
RICHARD C. LILLEHEI

The definition of shock has always been a source of great controversy among investigators in the field. This problem has stemmed in part from the lack of knowledge of the precise pathophysiology of shock. The various types of shock and its many presentations have also added fuel to the controversy. Finally, there has been a tendency for each investigator to define shock in terms of the particular aspect under investigation in that particular laboratory or hospital. Nevertheless, one definition of circulatory shock has come to be generally accepted: shock occurs when perfusion of the bodily tissues is inadequate to sustain normal physiologic function.

## ■ What are the causes of shock?

There are three basic types of circulatory shock: (1) cardiogenic, (2) hemorrhagic (traumatic or oligemic), and (3) septic. Anaphylactic shock is a systemic hypersensitivity reaction that can occur when an individual is exposed to a substance to which he has become highly allergic. Although such a reaction can produce some of the classic manifestations of circulatory shock (pallor, hypotension, obtundation), this form of circulatory collapse is usually not considered to be a form of true shock for several reasons. First, it is usually readily managed by the combination of transient circulatory and respiratory support and antihistamines. In addition, problems associated with the true shock states, such as coagulation disorders and pulmonary dysfunction, do not generally follow an episode of anaphylactic shock.

Cardiogenic shock occurs when the heart is unable to pump a sufficient volume of blood to the tissues. The most common antecedent event is a massive myocardial infarction, following which there is an inadequate amount of functioning myocardium to meet the circulatory needs of the body. Cardiogenic shock can also occur after open-heart surgery or secondary to severe congestive heart failure caused by coronary artery, valvular, or myocardial disease. Although heart disease is the leading cause of death in the United States today, cardiogenic shock is the second most common form of circulatory shock. Because of its genesis, this form of shock is prevalent in the middle and older age groups.

Hemorrhagic or hypovolemic shock is the most common type of circulatory collapse in our society. Profound hemorrhage is the usual etiology of this form of shock, but it can also occur in patients who become severely dehydrated. Hemorrhagic shock is seen in patients of all ages, but because the most frequent antecedent event is trauma, oligemic shock tends to be most prevalent in the younger, more active age groups.

Septic shock is the third most frequently encountered form of shock, but its incidence is on the rise. It occurs in all age groups, and since it is caused by an overwhelming systemic infection, the aged and debilitated are most commonly affected with this condition.

**Table 26-1.** Comparison of endotoxin and gram-negative shock

| | *Cause of shock* | |
|---|---|---|
| *Parameter* | *Endotoxins* | *Gram-negative bacteria* |
| Mean arterial pressure | Low | Normal-low |
| Central venous pressure | Low | Low |
| Total peripheral resistance | High | Low |
| Cardiac index | Low | High |
| Arterial $O_2$ tension | Normal | Low |
| Pulmonary arteriovenous admixture | Normal | High |
| Lactic acidemia | High | High |

Although often used synonymously, a distinction should be made between endotoxin shock and septic shock (Table 26-1). Endotoxin shock is a form of circulatory collapse produced in experimental animals by the systemic injection of endotoxin, a lipopolysaccharide derived from the cell wall of gram-negative bacteria. Septic shock occurs in man and can be produced by gram-negative or gram-positive bacteria, fungi, yeast, and possibly viruses. Most instances in man are caused by gram-negative bacteria.

## ■ What parameters are used to evaluate and treat patients in shock?

In the past shock was usually equated with hypotension. However, with the advent of the intensive care unit and the resultant close monitoring and supervision of critically ill patients, most investigators realized that there was more to circulatory collapse than simply a decreased blood pressure. As we have become increasingly more sophisticated in the management of these patients, a host of hemodynamic and metabolic disturbances besides hypotension are now recognized to occur.

The hemodynamic parameters most frequently employed to describe and treat shock are the mean blood pressure, the cardiac output or index, and the total peripheral vascular resistance. These variables are interrelated by the formula:

$$P = F \times R$$

where P is the mean arterial blood pressure, F represents the systemic blood flow (that is, cardiac output), and R is the total peripheral vascular resistance. Both the mean blood pressure and the cardiac output are directly measurable in the patient. The total peripheral resistance (TPR, in dynes-sec/cm$^5$), however, is a derived function, that is obtained using the expression:

$$TPR = \frac{\overline{BP} - RAP}{CO} \times 80$$

where $\overline{BP}$ is the mean arterial blood pressure, RAP is the right atrial pressure, CO represents the cardiac output, and 80 is the standard conversion factor in the formula.

Using these hemodynamic variables and other measurable parameters, many derived indices can be obtained that are useful in evaluating and treating the patient in shock. One of the most commonly employed functions is the systemic oxygen consumption (SOC, in ml/min), which is determined by the following expression:

$$SOC = CO \times (A_{O_2} - V_{O_2})$$

where $A_{O_2}$ and $V_{O_2}$ are the arterial and venous oxygen contents, respectively. The SOC indicates the amount of oxygen utilized by the body each minute and thus gives an indication of the aerobic metabolic state.

Another helpful variable in these patients is the arteriovenous oxygen difference, which is simply $A_{O_2} - V_{O_2}$. This value is indicative of not only the state of oxygen uptake by the tissues, but also the amount of tissue perfusion. Further manipulation of these parameters results in a formula describing the oxygen extraction ratio $\frac{(A_{O_2} - V_{O_2})}{A_{O_2}}$, the oxygen availability ($A_{O_2} \times CO$), and a number of other variables that help to describe the hemodynamic-metabolic status of the patient in shock.

## ■ What is the pathophysiology of shock?

Although in the late stages there are many similarities among the various types of shock, the fundamental pathophysiology early in shock differs with each form of circulatory collapse. Much remains to be learned about the genesis of each type of shock. The following is an account of what is presently known.

### *Cardiogenic shock*

With the advent of coronary care units during the past decade the incidence of death caused by arrhythmias has dropped sharply in the early postinfarction period.[1] However, there has been no change in the incidence of power failure and shock in these patients.[2] In fact, cardiogenic shock is more frequently encountered today, because the prevention of deaths from rhythm disturbances has increased the population at risk.

Cardiogenic shock occurs when there is an insufficient amount of residual functioning myocardium to adequately perfuse the body. A recent study by Page et al.[3] has demonstrated that approximately 40% or more of the left ventricular mass must be lost for shock to occur. This amount of destruction may occur either with a massive acute myocardial infarction or following a succession of smaller infarcts. There does not appear to be a crucial area of the left ventricle that is necessary for proper myocardial function,[4, 5] although some studies have demonstrated a high frequency of apical infarction in patients who develop shock.[3, 6] It is most likely that the total area of left ventricular damage is the determining factor in the possible subsequent development of shock.

Because of the association between the size of the infarct and the occurrence of cardiogenic shock,[7] there has been a recent renewal of interest in the concept of infarct extension. A number of studies have demonstrated an ischemic zone surrounding a fresh infarct.[3, 8] This perimeter of marginally viable or ischemic tissue has the potential to undergo necrosis, thereby extending the area of the original infarct. Reid et al.[9] have recently demonstrated that such infarct extension occurs in 85% of patients following acute myocardial infarction. Through such exten-

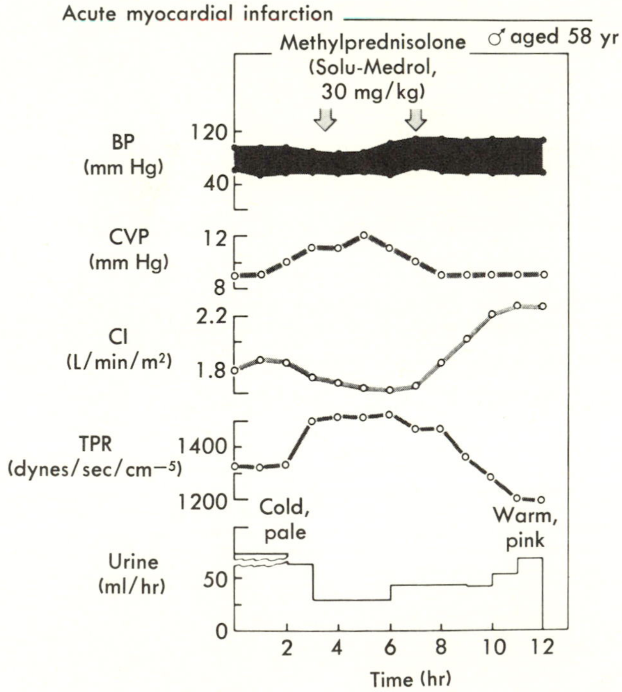


**Fig. 26-1.** Hemodynamic presentation of cardiogenic shock and the response to methylprednisolone (Solu-Medrol).

sion a patient may develop cardiogenic shock several days after the acute insult.

The initiating pathophysiologic event in cardiogenic shock is the acute inability of the heart to adequately perfuse the body. Cardiac output is markedly reduced because of a decrease in myocardial contractility[10] (Fig. 26-1). Coronary blood flow is reduced, and consequently myocardial oxygen extraction is high. Myocardial oxygen consumption can vary, but it is usually reduced. Because of the diminished supply of oxygen and nutrients, anaerobic metabolism occurs in the myocardium, as evidenced by excess lactate and lysosomal enzymes in the coronary sinus blood.[10, 11] Under the stimuli of hypoxia and acidosis the coronary arteries dilate in an attempt to divert blood to the ischemic myocardium.[12]

In addition to these myocardial responses to injury, a number of systemic compensatory changes occur when myocardial contractility is sufficiently reduced to cause a significant drop in the cardiac output (Fig. 26-1). With the fall in cardiac output the blood pressure initially declines. This reduction in the systemic perfusion pressure is detected by pressure-sensitive baroreceptors in the aortic arch and carotid sinus (Fig. 26-2). Through a combination of neurologic and humoral (epinephrine and norepinephrine) reactions mediated by the sympathetic nervous system, the body attempts to raise the systemic blood pressure in order to provide a sufficient head of pressure to adequatelv perfuse the organism. The net result of these neurologic and chemical inputs is an increase in the total peripheral vascular resistance, that is, systemic vasoconstriction in arterioles and venules (Fig. 26-3). We should note here that the increased total peripheral resistance further increases the ischemia of the heart by increasing the "afterload," or force required by the heart to expel blood from the left ventricle.

Despite the measurable increase in the total systemic vascular resistance, the caliber of *all* blood vessels is not reduced. Since the distribution of $\alpha$-receptors, which receive the com-

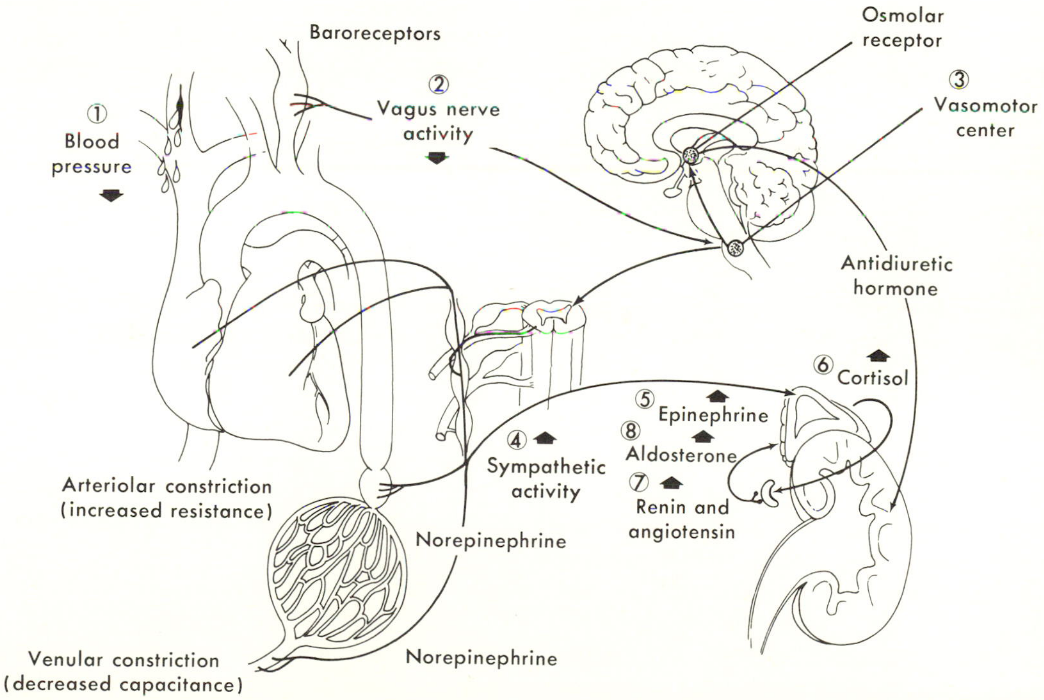


**Fig. 26-2.** Sympathoadrenal response to circulatory collapse. Circled numbers indicate sequence of events after initiation of sympathoadrenal response.

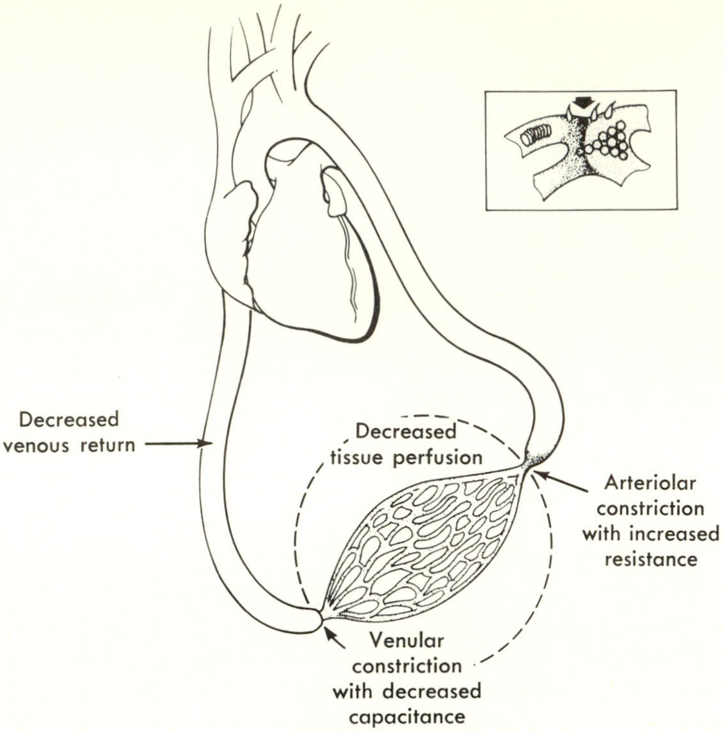


**Fig. 26-3.** Representation of the pathophysiology of ischemic anoxia in the capillary bed.

mands of the sympathetic nervous system, is not universal, some vascular beds are not constricted. The heart and brain, for example, contain few α-receptors, and the vessels supplying these vital organs are largely spared from the generalized vasoconstriction. Consequently, these organs preferentially receive more blood than other parts of the body during cardiogenic shock.

Shortly after the onset of the initial pathophysiologic changes the secondary effects of cardiogenic shock become evident. As a result of the heightened activity of the sympathetic nervous system and elevated levels of circulating catecholamines, the heart rate increases. Depending on the state of hydration of the patient and the magnitude of the pump failure, the central venous pressure and/or the pulmonary artery pressure may rise, and the patient may become dyspneic. Moreover, pulmonary arteriolar and venular constriction further impedes the flow of blood through the heart. The reduction in blood flow in the splanchnic circulation produces a drop in the urine output. Vasoconstriction in the cutaneous circulation, together with the generalized sympathetic discharge, produces a pale, cool, clammy quality in the skin. The poor perfusion of large areas of the body ultimately results in metabolic acidosis. In the majority of patients the respiratory system initially compensates for this acidosis, but with unrelenting circulatory collapse uncompensated metabolic acidosis eventually occurs.

The hallmarks of cardiogenic shock are therefore hypotension, low cardiac output, elevated peripheral vascular resistance, tachycardia, oliguria, and acidosis. The patient is cold, clammy, and often obtunded. Pulmonary edema is a common finding. The mortality in most series is in excess of 80%.[10]

### *Hemorrhagic shock*

Following the loss of more than 20% of the circulating blood volume, the signs of hypovolemic shock appear. Because of the reduction in the intravascular fluid volume, venous return to the heart is decreased.[13] The cardiac output consequently falls, and, mediated by the baroreceptor system, a sequence of physiologic compensatory events similar to that in cardiogenic shock occurs.

In order to maintain a systemic blood pressure sufficient to adequately perfuse the organism, the total peripheral vascular resistance rises.[14, 15] Through the combination of a reduction in cardiac output and a decrease in the caliber of the systemic blood vessels, blood flow to the splanchnic, pulmonary, cutaneous, and muscle beds is sharply reduced.[16-18] Because of the local autoregulatory mechanisms, however, not all organs are equally affected.[19] Blood flow in the kidney and liver is not depressed until late in the course of hemorrhagic shock.[18, 20-22] After an initial vasoconstrictor response the blood flow to the muscle mass rises as a result of autoregulatory "escape" from the sympathetic neurohumoral influence.[19] This competition between sympathoadrenal vasoconstriction and autoregulatory dilatation in various organs of the body is the normal physiologic compensatory mechanism that attempts to divert blood flow preferentially to the most vital organs. The net result is that in early hemorrhagic shock there is a redistribution of the cardiac output favoring the heart, brain, kidneys, and liver.[18]

The onset of oligemic shock also promotes the redistribution of body fluids in an attempt to increase the circulating intravascular volume. Interstitial fluid is transferred to the intravascular compartment at a rate approaching 1 L/hr.[23] Through the combination of a redistribution of renal blood flow within the kidneys and an increase in the circulating level of antidiuretic hormone (ADH), the renal excretion of water is markedly reduced.[24] Although the bowel is capable of normal secretion during early hypovolemic shock,[25] the dramatic reduction in superior mesenteric artery blood flow prevents this potential "third-space" fluid loss within the gastrointestinal tract. The entire organism therefore becomes oriented toward not only retaining fluid, but also transferring that fluid to the intravascular compartment.

These volume-regulating compensatory responses are capable of transiently sustaining life and even promoting survival if the duration of shock is brief. With continued blood loss or delayed or inadequate volume replacement, however, the pronounced systemic vasoconstriction and hypovolemia produce ischemia and stagnant hypoxia in the viscerocutaneous circulation. The results of this decreased systemic perfusion are anaerobic cellular metabolism, lactic acidosis, and cell death, all of which further compromise the organism (Fig. 26-4).

It has long been observed that myocardial function deteriorates in prolonged oligemic shock. The initial fall in cardiac output following hemorrhage is strictly caused by the reduction in venous return to the heart as a result of the loss of circulating blood volume. With persistent blood loss or inadequate treatment there is a further reduction in cardiac output as a result of the inability of the cardiovascular compensatory mechanisms (increased heart rate, increased peripheral resistance) to keep up with the loss of intravascular volume. Although there are individual variations, coronary blood flow essentially parallels the systemic flow pattern in hemorrhagic shock. Ultimately blood flow during systole far exceeds that in diastole, and coronary filling and flow become persistently reduced.[26] With the onset of ischemia, cardiac function begins to deteriorate, and myocardial oxygen availability and consumption fall.[27]

In addition to the detrimental effects of these coronary perfusion abnormalities on cardiac function, there is evidence that a myocardial depressant factor (MDF) may be present in the circulation of animals and man during hemorrhagic (and septic) shock.[28, 29] This peptide has been isolated from the venous effluent of the ischemic pancreas and has been shown to depress myocardial contractility. The existence of an MDF in shock is still quite controversial, however, since other investigators have either been unable to detect it or have attributed the myocardial depressant activity in shock serum to electrolyte disturbances.[30, 31] Regardless of the precise mechanisms involved, hemorrhagic shock

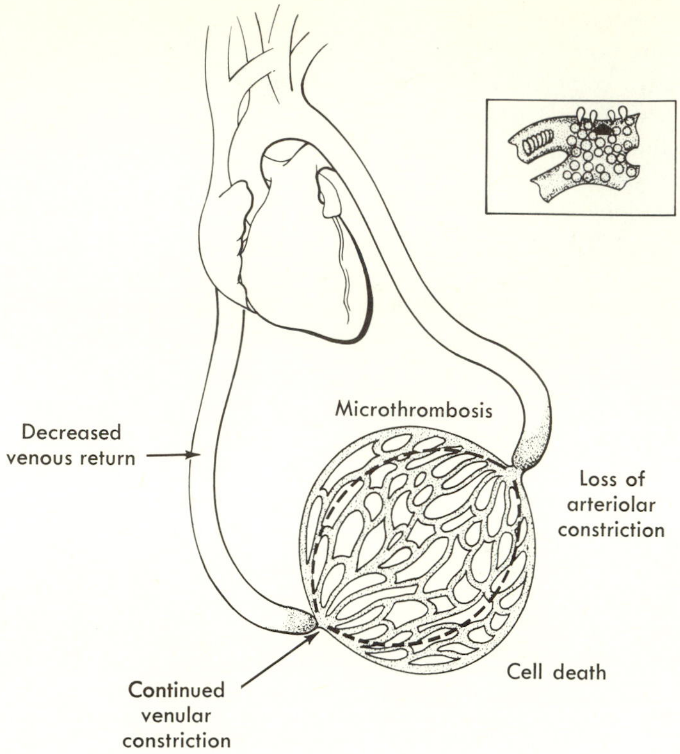


**Fig. 26-4.** Stagnant anoxia resulting from severe initial stress or prolonged shock states.

is associated with an absolute reduction in cardiac performance, especially late in the course of circulatory collapse.

During the past several years the cellular effects of hypovolemic shock have been extensively studied. Because the ultimate pathophysiology is similar, many of these findings also apply to cardiogenic shock.

An early effect of hypotension and hypoxia is the shift of cellular metabolism from aerobic to less efficient anaerobic metabolic pathways.[32] The end product of cellular metabolism thus changes from carbon dioxide and water to lactic acid. Hobler and Carey[33] have shown experimentally that in normotensive dogs excess lactate begins to accumulate when the arterial oxygen tension falls below 36 mm Hg. An abrupt decrease also occurs in the systemic oxygen consumption, reflecting the cellular utilization of anaerobic metabolic pathways. With hypotension superimposed on hypoxia even less oxygen is delivered to the cells, enhancing the rate of appearance of anaerobic metabolism.

Although anaerobic metabolism is capable of temporarily sustaining the majority of the cells of the body, it is much less efficient than aerobic metabolism. Thus tissue adenosine triphosphate (ATP) levels progressively decline with continued hemorrhagic shock.[34, 35] Because the cyclic nucleotides (cAMP, cGMP) are derived from ATP, their cellular concentrations also decline.[36] Since these cyclic nucleotides are thought to be the intracellular "messengers" that directly regulate the quality and quantity of cellular metabolic processes, the reduction in their generation has profound effects on cell function in general.

The combination of hypotension and hypoxia results in significant functional and morphologic changes in the intracellular organelles[37] (Fig. 26-5). Baue and Sayeed[38] found a reduction in the functional capacity of mitochondria in hemorrhagic shock. Not only was the oxidation of substrates reduced, but the efficiency of the electron transport system was also impaired. These authors

A

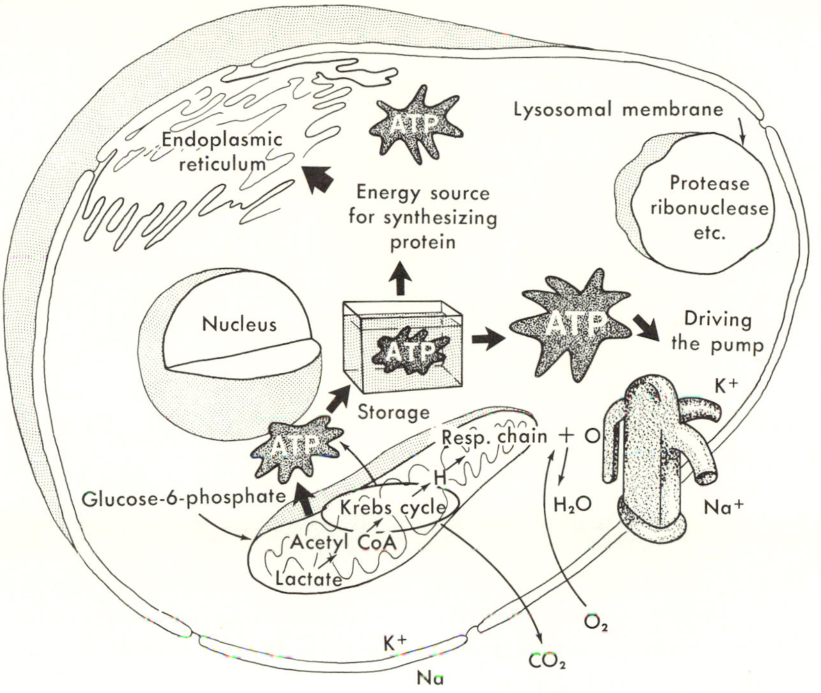


B

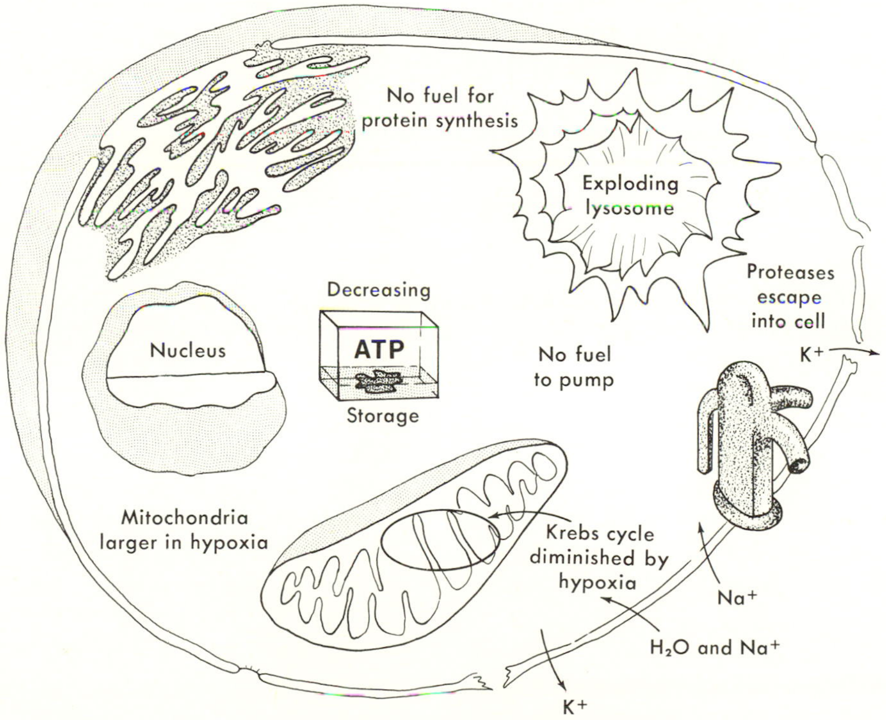


**Fig. 26-5. A,** Normal cell. **B,** Cell in shock.

demonstrated that mitochondrial concentrations of sodium and calcium increased, whereas the levels of potassium and magnesium decreased.[39] Since the changes in mitochondrial function are reversed by correction of these electrolyte abnormalities, it appears that electrolyte disturbances are intimately involved in the observed functional impairment of mitochondria during hypovolemic shock. The ultimate consequences of depressed mitochondrial activity are reductions in the tissue levels of the high-energy compound ATP as well as the intracellular messengers derived from ATP.

Another organelle profoundly affected during hemorrhagic shock is the lysosome. This structure becomes very fragile in the face of hypotension, hypoxia, or acidosis. With prolonged oligemic shock an increasing number of lysosomes rupture and discharge their contents into the cell. The concentration of these substances in the serum progressively rises with the duration of circulatory collapse.[40-42] Once released from the cell of origin, lysosomal enzymes may exert detrimental effects on the morphology and function of other cells and intracellular organelles.[43, 44] Although the primary site of lysosomal enzyme release during hemorrhagic shock is the gastrointestinal tract, substantial amounts have also been detected in the venous effluent from other splanchnic tissues.[40, 41] Regardless of the site of origin, these lysosomal enzymes have the potential to exert such adverse effects that they have been entertained as the controversial "shock toxin" that is common to all types of circulatory collapse and that determines irreversibility in shock.[45] At present, however, evidence is inconclusive for the existence of such a substance in all forms of shock.[46]

The observed changes in the structure and function of cells and intracellular organelles in hemorrhagic shock has been linked by membrane physiologists to profound alterations in the integrity of cell membranes. Studies by Cunningham et al.,[47] Shires et al.,[48] and Trunkey et al.[49] on skeletal muscle have shown increases in intracellular water and sodium and a decrease in potassium during hypovolemic shock. A concomitant decrease in extracellular fluid and an increase in interstitial potassium were observed. Associated with these changes was a marked reduction of the resting cell membrane potential, a decrease in the amplitude of the action potential, and a prolongation of both depolarization and repolarization times. Although the exact cause of these electrical changes during hemorrhagic shock is unknown, the results have been interpreted as reflecting either changes in the transport properties of muscle cells or a reduction in the efficiency of the active sodium pump. Similar data have been obtained in the kidney, connective tissue, and muscle by Essiet and Stahl[50] and in red blood cells by Johnson and Baggett.[51]

The pathologic cellular alterations in hypovolemic shock are abundantly reflected in the changes seen in many important clinical parameters used to evaluate and treat patients. The ultimate appearance of metabolic acidosis caused by the production of excess lactic acid by cells undergoing anaerobic metabolism has already been discussed. Depending on the state of the kidneys and the lungs, however, many patients seen in early hemorrhagic shock may have a normal blood pH or may even be slightly alkalotic as a result of adequate compensatory mechanisms, principally hyperventilation.[52] With prolonged circulatory collapse and the associated visceral vasoconstriction the compensatory ability of the kidneys is markedly reduced. In addition, the capacity for compensation of systemic acidosis by the lungs is severely restricted because of a number of changes that can occur in this organ during hemorrhagic shock. Thus with sustained shock acidosis is an almost universal finding.

Another systemic complication of oligemic shock is the appearance of coagulation abnormalities in an appreciable number of patients sustaining massive trauma.[53] The superimposition of sepsis on a traumatized patient makes the likelihood of coagulopathy even greater.[54] Although the coagulation changes can vary with the patient, the most frequent abnormalities include elevations in the prothrombin time and activated partial thromboplastin time and a depression of the platelet count. When coagulation factors are followed serially, decreased levels of factor V and plasminogen and increased amounts of fibrin degradation products are found, indicating the presence of intravascular coagulation abnormalities. Such coagulation abnormalities place the patient at a greater risk of spontaneous bleeding and microembolization. The latter can significantly contribute to both the hepatic and pulmonary dysfunction seen in patients after traumatic shock.[55, 56] Intravascular coagulopathy is not detectable in all traumatized patients, but when it does occur, there is a strong correlation between its magnitude and the severity of shock in the patient, suggesting that it plays a detrimental role.[57, 58]

The response of the endocrine system to hemorrhagic shock has been extensively investigated in recent years. The early release of epinephrine from the adrenal medulla and norepinephrine from the sympathetic nerve terminals has already been discussed. In addition to effecting compensatory cardiovascular changes, these substances exert profound biochemical effects on several organs. In experimental hemorrhagic shock in dogs there is a significant increase in systemic oxygen uptake when acidosis is prevented and a decrease if the pH is allowed to drop.[59] This enhanced oxygen consumption has been theoretically related to a catecholamine-induced acceleration of free fatty acid turnover.

Hyperglycemia, initially resulting from catecholamine-induced hepatic glycogenolysis, is a hallmark of traumatic shock. Blood glucose levels become elevated shortly after the onset of circulatory collapse and remain increased for several hours.[60] Serum insulin concentration, however, is low during oligemic shock in both experimental animals and man[60, 61] because of the depression of pancreatic insulin secretion[61, 62] by both hypotension and catecholamine stimulation. Thus the hyperglycemia of traumatic shock is related to the hepatic release of glucose and suppression of the normal insulin response to elevated serum blood glucose levels.

Although from the standpoint of cellular metabolism the increase in blood glucose is a potentially beneficial systemic response to stress, the lack of insulin prevents most of the circulating glucose from entering the cells to be available as metabolic fuel. To some extent this reduction in the availability of glucose as a metabolic substrate is compensated by higher levels of serum free fatty acids, which are the result of elevated concentrations of growth hormone during shock.[59, 63, 64] These fatty acids in the blood may be the source of fat emboli seen in the lungs and other viscera at autopsy of patients dying of shock without long bone fracture. The net result of these endocrine responses to hemorrhage, however, is a decrease in the amount of readily metabolizable substrates available to cells that have already been forced to resort to less efficient anaerobic metabolic pathways.

### *Septic shock*

In the face of an overwhelming infection a patient may suddenly experience a fever spike, mental confusion, tachypnea, oliguria, and tachycardia. The skin may be cool and clammy, or it may be warm and pink. Hypotension may or may not be present. The cardiac output is either normal or high, and the total peripheral vascular resistance is reduced. This constellation of signs and symptoms of septic shock in its early stage (Table 26-1) differs markedly from that following hemorrhage or myocardial infarction, although in later stages these differences tend to disappear.

Unlike cardiogenic or traumatic shock, septic shock appears to pass through at least three fairly distinct stages.[65-67] The usual initial presentation consists of a hyperdynamic cardiovascular and metabolic picture. The blood pressure is generally normal, and the cardiac output is high. Since hypotension is not a common feature in early septic shock, there is frequently a delay in the diagnosis of this condition. If one is attuned to the presenting symptoms, especially mental confusion, and the clinical setting of bacteremic shock, the diagnosis and treatment can be established quite early in the course of the disease.

The patient can remain in the early, hyperdynamic stage of septic shock for many hours before signs of deterioration appear. As shock progresses, the cardiovascular status changes to a normodynamic pattern. The heart rate remains elevated, but the cardiac output is in the normal range. The blood pressure is somewhat reduced, and the peripheral vascular resistance remains below normal. The patient continues to hyperventilate, and respiratory assistance is frequently necessary because of a progressively declining arterial $P_{O_2}$. The urine output remains low, and frank renal shutdown is common. This middle stage of bacteremic shock is usually of brief duration (several hours), and patients not responding to treatment soon experience profound cardiovascular decompensation.

Late, or preterminal, septic shock is almost invariably manifested by a hypodynamic cardiovascular picture, since cardiac insufficiency is the rule. It is in this stage of bacteremic shock that the "classic" signs and symptoms of circulatory collapse exist: hypotension, low cardiac output, and high total peripheral resistance. The heart rate continues to be elevated, and urine output is scanty at best. The stroke index, left ventricular stroke work, and other parameters of cardiac performance rapidly deteriorate. The central venous and pulmonary artery wedge pressures rise. Mechanical respiratory assistance is unable to correct either the profound hypoxia or the metabolic acidosis. Patients who remain in this decompensated state for more than a few hours fail to survive.

In addition to the hemodynamic differences between septic shock and cardiogenic and hypovolemic shock, there are striking metabolic differences that result from the cellular and systemic actions of bacteria and

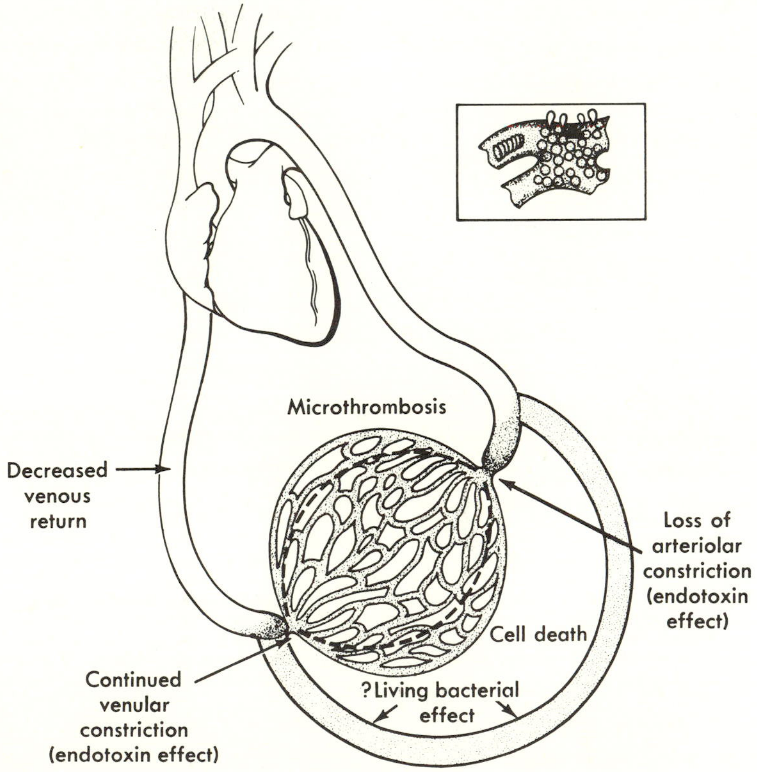


**Fig. 26-6.** Cellular anoxia in septic shock is associated with venular constriction and severe arteriovenous shunting thought to be caused by an inflammatory effect of living bacteria.

their toxins. A striking finding in patients seen in early septic shock is profound systemic vasodilatation, usually associated with a very high cardiac output. Although cellular metabolic factors may play a role in the genesis of the elevated cardiac index, thus making vasodilatation more apparent than real, most evidence indicates that the converse is true. In other words, it appears that the high cardiac index is primarily caused by the decreased systemic resistance in selected areas against which the heart has to pump.[68-70]

Another consistent finding during the early and middle stages of bacteremic shock is a decrease in the pulmonary and systemic arteriovenous oxygen difference indicative of shunting in these circulatory systems[66, 70] (Fig. 26-6). As a result of these shunts, vast areas of the body are not perfused with blood. These underperfused tissues soon become hypoxic, and anaerobic metabolism with lactic acid production ensues. Oxygen extraction and consumption decline, and metabolic acidosis occurs[71] (Fig. 26-7). As a result of specific depressant action(s) of endotoxin on carbohydrate metabolism, cellular glucose utilization is markedly reduced.[72, 73] Lysosomal enzymes become elevated in the systemic circulation and add further insult to the tissue injury caused by bacterial toxins and ischemia.[74]

Initially the lungs can compensate for the metabolic acidosis by reducing the arterial carbon dioxide tension. Thus patients in early septic shock are usually mildly alkalotic and hypocapnic. With time, however, bacterial toxins exert pronounced detrimental effects on pulmonary structure and function. Pulmonary edema and cytoplasmic swelling of alveolar type I and II cells are histologically evident early in bacteremic shock.[75, 76] These changes are caused in part by hypotension and by a direct action of endotoxin on pulmonary capillaries, resulting in an increase in membrane permeability.[77] The consequences of these pulmonary cellular changes are a decreased oxygen-diffusing capacity of the lung, a reduced pulmonary compliance, and an increase in the work of breathing. Systemic hypoxia occurs and is frequently resistant to increasing concentrations of oxygen in the

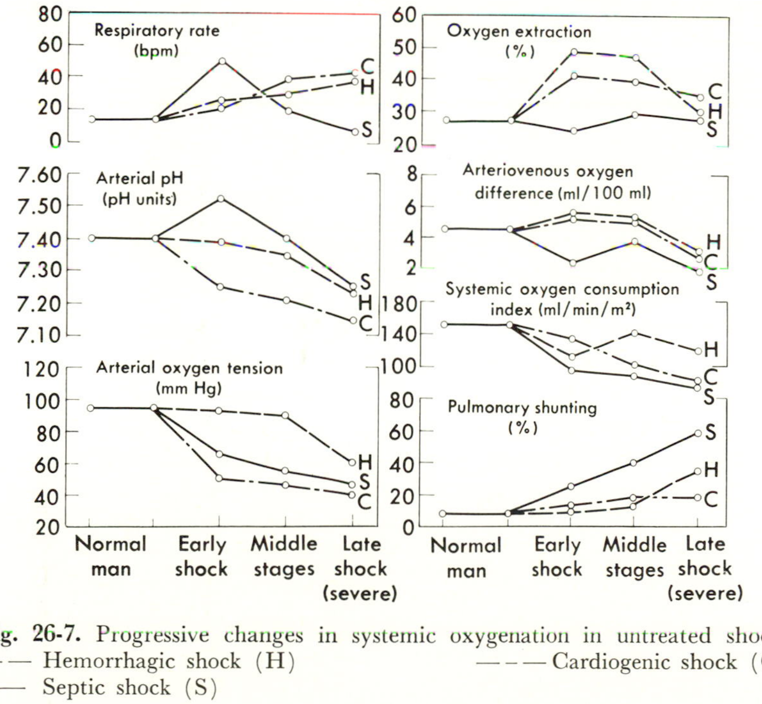


**Fig. 26-7.** Progressive changes in systemic oxygenation in untreated shock.
— — Hemorrhagic shock (H) — - — Cardiogenic shock (C)
—— Septic shock (S)

inspired air. The ability of the lungs to oxygenate blood is initially impaired, but ultimately the arterial $P_{CO_2}$ increases also. The net result of these pulmonary events is a reduction in the delivery of oxygen to the tissues. Anaerobic metabolism then supports these areas, and metabolic acidosis worsens.[78] As a result of the severe reduction in the functional capacity of the respiratory system, uncompensated metabolic acidosis occurs, leaving the patient in a preterminal state.[65]

In addition to the decreased ability of septic patients to extract sufficient oxygen from both the inspired air and the blood, there are adverse changes in the oxygen-carrying capacity of the blood. Red blood cell 2,3-diphosphoglycerate (DPG) concentration is reduced, and the oxyhemoglobin dissociation curve is shifted to the left.[79, 80] Thus hemoglobin has less tendency to release oxygen, and consequently the transfer of oxygen to the tissues being perfused is reduced. Intravascular coagulation, caused by fibrin deposition and platelet aggregation, and the ultimate deterioration of cardiac function, perhaps caused by an MDF released from the ischemic pancreas, further decrease the delivery of oxygen to the tissues.[81, 82]

In summary, current evidence strongly suggests that the basic pathophysiology of septic shock is markedly different from that in shock following hemorrhage or myocardial infarction. Whereas in the latter two forms of circulatory collapse hemodynamic alterations precede metabolic changes, in bacteremic shock cellular derangements apparently precede and may form the etiology of cardiovascular abnormalities. As a result of the combined effects of cellular and hemodynamic aberrations, however, the late stage of septic shock is remarkably similar to that found in hemorrhagic and cardiogenic shock, consisting of hypotension, vasoconstriction, low cardiac output, hypoxia, and acidosis.

## ■ What is shock lung?

A patient (S. L.) involved in a motor vehicle accident is rushed to the emergency room. On examination he is unconscious, has a fractured femur and pelvis, and is in shock with signs of intra-abdominal hemorrhage. There is no injury apparent on clinical or roentgenologic examination of the chest. After the initiation of resuscitative measures the patient is taken to the operating room, where he is found to have a ruptured spleen, a contusion of the pancreas, and a laceration of the left lobe of the liver. A splenectomy is performed, and the hepatic wound is oversewn. Following surgery the hypotension relents, and the patient is voiding satisfactory amounts of urine. He has received 5000 ml of crystalloid solution and 10 units of whole blood since the injury.

In the immediate postoperative period the patient's course is uncomplicated. The vital signs remain within normal limits, the mental status clears, and the patient is extubated. On the second postoperative day, however, the patient progressively develops agitation, dyspnea, tachypnea, and cyanosis. Blood gas determinations reveal a pH of 7.48, a $P_{O_2}$ of 50 mm Hg, and a $P_{CO_2}$ of 28 mm Hg. The chest x-ray film shows a diffuse, patchy infiltrate (Fig. 26-8). The patient is reintubated and placed on a volume respirator on 40% oxygen. During the ensuing 48 hours progressively higher inspiratory pressures and oxygen concentrations are required to maintain an adequate arterial oxygen tension. The chest roentgenogram reveals increasing consolidation, and the arterial oxygen tension remains reduced despite all resuscitative efforts. Now the blood pressure and cardiac output begin to fall, and the pulmonary artery wedge pressure rises. Death occurs on the morning of the fifth postoperative day. At autopsy the lungs are heavy and hemorrhagic and resemble liver on cross section. The cause of death is variously called acute respiratory distress syndrome, posttraumatic pulmonary insufficiency syndrome, or "shock lung."

Shock lung refers to a syndrome of symptoms and pathologic findings in patients who sustain major nonthoracic trauma. This syndrome has attracted a considerable amount of attention in recent years, because its incidence is apparently on the rise.[83] This increase is probably a result of the greater familiarity with the problem and thus more frequent diagnosis, as well as increasingly successful efforts in resuscitating patients who would have died earlier. Hence patients who formerly died in shock are now successfully supported through the acute event and are at risk from death resulting from such complications as acute renal failure, gastrointestinal bleeding, and pulmonary insufficiency. Currently patients dying from shock or mas-

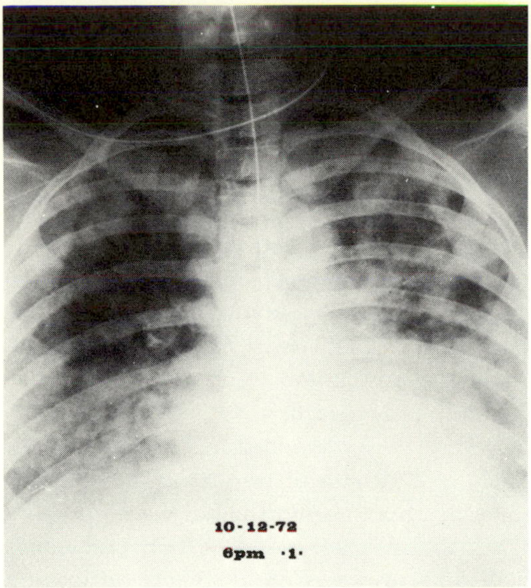


**Fig. 26-8.** Radiologic findings in posttraumatic pulmonary insufficiency syndrome.

sive trauma more frequently exhibit pathologic changes in the lungs than in any other organ.[84]

The diagnostic features of posttraumatic pulmonary insufficiency are marked respiratory distress and hypoxia (arterial oxygen tension less than 50 mm Hg) with associated pulmonary infiltrates and/or consolidation. The syndrome can occur with any type of severe injury or sepsis, with or without attendant shock. However, respiratory insufficiency following trauma is more common in patients who have shock and hypoxia when initially seen.[85] The syndrome is insidious in onset and thus is not usually diagnosed prior to the appearance of severe symptoms. The reported mortality in this condition is 50% to 90%.[86]

Besides hypoxia and tachypnea, several other systemic and pulmonary aberrations have been noted in patients with shock lung. The arterial carbon dioxide tension is generally normal or only slightly decreased because of the increased respiratory rate. Likewise, the pH is normal or slightly alkalotic in the early stages. The cardiac index and systemic oxygen consumption vary widely early in the course of the syndrome, but generally decrease with time. Virtually all patients exhibit reduced pulmonary compliance, increased physiologic dead space, increased pulmonary arteriovenous shunting, and abnormal ventilation-perfusion ratios.[87-89] In the few patients in whom pulmonary diffusing capacity was measured, it was reduced.[88]

The pathologic findings in the lungs vary with the duration of the syndrome. The initial changes consist of scattered petechial hemorrhages and areas of consolidation and atelectasis in the lower lung fields. Under light microscopy there is capillary engorgement, atelectasis, interstitial edema, and thromboemboli in the small pulmonary blood vessels.[87, 88] With time, hemorrhagic consolidation of the lung occurs. There is severe pulmonary venous congestion and interstitial edema with peribronchial, perivascular, and intra-alveolar hemorrhage. Ultimately the lungs grossly resemble liver. Microscopically there are hyaline membranes in the alveoli and diffuse hemorrhage, congestion, and bronchopneumonia.[87]

The etiology of posttraumatic pulmonary insufficiency is unknown, but a number of factors have been implicated. Certainly shock itself with the attendant acidosis, reduced pulmonary blood flow, and increased pulmonary vascular resistance (caused by arteriolar and venular vasoconstriction) plays a role.[90-93] However, low blood flow is not the sole cause, since the lung is capable of withstanding short periods of ischemia without apparent damage.[87, 94] Thromboemboli in the pulmonary vascular tree caused by intravascular coagulation and the administration of blood products has been implicated in the shock lung syndrome.[87] High levels of circulating catecholamines, histamine, and serotonin have also been entertained as factors.[95] Other investigators have stressed the injurious effects of fat emboli,[96, 97] since respiratory insufficiency following trauma is more common in patients sustaining long bone fractures.[85] The origin of the fat emboli may be from the marrow of long bone fractures but more likely is from the extensive fatty acid mobilization that occurs in severe stress.

Oxygen toxicity has also been cited as a contributing influence in the genesis of shock lung, since a large number of these patients have required mechanical respiratory support with high inspired oxygen concentrations from the time of injury.[98, 99]

The bulk of the recent investigative work on posttraumatic pulmonary insufficiency has been concentrated on the volume of IV fluids used in resuscitating traumatized patients. Virtually all patients who develop shock lung have received massive amounts of IV fluids and blood products, and the point has been raised that perhaps the syndrome is really an iatrogenic disease.[85, 100] Magilligan et al.[101] and Fulton and Fischer[102] showed in dogs that resuscitation from hemorrhagic shock with normal saline solution resulted in an increase in pulmonary extracellular water and pulmonary dysfunction, suggesting that the sodium load was the etiologic factor. With the use of hypertonic saline solution Fulton and Fischer[102] found that the functional and morphologic pulmonary changes were reduced, indicating that a large fluid volume increased the sodium-induced collection of fluid in the lungs. Although initial studies in baboons by Seigel and Moss revealed no functional pulmonary impairment following saline resuscitation from hypovolemic shock, subsequent work in their laboratory has demonstrated the accumulation of sodium and fluid in the pulmonary interstitium of these animals.[103-106]

Although excessive amounts of crystalloids are associated with respiratory insufficiency, massive blood replacement is also a factor in the genesis of pulmonary insufficiency.[83, 107] Dacron-wool filtration of infused blood decreases the pulmonary pathology by eliminating most of the platelet and leukocyte microaggregates,[108] but large amounts of even filtered blood may be injurious to the lungs.[109] In summary, the effects of the sympathoadrenal response to shock in the lung with arteriolar and venular vasoconstriction reduce its ability to tolerate large volumes of any IV replacement fluid.

In addition to controversy over the etiology of posttraumatic pulmonary insufficiency, there is also debate concerning the pulmonary pathology necessary to produce the syndrome. Both Bryant et al.[110] and Wilson et al.[111] reported functional respiratory impairment out of proportion to the morphologic changes observed in the lungs of dogs following hemorrhagic shock. These findings led them to conclude that the functional pulmonary changes were not significant in determining irreversibility in shock and that respiratory insufficiency was the result of vigorous resuscitation in the face of reversible pulmonary injury. Other investigators, however, have demonstrated marked functional and structural respiratory impairment resulting from hemorrhagic shock alone.[95, 111, 112] Henry et al.[113] found that pulmonary pathology progressively increased during the recovery period. Pulmonary congestion was the earliest change, and this picture progressed with time to peribronchial and perivascular edema and hemorrhage. Patchy atelectasis and consolidation occurred during the third and fourth hours after shock. These studies indicate that hemorrhagic shock itself can be responsible for creating significant damage to the lungs and that these other injurious factors are superimposed on the initial pathology caused by the shock or trauma.

From the data currently available a sequence of events can be outlined in the development of shock lung. With the onset of circulatory collapse both the systemic and pulmonary artery pressure and blood flow decline, and pulmonary vascular resistance increases. Because of these hemodynamic changes the distribution of pulmonary blood flow is altered so that the dependent portions of the lungs are preferentially perfused. With continued hypotension, pulmonary blood flow first shifts to the previously underperfused, less dependent areas and then is ultimately distributed throughout the lungs in a pattern similar to that in the preshock period.[114, 115] In response to the hypoperfusion and under the influence of hypoxia, histamine, and serotonin, the permeability of pulmonary capillaries increases, and fluid collects in the interstitium. There is also a loss of albumin that further increases edema through a decrease in the colloid osmotic pressure of the blood. Interstitial edema causes the lungs to become relatively stiff, and pulmonary compliance decreases while dead space increases. The combination of acidosis, edema, ischemia, and hypoxia promotes bronchoconstriction, which increases airway resistance and creates ventilation-perfusion abnormalities and pulmonary shunting.

With continued shock or overly vigorous resuscitation these early changes progress. The integrity of the pulmonary capillary endothelial membrane becomes disrupted, and interstitial edema increases. Pericapillary and peribronchial extravasation of red blood cells occurs. Scattered areas of atelectasis appear and increase the ventilation-perfusion defect. Destructive changes occur in types I and II alveolar cells, and surfactant synthesis is impaired.[116, 117] The consequent reduction in intra-alveolar surface tension accentuates the atelectasis and thus reduces the surface area available for gas exchange. The diffusing capacity for oxygen is reduced, and systemic hypoxia occurs. The decreased ability of the lungs to exchange gases also creates progressive hypercapnia, and uncompensated metabolic acidosis ultimately occurs. Acidosis compounds the pulmonary effects of hypotension, and a vicious cycle is created, which, if not interrupted, eventually destroys the lung and kills the patient. Superimposed on this basic shock-induced pulmonary pathology are the effects of microemboli from contused soft tissue, intravascular coagulation, and infused blood; fat emboli from coalescing fatty acids in the blood and/or extremity fractures; high oxygen concentrations in the inspired air; and fluid overload. These additional factors are capable of converting the initial, potentially reversible pulmonary changes to a state where shock lung becomes clinically evident.

## ■ What is the treatment of shock?

The proper management of the patient with circulatory collapse depends on an accurate initial assessment and frequent reassessment of the ongoing pathophysiologic processes. Although the specific treatment program varies with both the type of shock and the individual patient, the method of patient evaluation and many of the forms of treatment used are common to all forms of shock.

The initial step in evaluating the patient in shock is to obtain a good history and perform a thorough physical examination. As with any other disease, the history and physical examination will indicate the diagnosis in the majority of patients. Particular attention should be given to the respiratory status of the patient, and if necessary an airway and assisted ventilation should be employed.

Because of the possibility of sepsis as the cause of shock, all IV and urinary catheters and tubing should be removed, cultured, and replaced. A closed-drainage urinary catheter system is mandatory in order to reduce the incidence of subsequent urinary tract infection. Samples from blood, sputum, urine, and drainage tubes are obtained for gram stain and culture. An arterial catheter is inserted, usually into a brachial or radial artery, for accurate measurement of blood pressure and for use in determining cardiac output with dye dilution curves. In selected patients with cardiogenic shock a balloon-tipped catheter may be introduced into a major vein and advanced into the pulmonary artery. Blood samples are drawn for the determination of arterial gas concentrations, hemoglobin, leukocyte count, electrolyte levels, proteins, glucose levels, and clotting studies. An ECG and chest x-ray film are obtained, and the initial set of hemodynamic measurements is made.

Using this systematic approach to the evaluation of patients in shock, it is possible to establish the type of shock and to determine the hemodynamic and metabolic status of the patient within the first 30 to 60 minutes after the onset of circulatory collapse. The importance of obtaining such studies, which enable the practitioner to tailor the treatment to the patient's needs, cannot be overemphasized. In extremely urgent circumstances it may be necessary to forego some of these initial assessments and begin treatment more promptly. As soon as the patient's condition has stabilized, however, a complete hemodynamic and metabolic evaluation should be undertaken.

Since the basic pathophysiology of shock varies with the cause of the circulatory collapse, there are differences in the manner in which each type of shock is treated. As already indicated, attention should first be directed to the respiratory status of the patient, since potential pulmonary disturbances are an integral part of the picture in any form of circulatory collapse. As soon as proper steps have been taken to correct the respiratory and acid-base disturbances, other measures are initiated in line with the etiology of the shock.

### *Hemorrhagic shock*

In hypovolemic shock the basic defect is the lack of an adequate circulating blood volume, and the essence of treatment is the replacement of the patient's fluid losses, which in most instances involves whole blood (Table 26-2). Since some delay is experienced in obtaining properly matched blood for transfusion, the patient must be initially supported by nonerythrocyte-containing solutions. In the past there was considerable debate over not only the merits of colloid versus crystalloid solutions but also over the relative values of the various kinds of colloid and crystalloid solutions used. Much of this controversy has been resolved in recent years, and current evidence indicates that the patient in hemorrhagic shock can be hemodynamically supported during the initial phase of resuscitation with Ringer's solution, normal saline solution, low molecular weight dextran, or a 5% albumin solution.[118, 119] Furthermore, Reich and Eiseman[120] have demonstrated normal tissue oxygenation following resuscitation with Ringer's solution. Contrary to previous belief, the use of lactated Ringer's solution does not increase serum lactate concentration and contribute to metabolic acidosis.[118, 121]

**Table 26-2.** Treatment of traumatic shock

| *Condition to be corrected (restored)* | *Treatment* |
|---|---|
| Hypovolemia | Control of hemorrhage; blood plasma fractions, dextran, crystalloids |
| Stagnant anoxia, membrane integrity | Synthetic glucocorticosteroids (methylprednisolone, dexamethasone) |
| Oncotic pressure | Albumin |
| Oliguria | Furosemide |
| Hypoxemia | Respirator (volume type, positive end-expiratory pressure) |

Any of the solutions just mentioned are capable of supporting the patient in hypovolemic shock until matched blood becomes available. A balance of crystalloid and colloid is probably the best choice in order to avoid pulmonary congestion. Whatever type of fluid is used, warming of the fluid to at least room temperature prior to administration is of some benefit if the fluids are given rapidly.[122]

Although the immediate steps in the resuscitation of the patient in hemorrhagic shock are directed toward correcting the respiratory and circulatory deficits, another initial concern should be to discover and control the source of the fluid loss, in most instances bleeding. Pressure is applied to obvious external bleeding points. Surgery is usually required to control internal sites of hemorrhage. In patients with pelvic fractures and shock a G suit may significantly decrease blood loss and improve survival.[123] Whatever the source, it is imperative that any major bleeding be controlled early in order to reduce the duration of circulatory collapse and the likelihood of subsequent complications.

In patients where the source of bleeding is obscure, a peritoneal lavage using 1 L of 5% glucose instilled through a dialysis catheter may be of help. If the fluid that returns out the catheter is grossly bloody or if it contains more than 100,000 red blood cells/$mm^3$, then a laparotomy should be done to find the source of bleeding. Similarly, if the white blood cell count of the fluid is greater than 500 cells/$mm^3$, then a perforated bowel, stomach, or gallbladder may be the source of shock.

Although blood and IV fluids are the cornerstone of treatment, certain other maneuvers are helpful in both clinical and experimental hypovolemic shock. Exogenous glucose, for reasons that are not clear, improves hemodynamics and survival in oligemic shock.[124, 125] Glucagon increases the cardiac output and stroke volume and lowers the total peripheral resistance and the splanchnic resistance in experimental hypovolemic shock.[126] In addition, glucagon appears to stimulate the hepatic conversion of lactic, amino, and fatty acids to glucose, and it possibly increases ATP production.[127] We have not found glucagon to be a beneficial agent clinically. The administration of high-energy compounds (ATP-$MgCl_2$) is beneficial in experimental hemorrhagic shock,[128, 129] but the treatment has not been clinically evaluated. Phenoxybenzamine, by reducing peripheral resistance and improving renal blood flow, may be helpful in hypovolemic shock.[130]

In many instances of multisystem trauma merely restoring the blood volume may not be enough to successfully resuscitate the patient. Here the use of massive doses of glucocorticosteroids may correct hemodynamic and cellular disturbances of shock by a variety of effects,[131, 132] as shown in the following list:

*Effects of glucocorticosteroids in shock*

1. Restoration of vascular membrane integrity in lung, intestine, and forelimb
2. Stabilization of lysosomal membranes of lung, pancreas, liver, and kidney
3. Increases in visceral organ blood flow, cardiac index, coronary blood flow, oxygen consumption, and lactic acid metabolism
4. Decreases in sympathetic nerve transmission, arteriolar and venular resistance, platelet and leukocyte viscosity, extravascular lung water, myocardial infarct size, complement fixation by endotoxin, kinin production, and pulmonary arteriovenous shunting

We use 30 mg/kg of methylprednisolone sodium succinate (Solu-Medrol) given by IV route over a 10-minute period. This same dose may be repeated once or twice in the first 12 to 24 hours and then is stopped abruptly. This allows all the beneficial effects of these protean substances without producing any of the side effects that may come from chronic use.

More recently we have been using furosemide (Lasix) almost routinely in shock patients to improve urine output. Doses of 20 to 40 mg are given initially for oliguria or anuria, and if there is no response, 100 to 500 mg may be given. There are few if any harmful side effects of this potent diuretic, which helps prevent renal shutdown in shock with all the disastrous consequences of this problem.

In the treatment of hemorrhagic shock there are many agents that should probably be avoided. Formerly we believed that patients in hemorrhagic shock were always acidotic and that the administration of IV bicarbonate should be beneficial. However, recent studies have shown that there is less need for such agents, and these are now reserved for patients with a pH below 7.43.[133, 134]

Norepinephrine was formerly frequently used in the treatment of all forms of shock, but we now know that this potent vasoconstrictor causes damage to all the visceral organs, especially the lung and kidney.[130] Norepinephrine increases the mean systemic blood pressure at the expense of increasing vascular resistance and increases the work of the heart. Vasopressors more often improve the practitioner's sense of well-being than that of the patient, since the survival of patients in whom they are used is not improved. Dopamine, another catecholamine that increases blood pressure and lowers peripheral resistance, also does not improve survival in experimental hypovolemic shock.[135] Isoproterenol seems to have a limited potential in these patients, since its use is contraindicated in patients with heart rates in excess of 120 beats/min.

The essentials of the treatment regimen for hemorrhagic shock are therefore regulation of the respiratory and acid-base status, stopping the blood loss, appropriate volume replacement, and the use of large doses of methylprednisolone and diuretics. With early, vigorous treatment of hemorrhagic shock the mortality of this condition should be under 10%.[133, 134]

*Cardiogenic shock*

The basic defect in cardiogenic shock is an ineffective blood pump. The heart has suddenly become too weak to circulate a sufficient blood volume for the body's needs. The treatment of this form of shock therefore centers around attempts to improve the pumping ability of the heart (Table 26-3). There are two means by which this aim is currently accomplished: the administration of agents to increase the contractility of the myocardium and the use of measures designed to reduce the pressure against which the heart must pump blood (afterload).

The first step in resuscitation should always be directed at the regulation of the respiratory (and acid-base) status of the patient. The circulatory status is the next concern, since hypovolemia may occur in patients with cardiogenic shock.[136] Moreover, an optimum response to all other therapeutic maneuvers will not occur in the face of a circulatory deficit. The central venous and pulmonary artery pressures and urine output serve as guides to proper fluid replacement. In general the pulmonary artery wedge pressure should not be allowed to exceed 18 mm Hg, since overaggressive fluid therapy can promote pulmonary edema. The central venous pressure alone is not a reliable guide to fluid replacement in cardiogenic shock,[137] but when pulmonary artery wedge pressures are unavailable, the cautious use of the central venous pressure and urine output in gauging fluid administration is superior to the use of clinical judgment alone.

The treatment of cardiogenic shock primarily centers around the use of pharmacologic agents to assist the failing heart, but similar to the treatment of other forms of shock, considerable controversy has raged over the agent(s) that should be employed for this purpose. The arguments have primarily been concerned with the use of vasopressors vs vasodilators. Although the debate is by no means completely settled, there is ample evidence in the literature that vasopressors such as epinephrine, levarterenol, and metaraminol do not improve the survival of patients in cardiogenic shock.[138, 139] These agents do increase the blood pressure, but at the expense of an increased peripheral resistance with a consequent reduction in tissue perfusion and an increased oxygen demand on the already hypoxic myocardium. Positive inotropic agents such as glucagon and isoproterenol are also ineffective agents in the treatment of cardiogenic shock[140-142] (Fig. 26-9). Dopamine, a substance that increases blood pressure and cardiac output and reduces peripheral resistance, theoretically has promise, but has not been evaluated clinically.[143, 144] Digitalis should be used if congestive heart failure is present, but should not be administered prophylactically.

At the present time the most effective pharmacologic agents in the management of cardiogenic shock are the corticosteroids (Figs. 26-1, 26-10, and 26-11). A dose of 30 mg of methylprednisolone/kg or its equivalent is recommended, and this amount is administered as an IV bolus. In some cases it may be necessary to employ a positive inotropic agent such as isoproterenol to further augment the cardiac output, but these agents are used in the lowest concentrations and for

**Table 26-3.** Treatment of cardiogenic shock

| *Condition to be corrected (restored)* | *Treatment* |
|---|---|
| Hypovolemia | Plasma fractions, dextran, crystalloids, blood (occasionally) |
| Stagnant anoxia, membrane integrity, infarct size | Synthetic glucocorticosteroids (methylprednisolone, dexamethasone) |
| Oncotic pressure | Albumin |
| Oliguria | Furosemide |
| Pulmonary edema | Digitalis |
| Myocardial contractility | Glucagon, $\beta$-stimulators, $\alpha$-blockers |
| Hypoxemia | Respirator (volume type, positive end-expiratory pressure) |

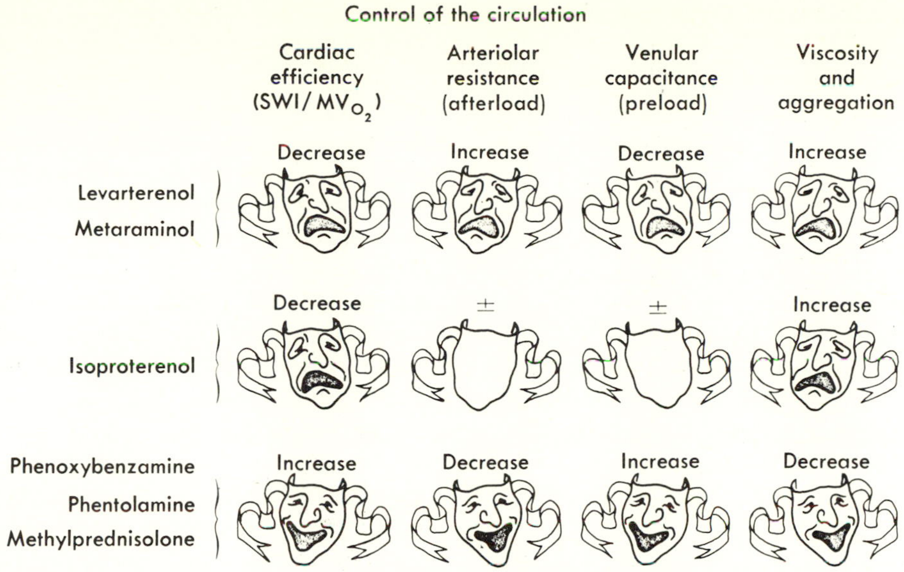


**Fig. 26-9.** Cardiac and systemic effects of drugs commonly used in the treatment of cardiogenic shock. SWI (stroke work index) = MSP (mean systolic pressure) − LVEDP (left ventricular end-diastolic pressure) × CI (cardiac index) ÷ Heart rate. $MV_{O_2}$, mean oxygen utilization.

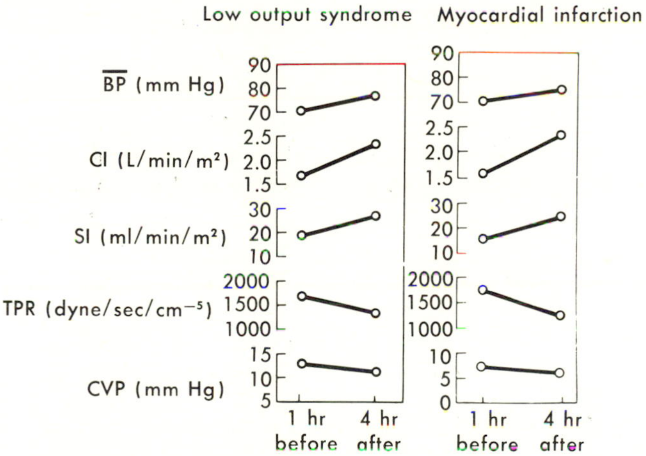


**Fig. 26-10.** Hemodynamic changes in cardiogenic shock following methylprednisolone administration (30 mg/kg).

the briefest time possible. Methylprednisolone has a stabilizing influence on cell membranes and causes peripheral vasodilatation. By decreasing afterload and/or by a direct myocardial effect, corticosteroids may decrease infarct size.[145] The use of massive doses of corticosteroids has increased the survival rate in both experimental and clinical cardiogenic shock from 20% to 60%.[146-149]

Patients who do not respond to pharmacologic agents are candidates for mechanical circulatory support. The mechanical assist devices basically fall into two categories: the series units, which reduce left ventricular pressure work, and the parallel devices, which decrease volume work. The intra-aortic balloon pump and the external counterpulsation machine are examples of the former. Each

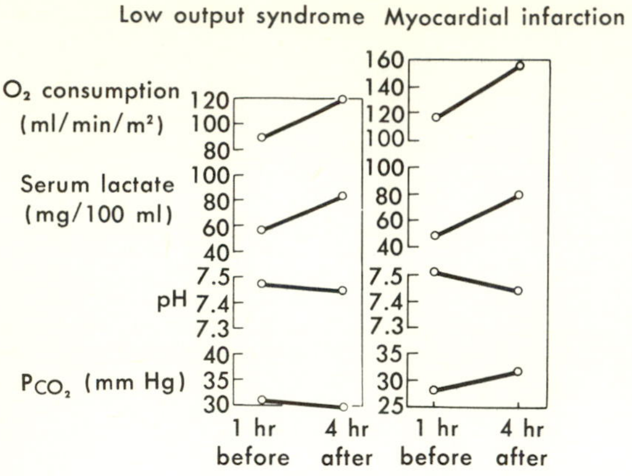


**Fig. 26-11.** Metabolic effects of methylprednisolone (30 mg/kg) in cardiogenic shock.

**Table 26-4.** Effect of intra-aortic balloon pumping on survival in cardiogenic shock

| | *No. of patients* | *Unable to insert balloon* | *Survival* | *%* |
|---|---|---|---|---|
| Acute myocardial infarction | 8 | 1 | 0 | 0 |
| Low output syndrome | 14 | 3 | 1 | 7 |
| Total | 22 | 4 | 1 | 5 |

**Table 26-5.** Influence of external counterpulsation on survival in cardiogenic shock

| | *No. of patients* | *Survival* | *%* |
|---|---|---|---|
| Acute myocardial infarction | 3 | 1 | 33 |
| Low output syndrome | 7 | 2 | 29 |
| Total | 10 | 3 | 30 |

machine acts to augment the systemic pressure and organ perfusion during diastole. In addition, by increasing the runoff during diastole, the heart has less of a pressure head against which it must pump during systole. Although both hemodynamic and metabolic improvement have been observed following the use of these series devices, survival has not been enhanced[150, 151] (Tables 26-4 and 26-5). Thus at present the series units are primarily used to support patients resistant to pharmacologic agents while the status of the coronary circulation is radiologically evaluated and, where feasible, until emergency aortocoronary bypass surgery is performed.[152] The parallel devices, which pump blood during systole and thereby reduce the volume handled by the left ventricle, are still beset with problems and not available for widespread clinical use.

The important concept in the use of mechanical circulatory assistance is to use these devices early in the course of shock rather than many hours or days later when many of the complications of shock, such as pulmonary and renal insufficiency, have occurred. Usually the clinician can determine in a few hours whether volume-drug-respirator support will resuscitate the patient. If not, the assistance devices should be used immediately.

### *Septic shock*

Unlike cardiogenic and hemorrhagic shock, the basic pathophysiologic defect in septic shock is unknown. These patients all have overwhelming systemic infections, but the mechanism by which the microorganisms produce shock is not clear. The uncertainties regarding the etiology and treatment of septic shock and the frequent failure to diagnose the condition in its early stages have contributed to the high mortality in the past. In recent years significant advances have been made in the treatment of this condition.

Once control of the patient's respiratory status has been accomplished, the circulatory needs should be evaluated (Table 26-6). Most of these patients are either absolutely or relatively volume deficient, and a large number will show considerable clinical improvement following the administration of IV fluids. Since anemia and defective tissue oxygenation are common in septic shock, the administration of blood or blood products is often necessary.[153, 154] Hypoalbuminemia is also a frequent finding, and if present, ap-

**Table 26-6.** Treatment of septic shock

| *Condition to be corrected (restored)* | *Treatment* |
|---|---|
| Hypovolemia | Plasma fractions, dextran, orystalloids, blood |
| Stagnant anoxia, membrane integrity, presence of anaphylatoxin (activated endotoxin) | Synthetic glucocorticosteroids (methylprednisolone, dexamethasone) |
| Oncotic pressure | Albumin |
| Oliguria | Furosemide |
| Congestive heart failure | Digitalis |
| Sepsis | Antibiotics |
| Arteriovenous admixture | Elimination of source |
| Hypoxemia | Respirator (volume type, positive end-expiratory pressure) |

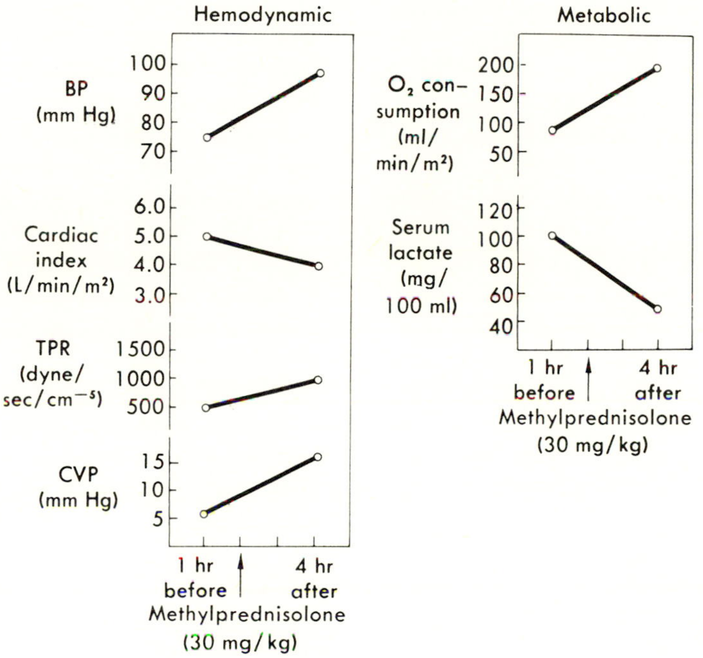


**Fig. 26-12.** Hemodynamic-metabolic effects of methylprednisolone (30 mg/kg) in septic shock.

propriate amounts of albumin should be given.[155] Concomitant with fluid therapy, large amounts of parenteral antibiotics should be given. Appropriate agents are used when positive cultures or smears are available. In the absence of a known pathogen we customarily employ the combination of cephalothin, gentamicin, and clindamycin in an attempt to provide coverage against the anaerobes and aerobes that are most commonly cultured from patients in septic shock. A localized infection should be drained if possible in order to prevent continued seeding of the patient's circulation with bacteria and their products.

As emphasized in the section on pathophysiology, the hemodynamic presentation of septic shock can be quite variable and is to a large extent dependent on the time at which the patient is seen after the onset of shock. Thus the use of cardiotonic and vasoactive agents can produce diverse effects in these individuals. Although various hemodynamic changes can be effected by the use of such agents, there is no evidence that in large series of patients survival is improved.[156]

**Table 26-7.** Results of corticosteroid therapy in septic shock

| | *Patients treated early* | *Patients treated late* | *Totals* |
|---|---|---|---|
| Survived shock | 25 (92.5%) | 10 (62.5%) | 35 (81.4%) |
| Died | 2 (7.5%) | 6 (37.5%) | 8 (18.6%) |
| Discharged or 30-day survivors | 15 (55.6%) | 3 (18.8%) | 18 (41.9%) |

Naturally certain individuals with specific complications such as arrhythmia or congestive heart failure are benefited by the judicious use of some of these drugs.

At present the best results in the treatment of septic shock have been obtained with the use of massive IV doses of corticosteroids in combination with the general supportive measures already described. Pharmacologic doses of the synthetic glucocorticosteroids improve both the hemodynamic and metabolic status of the septic patient (Fig. 26-12 and Table 26-3) and, more importantly, greatly enhance survival. With the advent of corticosteroid therapy, survival in bacteremic shock has risen from 20% to 35% to over 80%[157-159] (Table 26-7). Survival can exceed 90% if glucocorticosteroids are administered early in the course of septic shock.

### *Shock lung*

The treatment of posttraumatic pulmonary insufficiency deserves special comment, since this syndrome usually appears after the patient has been successfully supported through the acute stage of circulatory collapse. Although, as previously mentioned, the patient can experience a recurrence of circulatory collapse associated with the shock lung syndrome, shock is generally a preterminal event. The treatment of posttraumatic pulmonary insufficiency is therefore primarily concerned with reversing the pulmonary pathology and preventing the exacerbation of whatever histologic and physiologic abnormalities are already present.

Ventilatory assistance is essential in these patients, since the syndrome is associated with hypoxia, atelectasis, and a dramatic increase in the work of breathing. Because of the decreased compliance of the lungs, a volume respirator is used.[86] The inspired oxygen concentration ($F_{IO_2}$) is adjusted to maintain an arterial oxygen tension of around 80 to 100 mm Hg. Care should be taken to keep the $F_{IO_2}$ as low as possible in order to decrease the chance of superimposing the effects of oxygen toxicity on the injured pulmonary parenchyma.

In general these patients are fluid overloaded, and a marked improvement can occur following diuresis.[86] Sedation may be of some benefit because it allows the patient to follow the respirator more easily. Heparin is usually administered in order to reduce platelet aggregation, serotonin release, and intravascular coagulation.[86, 87] The judicious use of low molecular weight dextran may be of some benefit, since this material can reduce platelet adhesiveness and decrease the volume of extracellular lung water.[87] Antibiotics are administered to all patients with shock lung, since these individuals are particularly susceptible to infection. Massive doses of corticosteroids are used for their stabilizing effects on pulmonary cells, their ability to reduce platelet aggregation, and their favorable effects on pulmonary hemodynamics.[86, 87, 112]

This treatment regimen has produced a marked improvement in the survival of patients afflicted with posttraumatic pulmonary insufficiency[86] (Fig. 26-13). Patients who do not respond to these efforts are candidates for extracorporeal oxygenation, providing the pulmonary pathology is reversible. Although membrane oxygenators are still plagued with problems, some success in the treatment of shock lung has recently been reported.[160] As more experience with these devices is gained, the rate of patient salvage should improve considerably.

A

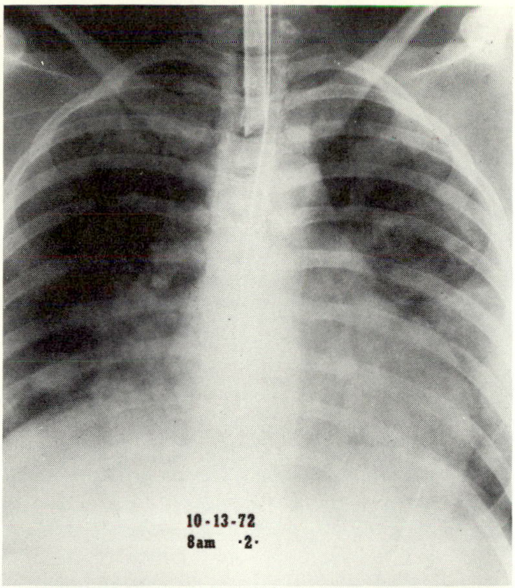


B

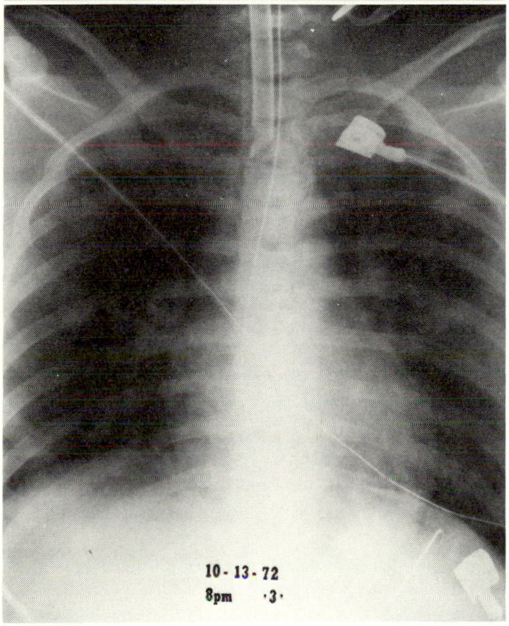


**Fig. 26-13. A,** Roentgenologic appearance of lungs 14 hours after initiation of treatment for shock lung. **B,** Chest x-ray film 24 hours after diagnosis and treatment of shock lung. There has been a remarkable clearing of the pulmonary infiltrate.

## SUMMARY

Shock occurs when tissue perfusion is inadequate to sustain normal physiologic function. The three types of circulatory collapse, in order of prevalence, are hemorrhagic, cardiogenic, and septic shock. The primary physiologic hallmarks of hypovolemic and cardiogenic shock are hypotension, vasoconstriction, and low cardiac output. The patient is cool, clammy, tachycardic, oliguric, and frequently acidotic. Patients in septic shock initially present with mental confusion, tachypnea, oliguria, and alkalosis. The blood pressure is usually normal, the total peripheral resistance is low, and the cardiac output is elevated. The pathophysiology of late bacteremic shock is similar to that of oligemic and cardiogenic shock. Anaerobic cellular metabolism is common in all types of circulatory collapse. Pulmonary insufficiency can occur with any form of shock, but it is most common after traumatic shock.

The treatment of circulatory collapse should be tailored to the type of shock and the needs of the patient. Adequate respiratory support and proper volume replacement are essential. Corticosteroids have an important place in the treatment of all types of circulatory collapse, since significant improvement in survival has been associated with their use. Various cardiotonic and vasoactive drugs may be useful, depending on the needs of the patient. With early, vigorous treatment the survival rates of hemorrhagic and septic shock can approach 90%, whereas that of cardiogenic shock is around 60%.

## REFERENCES

1. Sloman, G., Stannard, M., and Goble, H. J.: Coronary care unit: a review of 300 patients monitored since 1963, Am. Heart J. **75**:140-143, 1968.
2. Sobel, B. E.: The cardiac care unit in 1973, Hosp. Pract., Feb., 1973, pp. 115-124.
3. Page, D. L., et al.: Myocardial changes associated with cardiogenic shock, N. Engl. J. Med. **285**:133-137, 1971.
4. McQuay, N. W., Edwards, J. E., and Burchell, H. B.: Types of death in acute myocardial infarction, Arch. Intern. Med. **97**:1, 1955.
5. Malach, M., and Rosenberg, B. A.: Acute myocardial infarction in a city hospital. III. Experience with shock, Am. J. Cardiol. **5**:487, 1960.
6. Soloff, L. A.: Coronary artery disease and the concept of cardiac failure, Am. J. Cardiol. **22**:43, 1968.
7. Sobel, B. E., et al.: Estimation of infarct

size in man and its relation to prognosis, Circulation **46**:640, 1972.
8. Maroko, P. R., et al.: Precordial ST-segment mapping: an atraumatic method for assessing alterations in the extent of myocardial ischemic injury. The effects of pharmacologic and hemodynamic interventions, Am. J. Cardiol. **29**:223, 1972.
9. Reid, P. R., et al.: Myocardial-infarct extension detected by precordial ST-segment mapping, N. Engl. J. Med. **290**:123, 1974.
10. Mueller, H., Ayres, S. M., and Gregory, J. J.: Hemodynamics, coronary blood flow, and myocardial metabolism in coronary shock; response to l-norepinephrine and isoproterenol, J. Clin. Invest. **49**:1885, 1970.
11. Ricciutti, M. A.: Myocardial lysosome stability in the early stages of acute ischemic injury, Am. J. Cardiol. **30**:492, 1972.
12. Kirklin, J. W., and Archie, J. P.: The cardiovascular subsystem in surgical patients, Surg. Gynecol. Obstet. **139**:17, 1974.
13. Kerr, A. B., and Kirklin, J. W.: Changes in canine venous volume and pressure during hemorrhage, Surgery **68**:520, 1970.
14. Brobmann, G. F., et al.: Early regional vascular responses to hemorrhage and reinfusion in dogs, Surg. Gynecol. Obstet. **131**: 409, 1970.
15. Chien, S., and Usami, S.: Effects of hemorrhage on anesthetized dogs: role of the sympathetic system, Am. J. Physiol. **216**: 1322, 1969.
16. Barton, R. W., Reynolds, D. G., and Swan, K. G.: Mesenteric circulatory responses to hemorrhagic shock in the baboon, Ann. Surg. **175**:204, 1972.
17. Roding, B., and Schenk, W. G.: Mesenteric blood flow after hemorrhage in anesthetized and unanesthetized dogs, Surgery **68**:857, 1970.
18. Slater, G. I., et al.: Sequential changes in distribution of cardiac output in hemorrhagic shock, Surgery **73**:174, 1973.
19. Ludbrook, J.: The interaction between vasoconstriction and autoregulation after hemorrhage, Surg. Clin. North Am. **49**:637, 1969.
20. Selkurt, E. E.: Current status of renal circulation and related nephron function in hemorrhage and experimental shock. I. Vascular mechanisms, Circ. Shock **1**:3, 1974.
21. Stone, A. M., and Stahl, W. M.: Renal effects of hemorrhage in normal man, Ann. Surg. **172**:825, 1970.
22. Vanecko, R. M., Szanto, P. B., and Shoemaker, W. C.: Microcirculatory changes in primate liver during shock, Surg. Gynecol. Obstet. **129**:995, 1969.
23. Carey, L. C., Lowery, B. D., and Cloutier, C. T.: Hemorrhagic shock, Curr. Probl. Surg., p. 3, Jan., 1971.
24. Chien, S., and Usami, S.: Rate and mechanism of release of antidiuretic hormone after hemorrhage, Circ. Shock **1**:71, 1974.
25. Bacalzo, L. V., et al.: Effect of prolonged hypovolemic shock on jejunal fluid and sodium transport, Surg. Gynecol. Obstet. **134**:399, 1974.
26. Granata, L., et al.: Left coronary hemodynamics during hemorrhagic hypotension and shock, Am. J. Physiol. **216**:1583, 1969.
27. Heimbach, D. M., et al.: Myocardial blood flow and metabolism during and after hemorrhagic shock in the dog, Surg. Gynecol. Obstet. **137**:243, 1973.
28. Lovett, W. L., et al.: Presence of a myocardial depressant factor in patients in circulatory shock, Surgery **70**:223, 1971.
29. Lefer, A. M., and Spath, J. A.: Pancreatic hypoperfusion and the production of a myocardial depressant factor in hemorrhagic shock, Ann. Surg. **179**:868, 1974.
30. Wilson, J. M., Gay, W. A., and Ebert, P. A.: The effects of oligemic hypotension on myocardial function, Surgery **73**:657, 1973.
31. Wangensteen, S. L., Crampton, R. S., and Ferguson, W. W.: Myocardial depressant factor in cardiogenic shock, J.A.M.A. **228**: 1638, 1974.
32. Schumer, W.: Localization of the energy pathway block in shock, Surgery **64**:55, 1968.
33. Hobler, K. E., and Carey, L. C.: Effect of acute progressive hypoxemia on cardiac output and plasma excess lactate, Ann. Surg. **177**:199, 1973.
34. Chaudry, I. H., Sayeed, M. M., and Baue, A. E.: Depletion and restoration of tissue ATP in hemorrhagic shock, Arch. Surg. **108**:208, 1974.
35. Blackwood, J. M., et al.: Tissue metabolites in endotoxin and hemorrhagic shock, Arch. Surg. **107**:181, 1973.
36. Rutenburg, A. M., et al.: Adenosine 3′,5′-monophosphate metabolism in the liver in experimental hemorrhagic shock, Surgery **74**:660, 1973.
37. Holden, W. D., et al.: Ultrastructural changes in hemorrhagic shock, Ann. Surg. **162**:517, 1965.
38. Baue, A. E., and Sayeed, M. M.: Alterations in the functional capacity of mitochondria in hemorrhagic shock, Surgery **68**: 40, 1970.
39. Baue, A. E., Wurth, M. A., and Sayeed, M. M.: The dynamics of altered ATP-dependent and ATP-yielding cell processes in shock, Surgery **72**:94, 1972.
40. Clermont, H. G., Williams, J. S., and

Adams, J. T.: Liver acid phosphatase as a measure of hepatocyte resistance to hemorrhagic shock, Surgery **71**:868, 1972.
41. Clermont, H. G., and Williams, J. S.: Lymph lysosomal enzyme acid phosphatase in hemorrhagic shock, Ann. Surg. **176**:90, 1972.
42. Berman, I. R., et al.: Thoracic duct lymph in shock: gas exchange, acid base balance and lysosomal enzymes in hemorrhagic and endotoxin shock, Ann. Surg. **169**:202, 1969.
43. Bell, M. L., et al.: Role of lysosomal instability in the development of refractory shock, Surgery **70**:341, 1971.
44. Mela, L. M., Miller, L. D., and Nicholas, G. G.: Influence of cellular acidosis and altered cation concentrations on shock-induced mitochondrial damage, Surgery **72**: 102, 1972.
45. Tamakuma, S., et al.: Demonstration of a lethal endotoxemia of intestinal origin in refractory non-septic shock, Ann. Surg. **173**: 219, 1971.
46. Herman, C. M., et al.: The relationship of circulating endogenous endotoxin to hemorrhagic shock in the baboon, Ann. Surg. **179**:910, 1974.
47. Cunningham, J. N., Shires, G. T., and Wagner, Y.: Cellular transport defects in hemorrhagic shock, Surgery **70**:215, 1971.
48. Shires, G. T., et al.: Alterations in cellular membrane function during hemorrhagic shock in primates, Ann. Surg. **176**:288, 1972.
49. Trunkey, D. D., et al.: The effect of hemorrhagic shock on intracellular muscle action potentials in the primate, Surgery **74**:241, 1973.
50. Essiet, G. S., and Stahl, W. M.: Water and electrolyte content of tissues in hemorrhagic shock and surgical trauma, Surg. Gynecol. Obstet. **137**:11, 1973.
51. Johnson, G., and Baggett, C.: Red-cell fluid and electrolytes during hemorrhagic shock in the monkey, Ann. Surg. **178**:655, 1973.
52. Lowery, B. D., Cloutier, C. T., and Carey, L. C.: Blood gas determinations in the severely wounded in hemorrhagic shock, Arch. Surg. **99**:330, 1969.
53. String, T., Robinson, A. J., and Blaisdell, F. W.: Massive trauma, Arch. Surg. **102**: 406, 1971.
54. Hirsch, E. F., et al.: Coagulation changes after combat trauma and sepsis, Surg. Gynecol. Obstet. **133**:393, 1971.
55. Blaisdell, F. W., Lim, R. C., Jr., and Stallone, R. J.: Mechanism of pulmonary damage following traumatic shock, Surg. Gynecol. Obstet. **130**:1, 1970.
56. Nunes, G., Blaisdell, F. W., and Margaretten, W.: Mechanism of hepatic dysfunction following shock and trauma, Arch. Surg. **100**:546, 1970.
57. Altar, S., et al.: Intravascular coagulation: reality or myth? Surgery **68**:27, 1970.
58. Salzman, F. W.: Does intravascular coagulation occur in human shock in man? J. Trauma **8**:867, 1968.
59. Nahas, G. G., et al: Alterations in $O_2$ uptake following hemorrhage in dogs, Am. J. Physiol. **210**:1009, 1966.
60. Carey, L. C., Lowery, B., and Cloutier, C. T.: Blood sugar and insulin response of humans in shock, Ann. Surg. **172**:342, 1970.
61. Moss, G. S., et al.: Decline in pancreatic insulin release during hemorrhagic shock in the baboon, Ann. Surg. **175**:210, 1972.
62. Hiebert, J. M., McCormick, M. J., and Egdahl, R. H.: Direct measurement of insulin secretory rate: studies in shocked primates and postoperative patients, Ann. Surg. **176**:296, 1972.
63. Carey, L. C., Cloutier, C. T., and Lowery, B. D.: Growth hormone and adrenal cortical response to shock and trauma in the human, Ann. Surg. **174**:451, 1971.
64. Hanson, E. L., et al.: Response of glucose, insulin, free fatty acid, and human growth hormone to norepinephrine and hemorrhage in normal man, Ann. Surg. **177**:453, 1973.
65. MacLean, L. D., et al.: Patterns in septic shock in man—a detailed study of 56 patients, Ann. Surg. **166**:543, 1967.
66. Shoemaker, W. C., et al.: Use of sequential physiologic measurements for evaluation and therapy of uncomplicated septic shock, Surg. Gynecol. Obstet. **131**:245, 1970.
67. Siegel, J. H., Goldwyn, R. M., and Friedman, H. P.: Pattern and process in the evolution of human septic shock, Surgery **70**:232, 1971.
68. Wilson, R. F., et al.: Hemodynamic measurements in septic shock, Arch. Surg. **91**: 121, 1965.
69. Siegel, J. H., Greenspan, M., and Del-Guercio, L. R. M.: Abnormal vascular tone, defective oxygen transport, and myocardial failure in human septic shock, Ann. Surg. **165**:504, 1967.
70. Cohn, J. D., et al.: Arteriovenous shunting in high output shock syndromes, Surg. Gynecol. Obstet. **127**:282, 1968.
71. Duff, J. H., et al.: Defective oxygen consumption in septic shock, Surg. Gynecol. Obstet. **128**:1051, 1969.
72. Gimpel, L., Hodgins, D. S., and Jacobson, E. D.: Effect of endotoxin on hepatic adenylate cyclase activity, Circ. Shock **1**: 31, 1974.

73. Clowes, G. H. A., Jr., et al.: Energy metabolism in sepsis: treatment based on different patterns in shock and high output stage, Ann. Surg. **179**:684, 1974.
74. Clermont, H. G., Williams, J. S., and Adams, J. T.: Steroid effect on the release of the lysosomal enzyme acid phosphatase in shock, Ann. Surg. **179**:917, 1974.
75. Wilson, J. W.: Treatment or prevention of pulmonary cellular damage with pharmacologic doses of corticosteroid, Surg. Gynecol. Obstet. **134**:675, 1972.
76. Wilson, J. W.: Pulmonary factors produced by septic shock: cause or consequence of shock lung? J. Reprod. Med. **8**:307, 1972.
77. Motsay, G. J., et al.: Effects of massive doses of corticosteroids in experimental and clinical gram-negative septic shock. In Forscher, B. K., Lillehei, R. C., and Stubbs, S. S., editors: Shock in low- and high-flow states, Amsterdam, 1972, Excerpta Medica Foundation.
78. Schumer, W., and Sperling, R.: Shock and its effect on the cell, J.A.M.A. **205**:215, 1968.
79. Miller, L. D., et al.: The affinity of hemoglobin for oxygen: its control and in vivo significance, Surgery **68**:187, 1970.
80. McConn, R., and DelGuercio, L. R. M.: Respiratory function of blood in the acutely ill patient and the effect of steroids, Ann. Surg. **174**:436, 1971.
81. Milligan, G. F., et al.: Pulmonary and hematologic disturbances during septic shock, Surg. Gynecol. Obstet. **138**:43, 1974.
82. Wangensteen, S. L., et al.: Relationship between splanchnic blood flow and a myocardial depressant factor in endotoxin shock, Surgery **69**:410, 1971.
83. Schon, G. R., Delpin, E. S., and Millan, P. R.: Relationship of blood substitutes to pulmonary changes and volemia, Ann. Surg. **173**:504, 1971.
84. Martin, A. M., et al.: Pathologic anatomy of the lungs following shock and trauma, J. Trauma **8**:687, 1968.
85. Simmons, R. L., et al.: Respiratory insufficiency in combat casualties: IV hypoxemia during convalescence, Ann. Surg. **170**:53, 1969.
86. Geiger, J. P., and Gielchinsky, I.: Acute pulmonary insufficiency, Arch. Surg. **102**: 400, 1971.
87. Blaisdell, F. W., Lim, R. C., and Stallone, R. J.: The mechanism of pulmonary damage following traumatic shock, Surg. Gynecol. Obstet. **130**:15, 1970.
88. McLaughlin, J. S.: Physiologic consideration of hypoxemia in shock and trauma, Ann. Surg. **173**:667, 1971.
89. Germon, P. A., et al.: Shunting following trauma, J. Trauma **8**:724, 1968.
90. Kim, S. I., and Shoemaker, W. C.: Role of acidosis in the development of increased pulmonary vascular resistance and shock lung in experimental hemorrhagic shock, Surgery **73**:723, 1973.
91. Shapiro, B. J., Simmons, D. H., and Linde, L. M.: Pulmonary hemodynamics during acute acid-base changes in the intact dog, Am. J. Physiol. **210**:1026, 1966.
92. Gerst, P. H., et al.: The effects of hemorrhage on pulmonary circulation and respiratory gas exchange, J. Clin. Invest. **38**:524, 1959.
93. Sealy, W. C., et al.: Functional and structural changes in the lung in hemorrhagic shock, Surg. Gynecol. Obstet. **122**:754, 1966.
94. Buckberg, G. D., and Dowell, A. R.: The effects of hemorrhagic shock and pulmonary ischemia on lung compliance and structure in baboons, Surg. Gynecol. Obstet. **131**: 1065 1970.
95. Wyche, M. Q., et al.: Lung function, pulmonary extravascular water volume and hemodynamics in early hemorrhagic shock in anesthetized dogs, Ann. Surg. **174**:296, 1971.
96. Derks, C. M., and Peters, R. M.: The effect of shock and fat embolus on pulmonary mechanics and gas exchange, Surg. Gynecol. Obstet. **138**:413, 1974.
97. Derks, C. M., and Peters, R. M.: The role of shock and fat embolus in leakage from pulmonary capillary, Surg. Gynecol. Obstet. **137**:945, 1973.
98. Greenfield, L. J., McCurdy, W. C., and Coalson, J. J.: Pulmonary oxygen toxicity in experimental hemorrhagic shock, Surgery **68**:662, 1970.
99. Lee, C. J., Lyons, J. H., and Moore, F. D.: Cardiovascular and metabolic responses to spontaneous and positive-pressure breathing of 100 percent oxygen at one atmosphere pressure, J. Thorac. Cardiovasc. Surg. **53**: 770, 1967.
100. Collins, J. A.: The causes of progressive pulmonary insufficiency in surgical patients, J. Surg. Res. **9**:685, 1969.
101. Magilligan, D. J., et al.: Pulmonary intravascular and extravascular volumes in hemorrhagic shock and fluid replacement, Surgery **72**:780, 1972.
102. Fulton, R. L., and Fischer, R. P.: Pulmonary changes due to hemorrhagic shock resuscitation with isotonic and hypertonic saline, Surgery **75**:881, 1974.
103. Siegel, D. C., Cochin, A., and Moss, G. S.: The ventilatory response to hemorrhagic

shock and resuscitation, Surgery **72:**451, 1972.

104. Moss, G. S., et al.: Effects of saline and colloid solutions on pulmonary function in hemorrhagic shock. Surg. Gynecol. Obstet. **133:**53, 1971.
105. Moss, G. S., et al.: Morphologic changes in the primate lung after hemorrhagic shock, Surg. Gynecol. Obstet. **134:**3, 1972.
106. Moss, G. S., et al.: Effect of hemorrhagic shock on pulmonary interstitial sodium distribution in the primate lung, Ann. Surg. **177:**211, 1973.
107. Swank, R. L., Connell, R. S., and Webb, M. C.: Dacron wool filtration and hypotensive shock: an electron microscopical study, Ann. Surg. **179:**427, 1974.
108. Hallett, J. W., Sneiderman, C. A., and Wilson, J. W.: Pulmonary effects of arterial infusion of filtered blood in experimental hemorrhagic shock, Surg. Gynecol. Obstet. **138:**517, 1974.
109. Schloerb, P. R., et al.: Pulmonary edema after replacement of blood loss by electrolyte solutions, Surg. Gynecol. Obstet. **135:** 893, 1972.
110. Bryant, L. R., Trinkle, J. K., and Dubilier, L.: Acute respiratory pathophysiology after hemorrhagic shock, Surgery **68:**512, 1970.
111. Wilson, J. W., et al.: The lung in hemorrhagic shock, Am. J. Pathol. **58:**337, 1970.
112. Wilson, J. W.: Treatment or prevention of pulmonary cellular damage with pharmacologic doses of corticosteroid, Surg. Gynecol. Obstet. **134:**675, 1972.
113. Henry, J. N., et al.: A study of the acute and chronic respiratory pathophysiology of hemorrhagic shock, J. Thorac. Cardiovasc. Surg. **54:**666, 1967.
114. Tieffenbrun, J., and Shoemaker, W. C.: Sequential changes in pulmonary blood flow distribution in hemorrhagic shock, **174:** 727, 1971.
115. Tieffenbrun, J., Kim, S. I., and Shoemaker, W. C.: The relation of the distribution of pulmonary blood flow to lung function during hemorrhagic shock, Surg. Gynecol. Obstet. **138:**557, 1974.
116. Henry, J. N.: The effect of shock on pulmonary alveolar surfactant, J. Trauma **8:** 756, 1968.
117. Gilder, H., and McSherry, C. K.: Mechanisms of oxygen inhibition of pulmonary surfactant synthesis, Surgery **76:**72, 1974.
118. Lowery, B. D., Cloutier, C. T., and Carey, L. C.: Electrolyte solutions in resuscitation in human hemorrhagic shock, Surg. Gynecol. Obstet. **133:**273, 1971.
119. Moss, G. S., et al.: A comparison of asanguineous fluids and whole blood in the treatment of hemorrhagic shock, Surg. Gynecol. Obstet. **129:**1247, 1969.
120. Reich, M. P., and Eiseman, B.: Tissue oxygenation following resuscitation with crystalloid solution following experimental acute blood loss, Surgery **69:**928, 1971.
121. Coran, A. G., et al.: The effect of crystalloid resuscitation in hemorrhagic shock on acid-base balance: a comparison between normal saline and Ringer's lactate solutions, Surgery **69:**874, 1971.
122. Copping, J. W., Mather, G. S., and Winkler, J. M.: Physiologic responses to the administration of cold, room temperature, and warm balanced salt solutions in hemorrhagic shock in dogs, Surgery **71:**206, 1972.
123. Batalden, D. J., et al.: Value of the G suit in patients with severe pelvic fracture, Arch. Surg. **109:**326, 1974.
124. McNamara, J. J., et al.: Effect of hypertonic glucose in hypovolemic shock in man, Ann. Surg. **176:**247, 1972.
125. Gump, F. E., et al.: Exogenous glucose as an energy substrate in experimental hemorrhagic shock, Surg. Gynecol. Obstet. **136:** 611, 1973.
126. Bower, M. G., et al.: Hemodynamic effects of glucagon, Arch. Surg. **101:**411, 1970.
127. Schumer, W., et al.: Metabolic and microcirculatory effects of glucagon in hypovolemic shock, Arch. Surg. **107:**176, 1973.
128. Massion, W. H.: Value of high energy compounds in the treatment of shock, Am. J. Surg. **110:**342, 1965.
129. Chaudry, I. H., Sayeed, M. M., and Baue, A. E.: Effect of adenosine triphosphate–magnesium chloride administration in shock, Surgery **75:**220, 1974.
130. Bell, G., and Lister, G. D.: The effect of noradrenaline and phenoxybenzamine on the renal response to hemorrhage, Surg. Gynecol. Obstet. **130:**813, 1970.
131. Altura, B. M., and Altura, B. T.: Vascular actions of glucocorticoids and their relationship to protection in circulatory shock, Fed. Proc. **33:**394, 1974.
132. Kusajima, K., Wax, S. D., and Webb, W. R., Effects of methylprednisolone on pulmonary microcirculation, Surg. Gynecol. Obstet. **139:**1, 1974.
133. Cloutier, C. T., Lowery, B. D., and Carey, L. C.: Acid-base disturbances in hemorrhagic shock, Arch. Surg. **98:**551, 1969.
134. Collins, J. A., et al.: Acid-base status of seriously wounded combat casualties. II. Resuscitation with stored blood, Ann. Surg. **173:**6, 1971.
135. Dagher, F. J., Seaton, J. F., and Harrison, T. S.: Lack of effect of dopamine in ex-

perimental hypovolemic shock, Surg. Gynecol. Obstet. **130:**717, 1970.
136. Loeb, H. S., et al.: Hypovolemia in shock due to acute myocardial infarction, Circulation **11:**653, 1969.
137. Toussaint, G. P. M., Burgess, J. H., and Hampson, L. G.: Central venous pressure and pulmonary wedge pressure in critical surgical illness; a comparison, Arch. Surg. **109:**265, 1974.
138. Binder, M. J.: Effect of vasopressor drugs on circulatory dynamics in shock following myocardial infarction, Am. J. Cardiol. **16:** 834, 1965.
139. Dietzman, R. H., et al.: Relation of cardiac work to survival in cardiogenic shock in dogs, J.A.M.A. **199:**825, 1967.
140. Gunnar, R. M., et al.: Ineffectiveness of isoproterenol in shock due to acute myocardial infarction, J.A.M.A. **202:**64, 1967.
141. Deraney, M. F.: Glucagon? One answer to cardiogenic shock, Am. J. Med. Sci. **261:** 149, 1971.
142. Smith, H. J., et al.: Hemodynamic studies in cardiogenic shock: treatment with isoproterenol and metaraminol, Circulation **35:**1084, 1967.
143. Beregovich, J., et al.: Dose-related hemodynamic and renal effects of dopamine in congestive heart failure, Am. Heart J. **87:** 550, 1974.
144. MacConnell, K. L., et al.: The use of dopamine in the treatment of hypotension and shock, N. Engl. J. Med. **275:**1389, 1966.
145. Shatney, C. H., and Lillehei, R. C.: Effects of allopurinol and methylprednisolone and propranolol on experimental myocardial infarction site, Am. J. Cardiol. 1976. (In press.)
146. Schudl, S., Ascheim, R., and Killip, T.: Shock after acute myocardial infarction, Am. J. Cardiol. **26:**556, 1970.
147. Dietzman, R. C., Beckman, C. B., and Lillehei, R. C.: Pharmacologic and mechanical support for managing cardiogenic shock, Geriatrics **28:**69, 1973.
148. Dietzman, R. H., et al.: Corticosteroids as effective vasodilators in the treatment of low output syndrome, Chest **57:**440, 1970.
149. Motsay, G. J., et al.: Effects of corticosteroids on the circulation in shock: experimental and clinical results, Fed. Proc. **29:** 1861, 1970.
150. Beckman, C., et al.: Hemodynamic evaluation of external counterpulsation in surgical patients, Surgery **74:**846, 1973.
151. Scheidt, S., et al.: Intra-aortic balloon counterpulsation in cardiogenic shock, N. Engl. J. Med. **288:**979, 1973.
152. Mundth, E. D., et al.: Circulatory assistance and emergency direct coronary-artery surgery for shock complicating acute myocardial infarction, N. Engl. J. Med. **283:** 1382, 1970.
153. Siegel, J. H., Greenspan, M., and Del-Guercio, L. R. M.: Abnormal vascular tone, defective oxygen transport, and myocardial failure in human septic shock, Ann. Surg. **165:**504, 1967.
154. Milligan, G. F., et al.: Pulmonary and hematologic disturbances during septic shock, Surg. Gynecol. Obstet. **138:**43, 1974.
155. Vito, L., et al.: Sepsis presenting as acute respiratory insufficiency, Surg. Gynecol. Obstet. **138:**896, 1974.
156. Wilson, R. F., Sarver, E. J., and Rizzo, J.: Hemodynamic changes, treatment, and prognosis in clinical shock, Arch. Surg. **102:**21, 1971.
157. Neely, W. A., et al.: Septic shock: clinical, physiological, and pathological survey of 244 patients, Ann. Surg. **173:**657, 1971.
158. Weil, M. H., Shubin, H., and Biddle, M.: Shock caused by gram-negative microorganisms. Analysis of 169 cases, Ann. Intern. Med. **60:**384, 1964.
159. Winslow, E. J., et al.: Hemodynamic studies and results of therapy in 50 patients with bacteremic shock, Am. J. Med. **54:**421, 1973.
160. Hill, J. D., et al.: Prolonged extracorporeal oxygenation for acute post-traumatic respiratory failure (shock-lung syndrome) use of the bramson membrane lung, N. Engl. J. Med. **286:**629, 1972.

*chapter 27*

# Hepatic encephalopathy

**BERTRAM F. FELSHER**

Among the five major manifestations of severe liver disease—jaundice, ascites, hepatomegaly, variceal hemorrhage, and encephalopathy—only the latter two are urgently life threatening. Hepatic coma, an extreme form of encephalopathy, is the most common terminal event in patients with fulminant hepatitis or severe chronic liver disease. It is a frequent contributory or direct cause of death following variceal hemorrhage. Nevertheless, hepatic encephalopathy is potentially reversible. Thus knowledge of the clinical manifestations and treatment of hepatic encephalopathy is of paramount importance in the effective management of critically ill patients with liver disease.

## ■ What is the definition of hepatic encephalopathy?

Hepatic encephalopathy is the neuropsychiatric syndrome caused by liver disease. It has various manifestations but is essentially characterized by cerebral dysfunction. Several terms have been applied to this condition, including hepatic coma, hepatic precoma, portal-systemic encephalopathy, nitrogenous encephalopathy, and hyperammonemia. The term "hepatic failure" should not be used synonymously with hepatic encephalopathy, as the former refers to the existence of any overt clinical sign of hepatic dysfunction such as jaundice, which is not necessarily associated with encephalopathy.

## ■ What are the clinical manifestations of hepatic encephalopathy?

Hepatic encephalopathy comprises a broad clinical spectrum that ranges from almost undetectable mental impairment to unarousable coma (Table 27-1). The early manifestations usually consist of mild changes in memory, mood, and mental alertness. At this stage the patient may appear lethargic, apathetic, depressed, irritable, or euphoric. More advanced stages are marked by further deepening of the mental obtundation and the development of asterixis. Asterixis refers to the inability to sustain a prolonged muscular contraction and is usually demonstrated by having the patient hyperextend the hands with the arms outstretched, which produces a typical flapping motion ("liver flap"). A maniacal phase may intervene, especially in patients with fulminant hepatitis, that not infrequently leads to the inappropriate admission of the patient to a psychiatric unit.

Other common neurologic findings include slurred speech, dysphasia, ataxia, apraxia, rigidity, and hyperreflexia with ankle clonus. Less common late manifestations are involuntary movements of the face and limbs, hemi-

**Table 27-1.** Stages of hepatic encephalopathy

| *Stage* | *Clinical findings* |
|---|---|
| 1 | Mild confusion, euphoria or depression, slow mentation, blank expression, untidy, slurred speech, slight or no asterixis |
| 2 | Further obtundation, aberrant behavior, definite asterixis |
| 3 | Stuporous but arousable, marked confusion, incoherent speech, asterixis present if patient cooperative |
| 4 | Comatose, unarousable or responsive only to painful stimuli, usually no asterixis |

paresis, and positive plantar reflexes. Hepatic fetor, a musty "garliclike" breath odor, is a reliable sign of severe hepatic failure and therefore is frequently associated with encephalopathy.

In the last stage of encephalopathy the patient is deeply comatose and unresponsive to painful stimuli. Breathing is often stertorous. Preterminally there may be decerebrate rigidity and convulsions.

The course of encephalopathy varies according to whether the liver disease is acute or chronic. In acute cases usually the course is rapid and the ultimate outcome is reached within 10 days. In contrast, in patients with chronic liver disease, the course is ordinarily gradual, fluctuating, and lasts several days to a few weeks. Chronic encephalopathy is found only in patients with chronic liver disease who either have undergone a portacaval shunt operation or have unusually large natural portal-systemic anastomoses.

## ■ Are there any pathognomonic signs of hepatic encephalopathy?

The signs of mental impairment associated with hepatic encephalopathy are nonspecific. Other causes for cerebral dysfunction must be considered in the evaluation of patients with liver disease and apparent encephalopathy. Among these are subdural hematoma, brain tumor, brain abscess, hypoglycemia, acute alcoholic withdrawal, chronic alcoholic brain syndrome, and drug intoxication. Because localizing neurologic signs are unusual manifestations of hepatic encephalopathy, their appearance should suggest a space-occupying intracranial lesion. Hypoglycemia may be a complication of alcoholism, acute or chronic liver failure, and primary liver cell carcinoma. The tremor usually occurring in the alcoholic withdrawal syndrome is an important diagnostic feature. It is sometimes more difficult to decide whether the dementia and psychologic signs are produced by chronic alcoholism per se or result from hepatic failure. When these signs persist for several weeks despite appropriate therapy for encephalopathy in an alcoholic patient who had not previously undergone a portacaval shunt, chronic alcoholic brain syndrome is a more likely diagnosis even in the presence of obvious liver disease. If asterixis is present, the diagnosis of hepatic encephalopathy is strongly favored. The other less common causes of asterixis, namely, uremia, diabetic ketoacidosis, carbon dioxide narcosis, heart failure, and myxedema coma, are easily distinguished from hepatic failure.

## ■ What are the most useful tests for the diagnosis of hepatic encephalopathy?

There are no specific tests for hepatic encephalopathy. In patients with chronic liver disease the usual tests of liver function are not reliable indications of encephalopathy. However, in patients with acute hepatic necrosis a prothrombin activity of less than 10% is almost invariably associated with some degree of encephalopathy.

The employment of auxiliary tests may be helpful when signs of cerebral dysfunction are not clearly attributable to liver failure. The EEG pattern and levels of blood ammonia and cerebrospinal fluid glutamine provide electrophysiologic and biochemical data that may complement the clinical findings.

In a majority of patients with hepatic encephalopathy there is an abnormal EEG pattern characterized by bursts of high amplitude slow waves (1½ to 3/sec) occurring synchronously and beginning in both frontal areas. In later stages these slow (delta) waves spread and may eventually become generalized. The appearance of blunted triphasic activity interspersed with periods of flattening portends a fatal outcome in patients with acute hepatic failure. Usually as the patient's level of consciousness improves, the EEG changes revert to normal, but occasionally despite clinical remission, they persist for many days to several weeks. These EEG abnormalities can occur in other conditions associated with severe metabolic derangements and therefore are not specific for liver disease.

The blood ammonia determination, despite decreasing acceptance of its diagnostic applicability, remains as the most commonly employed biochemical test for hepatic encephalopathy. The lack of correlation of the blood ammonia level with the degree of hepatic encephalopathy is the primary reason for rejection of this test. Moreover, elevated levels may occur in patients with chronic liver disease in the absence of encephalopathy, and normal levels may be found in patients with advanced encephalopathy. It has been argued that a major cause for this absolute lack of correlation is the lag period required for the establishment of an equilibrium between peripheral tissue and blood ammonia. This disequilibrium is accentuated by a rise in blood pH that favors the conversion of the ammonium ion to free ammonia, which more readily passes through cell membranes. Thus the brain ammonia level, which is the actual determinant of CNS toxicity, will temporarily exceed the blood level. In addition, the neurologic expression of increased cerebral ammonia concentration may not occur immediately, accounting for a normal mental state in the face of elevated blood ammonia.

As a group, patients with liver disease show a poor correlation between the degree of encephalopathy and the level of blood ammonia. In the individual patient, however, if allowance is made for a lag period of as much as 72 hours, the ammonia levels reflect the state of consciousness. Therefore a persistently normal blood ammonia level is good evidence against encephalopathy and a change from an elevated to a normal value in conjunction with clinical improvement supports a diagnosis of encephalopathy. A normal adult value is approximately 100 $\mu$g/100 ml whether in the arterial or venous blood. However, even moderate physical activity of the forearm muscles may produce a substantial increase in the antecubital venous blood concentration. Furthermore, the ingestion of protein increases the blood ammonia level. It is therefore recommended that to avoid spurious results the determination of blood ammonia should be made on arterial blood with the patient in a rested, fasted state.

A more reliable test of hepatic encephalopathy is measurement of the cerebrospinal fluid glutamine level. This test appears to be better correlated with the degree of encephalopathy. It is unusual to find normal levels in patients with liver disease and any degree of encephalopathy. A value of 35 mg/100 ml is diagnostic of encephalopathy in patients with underlying liver disease but no respiratory failure, another cause for elevated glutamine levels. Recent studies suggest that the cerebrospinal fluid $\alpha$-ketoglutaramate concentration may be a more specific biochemical indicator of encephalopathy.

## ■ Are there any pathologic changes correlated with hepatic encephalopathy?

The morphologic changes found in the brains of patients with hepatic encephalopathy are nonspecific and appear to vary according to the duration of cerebral dysfunction. In patients with fatal acute massive hepatic necrosis and a telescoped course of coma, no neuropathology or only cerebral edema is found. In patients with chronic liver disease and a longer duration of encephalopathy, hypertrophy and hyperplasia of the protoplasmic astrocytes of the cerebral cortex are commonly found. More severe neuropathic changes, including neuronal degeneration in the brain and spinal cord, have been described in patients with very prolonged, severe irreversible hepatic encephalopathy. It is difficult to explain the clinical manifestations of hepatic encephalopathy on the basis of these observed pathologic changes. The clinical expression of this syndrome is more likely to be caused by biochemical rather than structural abnormalities.

## ■ What is the physiologic basis for hepatic encephalopathy?

Hepatic encephalopathy results from the metabolic disturbance produced by a combination of hepatic dysfunction and/or shunting of portal blood away from functional liver cells and into the systemic circulation. Portal-systemic shunting, whether from large extrahepatic anastomoses or functional shunts within the liver as a result of the imbalance of hepatocellular function and sinusoidal perfusion, rarely causes encephalopathy in the absence of underlying liver disease. Both of these mechanisms, however, act in concert to alter the metabolic exchange between liver and blood. This situation could lead to either a toxic accumulation of substances normally metabolized by the liver or a deficiency of factors produced by the liver that are necessary for normal cerebral function. Actually the latter hypothesis is virtually untested. On the other hand, there is abundant evidence supporting the concept of cerebrotoxicity.

A vast array of substances have been implicated in the pathogenesis of hepatic encephalopathy. This is not surprising considering the magnitude of the biochemical activity of the liver and the likelihood of multiple metabolic alterations occurring in the diseased liver. Thus elevated levels of various "candidate cerebrotoxins" have been found in the blood, cerebrospinal fluid, and urine of patients with encephalopathy. In most instances, however, supportive evidence of their pathogenic role was not obtained. Determination of the encephalopathogenic potential of these substances has been hampered by the lack of a suitable animal model. None of the chemical substances proposed thus far appears to be the sole cerebrotoxin causing encephalopathy. It is possible of course that the etiology of this condition is multifactorial. At the present time ammonia, short-chain fatty acids, and biogenic amines are the most likely circulating chemical mediators of encephalopathy.

Ammonia appears to play a prominent role in the pathogenesis of hepatic encephalopathy. Supporting this concept are the following lines of evidence: (1) Elevated blood and cerebrospinal fluid ammonia concentrations are found in most patients with hepatic encephalopathy. (2) Therapeutic measures designed to reduce hyperammonemia are clinically effective. (3) Administration of ammonia or its precursors to patients with liver disease or animals elicits the syndrome. (4) In children, hyperammonemic states caused by enzymic defects in the urea cycle are associated with a syndrome similar to hepatic encephalopathy.

In man the major source of ammonia is the intestines, where about 4 g is produced daily, and all but 50 mg is absorbed. This accounts for the five times greater concentration of ammonia in the portal vein as compared to the systemic circulation. About 85% (3.5 g) of the ammonia produced in the intestines is derived from urea secreted into the intestines and hydrolyzed by gastrointestinal ureases. An increased intake of protein leads to augmented ammonia production primarily by enhancing urea synthesis. Although most of this urease activity is of bacterial origin, a small fraction is contained within the intestinal mucosa. Of all the ammonia produced in the intestines, three fourths is derived from the colon and one fourth from the small intestine. A pH effect governing the transport of ammonia has been demonstrated for the colon but not the small intestine. That is, lowering the pH of the colonic contents reduces the absorption of ammonia ($NH_3$) because of the conversion to the less diffusible ammonium ion ($NH_4^+$).

Under normal conditions the ammonia absorbed from the gastrointestinal tract is taken up by the liver and then reconverted back to urea. In patients with liver disease ammonia may accumulate in the systemic circulation because of portal-systemic shunting as well as impaired hepatic synthesis of urea.

The new evidence suggesting that short-chain fatty acids, such as butyric, valeric, and octanoic acids, contribute to the cerebrotoxicity of hepatic encephalopathy is impressive. Further information is needed to better appreciate the pathogenic significance of these compounds.

A recent extension of the cerebrotoxic theory of hepatic encephalopathy is the displacement of normal neurotransmitters in the brain by amines acting as false neurotransmitters. This hypothesis is supported by the finding of elevated levels of octopamine in the blood and urine of patients with hepatic encephalopathy and in the brain of animals with experimentally induced hepatic coma. This amine is produced by the action of intestinal bacterial enzymes on ingested protein. It still remains to be proved that false neurotransmitters actually cause encephalopathy.

The precise biochemical effect of ammonia cerebrotoxicity is unknown. Available evidence indicates that ammonia probably is not a direct toxin but either interferes with cerebral energy metabolism or forms toxic compounds by reacting with cerebral metabolites. Whether the depletion of adenosine triphosphate (ATP) or $\alpha$-ketoglutarate, the decreased ratio of mitochondrial nicotinamide-adenine dinucleotide to its reduced form (NAD:NADH ratio), changes in the relative concentration of citric acid metabolites, or increased $\alpha$-ketoglutaramate levels is the ultimate biochemical mediator of ammonia toxicity remains to be shown. In contrast to ammonia, both the short-chain fatty acids and false neurotransmitters are direct neurotoxins.

In summary, the principal elements of hepatic encephalopathy are hepatic dysfunction and portal-systemic shunting. Ammonia, short-chain fatty acids, and biogenic amines are the most acceptable endogenous encephalopathogenic cerebrotoxins. The precise effect of cerebrotoxins on cerebral function is unknown.

## ■ What is the contribution to the development of hepatic encephalopathy by nonhepatic factors?

Besides the previously discussed primary determinants of hepatic encephalopathy, certain nonhepatic factors are known to promote the development of encephalopathy in patients with chronic liver disease. These are as follows:

*Common precipitating factors of hepatic encephalopathy*

- Azotemia
- Gastrointestinal hemorrhage
- Diuretics
- Drugs causing CNS depression
- Excessive nitrogenous intake
- Hypokalemic alkalosis
- Infection
- Constipation
- Rapid paracentesis

These factors by themselves are insufficient to cause the syndrome, but when superimposed on a background of underlying liver disease, they may precipitate or aggravate encephalopathy. In general these factors act by one of two physiologic mechanisms: (1) enhancing the cerebrotoxin (especially ammonia) level of the brain or (2) lowering the encephalopathic threshold of the cerebrotoxins. The cerebrotoxic level in the brain is raised by overproduction in nonhepatic sites as well as by local factors promoting entry into neuronal cells. The intake of nitrogenous substances, especially in the intestines, is a critical factor affecting ammonia and perhaps biogenic amine production. Thus increased dietary protein, ingestion of ammonium salts, and hemorrhage into the intestines are important secondary causes of encephalopathy. An additional cause for increased ammonia production is enhanced urea formation and secretion into the intestines because of protein degradation (starvation, infection, neoplasm) and azotemia. Constipation may cause increased intestinal absorption of ammonia. Potassium depletion and acidosis augment ammonia production from the kidneys. Any factor that causes hypovolemia and prerenal azotemia (diuretics, rapid paracentesis, blood loss) has the potential for precipitating encephalopathy. Hypokalemic alkalosis promotes the entry of ammonia into neuronal cells of the brain. Any factor that further compromises brain function (drugs, hypoglycemia, anoxia, carbon dioxide narcosis) may lower the encephalopathic threshold to ammonia or other cerebrotoxins. Tranquilizers, sedatives, anesthetics, and analgesics may precipitate or aggravate encephalopathy by causing CNS depression or anoxia. The deleterious effect of diuretics is attributable to multiple effects: transient hypovolemia with consequent azotemia and decreased hepatic or cerebral blood flow, potassium depletion and alkalosis, and increased renal ammonia production.

## ■ What is the conventional treatment of hepatic encephalopathy?

The rationale for the conventional therapeutic regimen for hepatic encephalopathy, which has been in effect for more than a decade, is reduction in the production and absorption of ammonia from the intestines and removal of precipitating factors. The first goal is accomplished by restricting dietary protein, cleansing the gastrointestinal tract with oral purgatives and/or high enemas, and reducing the fecal flora of urea-splitting bacteria with poorly absorbed antibiotics given orally or by retention enema. In general dietary protein is restricted to 0 to 20 g/day for acute encephalopathy, but in cases of chronic encephalopathy it is titrated according to the patient's clinical response. In cleansing the gastrointestinal tract an effective oral purgative is magnesium sulfate. It is preferable to use acidic cleansing enemas to minimize ammonia absorption. The most commonly used agent to reduce the fecal flora is neomycin, the total daily dose, including oral and rectal administration, being 2 to 3 g/day. It is best not to exceed this dose, as neomycin is absorbed slightly and excreted in the urine. It can cause oto- and nephrotoxicity as well as intestinal malabsorption, diarrhea, and staphylococcal enterocolitis. There is no evidence that the larger doses sometimes recommended are more effective. Alternatives to neomycin are other broad-spectrum antibiotics and nonabsorbable sulfonamides such as succinylsulfathiazole (Sulfasuxidine). These other antibacterial agents may be useful in cases of neomycin hypersensitivity or renal failure.

The common precipitating factors to be considered in every patient with hepatic encephalopathy are indiscretionary protein intake; hemorrhage in the gastrointestinal tract; diuretic therapy; renal failure; drugs that act on the CNS or are ammonia precursors, such as methionine; metabolic imbalances (especially hypokalemic alkalosis); infection (pneumonia, spontaneous peritonitis, or gram-negative septicemia); and constipation. Many of these factors can be eliminated. Variceal hemorrhage and functional renal failure (hepatorenal syndrome) are the least reversible of the precipitating factors and therefore commonly produce fatal hepatic coma.

In addition to these specific therapeutic measures, general supportive therapy for the other complications of hepatic failure such as coagulation defects, malnutrition, hypoglycemia, and hypoxemia, as well as provision of adequate caloric intake, should be instituted. Agitation should obviously not be treated with drugs. In cases of chronic active hepatitis the liver disease itself may be ameliorated by corticosteroid therapy.

■ **What are the newer or less conventional forms of treatment of hepatic encephalopathy?**

A more direct approach to reducing intestinal ammonia production has been the use of the urease inhibitor acetohydroxamic acid. Although preliminary studies showed reduction in the blood ammonia levels after oral administration of the drug to patients with encephalopathy, associated clinical improvement was not observed. In a similar vein, the transient induction of antibodies to urease was achieved by the injection of jack bean urease to patients with encephalopathy, but again clinical improvement did not consistently parallel the reduction in blood ammonia, and some toxic reactions were observed. The feeding of *Lactobacillus* in the attempt to replace the colonic flora with non-urease-producing bacteria is not by itself clinically effective but may be of some use as adjunctive therapy.

Lactulose, although only recently commercially available in the United States, has undergone several clinical trials here and abroad and appears to be at least as effective as neomycin in the treatment of acute as well as chronic encephalopathy. This agent is a synthetic disaccharide that is neither absorbed nor metabolized in the small intestine, but is converted by colonic bacterial enzymes to acetic and lactic acid, which causes acidification of the bowel contents. Its mechanism of action is thought to be related to the effect of fecal acidification in reducing ammonia and amine absorption as well as by its direct cathartic activity. This drug may be a useful substitute for neomycin in the treatment of patients with encephalopathy that is chronic or associated with renal failure.

Another approach to the treatment of

encephalopathy is reduction or neutralization of circulating cerebrotoxins. Dialysis, exchange transfusions, total body washout, and extracorporeal animal liver perfusion have not improved the survival rate in patients with encephalopathy caused by chronic liver disease or fulminant viral hepatitis. Preliminary studies suggest that exchange transfusions may be beneficial in the treatment of hepatic coma resulting from Reye's syndrome. Dramatic permanent reversal of hepatic coma has been reported in patients with fulminant toxin-induced hepatitis treated with the establishment of cross circulation to human volunteers. Ethical considerations limit the applicability of this rather heroic measure. An artificial liver would certainly be a more acceptable form of therapy. A major step in that direction was achieved by the recent studies showing that hemoperfusion through columns of activated charcoal effectively reverses hepatic coma in patients with acute or chronic liver disease.

In an attempt to counteract the possible effect of false neurotransmitters, levodopa, a precursor of dopamine, has been used in the treatment of hepatic encephalopathy. The results of the initial studies, although sparse, suggest a good effect. Unfortunately gastric irritation and bleeding and other side effects may limit its usefulness.

An extreme method to reduce the colonic formation of cerebrotoxins is colonic resection or bypass. The mortality rate for this procedure in patients with chronic liver disease is 25%. Therefore this treatment should be reserved only for patients with spontaneous, refractory, and chronic or recurrent encephalopathy present for at least 6 months and with otherwise good liver function. Good results have been reported for patients with postshunt encephalopathy.

Finally, the most direct and perhaps most dramatic form of treatment of hepatic encephalopathy is liver transplantation, which presently is still being developed and therefore reserved only for select patients with severe chronic liver disease. Hopefully further progress in the field of transplantation technology and immunotherapy will allow expansion of the indications for this treatment in the near future.

## BIBLIOGRAPHY

Conn, H. O.: Current diagnosis and treatment of hepatic coma, Hosp. Prac. **8**:65-72, 1973.

Gazzard, B. G., et al.: Charcoal haemoperfusion in the treatment of fulminant hepatic failure, Lancet **1**:1301-1307, 1974.

Kennedy, J., Parbhoo, S. P., MacGillivray, B., and Sherlock, S.: Effect of extracorporeal liver perfusion on the electroencephalogram of patients in coma due to acute liver failure, Q. J. Med. **42**:549-561, 1973.

Schenker, S., Breen, K. J., and Hoyumpa, A. M.: Hepatic encephalopathy: current status, Gastroenterology **66**:121-151, 1974.

Summerskill, W. H. J., and Wolpert, E.: Ammonia metabolism in the gut, Am. J. Clin. Nutr. **23**:633-639, 1970.

*chapter 28*

# Gastrointestinal bleeding

STEPHEN R. SEVERANCE

Hemorrhage from the gastrointestinal tract is a common and serious problem[1-8] accounting for at least 1% of all hospital admissions and ranking second only to cardiovascular disease as a reason for emergency hospitalization. The overall mortality from this condition ranges from 5% to 30%, but if only cases of *massive* bleeding (estimated loss of at least 20% of blood volume) are considered, the mortality ranges from 25% to 50%. Increased mortality is clearly related to delay in appropriate diagnosis and treatment. Therefore nowhere in the field of critical care is a well-organized, systematic, multidisciplinary approach more important. This chapter outlines such an approach.

## ■ What are the common causes of gastrointestinal bleeding?

The advent of fiberoptic endoscopy has greatly increased the accuracy of the diagnosis of gastrointestinal bleeding. Between 85% and 90% of gastrointestinal bleeding originates from a lesion proximal to the ligament of Treitz (*upper* gastrointestinal bleeding); another 5% to 10% from lesions distal to this point (*lower* gastrointestinal bleeding); and finally, in 5% to 10%, despite extensive diagnostic procedures, the exact site of bleeding cannot be established. Bleeding into the gastrointestinal tract may, in fact, originate from anywhere in the gastrointestinal tract, as well as from communicating (pancreas or biliary tree) or contiguous (aorta or spleen) organs. Potential sources of gastrointestinal bleeding are given in the following list:

*Sources of gastrointestinal hemorrhage**

- Upper gastrointestinal bleeding
  - Inflammatory
    - Duodenal ulcer
    - Gastritis
    - Gastric ulcer
    - Esophagitis
    - Stress ulcer
    - Pancreatitis
  - Mechanical
    - Hiatus hernia
    - Mallory-Weiss syndrome
    - Hematobilia
  - Vascular
    - Esophageal or gastric varices
    - Aortointestinal fistula
    - Hemangioma
    - Rendu-Osler-Weber syndrome
    - Mesenteric vascular occlusion
    - Blue nevus bleb
  - Systemic
    - Blood dyscrasias
    - Collagen diseases
    - Uremia
  - Neoplasms
    - Carcinoma
    - Polyps—single, multiple, Peutz-Jeghers syndrome
    - Leiomyoma
    - Carcinoid
    - Leukemia
    - Sarcoma
- Lower gastrointestinal bleeding
  - Inflammatory
    - Ulcerative colitis
    - Diverticulitis
    - Enterocolitis—regional (Crohn's disease), tuberculous, radiation, bacterial, toxic

*Modified from Sleisinger, M., and Fordtran, J.: Gastrointestinal disease: pathophysiology, diagnosis, and management, Philadelphia, 1973, W. B. Saunders Co.

Mechanical
- Diverticulosis

Neoplasms
- Carcinoma
- Polyps—adenomatous and villous, familial polyposis, Peutz-Jeghers syndrome
- Leiomyoma
- Sarcoma
- Lipoma
- Metastatic (melanoma)

Anomalies
- Meckel's diverticulum

Vascular
- Hemorrhoids
- Aortoduodenal fistula
- Aortic aneurysm
- Hemangioma
- Mesenteric thrombosis
- Hereditary hemorrhagic telangiectasia
- Blue nevus bleb

Systemic
- Blood dyscrasias
- Collagen diseases
- Uremia

Among these, four account for approximately 90% of upper gastrointestinal bleeding episodes: peptic ulceration (gastric or duodenal), diffuse erosion (esophagitis, gastritis, or duodenitis), esophageal varices, and gastroesophageal tears *(Mallory-Weiss syndrome)*. Peptic ulcer disease is by far the most common cause of gastrointestinal bleeding in this country.

One of these causes of upper gastrointestinal bleeding, the gastroesophageal tear, or Mallory-Weiss syndrome, deserves special mention. This lesion, usually the result of abrupt elevation of intra-abdominal pressure by forceful vomiting or other means, has been considered to be a very rare, nearly always catastrophic event invariably requiring surgery. However, recent studies[9, 10] employing fiberoptic endoscopy have proved this syndrome to be far more common than previously thought, accounting for 5% to 15% of cases of upper gastrointestinal hemorrhage. Furthermore, only one fifth of these patients require surgery, and a substantial number do not even require transfusion.[10]

## ■ What are the causes of lower gastrointestinal bleeding?

The necessity for time-consuming preparation limits the fiberoptic endoscopic localization of the site of lower gastrointestinal bleeding in the acute situation. Carcinoma of the colon, usually on the left side, remains the most common cause of rectal bleeding. This condition together with (in order of frequency) diverticulosis, ulcerative colitis, and polyps accounts for 90% to 95% of the cases. Interestingly, if analysis is restricted to those patients with bleeding severe enough to require transfusion, diverticulosis becomes most common, accounting for approximately 70% of the cases.[11]

## ■ What are the clinical features presented by patients with gastrointestinal bleeding?

Rectal bleeding and hematemesis or melena are the most common complaints of patients with lower and upper gastrointestinal bleeding, respectively. Hematemesis occurs in about one half to two thirds of patients with upper gastrointestinal bleeding. Blood exposed for a significant period of time to either acid or bacterial action turns black, explaining the frequent clinical observations of "coffee-ground" emesis or shiny black "tarry" stools (melena). Melena is almost always a sign of upper gastrointestinal bleeding, occurring in two thirds of such patients. Under normal conditions a minimum of approximately 100 ml of blood introduced into the stomach will produce melanotic stools. However, in conditions of diminished bacterial action (for example, neomycin therapy) or increased intestinal motility (blood within the gastrointestinal tract has a strong cathartic effect), upper gastrointestinal bleeding may result in the passage of actual red or more commonly "maroon-colored" blood via the rectum. Conversely, in conditions of stasis or diminished intestinal motility such as an obstructing carcinoma, lower gastrointestinal bleeding may produce black stools or so-called *pseudomelena.* Oral preparations containing either iron or bismuth may produce black stools in the absence of gastrointestinal bleeding. Such stools usually lack the shiny or tarry appearance produced by actual blood and yield a negative or weakly positive chemical reaction for blood. Truly melenic stool should invariably produce a strong (that is, 4+) chemical reaction for blood.

In addition to these overt symptoms of bleeding, approximately half of the patients with gastrointestinal bleeding will describe less specific symptoms such as weakness, faintness, fatigue, or abdominal pain. A few patients with acute and many with chronic bleeding present with one of these symptoms alone.

## ■ What specific information should always be obtained from the patient with gastrointestinal bleeding?

Ideally a complete traditional medical history and systems review should be obtained from every patient with gastrointestinal bleeding. Unfortunately the presence of severe bleeding or even shock may make this impractical early in the patient's hospital course. However, even under these circumstances there are a few pertinent questions that provide invaluable information and should never be omitted.

Any prior history of gastrointestinal disease or surgery should be noted. In Palmer's large series[12] nearly half the patients were already known to have a gastrointestinal lesion capable of producing bleeding. Such a history, while obviously very valuable, should not lead to diagnostic overcomplacency, since 40% of these patients were in fact bleeding from lesions other than those previously diagnosed.

Pain may suggest peptic ulcer, pancreatitis, or biliary disease (hematobilia); prior vascular surgery may lead to a diagnosis of aortoenteric fistula; and protracted wretching or vomiting of clear material *followed by* bloody emesis may indicate a gastric or gastroesophageal tear (Mallory-Weiss syndrome). Symptoms of liver disease should be sought, and careful questioning may be required to elicit a description of symptoms suggestive of bleeding diathesis. Although the symptoms of the more severe dyscrasias (for example, hemophilia) are commonly volunteered spontaneously, an almost forgotten difficult dental extraction may be the only clue to a mild one (for example, von Willebrand's disease).

Finally, and perhaps most important, a meticulous drug history is indispensable in any case of gastrointestinal bleeding. Salicylates and alcohol are by far the most common offenders, causing bleeding in their own right (that is, hemorrhagic erosive gastritis) as well as potentiating bleeding from independent lesions, especially peptic ulcer. More equivocal evidence has linked drugs such as indomethacin, phenylbutazone, corticosteroids, reserpine, nicotine, and the antimetabolites to either peptic ulcer formation, gastrointestinal bleeding, or both. The association of anticoagulants such as warfarin with gastrointestinal bleeding should be obvious. Less appreciated is the fact that the great majority of patients who bleed while on anticoagulant therapy do so from a distinct, usually independent anatomic lesion, for example, an ulcer or diverticulum.

When taking a drug history, it is important to recall that many nonprescription over-the-counter preparations, including innumerable aspirin-containing compounds, may not be classified as "medicines" by the patient and therefore may not be mentioned unless asked about specifically. Nowhere in the medical history is careful circumspection more important than in the detection of alcohol abuse. Witness the patient who is patently "tipsy" at 9:00 in the morning who drinks only "socially!" Questions regarding alcohol intake should always be casual and nonaccusatory in nature, possibly appended in an offhand manner to inquiries about nonprescription medications. When doubt exists, tactful questioning of family members is appropriate and may be helpful.

## ■ What elements of the physical examination are particularly useful in the evaluation of patients with gastrointestinal bleeding?

As in the case of the medical history, a complete examination is ideal, but not always immediately practical. The abdominal examination is obviously important, and the presence or absence of tenderness, peritoneal signs, succussion splash, or bruits as well as the relative activity of bowel sounds should be carefully noted. Hepatic or splenic enlargement, as well as other signs suggestive of liver disease or chronic alcoholism, such as palmar erythema, Dupuytren's contracture, spider telangiectasis, parotid enlargement, gynecomastia, and peripheral neuropathy, should be carefully sought.

The oronasopharyngeal area should never be overlooked in the physical examination. Silent bleeding in this area may be manifested by hematemesis alone (so-called *paradoxical hematemesis*) with unfortunate (and embarrassing!) consequences if not detected.

Some of the most useful clues, and seemingly the most easily overlooked, occur in the skin. A partial list of mucocutaneous disorders associated with gastrointestinal bleeding is reproduced here:

*Mucocutaneous disorders associated with gastrointestinal bleeding**

- Hereditary hemorrhagic telangiectasia
- Universal angiomatosis
- Blue rubber bleb nevus syndrome
- Multiple phlebectasia
- Pseudoxanthoma elasticum
- Ehlers-Danlos syndrome
- Homocystinuria
- Polyarteritis nodosa
- Atrophying papulosis of Degos
- Neurofibromatosis
- Kaposi's sarcoma
- Peutz-Jeghers syndrome
- Carcinoid syndrome

## ■ What is hereditary hemorrhagic telangiectasia?

The most common mucocutaneous disorder associated with gastrointestinal bleeding is hereditary hemorrhagic telangiectasia, or the Osler-Weber-Rondu syndrome.[13] The *telangiectasia* seen in this syndrome are dilated superficial capillary-venous vessels that may appear anywhere on the skin or in the mucous membrane of the gastrointestinal tract from the nasopharyngeal orifice to the anus. The telangiectasia may be restricted to the gastrointestinal tract with sparing of the skin, and unless suspected, they are easily missed on endoscopic examination. These lesions never appear on x-ray films. Although they appear to be hereditary, the lesions are not usually manifested until middle age. Bleeding tends to be chronic and seldom well-localized enough to be amenable to surgery. Oral iron therapy alone may be inadequate, and parenteral iron therapy may be necessary to maintain even a low normal hemoglobin level. *Acute massive bleeding* is uncommon in a patient with this disorder and should lead to a search for an associated localized arteriovenous malformation or an unrelated source of bleeding such as peptic ulcer.

## ■ How is the severity of bleeding most accurately assessed?

The rate of blood loss is as important as the total quantity lost in determining the clinical manifestations. Loss of more than half the circulating blood volume over a period of several weeks or months may produce only mild pallor and weakness, whereas the acute loss of 2 or 3 units of blood may result in syncope with many of the clinical signs of hypovolemia. The hypotension, tachycardia, mental confusion, clammy skin, and constricted veins of *shock* are reliable but rather insensitive signs, usually indicating relatively acute loss of at least 2000 ml of blood. Perhaps the most sensitive bedside indication of acute blood loss is *postural changes* in pulse or blood pressure, so-called *vasomotor instability*. Under normal conditions a change from the supine to the sitting or standing position initiates complex cardiovascular compensatory responses mediated by both neurogenic and humoral mechanisms that maintain blood pressure and pulse with minor changes. When hypovolemia caused by a deficit in blood or other fluids is present, these compensatory responses may be required to maintain normal blood pressure and pulse *even in the supine position*. In such a case, a change in position will result in abnormal changes in these values. The tilt test, utilizing a specially designed table

---

*Modified from UCLA Interdepartmental Conference: Ann. Intern. Med. **71**:993-1010, 1969.

to provide various angles of elevation, has been recommended as a sophisticated, although somewhat impractical, method of quantitating these changes. Nearly as much information may be obtained simply by determining blood pressure and pulse first in the supine and then in the sitting position. A drop in systolic pressure of 10 mm Hg or more or an increase of 20 beats/min or more in pulse indicates a minimum blood loss of 1000 ml in the average patient and even less in the older patient with diminished vascular tone. In the patient who already has hypotension in the supine position, this simple test adds little information and indeed may be dangerous.

## ■ How do hemoglobin or hematocrit values correlate with the results of blood loss?

The hemoglobin or hematocrit values immediately after acute blood loss, no matter how massive, will be virtually unchanged, since the blood remaining will be identical in composition to that lost. However, in an effort to restore intravascular volume, complex homeostatic mechanisms are initiated, resulting in renal conservation of fluid and electrolytes and in gradual shifts of fluid from extra- to intravascular compartments. These compensatory changes and the fall in hemoglobin and hematocrit that accompanies them are gradual, requiring more than 24 hours to be complete. *Hemoglobin and hematocrit are therefore unreliable indices of acute blood loss.* However, the IV infusions of fluid restore intravascular volumes as effectively and much more rapidly than the body's homeostatic mechanisms, and once fluids sufficient to eradicate any postural change in blood pressure or pulse have been infused, hemoglobin or hematocrit values reflect quantitative blood loss more accurately, each 4% drop in hematocrit reflecting a loss of approximately 1 unit of blood.

## ■ What initial diagnostic studies should be obtained?

A hemoglobin or hematocrit determination should be performed immediately. Stool and gastric aspirate, if not grossly bloody, should be tested for blood using guaiac or benzidine reagents. Complete blood count, urinalysis, and serum amylase, electrolyte, and liver function tests should be ordered. Assessment of the coagulation system is desirable in all patients and essential in any patient with liver disease or a history suggestive of a bleeding diathesis. Prothrombin and partial thromboplastin times, fibrinogen level, and platelet count or qualitative assessment of platelets on peripheral smear constitute an adequate coagulation "screen," with more sophisticated testing to elucidate any initial abnormalities. In addition, routine x-ray films of the chest and abdomen should be obtained. Because myocardial infarction, often "silent," occurs in 1% to 2% of patients with gastrointestinal hemorrhage, an ECG is indicated for older patients and those with coronary risk factors or massive bleeding. It is recommended that a gastrointestinal bleeding flow sheet similar to that shown in Fig. 28-1 be utilized at the bedside.

## ■ What should be included in the initial treatment of patients with gastrointestinal bleeding?

Since diagnostic procedures such as endoscopy or radiography are more hazardous when the patient's condition is unstable, the goal of initial treatment should be the *resuscitation* and stabilization of the patient's condition. IV therapy should be initiated using a large-bore (14- or 16-gauge) IV cannula (for example, Medicut or Intracath). A catheter for monitoring central venous pressure (CVP) should be placed in any patient with hypotension or shock and continued blood loss, and should be strongly considered in older patients or those with a history of cardiovascular disease in whom more than modest fluid and blood replacement is anticipated. In addition, oxygen therapy is indicated for any patient with hypotension or significant anemia. Most of these patients will be extremely apprehensive, and in all except those with definite shock, an appropriate sedative, such as phenobarbital, may be given parenterally. A vitamin K preparation such as phytonadione, 10 to 20 mg, may be given

The stomach and duodenum

Gastrointestinal bleeding: flow sheet

Date: 4/17/73

Clinical:

| Times: | 1 AM | 1 30 | 2 30 | | | | |
|---|---|---|---|---|---|---|---|
| Mental status | Confused | | clear | | | | |
| Pulse | 140 | 120 | 100 | | | | |
| Blood pressure Supine | 90/60 | 100/70 | 110/76 | | | | |
| Upright | — | 70/50 | 100/70 | | | | |
| CVP | 1 | 2 | 6 | | | | |
| Gastric lavage | bloody | brown | Clear | | | | |
| Stool | bloody | | 500 cc black | | | | |
| | | | | | | | |
| | | | | | | | |
| Laboratory: Hg/Hct | 7/20 | | 8.5/25 | | | | |
| WBC | 20,000 | — | — | | | | |
| BUN/creatinine | 45/1.8 | | | | | | |
| Prothrombin (sec) | 14 | | | | | | |
| Arterial pH and gases | | | | | | | |
| Blood electrolytes | NA 140 K 3.7 | | | | | | |
| Diagnostic: Note endoscopy | | | | | | | |
| barium studies, angiography, | Esophagoscopy NEG. | | | X-Ray D.U. | | | |
| string test, intubation, etc. | | | | | | | |
| | | | | | | | |
| Therapy: Blood products | — | 1500 Blood | whole → | | | | |
| Fluids (IV and PO) | 1000 Ringers | | | | | | |
| Electrolytes | " | | | | | | |
| Pharmacologic dose | 20 u. PiTressin | | | | | | |
| Tamponade with pressure | | | | | | | |
| Comments: | | | | | | | |
| | | | | | | | |

Name Bleeder, G.I.

Hosp. No. .000 000

**Fig. 28-1.** Flow sheet of stomach and duodenum. (Modified from Sleisinger, M., and Fordtran, J.: Gastrointestinal disease: pathophysiology, diagnosis and management, Philadelphia, 1973, W. B. Saunders Co.)

by IM or IV route to any patient with a prolonged prothrombin time. Since this medication is relatively harmless unless given in excessive dosages and requires several hours to begin generating prothrombin, it is not necessary to await laboratory results in patients with known cirrhosis, malnutrition from any cause, or a history of heavy salicylate use, which may also depress the prothrombin time.

Finally, a nasogastric tube should be placed in any patient with suspected upper gastrointestinal bleeding or with rectal passage of blood that is not clearly lower gastrointestinal in origin. Since a significant number of bleeding duodenal ulcers will present solely with rectal bleeding, this simple and harmless procedure may avoid considerable frustration and embarrassment!

Even in the presence of continuous bleeding from the duodenum, a closed pylorus may prevent the reflux of blood into the stomach, except at inconstant intervals. A significant number of lesions of the stomach that have stopped bleeding will rebleed early in the hospital course. Finally, distention as well as acidity aggravates the bleeding of erosive gastritis. For these reasons, except in the case of probable lower gastrointestinal bleeding, the nasogastric tube should not be removed following an initially negative aspiration, but rather taped in place and attached to intermittent or continuous suction for a period of several to 24 hours.

If the initial gastric aspirate is bloody or "coffee ground" in appearance, gastric lavage *(gavage)* using an iced solution should be begun. The purpose of this procedure is twofold. First, it reduces gastric blood flow by 50%[15] and will stop bleeding, at least temporarily, in approximately two thirds of patients with upper gastrointestinal hemorrhage.[12] Second, it allows removal of retained secretions, blood, and large clots, all of which interfere with the performance or interpretation of diagnostic procedures such as endoscopy or gastrointestinal x-ray films. Unfortunately this procedure may lose effectiveness if performed improperly. The most common mistake is the use of the relatively small nasogastric tube rather than a large tube (at least No. 36 French). A large tube is easier to position, less likely to become clogged, and allows removal of blood clots too large to pass through the small tube. Large double-lumen[16] or triple-lumen[17] tubes have been especially designed for this purpose, but in their absence an Ewald tube attached to a simple Y connector may be used. Using rubber tubing, one branch of the Y leads to an *irrigation bag* or similar receptacle for instillation of fluid, while the other branch leads to a pail or basin where the fluid may drain from the stomach by gravity. When one branch is in use, the other should be clamped with a hemostat. The tube is passed through the mouth or nose into the stomach and the patient placed in the prone or left lateral position at an angle of elevation that places the feet higher than the head. Proper positioning of the tube is then ensured by adjusting it until at least 40 ml of lavage solution can be aspirated after 50 ml is instilled.

Since varying degrees of absorption may occur during this procedure, there has been some disagreement over the recommended composition of the solutions used.[14] Very rarely, electrolyte abnormalities such as hyponatremia have been attributed to the use of iced *water* solutions, while the absorption of sodium chloride from *saline* solutions may lead to volume excess in susceptible patients who are not significantly volume depleted from bleeding. Isotonic sodium sulfate solutions have been used to minimize (although not eliminate) sodium absorption. In reality the choice of solution is probably irrelevant unless massive volumes are used in a patient with medical problems predisposing to fluid and electrolyte disturbances (for example, hyponatremia in the cirrhotic patient or volume overload in the patient with heart disease or renal failure). One or two liters of the solution chosen is placed over ice in a large basin, and approximately 300 ml at a time of the resultant mixture is instilled into the stomach. After each instillation the stomach is allowed to drain by simple gravity, but in order to dislodge blood clots, the tube should be irrigated frequently using a 50 ml irrigating syringe. Care should be taken to avoid unduly forceful suction, which may produce gastric artifacts difficult to distinguish from erosive gastritis if gastroscopy is performed later. Cessation of bleeding is indicated by a persistently clear or faint pink return from the stomach, and lavage should not be considered unsuccessful unless continued for a minimum of 1 hour without such clearing. Since iced lavage may cause shivering and discomfort, at times actually lowering the body temperature, the patient should be covered as warmly as possible during the procedure.

### ■ What type of fluid should be used for IV replacement in the presence of gastrointestinal bleeding?

Obviously the types and quantities of fluid used must be tailored to meet the specific needs of the individual patient. For example, the needs of the patient with minimum or slow bleeding and chronic congestive heart failure differ immensely from those of the patient with more rapid blood loss and preexisting dehydration from intractable vomiting.

In general IV therapy has two major objectives. The first is restoration of intravascular volume (reflected in blood pressure and pulse), which may be accomplished by infusion of either blood products or nonsanguineous fluids such as saline or albumin solutions. The second is restoration of oxygen-carrying capacity (reflected in the hemoglobin or hematocrit values), which can be accomplished solely through the use of blood products. Both practical and theoretical considerations govern the choice of preparations used to achieve these objectives. Practically speaking, the sophisticated methods involved in the modern "type and cross match" may require as much as an hour or more, making nonsanguineous solutions the mainstay of early resuscitation. In the small hospital with limited blood bank reserves or in the patient with a rare blood type, this delay may be even greater. In the rare circumstance of massive bleeding with shock and critically reduced oxygen-carrying capacity from the outset, *type-specific* blood can usually be provided in 10 minutes or less. If blood of the patient's specific type is not immediately available, O-negative blood may serve as the "universal donor" in this circumstance. A less important practical consideration is cost. A liter of saline solution costs a little over $1, a similar quantity of 5% albumin in saline solution over $50, and a unit of blood $25 to $50.[18]

In a more theoretical vein, studies in both man and animals have shown that acute blood loss is followed by a reduction not only in intravascular volume, but in extravascular volume as well, and that replacement of blood alone will not restore extravascular volume. Studies in experimentally bled animals have shown that animals treated with their lost blood plus nonsanguineous solutions such as saline or plasma solutions have twice the survival of those treated with the lost blood alone.[19] Similar, although less well-controlled, observations have been made in man.

The type of nonsanguineous solution to be used remains a subject of controversy.[18] *Crystalloid* solutions such as saline or Ringer's lactate solution have economy and relatively greater availability to recommend them. On the other hand, the recent theoretical implication of a fall in plasma oncotic pressure in the development of *posttraumatic respiratory insufficiency,* or *shock lung,* following the treatment of shock states has created a bias toward the use of *colloid* solutions such as albumin or plasma. Whether using crystalloid, colloid, or both, sodium bicarbonate should be added when systemic acidosis is present. In addition, solutions containing some glucose may be preferable in alcoholic patients, who occasionally develop hypoglycemia. (Dextrose-containing solutions may agglutinate the red blood cells in banked blood and therefore should never be infused simultaneously through the same IV line with blood.)

Blood may be administered in its whole form or as packed blood cells (with the plasma removed). Packed blood cells have the advantages of conserving other components such as plasma or clotting factors for use elsewhere and reducing the volume load for patients with marginal cardiac, renal, or liver function. In addition, packed blood cells contain considerably less ammonia than whole blood, possibly of importance in patients with severe liver disease. Whether whole blood or packed cells are used, transfusion therapy should be adequate not only to restore oxygen-carrying capacity sufficiently to maintain normal functions, but also to allow some reserve in case of recurrent blood loss. Under ordinary circumstances the return of the hematocrit to approximately 30% (or hemoglobin to about 10%) will achieve these objectives. Both packed cells and whole blood donated more than 24 hours before use are deficient in several clotting factors. Therefore every fifth or sixth unit transfused should be fresh (less than 24 hours old) whole blood. Banked blood is prevented from clotting by the addition of *citrate* to bind calcium, which is an essential factor in normal coagulation. For this reason, even though most hematologists believe that frank tetany will occur before ionized calcium is depressed sufficiently to effect clot formation, intermittent IV calcium infusion is a common practice during massive transfusion therapy.

Finally, the majority of commonly encountered clotting abnormalities will respond readily to adequate quantities, where indicated, of fresh-frozen plasma, platelet packs, or both. Clotting factor concentrates (for example, Konyne) carry an inordinate risk of hepatitis, may precipitate intravascular coagulation (especially in patients with liver disease),[20, 21] and therefore should rarely, if ever, be used.

## ■ What diagnostic approach should be followed to localize exactly the site of upper gastrointestinal bleeding?

A step-by-step systematic approach to the diagnosis of gastrointestinal bleeding has been devised[22] and should be extremely helpful as long as the importance of individualizing each case is remembered. The major diagnostic alternatives are barium contrast radiography, fiberoptic endoscopy, and selective or superselective abdominal arteriography.

With occasional dissent,[23] it is now generally agreed that barium contrast radiography, once the mainstay of diagnosis, has little if any diagnostic usefulness *in the presence of active upper gastrointestinal bleeding*. First, when compared with fiberoptic endoscopy, it is inaccurate, failing to detect many lesions even in well-prepared nonbleeding patients. For example, as many as 50% of esophageal varices,[24] 11% to 14% of benign gastric ulcers, 4% to 12% of gastric cancers, 6% to 17% of duodenal ulcers, and 50% of marginal ulcers are missed by the upper gastrointestinal series.[25] In unprepared patients with intraluminal blood and clots the degree of inaccuracy will be even greater. Although a special air contrast technique has recently been described for the detection of gastric erosions, gastric varices, and gastric or esophageal tears, these lesions will be detected by conventional barium studies in *less than 5%* of the cases. In addition, the detection of a lesion with bleeding potential on barium studies *does not establish that lesion as the site of present bleeding*. Among 1313 patients with upper gastrointestinal bleeding described by Palmer,[12] 2024 actual or potential bleeding lesions were found by endoscopy. More than 50% of the patients with cirrhosis, definite esophageal varices, and upper gastrointestinal bleeding were bleeding from a lesion other than the esophageal varices.[26, 27] Finally, contrast material in the intestinal tract precludes the effective use of fiberoptic endoscopy for several hours and of arteriography for 24 to 48 hours after a barium contrast study.

With rare exceptions,[28] gastroenterologists seem to agree that fiberoptic endoscopy is the diagnostic procedure of choice in the patient with active upper gastrointestinal bleeding and no contraindications to the procedure.[12, 29-31] Endoscopy is more fruitful if performed within the first 24 to 48 hours of hospitalization,[31] and properly performed should yield a positive diagnosis in over 80%

of the cases. The complication rate of the procedure is probably less than 1 in 300, with an overall mortality of less than 1 in 4000.[25]

There are relatively few contraindications to endoscopy. Since cooperation on the part of the patient is a prerequisite, it should not be performed in the combative or delirious patient. The comatose patient not only lacks cooperativeness but carries a higher risk of aspiration as well and should never undergo endoscopy unless endotracheal intubation has been performed. The patient's condition should always be stabilized prior to endoscopy, as morbidity and mortality are drastically increased in the presence of shock or vasomotor instability. Similarly, patients with acute cardiac or pulmonary conditions such as acute myocardial infarction or respiratory failure should not undergo endoscopy. Alternative diagnostic procedures should be strongly considered in cases of pancreatitis or possible perforated viscus, since either condition may be aggravated by endoscopy. Finally, since most institutions lack the facilities for actual sterilization of the endoscope itself, the procedure should be avoided if at all possible in cases of active tuberculosis or hepatitis B antigenemia.

The procedure may be carried out at the bedside or, more conveniently, in a specially equipped room. It should always be preceded by a thorough gastric lavage. Atropine or propantheline is administered parenterally prior to the procedure to reduce secretions and motility and minimize the risk of vagal reactions. Sedation should be adequate but minimal. Parenteral diazepam, phenobarbital, or meperidine (Demerol) alone or in various combinations has been used. The pharynx is usually anesthetized with a gargle of lidocaine viscous (2%) or anesthetic lozenges.

Examination following these preparations should disclose the precise lesion responsible for the bleeding in the majority of patients. In cases of torrential bleeding the lesion itself may be obscured by blood, and only the area involved can be stated with certainty. Conversely, bleeding may be slow enough to escape detection by conventional endoscopy. In the latter instances, examination using an ultraviolet light source immediately following the IV injection of fluorescin has been recommended.[32]

The most important complications of endoscopy are cardiorespiratory in nature, ranging from minor arrhythmias to apnea or cardiac arrest during the procedure. Rarely the instrument may perforate a viscus, most commonly the upper esophagus. An easily overlooked complication is pulmonary aspiration of gastric or oral secretions. One study[33] showed that variable quantities of radiopaque fluid introduced into the mouth during the examination were visible in the pulmonary tree on subsequent chest x-ray films in 25% of the patients. Fortunately none of these patients developed symptoms, but symptomatic aspiration has been reported.[34] The appearance of unexplained fever or respiratory symptoms following endoscopy should always suggest the possibility of this complication.

Selective or superselective arteriography should be considered in any case where endoscopy is contraindicated or fails to identify the site of bleeding. The current disagreement concerning its diagnostic efficacy probably arises from its use in cases where the rate of bleeding is insufficient for visualization. In the experimental animal, blood loss of at least 0.5 ml/min, the equivalent of less than 1 L/24 hr in man, was necessary for arteriographic visualization. Many clinical investigators, however, believe that blood loss of less than 2 ml/min or approximately 3 L/24 hr will seldom be demonstrated arteriographically.[35] Obviously, quantitating blood loss precisely in the average clinical situation is impossible. In one study[35] arteriography successfully localized the bleeding point in 85% of the patients receiving 5 units or more of blood in the 24 hours prior to study and in 80% of those manifesting shock at any time prior to examination.

The major complications of arteriography are vascular difficulties, including thrombosis, hemorrhage, and perforation. These can be minimized by careful assessment of the patient's clotting status prior to the procedure and by examination of the peripheral pulse both before and at frequent intervals after the maneuver.

## ■ What about the diagnosis of lower gastrointestinal bleeding?

The lower gastrointestinal tract is obviously more difficult to prepare for study than the upper. For this reason barium contrast radiology is even more difficult to interpret, and the exact role, if any, of fiberoptic endoscopy (colonoscopy) remains undefined. With few exceptions, the initial procedure should be proctosigmoidoscopy. If the history suggests the possibility of inflammatory mucosal disease such as ulcerative colitis or amebiasis, this procedure should be performed with minimum or no preparation to avoid the production of mucosal artifacts by enemas. Anoscopy, using a slotted instrument, should always precede sigmoidoscopy. Occasionally large internal hemorrhoids are seen and suspected as the site of bleeding but are not bleeding at the time of examination. In such a case, suspicion may often be confirmed simply by repeating the examination after asking the patient to "bear down" forcefully. Sigmoidoscopy should be performed whether anoscopy is positive or not. If no source of bleeding is observed, the presence or absence of blood coming from beyond the furthest penetration of the instrument should be noted. If sigmoidoscopy is nondiagnostic in the face of continued bleeding at a rate judged sufficient to allow visualization, arteriography should be considered.[36] As in the case with upper gastrointestinal bleeding, arteriography is of questionable value if barium contrast studies have been performed in the previous 24 to 48 hours. However, since bleeding from diverticula is commonly noted to cease following a barium enema,[37] barium contrast studies probably have a greater place in lower rather than upper gastrointestinal bleeding.

## ■ Other than iced lavage, what nonsurgical methods can be used to control bleeding?

The lack of any single consistently effective treatment is attested to by the multiplicity of those recommended.[38] With few exceptions, studies of these treatments have been uncontrolled. Usually the effectiveness of a given treatment in the initial control of bleeding is promising. Quite often, however, the incidence of recurrent bleeding or the number of patients eventually requiring surgery or another form of treatment is not clearly reported. Because many of the reported methods are new, the incidence of complication remains undefined. Especially for those procedures requiring special skill, the reported incidences of complications may vary widely from institution to institution.

Nowhere are these problems more apparent than in the treatment of bleeding esophageal varices. An effective method for at least temporary control of variceal bleeding is the infusion of pitressin, 20 units in 100 ml of dextrose and water, over a period of 20 minutes. The mechanism of this treatment is a reduction in portal blood flow. In one study[39] bleeding was arrested in over half of the patients so treated as compared to none in a control group treated with placebo injections. In the same study the overall mortalities of the treated and control group were 93% and 80%, respectively! Esophageal tamponade in some form or another has been used since 1930, and yet controversy over its effectiveness and safety still rages. For example, the reported incidence of major complications resulting directly from the use of the Sengstaken-Blakemore tube ranges from 8.6%[40] to 35%.[41] Deaths *directly attributable* to the use of the tube occurred in from 5.7%[40] to 22%[41] of the patients in whom it was used. Yet esophageal tamponade will arrest bleeding initially in 50% to 80% of the cases.

The major complications of esophageal tamponade are rupture or erosion of the esophagus, occlusion of the airway by the balloon, or aspiration of secretions resulting from inadequate drainage of the occluded esophagus. Each of these complications can be minimized by meticulous attention to the details of the procedure and a healthy respect on the part of all involved personnel for its malignant potential. Either a Sengstaken-Blakemore or a Linton tube may be used.

The Linton tube has a single large (400 cc) gastric balloon that is inflated in the stomach and drawn back snugly against the cardioesophageal sphincter by traction on the tube proximally. Lumens for aspiration distal to the balloon in the stomach and proximally in the esophagus allow for continuous monitoring of bleeding and aspiration of pooled secretions in the esophagus.

The Sengstaken-Blakemore tube has two balloons. The distal or gastric balloon holds only 200 cc and is designed less for tamponade than for simply anchoring the tube in its proper position. If bleeding continues once it is anchored snugly in place at the cardioesophageal junction, control is usually achieved by inflation of the proximal or esophageal balloon (Fig. 28-2). The volume in the esophageal balloon is less important than the pressure, which is measured by connecting its inflow tube to a sphygmomanometer and maintained at the minimum required to control bleeding, *no more than 40 mm Hg.* As with the Linton tube, a lumen distal to the gastric balloon allows monitoring of stomach contents. Difficulty in aspirating this lumen in either tube may be caused by its entrapment under the gastric balloon and may be corrected by deflating the balloon and readjusting the tube prior to reinflation. The Sengstaken tube has no lumen for esophageal aspiration and a regular Levine-type tube *must be passed for this purpose.* This second tube may be tied to the Sengstaken tube just above the esophageal balloon using suture material, or it may be passed separately through the opposite nostril.

The effectiveness and overall complication rate of these two tubes is probably very similar. The Linton tube has the advantage of being somewhat simpler to use and exerts its primary effect at the area most commonly involved in variceal bleeding—the cardioesophageal junction. The extra lumen for esophageal aspiration is an added convenience. (Sengstaken tubes with esophageal lumens are available, but considerations of size limit this extra lumen to an impractically small diameter.) The major disadvantage of the Linton tube is its greater dependency on

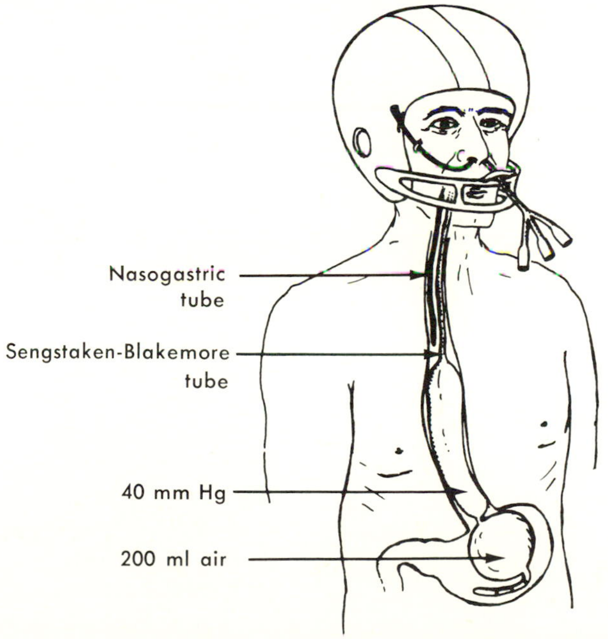


**Fig. 28-2.** Sengstaken-Blakemore tube in place. Both balloons inflated with nasogastric tube placed through external nares into a position just above esophageal balloon.

traction and, with it, a greater risk of erosion or pressure necrosis. The Sengstaken tube, on the other hand, carries a greater risk of respiratory complications such as airway occlusion or aspiration.

Whichever tube is used, it should be inserted by someone skilled in its use, preferably a gastroenterologist or surgeon. Each balloon should be tested by installing air prior to insertion. Smaller leaks can be detected by holding the balloon under water. To avoid the additional hazard of aspiration, topical anesthesia of the pharynx should be avoided when possible. The tube should be passed through the nose (preferably) or mouth *to its full length;* 50 to 100 cc of air instilled; and the balloon pulled up until the resistance of the cardioesophageal junction is encountered. The distance from mouth to cardioesophageal junction is amazingly constant from one individual to another, and if the tube is properly positioned, its 40 cm mark should be just visible at the patient's nose or mouth. At this point, unless bleeding is truly exigent, a plain x-ray film should be taken to assure proper positioning. The tube should then be advanced a few centimeters, the full quantity of air (200 cc for the Sengstaken, 400 cc for the Linton) instilled, and the balloon once again drawn snugly against the cardioesophageal junction, gentle traction then being applied.

The use of orthopedic gravity traction, although popular, is to be deplored. Should continued bleeding occur despite adequate traction on the gastric balloon, the esophageal balloon of the Sengstaken tube should be inflated. Channels to the balloon should be double clamped with rubber-shod clamps to avoid inadvertent use during subsequent irrigation. The patient should be in an intensive care area with constant observation for signs of respiratory embarrassment. A pair of scissors should be kept in a clearly visible spot near the bedside so that the tube may be cut should this occur. In addition to continuous suction on the esophageal tube, pharyngeal and tracheal suction should be performed as frequently as possible.

Some experts leave the balloon tubes inflated for only a few hours after hemostasis is achieved; others leave them for 24 hours. The tubes should never be inflated continuously for more than 24 hours.

### ■ What is the place of the selective arterial infusion of pitressin in the control of gastrointestinal bleeding?

The selective arterial infusion of pitressin, and less commonly epinephrine or propranolol, has been used successfully to treat bleeding not only from varices but from other sources in the upper[42] and lower[43] gastrointestinal tract as well. The relative effectiveness of the procedure has not been established. In the only controlled trial, bleeding was stopped for 24 hours or more in 71% of 28 patients with upper gastrointestinal bleeding treated with pitressin infusion, whereas only 28% of the control group stopped bleeding.[42] However, a high recurrence rate was reflected in the fact that cessation of bleeding for at least *5 days* occurred in only 25% of the pitressin-treated group and 16% of the control group. The overall mortality was the same in both groups, but many of the control group eventually received pitressin infusion after conventional therapy failed.

If treatment by selective pitressin infusion is elected, a catheter is placed in the superior mesenteric artery for bleeding from esophageal varices or the small intestine, in the celiac artery for gastric or duodenal bleeding, and in the superior or inferior mesentric artery for colonic bleeding. Two of these vessels have been infused simultaneously when continued bleeding is thought to be secondary to collateral blood flow.[42] After an initial arteriogram, infusion should be begun at a rate of 0.05 to 0.1 unit of pitressin/min and increased every few minutes until bleeding is controlled. Since *total occlusion* of the infused vascular system becomes more likely with increasing rates of infusion, the rate should not exceed 0.4 unit/min. For the same reason the possibility of arterial constriction of a dangerous degree should always be excluded by repeating the arteriogram after the necessary rate of infusion has been reached.

Common side effects of pitressin infusion include systemic arterial hypertension, bradycardia or other arrhythmias, and a reduction in cardiac output.[44] More serious complications include infarction of the perfused segment of intestine.[45] It has been suggested that the presence of hypotension or shock may make this complication even more likely. Since pitressin exerts a strong antidiuretic hormone–like effect, varying degrees of hyponatremia may occur. The administration of hypotonic solutions should be avoided and serum sodium measured frequently. The effect of reduced hepatic blood flow in cirrhotic patients treated with pitressin has not yet been determined.

## ■ What is the best treatment for hemorrhagic gastritis?

Hemorrhagic erosive gastritis poses a particular problem, since there is no completely satisfactory surgical approach should medical therapy fail. Fortunately bleeding will be arrested by iced lavage in nearly 90% of these patients. Several other methods have been reported to be successful in refractory gastric bleeding from gastritis or other causes. Bleeding was controlled in 23 of 25 patients treated with quantities of antacid sufficient to maintain gastric pH at 7.0 or above.[46] Intragastric administration of 8 or 16 mg of levarterenol in 100 or 200 ml of saline solution temporarily controlled bleeding in 7 of 13[47] and 11 of 12[48] patients, respectively. Levarterenol, 8 to 16 mg in 500 ml or more of saline solution, has also been administered intraperitoneally[48] with varying success in both upper and lower gastrointestinal bleeding. This technique has even been extended to *continuous* intraperitoneal infusion of levarterenol.[49] More anecdotally, a "thrombin cocktail" (also known as "magic mud") consisting of several thousand units of topical thrombin and a cup of Gelfoam mixed with antacid or saline solution may be instilled into the stomach. Gastric hypothermia, or cooling of the stomach by a cold alcohol solution run through a special intragastric balloon, has fallen into disrepute but still has its proponents.[50] Even a treatment as exotic as daily injections of human growth hormone has been alleged to control bleeding![51] Finally, intra-arterial pitressin infusion has been used almost as successfully in gastritis as it has in more localized lesions.[52]

## ■ When should surgical intervention be considered?

Obviously the answer to this question will depend on the general condition of the patient as well as the etiology of bleeding and its potential for surgical correction. Reported mortality for emergency surgery in peptic ulcer disease ranges from 10% to 25% as opposed to 50% to 75% for variceal bleeding.[53] Prediction of mortality through "indices"[53, 54] based on the presence or absence of various laboratory or clinical findings is of questionable value to the individual patient. In general a previous history of bleeding ulcer, recurrent bleeding during the current hospitalization, blood loss requiring 6 or more units of blood following the initiation of medical therapy, or continuous bleeding for 48 hours or more requiring 4 or more units of blood are all indications for surgical intervention in the duodenal ulcer patient. Criteria may be less strict for the patient with gastric ulcer, since many still consider surgery the treatment of choice for this condition whether bleeding is present or not. When considering surgery, it should be remembered that older patients or those with other conditions adding to surgical risk are also often those least likely to withstand the insult of unabated bleeding.

## ■ What new developments can be anticipated in the treatment of gastrointestinal bleeding?

With the increasing refinement of instruments a more definitive approach to specific lesions will become more and more feasible. Bleeding polyps have already been removed endoscopically from the upper gastrointestinal tract,[55] and endoscopic electrocoagulation has been used in the successful treatment of a variety of lesions.[56] Hemostasis has been achieved in the canine stomach using an endoscopically conducted laser beam, and human studies with this modality are projected in the near future.[57] In the field of arteriography, bleeding has been successfully controlled by embolization of the artery, supplying the bleeding site with the patient's own clotted blood.[58, 59]

## REFERENCES


1. Sleisinger, M., and Fordtran, J.: Gastrointestinal disease: pathophysiology, diagnosis and management, Philadelphia, 1973, W. B. Saunders Co.
2. U.C.L.A. Interdepartmental Conference: Diagnosis and management of gastrointestinal bleeding, Ann. Intern. Med. **71**:993-1010, 1969.
3. Dagradi, A. E.: Management of gastrointestinal bleeding, Am. J. Gastroenterol. **46**: 309-316, 1966.
4. Sedgwick, C. E., and Vernon, D. K.: Gastrointestinal bleeding: diagnosis and management, Surg. Clin. North Am. **48**:523-542, 1968.
5. Malt, R.: Control of massive upper gastrointestinal hemorrhage, N. Engl. J. Med. **286**: 1043-1046, 1972.
6. Palmer, E.: Upper gastrointestinal hemorrhage, J.A.M.A. **231**:853-855, 1975.
7. Crook, I.: Upper gastrointestinal bleeding, Ann. Surg. **175**:771-782, 1972.
8. Myren, J., and Semb, L. S.: New trends in diagnosis and treatment of upper gastrointestinal bleeding, Scand. J. Gastroenterol. **5**:415-416, 1974.
9. Dagradi, A., et al.: The Mallory-Weiss lesion: an endoscopic study of thirty cases, Gastrointest. Endosc. **13**:18-19, 1967.
10. Watts, H. D., and Adnurand, W. H.: Mallory-Weiss syndrome: a reappraisal, J.A.M.A. **230**:1674-1675, 1974.
11. Moen, R., et al.: Rectal hemorrhage: moderate and severe, Ann. Surg. **155**:794-805, 1962.
12. Palmer, E.: The vigorous diagnostic approach to upper-gastrointestinal tract hemorrhage: a 23-year prospective study of 1400 patients, J.A.M.A. **207**:1477-1480, 1969.
13. Holpern, M., Turner, A. F., and Citron, B. F.: Hereditary hemorrhagic telangiectasia, Radiology **90**:1143-1149, 1968.
14. Bryant, L. R., et al.: Comparison of ice water with iced saline solution for gastric lavage in gastroduodenal hemorrhage, Am. J. Surg. **124**:570-572, 1972.
15. Waterman, N. G., and Walker, J. L.: Effect of a topical adrenergic agent on gastric blood flow, Am. J. Surg. **127**:241-243, 1974.
16. Stempien, S. T., and Dagradi, A. E.: A double lumen tube for gastroesophageal lavage, Gastrointest. Endosc. **13**:26-27, 1966.
17. Tielman, P. R., and Yanek, S. X.: New tube for the diagnosis and treatment of upper gastrointestinal hemorrhage, Am. J. Surg. **127**:771-772, 1974.
18. Moss, G.: An argument in favor of electrolyte solution for early resuscitation, Surg. Clin. North Am. **52**:3-17, 1972.
19. Gillon, J., et al.: A bioassay of treatment of hemorrhagic shock, Arch. Surg. **93**:537, 1966.
20. Ratnoff, O.: Prothrombin complex preparation: a cautionary note, Ann. Intern. Med. **81**:852-853, 1974.
21. Lewis, M. D., et al.: Coagulation factor concentrates in the treatment of the hemorrhagic diathesis of fulminant hepatic failure, Gut **15**:993-998, 1974.
22. Hedberg, S. E.: Endoscopy in gastrointestinal bleeding: a systematic approach to diagnosis, Surg. Clin. North Am. **54**:549-559, 1974.
23. Allam, R. N., Dykes, B. W., and Toy, D. K.: Diagnostic accuracy of early radiology in acute gastrointestinal haemorrhage, Br. Med. J. **4**:281-284, 1972.
24. Dagradi, A. E., Skorneck, A. B., and Stempien, S. J.: The problem of diagnosis of esophageal varices: a radiologic and endoscopic study, Gastrointest. Endosc. **8**:2, 1961.
25. Cotton, P. B.: Fibreoptic endoscopy and the barium meal—results and implications, Br. Med. J. **2**:161-165, 1973.
26. Dagradi, A. E., Tan, D. J., and Stempien, S. J.: Sources of upper gastrointestinal bleeding in patients with liver cirrhosis and large esophagogastric varices, Am. J. Gastroenterol. **54**:458-463, 1970.
27. Waldran, R., et al.: Emergency endoscopy after gastrointestinal haemorrhage in 50 patients with portal hypertension, Br. Med. J. **4**:94-96, 1974.
28. Sandlow, L. J., et al.: A prospective randomized study of the management of upper gastrointestinal hemorrhage, Am. J. Gastroenterol. **61**:282-289, 1974.
29. Koton, R. M., and Smith, F. W.: Panendoscopy in the early diagnosis of acute upper gastrointestinal bleeding, Gastrenterology **65**: 728-734, 1973.
30. Sugawa, C., et al.: Early endoscopy, Arch. Surg. **107**:133-137, 1973.
31. Forrest, J. A., Finlayson, N. D., and Shearman, D. J.: Endoscopy in gastrointestinal bleeding, Lancet **2**:394-397, 1974.

32. Smith, B. H., and Berk, J. E.: Ultraviolet endoscopy in the diagnosis of upper gastrointestinal bleeding, Am. J. Gastroenterol. **60:** 549-556, 1973.
33. Prout, F. J., and Metreweli, C.: Pulmonary aspiration after fibre-endoscopy of the upper gastrointestinal tract, Br. Med. J. **4:**269-271, 1972.
34. Taylor, P. A., et al.: Pulmonary complications after oesophagogastroscopy using diazepam, Br. Med. J. **1:**666, 1972.
35. Stanley, R. J., and Wise, L.: Arteriography in diagnosis of acute gastrointestinal tract bleeding, Arch. Surg. **107:**138-144, 1973.
36. Casarella, W. J., et al.: Lower gastrointestinal tract hemorrhage: new concepts based on arteriography, Am. J. Roentgenol. Radium Ther. Nucl. Med. **121:**351-368, 1974.
37. Adams, J. T.: The barium enema as treatment for massive diverticular bleeding, Dis. Colon Rectum **17:**430-439, 1974.
38. Boyce, H. W.: Nonsurgical treatment for gastrointestinal hemorrhage, J.A.M.A. **231:** 1065-1066, 1975.
39. Merigar, T. C., Jr., Plotkin, G. R., and Davidson, C. S.: Effect of intravenously administered posterior pituitary extract on hemorrhage from bleeding esophageal varices, N. Engl. J. Med. **266:**134-135, 1962.
40. Bauer, J. L., Kreel, I., and Kark, A.: The use of the Sengstaken-Blakemore tube for immediate control of bleeding esophageal varices, Ann. Surg. **179:**273-277, 1974.
41. Conn, H. O., and Simpson, J. A.: Excessive mortality associated with balloon tamponade of bleeding varices, J.A.M.A. **202:**587-591, 1967.
42. Conn, H. O., et al.: Intraarterial vasopressin in the treatment of upper gastrointestinal hemorrhage: a prospective controlled clinical trial, Gastroenterology **68:**211-221, 1975.
43. Athanasoulis, C. A., et al.: Mesenteric arterial infusions of vasopressin for hemorrhage from colonic diverticulosis, Ann. Surg. **129:** 212-216, 1975.
44. Serinek, K. R., and Thomford, N. R.: Isoproterenol in offsetting adverse effects of vasopressin in cirrhotic patients, Ann. Surg. **129:**130-136, 1975.
45. Berardi, R. S.: Vascular complications of superior mesenteric artery infusion with pitressin in treatment of bleeding esophageal varices, Am. J. Surg. **127:**757-761, 1974.
46. Curtis, L. E., et al.: Evaluation of the effectiveness of controlled pH in management of massive upper gastrointestinal bleeding, Am. J. Surg. **125:**474-476, 1973.
47. Kiselow, M. C., and Wagner, M.: Intragastric instillation of levarterenol, Arch. Surg. **107:**387-389, 1973.
48. Douglass, H. O.: Levarterenol irrigation: control of massive gastrointestinal bleeding in poor-risk patients, J.A.M.A. **230:**1653-1657, 1974.
49. Oliveira, G. G., et al.: Long-term intraperitoneal infusion of norepinephrine in the control of massive bleeding from stress ulcers, Crit. Care Med. **2:**262-264, 1974.
50. Sandlow, L. J., and Spellberg, M. A.: Gastric hypothermia for control of upper gastrointestinal bleeding, Am. J. Gastroenterol. **59:**307-314, 1973.
51. Winamer, S. T., et al.: Beneficial effect of human growth hormone on stress ulcers, Arch. Intern. Med. **135:**569-571, 1975.
52. Athanasoulis, C. A., et al.: Intraarterial posterior pituitary extract for acute gastric mucosal hemorrhage, N. Engl. J. Med. **290:** 597-603, 1974.
53. Kim, U., et al.: Factors influencing mortality of surgical treatment for massive gastroduodenal hemorrhage, Am. J. Gastroenterol. **60:**24-35, 1974.
54. Wirthlein, L. S., et al.: Prediction of surgical mortality in patients with cirrhosis and nonvariceal gastroduodenal bleeding, Surg. Gynecol. Obstet. **139:**65-68, 1974.
55. Dagradi, A. E., Ruiz, R. A., and Alaama, A.: Endoscopic duodenal polypectomy, Am. J. Gastroenterol. **61:**379-382, 1974.
56. Papp, T.: Endoscopic electrocoagulation in upper gastrointestinal hemorrhage, J.A.M.A. **230:**1172-1173, 1974.
57. Dwyer, R. M., et al.: Laser induced hemostasis in the canine stomach, J.A.M.A. **231:**486-489, 1975.
58. Rosch, J., Dotter, C. T., and Brown, M. J.: Selective arterial embolization: new method for control of acute gastrointestinal bleeding, Radiology **102:**303-306, 1972.
59. Seto, R., et al.: Management of diffuse hemorrhage from gastric mucosa pathophysiology and microcirculatory responses in diffuse gastric hemorrhage controlled by arterial embolization, Int. Surg. **59:**103-105, 1974.

# *chapter 29*

# Respiratory management

BERNHARD A. VOTTERI

The recognition and treatment of respiratory dysfunction in critically ill patients makes up a major part of the work load of intensive care units. Advances in resuscitative methods and the treatment of acute renal failure have resulted in the survival of many patients through the early stages of acute disorders such as shock. In the later phases of resuscitation, respiratory failure has emerged as a leading cause of morbidity and mortality. Respiratory failure in such patients is usually a result of an acute derangement of ventilatory function and is thus distinguished from the general deterioration of pulmonary function seen in patients with chronic respiratory disease. The critically ill patient is often noted to have progressive failure of pulmonary gas exchange, which can be defined as failure to add oxygen to or remove carbon dioxide from venous blood. In such patients respiratory failure develops over a time frame of approximately moments to 24 or 48 hours. The goal of this chapter is to provide an introduction to the appropriate ventilatory management of such patients.

Multiple reports now attest to the efficacy of mechanical ventilatory support in acute respiratory failure. Mortality among patients treated for acute respiratory failure in critical care units has declined from 70% to as low as 20%.[1-3] Such increases in survival have been attributed to the development of well-equipped, well-staffed intensive care units where the systematic evaluation of patients for the detection of respiratory failure and the monitoring of cardiorespiratory function has permitted early comprehensive treatment of the critically ill patient.[1, 4-8]

## ■ What are the most common causes of acute respiratory insufficiency in intensive care units?

Acute respiratory failure is usually caused by one of the following disorders: adult respiratory distress syndrome, drug-induced ventilatory depression, impaired chest wall function caused by chest wall trauma or neuromuscular disorders, exacerbations of chronic obstructive pulmonary disease, and status asthmaticus.[2, 9]

Respiratory distress syndrome is the most common disorder requiring intensive pulmonary care. It has been conservatively estimated that 150,000 patients each year demonstrate this syndrome in the United States.[3] This disorder may follow surgical or accidental insults and is commonly associated with shock, cardiopulmonary bypass, fat embolism, viral and aspiration pneumonia, septicemia, inhaled or ingested toxins, oxygen toxicity, and CNS injury.[10-13] Ashbaugh and associates[10, 14] stated that patients with respiratory distress syndrome usually presented with severe dyspnea, tachypnea, and grunting respirations. Intercostal and suprasternal retractions were usually present, and cyanosis and hypoxemia responded poorly to oxygen administration. Progressive differences between alveolar and arterial oxygen tension (A-a $\Delta P_{O_2}$) could be demonstrated and was attributed to air space closure in areas where blood flow continued. This space closure was attributed to alveolar epithelial injury, reduced surfactant, altered surface tension, pulmonary capillary injury, and interstitial edema formation. Such closed air spaces could not be reopened and ventilated without generating high transpulmonary pressures and increasing inspiratory force. The resultant increase in the work of breathing required to maintain lung inflation ultimately leads to patient exhaustion; this was followed by generalized air space closure and increased shunting of blood that was reflected by progressive hypoxemia.

Most cases of the adult respiratory distress syndrome present the clinical picture of pulmonary edema, and increased lung water has been recognized in patients with this disorder. Indeed, the clinical separation of acute respiratory distress syndrome from left ventricular failure may be most difficult.[15] Pulmonary edema formation in adult respiratory distress syndrome usually develops in the presence of normal capillary wedge pressure and is not a result of cardiac dysfunction.[16] The pulmonary edema appears to result from a diffuse alteration of the pulmonary vasculature with a resultant increase in pulmonary capillary permeability and loss of plasma and fluid into the interstitial space.[17, 18] Recent reviews of the mechanisms of pulmonary edema point out that rapid protein losses into the interstitial space may follow pulmonary capillary and alveolar insults.[19, 20] Such alteration could readily explain the fulminant pulmonary edema often seen in adult respiratory distress syndrome.

### ■ What are the clinical signs of respiratory failure?

Although the signs of respiratory failure are frequently nonspecific and may simply involve restlessness and disorientation, other signs are frequently present, such as changes in the rate or pattern of breathing. Breathing may be rapid, shallow, labored, or associated with cough. The skin may be moist and appear cyanotic. Hypertension and tachypnea are often noted. Irritability, restlessness, sleeplessness, and/or coma may be present. It is now recognized that hypoxemia and acidemia are the major determinants of such symptoms and signs. The finding of any of the clinical signs just discussed is an urgent indicator for a more definitive diagnosis that can only be achieved by blood gas analysis. Without such studies, unrecognized hypoxic restlessness may lead to the administration of a sedative that may hasten progressive respiratory failure.

### ■ What is the definition of respiratory failure?

It is difficult to set forth a single definition of respiratory failure that is acceptable to all clinicians and physiologists. However, the following findings are most frequently accepted as evidence of respiratory failure: an inability to oxygenate arterial blood as shown by arterial oxygen tension ($P_{aO_2}$) of less than 50 torr while breathing room air with or without an impaired elimination of carbon dioxide as demonstrated by an elevation of arterial carbon dioxide tension ($P_{aCO_2}$).[2, 21]

### ■ Do all patients having respiratory dysfunction require mechanical ventilation for the control of respiratory failure?

Identifying respiratory failure does not invariably indicate a need for mechanical ventilatory assistance. Many patients who are in respiratory failure can be adequately supported by applying the full spectrum of respiratory care, consisting of the administration of controlled oxygen and humidified gases, intermittent positive pressure breathing (IPPB) treatments accompanied by chest physiotherapy and postural drainage, the use of bronchodilators, nasotracheal suctioning, bronchoscopy, and careful administration of IV fluids and diuretics.[5, 21] Despite such complete supportive care, as many as 50% of severely ill patients will nonetheless require prolonged artificial ventilation.[22, 23]

### ■ What are the criteria used in deciding to provide mechanical respiratory assistance?

Although attempts have been made to establish criteria for the use of continuous mechanical ventilation, these criteria are often modified to describe a specific pulmonary disorder in an individual patient.[2, 24] The need for mechanical ventilation is, however, obvious when sudden hypoventilation or prolonged apnea is demonstrated. More often the development of acute respiratory failure is not heralded by apnea. Instead, acute respiratory failure will usually be associated with progressive respiratory dysfunction, and arbitrary values must be established at which juncture intervention with airway control and mechanical ventilation will be undertaken. Such intervention is determined by reviewing serial objective measurements, including respiratory rate, tidal volume, vital capacity, maximum inspiratory force, A-a $\Delta P_{O_2}$, and $Pa_{CO_2}$.[2, 5] The A-a $\Delta P_{O_2}$ has been particularly useful in assessing the severity of deranged gas exchange.[11] Serial assessment of the chest x-ray film and intermittent measurement of tidal volume and airway pressure relationships during IPPB, or so-called effective compliance ($V_T/P$), is also useful.[5] Progressive worsening of all of these values despite full supportive respiratory care measures usually indicates the need for mechanical ventilatory support. Other measures that provide additional information about the adequacy of spontaneous ventilation and oxygenation include the measurement of the dead space:tidal volume ratio, lung compliance, and work of breathing.[5] Automated pulmonary measurement systems have recently been developed that permit rapid serial measurement of these variables. The use of such devices has made possible the early identification of the patient who will ultimately progress to overt respiratory failure.[24-26] Mechanical ventilation with control of the airway by endotracheal intubation will usually be required in the following situations: (1) acute respiratory failure associated with coma or progressive obtundation, (2) inability to raise $P_{a_{O_2}}$ above 40 torr in a cooperative patient who is breathing 100% oxygen, (3) drop in vital capacity to 15 cc or less/kg and maximum inspiratory force to less than 25 cm $H_2O$, and (4) progressive rise in $P_{a_{CO_2}}$.[2, 8]

Although the prophylactic use of mechanical ventilation has been promoted, its advantage over the initiation of mechanical ventilation after the monitoring of deteriorating pulmonary status has not been clearly established.[27, 28] Some experimental models of pulmonary aspiration and other forms of shock lung in animals suggest that morbidity and mortality may be reduced when mechanical ventilation is used prior to or during the induction of lung injury.[29-31] Many respiratory care units have applied prophylactic mechanical ventilation in situations where a high incidence of alveolar collapse, pulmonary shunting, reduced cough, and impaired secretion removal is expected.[12, 28, 32] Thus prophylactic mechanical ventilation has been recommended in the postoperative care of patients with cardiovascular or neuromuscular disorders.[33-35] It has also been used in the care of the severely traumatized patient, especially when flail chest or pulmonary contusion is demonstrated.[11, 36] Mechanical ventilation in the postoperative care of chronic obstructive pulmonary disease patients has also been effective in avoiding the development of acute respiratory failure.[5, 32]

### ■ What are the initial measures to be employed when sudden hypoventilation or prolonged apnea develop?

Immediate steps must be taken to improve alveolar ventilation and oxygenation. The mouth is cleared of secretions and foreign bodies, then mouth-to-mouth, mouth-to-airway, or bag mask resuscitation is immediately started, employing supplemental oxygen if available. Immediate attention is given to the observation of the chest for symmetrical movement with each bag mask inflation. It is unwise for the inexperienced worker to spend much time trying to insert an endotracheal tube, since most patients are well ventilated with a bag mask device. When the patient's ventilation has been stabilized, a definitive airway is established, and use of a ventilator is then started.[37] The ventilator is adjusted to provide adequate arterial oxygen and carbon dioxide tensions.

### ■ Is endotracheal intubation required to mechanically ventilate patients?

Endotracheal intubation is required whenever compromise of airway patency is recognized and in particular whenever the normal protective cough is diminished or inadequate tidal volume and vital capacity are demonstrated. When continuous mechanical ventilation is necessary, endotracheal intubation is employed to secure a protected airway.

## ■ Can intubation and mechanical ventilation be avoided by the use of narcotic antagonists and respiratory stimulants?

The action of narcotic antagonists such as naloxone is clearly defined.[38-40] When given in single, repeated doses or as continuous IV infusions, such antagonists reverse the effects of opiates such as morphine and reduce the level of respiratory depression. However, such drugs have transient action, and the effects of morphine frequently reappear. As a result, careful monitoring of the patient and judicious readministration of the drug antagonists are required. Nonetheless, such antagonists offer great value in drug-induced respiratory depression when the depressing agent is known. Unfortunately many episodes of ventilatory depression are a result of the abuse of multiple agents, and in such instances the depression is often ineffectively antagonized by naloxone. The use of respiratory stimulants has received renewed interest in the management of such drug-induced respiratory depression. It has been suggested that agents such as doxapram may reduce the duration and depth of such depressions; however, the need for definitive control of the airway is frequent nonetheless. Intensive nursing treatment and supportive care remain the treatment of choice in the management of multiple drug–induced ventilatory depression. Adequate provision for a definitive airway and a method to provide mechanical ventilation remain essential in treating such patients. The judicious use of specific antagonists offers an important adjunctive role. Respiratory stimulants such as doxapram may even be of value in reducing the duration of mechanical ventilation. However, further assessment of this drug is necessary before its proper role as a keystone in the management of such patients is established.[41]

## ■ Which is the initial airway of choice?

A cuffed endotracheal tube is preferred over tracheostomy as the initial airway in almost all patients requiring respiratory support. In most patients tracheostomy will be performed over a previously placed endotracheal tube if the period requiring mechanical ventilation is expected to be greater than 2 to 5 days. With meticulous care endotracheal tubes may, however, be left in place for a much longer period without serious sequelae.[42] Tracheostomy may be employed as an initial airway when facial burns or trauma makes an oral airway undesirable or impossible to pass.[43]

Nasotracheal intubation is frequently preferred by the patient and is better tolerated when it is anticipated that tracheal airway control will be required for greater than 12 to 24 hours, particularly in the patient who is alert. A properly placed nasotracheal tube can be more readily stabilized with less danger of accidental extubation and still permits appropriate mouth care. Nasotracheal intubation is technically slightly more difficult, and the additional length of the tube may lead to kinking as well as greater difficulty in tracheal and bronchial suction.[44, 45] Orotracheal intubation is usually employed in comatose patients, in short-term postoperative ventilatory management, and in cardiopulmonary emergencies, where it provides a quick and definitive airway.

## ■ What precautions should be observed during endotracheal tube placement?

Intubation is a period of great stress. It is usually accompanied by hypoxemia and increased catecholamine release. These factors lead to a high incidence of cardiac irregularities. Preparation of the patient with appropriate description of the method, local anesthetic, and application of the tube by experienced personnel with avoidance of laryngeal stimulation are essential to avoid complications. Prior to and during intubation, ventilation with high concentrations of oxygen is essential. The period of intubation itself should require less than 45 to 60 seconds. The tip of the endotracheal tube should be located 2 cm proximal to the carina in order that intubation of the right mainstem bronchus is avoided. If placement of the endotracheal tube tip is at or just below the carina, suctioning of the left mainstem bronchus is precluded, regional ventilation to the left lung is reduced, and accumulation of secretions and subsequent atelectasis soon follow.[7, 46]

■ **How can endotracheal tube placement be assessed?**

Both lung fields should be regularly auscultated to detect inadvertent endobronchial intubation. Auscultation should be repeated following movement of the patient, particularly flexion of the neck, which may advance the end of the tube beyond the carina. Unfortunately normal breath sounds and normal chest movement may be demonstrated despite right mainstem intubation with incomplete occlusion of the left bronchus. For this reason a postintubation chest x-ray film to determine tube position is mandatory. Regular evaluation of the tube should be undertaken to detect tube displacement and to identify obstruction against the tracheal wall. Patency of the tube can usually be assured by passing a large-bore catheter through the endotracheal tube. Definitive confirmation of satisfactory placement can, however, only be achieved by portable chest x-ray film or bronchoscopic evaluation.[47]

■ **How can patency of the airway be maintained?**

Following placement of an endotracheal tube, aseptic endotracheal suctioning is necessary to remove secretions in order that inspissated secretions do not coat and block the endotracheal tube and airway. The inspired gas is heated and humidified and airway temperature monitored in order to provide water content equivalent to 100% relative humidity at body temperature. The patient is turned regularly and chest percussion, vibration, and postural drainage are used to prevent the accumulation of secretions in dependent airways.[48-50] The volume and viscosity of sputum is assessed at the bedside. Tenacious secretions in the airway are a clue to infection or inadequate airway moisture. Although tracheal lavage with 2 to 4 ml washings of normal saline solution may be used to liquify secretions, this is rarely necessary if a heated humidifier is continuously used. The use of curved-tip catheters with fluoroscopic visualization permits the evacuation of persistent secretions.[44] If patency of the airway cannot be maintained as evidenced by loss of breath sounds and roentgenographic demonstrations of atelectasis or volume loss of the lung despite the use of frequent turning, chest percussion, and sighing, it may be necessary to perform fiberoptic bronchoscopy during continuous ventilation and thereby remove such secretions under direct visualization.[47, 51, 52]

■ **What are the hazards of endotracheal suctioning?**

The production of hypoxemia attended by cardiac irregularities and cardiac arrest by suctioning is well recognized. Oxygen supplementation and hyperinflation of the patient before and after suctioning is now practiced in many units and has markedly reduced the incidence of tachycardias.[53, 54] Lung collapse, alveolar hypoventilation, and hypoxemia can be avoided if the vacuum does not exceed 100 torr and application is limited to 15 seconds each time. In addition, the catheter diameter must not exceed half of the diameter of the endotracheal lumen; otherwise the vacuum would be directly applied to the peripheral airway.

■ **How frequently should endotracheal suctioning be performed?**

Suctioning should be performed only when necessary. Clinical assessment such as evaluation for the presence of breath sounds and/or the presence of coarse rales or rhonchi will frequently give a clue to the presence and location of airway secretions. Routine and frequent suctioning without indication is not recommended because of the risk of producing traumatic tracheal lesions as well as the need for the interruption of ventilation and the reduction in mean airway pressure with possible production of atelectasis. In addition, suctioning frequently intensified the patient's apprehension and feeling of helplessness.

### ■ What are the major hazards in the use of endotracheal tubes?

The hazards of tube displacement and bronchial intubation have already been mentioned. In addition, laryngeal and/or pharyngeal injury at the time of insertion should also be considered.[55, 56] Late developments include granuloma formation at the cords and tracheal cuff site. The pathogenesis of this injury has been attributed to endotracheal cuff–induced pressure necrosis of the mucosa, submucosa, and tracheal cartilage.[57-62]

### ■ How can tracheal cuff injury be prevented?

Endotracheal cuff injury can be minimized or entirely avoided by proper inflation of the high-compliance endotracheal tube cuffs. The cuff should be inflated only to the volume that provides a minimum leak at the required peak airway pressure. The use of the minimum occlusive volume (MOV) techniques and the monitoring of cuff volume inflation with maintenance of intracuff pressures of less than 30 cm $H_2O$ have proved to be important in reducing injury to the trachea.[58, 62] It should be recognized that intracuff pressures are transmitted directly to the tracheal wall by the compliant cuff. In a recent study intracuff pressures of greater than 90 torr were identified in patients where the MOV technique was employed without pressure monitoring.[63] When cuff pressure monitoring with a manometer and MOV are employed, continuous cuff inflation may be maintained without tracheal injury.[64, 65] Careful fixation of the endotracheal tube and avoidance of traction remain essential in avoiding traumatic tracheal injury. The use of flexible tubings and rotating joints as well as support of the inspiratory ventilator tube is necessary to achieve such protection.[5]

### ■ Is periodic cuff deflation necessary?

If proper cuff inflation technique is practiced, periodic cuff deflation is avoided and in fact condemned by some workers because deflation introduces the risk of tracheal-bronchial secretion aspiration, movement of tube, and reduced ventilation.[61] Cuff deflation would not appear to be necessary when high-compliance cuffs are employed or MOV inflation techniques are used.[65] If intermittent deflation is practiced, laryngeal secretions must be aspirated before deflation and tracheal-bronchial secretions immediately after deflation.[61] Cuff deflation during the positive pressure phase of inspiration may be of value in that the forcefully escaping gas expells oropharyngeal secretions that have collected above the cuff. Intermittent cuff reinflation also provides an opportunity to reevaluate intracuff volume, pressure, and MOV.

### ■ What are the acceptable levels of $P_{aO_2}$?

Although $P_{aO_2}$ is an important factor, it must be emphasized that the major factor in maintaining the integrity of cellular metabolism is adequate oxygen transport. Therefore the $P_{aO_2}$ must be considered in conjunction with cardiac output and ultimately tissue perfusion. When cardiac output and tissue perfusion are normal, it can be demonstrated that a $P_{aO_2}$ below 40 torr leads to marked changes in cerebral metabolism.[66] In critically ill patients with reduced cardiac output and compromised ability to increase cerebral blood flow caused by arteriosclerosis or heart disease, cerebral injury might be expected despite a $P_{aO_2}$ of 40 torr. Therefore a $P_{aO_2}$ less than 50 torr should be considered undesirable. In general a $P_{aO_2}$ of 60 to 80 torr is sought, since such a $P_{aO_2}$ provides adequate saturation of normal hemoglobin. In addition, if sudden major changes in ventilation-perfusion relationships created by suctioning or turning are expected, a $P_{aO_2}$ of 80 to 100 torr is desirable to provide some margin of safety.

Whereas the $P_{aO_2}$ defines the adequacy of arterial oxygenation, oxygen delivery to the tissues is assessed by measuring the saturation of mixed venous blood, ($S\bar{v}_{O_2}$), the arteriovenous oxygen difference, and blood lactate levels.[67-69] A $S\bar{v}_{O_2}$ of 60% or a $P\bar{v}_{O_2}$ of 35 torr or higher is desirable. The blood lactate level should be maintained below 2 mM/L.

## ■ What fraction of inspired oxygen ($F_{I_{O_2}}$) will provide a $P_{a_{O_2}}$ between 80 and 100 torr in a critically ill patient?

Recently multiple physiologic parameters that determine $P_{a_{O_2}}$ have been reviewed.[70-72] It was shown in critically ill patients that if hypoventilation, severe anemia, and reduced cardiac output were excluded as factors, the addition of unoxygenated venous blood, or so-called shunted blood, to the circulation was the most frequent and severe cause of hypoxemia.[2] In acute respiratory failure this shunting of blood was usually caused by venous blood passing through the capillaries of nonventilated or severely underventilated alveoli.[73] Such shunting can be estimated by $P_{a_{O_2}}$ determinations in the patient who is breathing a known concentration of oxygen. Often the magnitude of the shunt is assessed by determining the A-a $\Delta P_{O_2}$ while the patient is breathing 100% oxygen.[2, 11] Several investigators have recently reviewed the relationship between $F_{I_{O_2}}$ and $P_{a_{O_2}}$ in acute respiratory failure and have offered graphic simplification that aids in the selection of appropriate $F_{I_{O_2}}$ values after a shunt determination has been made. Such diagrams offer a practical approach to oxygen therapy and are regularly used in our unit.[74, 75]

To use such nomograms, an initial $F_{I_{O_2}}$ is arbitrarily chosen if previous blood gas determinations are not available. About 15 to 20 minutes later an arterial blood gas analysis is performed. The shunt diagram is then rechecked to rapidly select the next $F_{I_{O_2}}$ that will provide a $P_{a_{O_2}}$ of 70 to 90 torr. Thereafter regular arterial blood gas determinations are done to confirm the maintenance of an adequate $P_{a_{O_2}}$ during continuous mechanical ventilation. Meanwhile every effort is made to provide the optimum patterns of ventilation that will permit decreases in the $F_{I_{O_2}}$. The goal of therapy is to inflate collapsed air spaces and increase lung volume in order that the oxygenation of the blood can be achieved at a low inspired concentration of oxygen. It has been suggested that the use of high tidal volumes provides the optimum pattern of ventilation. Tidal volumes of 12 to 15 ml/kg delivered at a frequency of 10 to 14 respirations/min are usually recommended.[2, 76] In patients with disorders such as pulmonary edema and adult resipratory distress syndrome, peak airway pressures of greater than 40 cm $H_2O$ would often be required to achieve such high tidal volume. Recently Webb and Tierney[77] have cautioned against the use of high inspiratory pressure, since such ventilatory patterns have produced pulmonary edema and increased hypoxemia in animal studies. They have recommended that low frequency ventilation at peak inspiratory pressures of less than 30 cm $H_2O$ be employed when possible. The avoidance of high airway pressures is especially indicated when low end-expiratory lung volumes are expected. If hypoxemia progresses with such a ventilatory pattern and compliance decreases, they have favored the early use of positive end-expiratory pressure (PEEP) instead of progressive increases in tidal volume, airway pressure, and $F_{I_{O_2}}$.

That increases in lung volume and oxygenation can be achieved by the use of PEEP is now widely recognized.[10, 11, 13] It can be anticipated that the use of PEEP ventilation, or so-called continuous positive pressure ventilation (CPPV), will be widely applied to stabilize air spaces and thereby reduce the frequency with which high concentrations of inspired oxygen will be required in critically ill patients.

## ■ Does oxygen administration produce pulmonary injury?

High concentrations of oxygen are commonly used for extended periods of time in the care of critically ill patients with respiratory failure. In the past 10 years much attention has been directed to the finding that high partial pressures of inspired oxygen have a deleterious effect on the lung. Best known is the development of interstitial and alveolar edema during the breathing of pure oxygen. Weibel[78] has suggested that such lung abnormalities are a result of damage to alveolar epithelial and capillary endothelial cells, which are the cells that are directly exposed to the oxygen-rich atmosphere. When animals breathed pure oxygen for 48 hours, pronounced damage of the endothelial cells with marked thinning was evident. Such endothelial and alveolar alterations could permit an increased leakage of plasma protein and water into the interstitial and alveolar areas.[79-81]

The precise action of oxygen toxicity on lung function in the critically ill patient has been difficult to define, since shock and nonpulmonary trauma produce pulmonary lesions anatomically similar to the lesions of oxygen toxicity. Nonetheless, studies in man have revealed that significant lung dysfunction occurs in critically ill patients who are ventilated with 100% oxygen for long durations.[82, 83] Barber et al.[84] showed increased shuntlike effect, greater wasted ventilation, and heavier lungs in 100% oxygen-ventilated patients when compared to patients ventilated with air. Dysfunction became more evident with increasing exposure and was particularly marked after 40 hours of 100% oxygen breathing. Hyde and Rawson[85] described the development of patchy pulmonary infiltrates and progressive hypoxemia in patients who were ventilated with 83% to 91% oxygen. A reduction of inspired oxygen concentrations to less than 50% led to improvement as seen by chest x-ray films, pulmonary compliance, and oxygenation. Although such lung dysfunction was in part attributed to the ventilators that delivered the oxygen, recent laboratory studies in animals reveal that fatal pulmonary edema would develop in animals exposed to 100% oxygen irrespective of whether the animal was spontaneously breathing or was being mechanically ventilated.[86] Many other aspects of lung function and structure appear to be harmed by oxygen administration. Lung units that are distal to areas of airway closure become air free or atelectatic within 15 minutes of beginning 100% oxygen breathing.[87] Huber et al.[88] have shown that bacterial inactivation by alveolar macrophages is inhibited by the administration of pure oxygen for 48 hours. In addition, surfactant formation and mucus transport systems may be impaired by oxygen administration.[82, 89]

These problems created by exposure to oxygen dictate that patients should not be given unnecessarily high oxygen concentrations. However, fear of oxygen toxicity should not prevent the use of sufficiently elevated inspired oxygen concentration to provide adequate oxygenation. Withholding oxygen when the patient is severely hypoxemic for fear of oxygen damage may lead to the fatal complications of hypoxemia long before oxygen toxicity could become a real danger. The short-term administration of 50% to 75% oxygen to patients with cardiovascular failure has not been associated with major adverse effects on lung function.[90] Oxygen concentrations should be titrated to provide a $P_{aO_2}$ of 70 to 100 torr at the lowest $F_{IO_2}$.[91] If long-term oxygen administration proves to be necessary at an $F_{IO_2}$ of greater than 0.5 to 0.6, attention must be directed to improved patterns of ventilation and/or the use of PEEP.

## ■ What minute ventilation is required to provide adequate ventilation?

The minute ventilation required to maintain a given $P_{aCO_2}$ depends on the carbon dioxide production and the efficiency of ventilation.[5] Acute hypercapnia indicates that ventilation is not keeping pace with the metabolic production of carbon dioxide. When this happens, rapidly profound respiratory acidemia may occur. This situation requires therapeutic intervention to improve alveolar ventilation. In the critically ill patient increased carbon dioxide production and inefficient ventilation may demand twice the minute ventilation predicted for a normal man.[35, 92, 93] In the critically ill patient an initial tidal volume ($V_T$) of 12 to 15 ml/kg of body weight delivered at a frequency (f) of 10 to 14 respirations/min has been recommended.[12, 94] Large tidal volumes are chosen to improve the distribution of ventilation and reopen collapsed air spaces as well as increase alveolar ventilation. Such high minute ventilation may, however, lead to severe respiratory alkalosis unless alveolar ventilation is promptly controlled by appropriate adjustments of mechanical dead space, tidal volume, and breathing frequency.[95] Proper adjustment of dead space to provide the desired alveolar ventilation and $P_{aCO_2}$ can be established by the use of the Suwa nomogram.[76, 96] Some workers prefer to add 6-inch lengths of inspiratory tubing at 15-minute intervals and recheck end-tidal carbon dioxide or $P_{aCO_2}$. Within 15 to 20 minutes of such adjustments a repeat arterial blood gas analysis should be obtained.

Wasserman et al.[97] have also developed a ventilation nomogram that accurately predicts the change in $P_{aCO_2}$ induced by alterations in minute ventilation. This nomogram has been used for over 2 years in our unit and has permitted smooth control of the $P_{aCO_2}$ in a wide range of respiratory disorders. An alternate method of controlling $P_{aCO_2}$ is to blend 1% to 3% carbon dioxide into the inspiratory line of the mechanical ventilator while monitoring expired $P_{CO_2}$ or $P_{aCO_2}$.[98-100]

The rapidly progressive acidosis of acute respiratory failure must be distinguished from the slow elevation of $P_{aCO_2}$ compensated by renal generation of bicarbonate in patients with chronic obstructive lung disease states. Such hypercapnia may be regarded as a physiologically adaptive response to severe airway obstruction.[101] The treatment of patients with such compensated states of hypercapnia is largely centered on the use of controlled oxygen therapy. Artificial ventilation is usually delayed as long as possible while supportive measures are used. Only when progressive hypercapnia cannot be controlled by other measures is continuous ventilatory therapy applied.[102] In this instance hypercapnia should be reduced slowly, preferably at less than 10 torr/hr. Arterial pH should be monitored in order that alkalemia produced by the sudden removal of carbon dioxide can be prevented.[103] In order that acid-base derangements are rapidly identified, blood gas determinations should be performed within 30 minutes of initiating mechanical ventilation and within minutes of major alterations of ventilatory settings. Whenever the patient's condition deteriorates as evidenced by changes in heart rate, respiratory frequency, alterations in effective compliance, etc., repeat blood gas determinations are also appropriate. In the patient who is stable using mechanical ventilation, blood gas determinations may be reduced to every 12 hours. At a minimum, daily reassessments of blood gas levels should be performed for patients on continuous mechanical ventilation. The boxed material on p. 545 lists some of the orders required for initiating mechanical ventilation at Sequoia District Hospital. The guidelines prescribed by the primary physician are carried out by the critical care team, which consists of registered nurses experienced in respiratory care, respiratory therapists, laboratory technicians, and physical therapists. The team effort is coordinated by the head nurse and medical director who work closely with the primary physician.[104]

Monitoring of the alveolar ventilation has largely depended on serial arterial blood gas sampling; however, accurate control may eventually be achieved by continuous monitoring of intra-arterial $P_{CO_2}$. Safe, stable, intra-arterial $P_{CO_2}$ electrodes and pH and $P_{O_2}$ sensors have not been available. When sensors are developed, they could readily be coupled with an electronically equipped ventilator such as the Servo-Ventilator 900 to provide smooth control of $P_{aCO_2}$.

### ■ What are the complications of arterial puncture for obtaining blood gas samples?

The most common complications are pain at the puncture site and hematoma formation. This is particularly noted in patients who are receiving anticoagulants.[105, 106] Less common problems resulting from radial artery cannulation consist of peripheral embolization with Osler node formation, hand discomfort, and major ischemic episodes.[107] Up to 20% of the patients who are clinically free of arterial injury develop thrombosed radial arteries that recannulize.[105, 108] Despite these occasional complications from arterial

**SEQUOIA DISTRICT HOSPITAL INITIAL VENTILATION ORDERS**

1. Ventilation
   a. Establish minute ventilation, ($V_T \times f$) = (10 – 14 ml/kg), at 10-14 respirations/min.
   b. Adjust ($V_T - V_{DM}$)f using $V_D/V_T$ nomogram to provide a $P_{aCO_2}$ of ____ to ____ torr and a pH of ____ to ____.
2. Oxygenation
   a. Initial $F_{IO_2}$ = 0.70.
   b. Adjust $F_{IO_2}$ using shunt diagram to provide $P_{aO_2}$ of 60-100 torr.

Repeat blood gas determinations after each adjustment to provide stable values as previously.

3. Parameters to be monitored
   a. Continuously: ECG, rhythm and respiratory rate and pattern.
   b. Hourly: $V_T$, f, $V_T$/P, $F_{IO_2}$, inspiratory:expiratory ratio, cuff pressure, tempreature.
   c. Every 20 minutes: blood pressure and pulse.
4. Sighing
   a. Sigh up to 15-20 ml/kg when stiff lungs are present.
   b. Sigh every 30 minutes with volume at ________ ml.
5. Restrain hands until otherwise ordered.
6. Use upright portable chest x-ray films to visualize postintubation tube placement.
7. Perform continuous intake and output check and measure urine specific gravity every 8 hours.
8. Take daily weight: Yes ____ No ____
9. Use postural drainage and turn from side to side every 2 hr.
10. Submit tracheal aspirate for sputum gram stain and culture.
11. Perform suctioning and tracheal care as per Sequoia District Hospital guidelines.

blood sampling, it is generally agreed that arterial blood samples are essential in providing safe ventilator care.[109] Other sampling sites do not provide equivalent information. Central venous catheter blood samples are not suitable substitutes for arterial samples.[110] Arterialized capillary blood sampling, although safe and convenient, is relatively unreliable in assessing the $P_{aO_2}$ in patients with reduced perfusion. The insertion of plastic catheters into the radial artery either percutaneously or by direct exposure has facilitated both intermittent and continuous sampling of arterial blood and the monitoring of systemic arterial pressure.[108] This arterial cannula should be kept patent by the continuous infusion of heparinized solution. If flushing is done, this should be limited to a 3 ml bolus or less and the infusion should be slowly administered. Rapid infusions of 6 ml or greater cause predictable retrograde flushing to the subclavian arteries, a maneuver that may lead to cerebral embolization.[111] In order that the results of blood gas determinations yield the greatest information, a record of the tidal volume, respiratory rate, and $F_{IO_2}$ should be made at the time of sampling. All samples must be obtained under anaerobic conditions, and the sample should be stored in ice water if a delay is anticipated before analysis. Frequent calibration of the analytic equipment is necessary to ensure accurate results.

### ■ What is the purpose of the mechanical ventilator?

The goal of positive pressure mechanical ventilation is to improve the distribution of gas within the lungs, to reinflate partially collapsed segments of the lung, to maintain patency of the small airways, and to avoid disrupting pulmonary blood flow, thereby promoting adequate gas exchange. The basic principles underlying the use of ventilators have been provided by recent reviews.[35, 112-114] The crucial test, however, of a mechanical ventilator is its ability to provide adequate ventilation under conditions of increased airway resistance and reduced lung compliance in the patient.

## ■ What feature should be sought in a mechanical ventilator?

The type of ventilator to be used is largely a matter of personal preference and should be chosen in consultation with individuals knowledgeable in the use of mechanical ventilation devices. The ventilator should have an adequate driving force to permit the ventilation of patients with markedly increased airway resistance and reduced compliance. In critically ill patients it may be necessary to provide long-term ventilation at pressures exceeding end-tidal pressures of 50 cm $H_2O$ and minute ventilation of up to 20 L/min. The ventilator should be capable of delivering accurate tidal volume as well as providing measurement of the expired and inspired volumes. An airway pressure monitoring device that can identify disconnection or excess pressure is a mandatory feature. Mechanical ventilators that are not self-monitoring cannot be recommended for the modern respiratory care of the critically ill patient, since accidents caused by ventilator malfunction and tubing disconnection continue to occur.

Currently available ventilators that possess the necessary performance and monitoring features include the Bennett Volume Ventilator-MA-1, Engstrom 300, Ohio 560, Searle Adult Volume Ventilator, and Servo-Ventilator 900 (Elema-Schnonander). Several of these ventilators include desirable features such as removable patient circuits that are disposable or that can be autoclaved. Some of these devices can be controlled by servomechanisms. The Servo-Ventilator 900 can be programmed to adjust minute ventilation in response to alterations of $P_{ECO_2}$ or $P_{aCO_2}$. The place of this latter feature in continuous ventilation therapy awaits further clinical evaluation.

## ■ Why are volume-cycled ventilators frequently employed?

A volume-cycled ventilator is frequently chosen because it delivers a preset tidal volume despite marked variation in airway resistance or compliance. In addition, most volume ventilators can be adjusted to provide automated sighing. Pressure-cycled ventilators are less desirable because inspiratory gas flow delivery is limited by a preset pressure. In such ventilators tidal volumes show wide variations as a result of changes in airway resistance or compliance. Routine measures such as turning, suctioning, and coughing may be followed by marked reductions in tidal volume. Such unpredictable reductions in alveolar ventilation may then lead to significant hypoventilation with respiratory acidemia. Dangerous increases in alveolar ventilation may suddenly appear if compliance improves while a patient is ventilated in the control mode on a pressure-limited volume ventilator.[95, 115]

## ■ What ventilator settings are first selected?

When the patient is first placed on a ventilator, an effort should be made to provide small tidal volumes, low inflationary pressure, and rapid inspiratory gas flows, so that the inspiratory time occupies no more than one third of the entire respiratory cycle. If the patient shows no deleterious cardiovascular response to such initial settings, progressive increases in inspiratory volume and pressure as well as sustained pressure plateaus as necessary to achieve the desired distribution of ventilation can be chosen. If a clear reduction in arterial pressure, skin temperature, and urine flow suggest reduced cardiac output, it is likely that a circulatory deficiency exists. In such patients the repletion of intravascular volume may be necessary before increases in mean airway pressure and tidal volume can be undertaken.

## ■ Should the mechanical ventilator be set on the assist or the control mode to adequately ventilate the patient?

The administration of IPPB may be achieved either by setting the ventilator to follow the patient's spontaneous ventilatory effort and augment the tidal volume (assisted ventilation) or by cycling the ventilator automatically and thereby establishing a predetermined respiratory pattern for the patient (controlled). The assist mode is used on conscious or comatose patients who have normal, regular, and vigorous breathing patterns and who thereby maintain the $P_{aCO_2}$ in a desirable range. When complete apnea is present, the choice is obviously simple, in that controlled ventilation is necessary to ensure predictable gas exchange. Controlled ventilation is used in patients who are conscious or in a coma but who have apnea or are breathing very slowly or irregularly. Excessive tachypnea and flail chest are additional situations wherein controlled ventilation should be undertaken.[36] The conversion from assisted to controlled ventilation can usually be accomplished by increasing the $P_{aO_2}$ and lowering the $P_{aCO_2}$. Verbal reassurance of the patient is also important in these adjustments. If a rapid respiratory rate persists in the face of an adequate $P_{aO_2}$, $P_{\bar{v}O_2}$, and modest respiratory alkalemia, it may be necessary to employ drug therapy to control ventilation.

## ■ How is the patient who is fighting the ventilator managed?

When the mechanical ventilator cannot be synchronized with the patient's breathing, an immediate search should be undertaken to identify the presence of a mechanical derangement in the ventilatory inspiratory tubing or patient's airway. Factors such as kinked airway, airway obstruction, or displacement of the airway should be immediately excluded by clinical assessment. Observation should be made of chest wall movement, and the presence of breath sounds should be ascertained. Inspired oxygen concentration should be checked as well as tidal volume and airway pressures. Arterial blood gas analysis should be undertaken. During such assessment the patient should be supported by bag mask ventilation until the problem is identified. If hypoxemia is present, it should be relieved by appropriate adjustment of supplemental oxygen or ventilatory pattern. Other factors such as pain, confusion, or apprehension should be allayed, and slight increases in alveolar ventilation to appropriately adjust the $P_{aCO_2}$ should be made. Periodic sighing maneuvers or an increase of tidal volume with added mechanical dead space to stabilize the $P_{aCO_2}$ may ease the patient's fighting. If sedation is still necessary after these measures and a chest x-ray film has excluded mechanical factors such as pneumothorax, sedation can be achieved by the IV administration of 5 mg of diazepam over a 1- to 5-minute period while monitoring the patient's clinical and blood pressure response.[116] Many workers prefer the IV use of morphine sulfate, 2 to 10 mg, infused at 2 mg/min until adequate synchronization with the ventilator is achieved. If the use of opiates or diazepam is considered undesirable, nondepolarizing relaxants without ganglionic blocking activity such as pancuronium may be employed.

## ■ What airway pressures are maintained during mechanical ventilation?

The airway pressure employed is the airway pressure that will provide a predetermined tidal volume. This pressure, which is measured in the ventilator or can be measured at the mouth, will reflect alterations in airway resistance and lung compliance. In patients with low lung compliances airway pressures greater than 40 to 50 cm $H_2O$ would be required to deliver high tidal volume. On the other hand, in patients with high total compliance such as in emphysema, airway pressures as low as 10 to 15 cm $H_2O$ may be sufficient to provide the desired tidal volume.

## ■ When should negative phase ventilation be used?

The application of subatmospheric pressure to the airway (negative phase ventilation) reduces lung volume.[117] Reduced lung volume alters surface forces, makes alveolar units unstable, and leads to the collapse of alveolar units and terminal airways. These changes impair ventilation-perfusion matching and result in shunting of blood and progression of hypoxemia. Such adverse effects of negative phase ventilation preclude its use in the care of critically ill patients.

## ■ What is the purpose of the sighing maneuver?

Deep breathing, or sighing, maneuvers act to restore lung volume, reopen collapsed air spaces, and reduce hypoxemia produced by monotonous low tidal volume ventilation.[117,118] In addition, sighing maneuvers frequently relieve the patient's complaint of inadequate chest expansion.[119] Many ventilators are equipped with automatic devices that provide a deep breath at fixed intervals. Sighing volumes of 15 to 20 ml/kg are often administered at 15 to 30-minute intervals. Sighing can, however, be dangerous in patients with high lung volumes or in patients who require high mean airway pressures during tidal breathing. When sighing maneuvers are applied to such patients and in patients who are already receiving PEEP ventilation, increases in mean airway pressure may lead to alveolar rupture.[120] Webb and Tierney[77] have pointed out other risks of high pressure ventilation. Such observations call for a reexamination of the role of sighing maneuvers. Sighing is particularly hazardous and best avoided in patients with obstructive airway disorders who breathe at high lung volumes and utilize only the easily communicating airways.

## ■ Which variables should be monitored during mechanical ventilation?

Close clinical monitoring of the ventilated patient is mandatory. In addition, when patients are mechanically ventilated, the most useful variables to be measured include respiratory rate, expired tidal volume, airway pressure, inspired oxygen concentration, and end-expiratory $P_{CO_2}$ or $P_{aCO_2}$. The end-expiratory $P_{CO_2}$ has been found to be a useful rapidly available guide to the patient's $P_{aCO_2}$.[25] Recently the identification of altered lung compliance has been used as an early indicator of atelectasis, pneumothorax, pulmonary edema, or pulmonary emboli. Serial assessment of lung compliance has been of further use in the application of PEEP. During incremental increases in PEEP the lung volume expands until elastic limits are approached, at which point further increases in PEEP result in a sharp reduction in compliance. Such observations may indicate that the upper limits of PEEP have been reached.[25] Since mechanical ventilation may decrease cardiac output, hemodynamic measurements should also be assessed. Fluid balance must also be regularly monitored. The assessment of so many parameters plus hemoglobin, plasma, and urine osmolality, serum bicarbonate, base excess, etc., rapidly leads to the accumulation of an unmanageable data base. In order that the clinical events, drug administration, and objective measurements can be promptly assimilated and applied to clinical care, appropriate flow sheets should be developed for bedside use. Fig. 29-1 shows the flow sheet used in the care of critically ill patients at Sequoia District Hospital. This chart is mounted at the foot of the bed and subsequently folds and is accommodated by a standard-sized hospital chart. This single sheet replaces five or six redundant nursing and respiratory sheets, permits the entry of data at the bedside, and assures immediate accessibility to the patient's medical record. The continuity of nursing, respiratory therapy, and physician management is enhanced by such records.[121, 122]

## ■ What is the goal of PEEP ventilation?

The goal of PEEP is to improve systemic oxygen transport while delivering lower inspired oxygen concentrations. It is not sufficient to provide an increase in arterial oxygen alone. If arterial oxygen is increased by PEEP but cardiac output is reduced, less oxygen is in fact delivered to the tissues. An index of tissue oxygenation is obtained by examining mixed venous blood obtained from the pulmonary artery. Such sampling has been considerably simplified by the advent of the Swan-Ganz catheter.[123] The determination of the $S\bar{v}_{O_2}$ before and after the onset of PEEP is of distinct value in assessing changes in cardiac output as a result of the application of PEEP. Falls in $S\bar{v}_{O_2}$ during PEEP administration either suggest reduced cardiac output or increasing shunt as a result of the treatments. An optimum response to PEEP application will reveal increased $P_{aO_2}$

| | | | | | | | | | | | | |
|---|---|---|---|---|---|---|---|---|---|---|---|---|
| **Age:** ______ | | | | | | | | | | | | |
| **Hemodynamic status** | ECG | | | | | | | | | | | |
| | | | | | | | | | | | | |
| | Radial | | | | | | | | | | | |
| | Systemic: Cuff | | | | | | | | | | | |
| | Systemic: Gage S/D | | | | | | | | | | | |
| | Systemic: Gage mean | | | | | | | | | | | |
| | LA cm $H_2O$ / mm Hg | | | | | | | | | | | |
| | Venous cm $H_2O$ / mm Hg | | | | | | | | | | | |
| | PA: S/D | | | | | | | | | | | |
| | PA: Mean | | | | | | | | | | | |
| | C.O. (CI) | | | | | | | | | | | |
| **Preoperative weight:** ——— | Weight | | | | | | | | | | | |
| **Output** | Urine | | | | | | | | | | | |
| | | | | | | | | | | | | |
| | | | | | | | | | | | | |
| | Shift total | | | | | | | | | | | |
| **Fluid intake** | | | | | | | | | | | | |
| | | | | | | | | | | | | |
| | | | | | | | | | | | | |
| | | | | | | | | | | | | |
| | Shift total | | | | | | | | | | | |
| **Respiratory status** | Airway | | | | | | | | | | | |
| | Ventilation equipment | | | | | | | | | | | |
| | $\overline{V_T/P}$ | | | | | | | | | | | |
| | Respiratory rate | | | | | | | | | | | |
| | Inspiration:expiration | | | | | | | | | | | |
| | Cuff volume | | | | | | | | | | | |
| | $F_IO_2/O_2$ LPM | | | | | | | | | | | |
| | $P_{O_2}$ | | | | | | | | | | | |
| | pH | | | | | | | | | | | |
| | $P_{CO_2}$ | | | | | | | | | | | |
| | Base excess | | | | | | | | | | | |
| | Sampling time | | | | | | | | | | | |
| | Sampling site | | | | | | | | | | | |
| | Hemoglobin/Hematocrit | | | | | | | | | | | |
| | Sputum | | | | | | | | | | | |
| | | | | | | | | | | | | |
| **Neurologic status** | Level of consc. | | | | | | | | | | | |
| | Motor | | | | | | | | | | | |
| **Blood chemistry** | Time drawn | | | | | | | | | | | |
| | Test and result | | | | | | | | | | | |
| **Medications** | | | | | | | | | | | | |
| | | | | | | | | | | | | |
| | | | | | | | | | | | | |
| | | | | | | | | | | | | |
| | | | | | | | | | | | | |
| **Nursing notes** | | | | | | | | | | | | |
| | | | | | | | | | | | | |
| | | | | | | | | | | | | |

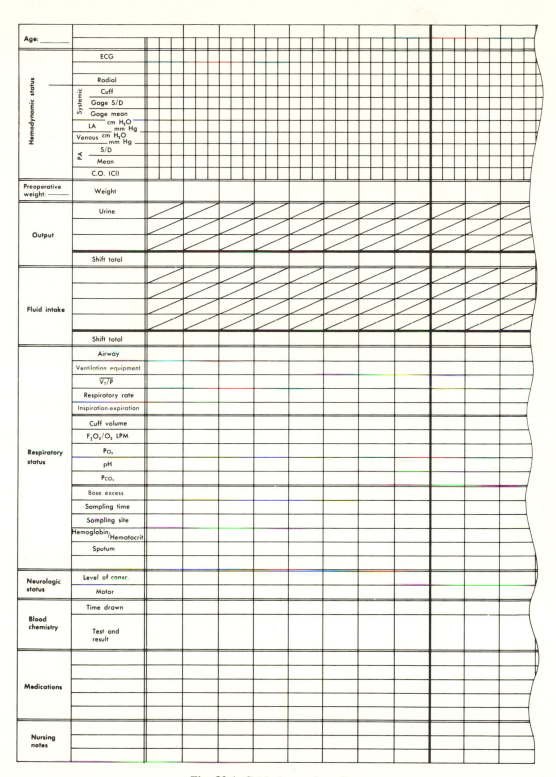

**Fig. 29-1.** Critical care flow sheet.

and $S\bar{v}_{O_2}$ in the face of $F_{IO_2}$ reductions.[2, 124, 125]

## ■ How is PEEP applied?

PEEP is produced in the airway by placing an impedance to outflow of the expired air. This can easily be achieved by attaching a large-bore tube to the exhalation port of the ventilator and then immersing the free end of the tubing in water to create the desired pressure of 2 to 15 cm $H_2O$. The airway pressure at end-expiration will therefore be determined by the column of water that must be displaced by the escaping gas. Accessory devices are now available on most ventilators to permit the application of variable pressures to the exhaled gas. In such cases airway pressure described by the manometer at end-expiration will be used as the guide for PEEP adjustment.

Increases in transpulmonary pressure achieved by the devices just described lead to the reinflation of previously underinflated or closed alveoli and terminal airways. In patients with decreased lung compliance and reduced lung volumes, increases in lung volume usually follow incremental increases in PEEP.[124]

## ■ When is PEEP used?

PEEP is employed when the $P_{aO_2}$ is less than 60 torr or showing a progressive decline while the patient is receiving $F_{IO_2}$ of 0.6 or higher by a closed system or when the functional residual capacity is less than half of normal despite appropriate adjustment of tidal volume and inspiratory:expiratory ratio, treatment of bronchospasm and cardiac failure, proper adjustment of fluid balance, frequent positional changes, and vigorous tracheal toilet.[14, 125, 126]

## ■ What is the optimum level of PEEP?

The optimum level of PEEP is determined by the response of the $P_{aO_2}$ to progressive increases in end-expiratory pressures. A $P_{aO_2}$ of 65 to 75 torr and $S\bar{v}_{O_2}$ of 60% on a $F_{IO_2}$ of 0.6 is desirable. The appropriate level of PEEP is established by the gradual application of increments of pressure at 2 to 4 cm $H_2O$ while reassessing the adequacy of cardiac output by monitoring blood pressure, pulse, skin temperature, and urine output and by analyzing $P\bar{v}_{O_2}$ and content. Suter et al.[127] demonstrated that the best PEEP level could be selected by monitoring compliance, a simple and nonintrusive measurement. Careful attention to airway pressure is necessary to confirm that the desired end-expiratory pressure is indeed achieved. PEEP effect is often lost if the patient inhales or exhales out of phase with the ventilator. In such instances the control of ventilation may be achieved by a temporary increase in oxygenation, reduction in $P_{aCO_2}$, or increases in sedation or neuromuscular block. In patients with low lung compliance, low lung volumes, adequate intravascular volume, and good cardiac function, a progressive rise of $P_{aO_2}$ is usually noted within minutes of the application of PEEP. $P\bar{v}_{O_2}$ and $S\bar{v}_{O_2}$ usually remain the same or rise. A PEEP of 20 cm $H_2O$ may need to be applied in order to increase the $P_{aO_2}$. In such patients it is frequently necessary to reduce tidal volumes in order to avoid the need for excessive high inspiratory airway pressures. The use of PEEP in a patient with obstructive airway disease is best avoided because of the risk of creating pneumothorax and decreasing cardiac output.[120]

If cardiac output falls during PEEP administration, PEEP should be reduced to the level best tolerated.[128] The reapplication of PEEP may be done later after the tidal volumes have been reduced and IV fluids, especially plasma, are administered. Supplemental measures to correct underlying disorders such as atelectasis, pneumonia, congestive heart failure, and/or fluid overload may subsequently permit the reduction of PEEP. If arterial oxygen tension has been improved by PEEP, priority should then be given to reducing the inspired oxygen to less than 60% oxygen. Once this is achieved, PEEP can slowly be reduced in increments of 1 to 2 cm $H_2O$. Arterial blood gas determinations should be monitored during the removal of PEEP, since lung volume reduction, air space closure, and hypoxemia may recur if the underlying disorder has been inadequately repaired. In particular the removal of PEEP in the hypervolemic patient may result in sudden increases in venous return, which may embarrass cardiac function in the patient with preexisting diminished myocardial contractility. The identification of left ventricular failure as a complicating factor in acute respiratory failure has been much facilitated by the use of the Swan-Ganz catheter.[15, 129] Once recognized and appropriately treated, rapid clearing of the left ventricular failure will permit reductions in PEEP and $F_{IO_2}$.

### ■ What are the circulatory effects of employing IPPB or CPPV?

Reduced cardiac output commonly occurs when high airway pressure is transmitted to intrathoracic blood vessels.[130] This may occur with IPPB or CPPV.[128, 131] The more compliant the lungs, the more profound will be the effect of airway pressure on the pulmonary and systemic circulation. If, in addition, intravascular volume has been depleted by blood loss, dehydration, or antecedent diuretic therapy, further decreases in cardiac output should be expected. Patients with compromised peripheral venous tone, such as those with idiopathic polyneuritis, spinal cord injury, or pretreatment with antihypertensives, ganglionic blocking medications, and opiates, will be particularly subject to reduction in cardiac output with increasing mean airway pressure. Reduction in cardiac output associated with the initiation of IPPB is most often seen when high inflation pressures are combined with a prolonged inspiratory phase of ventilation.[130] If, on the other hand, low tidal volumes, low mean airway pressures, and short duration of inflation are applied during the initiation of ventilation, circulatory adjustment may occur and may later permit marked changes in mean airway pressure without serious circulatory depression. The excessive elevation of PEEP may similarly produce reductions of cardiac output. However, careful incremental application of PEEP often increases output and may produce less circulatory disturbance than IPPB alone.[132]

### ■ Is there a risk of pneumothorax occurring in patients receiving PEEP?

Pneumothorax frequently occurs when patients receive mechanical ventilation, particularly when mean airway pressures are elevated and/or PEEP is applied.[46, 120, 133] Patients who run the highest risk of developing pneumothorax are those patients with underlying chronic obstructive pulmonary disease and/or emphysema in whom large tidal volumes and high inflation pressures are used. In such patients tidal volumes above 12 to 15 ml/kg and inflation pressures greater than 45 cm $H_2O$ are commonly associated with pneumothorax. The incidence of pneumothorax has been estimated to be approximately 15% to 30% in patients who are also receiving PEEP.[46, 120, 133] Some workers have observed subcutaneous emphysema and pneumothorax in 50% of patients who have been ventilated with PEEP.[22] To reduce such complications, measures to lessen the need for high airway pressures must be exploited. Such measures include the removal of secretions and the use of bronchodilators when airway obstruction is evident. The selective use of sedation and/or neuromuscular paralysis may reduce the need for high airway pressure in the struggling patient. Since pneumothorax occurs so commonly in ventilated patients, immediate recognition of this disorder is *essential*. The development of pneumothorax is frequently attended by the development of subcutaneous emphysema, tachycardia, diminished breath sounds, increased resonance to percussion, cyanosis, diaphoresis, and irregularities of the pulse.[120] Asynchronous chest movement and tracheal deviation may also be present. When these signs and symptoms are associated with rising peak airway pressure and sudden difficulty in ventilation of the patient, one should first conclude that a pneumothorax has developed. Since pneumothorax in the ventilated patient can lead to sudden death, a plan should be drawn up in advance to ensure prompt placement of the chest evacuation tubes, suction, and continuous decompression of any pneumothorax that may develop. As prolonged air leakage and delayed sealing of the pneumothorax may occur during PEEP ventilation, precautions should be exercised prior to the removal of tubes if the patient continues to require mechanical ventilation. Tubes should be patent, air leaks should have ceased, and the lungs should remain fully expanded for 48 hours prior to discontinuing the chest tubes. During the period of tube thoracostomy every attempt should be made to reduce mean airway pressures or to discontinue PEEP.[120]

### ■ When can the mechanically ventilated patient be returned to spontaneous breathing?

Techniques for assessing the patient's readiness for removal from the mechanical ventilator have recently been reviewed by Hodgkin et al.[134] It is generally agreed that the patient should be hemodynamically stable, reasonably alert, and coughing effectively. A spontaneous vital capacity of 15 cc/kg and a maximum inspiratory force of greater than 25 cm $H_2O$ are the most predictive indicators in assessing the patient's preparedness for the discontinuation of mechanical ventilation.[2, 134, 135] These measurements offer a useful means at the bedside for predicting the ability of the patient to be removed from the ventilator. Although arterial blood gas determinations are useful in establishing the stability of gas exchange while the patient is receiving mechanical ventilation, such stable values are not an accurate or good predictor of the ability of the patient to maintain adequate ventilation while breathing spontaneously. It is essential that oxygen supplementation be continued while the patient is off the ventilator to be certain that arterial hypoxemia does not supervene. In addition, deep breathing, chest physiotherapy, and tracheobronchial suctioning must be continued. The role of intermittent mandatory ventilation is currently being assessed and holds some promise in returning patients smoothly to spontaneous breathing.[136]

### ■ What place does extracorporeal oxygenation have in the management of respiratory failure?

Increasing attention has been directed to the use of extracorporeal oxygenation in the support of patients with acute respiratory failure who cannot be adequately oxygenated by the use of 100% oxygen employing volume-limited ventilation with PEEP incorporated into the circuit. The goal of therapy is to gain time for pulmonary recovery to occur. Current problems that need to be further explored before the efficacy of this method is clear include better guidelines for the selection of patients with potentially reversible pulmonary disorders and measures to control coagulation disorders and sepsis during prolonged bypass use.[137] The need for the total commitment of professional, technical staff, and ancillary services for days to weeks at a time limit this method to use by a small number of well-equipped centers.[138] It should be remembered that improvement in oxygenation is often outstanding with CPPV alone, and this mode of respiratory therapy should always be tried prior to consideration of the institution of extracorporeal oxygenation. Marked improvement in arterial tension without significant increases of the arterial-venous oxygen content difference may preclude the need for membrane oxygenator support.

### ■ What are common complications of continuous mechanical ventilation?

Alterations of alveolar ventilation frequently occur during continuous mechanical ventilation. Alveolar hypoventilation is usually a result of ventilator malfunction or changes in lung mechanics. Alveolar hyperventilation is also a hazard and is particularly noted in the patient who is being ventilated by a pressure ventilator that is set on a control mode. In this situation the improvement in pulmonary mechanics leads to marked increases in tidal volumes. Since the frequency of breathing is fixed, minute ventilation rapidly increases and respiratory alkalemia, dangerous cardiac arrhythmia, seizures, and death may follow.[95, 100, 115]

The accumulation of body and lung water is another frequent problem in acute respiratory failure. This syndrome has been characterized by positive water balance, radiographic changes suggestive of pulmonary edema, and impaired blood gas exchange in patients receiving prolonged artificial ventilation.[139] X-ray film changes of the lungs vary from localized to diffuse densities of the lungs. Positive water balance in acute respiratory failure is often unaccompanied by recognizable cardiac failure or elevated central venous or pulmonary artery wedge pressures. When left ventricular failure does supervene in respiratory failure, diagnosis by Swan-Ganz catheterization is useful in directing specific therapy.[15, 16, 129] Frequent and careful weighing as well as special attention devoted to fluid and salt intake and output are essential to avoid water imbalance. Regular assessment of plasma and urine osmolality will lead to early detection of this disorder. It should be recognized that a daily weight loss of approximately 500 g is expected in critically ill patients. It is frequently necessary to limit fluid administration for daily maintenance to 20 to 25 ml/kg/24 hr in patients who are mechanically ventilated to avoid positive water balance.[2, 139] Although contributions from humidifiers are not routinely measured, it should be understood that the humidifier is an additional source of water intake that may contribute up to 400 ml of water/day. The supplementary use of diuretic drugs may frequently prove necessary to maintain water and salt balance. Frequent changes of position are important in preventing the formation of pulmonary edema in dependent lung segments. Side-to-side changes are performed hourly.

### ■ What are the causes of infection during mechanical ventilation?

Hospital-acquired infection during ventilator therapy has been attributed to contamination of the humidifiers, respiratory tubing, and cleaning solutions. Cross contamination between patients by breaks in sterile tracheal suction apparatus has also been reported. The regular cleansing and sterilization of the patient's circuits and particularly humidifiers are important in preventing bacterial contamination of the airway from the ventilator circuit.[140] The use of aseptic suction techniques is important in preventing the inoculation of organisms into the airway. Despite meticulous techniques being employed, tracheal colonization by gram-negative bacilli frequently occurs. The development of fever, consolidation of the chest x-ray examination, and the identification of gram-negative organisms in the sputum suggest the appearance of a hospital-acquired gram-negative pneumonia.[141] Appropriate antibiotic treatment will frequently need to be started on a clinical basis, as the danger of septicemia with shock from these organisms is a major risk in the management of acute respiratory failure.

### ■ Is mental dysfunction encountered in the ventilated critically ill patient?

Mental dysfunction is often demonstrated in the ventilated patient and may appear as drowsiness, confusion, and inappropriate behavior with or without hallucinations. Such behavior may be more difficult to anticipate or to control than many of the complications that were discussed earlier. Inappropriate behavior may endanger the patient by leading to premature self-extubation with tracheal injury, fighting the ventilator, and other such complications. A plan for the early recognition of delirium has been suggested.[142] Investigation and correction of underlying metabolic abnormalities such as acidemia, hypoxemia, and electrolyte derangement should always be considered in patients demonstrating delirium. Environmental factors that deprive patients of sleep and remove patients from familiar contact should be avoided. The reassurance of seriously ill patients is important and is provided in large part by the constant presence of a careful, receptive, and knowledgeable staff. A nurse:patient ratio of 1:1 should be provided during continuous ventilation. Explanations and reassurance are given during suctioning, changing of tracheostomy, chest physical therapy, and other such bedside procedures. The use of a call bell or clicking mouth noises should be encouraged for use as signals to attract the staff's attention. Writing pads or laryngeal vibrations and periodic cuff deflation should be used to permit communication. Visits with the staff, psychiatric nurse, and family often permit and promote verbalization or expression of fears or hallucinations.[143]

Although specialized equipment and monitoring devices are important, it should be recognized that these are merely supplementary tools to be used by a knowledgeable staff. Attendants must be constantly present when a patient is on controlled ventilation, since transient disconnection of the tube, tube occlusion or displacement, or failure of the ventilator may prove to be rapidly fatal.

The staffing of the respiratory care unit should be made up of well-qualified critical care practitioners who have had clinical experience in respiratory care and cardiac monitoring. Ongoing critical care in-service education should be available to all personnel, and in addition, closely supervised bedside clinical experience should be provided to all new personnel.

Respiratory care protocols should be regularly reviewed with the staff and revision made during hospital joint practice committee meetings (meetings with physicians, nurses, and other allied health care personnel).

## REFERENCES


1. O'Donohue, W. J., Jr., Bake, J. P., Bell, G. M., Muren, O., and Patterson, J. L., Jr.: The management of acute respiratory failure in a respiratory intensive care unit, Chest **58**:603-610, 1970.
2. Pontoppidan, H., Geffin, B., and Lowenstein, E.: Acute respiratory failure in the adult, N. Engl. J. Med. **287**:690-698, 743-752, 799-806, 1972.
3. Respiratory Diseases Task Force: Report on problems, research approaches and needs, DHEW Pub. No. NIH 73-432, Washington, D.C., 1972, Department of Health, Education, and Welfare.
4. Bates, D. V.: Organization of intensive care units: results in cases of respiratory failure, Anesthesiology **25**:199-202, 1964.
5. Bendixen, H. H., Egbert, L. D., Hedley-Whyte, J., Laver, M. B., and Pontoppidan, H.: Respiratory care, St. Louis, 1965, The C. V. Mosby Co.
6. Bigelow, D. B., Petty, T. L., Ashbaugh, D. G., Levine, B. E., Nett, L. M., and Tyler, S. W.: Acute respiratory failure, experiences of the respiratory care unit, Med. Clin. North Am. **51**:323-340, 1967.
7. Safar, P.: Respiratory therapy, Philadelphia, 1965, F. A. Davis Co.
8. Seriff, N. S., Khan, F., and Lazo, B. J.: Acute respiratory failure: current concepts of pathophysiology and management, Med. Clin. North Am. **57**:1539-1550, 1973.
9. Campbell, D., Reid, J. M., Telfer, A. B., and Fitch, W.: Four years of respiratory intensive care, Br. Med. J. **4**:255-259, 1967.
10. Ashbaugh, D. G., Bigelow, D. E., Petty, T. L., and Levine, B. E.: Acute respiratory distress in adults, Lancet **2**:319-323, 1967.
11. Moore, F. D., Lyons, J. H., Pierce, E. C., Morgan, A. P., Drinker, P. A., McArthur, J. D., and Dammin, G. J.: Post traumatic pulmonary insufficiency, Philadelphia, 1969, W. B. Saunders Co.
12. Pontoppidan, H., Laver, M. B., and Geffin, B.: Acute respiratory failure in the surgical patient, Adv. Surg. **4**:163-254, 1970.
13. Safar, P., Grenvik, A., and Smith, J.: Progressive pulmonary consolidation: review of cases and pathogenesis, J. Trauma **12**: 955-967, 1972.
14. Ashbaugh, D. G., Petty, T. L., Bigelow, D. B., and Harris, T. M.: Continuous positive pressure breathing (CPPB) in adult respiratory distress syndrome, J. Thorac. Cardiovasc. Surg. **57**:31-41, 1969.
15. Unger, K. M., Shibel, E. M., and Moser, K. M.: Detection of left ventricular failure in patients with adult respiratory distress syndrome, Chest **67**:8-13, 1975.
16. Karliner, J. S.: Non-cardiogenic forms of pulmonary edema, Circulation **46**:212-215, 1972.
17. Robin, E. D., Carey, L. C., Grenvik, A., Blouser, F., and Gaudia, R.: Capillary leak syndrome with pulmonary edema, Arch. Intern. Med. **130**:66-71, 1972.
18. Katz, S., Aberman, A., Frand, U., Stein, F., and Faloys, M.: Heroin pulmonary edema: evidence for increased pulmonary capillary permeability, Am. Rev. Respir. Dis. **106**: 472-474, 1972.
19. Robin, E. D., Cross, C. E., and Zelis, R.: Pulmonary edema, N. Engl. J. Med. **288**: 239-246, 1973.
20. Staub, N. C.: State of the art review. Pathogenesis of pulmonary edema, Am. Rev. Respir. Dis. **109**:358-372, 1974.
21. Sykes, M. K., McNichol, M. X., and Camp-

bell, E. J. M.: Respiratory failure, Oxford, 1969, Blackwell Scientific Publications, Ltd.
22. Olcott, C., Barber, R. E., and Blaisdell, F. W.: Diagnosis and treatment of respiratory failure after civilian trauma, Am. J. Surg. **122:**260-268, 1971.
23. Safar, P., and Grenvik, A.: Multi-disciplinary intensive care, Mod. Med. **39:**92-99, 1971.
24. Peters, R. M., Hilberman, M., Hogan, J. S., and Crawford, D. A.: Objective indications for respiratory therapy in post-trauma and postoperative patients, Am. J. Surg. **124:**262-269, 1972.
25. Osborn, J. A.: Monitoring respiratory function, Crit. Care Med. **2:**217-220, 1974.
26. Peters, R. M., and Hilberman, M.: Respiratory insufficiency: diagnosis and control of therapy, Surgery **70:**280-287, 1971.
27. Macklem, P. T.: The indications for artificial ventilation are limited: controversies in internal medicine II, Philadelphia, 1974, W. B. Saunders Co.
28. Singer, M. M.: The advantages of an aggressive prophylactic approach: controversies in internal medicine II, Philadelphia, 1974, W. B. Saunders Co.
29. Camerson, J. L., Sebor, J., Anderson, R. P., and Zuidema, G. D.: Aspiration pneumonia; results of treatment with positive pressure ventilation in dogs, J. Surg. Res. **8:**447-456, 1968.
30. Stallone, R. J., Herbst, H., Cafferata, H. T., Blaisdell, F. W., and Murray, J. F.: Pulmonary changes following regional ischemia; response to treatment, Am. Rev. Respir. Dis. **98:**144, 1968.
31. Uzawa, T., and Ashbaugh, D. G.: Continuous positive-pressure breathing in acute hemorrhagic pulmonary edema, J. Appl. Physiol. **26:**427-432, 1969.
32. Lecky, J. H., and Ominsky, A. J.: Postoperative respiratory management, Chest **62**(suppl.):50S-57S, 1972.
33. Copperman, L. H., and Mann, P. E.: Postoperative respiratory care; a review of 65 consecutive cases of open-heart surgery on the mitral valve, J. Thorac. Cardiovasc. Surg. **53:**504-507, 1967.
34. Lefemine, V., and Harken, D. E.: Postoperative care following open-heart operations; routine use of controlled ventilation, J. Thorac. Cardiovasc. Surg. **2:**207-217, 1966.
35. Norlander, O. P.: The use of respirators in anesthesia and surgery, Acta Anaesthesiol. Scand. **30**(suppl.):5-74, 1968.
36. Roscher, R., Bittner, R., and Stockman, U.: Pulmonary contusions, clinical experience, Arch. Surg. **109:**508-510, 1974.
37. Standards for cardiopulmonary resuscitation (CPR) and emergency cardiac care (ECC), J.A.M.A. **227**(suppl.):833S-868S, 1974.
38. Buchner, H., Cimino, J. A., and Raybin, H. W.: Naloxone reversal of methadone poisoning, N.Y. State J. Med. **72:**2305-2309, 1972.
39. Foldes, F. F., Duncalf, D., Kuwabara, S.: The respiratory, circulatory and narcotic antagonistic effects of nalorphine, levallorphan and naloxone in anaesthetized subjects, Can. Anaesth. Soc. J. **16:**151-161, 1969.
40. Hasbrouck, J. D.: The antagonism of morphine anesthesia by naloxone, Anesth. Analg. **50:**954-959, 1971.
41. Fritz, H. W., and Rochester, D. F.: Respiratory stimulants and obstructed airways, N. Engl. J. Med. **288:**464-465, 1973.
42. Klaustermeyer, W. B., Winn, W. R., and Olson, C. R.: Use of cuffed endotracheal tubes for severe exacerbations of chronic respiratory airway obstruction, Am. Rev. Respir. Dis. **105:**268-275, 1972.
43. Selecky, P. A.: Tracheostomy: a review of present day indications, complications and care, Heart & Lung **3:**272-283, 1974.
44. Haberman, P. B., Green, J. P., Archibald, C., Dun, D. L., Horwitz, S. R., Ashburn, W. L., and Moser, K. M.: Determinants of successful selective tracheobronchial suctioning, N. Engl. J. Med. **289:**1060-1063, 1973.
45. Shapiro, A. G., and Walker, C. G.: Respiratory intensive care, Med. Clin. North Am. **55:**1217-1231, 1971.
46. Zwillich, C. W., Pierson, D. J., Creagh, C. E., Sutton, F. D., Schatz, E., and Petty, T. L.: Complications of assisted ventilation; a prospective study of 354 consecutive episodes, Am. J. Med. **57:**161-170, 1974.
47. Amikan, B., Landa, J., West, J., and Sackman, M.: Bronchofiberoscopic observation of the tracheobronchial tree during intubation, Am. Rev. Respir. Dis. **105:**747-755, 1972.
48. Bushnell, S. S., Bushnell, L. S., Reichle, M. J., and Skillman, J. J.: Respiratory intensive care nursing, Boston, 1973, Little, Brown and Co.
49. Gaskell, D. V., and Webber, B. A.: The Brompton Hospital guide to chest physiotherapy, Oxford, 1973, Blackwell Scientific Publications, Ltd.
50. Rie, M.: Physical therapy in the nursing

care of respiratory disease patients, Nurs. Clin. North Am. **3**:463-478, 1968.

51. Sackner, M. A.: Bronchofiberoscopy, Am. Rev. Respir. Dis. **111**:62-88, 1975.
52. Wanner, A., Landa, J. F., Nieman, R. E., Vevaina, J., and Delgado, I.: Bedside bronchofiberoscopy for atelectasis and lung abcess, J.A.M.A. **224**:1281-1283, 1973.
53. Shim, C., Fine, N., Fernandez, R., and Williams, M. H., Jr.: Cardiac arrhythmias from tracheal suctioning, Ann. Intern. Med. **711**:1149-1153, 1969.
54. Urban, B. J., and Weitzner, S. W.: Avoidance of hypoxia during endotracheal suction, Anesthesiology **31**:473-475, 1969.
55. Hawkins, D. B., Seltzer, D. C., Barnett, T. E., and Stoneman, G. B.: Endotracheal tube perforation of the hypopharynx, West. J. Med. **120**:282-286, 1974.
56. McGovern, F. H., Fitz-Hugh, G. S., and Edgeman, L. J.: The hazards of endotracheal intubation, Ann. Otol. Rhinol. Laryngol. **80**:556-564, 1971.
57. Blanc, V. F., and Tremblay, N. A.: The complications of tracheal intubation; a new classification with a review of the literature, Anesth. Analg. **53**:202-213, 1974.
58. Bryant, L. R., Trinkle, J. K., and Dubilier, L.: Reappraisal of tracheal injury from cuffed tracheostomy tubes; experiments in dogs, J.A.M.A. **215**:625-628, 1971.
59. Geffin, B., Grillo, H., Cooper, J., and Pontoppidan, H.: Stenosis following tracheostomy for respiratory care, J.A.M.A. **216**: 1984-1988, 1971.
60. Grill, H. C., Cooper, J. D., Geffin, B., and Pontoppidan, H.: Low-pressure cuff for tracheostomy tubes to minimize tracheal injury, J. Thorac. Cardiovasc. Surg. **62**:898-907, 1971.
61. Harley, H. R.: Laryngeal tracheal obstruction complicating tracheostomy or endotracheal intubation with assisted respiration, Thorax **26**:493-533, 1971.
62. Shelly, W. M., Dawson, R. B., and May, I. A.: Cuffed tubes as a cause of tracheal stenosis, J. Thorac. Cardiovasc. Surg. **57**: 623-627, 1969.
63. Cox, P. M., and Schatz, M. E.: Pressure measurement in endotracheal cuffs: a common error, Chest **65**:84-87, 1975.
64. Ching, N., and Nealon, T. F.: Cuff pressure measurements, Chest **66**:604-605, 1974.
65. Jenicek, J. A., Danner, C. A., and Allen, C. R.: Continuous cuff inflation during long term intubation and ventilation: evaluation of technique, Anesth. Analg. **52**:252-257, 1973.
66. Cohen, P. J., Alexander, S. C., Smith, T. C., Reivich, M., and Wollman, H.: Effects of hypoxia and normocarbia on cerebral block flow and metabolism in conscious man, J. Appl. Physiol. **23**:183-189, 1967.
67. Lee, J., et al.: Central venous oxygen saturation in shock; a study in man, Anesthesiology **36**:472-478, 1972.
68. Mithoefer, J. C., Holford, F. D., and Keighley, J. F.: The effect of oxygen administration on mixed venous oxygenation in chronic obstructive pulmonary disease, Chest **66**:122-132, 1974.
69. Tenny, S. M.: A theoretical analysis of the relationship between venous blood and mean tissue oxygen pressure, Respir. Physiol. **20**:283-296, 1974.
70. Barrocas, M., Nuchprayoon, C. V., Claudio, M., King, F. W., Danon, J., and Sharp, J. T.: Gas exchange abnormalities in diffuse lung disease, Am. Rev. Respir. Dis. **104**:72-85, 1971.
71. Snider, G.: Interpretation of the arterial oxygen and carbon dioxide partial pressure. A simplified approach for bedside use, Chest **63**:801-806, 1973.
72. West, J. B.: Ventilation/blood-flow and gas exchange, ed. 2, Philadelphia, 1970, F. A. Davis Co.
73. Hedley-Whyte, J., Laver, M. B., and Bendixen, H. H.: Effects of changes in tidal ventilation on physiologic shunting, Am. J. Physiol. **206**:891-897, 1964.
74. Benatar, S. R., Hewlett, A. M., and Nunn, J. F.: The use of iso-shunt line for control of oxygen therapy, Br. J. Anaesth. **45**:711-718, 1973.
75. Druger, G. L., Simmons, D. H., Levy, S. E.: The determination of shunt-like effects and its use in clinical practice, Am. Rev. Resp. Dis. **108**:1261-1265, 1973.
76. Suwa, K., Geffin, B., Pontoppidan, H., and Bendixen, H. H.: A nomogram for dead space requirement during prolonged artificial ventilation, Anesthesiology **29**:1206-1210, 1968.
77. Webb, H. H., and Tierney, D. F.: Experimental pulmonary edema due to intermittent positive pressure ventilation with high inflation pressures, protection by positive end-expiratory pressure, Am. Rev. Respir. Dis. **110**:556-565, 1974.
78. Weibel, E. R.: Oxygen effect on lung cells, Arch. Intern. Med. **128**:54-56, 1971.
79. Kapanci, Y., Weibel, E. R., Kaplan, H. P., and Robinson, F. R.: Pathogenesis and reversibility of the pulmonary lesions of oxygen toxicity in monkeys. II. Ultrastruc-

tural and morphometric studies, Lab. Invest. **20**:101-113, 1969.
80. Kaplan, H., Robinson, S., Kapanci, Y., and Weibel, E. R.: Pathogenesis and reversibility of the pulmonary lesions of oxygen toxicity in monkeys, clinical and light microscopic studies, Lab. Invest. **20**:94-100, 1969.
81. Kistler, G. S., Caldwell, P. R. B., and Weibel, E. R.: Development of fine structural damage to alveolar and capillary lining cells in oxygen poisoned rat lungs, J. Cell. Biol. **32**:605-628, 1967.
82. Burger, E. J., and Mead, J.: Static properties of lungs after oxygen exposure, J. Appl. Physiol. **27**:191-197, 1969.
83. Nash, G., Blennerhassett, J. B., and Pontoppidan, H.: Pulmonary lesions associated with oxygen therapy and artificial ventilation, N. Engl. J. Med. **276**:368-374, 1967.
84. Barber, R. E., Lee, J., Hamilton, W. K.: Oxygen toxicity in man; a prospective study in patients with irreversible brain damage, N. Engl. J. Med. **283**:1478-1484, 1970.
85. Hyde, R. W., and Rawson, A. J.: Unintentional iatrogenic oxygen pneumonitis—response therapy, Ann. Intern. Med. **71**: 517-531, 1969.
86. Nash, G., Bowen, J. A., and Langlinais, P. C.: Respiratory lung, a misnomer, Arch. Pathol. **91**:234-240, 1971.
87. West, J. B.: Pulmonary gas exchange in the critically ill patient, Crit. Care Med. **2**:171-180, 1974.
88. Huber, G., La Force, M., and Mason, R.: Impairment and recovery of pulmonary antibacterial defense mechanisms after oxygen administration, J. Clin. Invest. **49**:47a, 1970. (Abstract 149.)
89. Morgan, T. E., Finley, T. N., Huber, G. L., and Fiaklow, H.: Alterations in pulmonary surface active lipids during exposure to increased oxygen tension, J. Clin. Invest. **44**: 1737-1744, 1965.
90. Singer, M. M., Wright, F., Stanley, L., Roe, B., and Hamilton, W. K.: Oxygen toxicity in man; a prospective study in patients after open-heart surgery, N. Engl. J. Med. **283**:1473-1478, 1970.
91. Pontoppidan, H., and Berry, P. R.: Regulation of the inspired oxygen concentrations during artificial ventilation, J.A.M.A. **201**: 11-14, 1967.
92. Pontoppidan, H., Hedley-Whyte, J., Bendixon, H. H., Laver, M. B., and Radford, E. P.: Ventilation and oxygen requirements during prolonged artificial ventilation in patients with respiratory failure, N. Engl. J. Med. **273**:401-409, 1965.
93. Radford, E.: Ventilation standards for us in artificial respiration, J. Appl. Physiol. **7**: 451-460, 1955.
94. Bendixen, H. H.: Rational ventilator modes for respiratory failure, Crit. Care Med. **2**: 225-227, 1974.
95. Ayres, S. M., and Grace, W. J.: Inappropriate ventilation and hypoxemia as causes of cardiac arrhythmias. The control of arrhythmias without antiarrhythmic drugs, Am. J. Med. **46**:495-505, 1969.
96. Stoyka, W. W.: The reliability and usefulness of the Suwa nomogram in patients in respiratory failure, Can. Anaesth. Soc. J. **17**:119-128, 1970.
97. Wasserman, K., Selecky, P., and Ziment, I.: A graphical approach to assess $V_E$-$P_aCO_2$-$V_D/V_T$ relationship in patients on respirators, Am. Rev. Respir. Dis. 1976. (In press.)
98. Breivik, H., Grenvik, A., Millen, E., and Safar, P.: Normalizing low arterial $CO_2$ tensions during mechanical ventilation, Chest **63**:525-531, 1973.
99. Lipton, B., and Kahn, M.: Carbon dioxide and large volume ventilation in the management of patients undergoing cardiac surgery, Can. Anesth. Soc. J. **19**:49-59, 1972.
100. Mazzara, J. T., Ayres, S. M., and Grace, W. J.: Extreme hypercapnia in the critically ill patient, Am. J. Med. **56**:450-456, 1974.
101. Barach, A. L.: Hypercapnia in chronic obstructive lung disease—an adaptive response to low-flow oxygen therapy, Chest **66**:112-113, 1974.
102. Kettel, L. J., Diener, C. F., Morse, J. O., Stern, H. F., and Burrows, B.: Treatment of acute respiratory acidosis in chronic obstructive lung disease, J.A.M.A. **217**:1503-1508, 1971.
103. Safar, P., Nemota, E. M., and Severinghaus, J. W.: Pathogenesis of central nervous system disorder during artificial hyperventilation in compensated hypercarbia in dogs, Crit. Care Med. **1**:5-16, 1973.
104. Levine, B. E., Kravetz, H. M., Spotnitz, M., and Westfall, R. E.: The role of the community hospital in acute respiratory failure management, Chest **62**(suppl.): 10S-13S, 1972.
105. Bedford, R. F., and Wollman, H.: Complications of percutaneous radial artery cannulation; an objective prospective study in man, Anesthesiology **38**:228-236, 1973.
106. Mortensen, J. E.: Clinical sequela from arterial needle puncture, cannulation and incision, Circulation **35**:1118-1123, 1967.
107. Matthews, J. I., and Gibbons, R. B.:

Embolization complicating radial-artery puncture, Ann. Intern. Med. **75**:77-87, 1971.
108. Gardner, R. M., Schwartz, R., Wong, H. C., and Burke, J. P.: Percutaneous indwelling radial artery catheters for monitoring cardiovascular function. Prospective study of the risk of thrombosis and infection, N. Engl. J. Med. **290**:1227-1231, 1974.
109. Petty, T. I., Bigelow, D. B., and Levine, B. E.: The simplicity and safety of arterial puncture, J.A.M.A. **195**:693-695, 1966.
110. Phillips, B., and Peretz, D. I.: A comparison of central venous and arterial blood gas values in the critically ill, Ann. Intern. Med. **70**:745-749, 1969.
111. Lowenstein, E., Little, J. W., and Hing, H. L.: Prevention of cerebral embolization from flushing radial-artery cannulas, N. Engl. J. Med. **285**:1414-1415, 1971.
112. Egan, D. F.: Fundamentals of respiratory therapy, ed. 2, St. Louis, 1973, The C. V. Mosby Co.
113. Mushin, W. W., Rendau-Baker, L., Thompson, P. W., and Mapelson, W. W.: Automatic ventilation of the lungs, Philadelphia, 1969, F. A. Davis Co.
114. Rattenborg, C., and DeBorde, R.: Lung ventilation: function and principles, Inhalation Ther. **12**:48, 1967.
115. Kilburn, K. H.: Shock, seizures and coma with alkalosis during hyperventilation, Ann. Intern. Med. **65**:977-984, 1966.
116. Knapp, R. B., and Dubow, H. S.: Diazepam as an induction agent for patients with cardiopulmonary disease, South. Med. J. **63**:1451-1453, 1970.
117. Mead, J., and Collier, C.: Relation of volume history of lungs to respiratory mechanics in anesthetized dogs, J. Appl. Physiol. **14**:669-678, 1959.
118. Hedley-Whyte, J., Pontoppidan, H., and Laver, M. B.: Arterial oxygenation during hypothermia, Anesthesiology **26**:595-602, 1965.
119. Opie, L. H., Smith, A. C., and Spalding, J. M.: Conscious appreciation of the effects produced by independent changes of ventilation volume and end-tidal $PCO_2$ in paralyzed patients, J. Physiol. (Lond.) **149**:494-499, 1959.
120. Steier, M., Ching, N., Roberts, E. B., and Nealon, T. F.: Pneumothorax complicating continuous ventilatory support, J. Thorac. Cardiovasc. Surg. **67**:17-23, 1974.
121. Hilberman, M., and Peters, R. M.: A data collection system for intensive care, Crit. Care Med. **3**:27-30, 1975.
122. Kramer, S. G., Lipson, C. S.: Intensive care unit flow sheet, Surgery **67**:590-592, 1970.
123. Swan, H. J., Ganz, W., Forrester, J. S., Marcus, H., Diamond, G., and Chonette, D.: Catheterization of the heart in man with use of a flow-directed balloon-tipped catheter, N. Engl. J. Med. **283**:447-451, 1970.
124. Nicotra, M. B., Stevens, P. M., Viroslav, J., and Alvarez, A. A.: Physiologic evaluation of positive end-expiratory pressure ventilation, Chest **64**:10-15, 1973.
125. Sugerman, H. J., Rogers, R. M., and Miller, L. D.: Positive end-expiratory pressure (PEEP) indications and physiologic considerations, Chest **62**(suppl.):86S-94S, 1972.
126. Kumar, A., Falke, K. L., Geffin, B., Aldredgy, C. F., Laver, M. B., Lowenstein, E., and Pontoppidan, H.: Continuous positive-pressure ventilation in acute respiratory failure, effects on hemodynamics and lung function, N. Engl. J. Med. **283**:1430-1436, 1970.
127. Suter, P. M., Fairley, H. B., and Isenberg, M. D.: Optimum end-expiratory airway pressure in patients with acute pulmonary failure, N. Engl. J. Med. **292**:284-289, 1975.
128. Powers, S. R., Mannal, R., Neclerio, M. S., English, M., Marr, C., Leather, R., Ueda, H., Williams, G., Custead, W., and Dutton, R.: Physiologic consequences of positive end-expiratory pressure (PEEP) ventilation, Ann. Surg. **178**:265-272, 1973.
129. Stevens, P. M., Friedman, G. K., and Nicotra, M. B.: The value of flow directed intravascular catheters in cardiorespiratory failure, Am. Rev. Respir. Dis. **107**:1111-1112, 1973.
130. Cournand, A., et al.: Physiologic studies of the effects of intermittent positive pressure breathing on cardiac output in man, Am. J. Physiol. **152**:162-174, 1948.
131. Schapiro, M., and Daum, S.: Hemodynamics of the pulmonary circulation in patients on intermittent positive pressure breathing with a bird respiratory, Anesth. Analg. **53**: 31-38, 1974.
132. Colgan, F. J., Nichols, F. A., and DeWeese, J. A.: Positive end-expiratory pressure, oxygen transport and the low-output state, Anesth. Analg. **53**:538-543, 1974.
133. Kumar, A., Pontippidan, H., Falke, K. J., Wilson, R. D., and Laver, M. B.: Pulmonary barotrauma during mechanical ventilation, Crit. Care Med. **1**:181-186, 1973.
134. Hodgkin, J. E., Bowser, M. A., and Burton, G. G:. Respiratory weaning, Crit. Care Med. **2**:96-102, 1974.

135. Sahn, S. A., and Lakshminarayan, S.: Bedside criteria for discontinuation of mechanical ventilation, Chest **63**:1002-1005, 1973.
136. Downs, J. B., Klein, E. F., Desautels, D., Modell, J. H., and Kirby, R.: Intermittent mandatory ventilation; a new approach to weaning patients from mechanical ventilators, Chest **64**:331-335, 1973.
137. Divertie, M. B.: Extracorporeal oxygenation: a flower before the spring, Chest **66**: 343-344, 1974.
138. Mortensen, J. D.: Extracorporeal membrane oxygenation for pulmonary assist in patients with ARF, Chest **67**:129-130, 1975.
139. Sladen, A., Laver, M. D., and Pontopiddan, H.: Pulmonary complications and water retention in prolonged mechanical ventilation, N. Engl. J. Med. **279**:448-453, 1968.
140. Sanford, J. P.: Infection control in critical care units, Crit. Care Med. **2**:211-216, 1974.
141. Benner, E. J., Munzinger, J. P., and Chan, R.: Superinfections of the lung; an evaluation by serial transtracheal aspiration, West. J. Med. **121**:173-178, 1974.
142. Katz, N. M., Agle, D. P., DePalma, R. G., and DeCossee, J. J.: Delirium in surgical patients under intensive care, utility of mental status examination, Arch. Surg. **104**:310-313, 1972.
143. Fuhs, M., Rieser, M., and Brisbon, D.: Nursing in a respiratory intensive care unit, Chest **62**(suppl.):14S-18S, 1972.

*chapter 30*

# Instrument safety

**PAUL E. STANLEY**

All of recorded history indicates that man has been interested in the health of his neighbor and has always been ready to suggest favorite remedies for whatever the illness might be. One of the earliest of the recorded rules and regulations concerning the health of the individual as well as the health of the public is to be found in the early books of the Bible, the so-called Mosaic Law, which was written about 1500 B.C.

Some instrumentation was developed over the years, but it remained for men of the 20th century to bring forth modern medical devices. Referring to the results of developments, Dr. John D. Porterfield III, director of the Joint Commission on Accreditation of Hospitals, recently remarked that "the patient has somehow learned to expect the difficult to be routine, the impossible to be frequent, and the miraculous to be something only slightly less than frequent."[1] These changes are the result of the application of engineering and technology to health care and medical problems.

## ■ How has engineering affected nursing?

To a very great extent the responsibility for the safe use of medical instrumentation and equipment falls on the attending critical care technician. Usually a specialist in the operation of the ECG may be dispatched from the hospital's central services to connect a machine to a patient and take an ECG recording. The staff in the critical care unit will have training along similar lines.

But it is especially important for critical care practitioners to be aware of the technical changes that have occurred and are occurring. They should be informed not only of the medical implications of such developments, but of the safety factors involved. In addition, the development of new electromedical devices is so rapid that a continuing program of learning is needed. This chapter has been prepared as a partial step in this education.

## ■ How have engineering and technology made contributions to health care services?

As early as 1747 Benjamin Franklin observed that electricity passing through a muscle caused it to "convulse."[2] A few years later Fontana of Bologna discovered that electricity was involved in the functioning of the heart. It was in 1887 that Waller displayed the electrical activity of the heart,[3] but it was not until 1912 that Einthoven was able to produce a useful ECG.[4] Electronic medical devices were introduced late in World War II, and the computer is just now in operation in some hospitals. In 1969 about $25 million was spent on cardiac monitoring devices. In 1975 the figure was in the neighborhood of $75 million, with the total medical instrumentation sales approaching $750 million[5] (Fig. 30-1).

Tiny transistorized radios, instant-on color television sets, and microwave ovens are constant reminders of the contributions of electrical technology to the quality of our everyday lives. Similarly, the care of the ill has been aided by technologic advances that are the result of the application of engineering and technology to the problems of the diagnosis and treatment of diseases. Probably the effect has been more prominent in the care of critically ill patients than anywhere else. Cardiac monitors, cardiac pacemakers, respirators, and even automatic blood gas analysis instruments are but a few of the many devices

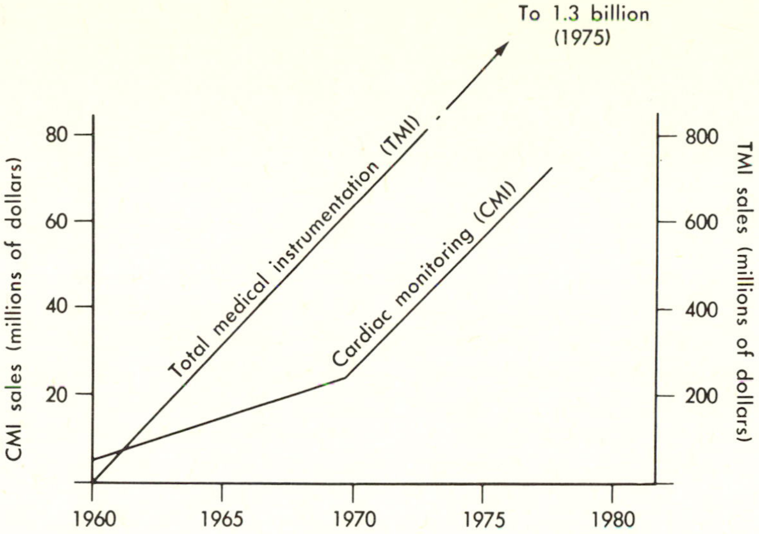


**Fig. 30-1.** Electronic medical device sales. CMI, cardiac monitoring instrumentation; TMI, total medical instrumentation.

now used or soon to be used in the critical care areas of the modern hospital.

While technologic advances provide assurance that critically ill patients will receive every possible assistance in their efforts to return to health, they also contribute problems.

## ■ How does instrumentation introduce problems?

In the home, problems arising from failure of one of the multitude of appliances are usually no more than nuisances. However, in a hospital critical care unit, device failure can bring discomfort, injury, or even death to the patient. These hazards are many but can be brought together in two general classes: instrument effectiveness and instrument system safety. It is therefore apparent that everyone in anyway associated with critical care should be well informed of the hazards as well as the benefits of the vast array of instruments and devices in current use.

## ■ What does the term "instrument effectiveness" mean?

Instrument effectiveness can be said to be simply that the data obtained from the meter readings are accurate and truly indicate what the practitioner who ordered the use of the instrument wanted. A precise reading of the oxygen content of the blood ($P_{O_2}$) is of no value if the desired information was the pH. Nor is a precise value of an average of the systolic and diastolic pressures of importance when the peak values of both are desired for the diagnosis of the condition. Whether or not a device does what it is intended to do may be described as its effectiveness.

## ■ What are some examples of effectiveness?

In the *Report of the Inter-Society Commission for Heart Disease Resources* (1971) it is pointed out that all models of one brand of defibrillator failed to deliver the energy indicated.[6] In a recent test program four defibrillators of identical make and model delivered from 55% to 93% of the indicated or stored energy, while another delivered 444 watt-seconds when set at the 400 watt-second level.[17]

If a patient should receive 400 watt-seconds of defibrillation energy, he may fail to respond to 55% of 400 (or 220) watt-seconds received from a faulty defibrillator. The result may be death—death caused by an ineffective device.

A similar condition has been known to

exist in pacemakers in that the figures on the dial have been found to not correspond to the current delivered by the device. In numerous instances "noise" or artifacts on the screen of a cardiac monitor obscure the ECG, thus making the monitor ineffective.

Such failure of instruments to perform effectively may be caused by poor design, poor maintenance, or improper use of the device. Because of the importance of continued effective and safe operation, both the engineer and the technician involved in the design, manufacture, and care of the devices are needed in hospitals to ensure that the medical devices used anywhere, and especially in critical care areas, perform their functions effectively and safely.

## ■ What is meant by the term "instrument safety"?

Although effective instrument or apparatus operation is of the utmost importance, no other hazards must ensue from the use of the equipment. The patient must not suffer electric shock, burns, undue pain, or other trauma caused by any part of the electromedical system in operation. This safety must extend to the operator and other personnel as well as to the patient.

The hazards from the unsafe operation or use of devices are many. Since most of the devices are electrically operated, electric shock is usually the hazard considered most likely to occur. It is important and will be reviewed at length, but electric devices may start fires or ignite explosive gas mixtures, or they may not function properly when there is "too little" electricity, that is, when the voltage is lowered, as during a "brown out." Many situations may occur that require engineering analysis for solution, and for that reason these will not be treated here. Since its analysis is quite straightforward, the electric shock hazard will be examined rather fully.

## ■ What is an electric current?

It is not the purpose of this chapter to discuss the whole of the science and engineering of electricity. One text dealing with the basics of electricity is given in the references.[7] However, a few of the principles can be expressed very briefly.

There are two requisites for the flow of an electric current: (1) a voltage source and (2) a closed circuit that includes the voltage source.

The character of the voltage source is determined in part by the potential difference between its two poles. For the dry cell flashlight battery this is 1.5 volts; the voltage of an x-ray unit will be in the thousands or even hundreds of thousands of volts. The symbol V is usually chosen to represent the magnitude of the voltage.

Also of importance in the voltage source character is its frequency. A *direct* current source is one that "pushes" continually in one direction. It may be said to be at 0 frequency as compared with an *alternating* current source, having a frequency greater than 0, most commonly, 60 cycles per second, or 60 hertz (Hz). The usual household supply and that of the hospital room is a 120 V, 60 Hz alternating current.

The character of the circuit is a bit more complicated and must be described in terms of three kinds of elements: resistance, inductance, and capacitance. These combine into an overall characteristic called impedance. For simplicity we shall use resistance only and will represent it by R. Current is represented by I (Fig. 30-2) and voltage by V. The relationship between these quantities is known as Ohm's law and is as follows:

$$I = \frac{V}{R}$$

The circuit may be closed by any conductor, including the human body; hence electric shock hazards occur.

Resistances (or impedances) may occur at many places in the circuit, and all must be taken into account in evaluating the possible hazards. One resistance component exists within the voltage source itself (Fig. 30-2). For example, a 1.5 V No. 6 dry cell will generate a current of more than 30 amps through an ammeter, which is essentially a

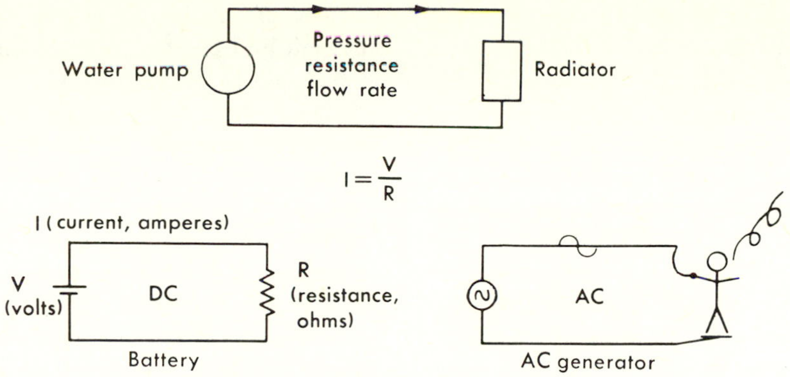


**Fig. 30-2.** Schematic of electric circuit.

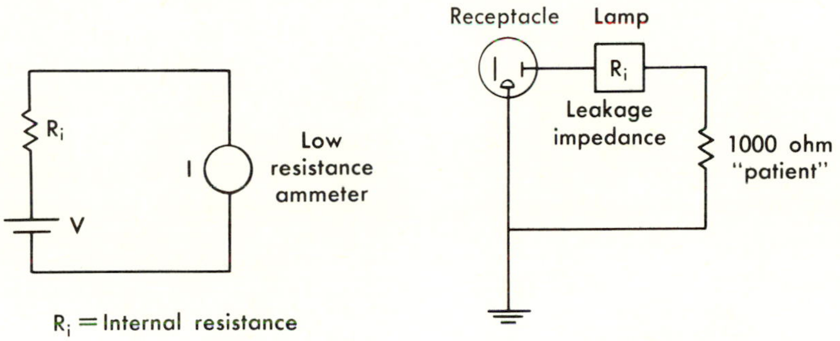


**Fig. 30-3.** Internal resistance and internal impedance.

short circuit. This means that the resistance of the cell is:

$$R_I = \frac{1.5}{30} = 0.05 \text{ ohm}$$

On the other hand, an AA size 1.5 V dry cell will generate less than 3 amps. This means its resistance is:

$$R_I = \frac{1.5}{3} = 0.5 \text{ ohm}$$

Fig. 30-3 illustrates a voltage source caused by "leakage" of an alternating current lamp. It has a voltage of 120 V, yet it will generate less than 1 microampere of current through a 1000 ohm "patient." By Ohm's law this means that the internal leakage resistance is 120 megohms (120 million ohms). This is so high that it will cause a voltmeter to read incorrectly, showing only 80 V or even less.

### *Body resistance*

It is to be noted that a "patient" was indicated as having a resistance of 1000 ohms. A precise value is very difficult to specify. With the use of needle electrodes and low voltage direct current, measurements seem to indicate that the body resistance may range from 100 to 1000 ohms, depending on the distance between the electrodes. A conservative value of 1000 ohms should be used in most calculations, especially when one of the electrodes may be a cardiac catheter.[8]

Skin resistance is a function of the thickness of the callous skin on the surface, the amount of other dead tissue, the oiliness of the surface, and the amount of moisture in the skin. For dry, calloused hands the skin resistance may be as high as 500,000 ohms. After scrubbing with soap and thorough soaking in water the same hand skin may drop to a resistance

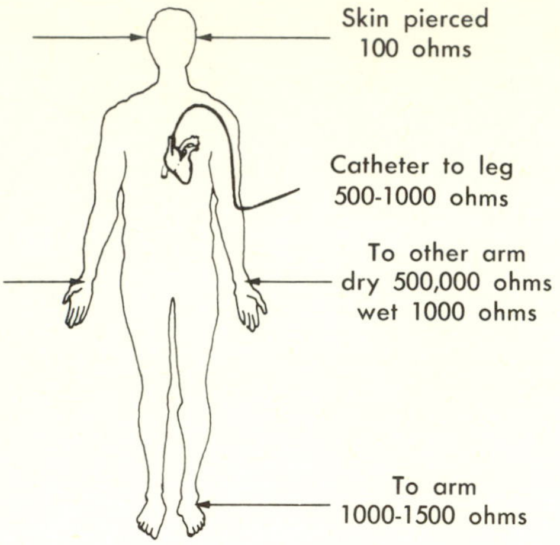


**Fig. 30-4.** Typical body resistance.

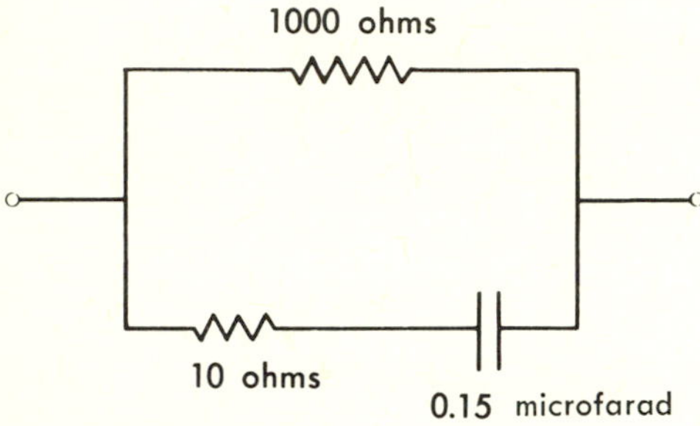


**Fig. 30-5.** The "patient" simulator.

of 500 to 1000 ohms or less. Similar low resistances may occur when the skin is cleansed with alcohol and covered with an electrode paste or lotion before attaching an ECG electrode, for example. Thus it is apparent that the body resistance, including skin, may be quite low, and that a value of 1000 ohms is a safe and conservative assumption for skin-to-skin-to-electrode resistance (Fig. 30-4).

The effect of frequency on the current flow and its physiologic reaction is simulated by paralleling the 1000 ohms with another resistor and a capacitor (Fig. 30-5).

## ■ How much voltage is dangerous?

A question often asked is, How much voltage is required to cause death or serious injury? The answer comes from the application of Ohm's law to the data just given on current and resistance. If the circuit through which the current passes runs from a cardiac catheter in the heart to a well-applied ground electrode on the right leg, the resistance can be seen to be of the order of 1000 ohms. If a current in excess of 50 microamperes is considered to be hazardous, 50 mV from a low impedance source would be a lethal voltage. On the other hand, for the calloused 500,000 ohm hands a voltage of 100 V would cause a very small current to flow and probably no harm would result. Of course when the voltage is several hundred volts, other effects such as burns occur; these are not to be considered here.

Since the hand-to-hand resistance may be as low as 1000 ohms and if 10 ma or so may cause sudden involuntary muscular reactions that could lead to a fall or other undesirable results, a potential difference of approximately 10 V could be considered hazardous.

## ■ What is electric shock?

Benjamin Franklin's analysis of the "convulsion" of the muscle caused by the flow of electricity through it has been alluded to. This is electric shock. In itself this electrical contraction of the muscles, if brief and not too violent, does little if any harm. Some pain may be felt and the experience is frightening, but little else. However, the conditions under which the shock occurs may result in other phenomena that are serious.

Two general categories of electric shock are recognized: (1) the macrocurrent or gross shock situation, wherein a current passes through the body of the subject and (2) the microcurrent shock, wherein a current passes directly through the heart wall from a conductor in the heart (Figs. 30-6 and 30-7).

## ■ What are macrocurrent shock hazards?

The macrocurrent shock may be considered as a stimulus causing an involuntary reaction (Fig. 30-8). Almost everyone jumps at the slightest shock. The threshold of sensitivity varies greatly with individuals, but for some persons currents as small as ½ ma will be unpleasant and may cause a reaction. Such

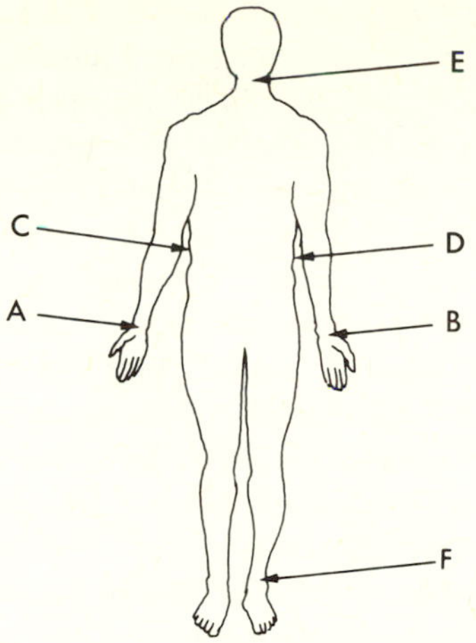


**Fig. 30-6.** Macrocurrent shock. Current flows between points on surface of body, for example, *A* to *F*.

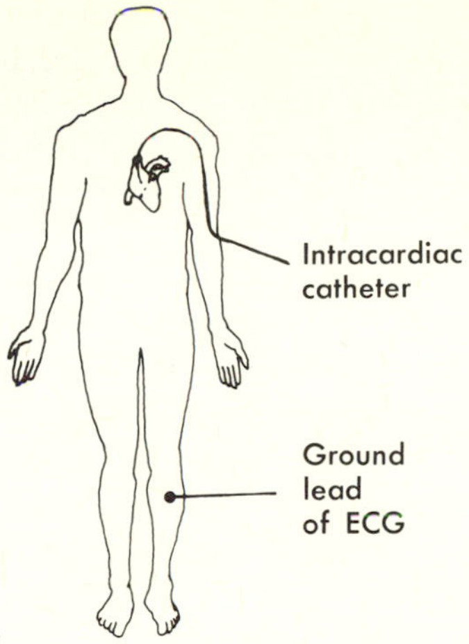


**Fig. 30-7.** Microcurrent shock. Current flows directly to heart through catheter to ECG ground lead.

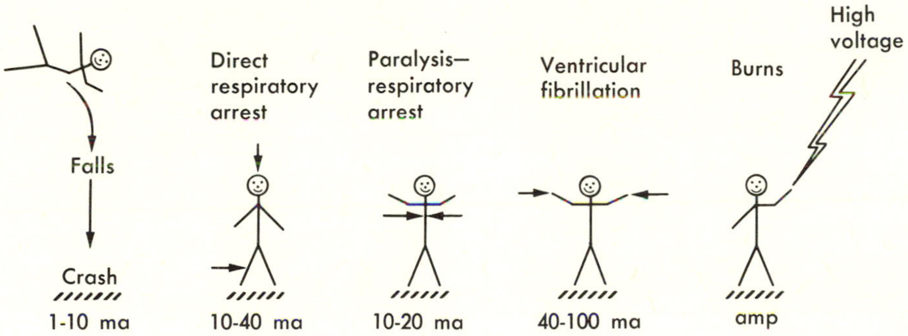


**Fig. 30-8.** Possible effects of gross or macrocurrent shock.

convulsive reactions have led to fatal falls, and it does not take much imagination to conceive of situations in the hospital wherein a reaction to shock could have serious consequences. Therefore it is included here as one of the several lethal effects of the electric current.

Dalziel conducted numerous experiments to determine perception and "let-go" currents.[9] Continued investigations have shown that for man the average current for which the subject can just let go is about 16 ma. If the current is only slightly larger than this value, the muscle "freezes" and the subject is unable to move the part of the body through which the current flows. The sensation is very painful, and if for no other reason than fright, there appears to be an almost complete paralysis of the body. Obviously if the current flow is through the chest muscles, respiration stops and the subject will undergo asphyxiation in a few minuets. If the circuit is broken in time, respiration will spontaneously begin again.

However, there is one form of respiratory arrest that may persist after the current ceases to flow. Called permanent respiratory arrest, it results when the current flows through the medulla of the brain where the respiratory control is centered. This means that the current must flow through the head and neck to some point on the body. Very little data exist concerning the magnitude of current that will cause this phenomenon, but it is probable that a current of a few milliamperes will be hazardous. Larger currents may cause permanent and often fatal damage to the nervous system.

Artificial respiration is the most obvious treatment for the person who has suffered permanent respiratory arrest. Here more than in any other circumstance prolonged respiratory assistance may result in recovery, even after several hours of seemingly useless effort.

Burns of electrical origin constitute a considerable hazard. Low frequency currents may produce deep burns that can lead to the loss of a limb or even to death. These are most likely to occur when the person comes in contact with a high voltage source, because quite large currents are required. However, electrical burn injuries do occur in the hospital because of the high frequency currents used in cautery and surgical procedures.

By far the largest portion of electrical deaths occur as a result of ventricular fibrillation.

## ■ How does electric shock cause ventricular fibrillation?

The heart consists of a large number of muscle cells that possess the properties of excitability, contractibility, and conductivity. Briefly, these arise from the electrolytic make-up of the cells, which results in a potential difference of some 90 mV between the inside and outside of the cell across the membrane that makes up the cell wall. An electrical stimulus (or even a mechanical or chemical stimulus) will cause a flow of ions across the cell wall, giving rise to the conductivity aspect, and will cause a contraction. The flow of ions is a current whose effect is observed on the body surface as one phase of the ECG. The current flow changes the potential difference across the cell wall and puts the cell in a "depolarized" state for a fraction of a second, after which it slowly repolarizes again.

In the right atrium of the heart there is a small mass of special tissue called the sinoatrial node that serves as a pacemaker for the heart. It has the property of self-excitation, so that about 70 times/min it sends out an electrical pulse that causes the muscles of the atria to contract in a wavelike manner. The result of this contraction forces the blood from the atria into the ventricles. When this wave reaches the group of cells known as the atrioventricular node, the accompanying electric currents trigger the node, causing it to send out a signal through highly conductive lines called the bundle of His and the Purkinje fibers to all parts of the ventricle muscles, causing them to contract and drive the blood out into the arteries.

The P wave of the ECG is the sum of the contraction and associated current flow of the atrial muscles of the heart. The QRS complex comes from the contraction of the ventricles, whereas the T wave is the repolarization of these muscles.

For a short time after a cell has been excited and contracts it is incapable of responding to further excitation. This is true of the ventricular muscles just after the QRS complex has been generated. However, soon after, in the S-T interval, some cells will be repolarizing, so that if an external stimulus is applied just about the time of the T wave, another contraction of the ventricles will occur. Such an action is called premature ventricular contraction (PVC). If the stimulus is a small 60 Hz current applied at this sensitive time, a series of PVC's may result. Often the frequency of occurrence of the PVC will increase, and the heart action degenerates into ventricular fibrillation. This is a state of random quivering of the heart muscle with no pumping action; hence unless the condition is corrected soon, death results.

If a flow of electric current occurs through the body, a small portion of it will pass through the heart and may cause the heart to fibrillate. This is the condition referred to as "macrocurrent shock" or macroshock because the magnitude of current required to produce harmful results is of the order a thousand times larger than the hazardous current level when there is a direct electrical connection to the heart muscle.

Because the mechanism of death from electric shock was not understood, especially when ventricular fibrillation appeared to have been induced, King at Columbia University undertook to conduct a systematized study of the problem.[10] During a 6-year period over a thousand animals, ranging in size from rabbits to calves and sheep, were subjected to carefully controlled electric shocks. Anesthetized animals were used, and starting with a small current, repeated shocks of increasing strength were applied until ventricular fibrillation resulted. The investigation resulted in a wealth of data, but only limited conclusions were drawn. Among them was the observation that once fibrillation was induced in a heart, it seldom, if ever, spontaneously reverted to normal action. Furthermore, the heart was found to be most sensitive if it was shocked between the termination of the T wave and the beginning of the QRS complex. Few conclusions were drawn as to the magnitude of current that would induce fibrillation. However, this work as extended by others in association with King remained the landmark in this area for some 20 years. Kouwenhoven and his associates at Johns Hopkins University, using more sophisticated measuring devices, carried on an investigation somewhat similar to King's, but with the objective of determining the minimum fibrillating current as an additional parameter.[11]

Dalziel at the University of California at Berkeley, as already noted, conducted a study of the magnitude of the just perceptible and the maximum let-go currents and developed a statistical technique for analyzing the results. He applied this technique to the King data and deduced from it a threshold fibrillating current for man that incorporated the concept that it was dependent on the weight of the man. Later, using Kouwenhoven data, Dalziel proposed the following equation:

$$I = \frac{K}{\sqrt{T}}$$

where I is the current in milliamperes, T is the time in seconds, and K is a constant (approximately 100 ma/sec$^{1/2}$). This leads to the conclusion that 100 ma flowing for 1 second from arm to arm in an adult will probably induce ventricular fibrillation.[12]

In some cases it appears that cardiac arrest occurs when large currents flow through the chest. This situation probably would require the current to flow for some minutes so that death occurs as a result of the cessation of circulation. There is some probability that, if the current flow is for just a second or so, the heart rhythm might start spontaneously after the current flow stops, somewhat in the manner observed after defibrillation.

Until relatively recent times, these macroshock situations were the only electric shock hazards against which care had to be taken.

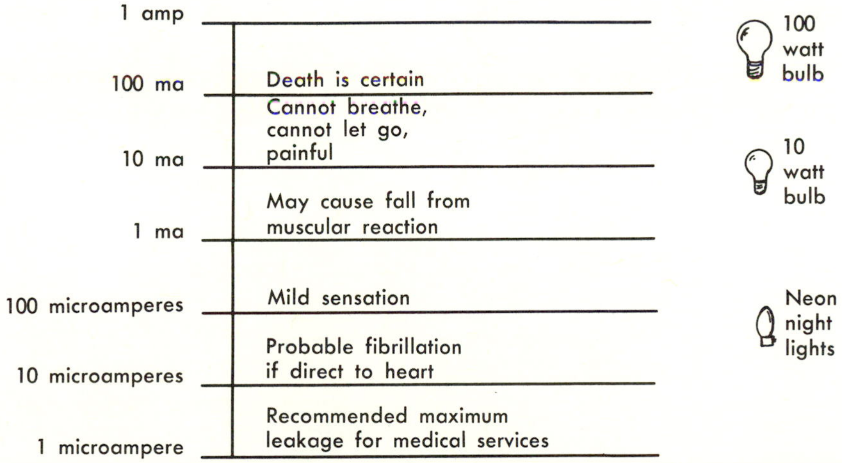


**Fig. 30-9.** Electric current shock hazard.

## ■ What is microshock?

When an electrical conductor connects directly to the heart wall, all of the current flowing in it will pass through the heart. The current required to cause fibrillation will be quite small, measured in millionths of amperes, or microamperes. This condition is called microshock, in contrast to macroshock, wherein the current is measured in thousandths of amperes, or milliamperes.

In 1962 Weinberg and associates published a report of studies of electric shock hazards in cardiac catheterization, concluding that currents as low as 35 microamperes could produce ventricular fibrillation in the dog when the current passed through the heart wall.[13] Other studies indicate that a current as low as 12 microamperes at 60 Hz has been known to produce fibrillation in the canine ventricle. One case is reported in which 180 microamperes produced fibrillation in a human being. More recently the evidence is that usually larger heart currents are required to produce fibrillation in human beings. However, in the interest of safety a value of 10 to 20 microamperes is considered to be the maximum safe current through the heart wall (Fig. 30-9).

## ■ How serious is the electric shock hazard?

There have been many articles about the hazards of electricity in hospitals and the number of fatalities that result. Most of them have no basis in fact. Although there are no hard data available, the number of fatalities caused by electric shock in hospitals is probably less than 10 annually. But even one is too many, because most, if not all, such accidents can be eliminated. The methods are relatively simple and will be discussed later.

## ■ Where do the hazards originate?

First, most electrical energy in the United States is provided by means of a two- (or three-) wire system in which one (or two) of the wires may be at or near ground potential and the other (the live conductor) at the line voltage—nominally 120 V. A current will flow through a circuit (or a human being) connected from the "live" wire to the ground, which may be either of the other circuit wires, or a water pipe, or a wet floor. Several possibilities exist for the development of a hazardous situation whenever electrical equipment is used on this electrical supply system.[14]

Second, an important consideration is that the electrical system, includes not only the instrumentation and devices but also the wiring of the building. If it is not installed properly, many hazardous conditions may result.

Third, the equipment used may be the source of the hazards. For example, a very common fault in electrical equipment is the failure of the ground connection in passing through the power cord. The design of many types of plugs is such that the ground wire breaks in the plug after a few months of use. When this happens, that piece of equipment is ungrounded and a hazard could exist.

A fourth hazard is generated if, because of wear and improper maintenance or because of a flaw in design or manufacture, the live wire is exposed or touches the ungrounded frame of a lamp, instrument, or bed. A person touching the electrically live wire or frame and ground will provide a conducting path through which a dangerous or lethal current may flow. Obviously the current could be large enough to be hazardous in the macroshock category. If the current passes through a catheter directly into the heart, death would almost certainly result.

Fifth, whenever two electrical conductors are in close proximity, a capacitive coupling exists between them. This means simply that it is possible for a small quantity of electric charge to pass through the insulation from one conductor to the other. If the voltage between the conductor is alternating, an alternating current will flow. Thus if one of the conductors is the hot wire of the electrical supply to a piece of equipment, a current will flow through the capacitive coupling to the frame and to ground through any available path. This path could be the human body. The current is called the leakage current and should be measured as it flows through a 1000 ohm resistance. Resistive and inductive coupling may also contribute to the leakage current.

A sixth source of hazardous electric shock is the failure of the personnel using the equipment to understand that misuse can result in danger. Most equipment offered on the market today is safe if well maintained and properly used. However, the simplest of devices can kill if faulty operation is not recognized or if the unit is misused.

A seventh hazard may be termed "intentional" for want of a better word. It is most likely to occur with children who put hairpins or paper clips into receptacle slots, but many persons "play" with electric devices and may do the wrong thing.

## ■ What are some examples of sources of hazards?

In one of the earliest reports of the induction of ventricular fibrillation by the flow of current through a catheter in the heart, Mody and Richings[15] found that the ground wire opened in the distribution box as the result of a loose screw. This could have been prevented by a good testing and maintenance program in the hospital.

In a second case sufficient voltage and low enough leakage impedance existed between the x-ray tube mounting over the table used in cardiac catheterization and the cable so that 25 microamperes would flow through 1000 ohms connected between them. The problem was that the ground wire had never been connected to the ground bus. Although some problems with 60 Hz noise had been observed during angiography, this condition had been allowed to go uninvestigated for the 3 years after the installation had been "completed" in the new hospital. Had a serious incident occurred, it could have been credited to poor workmanship and poor inspection and testing, but more importantly, to poor reporting of the problem on the part of the physicians and nurses.

In still another case an ECG was to be used in a regular hospital room. As a matter of course, the wall outlet was checked for polarity and ground continuity. The grounding wire was found to be broken, although it had been patent some time in the past. Inspection showed the wire had been nicked in removing the insulation, and building vibration had caused the failure. Here a testing procedure may have prevented a serious incident.

In a coronary care unit in which five of the eight patients had indwelling intracardiac catheters, all of the monitors had leakage currents in excess of 25 microamperes.[16] Pulsing in the leakage currents of up to 48 microamperes was observed on one monitor, evidently caused by a faulty grounding system and coupling between the monitor and other electric devices. This is an example of faulty design, but also of faulty testing and maintenance.

These are probably enough examples to give an indication of the varied nature of the problems that can arise from improper wiring of the hospital building accentuated by poor reporting and testing procedures.

Some hazards are equipment problems. They may arise from improper maintenance and use, but many will result from poor quality control or poor design on the part of the manufacturer of the instrument. Here are examples, some of them mere statements of observed facts.[16]

A leakage current of 120 microamperes was measured in the injector used in angiography. A recorder used in the cardiac catheterization laboratory had a leakage current of 45 microamperes. A leakage current of 5 ma was measured in ultrasonic generators used in the physiotherapy section. These are examples of poor design of the equipment. However, the shortcomings of the design can be offset by making certain that the grounding wires of the instruments are in good condition. This is a matter for the maintenance technicians to check regularly.

An example of the need for the engineer and technician to be involved in checking and replacing the plugs on the power cords of the instruments follows. One hospital engineer reported that a survey of 300 molded-on plugs cut off of hospital equipment such as electric beds, portable suction pumps, hypothermia machines, etc. revealed the following conditions on detailed examination: (1) Fifty-five percent of the plugs had no ground prong. The ground prongs had been removed because they were broken in "normal" hospital use or were bent and could not be inserted in receptacles. (2) Forty-five percent of the plugs had all three prongs apparently intact. Visual inspection showed *apparently* safe plugs.[17] When the plugs with apparently intact prongs were tested with a continuity meter, it was found that only 15% of the plugs were actually safe. Often when such a situation occurs in the critical care area, artifacts will be seen on the monitor. It becomes the duty of the practitioner to report it, but the best remedy is a good testing and maintenance program.

A final example of both faulty equipment and improper building wiring is that of a cardiac patient who was shocked sufficiently to be thoroughly frightened when he touched the pendant nurse call button. He was on a cardiac monitor. Investigation showed that the call button was not insulated but was grounded and the monitor was faulty in that it had a partial short on the live wire to the chassis and was not grounded. These are both design and maintenance faults.

But the users of the equipment are often at fault. Because the attached cord was too short, a two-wire extension was used for 2 months on an injector in angiography.[16] The leakage current on the injector was high, resulting in the ungrounded machine-induced fibrillation of a number of patients before the cause was detected and repaired. No physician, nurse, or technician should ever allow the use of a two-wire cord on an instrument that has a three-wire power cord. In another case an inexpensive two-wire extension cord was found on an ECG machine "because the regular three-wire cord would not work."

Two examples will suffice to show that several items may be involved. A 53-year-old patient was thrown into ventricular fibrillation when the control mechanism of the electrically operated bed was immerged in urine.[18] Analysis of this case revealed the following situation: The patient, having a mild left hemiparesis, had elevated the backrest of the electrically operated bed to the vertical position, leaving the control mechanism resting on the lap. While attempting to return the urinal to the bedside table with the paretic left arm, the patient lost control over the heavy bottle and spilled most of its content over the bed, thereby immersing the control mechanism in the urine. The control mechanism, in turn, carried current from a conventional 120 grounded power line to the motor operating the bed mechanism. The patient was connected to ground by one of the ECG monitor electrodes taped to the anterior chest wall, its connecting cable terminating at the chassis of the monitor grounded through the third wire of the power cord. Thus current from the control mechanism passed through the urine, the patient's buttocks, the chest electrode to the chassis of the monitor, and from there to ground via ground wire. Only the quick action of a resident who observed the appearance of a 60 Hz signal on the remote monitor at the nurses' station prevented the accident from becoming fatal.

In another case a 52-year-old male patient was on an external cardiac pacemaker connected to the power line. A transvenous bipolar catheter electrode was placed through the right jugular vein into the right ventricle of the heart. Later the patient was found dead. An examination revealed that the instrument grounding system (third prong) was eliminated by use of a 10-foot two-wire extension cord. Leakage current of the instrument (including the 8-foot three-wire power cord of the instrument and the 10-foot two-wire extension cord) measured 54 microamperes.[19]

This accident could have been avoided if (1) a three-wire, instead of a two-wire, extension cord had been used on the pacemaker, (2) the patient had no access to any conductor to ground, (3) the pacer lead had had a current-limiting device of 5 microamperes, or (4) a battery-powered pacemaker had been used. However, the primary cause was an improper procedure—the use of the two-wire extension cord.

An incident of the "intentional" type occurred in a pediatric ward when a child found a hairpin and inserted it into the "live" slot of a receptacle. He then tried to pull it out with his teeth. His nose touched the grounded metallic plate surrounding the receptacle, resulting in a circuit from the hairpin through the lips to the nose and the plate. He suffered severe burns of the mouth and lips.[18]

To sum up and repeat for emphasis, the electric shock incidents just reviewed were caused by one or a combination of the following: (1) poor design of the wiring system or equipment; (2) poor maintenance of the wiring system or the equipment; (3) improper use of a device; and (4) carelessness on the part of the designer, manufacturer, or user or lack of knowledge as to how to use the instruments.

These examples do not exhaust the list of ways in which electric shock accidents can occur. Instead they merely point out that the conditions that lead to shock are almost as varied as the number of possible combinations of people, devices, and wiring systems. They indicate that the only way to avoid accident is to be "eternally vigilant." However, certain basic principles can be applied that will help reduce the hazards of electric shock.

## ■ How is electric shock prevented?

From an earlier discussion it would seem that protecting a patient from the probability of electric shock is quite simple in principle. The reduction of hazardous currents can be achieved by:

1. Preventing a voltage difference from occurring in such a way that the patient or other person cannot close the circuit and thus allow a current to flow (Fig. 30-10, *A*)
2. Putting a high resistance in all circuits that could include the patient, thus reducing the current to less than hazardous levels (Fig. 30-10, *B*)

However, the implementation of these procedures is quite difficult, especially when the human factor is included.

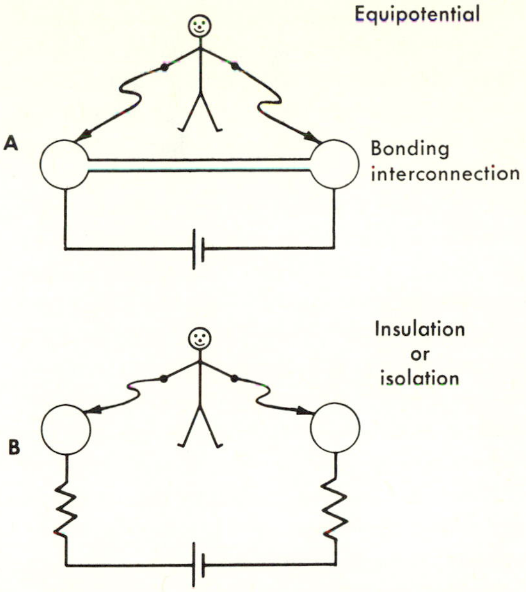


**Fig. 30-10.** Preventing electrical shock by, **A,** equipotential bonding or grounding or, **B,** inserting high resistance in circuit.

It has been pointed out that the values contributed by electric instruments far outweigh the hazards they introduce. Nevertheless, accidents do occur and they can result in discomfort, injury, or death to the patient, nurse, or physician, but almost all are preventable. To assist in the task of providing for conditions that will result in reasonable safety, many groups are working on codes and standards that help establish recommended safe practice. One of these, which is still a tentative standard, is *The Safe Use of Electricity in Patient Care Areas of Health Care Facilities.*[8]

A basic step to safety is to define the hazard to persons in terms of classes of risk, as follows:

Risk class I: staff and nearly well patients
Risk class II: seriously ill patients
Risk class III: patients with a conductor connected to their heart muscles

Risk class I comprises patients and other personnel without any debilitating disease. For such persons hazardous currents begin at the 1 ma level.

Risk class II includes patients who are critically ill, who may be sedated, or who may be connected to monitoring or other devices. For these patients all apparatus must have a leakage current of less than 100 microamperes.

Risk class III patients are those who have a low impedance electric conductor leading to the heart. It is very difficult to provide protection by electrical design for these patients. The basic protection for such patients is insulation of the exposed conductor terminal. When this is done, the risk class III patient becomes in reality a risk class II patient.

For risk class I persons all devices designed and manufactured in accordance with standards adopted by the electrical manufacturing associations and maintained by regular inspection and repair will be safe, if properly used. This will include having acceptable wiring in the area where such devices are to be used. The minimum wiring system is a three-wire grounded system with a ground conductor separate from the conduit.

For risk class II persons the acceptable wiring system combines the minimum with the grounding of exposed conductive surfaces such as water pipes and construction metal. Other large metal objects that may become electrically energized should also be connected to the common ground in the patient area. This system is referred to as an equipotential grounding system.

The equipotential grounding system may have additional features added, such as the insulation of all exposed metal or the use of isolated power systems. Further detail on the design and installation of such systems is appropriate to an engineering manual and will not be treated here. However, great care must be exercised in the use of equipment in the presence of the risk class II patient. Perhaps foremost is the assurance that the equipment is properly designed, that it is the right equipment for the purpose, and that it has been well maintained.

An important part of the purchase of any device is preparation of a set of specifications for it. These specifications should be prepared by a committee consisting of members of the medical and nursing staffs who will be involved in the use of the apparatus, and members of the engineering and technical staffs who can determine the electrical safety features of the device. Such a committee should determine the availability of repair and calibration services and many other features in addition to the medical functions that the device may fulfill.

If possible, the engineering members of the committee should have the opportunity to make prepurchase inspections and tests on the device, and the medical and user staff members should be permitted to check its operational features.

Once the device is ordered and received at the hospital, a series of inspections and tests should be established for it. These will include (1) preacceptance testing, (2) preventive maintenance procedures, (3) preuse testing under certain critical circumstances, (4) postrepair testing, and (5) postmisuse testing.[20]

To expand further on the preceding discussion, the first testing and inspection of a device may come when a unit has been brought to the hospital for demonstration and possible purchase. It should be there only on the approval of the appropriate engineer, who will have examined the specifications prior to the approval for demonstration. When it comes to the hospital, perhaps brought by a salesman, it should go directly to the engineer and engineering staff for acceptance testing. After this and only after this should it go to a floor to be used or demonstrated.

Much of the acceptance test procedure may be circumvented in some cases by the use of the work done in Philadelphia by The Emergency Care Research Institute.* However, this does not eliminate examination of a particular piece of equipment in a particular hospital.

*The Emergency Care Research Institute, 913 Walnut Street, Philadelphia, Pa.

One of the things to be looked for in this first test is how many little-used knobs are on the front panel—knobs that can disturb the functioning of the euipment if not correctly adjusted. For example, one moment of panic occurred in the open-heart surgery room when the patient's blood pressure as shown on the scope was very low. The actual situation was that the technician had turned the wrong knob, intending to raise the pattern on the screen. Instead the knob he turned unbalanced the pressure transducer bridge. Other prepurchase tests should include calibration frequency response where important. For example, a small square wave applied to an ECG machine can give a good indication of excessive filtering or damping in the recording part of the machine or its quality of performance.

Once the prepurchase acceptance tests are completed, the decision on what instrument or device to buy is made and the order placed, the engineering staff now waits for the arrival of the equipment. Once again, inspection and testing are in order. Equipment can be damaged in shipment, maybe not visibly, but as far as safety or performance is concerned. A dropped box may break a fuse holder in such a manner that the hot wire touches the ungrounded case, yet no damage may show externally.

Once the equipment is accepted and in use in the hospital, continued and regular preventive maintenance tests specifically designed for each device should be performed. Records of these tests and any corrective repairs made should be kept by the hospital.

Sometimes it becomes important to make tests that combine the characteristics of the power system and the instrumentation and to separate them if they combine in an adverse fashion. For example, I recently had occasion to test the leakage of a piece of equipment that the hospital planned to use on an isolated power system. The hospital tests showed the leakage exceeded the specifications by 50% and the engineer refused to accept the device. However, a test on the same unit made in the hall outside the electronics laboratory on a conventional grounded power supply showed a lower leakage current within specifications. The problem was in the very high leakage of the isolated system and the method of measurement.

Test protocols should include provision for testing immediately prior to any difficult and dangerous procedure such as cardiac catheterization and extensive surgery. These may be simple go–no go tests that can be performed by the nurse or medical technician, or they may be more instrumented measurements made by the medical equipment technician or engineer.

The remarks just made may seem to be more detailed and technical than necessary in a book such as this. However, since critical care practitioners are most involved with the use of all manner of electromedical devices, it is important that they be informed on what is required to have a safe, effective instrumentation system. This includes the acceptance of responsibility, specific tasks, participation in planning and implementation, and awareness and reporting.

### *Acceptance of responsibility for environment*

The most important thing critical care practitioners can do to ensure the safety of their patients as far as the instrumentation is concerned is to recognize that they must accept responsibility for the entire environment of the patient. This means that the patient must receive the best possible care with the minimum of discomfort commensurate with the situation. Obviously an electric shock, even a slight one, can not be tolerated, nor can burns, excessive pressures, or whatever unnecessary effects occur to disturb the patient.

### *Specific tasks*

To be involved in a continuing education program at the risk of repetition is the next most important thing critical care practitioners can do in the instrument safety field; this means to be informed. They should not only have studied these notes, but should have read some of the references listed in the bibliography. They should have read very carefully the operation manuals on the devices they are likely to be called on to use. They should give special attention to any precautionary notes in the operation manuals.

### *Planning and implementation*

Being involved in the planning and implementation of the instrumentation program is also important. Although architects and engineers are the usual sources for designs of hospitals, the medical and nursing staff are the users. In an area where the design and the installation of the instrumentation are such an important part of the functioning of the system, critical care practitioners should have input into the design. Furthermore, they should have an opportunity to plan the ways in which the system is to be used. This means they should ask for and accept membership on planning committees, safety committees, etc.

### *Awareness and reporting*

To recognize and report any incidents, observations, or accidents involving the instrumentation may be lifesaving. The observation of artifacts, stray "noise," extra-wide baseline, or any other effect on an oscilloscope or recording device may be an indication of possible hazardous conditions in electrical devices or they may merely mean that the electrodes are not making contact with the patient. In any case, their cause should be investigated, and if the problem is not immediately recognized and remedied, help should be obtained. The nursing supervisor and/or the engineer or technician should be called. The problem may be simple and the solution equally simple, but it could result in a fatality.

If a tingling sensation is felt, or someone thinks that it is, the occurrence should be reported to the technical staff and they should investigate it immediately.

Sometimes an instrument is dropped accidently or a fluid is spilled over it. Unless the device is a life-support instrument, it should be unplugged and the incident reported. Anyone may experience an accident, and there should be no penalty. But the failure to report it could be reason for severe penalty.

## SUMMARY

This chapter is in itself a brief summary of a subject that has blossomed into volumes of continuing growth. Briefly, the nature of electricity and its associated hazards have been reviewed. The prevention of accidents involving these hazards is the responsibility of many persons—engineers, manufacturers, hospital administrators, technicians, and nurses. For all these persons, and especially for the critical care practitioner, the whole safety problem can be summed up in two very brief statements:

1. Be informed.
2. Be involved.

## REFERENCES

1. Porterfield, J. D., III: To the defense of the system, hospitals, J. Am. Hosp. Assoc. **48:**49, 1974.
2. Smyth, A. H., editor: The life and writings of Benjamin Franklin, vol. 2, New York, 1905, Macmillan Publishing Co., Inc.
3. Waller, A.: On the electromotive changes connected with beats of the mammalian heart, and the human heart in particular, Trans. R. Soc. Lond. **180:**169, 1889.
4. Einthoven, W.: The different forms of the human electrocardiogram and their signification, Lancet **1:**853, 1912.
5. Engineering in the health care industry, Soundings **2:**No. 1, 1971.
6. Intersociety Commission for Heart Disease: Electronic equipment in critical care areas, Circulation **43:**A-97, 1971.
7. Karselis, T.: Descriptive medical electronics and instrumentation, Thorofare, N. J., 1973, Charles B. Slack.
8. Safe use of electricity in patient care areas of health care facilities, Standard 76BT, Boston, Mass., 1975, National Fire Protection Association.
9. Dalziel, C. F.: Threshold 60 cycle fibrillating currents, Trans. Am. Inst. Electrical Engineers **79:**667, 1960.
10. King, B. G.: Effect of electric shock on heart action with special reference to varying susceptibility in different parts of the cardiac cycle, Doctoral thesis, Columbia University, New York, 1934, Aberdeen Press.
11. Kouwenhoven, W. B., Knickerbocker, G. G., Chesnut, R. W., Milnor, W. R., and Soss, D. J.: A-C shocks of varying parameters

affecting the heart, A.I.E.E. Trans. E.E. **78:** 163, 1959.
12. Dalziel, D. F., and Lee, W. R.: Re-evaluation of lethal electric currents, I.E.E.E. Trans. IGA **4:**467, 1968.
13. Weinberg, D. L., Artley, J. L., Whalen, R. E., and McIntosh, H. D.: Electric shock hazards in cardiac catheterization, Circ. Res. **11:**1004, 1962.
14. Bruner, J. M. R.: Hazards of electrical apparatus, Anesthesiology **28:**396, 1967.
15. Mody, S. M., and Richings, M.: Ventricular fibrillation resulting from electrocution during cardiac catheterization, Lancet **2:**698, 1962.
16. Stanley, P. E.: Personal notes.
17. Lubin, D.: Molded-on attachment plug caps can create hazardous electrical situations in the hospital, report to the American Society of Hospital Engineers, Committee on Electrical Safety in Hospitals, 1968, American Society of Hospital Engineers.
18. Aronow, S., Bruner, J. M. R., Siegal, E. F., and Sloss, L. J.: Ventricular fibrillation associated with an electrically operated bed, N. Engl. J. Med. **281:**31, 1969.
19. Von der Mosel, H. A.: Accident case history, Med. Electronics Data **1:**74, 1970.
20. Stanley, P. E.: Safety in the electromedical equipment system, National Safety News **110:**No. 5, 71; No. 6, 90; **111:**No. 1, 87, 1975.

*chapter 31*

# Overview of critical care and the rehabilitative process

MILDRED LAWSON
EMILY S. HACKLER

Any change in a person's state of mental, physical, and social well-being precipitates anxiety. A serious interruption in this homeostasis constitutes crisis, and in any type of health crisis, critical care involving decisive and careful judgment is necessary if the patient is to survive. *Restoration of the person's homeostasis to a noncritical level is the primary goal of critical care.* However, rehabilitative care is needed to assist the patient to return to the precrisis level of homeostasis or to function at a maximum level consistent with the disease state.

Rehabilitation is an active and dynamic program that enables an ill or disabled person to achieve the greatest possible efficiency in his or her physical, emotional, social, and economic functions. Hence *the primary goal of rehabilitation is to restore the individual to a useful and meaningful life.*

The challenge in rehabilitation lies in the extent and variety of the disease-related and treatment-related disabilities presented and whether the patient's condition is to be "cured" or "controlled." Obviously the scope of acute illness and critical care does not allow discussion of every aspect of treatment and rehabilitation. Therefore generalized guidelines will be discussed to assist all members of the health care team to make significant contributions to the patient's rehabilitation plan, with emphasis on the problem-oriented concept of care planning and the team approach to rehabilitation.

Early and dynamic assistance for the patient's rehabilitation process will lessen or prevent some acute disabilities from occurring or becoming chronic, perhaps reducing the time needed for recovery or restoration as the patient goes through each phase of illness.[1] These phases of illness have been divided into the following four categories:

| | |
|---|---|
| Phase I | Acute illness, usually in critical care unit |
| Phase II | Inpatient hospital convalescence |
| Phase III | Convalescence at home |
| Phase IV | Recovery and maintenance |

Each phase will be explored with regard to immediate and long-term goals for rehabilitation and developing nursing care implications. The emphasis for nursing care will be placed on (1) observation of the patient; (2) coordination of the team efforts for the patient's rehabilitation; and (3) discharge planning, which includes patient-family education regarding the patient's disease and rehabilitation plans. Any plan for rehabilitation is incomplete without the educative process for patient and family. The critical care team may have the perfect program, but ultimately it is the patient and family who decide which goals are workable for them.

## ■ When does rehabilitation begin?

Rehabilitation begins in the first phase of the patient's care, often as early as the second day after admission into the critical care unit. Frequently short-term goals are set for the prevention of complications in the patient's recovery process. Once the first phase of illness is past, rehabilitation plans will include long-term goals in addition to the short-term goals and necessitates consideration of the following:

1. The patient's level of physiologic and psychologic functional ability
2. Whether the patient can be expected to return to previous health status without residual handicaps
3. Whether ongoing disease or handicap will persist
4. Whether or not there is increasing disability to be expected from progressing disease

## ■ How should the rehabilitation process be designed?

*Team approach (Table 31-1)*

Rehabilitation from critical illness should be a dynamic process resulting from the

**Table 31-1.** Functions of the team members

| *Team member* | *Function* |
|---|---|
| Primary physician | Responsible for obtaining initial data base: history, physical, and baseline laboratory studies<br>Directs diagnostic and therapeutic program<br>Directs and supervises team functioning<br>Teaches other team members, patient, and family |
| Physiatrist | Directs and supervises team functioning<br>Teaches other team members, patient, and family<br>Tests patient's physical functioning<br>Supervises patient's rehabilitation program |
| Nurse | Coordinates team activity and patient care<br>Interprets physician's instructions to patient and family<br>Conducts health teaching with patient and family<br>Makes community referrals |
| Physical therapist | Devises and supervises individual exercise programs within prescribed physical limits<br>Teaches the patient during prescribed exercise program and conducts gait training<br>Uses physical agents in restoration of bodily function after illness or injury<br>Recommends activities to save energy and alleviate boredom and depression |
| Occupational therapist | Trains and evaluates self-care<br>Trains and evaluates activities of daily living<br>Assesses upper and lower extremities, including strength and range of motion, sensory-motor, prevocational exploration, splinting, and work therapy |
| Social worker | Collects social data pertinent to rehabilitation goals<br>Counsels patient and family<br>Assesses social environment and acts as liaison between team and family<br>Assists in home placement of patient |
| Clinical psychologist | Conducts patient's psychologic evaluation<br>Participates in psychologic counseling and crisis intervention<br>Leads group therapy<br>Conducts stress interviews |
| Vocational counselor | Evaluates aptitude, ability, interest, and dexterity<br>Assesses physical requirements of former job<br>Helps patient set vocational goals<br>Arranges work tryouts in job settings<br>Makes referrals to community agencies and local workshops<br>Provides liaison between local employers and patients seeking jobs |

creative efforts of a team of health professionals dedicated to helping the patient achieve the greatest possible use of emotional, physical, social, and economic resources and educating the patient to manage problems. As in any collaborative effort, communication among the members of the team and with the patient is essential for a successful program. The physician is responsible for the management of the medical problems and for overall coordination of the team; however, it is the responsibility of the nurse to coordinate the various parts of the whole program on a day-to-day basis so that consultations, treatments, and basic care are individualized for the patient. The patient's record is the tool for communication between all members of the team.

### *Data base of patient information*[2, 3]

The physician's history, physical, and initial laboratory studies are one part of the data base. Other parts include evaluations by the nurse, physical therapist, occupational therapist, and social worker. Initial plans for rehabilitation (assessment, goal setting, implementation of plans for achieving goals, and patient-family education) are focused on problems noted in the initial data base. Evaluation of the plan of care, reassessment of goals, and alterations in the plan of care are based on subjective and objective data collected during each phase of the patient's illness.

***Subjective data.***[2, 3] There are many facets of a patient's personality that only the patient or family can provide. These facets are called "subjective" or "soft" data and include pain, habits of living, "feelings," and personal expectations (goals) for eventual recovery or methods of coping in the event total recovery is not expected. Without knowledge of these facets, goals that the staff may have set for the patient may be irrelevant or difficult to attain.

Personal interviews with the patient are essential to determine his own goals and to develop a "patient profile" from which realistic goals for the patient can be established. A complete patient profile requires both subjective and objective information about the patient's diagnosis, awareness of the condition, and personal habits. Age, economic status, and cultural background are also relevant data in preparing a meaningful patient care plan.

***Objective data.***[2, 3] Objective or "hard" data consist of factual information about the patient and are reflected in the patient's record as the physical examination, laboratory studies, special tests, observation (flow) charting, narrative charting, and consultation-evaluation sheets recorded by various members of the team. Objective data form the core on which assessments, goals, and patient plans of care are based, whereas subjective data obtained from the patient or family modify and individualize the plan of patient care.

### *Assessment of patient needs*

Interpretation of the subjective and objective data collected by all personnel working with the patient is summarized, and goals for care are established in terms of present and potential ability. The assessment of the patient's physiologic, psychologic, occupational, and financial potential must be periodically reviewed and reassessment made according to the patient's progress or regression.

Ideally the initial and periodic assessments are done in team conferences with the patient and significant family members present. It is not always possible for all members of the team to meet in conferences concerning every patient as often as desirable except when the patient is admitted to a rehabilitation unit. On intermediate care units and general wards it is the responsibility of the primary physician and the primary nurse to summarize accumulated data, assess the data, and restate goals for the patient.

*It is the moral and professional responsibility of every member of the team participating in the patient's recovery program to record the patient's progress or lack of progress in the patient's record.* This is the only way a permanent record can be maintained from which assessments of the patient's condition can be made, leading to goals and

## FUNCTIONAL STATUS REPORT*

Patient ______________________ Diagnosis ______________________
Date ______________________

**LIMB MOTION (passive or active)** *Admission*† | *Goal*‡ | *Discharge*† | *Signature*

1. Upper right function ______
2. Upper left function ______
3. Lower right function ______
4. Lower left function ______

**EXERCISE PRESCRIPTION**

**ACTIVITIES OF DAILY LIVING**

5. Eating/feeding ______
6. Personal hygiene ______
7. Grooming ______
8. Bowel management ______
9. Bladder management ______
10. Skin management ______
11. Bed activities (rolling, sitting) ______
12. Dress ______
13. Transfers ______
14. Wheelchair activities ______
15. Ambulation (assisted or independent) ______
    a. Assistance device ______
    b. Distance ______
    c. Duration ______
16. Stairs, curbs, ramps ______
17. Homemaking ______
    a. Meals ______
    b. Child care ______
    c. Usual cleaning chores ______

**COMMUNICATION AND PSYCHO/SOCIAL ACTIVITIES**

18. Reading (graphic comprehension) ______
19. Understanding spoken language ______
20. Language expression ______
21. Writing ______
22. Speech intelligibility ______
23. Attention (concentration) ______
24. Cognition ______
25. Orientation ______
26. Emotional reaction ______
27. Family/environmental interaction ______
28. Vocational ability ______

**MEDICAL MANAGEMENT**

29. Pain ______
30. Self-medication ______
31. Medical problems other than diagnosis ______
32. Other problems (treatments) ______

Physician ______ Speech pathologist ______
Primary nurse ______ Social worker ______
Psychologist ______ Occupational therapist ______
Vocational counselor ______ Physical therapist ______

*Patterned after form used at University of California Irvine Medical Center, Orange, Calif.
†Charted by predetermined code.
‡Cross referenced with boxed material on p. 581.

plans of care for the management of the patient's physical, social, and mental problems created by the disease.

The boxed material on p. 579 is one type of summary sheet that may help practitioners make more comprehensive assessments, both objectively and subjectively, of patient care needs. Obviously each patient is unique; therefore each patient's assessment will depend on the findings the practitioner makes in the analysis of the data collected.

### *Problem list and initial plan of care*[2, 3]

Persons are admitted to hospitals because they have problems. The complete data base depicts these problems as does ongoing subjective and objective information obtained during the various phases of the patient's rehabilitative process. It is therefore logical to organize the patient plan of care from a problem-oriented base. *These are the patient's problems—not problems that the staff incur in solving or coping with the patient's problems.*

From the data base a list of the patient's problems is itemized numerically, not necessarily in order of importance, but as they appear in the original and ongoing subjective and objective information obtained about the patient. This master list of problems is kept in front of the patient's chart and becomes a permanent part of the record.

The physician's initial plan of care is written from the problem list with diagnostic, therapeutic, and educational aspects of problem solving included for every problem.

### *Problem list and care plan*

Problems specific to the patient's long-term care and rehabilitation are taken from (or added to) the master problem list, and a plan of care is built around the problem. The boxed material on p. 581 outlines a logical sequence of recording the plan of care that is written in the form of diagnostic, therapeutic, and educational orders. This form is designed for convenience of use by all team members and is to be read at the start of conferences in much the same manner as "minutes of the meeting," updated as necessary, and then continued in use until the next meeting and/or reassessment. This constitutes the plan of care. It is not a "medical plan of care" or a "nursing care plan"; rather, it is a *patient plan of care.*

In no other area of care is the patient plan of care more important than in rehabilitation efforts where multidisciplinary care must be coordinated to the patient's maximum benefit. Time is crucial in most areas of rehabilitation, and prompt planning for treatment will eliminate or minimize complications that might ensue during the course of recovery such as decubiti, contractures, problems in performing activities of daily living, and emotional deterioration secondary to inactivity and depression.

The problem list and care plan is a tool for the coordination of patient care and provides rapid communication to all members of the team, including the patient. Ideally the plan is kept at the patient's bedside while an inpatient and becomes a permanent part of the record when the patient is discharged.

### *Progress notes*

The problem list and care plan, although comprehensive, does not eliminate the need for daily, or frequent, progress notes to indicate the effectiveness of the patient plan of care. One process enhances the other in that progress notes are referenced from the patient's problems and the patient plan of care is reassessed from the progress notes recorded by the various team members.

Progress notes should be dated, identified by problem number and name, and recorded by the *"SOAP"*[3] method of narrative recording, as shown on p. 582.

## ■ What constitutes a problem?

A problem is anything that requires diagnostic, therapeutic, or educational action presently (active problem) or in the past (inactive problem) as defined subjectively (by the patient) or objectively (by the observer).[3]

Specifically the practitioner may identify visual-perceptual difficulties in the stroke patient that will influence the direct care given

**PROBLEM LIST AND CARE PLAN***

Patient ______________________________ Date ______________

Diagnosis ______________________________

Problem No. ________ Problem name *Right CVA*

*a. Left hemiparesis*

*b. Dysphagia*

*c.*

*d.*

**SUBJECTIVE INFORMATION**

Soft data—information obtained from the patient/family/significant others

**OBJECTIVE INFORMATION**

Hard data—information obtained from tests, special procedures, observation, etc.

**ASSESSMENT**

May be a statement of the patient's potential for recovery (initial assessment) or a statement of patient progress or lack of progress (ongoing assessments)

**GOALS**

Stated in terms of expected outcome

**PLAN**

1. Patient/family education: summary of educational objectives, method of meeting objectives
2. Orders†

| *Date* | *Diagnostic procedures* | *Date* | *Therapeutic procedures* |
|---|---|---|---|
| | Things done *to* the patient, for example, laboratory studies, special procedures and tests, vital signs, temperature, intake and output, consultations | | Things done *for* the patient, for example, comfort, safety, medications, activity, patient preferences for basic care, diet, etc. |

*Problems specific to the patient's rehabilitation taken from the "master problem list."

†Orders to be continued on supplementary order sheet until date of next conference and/or reassessment.

| | |
|---|---|
| Date ________________ | |
| Problem No. ________ | Name ________________ |
| **SUBJECTIVE** | What the patient says about the problem |
| **OBJECTIVE** | What the observer sees in the problem |
| **ASSESSMENT** | The observer's interpretation of the patient's problem, considering subjective and objective findings and usually stated (in terms of rehabilitation) as patient progress or lack of progress |
| **PLAN** | Extended to include what the observer did to help the patient as well as future plans for solving the problem |

as well as the teaching planned for the family, or the practitioner may identify a socioeconomic problem in a young cardiac patient that will affect the priorities established in working with the patient. Social, emotional, and economic problems are often urgent matters to be resolved when the patient is in an active rehabilitation setting; nevertheless, the practitioner must be alert to these problems in the early management of critically ill patients. Properly identifying only the physical problems and assigning them to a problem list is an incomplete exercise, because the total patient and the family must be considered if the problem is to be solved at its highest level of resolution.

## ■ What problems are specific to rehabilitation?

### *Physical impairment*

When considering the rehabilitation needs of the acutely ill patient, those caring for the patient will encounter many levels of problems. First, there is a need to assess the physical patient care needs because this assessment will help prevent secondary complications caused by the acute health problem. It will also help to determine if the patient will require other types of special therapy such as physical therapy, occupational therapy, or speech therapy. In the case of the stroke patient, the practitioner should be expected to provide range of motion therapy for the afflicted extremities and also to help identify whether the patient will benefit from evaluation by a special therapist. In the case of the patient recovering from myocardial infarction, it is important that the physical activity component of rehabilitation be carefully assessed, supervised, and advanced as the patient regains strength. Early involvement in an active therapy program is of the utmost benefit to all patients. All stroke victims who have disability, regardless of how minimal, and all patients recovering from myocardial infarction, regardless of how severe, should be given the benefit of a complete rehabilitation evaluation.

### *Emotional difficulties*

Another problem to be managed is in the area of the emotional impact of the disease on the individual. Heart disease and stroke have profound effects on the patient and family. Often the patient has impaired body image perception, but those close to him also suffer from the same "role-change shock." The strong man who has been the undisputed head of the household or the woman who has been a wife, mother, and/or full-time employee in an outside job will have problems accepting himself or herself in a diminished role. The same stages of grief experienced over loss of a loved one can be experienced by the patient over loss or change of self-image.

At the same time significant others in the patient's life may experience grief over loss of the patient as they have perceived him or her. Initial shock followed by denial, anger, regression, and depression is hopefully resolved into acceptance. Lack of acceptance may take the form of hypochondriasis and invalidism, whereas healthy acceptance will become apparent by the patient's willingness to learn to live at his or her maximum potential, whatever that may be. Patients achieve this latter state of acceptance more easily with the assistance and support of staff and family who have carefully identified patient problems and planned care.

### *Financial concerns*

The cost of medical care is a major problem for many patients who find themselves facing financial disaster after surviving the acute episode of major illness. This type of problem shares an equal footing with problems of a physical nature, because the patient will not improve unless his mind is comfortable in knowing that the costs for health care can be handled. A social worker can begin to counsel the patient and family in methods of coping with financial problems even in the acute phase of illness. Solutions to this kind of problem often lie in referring the family to the proper financial assistance program.

### *Vocational readjustments*

The fourth concern in the early management of the acutely ill cardiac or stroke patient is vocational rehabilitation. If the patient is an active person who is interested and capable of returning to work, referral to vocational rehabilitation is important. Patients will receive counseling about returning to their previous type of employment or consultation about job retraining. Often many physical problems of an ill individual will be made manifest by the presence of an underlying financial problem or job insecurity. The alert practitioner will recognize these problem areas in making assessments early in the patient's hospitalization.

### *Resocialization*

The phase of resocialization of patients is also significant. After survival of an acute health care problem, patients return to the community to face the monumental task of reorganizing life in a meaningful way and at the same time living within the restraints placed on them by their disease. The term "resocialization" denotes the patient's reintegration into family and community life. Basically resocialization provides the afflicted person with experiences that enable him to regain confidence and self-respect despite the presence of physical disabilities or language disorders. Resocialization helps the victim of illness to visualize himself as a person rather than as a patient. More specifically, it means meeting and communicating with people other than family members or those responsible for physical care, for example, learning to use public buildings and transportation, going to the store and being able to purchase needed goods with confidence, or eating in a restaurant without undue embarrassment.[4]

Regardless of a person's age, vocational potential, or sex, the return to a home and community life requires consideration from the health professionals. Unless an individual is helped to find quality in life, most of the life-saving measures used during the critical care phase have been purposeless.

## ■ How do phases of illness and goals for patient rehabilitation interphase with nursing care?

| | *Phase I: Acute illness* |
|---|---|
| Where? | 1. Usually in acute care units<br>2. Sometimes "specialed" by private duty nurses on general hospital ward |
| Immediate goals | 1. Life-saving<br>a. Coping with emergency situations<br>b. Prevention of complications of the primary illness |
| Long-term goals | 1. Life-supporting<br>a. Emotional support to patient and family; help in preservation of home, family, and social relationships<br>b. Minimizing of potentially harmful physiologic and psychologic effects of bed rest and prevention of secondary complications to the primary illness |

c. Beginning of patient/family education regarding patient's illness

Nursing implications
1. Specialty training, including cardiopulmonary resuscitation
2. Knowledge of interrelatedness of disease to all organ systems of the body and complications as a result of the primary disease
3. Protection of patient as much as possible from emotional stress during the acute phase of illness but awareness of psychosocial problems the illness has caused, with immediate help in the form of sedation, but help of a more permanent nature included
   a. Being a good listener
   b. Obtaining and giving information to patient and family about the illness
   c. Providing realistic and truthful reassurance whenever possible
4. Understanding of undesirable effects of prolonged bed rest and problems, including deconditioning with impaired orthostatic tolerance, venous thrombosis, atelectasis, and psychologic depression and anxiety
   a. Raising patient to sitting position slowly at least twice per shift unless contraindicated by physician
   b. Passive range of motion therapy for all extremities at least once per shift unless contraindicated by physician; consultation with physical therapist obtained if possible
   c. Support stockings (Teds or Ace wraps) for legs
   d. Encouragement of patient to deep breathe several times per shift and turn side to side
   e. Explanation of why bed rest is necessary and plans for progressive activity to help allay psychologic depression of inactivity and fear of being helpless forever
5. Patient/family education
   a. Orientation of patient to the acute care unit, informing patient and family of visiting restrictions necessary for rest and recovery
   b. Orientation of patient to diagnosis, treatment, and rehabilitation plans as soon as possible
   c. Preparation of patient for transfer to an area of less acute care, including an explanation of new ward or unit and introduction to practitioner who will give or be responsible for most of patient's care after transfer

### *Phase II: Hospital convalescence*

Where?
1. Intermediate care unit
2. General wards
3. Rehabilitation unit

Immediate goals
1. Prevention of exacerbation or complications of the primary illness
2. Continuation of emotional support for patient and family, working toward resolution of psychosocial problems brought about by patient's illness
3. Continuation of prevention of the harmful effects of bed rest
4. Continuation of patient/family health teaching

Long-term goals
1. Increase in functional capacity to a level that will allow reasonable self-care after discharge
2. Patient/family understanding of disease state to degree that good health habits are understood and started for family unit
3. Patient/family adaptation to the patient's chronic disease and/or residual handicaps as a result of the disease
   a. Psychologic adjustments
   b. Physical adjustments
4. Patient/family participation in an ongoing rehabilitation program after discharge from the hospital

Nursing implications
1. Preparation to receive patient from the acute care unit or area of intermediate care
   a. Meeting the patient before transfer
   b. Talking with practitioner in acute care or intermediate care unit who has been giving most of patient care
   c. Consultation with patient's primary physician
   d. Meeting and talking with family of patient
   e. Review of patient record and upgrading or commencement

of progressive patient plan of care
2. Close observation of patient
   a. Basic knowledge of patient's disease to enable recognition of relapse or complications and the effects of progressive activity—whether too much or too little
   b. Recognition of signs of withdrawal or depression and appropriate steps taken to help patient
3. Establishment of "caring" relationship with patient and family
   a. As much direct patient care as possible given
   b. Maintenance of "open-line" communication between patient and family by frequent counseling and listening sessions
   c. Role as "patient's advocate"
4. Recognition of problems that may be helped by other members of the rehabilitation team and promotion of consultations
5. Coordination of rehabilitative efforts of all team members, individualizing to patient's needs and preferences as much as possible
6. Patient/family education
   a. Orientation of patient and family to the new area of care with regard to visiting hours, who is responsible for care, and suggestions for family involvement in helping patient recover
   b. Enlargement of orientation of patient to the diagnosis, treatment, and rehabilitation plans, including patient's family
   c. Preparation of patient psychologically for discharge from the hospital
7. Discharge planning
   a. Consultation with primary physician
   b. Visit by nurse, social service worker, or public health nurse to home or nursing care facility before discharge to ensure adequacy of facility for patient's ongoing care
   c. Arrangements for transportation from home to hospital for clinic appointments and outpatient rehabilitation
   d. Appointments made as necessary with physician, speech therapist, occupational therapist, physical therapist, etc., to ensure patient's continuation in a rehabilitation program
   e. Arrangement for public health nurse to visit patient at home to evaluate care and physical condition
   f. Encouragement provided to patient and family to ask questions and to feel free to call and ask for more information if problems develop after discharge

***Phase III: Outpatient convalescence***

| | |
|---|---|
| Where? | 1. At home<br>2. At nursing care facility |
| Immediate goals | 1. Regaining of strength by gradually increasing amount of physical activity<br>2. Help for patient to achieve the maximum physical fitness possible compatible with the disease<br>3. Retardation or arrest of the disease process with continued medical care and patient education<br>4. Improvement in vocational rehabilitation possibilities for patients whose jobs require relatively high energy expenditure<br>5. Enhancement of self-image and sense of well-being |
| Long-term goals | 1. Resocialization of patient<br>2. Return to work |
| Nursing implications | 1. Hospital<br>a. Communication with patient to clarify home care instructions<br>b. Communication with public health nurse regarding follow-up home visit with patient<br>2. Community<br>a. Public health nurse or visiting nurse to assist patient with home care or obtain consultation with therapists and/or treatment as necessary<br>3. Clinic<br>a. Review of patient's record and additions to record to indicate patient's progress |

b. Provision of psychologic support to patient and family with clarification of home care instructions and continuation of health care teaching

*Phase IV: Recovery and maintenance*

| | |
|---|---|
| Where? | 1. At home |
| Long-term goals | 1. Control of health problems<br>2. Maintenance of physical functional capacity<br>3. Maintenance of occupational productivity and improvement of general quality of life |
| Nursing implications | 1. Same as phase III except on less frequent basis |

## SUMMARY

The challenge of rehabilitation lies in its potential to restore ill and disabled persons to a functional and meaningful existence. It requires commitment to this concept by the total health care team, along with a well-organized system for communicating and coordinating rehabilitation plans with each member of the team. The *problem-oriented medical record* provides the most comprehensive and consistent method of communication via the patient record. The practitioner having primary responsibility for patient care is the individual on the team with the greatest opportunity to coordinate these rehabilitation efforts beginning with admission to the critical care unit and continuing in the subsequent phases of recovery until the patient is discharged to the community.

Obviously the first step in rehabilitation lies in recognizing and anticipating disabilities that can result from the disease process. Prompt attention in the form of prevention as well as rehabilitation therapy can reduce the degree of disability and the time needed for recovery and perhaps retard progress of the disease state. Early assistance in helping the patient adjust to physical, emotional, social, economic, and vocational stresses incurred cannot be overemphasized. This all-encompassing approach to patient care implies the utilization of innovative methods in meeting both the short- and long-term needs of patients. Furthermore, it requires health professionals of many disciplines to work cooperatively so that the patient is restored to maximum mental and physical function.

It should be remembered that there are few absolutes in the field of rehabilitation. Although the multidisciplinary approach is desirable, the unavailability of some of the team members should not preclude rehabilitation efforts. Often with good plannning it is possible for the physician, nurse, patient, and family to achieve some of the goals of rehabilitation. Any successful rehabilitation includes the patient's goals and an educative process so that the patient is cognizant of his own abilities and responsibilities. The patient must be involved in establishing the goals for recovery. He must be aware of his physical limitations and how they can best be modified so that he can function comfortably and safely in an environment best suited to meet his needs.[5]

> The hopes of men and women who are seeking rehabilitation are an example to us. We may put our own hopes into their success. That is primarily what rehabilitation is. The whole elaborate complex of agencies, services, buildings, people and things is not rehabilitation. Rehabilitation is the extending of a hand when a hand is needed, so that the first step, and the second step, and the third step may be taken . . . until finally, the hand is no longer required and the person can manage to take the steps on his own. It is then that commitment involves letting go of the hand, saluting the accomplishment and independence of the person, and turning to the next one whose hand is extended in need.*

*From Turiello, A. M.: Rehabil. Lit. **31**:No. 5, 1970.

## REFERENCES

1. American Heart Association, Committee on Exercise: Exercise testing and training of apparently healthy individuals: a handbook for physicians, New York, 1972, The Association.
2. Weed, L. L.: Medical records, medical education and patient care, Cleveland, 1971, Press of Case Western Reserve University.
3. Hurst, J. W., and Walker, H. K.: The problem oriented system, Medcom learning systems, New York, 1972, Medcom Press.
4. Hackler, E., and Howell, A. T.: Resocializing the stroke patient . . . by trained volunteers, Nurs. Outlook **12**:73, 1972.
5. Turiello, A. M.: A commitment to service in rehabilitation, a statement of a philosophy, Rehabil. Lit. **31**:No. 5, 1970.

*chapter 32*

# Physical assessment and rehabilitation of the patient recovering from stroke

EMILY S. HACKLER

Recovery from stroke is a complex process. Language disorders, physical disability, confusion, depression, and social chaos often accompany this dreadful disorder. Solutions to these catastrophic effects require concentrated and coordinated efforts of the rehabilitation team, the patient, and the family.

Basically recovery from stroke is dependent on its cause, the extent of brain damage, and the motivation of the patient. However, in order to achieve the optimum function of each ptaient, a thorough rehabilitation evaluation is essential. In addition to the medical and nursing evaluation, it is imperative that the physical therapist, occupational therapist, speech pathologist, social worker, and vocational counselor fully contribute in determining the direction of the therapeutic program.

The objective of this material is to present critical care practitioners with an overview of stroke and to demonstrate the necessity of a multidisciplinary approach in planning and implementing an adequate rehabilitation program.

## ■ What is a stroke?

The American Heart Association defines a stroke as something that occurs when the blood supply to a part of the brain is reduced or cut off and, as a result, the nerve cells in that part of the brain cannot function. When this happens, the part of the body controlled by these nerve cells cannot function either. The result of a stroke may be weakness, loss of feeling in or paralysis of one side of the body, difficulty with vision, inability to walk, and difficulty in speaking or understanding. These effects may be very slight or very severe, temporary or permanent.[1] The etiology of the stroke syndrome listed in Klassen[2] includes the following criteria:

I. Vascular causes
- A. Ischemia and infarction
  1. Atherosclerosis in neck vessels and intracranial arteries
     a. With thrombosis
     b. Without thrombosis
  2. Thrombosis without atherosclerosis
     a. Arteritides, for example, collagen disorders
     b. Trauma to neck arteries
     c. Hematologic disorders, for example, polycythemia, sickle cell anemia
     d. "Hypercoagulable" states, for example, pregnancy, contraceptive medication
  3. Embolism
     a. Cardiac, for example, atrial fibrillation, mural thrombus, endocarditis (septic and marasmic)
     b. Atherosclerotic, for example, from neck arteries
     c. Paradoxical
  4. Systemic hypotension
     a. Drug induced
     b. Cardiac in origin
     c. Shock
     d. Idiopathic postural
- B. Intracerebral hemorrhage
  1. Hypertensive
  2. Rupture of congenital aneurysm or vascular malformation
  3. Bleeding disorder

- C. Venous sinus thrombosis associated with infection, dehydration, "hypercoagulable" states (postpartum, postoperative)
- II. Nonvascular causes
  - A. Intracranial mass lesions
    - 1. Trauma
      - a. Subdural hematoma
      - b. Extradural hematoma
      - c. Intracerebral hematoma
      - d. Cerebral edema
    - 2. Tumor
      - a. Primary, for example, glioma, meningioma
      - b. Metastatic
    - 3. Infection
      - a. Abscess
      - b. Meningitis
  - B. Degenerative disorders
    - 1. Multiple sclerosis
  - C. Metabolic disorders
    - 1. Hypoglycemia
    - 2. Electrolyte and acid-base disorders
    - 3. Hepatic and renal failure
    - 4. Postictal

## ■ What are the phases of stroke recovery?

Unlike most acute diseases that resolve in short periods of time, recovery from stroke requires months and sometimes years of hard work on behalf of the patient. Early assessment and prompt treatment of the disabilities are the keys to successful long-term rehabilitation. Table 32-1 indicates the generalized predictions of early recovery and the types of care and health personnel needed to provide essential services.

## ■ How is the stroke patient evaluated?

Because the disabilities caused by stroke are variable as a result of the extent of brain damage in each patient, there are several cardinal areas to observe.

### *Cognitive abilities*

First, it is important to establish the cognitive powers of the stroke patient. Is he able to follow verbal instructions and is he oriented to his environment? If an individual cannot respond appropriately to verbal commands, is he able to comprehend pantomime instructions? The practitioner responsible for a stroke patient's care should determine this as early as possible when providing care. This can be accomplished, to a limited extent, by asking the patient to perform tasks such as raising an arm or pointing to an object. The practitioner should avoid asking yes or no questions because this may provide inadequate data. Many patients will respond with a nod or merely guess the answer, but they will do so in a seemingly appropriate manner, thus leading the practitioner to believe the question was answered correctly.

The importance of identifying the level of comprehension is to ensure that a reliable care plan can be established to encourage the patient's participation in his own care as early as possible. It also will serve to eliminate misapprehensions about the patient's functional status at the outset. Often a patient who fails to cooperate with instructions to help himself is misinterpreted as an individual who is resistant to participating in his program. In reality, it probably indicates that he is not comprehending or processing incoming verbal stimuli.

Although the practitioner should attempt to identify the cognitive level of each patient early in the hospitalization, it must be remembered that the occupational therapist, speech pathologist, and psychologist possess special testing techniques that should be utilized to establish an accurate assessment.

### *Motor function*

What can the stroke patient do voluntarily and selectively for himself? Is he able to move his extremities, feed himself, transfer independently, stand, or walk? All of these skills require motor function and are essential for an individual to accomplish if he is expected to assume any degree of self-care. If an individual has sustained paralysis on one side of the body (hemiplegia), he will have difficulty standing, walking, or sitting. The practitioner must be alert to the complications of immobile extremities and quickly establish a routine of passive exercise to prevent encapsulations and contractures. Spasticity is common; therefore it is essential that the extremity be ranged only to the point of resistance.

Hemiplegic patients should not be allowed to lie on the affected side because it pre-

**Table 32-1.** Comprehensive stroke care and natural neurologic pattern of recovery in cerebral vascular disease*

| *Stage* | *Time* | *Clinical symptoms* | *Level of care* | *Health professionals* |
|---|---|---|---|---|
| I: flaccid or flail | Onset to 72 hr | No tendon reflex, no resistance to passive movements | Nursing care and prevention of pressure areas, contractures, edema, painful shoulder, malnutrition; preparation for independence, involving bed exercises, dangle or up in chair for sitting tolerance, beginning self-care (bed activities) | Acute facility personnel, physician, nursing personnel, dietitian, social service workers, physical therapist/bedside, speech evaluation specialist |
| II: spasticity | 24 hr to 1 mo† | Hyperactive tendon reflex, presence of exaggerated activity (withdrawal) | Nursing care and continuance of preventative measures with special attention to prevention of contractures; higher level of independence, with learning of safe transfer, assisted ambulation, self-care in bathroom | Acute or extended care facility personnel, physician, nursing personnel, physical therapist, occupational therapist, speech therapist, social service workers, family counselors, dietitian |
| III: synergy‡ | 2-3 weeks | Presence of patterned stereotyped movements set off by voluntary movement in proximal muscle groups | Nursing care and continuation of observation for developing secondary disabilities, range of motion development (passive and active) | Acute or extended care facility personnel, physician, nursing personnel, physical therapist, occupational therapist, speech therapist, social service workers, family, visiting nurse, psychologist |
| IV: near normal with some weakness, incoordination | 1 week to 6-8 mo§ | Variety of voluntary movements under control | Nursing care minimal if patient is alert | Physician, outpatient therapy personnel, physical therapist, occupational therapist, speech therapist |

*From Memorial Hospital of Long Beach: Comprehensive stroke care, Long Beach, Fla., 1970, Regional Medical Program, Area VIII.

†If patient remains in first two stages more than 6 months, prognosis for recovery of muscle function in the involved extremities is doubtful.

‡Patient can initiate some fixed patterned movements.

§Average therapy time is 6 months except for recovery of speech. Most patients reach maximum functional level 3 to 6 months from onset, except for speech recovery.

disposes to subluxation of the joint. Proper positioning, range of joint motion therapy, and appropriately selected slings will help prevent these disabilities. Patients who do not receive early skilled care may incur irreversible and permanent disability that will prevent them from functioning at their most efficient level.

Again, the nurse is an important member of the health team because on the patient's admission to the hospital, early observations and plans for care are vital in preventing complications of restricted joint function. However, the occupational therapist and physical therapist are key people in providing a reliable assessment of muscle strength and joint action potential.

### *Language disorders*

It is important for health professionals, especially nurses, to recognize that language entails more than "talking." It encompasses an individual's ability to speak, read, write, and identify objects in the environment. Often the stroke patient loses the ability to talk (aphasia), but is also unable to perform the aforementioned tasks. In essence, the entire communication system has been short-circuited by the stroke. Essentially his thoughts and desires become locked within his head, and his level of frustration at not being able to communicate escalates. If this problem is not identified, it impedes his ability to function effectively in all aspects of daily living.

The patient and family are often confused and frightened by this occurrence. They need education about aphasia, its cause, and its treatment. The need for a speech pathologist to work with the patient is urgent. Under the guidance and supervision of the pathologist, the critical care practitioner and family can begin to reinforce appropriate methods of stimulating language. They can help the patient to establish techniques in communication that will enable more effective and independent functioning. Rather than expecting the patient who has an expressive aphasia to verbally express his thoughts, they will help him identify alternate methods of communicating, such as pointing or using pantomime gestures. The need for the speech pathologist to guide and direct this type of activity on behalf of the patient cannot be overemphasized.

### *Visual perceptual awareness*

Following a stroke, the patient may have difficulty in perceiving the world around him. Although the world does not change, the ability to visually or perceptually interpret data may be impaired in accordance with the site of insult to the brain, resulting in disruption of sensory integration. The patient not only suffers a loss of control of body functions, but he no longer perceives the world in a logical manner.

Perception is the ability to integrate and interpret messages from our internal and external environment. This ability is the result of combined activities of end-organs, peripheral nerves, tracts and ganglia, and the integrative sensory cortex. In general the sensory input of the person with brain damage is disturbed at the integrative level.[3]

Simple tasks such as identifying articles of clothing or eating utensils or determining verticality become overwhelming obstacles in participating in the activities of daily living. It appears that the person with left hemiplegia has greater difficulty with sensory integration. The degree of perceptual loss cannot be correlated with the person's physical ability.[3] The patient with left-sided involvement tends to exhibit a denial to his affected side, lacks feeling, and frequently is unaware of where his limbs are placed in relation to the rest of his body. Often he will dress only the unaffected side and leave the affected parts unattended.

The alert practitioner should anticipate some of the needs of the patient with visual perceptual disorders. An attempt should be made to create a safe environment by placing objects within reach of the unaffected extremity. Also, because the judgment of these patients is impaired, the practitioner should remind patients to lock their wheelchairs and give heed to their affected extremities. Family members should be educated to help patients in the same manner.

Hemianopia is another problem in the category of visual-perceptual disturbances. This is a deficit that causes blindness in half of the visual field of both eyes and classically is identified when a patient is observed eating food from only one side of his tray. The bedside practitioner, as a primary resource to the patient, should strive to maintain an environment conducive to stimulating him to function independently within the limitations of the disability. Placement of objects in the range of his visual field will make the patient aware of what is available to him. Furthermore, it is important to remind the patient to look in the direction of his affected side because he does not perceive objects in the blind half of his visual field and, as a result, bumps into doors and furniture. Patients with this type of complication will benefit from occupational therapy programs to improve body image awareness.

## ■ Why is reality orientation important?

Confusion is often a disturbing symptom of stroke to the patient and the family. The practitioner is in an ideal position to establish a reality orientation program that will help the patient relate to surroundings. The practitioner should be concerned about preventing sensory deprivation in the patient who has motor, sensory, and proprioceptive loss because he is receiving distorted feedback from the environment.[4] Disorientation at night often becomes a serious problem because the darkened room is devoid of sensory stimuli. Use of a small night light may help alleviate this particular problem.

Other methods of orientating the patient to the present world include the use of large calendars and clocks. These will help him become aware of the date and time. Also, all staff members should introduce themselves by name each time they approach the patient and remind him of what he is expected to do for himself. It is helpful for family members to bring the patient his favorite articles of clothing and pictures of familiar people who are special in his life. A radio or television near the patient's bedside can offer an excellent source of sensory input if used judiciously. Overuse of these appliances should be discouraged, however, because they may become a factor that will limit the patient from having other sensory integration experiences.

## ■ How does a program in activities of daily living begin?

An *activity of daily living* (ADL) program begins when a patient is asked to turn himself in bed, feed himself, or bathe himself. As time progresses and the patient increases his strength and activity tolerance, the patient will be required to assume more responsibility for himself. He should dress himself, put on his own braces, ambulate unassisted, and be responsible for his own hygiene program. The goal of a planned ADL program is to give the patient the appropriate skills so that he can care for himself as much as possible when he is returned to the community.

The ADL program is designed and initiated early in the patient's hospitalization with the goal of meeting the long-term self-care needs of the individual so that he can perform successfully when he returns to his home or to work. Despite the endeavors of the rehabilitation staff to anticipate the home care needs, the patient confronts his "moment of truth" when he is on his own and is expected to function under his own power, at whatever level that may be. Home visits by a public health nurse are essential so that the patient will have the necessary support from this member of the health team.

In summary, practitioners who work with stroke patients require a heightened awareness of the vicissitude of motor, sensory, and proprioceptive disorders that occur. Although their roles are vitally significant because they are responsible for providing most of the patients' direct physical care, it is the coordinated efforts of the rehabilitation team that are required to meet the comprehensive needs of persons afflicted with stroke.

## REFERENCES

1. American Heart Association: Facts about stroke, New York, 1968, The Association.
2. Klassen, A. C.: The stroke syndrome: diagnostic procedures, Med. Times **97**:No. 5, 1969.
3. Burt, M. M.: Perceptual deficits in hemiplegia, Am. J. Nurs. **70**:No. 5, 1970.
4. Wingerson, E.: Occupational therapy and the team trauma patient, 1974, American Congress of Rehabilitation.

*chapter 33*

# Physical assessment and reconditioning of the patient recovering from myocardial infarction

MILDRED LAWSON

For the patient recovering from myocardial infarction there is serious risk in the sudden, nonregulated, and injudicious use of strenuous exercise. But it is a risk that can be minimized or eliminated through proper evaluation, preliminary testing, and the individualized prescription of exercise programs. Activity during each phase of the patient's illness is systematically prescribed by the physician and supervised or monitored by the physician or well-trained allied health personnel.[1]

At least three methods have been suggested for prescribing activity for cardiac patients: (1) in accordance with the "cardiac status and prognosis" method of classification of the New York Heart Association (Table 33-1), (2) according to energy expenditure lists, and (3) in accordance with ECG recordings during activity stress testing.[2]

As recovery progresses, the specific activities performed and the immediate objectives of the exercise plan may change, but the general principles of exercise evaluation, prescription, and training will apply during all phases of recovery and maintenance.

## ■ What is physical fitness?

Physical fitness has been defined as "the ability to carry out daily tasks with vigor and alertness; without undue fatigue and with ample energy to enjoy leisure-time pursuits and to meet unforeseen emergencies."[3] The body's maximum oxygen uptake during physical effort is a measure of physical fitness and is known as the $V_{O_{2max}}$, or aerobic capacity. It decreases with advancing age, disease, and deconditioning, but can usually be increased with a program of physical reconditioning.[1, 4]

## ■ What are the physiologic principles of exercise?

Physical activity depends basically on the ability of individual muscle cells to carry out the many metabolic steps that terminate in the oxidation (burning) of food particles and the liberation of heat (energy). Food, oxygen, and aerobic (oxygen-using) enzymes located in the mitochondria of each muscle cell combine to produce carbon dioxide ($CO_2$), water ($H_2O$), and heat (energy). The major source of energy fuel is derived from fat and carbohydrate food intake, which is burned (oxidized) as needed or stored in adipose tissue.[4]

Unlike fuel, oxygen cannot be stored in the body. The oxygen demands of activity must be met by an increase in oxygen intake, transport, delivery, and utilization. The maximum amount of oxygen that can be transported from the lungs to the working muscles determines the amount or level of exercise.

An increase in total body oxygen consump-

**Table 33-1.** Classification of patients with heart disease*

| *Class* | *Cardiac status†* | *Prognosis‡* |
|---|---|---|
| I | 1. Uncompromised | 1. Good |
| II | 2. Slightly compromised | 2. Good with therapy |
| III | 3. Moderately compromised | 3. Fair with therapy |
| IV | 4. Severely compromised | 4. Guarded despite therapy |

*Modified from New York Heart Association, Inc.: Diseases of the heart and blood vessels—nomenclature and criteria for diagnosis, Boston, 1973, Little, Brown & Co.

†Cardiac status should reflect an overall assessment based on a consideration of etiologic, anatomic, and physiologic diagnoses.

‡Prognosis should be based on an assessment of the potential effects of optimal current medical and surgical therapy.

tion is made possible by increases in pulmonary ventilation, cardiac output, and oxygen extraction by the tissues. Greater cardiac output is the result primarily of accelerated heart rate and, to a lesser extent, greater stroke volume.[1]

## ■ How is energy expenditure expressed?

### *Calorie*

The large calorie (kilocalorie) of energy represents the heat (energy) required to raise the temperature of 1 kg of $H_2O$ from 0° to 1° C. A person lying quietly in the resting state consumes approximately 1 calorie of energy (or 200 cc $O_2$/min). Calorie expenditure may be adjusted for time or rate of utilization and expressed as calories per hour or calories per minute, or it may be adjusted for the size of the individual and expressed as calories per square meter of body surface area or as metabolic units.[4]

### *Metabolic unit*

A person sitting quietly at rest consumes 1 metabolic unit (MU or met) of energy, which is considered to be approximately 3.5 cc $O_2$/kg of body weight/min. Energy expenditure for various activities is stated in multiples of the basal expenditure.[5] For example, a 50 kg person uses 175 cc $O_2$/min (1 met) sitting quietly at rest (50 × 3.5). Exercise requiring 1000 cc $O_2$ would require 5.6 mets of energy expenditure for that person (1000 ÷ 175).

The literature abounds with results of studies determining the amounts of $O_2$ required to perform various functions. The $O_2$ requirement for any function is the same for all persons. But persons differ in individual $V_{O_{2max}}$ capacity, and $V_{O_{2max}}$ is affected by disease and inactivity. The physician having primary responsibility for the patient will determine what energy expenditure is appropriate for the patient. The activity level will then be kept at that level or lower.

The New York Heart Association Cardiac Classification (Table 33-1) can be correlated with energy expenditure according to Turrell and Hellerstein, as follows[2]:

| *Class* | *Calories/min* |
|---|---|
| I | 4.0 to 6.6 |
| II | 2.7 to 4.0 |
| III | 1.5 to 2.7 |
| IV | Less than 1.5 |

Table 33-2 lists various activities with the required caloric expenditure. When developed, such lists can be used in much the same manner as diabetic food exchange lists. Activity is prescribed by matching the patient's functional capacity with activities requiring the recommended calorie expenditure or less.

## ■ What is the sequence of progressive activity following myocardial infarction?

The activity component of the patient care plan must be designed to provide a supervised progressive increase in activity for the patient that takes him from total dependency on admission to the coronary care unit to

**Table 33-2.** Caloric expenditure or metabolic equivalents of energy required for miscellaneous activities for 70 kg man*

| *Activity* | *Cal/min* | *Mets* | *Activity* | *Cal/min* | *Mets* |
|---|---|---|---|---|---|
| *Industrial* | | | *Hospital* | | |
| Watch repairing | 1.6 | 1.5 | Bed rest | 1.0 | 1 |
| Radio assembly | 2.7 | 2.5 | Sitting | 1.2 | 1 |
| Sewing/machine | 2.9 | 2.5 | Dangling feet, 5 min | 1.5 | 1 |
| Bricklaying | 4.0 | 3.5 | Standing/relaxed | 1.4 | 1 |
| Plastering | 4.1 | 3.5 | Eating | 1.4 | 1 |
| Wheeling barrow, 115 lb/ 2.5 mph | 5.0 | 4.0 | Conversing | 1.4 | 1 |
| | | | Dressing/undressing | 2.3 | 2 |
| Carpentry | 6.8 | 5.5 | Washing hands/face | 2.5 | 2 |
| Mowing lawn/hand | 7.7 | 6.5 | Using bedside commode | 3.6 | 3 |
| Felling tree | 8.0 | 6.5 | Walking, 2.5 mph | 3.6 | 3 |
| Shoveling | 8.5 | 7.0 | Showering | 4.2 | 3.5 |
| Ascending stairs, 17 lb load/ 27 feet/min | 9.0 | 7.5 | Using bedpan | 4.7 | 4 |
| | | | Walking downstairs | 5.2 | 4.5 |
| | | | Walking, 3.5 mph | 5.6 | 5.5 |
| *Recreational* | | | Propulsion/wheelchair | 2.4 | 2 |
| Painting/sitting | 2.0 | 1.5 | Ambulation/braces, crutches | 8.0 | 6.5 |
| Playing piano | 2.5 | 2 | | | |
| Driving car | 2.8 | 2 | *Housework* | | |
| Canoeing, 2.5 mph | 3.0 | 2.5 | Sewing/hand | 1.4 | 1 |
| Horseback riding/slowly | 3.0 | 2.5 | Sweeping floor | 1.7 | 1.5 |
| Playing volleyball | 3.0 | 2.5 | Sewing/machine | 1.8 | 1.5 |
| Bowling | 4.4 | 3.5 | Polishing furniture | 2.4 | 2 |
| Cycling, 5.5 mph | 4.5 | 3.5 | Peeling potatoes | 2.9 | 2.5 |
| Running | 5.0 | 4 | Scrubbing/standing | 2.9 | 2.5 |
| Swimming, 20 yd/min | 5.0 | 4 | Washing small clothes | 3.0 | 2.5 |
| Jogging, 5 mph | 5.6 | 7-9 | Kneading dough | 3.3 | 2.5 |
| Walking briskly, 3½-5 mph | 5.6 | 5-7 | Scrubbing floors | 3.6 | 3 |
| Dancing | 5.5 | 4.5 | Cleaning windows | 3.7 | 3 |
| Gardening | 5.6 | 4.5 | Making beds | 3.9 | 3 |
| Playing tennis | 7.1 | 6 | Ironing/standing | 4.2 | 3.5 |
| Riding horse/trotting | 8.0 | 6.5 | Mopping | 4.2 | 3.5 |
| Spading | 8.6 | 7 | Hanging wash | 4.5 | 3.5 |
| Skiing | 9.9 | 8 | | | |
| Playing squash | 10.2 | 8.5 | | | |
| Cycling, 13 mph | 11.0 | 9 | | | |

*Modified from Zohman, L. R., and Tobis, J. S.: Cardiac rehabilitation, New York, 1970, Grune & Stratton, Inc.

functioning at the maximum physical level compatible with his functional and therapeutic classification following the myocardial infarction.

Table 33-3 offers an outline that may be used for general guidelines in progressive activity, but it must be emphasized that there is no one plan that can be predetermined. The plan must be individualized for each patient. Further emphasis is placed on the following factors:

1. The physician with total responsibility for the patient must make the decision as to the level of activity in which the patient may participate and when he may advance to a higher level of activity.

2. Physical therapists, if available, may be responsible for supervising the progressive increase in activity permitted the patient during his stay in the hospital. Usually, however, it is the nurse who performs this task. The physical therapist or nurse is responsible for observing and inquiring about the presence of any complications or any unstable situation

**Table 33-3.** Progressive activity program*

| *Phase* | *Activity level†* | *Approximate time‡* | *Activity* | *Contraindications* | *Precautions* |
|---|---|---|---|---|---|
| I: acute illness (critical care unit) | 0 | Admission | Approximate energy expenditure = 1.0 calorie/min or 1 met<br>Complete bedrest without activity until pain remits | | Cardiac monitor<br>Avoid activity<br>Avoid emotional stress<br>Avoid Valsalva maneuver<br>Light diet |
| | 1 | Day 2-3 | Approximate energy expenditure = 1.0-1.5 calories/min<br>Begin feeding self<br>Bed rolled up 45 degrees to comfort; elbows supported<br>Passive exercise, range of motion to extremities<br>Bedpan | Heart rate should not exceed basal heart rate<br>Signs of shock or congestive heart failure<br>Pain<br>Tachycardia<br>Ventricular arrhythmias | All activity with assistance<br>Cardiac monitor<br>Avoid emotional stress<br>Light diet<br>Begin teaching |
| | | Day 4-5 | Begin active and resistive foot exercises<br>Partial morning care—washing face and hands, brushing teeth—while in bed with elbows supported<br>Bedside commode<br>Visitors—members of immediate family only, one at a time for 5 min, 1-2 times/day | Strong emotional reaction | Screen and limit visitors |
| II: early hospital convalescence | | | | | |
| 1. Intermediate care unit | 2 | Day 6-7 | Approximate energy expenditure = 1.5-3.0 calories/min or 1.5-4.0 mets<br>Continue previous activities<br>Dangle feet over side of bed (feet supported with foot stool) for meals<br>Sponge bath in bed, practitioner to wash feet and back<br>Bedside hygiene<br>Active range of motion | Heart rate should not exceed basal rate (>10)<br>Same as level 1 | All activity with supervision and assistance<br>Cardiac monitor<br>Avoid Valsalva maneuver<br>Regular or low salt diet<br>Avoid chilling<br>Continue teaching<br>Involve patient with plan of care |

*From Lawson, M.: Progressive coronary care, Heart & Lung **1**:243-245, 1972.

†The energy level that the therapist or practitioner will be permitted to carry out should be equal to or *less* than the amount the physician permits the patient to do on an intermittent basis. Activity levels are patterned after, but do not correspond to, those listed by Cain and associates.[6]

‡No activity can be assigned according to the day of illness. The schedule must be individualized for each patient. The approximate days are listed to be guidelines only.

*Continued.*

**Table 33-3.** Progressive activity program—cont'd

| *Phase* | *Activity level* | *Approximate time* | *Activity* | *Contraindications* | *Precautions* |
|---|---|---|---|---|---|
| II: early hospital convalescence—cont'd<br>1. Intermediate care unit—cont'd | | | Sit up in chair with feet elevated 30-60 min in evening | | |
| | | | Visitors—members of immediate family, two at a time, 10-15 min twice daily | Strong emotional reaction | Counseling, teaching, restricting visitors if necessary |
| | | Day 8-9 | Up in chair 2-3 times daily, 30 min-1 hr, bedside<br>Begin dressing self, changing gown | | |
| | | | Walk to bathroom with assistance<br>Walk to chair with assistance | Faintness<br>Diaphoresis<br>Dyspnea<br>Pain<br>Tachycardia<br>Bradycardia<br>Ventricular arrhythmias | Telemetry<br>Cardiac monitoring if available; otherwise, take pulse before and after activity |
| | 3 | Day 10-14 | Approximate energy expenditure = 3.0-4.0 calories/min for limited times | Heart rate should not exceed basal heart rate (>15) | All new activity with supervision and assistance |
| | | | Bathe in tub in morning<br>Dressing, shaving, combing hair, etc., while standing<br>Walk in hall (50 feet) one time at average walking pace in evening | Same as level 2 | Stay with patient during bath<br>Telemetry monitoring or taking pulse before and after activity |
| 2. General ward or inpatient rehabilitation unit | 4 | Day 15-16 | Approximate energy expenditure = 3.0-4.0 calories/min for longer periods of time | Heart rate should not exceed basal heart rate (>20) | Teach patient to take own pulse; pace self |
| | | | Continue walking length of hall (50 feet) 2-3 times daily at normal walking pace<br>May have visitors other than immediate family | Same as for previous levels | |
| | 5 | Day 17-18 | Approximate energy expenditure = 4.0-5.0 calories/min | Heart rate should not exceed basal heart rate (>25) | Same as for levels 3 and 4 |
| | | | Walk length of hall 2 times<br>Lateral side bending and trunk twisting, 2 times each side | Same as for previous levels | Exercises are to be spaced over waking hours; all exercises determined by pulse rate |

**Table 33-3.** Progressive activity program—cont'd

| *Phase* | *Activity level* | *Approximate time* | *Activity* | *Contraindications* | *Precautions* |
|---|---|---|---|---|---|
| | | | Flexion and extension activities of upper extremities and trunk while in standing position | | |
| | | Day 19-21 | Shower | | |
| | | | Lateral side bending 5 times | | |
| | | | Walk length of hall, walk up 2 steps and down 2 steps | | |
| | | Day 18-21 | Patient discharged to home | | Public health nurse referral for home visit |
| III: convalescence at home | | | | | |
| 1. Early | 5 | Week 4-6 | Approximate energy expenditure and activity same as during level 5 in hospital until return to clinic | | |
| | | | Beginning slowly, daily walks on level surface | Angina<br>Dyspnea<br>Faintness<br>Erratic pulse<br>Rapid pulse<br>Fatigue<br>Pedal edema<br>Emotional upset | Walk with someone else<br>Pace self |
| | | Week 6-8 | Clinic visit | | |
| | | Week 8-10 | Physician may order treadmill or Master's two-step stress testing | Pericarditis<br>Endocarditis<br>Valvular disease | |
| | | | Return to light work, part-time | | |
| 2. Late | 6 | Week 10-12 | Caloric expenditure according to diagnosis and cardiac functional classification | Heart rate not to exceed 60%-70% of predicted maximal heart rate | Short rest periods during day<br>Avoid emotional stress<br>No smoking |
| | | | Continue daily walks and moderate exercises | Same as for level 5 | Dietary moderation<br>Avoid sudden exercise or competitive efforts |
| | | | Work to tolerance | | |
| IV: recovery and maintenance | | Week 12-24 | Sexual intercourse (approximately same caloric expenditure as climbing two flights of stairs, 15 steps) | | Counseling |

*Continued.*

**Table 33-3.** Progressive activity program—cont'd

| *Phase* | *Activity level* | *Approximate time* | *Activity* | *Contraindications* | *Precautions* |
|---|---|---|---|---|---|
| IV: recovery and maintenance—cont'd | | | Begin physical fitness program<br>1. Stress test<br>2. Supervised exercise program | After heavy meal<br>Fatigue<br>Anger or tension<br>Pain<br>Pericarditis<br>Endocarditis<br>Valvular disease<br>Hypertension | Physician in attendance for supervised exercise<br>Family taught cardiopulmonary resuscitation<br>Patient/family education |
| | | | 3. Unsupervised exercise program | | |

before proceeding with the prescribed activity. No activity will be undertaken if the patient is having chest pain, marked dyspnea, dizziness, or faintness. Other contraindications include tachycardia, bradycardia, or significant arrhythmias.

3. ECG monitoring by telemetry is desirable, but not essential. The patient's pulse can be taken prior to, during, and immediately following activity, with any marked change of rate or regularity being documented immediately by a full 12-lead ECG.

4. Until the patient has shown a tolerance for the prescribed activity, he should not be left unattended.

5. Patients can be taught to pace their own activity by taking the pulse and by recognizing when to limit or stop activity. Having the patient perform a large portion of his personal care (under supervision) before discharge is one test for safely increasing the amount of activity for the patient. This reinforces the patient's belief that his myocardial infarction has not made an invalid of him.

## ■ What are the principles of the exercise prescription?

Exercise is potent therapy and, as with any treatment or drug, it must be used with respect if its benefits are to be realized and if undesirable side effects are to be avoided.

To achieve the desired degree of cardiorespiratory conditioning, exercises are prescribed that produce sustained increases in metabolic, cardiovascular, and respiratory function. Examples of these include vigorous walking, bicycling, swimming, jogging, running, and rope jumping. Limited patients or those just beginning an exercise program often begin with a progressive walking program. This has the advantage of being exercise that can be done alone after the safe target heart rate has been established and pulse taking techniques have been taught to the patient.

The rehabilitation team can work with patients on an outpatient basis, providing a semi-supervised program by checking the patient's progress weekly. In addition to being a morale booster for the patient, it enables the team to pick up any program that may be developing and refer the patient back to the physician.

Factors to be considered in the prescription of exercise, in addition to the patient's functional ability, are the type of exercise and the intensity, duration, and frequency of the exercise, as outlined in the diagram on p. 599.

### *Type of exercise*

The success or failure of a conditioning program for the patient will depend ultimately on the motivation of the patient; his interests and how much he believes the program will help him will determine how hard he works at making the program a success. To

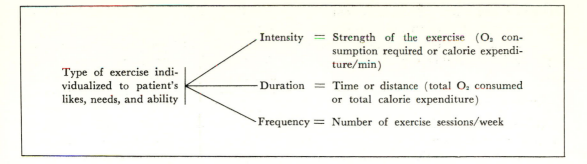

Type of exercise individualized to patient's likes, needs, and ability

- Intensity = Strength of the exercise ($O_2$ consumption required or calorie expenditure/min)
- Duration = Time or distance (total $O_2$ consumed or total calorie expenditure)
- Frequency = Number of exercise sessions/week

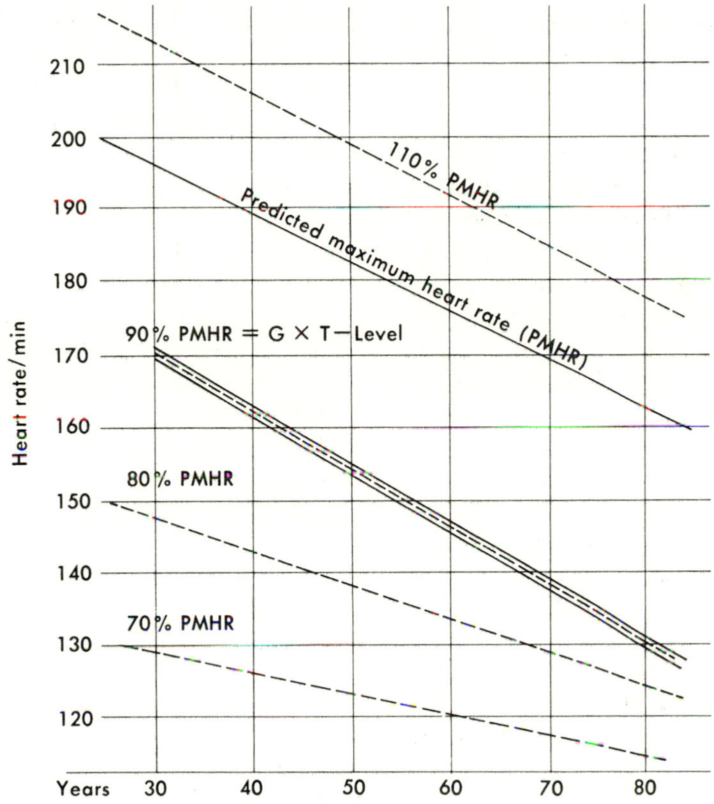


**Fig. 33-1.** Maximum heart rate according to age and percentage of maximum heart rates for the graded exercise test (GXT). (Courtesy Alan R. Bures, M.D., University of California, Irvine, College of Medicine, Irvine, Calif.; modified from Sheffield, L. T., Holt, J. H., and Reeves, T. J.: Circulation **32:**Oct. 1965.)

enhance the chances of success, the patient should be well informed as to the benefits of the exercise prescription, and the exercises should be individualized to the patient's interests and capabilities, including age, sex, and body type as factors.

### *Intensity of exercise*

Heart rate is the best indicator of the intensity of exertion, since it is directly related to $O_2$ consumption and calorie expenditure and it is easily determined. The training heart rate for the patient is figured roughly as 70% to 80% of the maximum heart rate predicted (Fig. 33-1). Maximum heart rate represents the limit of the patient's oxygen uptake ($V_{O_{2max}}$) and is rarely the target rate in stress tests. $V_{O_{2max}}$ decreases with advancing age, disease, and deconditioning, along with parallel decreases in maximally attainable heart rate and cardiac output; these factors must be taken into consideration in determining desirable heart rates (intensity) for the physical conditioning of the patient.

### *Duration of exercise*

Duration and intensity of exercise go hand-in-hand, since an increase in one requires a decrease in the other. Exercise duration can be prescribed in terms of time or distance (minutes or miles) or in terms of total $O_2$ consumed or total calories expended.[4]

### *Frequency of exercise*

Two to three exercise sessions per week are usually prescribed for patients beginning a program and for those of low fitness.[7] As training progresses and as fitness improves, exercise should become more frequent, probably daily or every other day. However, adequate recovery time from the exercise should be allowed; the body needs time to respond to exercise and some patients require more than 24 hours to adjust.

## ■ What is the purpose of stress testing?

The objective of exercise stress testing is to determine the patient's cardiopulmonary functional capacity so that the prescribed exercise program does not exceed the patient's functional ability. Other objectives for stress testing include the evaluation of responses to conditioning and increased individual motivation for adhering to the exercise program.

## ■ What is the method of stress testing?

Several tests are used to determine exercise capacity; the most widely used are the Master's two-step, the treadmill, and the bicycle ergometric tests.[1, 4] The type of test is chosen by the physician according to the data to be collected and the level of fitness of the patient. Cost and space are also factors in the selection of equipment.

Exercise tests may be single or multistage. In the single stage test the work load is held constant throughout; in the multistage test it is increased at regular intervals until the end point is reached. End points may be aimed at maximum or submaximum performance. In a submaximum test the patient does not attain his top performance or functional aerobic capacity but stops at some arbitrary end point such as a predetermined target heart rate based on his age and activity adjustments. Mandatory end points may be imposed by dyspnea, chest pain or cerebral dysfunction, pathologic ECG changes, or inappropriate blood pressure response (a decline in systolic pressure or failure of pressure to rise during increasing exercise). Submaximum testing is terminated at the appearance of any one of these symptomatic or dysfunctional end points or of any other signs of poor exercise tolerance.[1]

Although the American Hospital Association Committee on Exercise[1] believes that a multistage test should be supervised by a physician, the rehabilitation team members may be expertly trained to administer the test with a physician readily available. The team members (skilled in cardiopulmonary resuscitation) would be constantly observing the ECG oscilloscope, blood pressure, heart rate, and the patient for any untoward clinical signs. Other precautions include having resuscitation equipment and drugs easily accessible. A history, physical examination, and resting ECG are taken prior to the patient's undergoing exercise stress testing.

In performing any stress test the patient should be rested and in the fasting state. He should be instructed in the procedure and even exercised a few seconds for familiarization with the apparatus before ECG lead application. ECG and blood pressure recordings are made in the supine and then in the upright position to detect orthostatic influences. The patient is then exercised. ECG and blood pressure recordings are made every third minute during exercise, standing immediately after exercise, immediately after lying supine, and at 2, 4, and 6 minutes after exercise.[8]

## ■ What ECG changes constitute a positive test?[4, 7, 10]

Characteristic horizontal S-T segment depression in a postexercise supine record constitutes an abnormal response. Slight "terminal dipping" of the S-T segment with a late

## REPORT OF STRESS PERFORMANCE AND THE PATIENT'S EXERCISE PRESCRIPTION*

Name ______________________ Test No. ______________________
Age ________ Sex ________ Date ________ Previous test ______________________
Attending physician ______________________

**STRESS TEST PERFORMANCE**

__________ Highest heart rate (HR)/min
__________ Predicted maximum HR/age
__________ % of predicted maximum HR
__________ Exercise capacity/fitness
__________ Maximum mets capacity

At HR of __________/min
__________________ symptoms
__________________ ECG change
(1.0 met = Approximate energy use at rest)

**YOUR ACTIVITY LEVEL SHOULD BE**

__________ Minimal (up to 2.0 mets)
__________ Very light (less than 3.0 mets)
__________ Light (3-5 mets)
__________ Moderate (5-7 mets)
Usual daily activities
__________ Heavy (7-9 mets)
__________ Very heavy (over 9.0 mets)

*Always* start one level lower.
Relate activity/exercise to pulse response.

**YOUR EXERCISE PRESCRIPTION**

*Type* Select your appropriate activity level (see mets chart)
__________ Start and follow a *daily walk* program.
__________ Use home bicycle exerciser.
__________ Join group exercise program.
__________ Perform own sports activities.
__________ Other: ______________________

*Intensity* Monitor with *10 sec* pulse rates.
Always start count as "*zero*—1—2—"
Target training range
__________ Target (70%)
__________ Upper limit (85%, do *not* exceed)
Recovery time __________ min (minimum cool-down time)

*Duration* Exercise at least 30 minutes each session.

*Frequency* Perform a minimum of three times a week in order to secure and maintain a desirable degree of fitness training.

**REDUCE/ELIMINATE YOUR CORONARY RISK FACTORS**

__________ Reduce overweight.
__________ Do not smoke.
_____x_____ Exercise regularly.
__________ Reduce high cholesterol or % fat in diet. (Check with physician.)
__________ Control high blood pressure. (Check with physician.)
_____x_____ Have regular medical check-ups.

This exercise prescription should be reevaluated after __________ months.
Comments:

______________________
Physician's signature

*Courtesy N. Nequin, M.D., Cardiac Rehabilitation and Coronary Risk Reduction Programs, Swedish Covenant Hospital, Chicago, Ill.

## ACTIVITY LEVEL EQUIVALENTS*

Maximum met capacity __________ Starting met level __________
(Stay below upper limit pulse rate.)

**STRESS TEST**

| Stage | 0 | ½ | I | II | III | IV |
|---|---|---|---|---|---|---|
| Mets | 1.8 | 3 | 5 | 7 | 9-10 | 13-14 |

**ACTIVITY LEVEL CHART (measurement in mets)[1]**

| | *Level* | | | | | |
|---|---|---|---|---|---|---|
| *Activity* | *Minimal (1.6-2.0)* | *Very light (3)* | *Light (3-5)* | *Moderate (5-7)* | *Heavy (7-9)* | *Very heavy (9.0)* |
| Self-care (home) | Wash/shave<br>Dress<br>Desk work<br>Writing<br>Dishes | As in minimal<br>Drive car | Clean windows<br>Rake<br>Wax floor<br>Paint | Light gardening<br>Lawn mowing/hand, level<br>Climb stairs slowly | Saw wood<br>Heavy shoveling | Carry loads up stairs[3]<br>Climb stairs quickly |
| Work | Hand sew<br>Watch repair | Sitting<br>Clerical<br>Assembler<br>Store clerk<br>Bartender<br>Drive truck[2]<br>Crane operator[2] | Stock shelves<br>Move light objects<br>Light welding<br>Light carpentry[3]<br>Machine assembly<br>Auto repair | Carpentry, exterior home building[3]<br>Move objects, 45-65 lb[3]<br>Drills | Tend furnace[3]<br>Dig ditches[3]<br>Move objects, 85-100 lb[3] | Lumberjack[3]<br>Heavy laborer[3] |
| Play | Sitting | Shuffleboard<br>Horseshoes<br>Bait casting<br>Billiards<br>Walk at 2 mph | Dancing (waltz)<br>Golf<br>Table tennis | Badminton<br>Tennis (doubles)<br>Snow skiing<br>Sex[2, 4] | Canoeing[3]<br>Fencing<br>Paddleball<br>Tennis (singles) | Handball<br>Squash<br>Ski touring<br>Basketball |
| Physical conditioning | Walk at 1.5 mph level | Stationary bicycle, low resistance<br>Very light calisthenics | Walk at 3 mph<br>Level bicycling at 6 mph<br>Light calisthenics | Walk at 3½-5 mph<br>Bicycling at 9-10 mph<br>Swim breast stroke | Jog at 5 mph<br>Swim crawl stroke<br>Rowing machine | Run at 6 mph<br>Bicycle at 13 mph or steep hill<br>Rope jumping |
| Goal (total distance) | | | Walk 1 mile | + Jog ½ mile | + Jog 1 mile | + Jog 2 miles |
| Group program | Starter (individual) | Hospital outpatient | Hospital outpatient | Hospital-based YMCA (YWCA) | Hospital-based YMCA (YWCA) | YMCA (YWCA) |
| Duration | | 8 weeks | Same | 10 weeks | Same | Maintenance adult fitness |
| Program | A | B | | C | | D-E |

*Courtesy N. Nequin, M.D., Cardiac Rehabilitation and Coronary Risk Reduction Programs, Swedish Covenant Hospital, Chicago, Ill.

[1]Modified from Haskell and Wenger.[9]

[2]May have added psychologic stress that would increase work load on the heart.

[3]May produce higher work load on the heart because of use of arms or isometric exercise.

[4]For sex, maximum met level is 5.0, usually for less than 30 seconds, with 3.7 mets during the pre- and postorgasmic periods.

## BASIC EXERCISE GUIDELINES FOR THE PATIENT*

1. Definitions
   Resting pulse rate (RPR): Pulse count taken at rest with patient supine (awake), sitting, or standing (relaxed).
   Working heart rate (WHR): Pulse count at the height of exercise; if constant monitor is not used, the 10-second pulse count immediately after stopping exercise.
   Exit pulse rate (EPR): Pulse count at the end of exercise session. This should always be 18 beats/10-second count *or lower* before leaving the exercise area.
2. If your WHR exceeds the *upper limit,* the exercise was too much for you. Slow down either by decreasing the intensity or the duration of exercise.
3. A correct exercise session should consist of three periods:

| *Warm-up* | *Exercise* | *Cool-down* |
|---|---|---|
| 5-10 minutes | 15-30 minutes or more | 5-15 minutes or as directed |

4. Like any other medication, exercise may have some side effects: prolonged fatigue, muscular strain, joint pains, and symptoms referable to the heart. Discuss any problems with your physician or the physician in charge of the group program.
5. *Do not* exercise within 2 hours of a heavy meal. Avoid extremes of hot or cold temperatures; wear a mask or scarf across your face during cold weather, and do not use the sauna or whirlpool after exercise.
6. Keep a *daily log* of your exercise sessions, recording RPR, WHR, EPR, the type of exercise and duration, and any symptoms. Discuss this record periodically with the physician.
7. Mets equivalents
   1.0 Supine, rest, awake; sitting quietly, standing relaxed
   1-2 Exercise capacity for the first week after heart attack
   3.0 Exercise capacity at end of average hospitalization
   5-6 Walking treadmill at 3-4 mph; climbing stairs; sex
   8-9 Maximum capacity for a recovered heart attack victim
   12 Maximum capacity for a normal but untrained young man
   20 Maximum capacity for trained athletes
8. "Train, don't strain."
9. *Exercise for your life, for life.* But exercise is *not* the total answer to rehabilitation.
   Reduce to ideal weight.
   Stop smoking.
   Lower cholesterol and triglycerides.
   Control high blood pressure.
   Modify tension, deadlines.
   See your physician regularly.

*Modified from Haskell, W. L. Courtesy N. Nequin, M.D., Cardiac Rehabilitation and Coronary Risk Reduction Programs, Swedish Covenant Hospital, Chicago, Ill.

upright T wave and prolongation of the Q-T interval completes the typical finding and may allow a positive interpretation occasionally, even in the presence of less than some arbitrary degree of horizontal S-T segment depression.

An increased heart rate, slight shortening of the P-R interval, peaking of the P wave, and increases or decreases in T wave amplitude are normal findings. A slight change in intraventricular conduction, inversion of T waves, or depressed but upward sloping S-T segments are classified as borderline responses.

The test may not be interpreted in the presence of right or left bundle branch block. Furthermore, preexistent S-T segment abnormalities make further S-T segment changes difficult to interpret. Wolff-Parkinson-White syndrome negates the value of the test as does the presence of digitalis, quinidine, hypokalemia (with ST-T changes), excessive thyroid medication, or ST-T changes occurring while standing before the test.

## REFERENCES


1. American Heart Association, Committee on Exercise: Exercise testing and training of apparently healthy individuals: a handbook for physicians, New York, 1972, The Association.
2. Turrell, D. L., and Hellerstein, H. D.: Evaluation of cardiac function to specific physical activities following recovery from acute myocardial infarction, Progressive Cardiovascular Disease **1**:237, 1958.
3. Sharkey, B. J.: Physiological fitness and weight control, Missoula, Mont., 1974, Mountain Press Publishing Co.
4. Zohman, L. R., and Tobis, J. S.: Cardiac rehabilitation, New York, 1970, Grune & Stratton, Inc.
5. Wingerson, E.: Occupational therapy and the head trauma patient, San Francisco, 1974, American Congress of Rehabilitation.
6. Cain, H. D., Frasher, W. G., Jr., and Stivelman, R.: Graded activity program for safe return to self-care after myocardial infarction, J.A.M.A. **177**:111, 1961.
7. Lawson, M.: Progressive coronary care, Heart & Lung **1**:240, 1972.
8. Bures, A. R.: Exercise electrocardiography, Heart Bull. **19**:No. 1, 1970.
9. Haskell, W. L., and Wenger, N. K.: The exercise prescription, network for continuing medical education, Jan., 1974, unpublished data.
10. Detry, J.-M. R.: Exercise testing and training in coronary heart disease, Baltimore, 1973, The Williams & Wilkins Co.


## BIBLIOGRAPHY FOR CHAPTERS 31-33


American Heart Association: Facts about stroke, New York, 1968, The Association.

American Heart Association, Committee on Exercise: Exercise testing and training of apparently healthy individuals: a handbook for physicians, New York, 1972, The Association.

Brown, E. L.: Newer dimensions of patient care, New York, 1965, Russell Sage Foundation.

Bures, A. R.: Exercise electrocardiography, Heart Bull. **19**:No. 1, 1970.

Burt, M. M.: Perceptual deficits in hemiplegia, Am. J. Nurs. **70**:No. 5, 1970.

Cunningham, D. A., and Rechnitzer, P. A.: Exercise prescription and the postcoronary patient, Arch. Phys. Med. Rehabil. **55**:July, 1974.

Detry, J.-M. R.: Exercise testing and training in coronary heart disease, Baltimore, 1973, The Williams & Wilkins Co.

Dies, C.: Personal communication, 1975.

Fletcher, G. F., and Cantwell, J. D.: Exercise and coronary heart disease, role in prevention, diagnosis, treatment, Springfield, Ill., 1974, Charles C Thomas, Publisher.

Foltz, J. R., and Deck, E. S.: A sociological framework for patient care, New York, 1966, John Wiley & Sons, Inc.

Friedman, M., and Rosanman, R. H.: Type A behavior and your heart, New York, 1974, Alfred A. Knopf, Inc.

Hackler, E., and Howell, A. T.: Resocializing the stroke patient . . . by trained volunteers, Nurs. Outlook **12**:73, 1972.

Hall, L., and Alfano, G.: Incapacitation or rehabilitation? Am. J. Nurs. **64**:No. 11, 1964.

Hurst, J. W., and Walker, H. K.: The problem oriented system, Medcom learning systems, New York, 1972, Medcom Press.

Jackson, J., Sharkey, B. J., and Johnston, L. P.: Cardiorespiratory adaptations to training at specified frequencies, Res. Q. Am. Assoc. Health Phys. Educ. **39**:295, 1968.

Klassen, A. C.: The stroke syndrome: diagnostic procedures, Med. Times **97**:No. 5, 1969.

Larsen, O. A., and Malmborg, R. O., editors: Coronary heart disease and physical fitness proceedings of a symposium held in Copenhagen, September 2-5, 1970, Baltimore, 1970, University Park Press.

Lawson, M.: Progressive coronary care, Heart & Lung **1**:240, 1972.

Lawson, M.: A nursing adaptation to the problem oriented medical record, unpublished data, 1974.

The Lippincott manual of nursing practice, Philadelphia, 1974, J. B. Lippincott Co.

Manthey, M., and Kramer, M.: A dialogue on primary nursing, Nurs. Forum **9**:No. 4, 1970.

Manthey, M., Diske, K., Robertson, P., and Harris, I.: Primary nursing, Nurs. Forum **9**: No. 1, 1970.

Memorial Hospital of Long Beach: Comprehensive stroke care, Long Beach, Fla., 1970, Regional Medical Program, Area VIII.

Milhous, R. L.: The problem oriented approach to rehabilitation medicine, In Walker, H. K., Hurst, J. W., and Woody, M. F., editors: Applying the problem oriented medical system, Medcom medical update series, New York, 1973, Medcom Press.

Naughton, J. P., Hellerstein, H. D., and Mohler, I. C., editors: Exercise testing and exercise training in coronary heart disease, New York, 1973, Academic Press, Inc.

Nequin, N. D.: Unpublished data, 1974.

Redman, B. K.: The process of patient teaching in nursing, ed. 2, St. Louis, 1972, The C. V. Mosby Co.

Rutledge, K. A.: The professional nurse as primary therapist: background, perspective and opinion, J. Operational Psychiatry **5**:No. 2, 1974.

Sarno, J., and Sarno, M. T.: Stroke: the condition and the patient, New York, 1969, McGraw-Hill Book Co.

Sharkey, B. J.: Physiological fitness and weight control, Missoula, Mont., 1974, Mountain Press Publishing Co.

Smith, G. W.: Care of the stroke patient, New York, 1967, Springer Publishing Co., Inc.

Tobis, J. S.: Personal communication, 1975.

Turiello, A. M.: A commitment to service in rehabilitation, a statement of a philosophy, Rehabil. Lit. **31**:No. 5, 1970.

United States Department of Health, Education, and Welfare, Social and Rehabilitation Services: A survey of medicine and medical practice for the rehabilitation counsellor, Washington, D.C., 1969, Rehabilitation Services Administration.

Weed, L. L.: Medical records, medical education and patient care, Cleveland, 1971, Press of Case Western Reserve University.

Whipple, G. H., Peterson, M. A., Haines, V. M., Learner, E., and McKinnon, E.: Acute coronary care, Boston, 1972, Little, Brown & Co.

Wingerson, E.: Occupational therapy and the head trauma patient, San Francisco, 1974, American Congress of Rehabilitation.

Zohman, L. R., and Tobis, J. S.: Cardiac rehabilitation, New York, 1970, Grune & Stratton, Inc.

# Glossary

**A-a$\Delta P_{O_2}$** Difference between alveolar and arterial oxygen tension.

**abortion** Premature expulsion from the uterus of the products of conception.

**abruptio placentae** Premature detachment of a normally implanted placenta occurring in the region of maternal transdecidual arterial blood supply and attended by maternal systemic reactions in the form of shock, oliguria, and fibrinopenia.

**accelerated conduction** Conduction that is faster than expected.

**accelerated pathway** Portion of the conduction system that transmits impulses more rapidly than normal.

**acetylcholine** Ester of choline that causes vasodilation and increased flow.

**ACH** See *Acetylcholine.*

**acidosis** Chemical state of the blood and body fluids that occurs when there is excess acid or a deficiency of alkali. This may occur in a variety of disease states, but is a common concomitant of kidney failure.

**ACTH** See *Adrenocorticotropic hormone.*

**activated charcoal** Charcoal treated with steam, air, carbon dioxide, oxygen, zinc chloride, sulfuric acid, phosphoric acid, or a combination of these substances at temperatures ranging from 500° to 900° C to increase its absorptive powers. It has been estimated that 1 ml of charcoal, finely divided, possesses a total surface area of approximately 1000 $m^2$; used as a general purpose antidote.

**adenosine triphosphate** Enzyme found in all cells. When this substance is split by enzyme action, energy is produced.

**ADH** See *Antidiuretic hormone.*

**adrenal cortex** Outer layer of the adrenal gland; secretes corticosteroids.

**adrenal medulla** Inner layer of the adrenal gland; secretes catecholamines.

**adrenergic receptors** Term applied to nerve fibers that, when stimulated, release epinephrine at their endings.

**adrenocorticotropic hormone** Corticotropin.

**aerobic capacity** Greatest amount of oxygen that can be transported from the lungs to the working muscles; also known as maximum oxygen uptake ($V_{O_{2max}}$).

**akinesia** Complete or partial loss of muscle movement.

**albumin** Group of simple proteins.

**albuminuria** Presence of protein (albumin) in the urine. Most commonly this represents an abnormal situation but may not be specific. The test for albumin in the urine serves as a screening test for kidney disease.

**aldosterone** Hormone secreted by the adrenal cortex that promotes sodium retention and potassium excretion.

**Allen's test** Test performed by compressing both the ulnar and radial arteries and having the patient repeatedly make a fist, then either the radial or the ulnar artery is released. If the hand fails to blush after release of one artery, this signifies lack of patency to the palmar arch.

**allograft** Autograft.

**$\alpha$-receptors** Sympathetic nerve terminals in certain blood vessels that promote vascular smooth muscle contraction.

**alternating current** Electric current that reverses its direction at regularly recurring intervals, the frequency being determined by the frequency of the alternator supplying the current and the successive half waves being similar in shape and area.

**alveolar ventilation** Calculated volume of ventilation that is effective in gas exchange.

**alveoli** Small hollows or cavities; air cells of the lung.

**analgesia** Absence of painful sensation in a particular area.

**anaphylaxis** Hypersensitive state of the body with respect to a foreign protein or drug.

**aneurysm** Localized abnormal dilation of a blood vessel caused by congenital defect or weakness of the wall of the vessel.

**angina pectoris** Clinical term for a condition caused by disease of the coronary arteries. The usual symptoms are paroxysmal pain accompanied by a sense of constriction about the chest.

**angiocardiography** In radiology, the visualization

of blood vessels by injection of a nontoxic radiopaque substance.

**anoxia** Lack of oxygen supply to the tissues.

**antibody** Protein substance developed by the body usually in response to the presence of an antigen.

**anticoagulant** Agent that prevents or delays blood clotting.

**antidiuretic hormone** Vasopressin; promotes water retention.

**antigen** Substance that induces the formation of antibodies.

**aortic** Pertaining to the large vessel arising from the left ventricle and distributing, by its branches, arterial blood to every part of the body.

**aortic stenosis** Narrowing of aorta or its orifice because of lesions of the wall with scar formation, infection as in rheumatic fever, or embryonic anomalies.

**aortocoronary–saphenous vein bypass** Surgical procedure using the saphenous vein segment as a conduit to transport blood from the ascending thoracic aorta to the coronary artery, bypassing obstructions in the coronary artery.

**Apgar score** Number assigned at birth assessing the condition of the infant; based on color, heart rate, respiratory rate, muscle tone, and responsiveness.

**apnea** Absence of respiration for a period greater than 10 seconds, producing hypoxia and bradycardia in the neonate; cessation of breathing.

**aponeurosis** Flat fibrous sheet of connective tissue that serves to attach muscle to bone or other tissues at their origin or insertion.

**arborization** Interlacing; ramification; applied to nerve processes, terminations, fibers, and arterioles. A structure having the conformation of a tree.

**arrhythmia** Absence of rhythm; irregularity.

**arteriotomy** Incision of an artery.

**arteriovenous oxygen difference** Difference between the oxygen content in the arterial and venous circulations.

**arteriovenous shunt (hemodialysis)** Direct connection between an artery and a vein surgically created by a conduit that protrudes through the skin.

**arteriovenous shunting** Passage of blood from the arterial circulation to the venous circulation without transit through the capillaries.

**artifacts** ECG and EEG waves that arise from sources other than the heart or the brain.

**artificial pacemaker** Electronic device used to stimulate the heart electrically so that it will depolarize.

**assessment** Observer's opinion of the patient's mental, physical, or social status or progress or lack of progress from therapeutic and educational assistance based on subjective and objective information.

**assisted ventilation** Mechanical ventilation in which the initiation of each breath is by the patient's spontaneous inspiratory effort.

**asystole** Lack of normal cardiac contraction.

**atelectasis** Collapse or nonexpansion of the alveoli, segment, lobe, or total lung.

**ATP** See *Adenosine triphosphate.*

**atresia** Pathologic closure of a normal anatomic opening, or congenital absence of the opening.

**atrial fibrillation** Rapid irregular atrial depolarization (300 to 700 beats/min).

**atrial flutter** Rapid regular atrial depolarization with fusing of the "f" and T waves (atrial repolarization) (280 to 340 beats/min).

**atrial tachycardia** Rapid atrial rhythm (100 to 260 beats/min) from an ectopic focus; may be sustained or paroxysmal.

**atrioventricular block** Pathologic delay in atrioventricular conduction.

**atrioventricular junction** Specialized conducting tissue of the AV node, bundle of His, and common AV bundle.

**autograft** Skin (or tissue) taken from one area of the body for transplant to another area.

**autologous grafts** Tissue, usually skin, that is moved from one part of the body to another site on the same individual.

**autonomic nervous system** Part of the nervous system that is concerned with control of involuntary body functions.

**A-V** See *Arteriovenous.*

**AV** See *Atrioventricular.*

**axon** Process of a neuron that conducts impulses away from the cell body.

**azotemia** Elevation of blood urea concentration.

**Babinski reflex (plantar extensor sign, sign of the toe)** Pathologic reflex involving extension of the great toe of the foot occurring when a stimulus is applied to the sole of the foot, the calf, or the anterior tibial region. This signifies a lesion in the spinal cord above the lumbar level or in the brain.

**baroreceptors** Pressure-sensitive nerve terminals in certain blood vessels that send signals to the brain when the systolic blood pressure falls.

**basophil** Type of white blood cell thought to bring anticoagulant substances to inflamed tissues.

**Battle's sign** Presence of ecchymosis over a mastoid process, which signifies a petrobasilar fracture.

**$\beta$-adrenergic blocker** Sympathomimetic (adrenergic) drugs stimulate $\alpha$- and/or $\beta$-receptors. Some of the effects of stimulating a $\beta$-receptor are (1) stimulation of the heart, (2) dilation of blood vessels, and (3) dilation of the bronchial musculature. A $\beta$-adrenergic *blocker* reverses these effects.

**bicarbonate precursor** Sodium lactate injection, used in the treatment of metabolic acidosis, that is metabolized in the body to sodium bicarbonate.

**bioavailability** Amount of drug released from a drug formulation for absorption into the circulation.

**bipolar** Having or involving the use of two poles.

**bougie** Slender cylinder for introduction into the cervical canal.

**bradycardia** Abnormally slow heart rate; in the neonate, less than 90 beats/min.

**bronchopulmonary dysplasia** Chronic fibrotic lung disease; in the neonate, produced by exposure of the lung to high oxygen concentrations, usually 70% for more than 2 days.

**bronchospasm** Spasmodic narrowing of the bronchi.

**bundle branch block** Partial or complete block of one or more of the ventricular bundle branches.

**bundle of His** Group of fibers; an atrioventricular fasciculus.

**calculus** Refers to the formation of a stone or "rock"; in the case of the kidney and urinary tract, is called renal or urinary calculus.

**calorie (kilocalorie)** Heat unit; the amount of heat required to raise the temperature of 1 kg of water from 0° to 1° C; also known as the large calorie and is used in the study of metabolism. The small calorie is the amount of heat required to raise the temperature of 1 g of water 1° C and is one one-thousandth of the large calorie.

**calyx** Any cuplike division of the kidney pelvis.

**capillaries** Network of vessels between the arterioles and the veins. Oxygen and nutritive materials diffuse through the walls into the tissues, and carbon dioxide and waste products from the tissues enter the circulatory system.

**cardiac arrhythmia** Irregular heart action caused by disturbances, either physiologic or pathologic, in the discharge of cardiac impulses from the sinoatrial node or their transmission through conductile tissue of the heart.

**cardiac decompensation** Inability of the heart to maintain adequate circulation.

**cardiac output** Blood volume in liters ejected per minute by the left ventricle.

**cardiac plexus** Cardiac nerves beneath the arch of the aorta.

**cardiac tamponade** Compression of the heart caused by a collection of fluid in the pericardial sac.

**cardiodynamics** Study of the forces involved in the heart's action.

**cardiogenic** Having origin in the heart itself.

**cardiogenic shock** Condition that interferes with function of the heart as a pump, producing shock.

**cardiotonic** Substance that stimulates the heart to improve its muscular tension.

**cardioversion** Procedure of delivering a countershock to the heart that is programmed to occur after the impulse for depolarization has spread across the atrium. The purpose is to interrupt an abnormal rhythm so that the normal rhythm can take over.

**carotid sinus (body)** Collection of vagal cells near the bifurcation of the carotid artery that are sensitive to pressure and carbon dioxide content of the blood. Massage of these bodies stimulates the vagus and may slow the atrial heart rate.

**cartilage** Type of dense connective tissue consisting of cells embedded in a ground substance.

**cast (in urinary sediment)** Cylindric structure that may be seen in the urine when viewed through the microscope. The number and type of casts present are helpful in indicating the type of kidney disease present.

**catecholamines** Epinephrine, norepinephrine, and similar compounds that have sympathomimetic actions.

**causalgia** Form of pain, usually severe, in which a usually nonpainful stimulation is perceived as extremely painful. It is spontaneous and usually has a burning quality. This is usually seen in lesions of the CNS and also in proximal portions of damaged nerve roots. In its later stages the involved extremity is pale and cold and may respond favorably to sympathetic blockage.

**cell** Unit of structure of all animals and plants; the physical basis of all life processes.

**cerebral vascular disease** Disease of the blood vessels of the brain.

**chemoreceptor** Sense organ or sensory nerve ending that is stimulated by a chemical substance.

**cholinergic** Term applied to nerve endings that liberate acetylcholine.

**chordae tendineae** Tendinous cords that join the papillary muscles of the heart with the valves.

**chronotropic** Affecting the rate of muscular contraction; term used to describe the cardiac-slowing effect of impulses in certain fibers of the vagus nerve.

**chyle** Milklike contents of the lacteals and lymphatic vessels in the intestine; consists of the products of digestion.

**cicatrix** Scar tissue caused by a predominance of white collagen fibers.

**cilia** Hairlike processes projecting from epithelial cells.

**cineangiography** Part of the process of cardiac catheterization and angiography that utilizes frames taken at a rapid rate to show movement of the structures and contrast media.

**cisternae** Reservoirs or cavities.

**claudication** Weakness of the legs accompanied by cramplike pains in the calves caused by poor circulation of the blood to the legs.

**clearance** Pertains to measurement of renal function and indicates the volume of blood from which a substance (for example, creatinine or urea) is completely removed in a given unit of time (for example, a minute or day) by the kidneys.

**clonus** Jerking repetitive movement of a muscle when it is forcibly stretched. Generally performed at the ankles, this indicates a lesion above the lumbar level, either in the spinal cord or brain.

**coarctation of the aorta** Constriction of the aorta.

**cold caloric irrigation** Technique of testing integrity of brain stem function carried out by irrigating the external auricular canal of the patient with cold saline solution while the head is flexed at approximately 30 degrees after checking the patency of the ear canal. Stimulation of the labyrinth produces jerky, regular movements of the eyes in the normal patient. Absence may signify damage at the pontine level of the brain stem.

**collagen** Fibrous insoluble protein found in the connective tissue.

**collateral circulation** Circulation carried on through secondary channels.

**colloid** Dissolved proteins of the plasma and interstitial fluids.

**conduction** Transmission of an impulse from one part of the heart to another.

**congestive heart failure** (**decompensation, cardiac or myocardial insufficiency**) Not a disease entity, but a *syndrome* resulting from many forms of heart disease; a condition that occurs when the heart fails to circulate the optimum amount of blood required by the body. One or both of the ventricles may fail. There is an inadequate emptying of the chambers of the heart.

**continuous positive airway pressure** Mechanism of gas delivery (under pressure) to the alveoli used to maintain inflation of the alveoli during expiration in the presence of atelectasis.

**continuous positive pressure ventilation** Positive end-expiratory pressure applied to the airway during mechanical ventilation.

**contralateral** Opposite side of a point of reference.

**controlled ventilation** Mechanical ventilation in which the autonomic cycling device in the ventilator initiates inspiration.

**convalescence** To recover health gradually; the interim between acute illness and recovery.

**coronary occlusion** Obstruction of the lumen of the coronary artery caused by atheroma, thrombus, or embolus.

**coronary thrombosis** Formation of a clot in some portion of the coronary arteries, which supply blood to the heart muscle, resulting in obstruction of the artery, which may result in infarction (necrosis) of the area of the heart supplied by the occluded vessel.

**corticosteroids** Hormones secreted by the adrenal cortex.

**corticotropin** Hormone secreted by the anterior pituitary that stimulates the adrenal cortex; adrenocorticotropic hormone.

**cortisol** The principal glucocorticoid secreted by the adrenal cortex; hydrocortisone; 17-hydroxycorticosterone.

**cortisone** Glucocorticoid that resembles cortisol.

**CPAP** See *Continuous positive airway pressure.*

**CPPV** See *Continuous positive pressure ventilation.*

**crepitation** Crackling feeling or sound commonly used to describe the condition that results when air escapes into the tissue.

**crescendo angina** Refers to increased frequency, provocation, or change in intensity or character of anginal discomfort and usually associated with ischemic ECG changes.

**crystalloid** Noncolloid substance able to pass through a semipermeable membrane; forms true solution.

**current** Movement of positive or negative electric particles (as electrons) accompanied by such observable effects as the production of heat, of a magnetic field, or of chemical transformations.

**cyanosis** Bluish coloration of the skin and mucous membranes that accompanies inadequate oxygenation of the blood to the tissues.

**cytomegalic inclusion disease** Transplacentally acquired viral infection. Mothers are asymptomatic. Infants may be asymptomatic but may be affected by deformity or may die.

**cytoplasm** That portion of the protoplasm other than the nucleus.

**data base** Information necessary for complete patient care; includes the chief complaint, history of the present illness, patient profile, history, and physical and laboratory tests.

**decerebrate posturing** Position of the extremities of a patient, generally comatose, in which the arms are extended and internally rotated and the legs are extended with the feet in forced plantar flexion, caused usually by compression of the brain stem at lower levels.

**decorticate posturing** Position of the extremities in a comatose patient (although not necessarily as deeply unconscious as the decerebrate patient), in which the upper extremities are flexed at the elbows and at the wrists. The legs may be flexed. Decerebrate and decorticate positions are generally produced by the application of painful stimulation to the comatose patient. Decorticate posturing indicates a lesion higher in the brain stem in a mesencephalic region.

**default** Failure of an impulse to occur or to be transmitted when it would be expected to do so.

**defibrillator** Machine used to deliver an electric charge to the heart; also termed a depolarizer.

**dendrite** Branched protoplasmic process of a neuron that conducts impulses to the cell body.

**depolarize** To prevent, decrease, or remove polarization of (as a dry cell) by adding a substance that prevents the accumulation of reaction products.

**dermis** Skin.

**diabetes insipidus** Disorder caused by deficiency of, or renal unresponsiveness to, antidiuretic hormone (vasopressin).

**diabetes mellitus** Disease characterized by a deficiency of insulin, relative or absolute, and hyperglycemia.

**dialysis** Diffusion of dissolved particles from one fluid compartment to another across a semipermeable membrane.

**dialysis disequilibrium syndrome** Syndrome occurring as a result of dialysis; may be manifest by cerebral and other neurologic disturbances, cardiac arrhythmia, and pulmonary edema and is caused by a rapid change in extracellular fluid composition as a result of dialysis.

**dialysis fluid** Solution flowing on the opposite side of the semipermeable membrane to blood.

**diaphoresis** Profuse perspiration.

**diastole** Normal period in the heart's cycle during which the muscle fibers lengthen, the heart dilates, and the cavities fill with blood.

**DIC** See *Disseminated intravascular coagulation.*

**diencephalon** Second portion of the brain or that lying between the telencephalon and the mesencephalon.

**diffusion** Process whereby different gases interpenetrate and become mixed as a result of their constant molecular motion.

**direct current** Electric current flowing in one direction only and substantially constant in value.

**disability** Absence or impairment of physical, intellectual, or financial fitness.

**disseminated intravascular coagulation** Hemorrhagic disease characterized by gross intravascular clotting, consumption of coagulation factors, and excessive bleeding.

**diuresis (dried out)** Increased excretion of urine.

**diuretic** Any drug or substance that increases the flow of urine. Such substances are used medically to rid the body of excess salt and water that accumulate in certain kidney diseases, heart failure, and liver disease.

**Doppler principle** Observation that the pitch of a whistle on a rapidly moving body, like a locomotive, is higher when the body is approaching the listener.

**DPT vaccine** Diphtheria-pertussis-tetanus vaccine.

**dynamic** Active, as opposed to static; pertaining to the process of change.

**dyskinesia** Defect in voluntary movement.

**dyspnea** Shortness of breath, difficult breathing.

**dysrhythmia** Disturbance of rhythm, as abnormality of rhythm in speech, or disturbance or irregularity in the rhythm of the brain waves as recorded by electroencephalography.

**ecchymosis** Extravasation of blood under the skin.

**ectopic pregnancy** Pregnancy outside of the uterus, usually in the fallopian tube.

**effective compliance** Ratio of tidal volume to peak airway pressure.

**elastin** Protein forming the principal substance of yellow elastin tissues.

**electrode** Contact for introduction or detection of electrical activity.

**embolectomy** Removal of an embolus through an incision in the blood vessel wall.

**embolism** Occlusion of an artery by an embolus.

**embolized atheroma** Embolized fat particle lodged in a vessel.

**embolus** Bit of matter foreign to the bloodstream that may lodge in some vessel and obstruct the circulation to the area served by the vessel.

**emphysema of the lung** Condition in which the alveoli become distended and destroyed.

**endarterectomy** Surgical removal of atheromatous material from the intima of an artery.

**endocarditis** Inflammation of the lining membrane of the heart or endocardium.

**endocardium** Inner lining of the heart.

**endoneurium** Delicate connective tissue sheath that surrounds nerve fibers.

**endotoxin** Cell wall toxin produced by gram-negative bacteria.

**enzymes** Catalytic substance formed by living cells and having a specific action in promoting a chemical change.

**eosinophil** Leukocyte cell that stains readily with acid stain.

**epicardium** Inner layer of the pericardium.

**epimysium** Outermost sheath of connective tissue that surrounds a skeletal muscle.

**epinephrine** Catecholamine secreted by the adrenal medulla; adrenaline. It stimulates $\beta$-adrenergic responses.

**epineurium** General connective tissue sheath of a nerve.

**epithelium** Layer of cells forming the epidermis of the skin.

**erythropoietic factor** Substance produced primarily by the kidney that directly or indirectly stimulates the bone marrow to produce red blood cells. This substance may be increased in certain kidney diseases, leading to an excess of red blood cells (erythremia), or decreased in others, leading to a deficiency of red blood cells (anemia).

**escape interval** Interval between a normal impulse and an escape focus; usually applies when there is a default.

**eschar** Slough or scab (layer) of dead skin or tissue.

**ethanolism** Alcoholic condition or condition involving alcohol.

**expressive aphasia** Impairment in the formulation and/or expression of language.

**extracorporeal circulation (pump perfusion, pump bypass)** Circulation that takes place outside the body, as by the use of a mechanical pump and oxygenator.

**extrasystole** Premature impulse from a focus other than the sinus node.

**f waves** Either fibrillation or flutter waves.

**$F_{IO_2}$** Inspired oxygen; expressed as a fraction.

**factor VII** Proconvertin, stable factor, or serum prothrombin conversion accelerator; with calcium, is involved in the extrinsic system of prothrombin activation by converting tissue thromboplastin to an active product.

**factor XII (Hageman factor)** By reacting with foreign products in the circulation and factor XI (plasma thromboplastin antecedent), produces a contact activation product that starts the intrinsic system of prothrombin activation.

**fascia** Fibrous membrane that unites the skin with underlying tissue.

**fasciculus** Bundle of nerve or muscle fibers.

**fasciotomy** Incision of a fascia.

**fibril** Small filamentous structure that is often the component of a cell.

**fibrillation** Twitching or quivering of the muscle cells.

**fibrin** Insoluble protein of a blood clot.

**fibrinogen** Soluble protein in the blood plasma that, by the action of thrombin, is converted into fibrin.

**fibrinogenopenia** Condition in which there is a decreased amount of fibrinogen in the blood.

**fibrinolytic** Agent that has the ability to dissolve a blood clot.

**fibroblast** Any cell or tissue from which connective tissue is developed.

**focal motor signs** Refers to the presence of either spastic or flaccid weakness, or clonus in a single area, which implies a lesion at one point in the CNS.

**frequency** Number of complete alterations per second of an alternating electric current; the number of sound waves per second produced by a sounding body (as a tuning fork); the number of complete oscillations per second of the electric or magnetic component of an electromagnetic wave.

**funiculus** Division of the white matter of the spinal cord consisting of fasciculi or fiber tracts.

**GABA** See *γ-Aminobutyric acid.*

**gallop rhythm** Abnormal heart rhythm having three sounds/cycle, resembling in sound the gallop of a horse.

**γ-aminobutyric acid** Amino acid found in small amounts in some proteins.

**gamma globulin** Protein formed in the blood. Ability to resist infection is related to concentration of such proteins.

**ganglion** Mass of nervous tissue composed principally of nerve cells and lying outside the brain and spinal cord.

**gestational age** Age of the fetus as calculated from the time of conception: preterm, less than 38 weeks; term, 38 to 42 weeks; postterm, more than 42 weeks.

**GFR** See *Glomerular filtration rate.*

**glia cells** Nonnervous or supporting tissue of the brain and/or spinal cord.

**globulins** Group of simple proteins soluble in neutral solutions of salts of strong acids with strong bases.

**glomerular filtration rate** Expression of the quantity of glomerular filtrate formed each minute in all nephrons of both kidneys.

**glomerulonephritis** General name given to diseases that are characterized by inflammatory or other anatomic changes in the renal glomerulus; often the result of an allergic or autoimmune reaction of the glomeruli of the kidney to a streptococcal infection in the body.

**glomerulus** Tuft of capillaries invaginated into the first part of the kidney tubule where filtration of blood (plasma water) takes place.

**glucagon** Hormone secreted by the alpha cells of the pancreatic islets that raises the blood glucose level.

**glucocorticoids** Adrenocortical hormones that promote gluconeogenesis and thus raise the blood sugar.

**glycogenolysis** Breakdown of glycogen to glucose.

**goals** Expected outcome as a result of diagnostic, therapeutic, and educational management of the patient's problems: short-term, immediate or day-to-day; long-term, overall or ultimate outcome expected.

**Golgi apparatus** Network of irregular wavy threads present in the cytoplasm of all nerve cells and many other cells.

**graft** Skin or other living substance inserted into a similar substance for attachment and growth into an integral part of the original substance.

**ground** In electricity, to connect (an electrical

conductor) with the ground, which becomes part of the circuit, as to *ground* a wire.

**growing fracture** Fracture, usually linear, of which the x-ray film appearance shows a separation of the fracture edges with the passage of time. This usually indicates a tear of the dura at the time of the injury with gradual pulsatile expansion of the arachnoid through the fracture, forcing the edges apart.

**gumma** Soft tumor of the tissues characteristic of the tertiary stage of syphilis.

**handicap** Any disadvantage that makes success more difficult.

**hard data** Information about the patient that can be observed or measured, as in laboratory data, special tests, or procedures; also referred to as objective data.

**health care team** Group of professionals and paraprofessionals working together to give and promote health care.

**heart block** Interruption in the conduction of the electrical impulse through the atrioventricular node.

**hematocrit** Volume of erythrocytes packed by centrifugation in a given volume of blood.

**hematuria** Presence of red blood cells in the urine; may be gross or microscopic.

**hemianopia, homonymous** Defective vision or blindness in half of the visual field.

**hemiplegia** Paralysis of one side of the body.

**hemodialysis** Removal of certain elements from the blood by virtue of differences in the rates of their diffusion through a semipermeable membrane while the blood is being circulated outside the body.

**hemodynamics** Study of the factors affecting the flow and force of the circulating blood.

**hemoglobinuria** Presence of hemoglobin in the urine.

**hemolysis** Rupture of erythrocytes with release of hemoglobin into the plasma.

**hemopericardium** Collection of blood within the fibroserous pericardial sac that surrounds the heart.

**hemostasis** Arrest of the escape of blood by either natural or artificial means.

**hemothorax** Accumulation of blood within the thorax, usually in pleural cavity.

**Henle's loop** U-shaped portion of the renal tubule.

**heparin rebound** Phenomenon of reactivation of heparin effect (after neutralization with protamine sulfate) occurring from 5 minutes to 5 hours after neutralization.

**hepatomegaly** Enlargement of the liver.

**hepatotoxic** Destructive to liver cells.

**Hering-Breuer reflex** Reflex inhibition of inspiration resulting from stimulation of pressoreceptors by inflation of the lungs.

**Hertz** Unit of frequency of a periodic process equal to 1 cycle per second.

**heterografts** Tissue transplanted from one species to another.

**hilus** Depression or recess at exit or entrance of duct into a gland.

**histamine** Amine substance found in the body wherever tissues are damaged.

**histiocyte** Cell present in all loose connective tissues that exhibits marked phagocytic activity.

**homeostasis** Process of maintaining equilibrium; the maintenance of steady states in the organism by coordinated physiologic processes.

**homografts** Transfer of tissue from another individual of the same species.

**hyaluronidase** Enzyme that depolymerizes hyaluronic acid to increase the permeability of connective tissue.

**hydrostatic pressure** Pertaining to the pressure of liquids in equilibrium and that exerted on liquids.

**hypalgesia** Refers to a painful stimulus being perceived but not to the same degree as it would be normally.

**hyperbilirubinemia** Excessive accumulation of bilirubin in blood and tissue; presents the risk of kernicterus in the newborn.

**hypercapnia** Increase in carbon dioxide content.

**hyperemesis gravidarum** Severe vomiting during pregnancy, usually during the first trimester, often accompanied by marked and prolonged nausea.

**hyperemia** Increase in blood flow.

**hyperkalemia** Elevation of potassium level in blood serum above 5.5 mEq/L.

**hypernatremia** Elevation of the sodium concentration in the blood serum above 145 mEq/L.

**hypertension** Elevation of blood pressure above the normal range.

**hypertrophy** Increase in size of an organ or structure that does not involve tumor formation.

**hypervolemia** Increase above normal in the volume of circulating blood or blood components.

**hypocalcemia** Abnormally low level of serum calcium.

**hypocapnia** Lack of carbon dioxide in the blood.

**hypochloremia** Decrease in the chloride level in the blood serum below 95 mEq/L.

**hypodermis** Subcutaneous layer of skin.

**hypoglycemia** Abnormally low blood sugar concentrations.

**hypokalemia** Decrease in the level of potassium in the blood serum below 3.5 mEq/L.

**hyponatremia** Decrease in the level of sodium in the blood serum below 135 mEq/L.

**hypotension** Blood pressure below the normal range.

**hypothalamus** Region of the brain adjacent to the pituitary. It secretes hormones or factors that are closely concerned with the regulation of pituitary function.

**hypothermia** Subnormal temperature of the body.

**hypovolemia** Decrease below normal in the volume of circulating blood or blood components.

**hypoxemia** Low oxygen tension of the blood.

**hypoxia** Lack of adequate amount of oxygen in inspired air such as occurs at high altitudes; reduced oxygen content or tension.

**iatrogenic** Occurring as a result of medical or surgical treatment.

**immunoglobulins** Body proteins capable of acting as antibodies.

**impedance** Apparent opposition in an electric circuit to the flow of an alternating current that is analogous to the actual electrical resistance to a direct current and that is expressed as the ratio of the effective electromotive force to the effective current.

**inborn error of metabolism** Genetic biochemical disturbance with enzyme deficits that results in metabolic pathology.

**infarct** Area of tissue death caused by lack of adequate blood supply.

**infarct extension** Enlargement of an original area of myocardial infarction caused by the death of cells in the marginally ischemic zone.

**infarction** Interruption of circulation to an area with actual irreversible destruction of cerebral tissue.

**inferior vena cava** Vein that carries blood from the lower part of the body to the right atrium.

**initial plan of care** Medical plan of care prepared by the physician.

**inotropic** Affecting the force of muscular contractions.

**inotropic agent** Substance that increases myocardial contractility.

**inspissation** Process of becoming dry or thick by evaporation.

**insulin** Hormone secreted by the beta cells of the pancreas that promotes the utilization of glucose.

**integument** Covering, such as the skin.

**intermittent positive pressure breathing** Principle used in the operation of certain types of respirators.

**internal mammary artery bypass** Surgical procedure using the internal mammary artery in situ proximal and still attached to the subclavian artery, using the distal end to anastomose to the coronary artery beyond the coronary artery obstruction.

**internuncial neuron** Connecting neuron in a neural pathway.

**interstitial** Area between the cells and the intravascular area.

**intima** Endothelium that lines the blood vessels.

**ions** Free electron or other charged subatomic particle.

**IPPB** See *Intermittent positive pressure breathing.*

**ipsilateral** Same side as point of reference.

**ischemia** Insufficient blood supply to an area to maintain normal muscle function.

**joule** From James Prescott Joule, English physicist; metric-kilogram-second unit of work or energy. Adopted in 1948 as the unit of heat.

**junctional extrasystole** Extrasystole arising from atrioventricular junction.

**junctional rhythm** Rhythm originating in the atrioventricular junction.

**junctional tachycardia** Tachycardia (greater than 70 beats/min) originating in the atrioventricular junction, that is, the atrioventicular node, bundle of His, or common bundle.

**keloid** New growth of skin, that is, scar tissue, caused by a colloidal disorder.

**keratinization** Process by which the epithelial cells that are exposed to the external environment lose their moisture content and are replaced with a horny substance.

**kernicterus** Condition with severe neural symptoms associated with high levels of bilirubin in the blood. It is characterized by deep yellow staining of many areas of the brain accompanied by widespread destructive changes.

**labile** Subject to much variation.

**lacteals** Lymphatics that originate in the villi of the small intestine.

**laminaria** Dried seaweed that swells on the absorption of water.

**large for gestational age** Refers to infant whose weight is above the 90th percentile.

**leukocytes** White blood corpuscles that are markedly phagocytic.

**lidocaine** Short-acting antiarrhythmic drug especially effective in ventricular arrhythmias.

**ligamentum nuchae** Upward continuation of the supraspinous ligament.

**long tract signs** Includes such signs as clonus, spasticity of muscles, plantar extensor sign, and possible bladder involvement and signifies a lesion generally of the mid- or upper spinal cord or brain.

**lumen** Passageway inside a blood vessel or other tubular organ.

**lung compliance** Degree of distensibility of the lung; volume increase per unit of distending pressure increase.

**lymph** Alkaline body fluid formed in tissue spaces all over the body.

**lymphatic** Pertaining to the lymph; a vessel conveying lymph.

**lymphocyte** Lymph cell or white blood corpuscle without cytoplasmic granules.

**lysosome** Enzyme present in cell fluid that digests substances brought in by phagocytes; an intracellular organelle containing autodigestive enzymes.

**malpighian corpuscle** Spherical body (renal corpuscle) found in the cortex of the kidney.

**mast cells** Connective tissue cells that produce histamine and heparin.

**master problem list** Permanent list of patient problems, current and resolved. List is kept in front of the chart and serves as a "table of contents."

**maximum inspiratory force** Negative pressure measured in centimeters of water at the airway of a patient who is inspiring maximally against an obstruction.

**maximum oxygen uptake** Greatest amount of oxygen that can be transported from the lungs to the working muscles; also known as aerobic capacity or $V_{O_{2max}}$.

**mediastinitis** Inflammation of the mediastinum.

**mesencephalon** Midbrain.

**mesenchymal cells** Diffuse network of cells forming the embryonic mesoderm.

**mesoderm** Primary germ layer of the embryo lying between the ectoderm and the entoderm.

**mesothelium** Layer of cells that line the body cavities.

**metabolic acidosis** Deficiency of base bicarbonate ions that results in a lowered capacity of the blood for buffering and an excessive hydrogen-ion concentration in the body fluids with a decrease in plasma pH below 7.35.

**metabolic alkalosis** Excessive concentration of base bicarbonate ions with a deficit of hydrogen ions in the body fluids that results in an increase of the plasma pH above 7.45.

**metabolic equivalent** Heat unit, abbreviated MU or met; the energy expenditure for various activities stated as multiples of the basal metabolic expenditure; commonly accepted as approximately 3.5 cc $O_2$/kg of body weight/min.

**metabolism** Sum of the physical and chemical changes that occur within the body.

**metaplasia** Conversion of one kind of tissue into another.

**microampere** One millionth of an ampere.

**microthermy (diathermy)** Heating units used for physiotherapy; heat generated by conversion of radio waves with energy given off as heat.

**microwave** Very short electromagnetic wave.

**milking (stripping) chest tubes** Process of compression to the chest tubes beginning at the upper portion of the tubes and working down to the chest bottles to evacuate clots and drainage.

**mineralocorticoids** Adrenocortical hormones that promote sodium retention and potassium excretion.

**minimal occlusive volume** Volume of endotracheal cuff inflation that still permits a minimum airway leak during the inspiratory phase of ventilation.

**minute ventilation** Total ventilation per minute measured by expired gas collection for 1 to 3 minutes.

**miosis** Excessive contraction of the pupil.

**mitochondria** Intracellular organelles involved in cellular oxidation.

**mitral regurgitation** As a result of failure of the valve to close completely, blood is allowed to flow back into the auricle.

**MOV** See *Minimal occlusive volume.*

**mucolytic** Tending to dissolve or liquefy mucus.

**mural thrombus** Blood clot originating from a diseased area of the endocardium.

**myelin sheath** Fatty semifluid covering of a nerve fiber that serves to insulate the fiber and to speed the rate of impulses.

**myocardial infarction** Area of necrosis (death of tissue) in the myocardium caused by lack of blood supply resulting from obstruction of the circulation to the heart muscle.

**myocarditis** Inflammation of the cardiac muscular tissue.

**myocardium** Muscular wall of the heart that lies between the endocardium on the inside of the heart and the epicardium on the outside of the heart.

**myxedema** Hypothyroidism; a disease caused by deficiency of thyroid hormones.

**nanograms** One billionth ($10^{-9}$) of a gram; abbreviated ng; also called a millimicrogram.

**natural pacemaker** Any pacing site in the heart.

**necrosis** Tissue death.

**neonate** Any infant less than 28 days old.

**nephron** Functional unit of the human kidney, of which there are more than 1 million in each kidney.

**nephrotoxic** Quality of being toxic or destructive to kidney cells.

**neuron** Nerve cell that is the structure and functional unit of the nervous system.

**noise** Unwanted signal that enters an electronic system.

**norepinephrine** Catecholamine secreted by the adrenal medulla and sympathetic nerve endings and found also in the brain. It stimulates $\alpha$-adrenergic responses.

**nucleus** Vital body in the protoplasm of the cell.

**nystagmus** Jerky movements of the eyes seen on voluntary or involuntary gaze, particularly with cerebellar and brain stem lesions.

**objective data** Information about the patient that can be observed or measured as in laboratory data, special tests, or procedures; also referred to as hard data.

**obstructive uropathy** Any condition that leads to obstruction of the flow of urine. Such obstruction may lead to impairment of kidney function and an increased incidence of urinary infection.

**oculocephalic reflex (doll's eye maneuver)** Technique of testing integrity of brain stem function in which the patient's head is jerked to one side and then to the other. In a normal individual the eyes will conjugately lag behind the head movement and then slowly assume the midline position. Failure of the eyes to either lag properly or revert back to the midline indicates a lesion on the ipsilateral side at the brain stem level.

**ohm** Practical meter-kilogram-second system unit of electrical resistance that is equal to the resistance of a circuit in which a potential difference of 1 V produces a current of 1 amp to the resistance in which 1 watt of power is dissipated when 1 amp flows through it; is taken as standard in the United States.

**Ohm's law** Law in electricity that holds that the strength or intensity of an unvarying electric current is directly proportional to the electromotive force and inversely proportional to the resistance of the circuit.

**oligemia** Hypovolemia or reduction in circulating intravascular volume.

**oligodendrocytes** Neuroglial cells having few and delicate processes.

**oliguria** Low urine output.

**opisthotonus** Form of tetanic spasm in which the head and heels are bent backward and the body bowed forward.

**organ** Collection of tissues organized for the performance of a given function.

**organelle** Cytoplasmic substance that performs a definite function.

**osmolarity** Characteristic of a solution determined by the ionic concentration of the dissolved substance per unit of solvent.

**osmosis** Diffusion of a substance through a semipermeable membrane.

**osmotic pressure** Pressure generated across a semipermeable membrane separating two solutions of different concentration.

**oxidation** Originally, the process of combining with oxygen; currently, an increase in the positive valence of an element (or a decrease in negative valence) occurring as a result of the loss of electrons. Each electron so lost is taken on by some other element, thus accomplishing a reduction of that element.

**$P_{aCO_2}$** Arterial carbon dioxide tension.

**$P_{aO_2}$** Arterial oxygen tension; expressed in torr.

**$P_{IO_2}$** Partial pressure of inspired oxygen.

**$P_{\bar{V}O_2}$** Oxygen tension of a blood sample obtained from the pulmonary artery (mixed venous blood).

**pacemaker** That area, organ, or instrument that initiates the impulse for heart depolarization.

**pancarditis** Inflamed condition involving all the structures of the heart.

**papillae** Small, nipplelike protuberances.

**papillary muscles** Muscle fibers in the ventricular walls to which the chordae tendineae are attached.

**paradoxical pulse** Pulse that decreases or disappears during inspiration.

**parasympathetic system** Craniosacral division of the autonomic nervous system.

**parasympatholytic agent** Drug that opposes the parasympathetic (cholinergic) nervous system.

**paresthesia** Abnormal perception of a sensation.

**partial bypass** Establishment of circulation in which the heart is pumping and maintaining a portion and the remainder of the circulation is performed by mechanical means.

**partial pressure** Pressure of one gas in a mixture.

**passive exercise** Movement of a body part of a patient without the voluntary participation of the patient.

**patent ductus arteriosus** Patency of the duct between the pulmonary artery and the aorta that exists in fetal life but that should close between the third month and the first year of life.

**patient's plan of care** Plan of care coordinated to include the plans for the patient's care by all members of the health care team.

**PEEP** See *Positive end-expiratory pressure.*

**perception** Ability to integrate and interpret messages from the internal and external environment. It is the combined result of activities of end-organs, peripheral nerves, tracts and ganglia, and the integrative sensory cortex.

**percutaneous** Performed through the skin without an incision.

**perforation** Hole or break in the containing wall of an organ.

**perfusion** Passage of a fluid, especially the passage of blood through the vessels of an organ or area.

**pericardiocentesis** Surgical aspiration of fluid from the pericardial sac.

**pericarditis** Inflammation of the fibroserous sac that surrounds the heart.

**perineurium** Connective tissue sheath investing a fasciculus or bundle of nerve fibers.

**periodic breathing** Prolonged interval between respirations (10 seconds) that is self-resolving and does not result in hypoxia or bradycardia.

**peripheral embolic phenomena** Clinical signs and symptoms of an embolus in a peripheral vessel.

**peripheral resistance** Resistance to the flow of blood that is determined by the tone of the vascular musculature and the diameter or caliber of the vasculature.

**peripheral vascular disease** Disease of any of the blood vessels outside the heart, usually referring to the blood or lymph vessels of the extremities.

**peritoneal dialysis** Process wherein the patient's peritoneal membrane is used for the same purpose that a hemodialysis apparatus (artificial kidney) is used, that is, for the removal of desired solutes from the body.

**phagocytosis** Ingestion and digestion of bacteria and particles by phagocytes.

**pharmacokinetics** Study of the rate of absorption, distribution, metabolism, and excretion of drugs.

**phlebitis** Inflammation of a vein.

**phlebothrombosis** Development of venous thrombi in the absence of antecedent inflammation of the vessel wall.

**phlegmasia cerulea dolens** Acute fulminating form of deep venous thrombosis with pronounced edema and severe cyanosis of the extremity.

**phonocardiogram** Mechanical or electronic registration of heart sounds.

**physiatrist** Physician who tests the patient's physical functioning and supervises the rehabilitation program.

**physical fitness** Ability to carry out daily tasks with vigor and alertness, without undue fatigue, and with ample energy to enjoy leisure time pursuits and to meet unforeseen emergencies.

**pineal gland** Structure in the midline of the brain behind the third ventricle that in many individuals may be calcified; serves as a convenient marker on plain x-ray films. A mass lesion on a particular side will often produce a shift of the pineal gland toward the opposite side.

**pinocytosis** Absorption of liquids of phagocytic cells.

**placenta previa** Placenta that develops in the lower uterine segment in the zone of dilatation, so that it covers or adjoins the internal cervical os.

**plasma** Liquid part of lymph and blood.

**plasma cell** Cell found in bone marrow and loose connective tissue.

**pneumothorax** Collection of air or gas in the pleural cavity caused by perforation of the chest wall, which may result in collapse of the lung.

**polarity** Particular either positive or negative state (as of a body) with reference to the two poles or to electrification.

**polycystic kidney disease** Inherited disease that results in the encroachment of normal kidney tissue by the gradual growth of many cysts in each kidney, leading to kidney failure and high blood pressure.

**positive end-expiratory pressure** For most patients, positive pressure is only given during the *inspiratory* phase of respiration. For patients such as those with shock lung syndrome, *positive end-expiratory pressure* has been used.

**potential difference** Difference in electric potential between two points that represent the work involved in the energy released in the transfer of a unit quantity of electricity from one point to another.

**P-R interval** Period from the onset of the P wave to the onset of the QRS complex.

**preeclampsia** Disease in which hypertension, edema, and/or proteinuria occur after the twenty-fourth week of pregnancy or in the early puerperium. In severe forms coma or convulsions (eclampsia) may occur.

**premature contraction** Any contraction of the ventricle or atrium that occurs early with respect to the dominant rhythm.

**premature impulse** Any impulse that occurs early with respect to the dominant rhythm.

**premature rupture of membranes** Spontaneous rupture of the amniotic sac prior to the onset of labor.

**pressure ventilator** Ventilator in which gas delivery is limited by a predetermined pressure.

**primary nurse** Nurse who has primary responsibility for planning, giving, or supervising the care of the patient and is held accountable for such responsibility.

**priming of artificial kidney** Preparation of artificial kidney for dialysis.

**problem** Anything that requires diagnostic, therapeutic, or educational action immediately (active problem) or in the past (inactive problem) as defined subjectively (by the patient) or objectively (by the observer).

**problem-oriented medical record** Tool of the problem-oriented medical system. It is organized around the patient's problems and is a lasting record of the diagnostic, therapeutic, and educational approaches (relative to each problem) that have been utilized to assist the patient.

**proprioceptive** Receiving stimuli within the tissues of the body, as within muscles and tendons.

**prostaglandins** Naturally occurring substances, first found in the semen of man and sheep and subsequently found also in menstrual fluid, that cause strong contraction of smooth muscle and dilation of certain vascular beds.

**protoplasm** Living substance of the cell that constitutes the physical basis of all living activities.

**pulmonary compliance** Reflection of the elasticity (expansibility) of the lungs.

**pulmonary hypertension** Elevation of pulmonary pressures.

**pulsatile** Characterized by a rhythmic pulsation.

**pulse pressure** Difference between systolic and diastolic blood pressure.

**Purkinje fibers** Atypical muscle fibers lying beneath the endocardium of the heart that form the impulse-conducting system of the heart.

**pyelogram (urogram)** X-ray study whereby the kidneys and urinary tract can be visualized by either injecting an x-ray radiopaque material into a patient's veins (intravenous pyelography) or by introducing the same substance directly into the urinary tract (retrograde pyelography).

**pyelonephritis** Inflammation of the kidneys and renal pelvis. This implies infection with bacteria and is associated with anatomic abnormalities of the urinary tract.

**pyoderma** Purulent skin disease.

**pyrogenic reaction** Syndrome manifested by pyrexia that may be accompanied by rigor and is caused by a reaction to proteins foreign to the patient.

**pyuria** Presence of pus in the urine.

**Queckenstedt's test** Technique applied to determine if a complete block exists in the spinal canal; also used to determine if there is obstruction of a lateral sinus. The test is performed by initiating jugular compression while a lumbar puncture needle is present and connected to a manometer. A rise and fall of the spinal fluid column indicates that there is a lack of complete obstruction in the spinal column. When applied unilaterally, its presence indicates patency of the ipsilateral sinus. Its failure to rise when one side is compressed while it does rise when the other side is compressed indicates an obstruction of that lateral or transverse sinus.

**Quincke's pulse** Capillary pulse caused by a high pulse pressure; seen classically in aortic regurgitation and elicited clinically by applying light pressure to a fingernail.

**rale** Abnormal sound heard in auscultation of the chest produced by passage of air through the bronchi, which contain secretion or exudate or which are constricted by spasm or a thickening of their walls; may be heard on either inspiration or expiration.

**Ranvier's nodes** Constrictions in the medullary substance of a nerve fiber at more or less regular intervals.

**rate** Number of impulses per unit time, usually per minute.

**receptive aphasia** Sensory aphasia; impairment in the comprehension of language.

**receptor** Group of cells functioning in the reception of stimuli.

**reconstitution** Continuous repair of progressive destruction of tissues.

**recovery** Restoration from illness.

**red infarct** Pathologic change that occurs in the brain that has first been rendered ischemic by lack of blood and then, with restriction of blood flow, diapedesis of red blood cells occurs into the parenchyma of the brain without actually producing a well-formed hematoma, only infiltration of red blood cells.

**rehabilitation** Restoration to a disabled individual of maximum independence commensurate with limitations by developing residual capacities. It implies prescribed training and employment of many different methods and professional workers.

**renin** Hormone produced by the juxtaglomerular cells of the kidneys. It regulates aldosterone secretion by the adrenal cortex and raises blood pressure.

**resistance** Property of a body whereby it opposes and limits the passage through it of a steady electric current.

**resocialization** Patient's reintegration into family and community life following critical and/or long-term hospitalization.

**resolution** Subsidence of problems.

**respiratory acidosis** Inadequate pulmonary ventilation with retention of carbon dioxide and an increase in carbonic acid.

**respiratory alkalosis** Decrease in the carbonic acid concentration of the extracellular fluid caused by hyperventilation, which blows off carbon dioxide.

**respiratory distress syndrome** Lung disease of the preterm infant characterized by atelectasis of the alveoli.

**reticular** Meshed or in the form of a network.

**retrograde** To travel in a reverse direction.

**revascularization** Surgical means of reconstituting vascularization to the heart, organ, or vessel being replaced; usually done by a bypass procedure.

**rhythm** Relationship of one impulse to its neighbors.

**ribosome** Submicroscopic ribonucleoprotein particle attached to the endoplasmic reticulum of cells; the site of protein synthesis in cytoplasm.

**rouleaux** Grouping of red blood corpuscles whose formation resembles a pile of coins.

$S_{aO_2}$ Percent saturation of arterial blood.

$S_{\bar{v}O_2}$ Percent saturation of mixed venous blood.

**saltatory conduction** Skipping from node to node.

**Schwann cells** Cells of ectodermal origin that comprise the neurilemma.

**sclerosis** Thickening or hardening.

**semipermeable membrane** Barrier to substances above a specific size but allowing passage of substances below that size.

**sensory deprivation** Decrease in sensory stimulation (sight, sound, touch, and smell) caused either by injury to the brain or lack of dynamic environment.

**septicemia** Active bacterial infection of the bloodstream.

**shock** State of inadequate tissue perfusion that results from a decreased effective circulating blood volume.

**shock lung** Syndrome of pulmonary insufficiency following shock.

**shoulder subluxation** Separation of humeral head out of the glenoid cavity resulting in pull on the soft tissue of the joint.

**shunt** Diversion.

**Silverman-Anderson score** Scoring device for assessing degree of respiratory distress.

**sinus bradycardia** Sinus rate of less than 60 beats/min in the adult.

**sinus pacemaker** Primary initiator of a normal cardiac depolarization; located in the right atrium.

**sinus tachycardia** Sinus rate of 100 or more beats/min in the adult.

**small for gestational age** Refers to infant whose weight is below the 10th percentile.

**soft data** Information that only the patient or family can provide, including pain, habits of living, and "feelings"; also referred to as subjective data.

**splanchnic** Pertaining to the intra-abdominal viscera.

**Starling's law of the heart** Force of the heart beat is determined primarily by the length of fibers comprising its muscular wall.

**status epilepticus** Condition in which seizure activity continues for several minutes or hours or consists of interrupted seizures separated by short periods of relative quiet.

**stratum corneum** Outermost horny layer of the epidermis.

**stratum germinativum** Innermost layer of epidermis that divides to replace the rest of the epidermis as it wears away.

**stratum granulosum** Layer of cells found in the epidermis of the skin between the stratum germinativum and stratum lucidum.

**stratum lucidum** Translucent layer of epidermis lying between the stratum corneum and stratum granulosum.

**stenosis** Constriction or narrowing of a passage or orifice.

**stereotaxis** Method of precisely locating areas in the brain.

**stroke volume** Amount of blood ejected by the left ventricle at each beat.

**stroma** Foundation supporting tissues of an organ.

**subdural hygroma** Fluid collection between the dura and the arachnoid resulting from a tear in the arachnoid whereby spinal fluid leaks out into the subdural space.

**subjective data** Information that only the patient or family can provide, including pain, habits of living, and "feelings"; also referred to as soft data.

**superior vena cava** Vein that carries blood from the upper part of the body to the right atrium.

**supernatant** Clear liquid remaining on the top after a precipitate settles.

**supine hypotensive syndrome** Hypotension characterized by abnormally low blood pressure when the patient is lying down on the back.

**surfactant** Chemical produced by alveolar cells that is responsible for maintaining intra-alveolar surface tension.

**Swan-Ganz catheter** Catheter with an inflatable balloon tip that can be manipulated into a peripheral pulmonary artery to measure pressures in the pulmonary artery.

**sympathetic nervous system** Division of the autonomic nervous system.

**sympathomimetic agent** Adrenergic agent; a drug whose action mimicks that of the sympathetic (adrenergic) nervous system.

**synapse** Innervation of one neuron by another.

**syndrome** Group of symptoms that occur together and are given a name to identify the specific combination of symptoms.

**systemic oxygen consumption** Amount of oxygen consumed by the body per minute.

**system** Collection of organs that act together in the performance of a given function.

**systole** That part of the heart cycle in which the heart is in contraction, that is, when the myocardial fibers are tightening.

**T tube** Apparatus for connecting humidified oxygen to the endotracheal tube to which a spirometer can be attached for the evaluation of tidal volume and the appropriate removal of the endotracheal tube.

**tachycardia** Rapid heart rate over 100 beats/min; over 180 beats/min in the neonate.

**tachyphylaxis** Decreasing responses to a drug that follow consecutive injections made at short intervals.

**tachypnea** Rapid respiratory rate.

**telencephalon** Embryonic endbrain of the prosencephalon from which the cerebral hemispheres, corpora striata, and rhinencephalon develop.

**teratogenic** That which produces fetal deformity.

**tetralogy of Fallot** Combination of four defects: (1) ventricular septal defect, (2) pulmonic stenosis, (3) right ventricular hypertrophy, and (4) overriding of the aorta. (Aorta branches out from just above the ventricular septal defect instead of the left ventricle, so it receives blood from both ventricles.)

**thermoneutral environment** Environment that keeps body temperature at an optimum point at which the least amount of oxygen is consumed for metabolism.

**thoracostomy** Incision of the chest wall with maintenance of the opening for the purpose of drainage.

**thrombin** Enzyme in the blood derived from prothrombin that is responsible for the conversion of fibrinogen into fibrin.

**thrombolytic** Causing the dissolution of a blood clot.

**thrombophlebitis** Accumulation of a blood clot within a vein accompanied by inflammation.

**thrombus** Blood clot inside a blood vessel or chamber of the heart that remains at the place of its formation.

**thyrocalcitonin** Hormone that lowers the blood calcium level; secreted by the parafollicular cells of the thyroid gland.

**thyroxine** Hormone secreted by the thyroid gland that increases oxygen consumption and thus increases metabolic rate.

**TIA** See *Transient ischemic attack.*

**tissue** Collection of similar cells that act together in the performance of a particular function.

**tokodynamometer** Instrument for measuring uterine contractions.

**torr** Abbreviation for torricelli scale; 1 torr is equal to 1 mm Hg and is used in expressing the partial pressure of a gas.

**torticollis** Contracted state of the cervical muscles producing a twisting of the neck and an unnatural position of the head.

**total peripheral resistance (afterload)** Degree of constriction of the systemic blood vessels.

**toxicity** Harmful quality.

**transected** Cross section; cutting across.

**transient ischemic attack** Form of minor stroke in which a patient manifests focal neurologic signs caused by temporary interruption of blood flow to an area of the brain that is temporary and reverts within several hours, usually less than 6. Persistence of symptoms indicates infarction of a particular area.

**tricuspid atresia** Absence of the opening between the right atrium and right ventricle.

**triiodothyronine** Hormone secreted by the thyroid gland that resembles thyroxine.

**trismus** Motor disturbance of the trigeminal nerve, especially spasm of the masticatory muscles with difficulty in opening the mouth (lockjaw).

**tropocollagen** Fundamental units of collagen fibrils obtained by prolonged extraction of insoluble collagen with dilute acid.

**tubular necrosis** Death of the cells of the small tubes of the kidneys resulting from disease or injury.

**tunica** Enveloping or covering membrane.

**tunica adventitia** Outer coat of an artery or any tubular structure.

**tunica intima** Lining coat of an artery.

**tunica media** Middle muscular coat of an artery.

**ultrafiltration** Filtration under pressure through filters with minute pores; results in removal of water by the artificial kidney.

**uncal herniation** Process whereby the medial portion of the temporal lobe protrudes over the tentorial edge in cases of increased intracranial pressure, particularly from the temporal side. Progression of this process causes pressure directly on the brain stem after first putting pressure on the third cranial nerve. The sign of uncal herniation is a dilated pupil on the side of the herniation.

**underwater seal (water trap)** Situation where the tube that exits from the patient's chest cavity is placed under water to allow the outflow but no ingress of air, thus establishing a one-way valve.

**uremia** Clinical state produced when severe functional impairment of the kidneys exists.

**$V_{DM}$** Mechanical dead space; the volume of gas contained in inspiratory tubing that does not participate in gas exchange.

**$V_T$** Tidal volume; the volume of gas inspired or expired.

**Valsalva's maneuver** Attempt to forcibly exhale with the glottis, nose, and mouth closed. If the eustachian tubes are not obstructed, the pressure on the tympanic membranes will be increased. Maneuver can also be done with just the glottis closed, but only the intrathoracic pressure will be increased. The maneuver may cause increased intrathoracic pressure, slowing of the pulse, decreased return of blood to the heart, and increased venous pressure.

**valvular** Pertaining to, affecting, or of the nature of a valve.

**valvular insufficiency** Inadequate or incomplete closure of a valve that permits a backflow of blood in the wrong direction.

**valvulitis** Inflammatory process of the heart valves. Valves may be impaired to the extent that they close incompletely or do not open completely.

**vasculitis** Inflammation of a vessel.

**vasoconstrictor** Agent that increases the diameter of blood vessels by producing relaxation of the smooth muscles in the walls of the vessels; a drug that decreases total peripheral resistance.

**vasopressin** Antidiuretic hormone secreted by the hypothalamus and posterior pituitary gland. It promotes the renal reabsorption of water.

**vasopressor** Drug that increases total peripheral resistance.

**ventricular extrasystole** Extrasystole arising from the ventricle.

**ventricular fibrillation** Disorganized rapid and ineffective ventricular depolarization.

**ventricular hemiblock** Block of only one division of the left bundle branch, that is, either anterior superior or posterior inferior hemiblock.

**ventricular septal defect** Opening in the ventricular system.

**ventricular tachycardia** Tachycardia originating from the ventricular Purkinje system.

**ventriculotomy** Incision of a ventricle of the heart.

**ventilation-perfusion defect** Occurs when areas of the lung receive inspired air but no blood, or vice versa.

**visual verticality** Perception of the visual upright.

**voltage** Electric potential or potential difference; expressed in volts.

**voltmeter** Instrument (as a galvanometer) for measuring in volts the differences of potential between different points of an electric circuit.

**volume ventilator** Ventilator that delivers a predetermined volume of gas with each cycle.

**wallerian degeneration** Degeneration of a nerve fiber that has been severed from its cell body.

**watt** Unit of electric power, being the work done at the rate of 1 joule/sec. It is equivalent to a current of 1 ampere under a pressure of 1 V.

**wedge pressure** Pulmonary or capillary pressure measured at cardiac catheterization by wedging the cardiac catheter in the most distal pulmonary artery branch. It reflects mean left arterial pressure.

**Wenckerbach block** Type of second-degree block characterized by a changing relationship between input, for example, P wave, and output, for example, QRS complex. In atrioventricular Wenckebach block there is a gradual increase in the P-R interval until a nonconducted impulse occurs.

**zymogen** Inactive precursor that is converted to an active enzyme by the action of acid, another enzyme, or some other means.

# Index

E

**M**

## P

**T**